Occupational and Environmental Infectious Diseases

Epidemiology, Prevention, and Clinical Management

Occupational and Environmental Infectious Diseases

Epidemiology, Prevention, and Clinical Management

EDITED BY

Alain J. Couturier, MD, MS

Executive Medical Director
Occupational Health Network
South Bend, Indiana

OEM Press
Beverly Farms, Masschusetts

OEM Press
8 West Street
Beverly Farms, MA 01915
1-800-533-8046

ISBN 1-883595-27-4

Printed in the United States of America

5 4 3 2 1

Library of Congress Catalog Card Number: 00–037443

To my family—my wife, Debra, and sons, Nicholas and Alexander.

Without your loving support, I could not have accomplished this project.

Contents

Contributors

Andrew W. Artenstein, MD
Assistant Clinical Professor
Brown University School of Medicine
Providence, RI
Hawthorn Medical Associates, Inc.
New Bedford, MA

Bruce A. Barron, MD, MS
Clinical Assistant Professor of Environmental Medicine
University of Rochester School of Medicine and Dentistry
Rochester, NY

Jay A. Brown, MD, MPH
Medical Director
Center for Occupational Health
Bloomington Hospital
Bloomington, IN

Karin E. Byers, MD, MS
Assistant Professor of Medicine
Allegheny General Hospital
Pittsburgh, PA

Susan O. Cassidy, MD, JD
Health and Disability Consulting
Madison, CT

Alain J. Couturier, MD, MS
Executive Medical Director
Occupational Health Network
South Bend, IN

Lori Checkley, MD
Associate Director
Family Practice Residency
St Joseph Medical Center
South Bend, IN

Roy L. DeHart, MD, MPH
Professor and Chairman
Department of Family and Preventive Medicine
University of Oklahoma College of Medicine
Oklahoma City, OK

Diane Dickerson, RN, BS, COHN-S
Employee Health Nurse
Employee Health Services
Inova Alexandria Hospital
Alexandria, VA

Daymon Evans, MD, MPH
Medical Director, Employee Health Services
Community Hospitals of Indianapolis
Indianapolis, IN

Elissa Ann Favata, MD
Executive Medical Director
Environmental and Occupational Health Associates
Cherry Hill, NJ
Clinical Assistant Professor
Department of Environmental and Community Medicine
UMDNJ-Robert Wood Johnson Medical School
Piscataway, NJ

Jean Spencer Felton, MD
University of California, Irvine
Irvine, CA

Philip E. Fisher, MD
St Joseph's Medical Center
South Bend, IN

Robert C. Godefroi, MD, MPH
Medical Director
Andover, MA

Michael D. Goldstein, MD, MPH
Adjunct Assistant Professor
Department of Environmental and Community Medicine
Robert Wood Johnson Medical School
Langhorne, PA

Peter P. Greaney, MD
Medical Director
Work Care
Orange, CA

Tee L. Guidotti, MD, MPH
Professor and Chair
Department of Environmental and Occupational Health
George Washington University Medical Center
School of Public Health and Health Services
Washington, DC

Gerri S. Hall, PhD
Adjunct Associate Professor
Ohio University
Staff, Department of Clinical Pathology
Cleveland Clinic Foundation
Cleveland, OH

Harold E. Hoffman, MD, CCFP
Adjunct Professor
Occupational Health Program
Public Health Sciences Department
University of Alberta
Edmonton, Alberta, Canada

Robert P. Hurley, MD
Medical Director
Comp Care
Roswell, NM

Jeffrey G. Jones, MD, MPH, MS
Medical Director
St Francis Traveler's Health Center
Indianapolis, IN

Geoffrey A. Kelafant, MD, MSPH
Medical Director, Occupational Health Services
Sarah Bush Lincoln Health Center
Mattoon, IL

Ellen R. Kessler, MD, MPH
Medical Director
Inova Occupational Health
Inova Health System
Fairfax, VA

Timothy J. Key, MD, MPH
Department of Family and Community Medicine
Division of Occupational and Environmental Medicine
School of Medicine
University of Alabama at Birmingham
Birmingham, AL

Paul C. Levy, MD
University of Rochester Medical Center
Strong Memorial Hospital
Pulmonary and Critical Care Unit
Rochester, NY

Cynthia R. Lewis-Younger, MD, MPH
Assistant Director
Occupational Health Clinic
Rocky Mountain Center for Occupational and Environmental Health
Assistant Professor
University of Utah School of Medicine
Salt Lake City, UT

Daniel R. Lucey, MD
Associate Professor of Medicine
Uniformed Services
University of the Health Sciences
Bethesda, MD

Boris D. Lushniak, MD, MPH
Medical Officer/Dermatologist
Centers for Disease Control and Prevention
National Institute for Occupational Safety and Health
Cincinnati, OH

Daniel J. Martin, MD
Director of ICU/CCU
St Luke's Hospital
New Bedford, MA

Robert J. McCunney, MD, MPH
Director, Environmental Medical Service
Massachusetts Institute of Technology
Cambridge, MA

Freddy G. McMurry, MD, MPH
Assistant Medical Director
Occupational Health Group
Decatur, AL

John D. Meyer, MD, MPH
Institute of Occupational and Environmental Health
West Virginia University School of Medicine
Morgantown, WV
Centre for Occupational and Environmental Health
University of Manchester
Manchester, United Kingdom

Daniel A. Nackley, MD, MSc
Attending Physician in Occupational Medicine
Allegheny General Hospital
Pittsburgh, PA

Harry M. Neill, CIH
Vice President
1 Source Safety and Health, Inc.
Exton, PA

Andrew Nickelson, MD
Medical Director
Occupational Health Network
Three Rivers, MI

Wendell H. Perry, DO
Staff Physician
Occupational Health Network
South Bend, IN

Lou Ellen Phillips-Smith, PhD
Senior Manager/Study Director
Watson Laboratories, Inc.
Salt Lake City, UT

Robert S. Rhodes, MD, MPH
Associate Professor of Medicine
Johns Hopkins University College of Medicine
Baltimore, MD
Associate Professor
Occupational and Community Medicine
State University of New York, Buffalo
Regional Director of Health Services
General Motors Corporation
Buffalo, NY

Victor S. Roth, MD, MPH
Assistant Clinical Professor
The University of Michigan Occupational Health Services
Staff Physician, M-Works
Ann Arbor, MI

Jonathan S. Rutchik, MD, MPH
Occupational Neurology Consultant
New York, NY

Brian S. Schwartz, MD, MS
Associate Professor and Director
Division of Occupational and Environmental Health
The Johns Hopkins School of Hygiene and Public Health
Baltimore, MD

Janet M. Serkey, RN, ICP, JD
Infection Control Proctimer
Department of Infection Control
Cleveland Clinic Foundation
Cleveland, OH

Lynn G. Stansbury, MD
Staff Physician
National Institutes of Health
Occupational Medicine Service
Bethesda, MD

Gregg M. Stave, MD, JD, MPH
Assistant Consulting Professor
Division of Occupational and Environmental Medicine
Duke University Medical Center
Durham NC
Director, Corporate Health
Glaxo Wellcome, Inc.
Research Triangle Park, NC

Marion Swinker, MD, MPH
Director
Office of Prospective Health
East Carolina University School of Medicine
Greenville, NC

David R. Trawick, MD, PhD
Pulmonary and Critical Care Medicine
University of Rochester Medical Center
Rochester, NY

Randall L. Updegrove, MD, MPH
Medical Director
Corporate Care/Occupational Medicine
Providence, RI

Mark J. Utell, MD
Professor of Medicine and Environmental Medicine
Director, Pulmonary and Occupational Medicine Divisions
University of Rochester Medical Center
Rochester, NY

Stephen F. Wintermeyer, MD, MPH
Clinical Assistant Professor of Medicine
Division of Pulmonary, Allergy, Critical Care and Occupational Medicine
Indiana University School of Medicine
Indianapolis, IN

Eric P. Wohlrab, MD, MPH, MS
Medical Director
La Porte Horizon Center
La Porte, IN

Chin S. Yang, PhD
President
P&K Microbiology Services, Inc.
Cherry Hill, NJ

Carl N. Zenz, Jr., MD
Corporate Medical Department
Universal Oil Products, Limited Liability Corporation
Des Plaines, IL

Foreword

Illnesses such as heptitis B, Lyme disease, and zoonoses are examples of some infectious diseases that can be contracted by people who work in certain settings. In the United States, over 100 infectious diseases must be reported to state health departments. Workers may be at risk for contracting infectious diseases in the workplace because of people with whom they come in contact on the job, the work environment, or the job itself.

In the United States, working with people or in the delivery of care to others, including the activities of the nearly 10 million health care workers, presents the greatest risk for occupationally acquired infectious disease. However, the environment in which one works also plays a major role, whether the job duties are conducted indoors or outdoors. The geographic location of the job may also present certain indigenous risks. Legionnaires' disease, mosquito-borne infections, and various types of fungal infections associated with different soils are among the notable examples of environmental risks for infectious diseases. Last, but no less important, are specific aspects of the job that pose risks for infectious illnesses, including the handling of animals, infectious agents, and various other materials such as raw sewage.

The adverse impact of infectious illnesses on any enterprise, including businesses and nonprofit and governmental organizations, can be significant. In fact, recent studies have focused on certain types of occupational illnesses such as influenza and their effect on productivity, measured primarily by absenteeism. Clearly, the prevention, control, and treatment of occupational infectious diseases are important responsibilities of occupational health professionals.

This book is logically organized into three basic sections: Fundamentals, Diseases, and Unique Problems and Settings. Chapter topics range from the clinical evaluation of infectious diseases and appropriate vaccinations to infections as common as hepatitis A or as rare as occupational rabies. The topics are diverse and include a fascinating history of occupational infectious diseases, special precautions for pregnant workers, and some of the unique challenges associated with globally emerging infectious diseases, emerging microbial agents of the indoor environment, and biologic warfare.

Supporting the text are excellent tables, regulatory agency guidelines, and peer-reviewed references. The practical focus of the book holds particular appeal for those readers seeking information on vaccinations and vaccination schedules and dosages as well as appropriate work restrictions in the face of infectious disease in the workplace.

Dr. Couturier, with whom I have had the pleasure of working at the Massachusetts Institute of Technology for a four-month period during his residency training in occupational medicine, has been extremely enthusiastic about, and committed to, this book since its inception. He has assembled a group of authoritative and motivated authors who obviously shared his vision of producing a comprehensive source of information on this important aspect of occupational medical practice. This book should fill a void in the literature and serve as a practical guide for occupational health professionals, especially physicians and nurses, who care for working people worldwide.

Robert J. McCunney, MD, MPH

Preface

The practice of occupational and environmental medicine encompasses a vast array of clinical and nonclinical disciplines. Nowhere is this more evident than in the realm of the identification, prevention, and management of workplace and environmental infectious diseases. In this realm, the disciplines of epidemiology, microbiology, immunology, molecular genetics, pharmacology, ecology, industrial hygiene, and biostatistics are interwoven with family practice, internal medicine and all of its subspecialties, and preventive medicine.

While it is unlikely that any one practitioner would be involved in all of these disciplines simultaneously, it is not uncommon for the occupational health professional to have to synthesize the diverse bodies of knowledge that comprise these disciplines when risk management strategies are being devised and implemented. Unfortunately, this information is often scattered among different resources and is therefore difficult to retrieve. In the midst of physicians' ever-burgeoning time demands, it is the goal of this comprehensive yet practical textbook to reduce this burden. With this in mind, this book is organized into three distinct sections.

The first section provides the fundamental framework for understanding the epidemiology, prevention, and management of infectious diseases related to occupational and environmental factors—from the history, laboratory evaluation, and etiology and epidemiology of infectious diseases to high-risk occupations, legal issues, available vaccines, medical surveillance, and worker training and education. In particular, the chapter on etiology and epidemiology of infectious disease was designed to serve as a resource for studying for that section of the American Board of Preventive Medicine Certifying Examination as well as a review for medical students, residents, fellows, and practicing clinicians.

The second section, which is devoted to specific infectious diseases, constitutes the bulk of the book; the chapters are generally organized in a sequential fashion by organ-system involvement. The rationale for this approach is to reflect and conform to the workers' compensation system, which typically codifies illnesses by organ system, as well as to follow in logical sequence those medical specialities and subspecialties involved in the care of these patients.

The third and last section of the book is devoted to unique workplace settings and problems requiring special approaches to infectious disease prevention and management. Separate chapters are devoted to the special considerations related to work in health care, laboratory, and sewage facilities. In addition, there are chapters on infectious disease issues for pregnant workers and for employees who work with animals (occupational zoonoses). The last three chapters of the book highlight globally emerging infectious diseases, emerging microbial diseases of the indoor environment, and biologic warfare, which threaten not only workers but also the global community.

It is beyond the scope of this book to cover separately and comprehensively all occupational and environmental conditions that pose risks for the transmission of infectious diseases. However, it is its goal to provide a logical framework to more effectively address and facilitate the identification, prevention, and management of occupationally and environmentally related infectious diseases wherever they may occur in our increasingly global economic community.

This textbook would not have been possible without the expertise, hard work, and dedication of its many contributors. I wish to extend my sincere gratitude to all of them. My thanks also goes to Curtis Vouwie, Publisher of OEM Press, to whom I am indebted for his encouragement and support throughout this project, from its conception to its birth as a bound book. Kathy O'Brien, whose editorial skills transformed the raw manuscript into a polished publication, deserves very special thanks, as do Marty Tenney, who designed the book and so ably managed its production, and Linda Scott and Karla Goethe, whose professional expertise were also indispensable to the publication process.

AJC

I / Fundamentals

1 / History of Occupational Infectious Diseases

Jean Spencer Felton

> There are many handicrafts and arts which cause those who exercise them certain pains and plagues.
>
> —*Hippocrates*

Populations today are on the move, enabled by advances in transportation and motivated by the many impacts of modern communication. Diseases previously believed to be localized geographically now spread worldwide and affect labor forces everywhere. A look into centuries past reveals the ubiquity of a broad variety of physical disorders occasioned by the inroads into the human body of a diversity of microorganisms.

The rise of terrorism, the fear of biologic warfare, the emergence of new diseases, the resistance of certain pathogens to antibiotics, and the increased frequency of natural disasters have changed the perception of both old and new disease agents. The rise in prison populations, the influx of immigrants from countries where numerous infectious diseases are endemic, and the continuing demands of business travel have fused to a great extent the long-held separateness of occupational and nonoccupational illnesses. The invasion of the business sector by communicable diseases has muddied workers' compensation coverage, often making judgments of job relatedness extremely difficult.

The Pre-Industrial Age

Plagues of one disease entity or another have been recorded for centuries, even though their causes were unidentified. Thucydides, considered the greatest historian of antiquity, as early as 430 BC described an epidemic that ravaged Athens, thus strongly influencing the outcome of the Peloponnesian War [1]. The pestilence, presumably starting in Ethiopia, traveled to Egypt and then was carried by ship across the Mediterranean to Athens, bringing death to possibly two thirds of the population, and a disastrous breakdown of the citizens' and military forces' morale, the frequent concomitant of pandemics [2]. A second epidemic struck a military force led by Pericles. This epidemic is believed to have been a highly malignant form of scarlet fever, or bubonic plague, typhus, smallpox, measles, or anthrax of extraordinary virulence [3].

Biblical references to individual and mass illnesses are numerous. In Exodus, one learns that the waters of the Nile "were turned to blood," "flies" appeared, as did "lice," and a "cattle murrain," "boils," "hail," "locusts," and "darkness" [4]. The book of Leviticus offers clear diagnoses of leprosy, gonorrhea, and leukorrhea, along with specific directions concerning segregation of the patient, burning of bedclothes, and disinfection [5]. Forewarnings of cholera epidemics, related to polluted water and contaminated foodstuffs, are rife in Leviticus in its references to the dangers of "unclean" cooking vessels, "flying creeping" things, and animal carcasses [6].

Plagues persisted through the years, and the returning Crusaders in the eleventh, twelfth, and thirteenth centuries brought leprosy to Europe, where the disease had always been endemic but at low levels. The number of lepers increased tremendously in Europe during the Middle Ages, although the stigmatization of leprosy was mistakenly attached to a variety of other dermatologic disorders. While not all were contagious, people called *lepers* were completely ostracized from society; distinctive clothing to identify them became mandatory, and their segregation was strictly imposed in places of public assembly or worship [7]. An unwelcome "import" brought back to Europe by the Crusaders was the Black Death, or bubonic plague. Oddly, the fierce Tartars, with some understanding of this scourge's contagion, after attacking a city in the southeast Crimea, upon their departure catapulted into the city corpses of soldiers who had died of plague [8].

In the years between 540 and 1666, there were three great pandemics: The plague of Justinian in the years 540–590, the Black Death of 1346–1361, and the pandemic that raged in Europe from 1665 to 1666 and produced the Great Plague of London [9]. At some point during the first and last of these three, the mode of transmission in pandemics changed from the rat-flea-man cycle of bubonic plague to the predominantly more severe pneumonic form of the disease.

Although the belief that the miasma arising from the Earth was the cause of disease was prevalent as late as the seventeenth century, a century earlier, in 1546, Fracastoro identified contagion as the principal factor responsible for the rise and spread of epidemic disease, a conclusion reached after his study of plague, typhus fever, syphilis, and other communicable disorders [10]. His treatise *De Contagione eet Contagiosis Morbis et Eorum Curatione* is the first scientific statement on the true nature of contagion and the transmission of diseases by "germs" [11]. This work was translated into English by Wilmer Cave Wright [12], who was later encouraged to translate Ramazzini's classic work into English, thus making it the standard contemporary reference and Ramazzini the so-called Father of Occupational Medicine. Further, it was Fracastoro who introduced *syphilis* as the first designation given the disease; the term was derived from the name of a shepherd infected with the disease who figured in a medical poem Fracastoro wrote in 1530 [13].

It was Antony van Leeuwenhoek (1632–1723), a linen draper in Delft who developed the microscope, who initially observed bacteria and other microscopic organisms. He described forms known today as *cocci*, *bacilli*, and *spirilla* [14] but did not make a connection between these "little animals," as he referred to them, and disease. Although there were suggestions concerning this relationship, it was not until the 1830s and 1840s that the germ theory of disease was revived on the basis of new evidence [15]. An early connection between infectious disease and work emerged about the same period. *Fever* was a portmanteau term used for typhoid, typhus, and relapsing fevers. Severe outbreaks of these infections were seen in the early decades of the nineteenth century in Ireland, then in Scotland and England. There was awareness of an economic deficit, as these disorders affected workers. Each individual, it was estimated, lost an average of six weeks of employment, and for nearly 13,000 patients at the Glasgow Fever Hospital, this totaled £29,004. Added to this sum was the cost of medical and nursing care at £1 per patient. The funeral costs for some and provision for the surviving widows and orphans further raised the debit, all of this stimulating action toward a better public health [16].

Occupational medicine, as a discrete medical discipline in the health care world, was not given substance until 1700, when Bernardino Ramazzini of Modena, Italy, produced the first edition of *Diseases of Workers*. Although sparse writings had appeared earlier, it was this *De Morbis Artificum Diatriba* that offered a view of the work-related illnesses seen in over 50 distinct trades and occupations. As mentioned previously, it was Wright's excellent translation that made this work available to the English-speaking world, despite earlier literary appearances in that language [17].

Infectious diseases had yet to be identified in microbiologic terms, but Ramazzini did write of the hazards of military service. "[A]rmies are almost always decimated by some malignant epidemic. Camp fevers . . . and other fatal and contagious diseases are famous or rather infamous" [18]. He cites a Greek military surgeon who, apart from wounds, classifies camp diseases as malignant fever or dysentery and concluded that "the morbific seed of malignity that breeds and fosters camp fever is harbored in corrupt and polluted air" [19]. Sailors and seafarers were subject to "malignant and pestilential fevers" [20] and hunters experienced "day cholera" [21]. Common to many trades, Ramazzini indicates, is terminal "consumption," as seen in glass workers [22], wet nurses [23], stone cutters [24], and silk carders [25]. He cautions of laundresses' contact with "a thousand kinds of filth from persons . . . polluted with the French disease [syphilis]" and writes that treatment should "dislodge the gross humors" [26].

It cannot be said that the terms used in Ramazzini's day are the equivalents of today's nosology, but the clinical descriptions of various fevers do parallel some of our current infectious disorders. Not clarified, of course, is the source of the organisms—fellow workers, fomites, the environment, or impaired personal hygiene? In view of the working conditions of the times, it may be concluded that many of the disease states indicated were inherent in these early jobs.

The Industrial Age

Although the calendar marks with stunning accuracy the passage of time, the name given a particular historic era is arbitrary and usually imposed by social historians long after the beginning of an era. In the mid-nineteenth century, at the beginning of what came to be called *The Industrial Age*, many inventions of power machinery, such as Watt's steam engine and Cartwright's power loom, led to changes in the processes used to produce goods. As the eminent British sociologist Arnold Toynbee expressed, "It was by these discoveries that population was drawn out of cottages in distant valleys by secluded streams and driven together into factories and cities" [27]. Or, as stated by his equally famed nephew, Arnold Joseph Toynbee, the period was characterized by "[t]he deliberate application of science to technology" [28].

The term *Industrial Revolution* was coined by the French in the 1830s to describe the change from an agrarian economy to an industrial one in which goods were produced in city factories by machines of mass production. The movement of the masses from farms to cities began in the 1700s in Britain, for the country was then free from wars [29]. The significance of this relocation in regard to infectious disease lies in the sudden congestion in cities of great numbers of persons accustomed to farm living. With the crowding came long hours of work, child labor, the absence of sanitary measures, the creation of slums, the appearance of occupational diseases, and, indubitably, the loss of health or life to the invasion of as yet unidentified microorganisms.

The early observers of the interaction of work and health began to see, as did Ramazzini in his day, the devastating effects on workers, whether artisans, laborers, or professionals. One of the first physicians to be concerned with the adverse effects of labor was Charles Turner Thackrah, "born . . . into a society which was distinguished by the profound juxtaposition of wealth and poverty which prevailed at the time" [30]. His work, *The Effects of Arts, Trades, and Professions*, appeared in 1832 [31]. Thackrah died of chronic pulmonary tuberculosis, as did such notable contemporaries as John Hunter and John Keats [32]. The disease was then a common fatal infection of dissecting-room students. Thackrah published early on the subject of cholera and later wrote about sexually transmitted diseases, "I scarcely need advert to the diseases of the genital organs more frequent in soldiers and sailors than in most classes of society" [33]. He noted also that sugar refiners died of tuberculosis [34] and that surgeons and accoucheurs were predisposed in the discharge of their professional duties to the absorption of "syphilitic poison" and its ultimate lethal effects [35]. The latter observation was made long before the identification of the causative *Treponema pallidum* by the microscopist Schaudinn in 1905 [36].

The Factory System and Its Ills

The growth and multiplication of factories continued at a rapid pace during the early nineteenth century, accompanied by the deleterious effects on workers, both adults and children. Although the presence of illness among factory employees was noted by the factory owners and physicians of the day, etiologic clarity was lacking. A practitioner of the period, when asked his opinion concerning the medical effects produced by the hours of labor, responded, "The first effects appear to be upon the digestion, the appetite suffers, the digestion is impaired, and consequent emaciation and debility are induced. Scrofulous diseases are common . . ." [37]. Medical opinions differed as to causation by various exposures in factory settings, some physicians even believing that work in certain plants was actually beneficial and cured disease. Because of the endemicity of so many of the infectious diseases in urban areas, it would be difficult to differentiate an occupational disease from a contagious disorder rampant in the community or to identify "cotton-consumption" or "cotton inflammation of the lungs" [38] specifically as today's byssinosis, or byssinosis compounded by tuberculosis. Were the diseases brought into the factories from the totally unsanitary living areas or were the pneumoconioses that were produced in the manufacturing processes worsened by the endemic "scrofula" of the cities [39]?

A nineteenth century description of a worker implies a body subject to the invasion of any infectious agent: "These artisans are frequently subject to a disease, in which the sensibility of the stomach and bowels is morbidly excited; the alvine secretions are deranged, and the appetite impaired. Whilst this state continues, the patient loses flesh, his features are sharpened, the skin becomes pale, leaden colored, or of the yellow hue which is observed in those who have suffered from the influence of tropical climates." Following are "the horrors of a disordered imagination, . . . gloomy apprehension, the deepest depression, and . . . despair" [40]. Of the many conditions presdisposing to "contagious disease," "extreme labor" and its consequent physical exhaustion were cited [41].

As the nineteenth century approached its close, discerning physicians began to document the afflictions arising in industry. One of the early practitioners concerned with factory medicine was John Thomas Arlidge, whose monograph appeared in 1892 [42]. This magnum opus fell into almost complete oblivion for about 50 years. Like so many dedicated specialists in occupational medicine, Arledge was ostracized "for what was considered to be illegitimate interference with deplorable factory conditions which he had ample opportunity to observe as a certifying factory surgeon for Stoke, Longton, and Fenton" [43]. In his discussion of organic dust of an animal nature and the manufacture of wool, he wrote of anthrax, then called *wool-sorters' disease*. The rapidity of the disease course was noted; in some instances, death ensued in 19 hours. Of interest, also, was the case of a mohair sorter's wife, who had not been within half a mile of the mill but developed fatal anthrax of the face [44].

An important tome edited by another British physician, Thomas Oliver, and published in 1902, included an extensive discussion of infectious diseases associated with work [45]. A full chapter was devoted to the diseases of soldiers, including malaria, dysentery, typhoid fever, and cholera. The author of the chapter, John R. Dodd of the Royal Army Medical Corps, pointed out that in the Crimean War, three times as many British troops died of sickness as those who died at the hands of the Russians. Further, because of the accompanying illnesses, he referred to the Ashanti Expeditions into West Africa as *doctors' wars* [46].

Seamen were subject to malaria, yellow fever, dysentery, cholera, plague, and "phthisis." Regrettably, men were allowed to "sign on" as mariners with no inquiry as to their physical fitness for the occupation [47]. Among stable personnel, glanders and its more chronic and constitutional lymphatic form, farcy, were noted, along with tetanus and rabies. Anthrax, vaccinia, tuberculosis, tinea, foot and mouth disease, diphtheria, actinomycosis, and trichinosis were some of the zoonoses to which animal handlers were subject [48].

Upholsterers occasionally had to remake used mattresses, and it was found that when "mattresses have become fouled in places by discharges from patients suffering from infectious diseases, considerable risk is incurred by those who by hand teaze the contents of such bespoiled bedding" [49].

In these late years of the nineteenth century, various legislative actions were taken in England, raising the allowable age at which children could be employed, giving greater power to central authority in the regulation of certain trades, and extending the coverage provided by earlier workers' compensation acts. Oliver, in his 1908 text, expressed some cynicism about the laws passed. He wrote, "In this country industrial legislation is based upon experience and expediency, so that no sooner is an Act in operation than its weak points become apparent and a fresh Act is required to remedy defects and remove flaws, but it too generally ends in introducing controversial matter and in providing employment of lawyers and doctors" [50]. A lengthy chapter was devoted to "Diseases Due to Parasites and Micro-Organisms," much of the discussion relating to ankylostomiasis, particularly because the infestation affected numerous miners in the construction of the St. Gothard Tunnel in Switzerland. In connection with the spread of the illness, Oliver commented that, "Probably one diseased and thoughtless miner is capable of infecting a mine owing to the myriads of ova passed in his stools" [51]. The military were similarly stricken by hookworm disease.

Hospital nurses worked in hazardous conditions, as the infirmary wards were poorly ventilated. Many of the nurses suffered from "hospital throat," and those attending patients with infectious diseases could acquire the disorder. Small finger wounds became infected with resulting bacteremia, and tuberculosis was transmitted to the attendant staff through bad handling of the patients' sputum. Physicians ran comparable risks through their "treatment of abscesses and foul wounds in operation" [52].

American Workers

It was noted in the Memorial of Occupational Diseases sent to President Taft in June 1910 by the First National Conference on Industrial Diseases that nearly all of the standard reference works on occupational diseases were prepared by English or Continental authorities [53]. To fill this gap, a work was undertaken by Dr. W. Gilman Thompson of Cornell University Medical College in New York. *The Occupational Diseases*, published in 1914, was directed not only to physicians but to those individuals in various manufactures or trades "in which the health of the workman is closely related to problems of efficiency and humanitarian effort" [54]. Thompson had published extensively before, had established clinics dedicated to occupational disease, and was active on the visiting staffs of New York's largest hospitals.

He, like others, was concerned with tuberculosis and its high mortality among workers [55], and, in his discussion of diseases due to irritant substances, included a section titled "Germs." Ankylostomiasis, anthrax, foot and mouth disease (aphthous fever), glanders, and farcy were reviewed, as was the "septicemia" incurred by those handling "putrid or decomposing animal products" [56], such as in the making of bone fertilizers from the carcasses of dead horses. Not touched on previously was localized tuberculosis (verruca necrogenica) of the hands and forearms of butchers inoculated through the handling of tuberculous cattle [57]. Thompson advocated the early treatment of syphilis (not necessarily occupationally acquired disease), since lead poisoning in a patient with syphilis could present "symptoms of unusual gravity" [58].

Dr. George M. Price of New York was closely involved in sanitation controls within the clothing industry and by 1914 believed that tuberculosis was the main end result of the transmission of microorganisms via coughing, sneezing, salivation, and the like, in the workplace. He felt that tubercle bacilli were ubiquitous in all industrial plants and that workers already suffering from pulmonary infections or those with dust-laden lungs had no immune resistance to "tuberculous phthisis" [53].

Building on American experience was not easy, for Dr. George M. Kober of Washington, DC, refused a publishers' request in 1911 to produce a book on occupational diseases because "the scarcity of statistical data in reference to disease and accident-hazards in the various occupations in this country, had compelled him in his former writings to get most of his facts from Europe and the State of Massachusetts" [59]. However, 1916 saw the production of Kober and Hanson's nearly 1,000-page volume which sold for $8.00 [60]. Anthrax and pulmonary anthrax were reviewed at length [61], and a separate chapter titled "Parasites and Occupation," was included. In the chapter, malaria, amebic dysentery, uncinariasis, filariasis, trichinosis, infestation with ascaris lumbricoides, and schistosomiasis were assessed as occupational diseases [62]. The occupational devastation caused by malaria was described as having "been the greatest obstacle to colonization of the tropics by the white race; it has transformed fertile, rich and populous regions into lonely wastes; it has rendered the development of valuable natural resources impossible and by decimating armies has defeated the highest hopes of nations in critical struggles" [62]. The French failure in the construction of a canal in Panama gives substance to this observation. Tuberculosis was discussed as a disease resulting from the continuous and considerable exposure to industrial dust [63].

World War I

Although there had been epidemics of influenza throughout history—in 412 BC, Hippocrates chronicled a flu-like disease that obliterated an Athenian army [64]—none manifested the mortality of the scourge of 1918. The disease hit the New World in 1647, coming from Valencia, Spain, and was promptly dubbed *Spanish influenza* ("influence" in Italian). Later, in 1918, the disease had killed more people within days than all of the World War I armies in four years of fighting. By December, 500,000 Americans had perished, and nearly 20,000,000 had contracted the disease. Attending nurses and volunteers died alongside the patients in their care. The epidemic started on March 11th at Fort Riley, Kansas, and soon after the first patient was stricken, there was an explosive outbreak [65]. Influenza spread throughout Europe after our troops landed in France; 132 cases were reported within 12 days of their arrival. The outbreak was rampant on ships and trains and in army camps and naval hospitals, where people were together in close proximity. An army transport landing troops in England soon had 2,300 ill with influenza, 119 of whom died. Tightly packed troop compartments provided unmatched "culture" conditions for the disease-causing pathogen. After rampaging through the Western world, the disease struck Asia.

In the United States, worker after worker succumbed in the Quincy, Massachusetts, shipyards. Dozens of army camps were affected and medical care did not alter the spread of the epidemic. Masks were ordered for universal wear; this writer remembers having to don a mask whenever leaving his house in San Francisco, where one fourth of California's 40,000 cases occurred. All industries were losing employees to influenza: Washington's federal agencies, packing plants, street transportation, East Coast and Gulf Coast shipyards, gold and coal mines, hospitals, and plantations. Public gathering places were closed. All manner of treatment modalities and cures were proffered without effect.

The Navy had been hit badly, with 120,000 of its personnel—one fourth of its total—being stricken, 5,000 dying. The Army, 10 times the size of the other service, lost 25,000. Residents of Dublin died at a rate of 250 a day [66]. When the Armistice was signed in November, the siege slackened. But at its height, one health department was advised, "Hunt up your woodworkers and cabinetmakers and set them making coffins." Later, "Then take your street laborers and set them to digging graves" [67]. With more than 25 million Americans infected, perhaps a billion worldwide, the direct U.S. economic losses were estimated at $3 billion, but it is believed that the epidemic ultimately cost the United States alone 10 million years in productive lives cut off at their prime [67]. Was the pandemic one of occupationally incurred infectious disease because fellow workers transmitted the illness? Was it a community epidemic unrelated to work? Servicemen were workers. Health care personnel were workers. Family members were workers. While the insurance payments going to policyholders were high, no exact data seem to be available that would divide the morbidity or mortality into job-relatedness or nonoccupational illness. It is hoped that no comparable epidemiologic "opportunity" to help answer these questions will arise again.

Between the Wars

In 1920, Dr. Harry E. Mock, a medical officer in World War I and afterward, Chief Surgeon (Medical Director) of Sears, Roebuck & Company in Chicago, amassed the collective knowledge of occupational medicine current at that time in his book *Industrial Medicine and Surgery* [68]. By then, the infectious diseases previously described had become common knowledge. In a 15,000-employee company in Chicago, 44 cases of infectious disease were encountered, including mumps (22), scarlet fever (9), diphtheria (6), measles (4), erysipelas (2), and varicella (1) [69].

Typhoid fever and smallpox were discussed, with emphasis placed on preventive vaccination.

Mock indicated that the combating of venereal diseases among employees had been woefully neglected by the majority of physicians in industry. Accounting for this lack of attention were the indifferent attitude that the medical profession had always assumed toward prevention of these diseases and the fact that the employees so affected, when discovered, were discharged. Mock advocated an emphasis on employee education, and some statements selected from a poster used for this purpose are of interest [70]:

- Prevention: (1) Keep away from prostitutes, both professional and non-professional. (2) Sexual intercourse is not necessary to physical and mental health. (3) Antiseptic washes . . . are not always reliable.
- Beware of advertising specialists who claim to cure "nervous debility" and "private diseases of men." Advertising specialists get large sums of money for "diseases" which do not exist.
- What to do (apart from reporting to a physician). Do no worry. Lead a vigorous, healthful life and forget about sex matters. Be consistent and adopt the same standard of sexual conduct for yourself that you expect of women.

In light of contemporary responses by the media to matters sexual and today's advertising emphasis on sex to sell everything and anything, one can conjure up employees' reactions to these precautions of 1920.

Tuberculosis in industry was faced by Mock and other physicians of the period, and they advocated avoiding overcrowding in the workplace, improving ventilation, removing dust, and examining employees. Discussed at length were the industrial pneumoconioses that predisposed to the acquisition of tuberculosis. Frequent examination, provision of sanatorium care, visiting nurse services, and re-employment of the healed employee were strongly advocated [71].

Last, concern was expressed regarding the Americanization of foreign employees and the industrial physician's role in such a program. The same points arise today: standard of living, language barriers, crowding in urban ethnic or national enclaves, inadequate wages, and the like. Mock advised bilingual posters, education, instruction regarding personal hygiene and sanitation, and access to medical care [72].

Sir Thomas M. Legge was Britain's first Medical Inspector of Factories, assuming the post in 1898. Early on, he directed his attention to anthrax [73], but most of his career was devoted to the industrial diseases arising from contact with workplace metals, dusts, organic compounds, and the usual broad variety of other toxic substances. In the work published posthumously, Legge reviewed the hazards of anthrax and tetanus and gave consideration to silicosis accompanied by tuberculosis. He wrote, "Stress is rightly laid on the fact that the bacillus tuberculosis, whether in the lung before the onset of the damage, during it, or entering after, is of paramount importance in influencing unfavorably the subsequent development of the disease" [74]. In addition, he noted the undue incidence of phthisis among persons employed in brass-working [75].

Late in the 1930s, Dr. H. M. Vernon, long identified with occupational medicine, produced a somewhat broader text emphasizing "health" as a goal as well as touching on anthrax in woolsorters [76], the high death rate in laundry workers from tuberculosis [77], and the combination of silicosis and tuberculosis [78,79].

World War II

The production of armaments and material needed for World War II led to the conversion of many peacetime plants and the construction of new facilities throughout the Allied countries. Women, the disabled, and older personnel were added to company rosters, and because of the burgeoning of manufacturing sites, occupational health services were added to worker rosters, not only because of the increased labor force—coming from all areas—but because of the use and production of innumerable toxic materials. By this time, many protective vaccines had been developed, and a broad variety was being administered to military personnel and some to civilian workers. The unidentified plants of the Manhattan District Project focused medical attention on the possible effects of exposure to radioactive sources—"the product"—rather than on specific groups of diseases. In the *Manual of Standard Practices for Industrial Nurses* used at the Hanford Engineer Works in Richland, Washington, however, two of the indicated procedures involved "communicable disease regulations" and "reportable diseases" [80]. No details have remained for review.

Acceptance into the armed services during the early phases of World War II was in keeping with some stringent physical standards. Active tuberculosis in the Army during those years was 1.24 per thousand, about one ninth that of World War I. Potential Army inductees who had venereal disease (syphilis) were classified as limited service, but none of these were actually inducted until July 1942. Gonorrhea was considered a remedial defect and such registrants were temporarily deferred until cured. With a liberalization of standards, somewhat over 200,000 registrants with venereal disease were inducted [81]. Men with other acute infectious diseases were deferred until recovery, without disqualifying sequelae. Certain parasitic infections were allowed in registrants, and treatment was initiated, but filariasis, trypanosomiasis, amebiasis, and schistosomiasis were causes for rejection [82].

Many of the immunizations given service personnel predated World War II, but the vaccinations performed also included typhoid-paratyphoid, smallpox, tetanus, yellow fever, cholera, plague, typhus, influenza, and Japanese B encephalitis. Protection for special situations included diphtheria and Rocky Mountain spotted fever immunizations. Human immune serum globulin was used for passive protection against measles and viral hepatitis, and extremely rarely, scarlet fever streptococcus toxin was administered to certain health care personnel [83].

The status of occupational medicine at the time of World War II was expressed by Cook [84] in this manner: "[The] principles of democracy and of economics had integrated industry, labor, and hygiene, at least in the United States, and raised all three to a national level of mutual concern. Research in this area had developed sufficiently for its emphasis to change from inquiry into causes of occupational disease to the anticipation and correction of hazardous conditions."

A wartime publication by Clarence O. Sappington, a prolific writer of the period, was one of the few monographs covering all aspects of occupational medicine until the freshet of monographs appeared after the passage of the Occupational Safety and Health Act in 1970. Sappington remarked that both localized and systemic infections are frequently of occupational origin and listed some 14 disorders and the workers in whom such diseases may be found. For example, he cited psittacosis (bacteriologists, parrot, and parakeet handlers) and tetanus (farmers, slaughterhouse, and packinghouse workers) [85].

The Postwar Years

During the postwar years, Dr. Rutherford T. Johnstone, a highly respected occupational medicine pioneer in southern California, wrote extensively, producing two textbooks, probably the only ones available to students for many years. While the first, bearing the date of 1948, covering primarily occupationally hazardous materials, tuberculosis was treated as a work-related disease, apart from the disorder in some health care workers and in workers exposed to free silicon dioxide, a relationship alluded to earlier [86].

In Johnstone's second work, an entire chapter reviewed infectious occupational diseases and addressed the question of their rising out of, and in the course of, employment. The diseases discussed included brucellosis, tularemia, anthrax, erysipeloid, psittacosis, Q fever, equine encephalomyelitis, and mite dermatitis. Those specific infections acquired from a contaminated work environment encompassed histoplasmosis, coccidioidomycosis, blastomycosis, creeping eruption, tetanus, leptospirosis, and schistosomiasis. In summary, Johnstone indicated that "under special circumstances, the infections of ordinary life may become occupational diseases" [87].

The Later Decades of the Twentieth Century

In 1955, the dean of occupational physicians in Great Britain, Dr. Donald Hunter of the London Hospital, produced the first edition of his eponymous classic, the most recent appearing in 1994. Even in the seminal work, Hunter included a heavily illustrated chapter titled "Occupational Diseases Due to Infections," naming most of the illnesses described by earlier writers. In recent editions, an entire section is devoted to diseases associated with microbiologic agents (bacteria, viruses, biotechnologic hazards), with emphasis on laboratory acquired infections [88]. While allusions to the infectious diseases potentially acquired by a work force are still touched on in contemporary writings, new fears have arisen throughout the world, occasioned by serious epidemics, contacts with affected populations from endemic areas, and the sequelae of natural disasters. History blends irrevocably into the present as it is learned that infectious disease mortality has been increasing in the United States [89]. These disorders currently are recognized as having an industrial presence, and special attention is now being directed toward health care workers [90–96].

New infectious diseases are emerging and certain of the once-conquered illnesses are reappearing [97–99]. Some of the determinants in the recrudescence of the old and the arrival of the new are global warming, human migration, population increases, deforestation, poverty, disruption of environmental habitats, the emergence of antibiotic-resistant bacteria, the increase in international travel, and the lack of precautions in many almost-primitive health care facilities [100].

Different work groups, such as the military, the Coast Guard and international relief personnel, are being exposed to communicable diseases through the extension of aid to refugees and the rescue of migrants [101–103]. The potential for infectious spread is also seen in day care centers [104], in competitive sports [105], and following natural disasters [106]. The emergence of Ebola hemorrhagic fever, the continuing HIV epidemic, the variant of Creutzfeldt-Jakob disease in the United Kingdom, and the effects of the invasion of *Hantavirus* pale in comparison to the potential for mass casualties through bioter-rorism. Biologic warfare technology can involve the use of anthrax spores, botulinum toxin, aflatoxin, or a modified *Yersinia pestis*, the plague bacterium [107]. The medical effects of biologic terrorism can be extreme [108], and as noted by one who conducts studies of agents of terrorism, "Biological weapons are . . . not detected by methods used for explosives and firearms, such as metal detectors and x-ray devices. Moreover, because the first indication of an attack is likely to be hours to days after exposure—when people first begin to develop disease symptoms—the perpetrators can be long gone from the scene before health and law enforcement authorities are aware there is a problem" [109].

American troops have already been given anthrax vaccine in Bosnia [110], Russia has an altered form of anthrax [111], and Iraq reputedly has 2,000 gallons of anthrax [112].

That there is some fear among health care workers of the contagion of infectious diseases—even at the individual, let alone mass, level—is evident in the reluctance of physicians and nurses to perform mouth-to-mouth resuscitation (MMR). Of the physicians, 45%, and of the nurses, 80%, would refuse to do MMR on a stranger. Between 18% and 25% of the two groups would not conduct MMR on a child [113]. In a second study, 82% of the nearly 1,000 persons queried were at least "moderately" concerned about disease transmission in the performance of bystander MMR [114].

Further fear within the United States stems from terrorist activities carried out in the form of the contamination of food with microbiologic agents. Deliberate inoculation of foodstuffs resulted in type 2 *Shigella dysenteriae* infection and salmonellosis in health care workers. The act was initiated by a religious cult in one instance and by someone with laboratory skills in the other [115,116].

The military view is expressed succinctly: "The possibility that biological weapons will be used against us is no longer unthinkable. Until recently, medical officers and other healthcare practitioners may have considered this topic more suitable for academic than practical pursuit. The fact is, however, that biological agents have been used as weapons since antiquity, and the threat that modern weapons will be used is real" [118].

In a summation of bioterrorism, it can be concluded, as set forth in a federal report, that "no government spending priorities for combating terrorism have been set, and no federal entity exists to channel resources where they are most needed and to prevent wasteful spending resulting from unnecessary duplication of effort" [116].

The Future

Concerns about infectious diseases contracted in the workplace have coursed from minimal interest in common disorders brought by workers to their workplaces, to an acceptance of some illnesses as concomitants or sequelae of many industrial exposures. While knowledgeable occupational health practitioners can inform or educate those persons whose daily tasks involve contact with pathogenic agents, there is not sufficient professional resources available to reach the solitary, immigrant, or remote workers subject to disease acquisition. Possibly, only through a symbiotic collaboration between occupational medicine and public health practitioners will infectious disease disappear from the workplace. The old and the new in infectious diseases will remain until an international surveillance system is implemented to enable the mobilization of an effective global response when infectious outbreaks occur. May historic transmittable diseases be eliminated from contemporary worksites and may the fears of world contamination be replaced by international understanding and cooperation.

References

1. Petersen EA, Mandel RM. Infectious diseases: old diseases return and new agents emerge. *Arch Intern Med* 1995;155:1571–2.
2. Cartwright FF. *Disease and History.* New York: Thomas Y. Crowell, 1972. P 7.
3. *Ibid*, p 8.
4. Exodus 7–10; Keller W. *The Bible As History* (2nd Rev Ed). New York: William Morrow, 1981. P 124.
5. Leviticus 13–15; Anon. The bible and medicine. *MD* 1978;22:87–99.
6. Leviticus 11:3–47; Brim CJ. *Medicine in the Bible: The Pentateuch.* New York: Froben Press, 1936. Pp 124–5.
7. Lyons AS, Petrucelli J II. *Medicine: An Illustrated History.* New York: Harry N. Abrams, 1978. P 345.
8. *Ibid*, p 349.
9. Ref 2, *supra*, pp 31–2.
10. Rosen G. *A History of Public Health.* New York: MD Publications, 1958. P 105.
11. Fracastoro G (Lat. Hieronymus Fracastorius). *Webster's New Biographical Dictionary.* Springfield, MA: Merriam-Webster, 1983. Pp 365–6.
12. Fracastorii H. *De Contagione et Contagiosis Morbis et Eorum Curatione*, Libri III. (*Contagion, Contagious Diseases, and Their Treatment*). Translation and notes by W. C. Wright. New York: G.P. Putnam's sons, 1930.
13. *Dorland's Illustrated Medical Dictionary*, 28th Ed. Philadelphia: Saunders, 1994. Pp 660, 1646.
14. Ref 10, *supra*, p 107.
15. Ref 10, *supra*, pp 108–9.
16. Ref 10, *supra*, p 212.
17. Ramazzini B. *De Morbis Artificum Diatriba.* (*Diseases of Workers.*) The Latin text of 1713. Revised, with translation and notes by Wilmer Cave Wright. Chicago: University of Chicago Press, 1940.
18. *Ibid*, p 359.
19. *Ibid*, p 363.
20. *Ibid*, p 465.
21. *Ibid*, p 473.
22. *Ibid*, p 65.
23. *Ibid*, p 195.
24. *Ibid*, p 249.
25. *Ibid*, p 261.
26. *Ibid*, p 255.
27. Toynbee A. *The Industrial Revolution of the 18th Century in England.* New York: Humboldt, 1890. P 15.
28. Toynbee AJ. *A Study of History* (rev, abridged). New York: American Heritage, 1972. P 62.
29. Cooke J, Kramer A, Rowland-Entwistle T. *History's Timeline* New York: Crescent Books, 1981. P 162.
30. Cleeland J, Burt S. Charles Turner Thackrah: a pioneer in the field of occupational health. *Occup Med* (Oxford) 1995;45:285–97.
31. Thackrah CT. *The Effects of Arts, Trades, and Professions and of Civic States and Habits of Living, on Health and Longevity with Suggestions for the Removal of Many of the Agents Which Produce Disease, and Shorten the Duration of Life* (2nd Ed, greatly enlarged). London: Longman, Rees, Orme, Brown, Green & Longman, 1832. Reprinted with a biographical essay: Meiklejohn A. *The Life, Work and Times of Charles Turner Thackrah, Surgeon and Apothecary of Leeds (1795–1833).* London: E. & S. Livingstone, 1957.
32. *Ibid* (Meiklejohn), p 9.
33. *Ibid* (Thackrah), p 22.
34. *Ibid*, p 135.
35. *Ibid*, p 175.
36. Garrison FH. *An Introduction to the History of Medicine* (4th Ed). Philadelphia: Saunders, 1929. P 708.
37. Noble D. *Facts and Observations Relative to the Influence of Manufactures upon Health and Life.* London: John Churchill, 1843. P 5. (Reprinted facsimile by Irish University Press, Shannon, Ireland, 1971.)
38. *Ibid*, p 27.
39. *Ibid*, p 75.
40. Kay JP. *The Moral and Physical Condition of the Working Classes Employed in the Cotton Manufacture in*

Manchester. London, James Ridgway, 1832. Pp 11–2. (Reprinted facsimile by Irish University Press, Shannon, Ireland, 1971.)
41. *Ibid*, p 13.
42. Arlidge JT. *The Hygiene Diseases and Mortality of Occupations*. London: Percival, 1892.
43. Posner, E. John Thomas Arlidge (1822–99) and the potteries. *Br J Ind Med* 1973;30:266–70.
44. Ref 42, *supra*, pp 411–5.
45. Oliver T. *Dangerous Trades: The Historical, Social, and Legal Aspects of Industrial Occupations as Affecting Health, by a Number of Experts*. London: John Murray, 1902.
46. Dodd JR. Diseases of soldiers at home and abroad. In: *Ibid*, pp 166–81.
47. Collingridge W. Health in the marine service. In: Ref 45, *supra*, pp 182–9.
48. Power D. Agriculture; horses; cattle. In: Ref 45, *supra*, pp 232–49.
49. Oliver T. Miscellaneous trades—upholsterers' occupation. In: Ref 45, *supra*, pp 789–90.
50. Oliver T. *Diseases of Occupation from the Legislative-Social, and Medical Points of View*. London: Methuen, 1908. P xvi.
51. *Ibid*, p 319.
52. *Ibid*, pp 345–6.
53. Price GM. *The Modern Factory: Safety, Sanitation and Welfare*. New York: John Wiley & Sons, 1914. P 409.
54. Thompson WG. *The Occupational Diseases: Their Causation, Symptoms, Treatment and Prevention*. New York: D. Appleton, 1914. P v.
55. *Ibid*, pp 53–8.
56. *Ibid*, pp 449–61.
57. *Ibid*, p 594.
58. *Ibid*, p 606. [Interesting relationship.]
59. Kober GM, Hanson WC (eds). *Diseases of Occupation and Vocational Hygiene*. Philadelphia: P. Blakiston's Son, 1916. P xiv.
60. SDL Review of *Diseases of Occupation and Vocational Hygiene* by George M. Kober and William C. Hanson. *Am Labor Leg Rev* 1917;7:226–7.
61. Kober GM, Hanson WC (eds). *Diseases of Occupation and Vocational Hygiene*. Philadelphia: P. Blakiston's Son, 1916. Pp 158–72.
62. *Ibid*, pp 173–86.
63. *Ibid*, pp 777–88.
64. Hoehling AA. *The Great Epidemic*. Boston: Little, Brown, 1961. P 4.
65. *Ibid*, pp 14–5.
66. *Ibid*, pp 186–9.
67. Fincher J. America's deadly rendezvous with the "Spanish Lady." *Smithsonian* 1989;19:130–45.
68. Mock HE. *Industrial Medicine and Surgery*. Philadelphia: Saunders, 1920.
69. *Ibid*, p 194.
70. *Ibid*, pp 196–200.
71. *Ibid*, pp 429–60.
72. *Ibid*, pp 769–75.
73. Colis EL. Sir Thomas Morison Legge, C.B.E., M.D., D.P.H. *J Ind Hyg* 1932;14:235–6.
74. Henry SA. Legge's *Industrial Maladies*. London: Oxford University Press, 1934. Pp 30, 32, 185–6.
75. *Ibid*, p 317.
76. Vernon HM. *Health in Relation to Occupation*. London: Oxford University Press, 1939. Pp 242–3.
77. *Ibid*, p 317.
78. *Ibid*, pp 233–6.
79. Vernon HM. To what extent is the health of industrial workers dependent on occupation? *Occup Psychol* 1939;13:10–24.
80. Cantril ST. Industrial medical program—Hanford Engineer Works. In: Stone RS (ed), *Industrial Medicine on the Plutonium Project: Survey and Collected Papers*. New York: McGraw-Hill, 1951. Pp 289–307.
81. Coates JB, Hoff EC (eds). *Medical Department, United States Army: Preventive Medicine in World War II*, Vol III, *Personal Health Measures and Immunization*. Washington, DC: Office of the Surgeon General, Department of the Army, 1955. Pp 5–7.
82. *Ibid*, p 5.
83. *Ibid*, pp 271–341.
84. Cook WL Jr. Occupational health and industrial medicine. In: Anderson RS, Hoff EC, Hoff PM (eds), *Medical Department, United States Army: Preventive Medicine in World War II*, Vol IX, *Special Fields*. Washington, DC: Office of the Surgeon General, Department of the Army, 1969. Pp 101–201.
85. Sappington, CO. *Essentials of Industrial Health*. Philadelphia: Lippincott, 1943. Pp 193–4.
86. Johnstone RT. *Occupational Medicine and Industrial Hygiene*. St. Louis: Mosby, 1948. Pp 402–11.
87. Johnstone RT, Miller SE. *Occupational Diseases and Industrial Medicine*. Philadelphia: Saunders, 1960. Pp 252–9.
88. Raffle PAB, Adams PH, Baxter PJ, et al (eds). *Hunters Diseases of Occupations*, 8th Ed. Boston: Little, Brown, 1994. Pp 545–76.
89. Pinner RW, Teutsch SM, Simonsen L, et al. Increasing U.S. mortality from infectious diseases. *JAMA* 1996;275:1400.
90. Clever LH. AIDS & bloodborne diseases in the workplace. In: LaDou J (ed), *Occupational Health and Safety*, 2nd Ed. Itasca, IL: National Safety Council, 1994. Pp 329–44.
91. Gantz NM. Infectious agents. In: Levy BS, Wegman DH (eds), *Occupational Health: Recognizing and Preventing Work-Related Disease*. Boston: Little, Brown, 1995. Pp 355–79.
92. Garibaldi R, Janis B. Occupational infections. In: Rom WN (ed), *Environmental and Occcupational Medicine*, 2nd Ed. Boston: Little, Brown, 1992. Pp 607–17.

93. Garner JS, Simmons BP. CDC guidelines for isolation precautions in hospitals. In: *Guidelines for Protecting the Safety and Health of Health Care Workers.* Atlanta: Centers for Disease Control, National Institute for Occupational Safety and Health, Division of Standards Development and Technology Transfer, 1988. Appendix 8, Pp A8-1–A8-84.

94. Lowenthal G. Occupational health programs in clinics and hospitals. In: Zenz C, Dickerson OB, Horvath EP Jr. (eds), *Occupational Medicine*, 3rd Ed. St. Louis: Mosby, 1994. Pp 875–82.

95. Weeks JL, Levy BS, Wagner GR (eds). *Preventing Occupational Disease and Injury.* Washington, DC: American Public Health Association, 1991. Pp 650–2.

96. Williams WW. Guideline for infection control in hospital personnel. In: *Guidelines for Protecting the Safety and Health of Health Care Workers.* Atlanta: Centers for Disease Control, National Institute for Occupational Safety and Health, Division of Standards Development Technology Transfer, 1988. Appendix 8, Pp A8-85–A8-109.

97. Patz JA, Epstein PR, Burke TA, et al. Global climate change and emerging infectious diseases. *JAMA* 1996; 275:217–23.

98. Johnson RT. Emerging viral infections. *Arch Neurol* 1996;53:18–22.

99. Peterson EA, Mandel RM. Infectious diseases: old diseases return and new agents emerge. *Arch Intern Med* 1995;155:1571–2.

100. Stoeckle MY, Douglas G Jr. Infectious diseases. *JAMA* 1996;275:1816.

101. Marfin AA, Moore J, Collins C, et al. Infectious disease surveillance during emergency relief to Bhutanese refugees in Nepal. *JAMA* 1994;272:377–81.

102. Gunby P. Military medicine undertakes peacetime mission, aiding in processing those fleeing from Haiti. *JAMA* 1994;272:191–2.

103. Gunby P. Rescuers of migrants require protection. *JAMA* 1994;22:422.

104. Thacker SB, Addiss DG, Goodman RA, et al. Infectious diseases and injuries in child day care—opportunities for healthier children. *JAMA* 1992;268:1720–6.

105. Goodman RA, Thacker SB, Solomon SL, et al. Infectious diseases in competitive sports. *JAMA* 1994;271: 862–7.

106. Emerging infectious diseases: coccidioidomycosis following the Northridge earthquake—California, 1994. *Arch Dermatol* 1994;130:555–6.

107. Stephenson J. Confronting a biological Armageddon: experts tackle prospect of bioterrorism. *JAMA* 1996;276:349–51.

108. Goldsmith MF. Preparing for medical consequences of terrorism. *JAMA* 1996;275:1713–4.

109. Eifried G, cited in Ref 107, *supra.*

110. Gunby P. Military stays in Bosnia: vaccinates for anthrax. *JAMA* 1998;279:260–1.

111. Reichmann D. New Russian anthrax strain might defeat U.S. vaccine. *Press Democrat* (Santa Rosa) Feb 14, 1998. P A9.

112. Lederer EM. Iraq's arsenal may still include deadly chemicals, countries say. *Press Democrat* (Santa Rosa) Feb 15, 1998, P A16.

113. Brenner BE, Kauffman J. Reluctance of internists and medical nurses to perform mouth-to-mouth resuscitation. *Arch Intern Med* 1993;153:1763–9.

114. Locke CJ, Berg RA, Sanders AB, et al. Bystander cardiopulmonary resuscitation: concerns about mouth-to-mouth contact. *Arch Intern Med* 1995;155:938–43.

115. Kolavic S, Kimura A. An outbreak of *Shigella dysenteriae* type 2 among laboratory workers due to intentional food contamination. *JAMA* 1997;278:396–8.

116. Torok T, Tauxe T. A large community outbreak of salmonellosis caused by intentional contamination of restaurant salad bars. *JAMA* 1997;389–95.

117. Combating terrorism: spending on government-wide programs requires better management and coordination. GAO/NSIAD-98-39, December 1, 1997.

118. Eitzen EM Jr, Takafuji ET. Historical overview of biological warfare. In: Sidell FR, Takafuji ET, Franz DP (eds), *Medical Aspects of Chemical and Biological Warfare.* Washington, DC: Office of the Surgeon General, 1997. Pp 415–23.

2 / Clinical Laboratory Evaluation of Infectious Diseases

Gerri S. Hall, Janet M. Serkey, and Lou Ellen Phillips-Smith

The clinical microbiology laboratory plays a key role in aiding internists, family physicians, surgeons, and infectious disease specialists with the diagnosis of infectious diseases in their patients. The role of the microbiology laboratory is more than culturing specimens. It involves the development of guidelines on the appropriateness of specimens for infectious disease analysis and the methods for collecting these specimens, direct microscopic evaluations of specimens, rapid testing for the presence of an infectious disease agent, when available [1], interpretation of results of direct observations, cultures and rapid testing and, when applicable, the susceptibility testing of isolated organisms to determine what antibiotics or other drugs may be appropriate for use—or at best, the ones to which the isolates may be resistant [2–4].

This chapter gives an overview of what assistance clinical microbiologists can provide health care professionals for the diagnosis of infectious diseases. For clinical practicality, the chapter is organized by specimen or body system. In addition, some generalizations about newer, emerging technologies are made.

Specimen Collection

BLOOD CULTURES

When a patient is suspected of having bacteremia or fungemia, the appropriate specimen to collect is a blood culture. The optimum amount of blood to be drawn is 20 mL, which is usually distributed into two different bottles or sources of media for growth of both bacteria and fungi. The 20 mL is collected using aseptic technique, which requires thorough cleansing of the area around the needlestick with Betadine and alcohol or another disinfectant. The area should not be manipulated after cleansing, but rather the needlestick done after the area has been cleaned. Methods for skin antisepsis prior to venipuncture vary from hospital to hospital, but the basic principles are similar. After a vein is palpated, the area around the vein is scrubbed with 70% alcohol for 30 seconds, followed by application of an iodine solution for 30–60 seconds. Application of alcohol alone for longer than 30 seconds may be necessary if a patient is hypersensitive to iodine. The bottle tops are cleansed with alcohol or iodine before venipuncture is performed.

Some labs inoculate bottles of blood culture media, and the results are read visually by the technologists over a period of five to seven days. A positive test result is determined by turbidity, hemolysis, or other visible changes. Some labs use a lysis centrifugation method (Isolator, Wampole Laboratories, Cranbury, NJ) alone or in conjunction with blood culture bottles. The Isolator may increase the yield of certain bacteria, such as staphylococci and fungi. For the culture of blood, most laboratories today use one of the "automated" blood culture systems: BacT/Alert (Organon Teknika), Bactec 9240 (Becton Dickinson, Sparks, MD), or Difco ESP (Trek Diagnostics, Westlake, Ohio). For each of these systems, labs determine whether they will inoculate one anaerobic blood culture bottle and one aerobic bottle or place all of the blood into two aerobic bottles. In addition, one or both bottles may contain a type of resin—or antibiotic removal materials—so that organisms may grow even if the patient has already been placed on antibiotics for empiric therapy. When sent to the lab, the blood culture bottles are placed onto the appropriate instrument, and for the next four to seven days, readings are taken to determine growth of an organism in each of the bottles. When a culture is positive, smears are prepared for examination by means of Gram's stain. The smear results are reported to the clinician by phone to give a rapid answer about what might be present in the blood of a patient. For bacteria, blood cultures are usually positive within the first 12 hours or less, and for fungi, within the first 24 hours or less. The blood culture systems used today allow for recovery of most common bacteria and fungi; however, there are some organisms that are not expected to be recovered from routine blood culture, including bacteria such as *Bordetella pertussis*, *Legionella pneumophila*, *Fransicella tularensis*, and possibly *Brucella* and *Bartonella* species. In addition, most of the automated systems may not provide 100% recovery of the dimorphic fungi, especially *Histoplasma capsula-tum* or *Blastomyces dermatitidis*. The reason for this may be the length of incubation needed for these fungi to be cultured and not the media or "system." If any of these agents are suspected, the lab should be informed before the blood is collected.

After organisms are isolated from a blood culture, they are assessed for genus and species identification, often followed by susceptibility testing. Laboratories are presently making more of an effort to aid the clinician in detection of possible lab contaminants, since the cost of identifying and treating potential contaminants is high [2,4]. In general, these contaminants include coagulase-negative staphylococci (CNS), viridans streptococci, *Propionibacterium acnes*, and *Bacillus* species. Any one of these organisms may indeed be the true pathogen in certain situations, but its isolation from a single blood culture does not necessarily indicate that the organism is the agent causing illness. After a short period of time, if a blood culture for another organism is positive in the same patient, one needs to reconsider whether the first positive culture truly indicates the pathogen. Generally, less than 3% of all blood cultures performed yield these contaminants if proper aseptic techniques are employed in the collection process [5,6]. The percentage should be monitored by the lab in order to quickly recognize any problems with increased contamination so that efforts to reduce this can be implemented in a timely fashion. Possible reasons for contamination include the improper cleaning of sites before collection of blood, improper disinfection of the ports used to inject blood into blood culture bottles, or improper handling of bloods once they reach the lab. Of all the blood cultures sent to any one lab, only about 10% of them are positive for any bacteria or fungi; most blood samples drawn are negative [5–7].

Transport of blood cultures to the lab should be done as quickly as possible, and bottles that contain blood should not be refrigerated before or during transport. If a blood culture is positive and the patient is placed on appropriate antibiotics, the need for subsequent "test-of-cure" blood cultures is debatable. If further cultures are performed, the blood sample should be drawn at least four to five days later, unless the patient does not appear to be responding, in which case repeat cultures should be performed to be certain another source of bacteremia has not occurred. If the lab utilizes bottles that contain resins, even if the patient is being treated appropriately, the sample may stay positive for a few days longer than anticipated because the resin may inactivate the antibiotic, allowing growth of the organisms in vitro. This appears to occur most often when the pathogen is *Staphylococcus aureus* or coagulase-negative staphylococci [5–7].

URINE TESTING

The processing of a urine sample for the diagnosis of urinary tract infection is one of the most commonly performed microbiologic assays. Labs usually receive more urine specimens than any other single specimen. Collection of urine is believed to be simple; however, its collection can be fraught with many contamination problems. Females and males need to be instructed in the proper collection of a urine sample [1,8]. If the area around the urethra is not well cleaned before collection, especially in the female patient, then the resultant positive urine culture may contain contaminating skin or normal urethral flora and not the pathogen. Mid-stream urine collection is ideal and, if done properly, will usually yield the pathogen if one is present in a quantity of about 10^5 CFU/mL or greater [4]. Lesser quantities may be clinically significant, depending on the organism and the host. Some laboratories may use one of a variety of screening techniques to determine the likelihood that the urine contains significant quantities of an organism. These include Gram's stain of unspun urine, bioluminescence measurement of bacterial adenosine triphosphate (ATP), and dip-stick techniques for determination of presence of pyuria and/or nitrates. If a screen is used, those samples that screen negative are disposed of and not cultured. If positive, a culture is performed. The culture involves plating 0.001 mL of the urine onto one each of blood agar and gram-negative selective media (Maconkey's agar), incubating for 24 hours followed by identification of resultant colonies. Usually, each lab sets up its own guidelines for full identification and susceptibility testing, based on the presence of one organism versus more than one in a quantity of 10^5 CFU/mL or greater.

If the patient is catheterized, it is inadvisable to collect the specimen from the Foley catheter bag; rather, it can be collected from the catheter after disinfection of the catheter port. Collection of a suprapubic aspirate from the bladder ensures sterile collection of the urine, and thus anything that grows is considered significant, regardless of the colony count [3,4].

If urine is being collected for the diagnosis of *Chlamydia trachomatis* or *Neisseria gonorrhoeae* for a patient suspected to have a sexually transmitted disease, the urine tested should be the first voided urine, without any prior cleaning of the urethral area, and should be collected at least one hour after the last urination. Cultures of urine for *C trachomatis* or *N gonorrhoeae* are insensitive for detection, but amplification techniques yield sensitivities equivalent to the urethral specimen in the male and nearly as sensitive as the cervical sample from the female.

RESPIRATORY TRACT SPECIMENS

Upper Respiratory Tract

Diagnosis of upper respiratory tract bacterial infection requires the collection of a throat specimen or, for viral isolation or detection, a nasopharyngeal specimen for microscopic examination. Bacterial throat cultures are usually collected only for the detection of group A streptococci or, in specific cases, for isolation of *N gonorrhoeae* or *Corynebacterium diphtheriae* (when the patient has pseudomembrane in the throat). Other bacterial organisms often represent only normal oral flora or carrier states and should not routinely be searched for or reported, if found [8,9].

For the detection of viruses, such as respiratory syncytial virus (RSV), influenza and parainfluenza viruses, adenoviruses, and cytomegalovirus, throat cultures or culture of nasopharyngeal aspirates are appropriate. Often, a panel of the various viral pathogens is searched for by culture, or more commonly, by antigen detection methods, which provide more rapid results [10–12].

Lower Respiratory Tract

For the diagnosis of pneumonia, sputum for culture is often considered the most appropriate specimen. Unfortunately, sputum collection is problematic. Often, patients merely "spit" oral material into the container instead of providing a good specimen that is representative of the lower respiratory tract. Even with a properly collected sputum sample, normal oral flora organisms are likely to be detected because the sputum has to come through the oral cavity during collection. With the use of Gram's stain to determine the quality of the specimen, labs should be able to inform the physician of the probability that the specimen is in fact sputum from the lower respiratory tract and therefore should provide adequate and significant clinical information when cultured [9,13,14]. Gram's stain may also be used to predict the presence of an infectious agent, such as *Streptococcus pneumoniae*, if predominant organisms are of a consistent morphology with this diagnosis. If Gram's stain demonstrates bacteria that are predominantly consistent in appearance with *Neisseria* or *Haemophilus* species, then cultures can be appropriately plated to detect the presence of one of these organisms. If the physician suspects organisms such as *Legionella* species, *Mycoplasma pneumoniae*, *Chlamydia pneumoniae*, or *Mycobacterium tuberculosis*, specific requests for culture of these organisms need to be made at the time of ordering, before cultures are processed. Likewise, if fungal organisms are suspected, especially *Histoplasma capsulatum* or *Blastomyces dermatitidis*, the lab should be informed of this so that correct media and incubation conditions are used. Requests for anaerobic culturing of the sputum will be rejected, because every sputum sample contains anaerobic bacteria because of the large numbers of such organisms in the oral cavity as part of the normal flora. If anaerobic pneumonia is in the differential diagnosis, i.e., a diagnosis of aspiration pneumonia or empyema is being entertained by the clinician, Gram's stain of the sputum consistent with the presence of anaerobes (i.e., a good quality specimen with polymorphic bacterial morphologies) should yield the information the clinician needs without performing anaerobic culture.

In addition to sputum testing, the bronchoalveolar lavage (BAL) to obtain lung secretions for the detection of pneumonia has become very popular [15]. Saline is instilled into the alveolar spaces with a bronchoscope and then the fluid, along with lung secretions, is removed via an endoscope. Culture of this fluid may increase the yield of the pathogens over that detected by sputum culture. For the diagnosis of *Pneumocystis carinii* pneumonia (PCP), the specimen obtained by BAL is far superior to the sputum sample, even an induced sputum [16,17]. Transtracheal aspirates, if collected appropriately and not merely through a tracheal or bronchial tube, are appropriate samples for determination of the causative agents of pneumonia.

If all of the above-mentioned specimens are inconclusive and a definitive diagnosis has not been made, open lung biopsy may be required. Since the lung is a sterile site, any organism detected may represent the pathogen involved in the pneumonia. Again, if organisms such as *Legionella pneumophila*, *Mycobacterium tuberculosis* or other mycobacterial strains, dimorphic fungi, or other fastidious organisms are being considered, then the physician should alert the lab and request that specific media be plated for their recovery.

CEREBROSPINAL FLUID

For determination of agents of bacterial, viral, or fungal meningitis, a properly collected cerebrospinal fluid (CSF) specimen is the specimen of choice. To reduce the chance of skin contaminants, usually the second or third collected specimen tube should be sent to the microbiology lab [18]. Gram's stain and culture for potential pathogens should be performed and the results of the Gram's stain called in immediately to the physician if they are positive. Requests for bacterial antigen tests (BAD) (described in serologic section) should be honored only after consultation with the lab. BAD assays are commercially available for detection of *S pneumoniae*, *H influenzae*, and *N meningitidis*. These tests may provide additional useful information when the patient has community-acquired pneumonia and has been given antibiotics prior to collection of a CSF specimen, possibly reducing the chance for growth of the pathogen. The sensitivity of most bacterial agent assays is no better than that of Gram's stain and may result in false-positive findings [19,20]. On the other hand, the request for a cryptococcal antigen assay is appropriate for all cases of suspected fungal meningitis, since the sensitivity of this assay for this disease is greater than 90% and its specificity is almost 100% [21].

Diagnosis of aseptic meningitis may be made clinically; if cultures are requested, the most commonly performed is that for enterovirus. Isolation of herpes simplex virus (HSV) from the CSF has a sensitivity of less than 5%, and if CSF is to be processed for detection of HSV, an amplification assay, such as polymerase chain reaction (PCR), should be requested [22].

WOUND SPECIMENS

The sampling of wounds for the diagnosis of wound infections is difficult to perform appropriately. Swabs are not appropriate collection devices [7,8]. Because of their small size, they sample only a small area for collection of adequate samples; they are not adequate for obtaining samples for anaerobic culturing; and they provide only surface screening of the wound, which often misses the site of the real infection deeper in the wound. Aspirate or biopsy specimens should be obtained, if possible. First, the area needs to be cleaned prior to specimen collection in order to decrease the amount of normal skin flora in the collection. In areas where aspirates are difficult to obtain, a small amount of nonpreserved saline can be injected into the wound first and then the contents drawn back into the syringe, along with the infected material.

GENITAL SPECIMENS

For cases of suspected sexually transmitted diseases, urethral specimens (from males) and cervical/urethral specimens (from females) should be collected after excess mucus is cleaned from the area [23]. Appropriate transport media for *Chlamydia* include M-4 or 2-SP, and the specimens should be collected with a calcium alginate other than a cotton-tipped swab. The use of wooden-tip swabs should be avoided, since these may inhibit the growth of *Chlamydia trachomatis* [24]. For isolation of *N gonorrhoeae*, a culturette type of swab, sent immediately to the lab after sample collection, or plating of the samples onto appropriate selective media, performed at the clinic office, is required. Amplification methods for the diagnosis of these two infectious agents are the preferred method in many labs, since they have been shown to be more sensitive, especially for the detection of *C trachomatis*. Each of the manufacturers of amplification assays provides a specific collection and transport kit for their specific assay, and this should be used when applicable [23,24].

If other organisms are suspected, such as *Haemophilus ducreyi*, a specific request needs to be reported to the lab. If a chancre is present and *Treponema pallidum* (syphilis) is in the differential diagnosis, the material within the chancre can be sent to the lab for darkfield examination, provided it is delivered immediately, before the specimen is allowed to dry. If vaginitis is the clinical diagnosis, *Candida* species and *Trichomonas vaginalis*, if present, can be detected by means of direct microscopic exams for budding yeast, with or without pseudohyphae, or motile trichomonads, respectively. In addition, use of a "scored" Gram's stain for detection of the presence of lactobacilli (as evidence of normal flora) or increased numbers of *Gardnerella vaginalis* (as evidence of bacterial vaginosis) should be performed. There is a nucleic-acid probe that can be used for detection of all three entities (AFFIRM, Becton Dickinson, Sparks, MD); this is discussed in a later section of this chapter [27].

STOOL SPECIMENS

Gastroenteritis may be caused by enteric bacterial pathogens, parasites, mycobacterial organisms (in the case of HIV disease), viral pathogens, or the toxins of *Clostridium difficile*. Fungi rarely cause gastroenteritis but may be present in stool specimens if the focus of the fungal disease is gastrointestinal or if the disease is disseminated.

To detect the causative pathogen, a stool sample is sent to the lab with specific requests. If an enteric pathogen is being sought, the lab will plate the stool for isolation of *Salmonella* species, *Shigella* species, and *Campylobacter* species. Many labs also provide a means of detection of *E coli* 0157:H7 (enterohemorrhagic *E coli*) in all stools, only bloody stools, or upon specific request. If other organisms such as *Yersinia enterocolitica*, *Vibrio* species, or *Aeromonas* species are being sought, specific requests must be conveyed to the lab. The detection of ova and parasites (O&P), as evidence of parasitic enteritis, is done by means of direct microscopic examination of unstained and stained preparations or by means of antigen detection reagents that specifically identify *Giardia lamblia*, *Cryptosporidium* species, and/or *Entamoeba histolytica* [26–28]. Processing of stools for enteric bacterial pathogens or parasites should be performed on outpatients and patients who have been in the hospital for less than three days. After longer hospitalizations, any development of diarrhea or gastroenteritis is invariably caused by other than enteric bacterial pathogens or parasites [29–31]. In general, three specimens are usually necessary for optimal detection of parasites and/or enteric pathogens. If *Mycobacterium avium-intracellulare* is suspected, a specific request must be conveyed to the lab, and results may require up to two to three weeks. Detection of the toxins of *C difficile* by means of enzyme immunoassay (EIA) or tissue culture or isolation of the organism and detection of the toxins in the isolates, is the way in which *C difficile* diarrhea is diagnosed in the lab. The disease is a clinical disease and the lab merely supports the diagnosis. The request for *C difficile* detection is appropriate for inpatients and outpatients, regardless of their time in the hospital prior to development of diarrhea [32]. For detection of viral agents in stool, direct antigen assays or electron microscopy for specific agents are usually employed [33]. For children, antigen assay for the detection of rotavirus is often the initial request for diagnosis of diarrhea [34].

BODY FLUIDS AND TISSUES

Body fluids and tissues need to be collected in a sterile fashion and sent immediately to the lab. Routine bacterial cultures detect most bacterial pathogens; fungal and viral cultures need to be specifically requested if a fungus or virus is thought to be a possible pathogen. If the specimen is collected in surgery, that information should be written on the request for culture sent to the lab.

ANAEROBES

If the clinician suspects anaerobic bacteria, a specific request for anaerobic culture must be sent to the lab. Certain specimens are unacceptable for anaerobic culturing. This includes those from sites at which anaerobes are part of the normal flora and thus the significance of their isolation could not be interpreted, namely sputum, throat swabs, vaginal swabs, feces, or saliva [8]. Specimens such as urine or cerebrospinal fluid often are not processed for anaerobes because the incidence of anaerobic infections at these sites is very low. Exceptions are made when all other more common etiologies have been exhausted and in other specific situations after consultation between the lab and the clinician. Anaerobic culturing of appropriate sites involves collection of aspirates, tissues, or body fluids, which are transported to the lab quickly and in appropriate anaerobic vials or containers. Swabs are inadequate for the isolation of anaerobes and should be discouraged or rejected. Gram staining of the specimens is essential for interpretation of anaerobic cultures and often provides useful information as to the adequacy of the specimen and hence significance of the isolates(s). Most anaerobic infections are polymicrobial, that is, composed of both aerobes and anaerobes.

Microscopic Identification of Microbial Pathogens

Gram's stain remains the mainstay of microscopic examination of microbial pathogens. It is relatively easy to perform; however, accurate reading and interpretation of the results requires a trained technologist or physician. The adequacy of the specimen can usually be judged from the Gram's stain as well as the quantities and morphology of the organisms seen. Acid-fast smear (AFB) assists in the rapid detection of mycobacterial organisms. It should be performed on concentrated specimens, and labs should be capable of reporting the results of AFB smear within the first 24 hours of receiving a specimen. *Nocardia* species and potentially *Rhodococci* species and some parasites, including *Cryptosporidium* species and *Cyclospora* species, are also partially acid-fast positive. These stains also require trained personnel for accurate analysis.

Toluidine blue stain, silver stain, calcofluor white fluorescent stain, or Giemsa stain can be used for the detection of *Pneumocystis carinii* [35]. In most labs, the calcofluor fluorescent wall stain is also used for the detection of fungal organisms, directly in clinical specimens, as a replacement for the KOH or wet mount, but calcofluor white stain provides a more sensitive and often more specific approach to the microscopic examination of fungal organisms.

In addition to microscopic examination of specimens, a number of serologic techniques for detection of antigens can be used for more rapid detection of bacterial and viral agents. The specimen is homogenized and/or a touch prep is made on a slide and an antibody tagged with a fluorescent or colored label is added to the specimen. The resultant fluorescent or colored product is read by microscope or colorimeter, respectively. Serologic detection of antibodies enables the rapid detection of the etiologic agent and may decrease the need for culture, depending on the specificity of the antibody and the need to identify polymorphic pathogens. Such antigen detection methods are discussed in more detail later in this chapter.

Culture

Culture remains the "gold standard" for detection of most pathogenic organisms. Agar and broth bacterial cultures are set up for most clinical specimens and incubated for 24 hours or more, depending on the suspected organism. In addition to often being the most sensitive method of detection, cultures may also be necessary for studying the epidemiology of a group of isolates or for performing susceptibility assays to detect resistance. In general, culture takes longer than other rapid molecular methods but may provide the most specific means of identification of the pathogen(s) involved. The media that is used in the lab should be planned by the laboratory technologists to provide for isolation of the most common species of bacteria and fungi. In cases in which an "unusual" pathogen is being considered, clinicians should inform the lab of this so that appropriate processing and/or culture media can be utilized. An example of this would be a patient in whom *Bartonella* species is being considered. *Bartonella* species may require a nonautomated blood culture method for isolation of the organism and may require longer than the four to five days presently required by most labs for the detection of agents of bacteremia or fungemia. If a physician considers *Zygomycetes* in the differential, informing the lab before processing occurs will ensure proper specimen handling. *Zygomycetes* may be fragile in specimens, and if it is macerated, ground, or otherwise homogenized, the yield may be low. If the specimen is teased apart and handled gently, the recovery of a *Rhizopus* species or other *Zygomycetes* is more likely [8].

Identification of Bacteria, Fungi, and Viral Agents

Identification of bacteria after isolation on agar or in broth requires use of conventional biochemical and microscopic tests. The biochemical tests may be performed in tubes, on plates, or in microtiter plates. Methods are available for manual or automated procedures, which require hours to days for completion. How far one proceeds with the specific identification is determined by the specimen site and absence or presence of multiple organisms. Most bacterial identifications are complete in less than 2 days of isolation. More fastidious bacteria may require longer turnaround times, and in some cases, the isolates may have to be sent out to reference labs for complete and specific identification. For mycobacterial isolates, genetic probes are most often used for rapid identification of the more common *M tuberculosis complex* and *M avium-intracellulare* complex isolates. For those isolates, which are probe negative, more conventional biochemicals or methods of high-performance liquid chromatography (HPLC) or sequencing are used. The latter methods often must be performed at reference labs.

Identification of yeast is similar to that of bacteria, requiring microscopic examination and biochemical differentiation. For identification of molds, there are not many available biochemical tools; thus, microscopic exam of organisms on a variety of fungal media is required. This usually requires expertise in such identification and/or sending of the isolates to a reference lab. Identification of yeast usually requires four to five days after isolation; turnaround time for molds differs, depending on the species, but is usually accomplished, at least to a genus level, in one to two weeks after isolation.

Identification of a virus requires determination of the specific cytopathic effect (CPE) in specific tissue cultures or identification of antigens by specific monoclonal antibodies. In many labs, molecular techniques utilizing probes, amplification, or in-situ hybridization have replaced more conventional methods of viral identification.

Molecular Methods for Detection or Specific Identification of Infectious Disease Agents

Use of DNA techniques in a wide variety of applications probably represents the major emerging technology in the microbiology lab today. There are commercially available culture confirmation probes for the rapid identification of *Mycobacterium* species (*M tuberculosis complex*, *M aviumintracellulare* complex, *M gordonae*, and *M kansasii*); fungal isolates (*Histoplasma capsulatum*, *Blastomyces dermatitidis*, and *Coccidioides immitis*); bacteria such as *Haemophilus influenzae*, *Campylobacter* species, and viral agents. These probes can be used to confirm the cultural identification of the above organisms in less than three hours, from the beginning of the procedure to completion. However, these probes are not sensitive enough to use directly on clinical specimens [36–38].

A breakthrough in rapid identification occurred when some of the probes that were being commercially developed were applied to detection of organisms directly within the respiratory, genital, or other specimen with a sensitivity approaching the more conventional culture methods. There are commercially available probes for direct detection of *Chlamydia trachomatis* and *Neisseria gonorrhoeae* in cervical or urethral specimens (PACE, Gen-Probe, San Diego, CA) [39]; for identification of the three most common agents of vaginitis (i.e., *Trichomonas vaginalis*, *Candida* species, and *Gardnerella vaginalis*) (AFFIRM, Becton Dickin-son, Sparks, MD) [25]; for direct detection of group A streptococcus in throat-swab specimens (Gen-Probe) [40]; and for detection of viral agents (e.g., HIV, CMV, EBV) in clinical specimens [36]. In addition, there are more probes available in research formats.

More recently, labs have become inundated with developments in the arena of amplification. Amplification techniques enable the lab to achieve sensitivities within clinical specimens equal to or better than culture and much more rapidly. Amplification increases the number of nucleic acid copies in a specimen to millions in a very short period of time (often less than 5 hours) [41,42]. With this potential, at first it appeared that amplification would take over all microbiologic conventional methods. Since its introduction, however, it is obvious that these techniques, although excellent in some areas, may not always be preferable. However, amplification has become very successful in the identification of organisms for which culture methods are long and tedious, for which there may be no available culture methods, or for which the need to know the answer very rapidly overrides the costs that might be involved in the use of molecular methods.

The manufacturing companies that have provided commercially available "kits" laboratories can use to perform amplification on clinical specimens have done a great job in providing "cookbook" formats for performing these molecular techniques. The detection of *C trachomatis* in genital specimens is done by means of one of three amplification methods: Ligase Chain Reaction (LCx, Abbott Laboratories), Polymerase Chain Reaction (Amplicor PCR, Roche Molecular Systems), or Transcription Mediated Amplification (TMA, Gen-Probe, Inc.) [23,43] and Strand Displacement Amplification (SDA, Becton Dickinson Microbiology Systems). LCx can also be used for the simultaneous detection of *N gonorrhoeae* and *C trachomatis.* Urine can be the sample for detection of both sexually transmitted disease etiologies by LCx, with sensitivities that approach or equal that of cultures. TMA and PCR will also have these assays available soon. In the future, other companies will also have their versions of amplification for *C trachomatis* and *N gonorrhoeae*.

For the detection of *M tuberculosis* complex directly in clinical specimens, two amplification methods are currently available commercially: TMA and PCR [44–46]. Both can be performed on respiratory specimens that are AFB-smear positive from patients who have never been previously diagnosed with tuberculosis. The FDA put these specific restrictions on their use. The assays require about five hours to perform and thus provide a very specific, rapid answer in order to help clinicians more appropriately treat suspected cases of tuberculosis and put TB patients in isolation more quickly to prevent further spread of the disease. These assays are, however, expensive to perform [37,47].

Although not commercially produced, amplification methods are available for a wide variety of agents. They are performed in research labs or are offered by commercial companies for detection of, for example, *Bordetella pertussis, Chlamydia pneumoniae*, *Mycoplasma pneumoniae*, and

Bartonella henselae. Amplification methods are also available for detection and determination of the viral load for diseases such as HIV, HCV, CMV, and HSV (in cerebrospinal fluid) [22,48, 49]. One manufacturer, Digene, provides an assay for human papillomavirus (HPV), which, although not truly an amplification procedure, yields results with a sensitivity equivalent to that of amplification [50].

The use of sequencing to detect and/or identify infectious disease agents from agar or broth cultures, or directly within clinical specimens following amplification, has become more available to clinical labs. Although sequencing is for the most part still in the research arena, it may in time become a more widely available technique in many labs.

Genetic typing of isolates by techniques such as pulsed-field gel electrophoresis (PFGE) is being utilized to determine the relatedness of bacterial or fungal isolates. This is particularly useful in the epidemiologic analysis of outbreaks or cluster cases of unusual organisms. There are a number of hospital labs and reference labs that provide these services.

Serologic Evaluation for Diagnosis of Infectious Diseases

The formation of antibodies during the process of infection can be detected in the sera of patients, and this detection can be used as a diagnostic tool for the laboratorian and clinician. In general, two specimens of serum should be submitted to the lab for serologic evaluation: one drawn during the peak, or acute, stage of the infectious process and the other during the convalescent phase, which is usually two to four weeks or more after the acute sera was drawn. Both specimens should be tested simultaneously in order to ensure that titer differences are due to the samples and not to variability in testing procedures [51].

Accurate demonstration of a positive serologic response usually requires a four-fold rise or decline in the titer between the acute and convalescent assay results. In addition, demonstration of IgM antibodies with or without IgG antibodies suggests acute infection; presence of IgG alone may indicate present or past infection. Not all infectious disease syndromes have reliable IgM assays that are available, however. Detection of IgG antibodies may also be used to determine the immune status of an individual and hence presumed protection from infection by certain agents. This might include detection of IgG for rubella, cytomegalovirus, or varicella-zoster virus. There are also screening antibody tests that have been developed; their purpose is to screen blood or blood products for the presence of viral agents, including hepatitis viruses, HIV, and CMV.

There are many methodologies that are available to the laboratory for the detection of antibodies specific for a disease. The more commonly employed methods include enzyme immunoassays (EIA), complement fixation (CF), immunodiffusion (ID), indirect immunofluorescence antibody (IFA), indirect hemagglutination assay (IHA), or radioimmunoassay (RIA).

There are some infectious diseases for which serology remains the primary mode of diagnosis because culture is unavailable or requires lengthy incubations or methods not available to most labs. This includes the diagnosis of *Chlamydia pneumoniae* [52], *Mycoplasma pneumoniae* [9], and *Bartonella henselae* [53]; *Rickettsial diseases* [11] such as spotted fevers; *Treponema pallidum* and *Ehrlichia* species [54]; Lyme disease [55]; and a number of viral entities. For some pathogens, such as *Legionella pneumophila*, there are culture methods; however, alone they are often not sensitive enough to provide adequate diagnosis and must be used in combination with serologic studies for maximum efficacy.

For the diagnosis of fungal and parasitic disease, detection of antibodies affords a complement to culture and microscopic examinations, respectively. Serologic studies complement culture of the systemic dimorphic fungi *Histoplasma capsulatum*, *Blastomyces dermatitidis*, and *Coccidioides immitis* [56]. Serology for *E histolytica* and *Toxoplasma gondii* are often more sensitive than the respective microscopic modalities or culture [57,58].

Table 2-1 lists some serologic methods and the diseases or organisms for which they are often used.

Table 2-1
Serologic Assays for Infectious Disease Agents

Organism/Disease	Methods	Comments
Bacterial Agents		
Bartonella henselae	IFA, EIA	For diagnosis of bacillary angiomatosis (BA) in HIV or cat-scratch disease.
Borrelia burgdorferi	DFA, EIA; Western blot test	For diagnosis of Lyme disease, CDC recommends confirmation of EIA or DFA with Western blot test; indeterminates are frequent; false-positive results in areas of low prevalence are common.
Legionella pneumophila	IFA	Four-fold rise in titer to 1:128 or single titer of > 1:512 is diagnostic.
Mycoplasma pneumoniae	CF, EIA	Presence of IgM antibodies better than IgG for diagnosis of acute infection.
		Cold agglutinins often positive but nonspecific.
Streptococcus pyogenes	ASO, anti-DNase B	Used for the diagnosis of sequelae of pharyngitis or group A streptococcal skin infections.
Chlamydia pneumoniae	MIF	IgM > 1:16 or IgG > 1:512; four-fold rise in titer is more specific.
Chlamydia trachomatis, LGV	MIF	IgM > 1:32 and IgG > 1:2,000 is diagnostic.
Chlamydia psittaci	MIF	Four-fold rise in titer most reliable for diagnosis.
Francisella tularensis	Microagglutination	> 1:60 suggestive; four-fold rise in titer most reliable; EIA in development.
Ehrlichia sp	IFA	Four-fold rise in titer, with baseline of 1:80 is diagnostic; assays not widely available.
Treponema pallidum	VDRL, RPR	Nonspecific screening tests; VDRL preferred for CSF testing.
	FTA-ABA, MHA-TP	Specific treponemal tests; confirmatory assays.
Leptospira sp	Microagglutination	EIA being developed.
Rickettsia rickettsii	IFA, EIA	> 1:64 positive for Rocky Mountain spotted fever.
	LA	Positive only during acute infection.
Fungal Agents		
Histoplasma capsulatum	ID, CF, EIA	H & M bands on ID; *H* = acute infection; *M* = acute or past.
		CF: > 1:8 suggestive.
		May cross-react with *Blastomyces* or *Coccidioides immitis.*
Blastomyces dermatitidis	ID, CF, EIA	CF: > 1:8 suggestive.
		May cross-react with *Blastomyces* or *Coccidioides immitis.*
Coccidioides immitis	CF, ID	≥ 1:16 suggestive.
Cryptococcus neoformans		Not usually helpful.
Aspergillus sp	CF, ID	Number of bands on ID may suggest extent of invasive disease but may be nonspecific for diagnosis.
Candida sp		Not useful for diagnosis of invasive disease.
Zygomycetes		Not widely available.

Table 2-1 (continued)

Organism/Disease	Methods	Comments
Parasites		
Entamoeba histolytica (amebiasis)	EIA, IHA	IHA ≥ 1:256. 95% with extra-GI disease; 70% with GI only.
Ascaris lumbricoides (ascariasis)	EIA	≥ 1:32
Chagas' disease	CF, IHA	≥ 1:8; 1:64
Cysticercosis	IHA	≥ 1:64
Echinococcosis	IHA	≥ 1:256
Fascioliasis	IHA	≥ 1:128
Filariasis	IHA	≥ 1:128
Leishmaniasis	IFA	≥ 1:16
Paragonimiasis	CF	≥ 1:8
Pneumocystosis	IFA	≥ 1:16
Schistosomiasis	IFA	≥ 1:16
Strongyloidiasis	IHA	≥ 1:64
Toxocariasis	EIA	≥ 1:32
Trichinosis	Bentonite flocculation	≥ 1:16
Toxoplasma gondii	IFA, EIA	IgM = past or present infection. IgM = active primary infection.
Plasmodium sp	IFA	≥ 1:64 for diagnosis of malaria.
Viral Agents		
Adenovirus	CF, EIA	
Arbovirus	IFA CF, HI, EIA	IgM and IgG; CSF and serum. Four-fold rise in titer best for diagnosis.
CMV	CF, IHA, EIA, IFA	
EBV	Heterophile, EIA EIA, RIA, CF	IgM and IgG for Viral Capsid (VCA). For immune status; also for stage of infection.
Hepatitis A	RIA or EIA	IgM anti-HAV = active infection.
Hepatitis B	RIA or EIA	HBsAg, anti-HBs, and anti-HBc donor screening.
Hepatitis C	EIA	
Hepatitis D	RIA	HBsAG, anti-HDV, and IgManti-HD determines disease state and provides total anti-HEV and IgM anti-HEV.
Hepatitis E	Western blot test, EIA, heterophile agglutination, HI, IFA, CF	
HIV	EIA, Western blot test	Positive EIA: repeat EIA and if still positive perform Western blot test for confirmation.
HSV	CF, IHA, EIA, IFA	Not very useful for diagnosis.
VZV	IFA, FAMA	For immune status; also for stage of infection.
Influenza A and B	CF, HAI	
Measles virus	HI, EIA, IgM by IFA	Four-fold rise for diagnosis.
Mumps virus	IFA, EIA, HAI	
Parainfluenza I, II, III prognostic information	HAI, CF, EIA	
Rabies	IFA, RFFIT	For diagnosis and immune status.
Rubella virus	EIA, IgM by EIA, LA	Four-four rise highly suggestive; Western blot test for diagnosis.

Abbreviations: *ASO* = antistreptolysin O antibody; *CF* = complement fixation; *DFA* = direct fluorescent antibody; *EIA* = enzyme immunoassay; *FTA-ABS* = fluorescent treponemal antibody-absorption; *HI* = hemagglutination inhibition; *ID* = immunodiffusion; *IFA* = indirect fluorescent antibody; *IHA* = indirect hemagglutination antibody; *LA* = latex agglutination; *Microagg* = microagglutination assay; *MIF* = microimmunofluorescence; *MHA-TP* = microhemagglutination-treponemal; *RIA* = radioimmunoassay; *RPR* = rapid plasma reagin; *VDRL* = Venereal Disease Research Laboratory.
Based on data from references 9, 11, 52–58.

Antigen Detection

To provide a more rapid diagnosis than culture provides, detection of antigens of the infectious agent directly in the clinical specimen may be utilized. For *Legionella pneumophila*, use of direct fluorescent antibody stain (DFA) for detection of antigens of *L pneumophila* serogroup 1 is commercially available and provides direct examination of, for example, sputum, bronchoalveolar fluid and cells, or lung tissue for making the diagnosis. DFA's sensitivity is only about 70–75% but combined with culture of the organism and serologic evaluation, it may provide increased sensitivity for detection of this pathogen. Detection of antigens in urine, rather than in the serum or at a body site, may be effective for diagnosis. Such is the case for detection of urinary antigens of *L pneumophila* [59] and *Histoplasma capsulatum* [60,61] in the diagnosis of legionnaires' disease and histoplasmosis, respectively. Detection of antigens may denote acute disease; however, with some antigen assays, this detection may indicate prior infection with the specific organism, because antigen excretion may extend well past the stage of acute disease. Table 2-2 provides information about some of the available antigen-detection assays. Table 2-3 summarizes the methods for detection of the organisms most commonly encountered occupationally.

Antimicrobial Susceptibility Testing

Most laboratories perform antimicrobial susceptibility testing routinely or on a request basis. For bacteria commonly isolated from blood, urine or CSF specimens, for example, each lab has the option of performing qualitative assay (Bauer-Kirby) or quantitative assay (MIC or E-Test assay). The choice of assay is often based on the methods available to the laboratory and the demands of the physicians it supports.

The Bauer-Kirby test employs uses of agar plates, onto which selected isolates are inoculated in a "lawn of growth" and upon which disks of specific antibiotic concentrations are applied. The plates are incubated, usually overnight, and on the following day, "zones of inhibition" (in millimeters) are recorded for each drug. The larger the zone that is found, the more susceptible the organism is to the drug being tested. There are standard methods for performing the assay in regard to media used, inoculation size, and concentration of disks [62,63].

The minimum inhibitory concentration (MIC) test can be performed in agar plates with varying concentrations of specific drugs, each plate containing one concentration of one drug, or they may be done in large tubes of broth (macrotube dilution) or in small volumes of broth in microtiter trays (microbroth dilutions). Regardless of the manner in which the test is performed, the results are read as the lowest concentration of each drug that inhibits the organism from growing, after overnight incubation.

For either the Bauer-Kirby or MIC assay, the results are coded as *S* = susceptible; *I* = intermediate; or *R* = resistant.

In addition to these interpretative criteria, if the MIC is performed, numbers in micrograms per milliliter (μg/mL) are also given to indicate the concentration that actually inhibited the organism.

Some labs perform a test called the *E-test*, which employs a strip, rather than a disk, that has been impregnated with a graded concentration of the antibiotic to be tested. These strips are placed on the top of an agar plate that has been seeded with the organism to be tested. When read, the place where the organism growth crosses a specific concentration of the drug on the strip is read as the MIC. The area of no growth around these strips resembles an ellipse rather than a circle. Use of the E-test is increasing, especially in small labs that infrequently perform susceptibility tests and those that test fastidious organisms, for which the MIC or Bauer-Kirby tests are not available or not rapidly accessible to the lab for that specific organism. The National Committee on Clinical Laboratory Standards (NCCLS) has set standard protocols for susceptibility testing procedures and interpretations.

The minimum bactericidal assay (MBC) is less often performed in laboratories but, when done, requires determination of not only the inhibitory level but also the actual killing capability of the drug in question. MBC can be determined only if a prior MIC test has been performed. Samples

Table 2-2
Antigen-Detection Assays for Specific Agents

Agent/Disease	Assay	Specimeen	Comments
Bacterial Agents			
Chlamydia trachomatis	DFA	Cervical or urethral	Can determine quality of specimen; less sensitive than amplification.
Legionella pneumophila	DFA EIA	Respiratory secretions Urine	About 70–75% sensitivity.
Group A streptococcus	EIA, LA	Throat swab	80% sensitivity; > 100% specificity. Best for serogroup I infections, which are the majority.
	OIA	Throat swab	> 85% sensitivity.
Bordetella pertussis	IFA	Nasopharyngeal specimen	Sensitivity equal to or greater than culture.
Clostridium difficile toxins	LA, EIA	Stool	Sensitivity may be less than that of cytotoxin B assays. Questionable specificity with some assays.
Fungal Agents			
Cryptococcus neoformans	LA, EIA	CSF, sera	> 90% sensitivity compared to culture.
Histoplasma capsulatum	EIA	Urine, CSF	Good for disseminated histoplasmosis.
Candida sp	LA	Sera	Specificity for invasive disease: controversial in literature.
Pneumocystis carinii	DFA	Respiratory secretions	May be more specific than other stains.
Parasites			
Giardia lamblia	EIA, DFA	Stool	
Cryptosporidium sp	EIA, DFA	Stool	
Entamoeba histolytica	EIA	Stool	May allow for differentiation of pathogenic vs. nonpathogenic species.
Viral Agents			
HIV	p24 antigenemia	Sera	Antigenemia detected.
CMV	Antigenemia	Sera	Antigenemia assay.
Rotavirus	LA, EIA	Stool	Preferred method.
RSV	DFA, EIA	Nasopharyngeal	Preferred method.
Adenovirus	IFA	Respiratory secretions	Preferred method over culture; often combined in viral respiratory culture.
	LA	Stool	Serotype 40/41.
Influenza	IFA, EIA, LA	Respiratory secretions	Preferred method over culture; often combined in viral respiratory culture.
Parainfluenza	IFA, EIA, LA	Respiratory secretions	Preferred method over culture; often combined in viral respiratory panel.

Abbreviations: *DFA* = direct fluorescent antibody; *EIA* = enzyme immunoassay; *LA* = latex agglutination; *IFA* = indirect fluorescent antibody; *OIA* = optical immunoassay.
Based on data from references 16, 26–28, 32, 34, 48, 59–61, 65–73.

Table 2-3
Methods and Specimens for Some of the Organisms Likely To Be Encountered Occupationally

Agent	Specimen	Culture	Other	Serology
Bacteria				
Bartonella sp [64]	Blood; skin biopsy	Yes: requires special media		Preferred method
Borrelia burgdorferi [52]	Sera	Rarely		
C trachomatis	Genital discharge	Yes: tissue culture	DFA, EIA, Probes, Amp	Preferred method for LGV
Brucella sp	Blood; bone marrow	Yes: requires special media		Not specific
C pneumoniae [30]	Respiratory sera	Not widely available	Amp	MIF
C psittaci	Respiratory secretions	Difficult		Yes: MIF, CF
C trachomatis	Urine	No	Amp	
Ehrlichia sp [8]	Sera	No		Preferred method
F tularensis				
Legionella pneumophila	Tissue; respiratory secretions;other sites	Yes: requires special media	DFA	Yes: IFA
Legionella pneumophila	Blood	Yes: rarely		
Legionella pneumophila	Urine		EIA antigen [45]	
Leptospira sp	Blood in acute phase; urine later	Yes: requires special media	Darkfield exam	Yes: EIA, Agg
M hominis	Genital discharge; urine; tissue; fluids	Yes		N/A
Mycobacterium sp	Respiratory secretions; blood; other	Yes: with smear	Amp for MTB [23,28,67]	Not widely used in U.S.
P multocida	Wound; blood	Yes		N/A
S moniliformis	Blood	Yes: requires special media		Yes: agg
Spirillum minor	Wounds; nodes; skin	No	Darkfield exam	
Treponema pallidum	Genital discharge	No	Darkfield exam	Preferred method
M pneumoniae	Respiratory secretions	Yes: insensitive	Amp*	Yes: CF, EIA
Y pestis	Node; respiratory secretions	Yes		
Fungi				
Aspergillus sp	Any site	Yes: with stains		Yes: ID, CF; more in development
B dermatitidis	Respiratory secretions; blood; skin; other	Yes: with smears		Yes: CF, EIA, ID
C immitis	Respiratory secretions; CSF; skin; other	Yes: with smears	Hazardous to work with in lab	Yes: ID, CF, ? EIA in development
Dermatophytes	Skin; hair; nails	Yes: with stains	Urine and CSF antigen	Yes: ID, CF, EIA
H capsulatum	Bon marrow; respiratory secretions; blood; tissue; fluids	Yes: with smears	Urine and CSF antigen assays [80,81]	Yes: ID, CF, EIA
Malassezia sp	Skin; blood	Yes: many species require oil for growth		N/A
Other molds	Any site	Yes: with stains	Must distinguish pathogen from saprophyte on clinical basis	Not widely used, except for *Zygomycetes*
P brasiliensis	Skin; respiratory secretions	Yes		Yes: cross-reacts with *B dermatitidis*

Table 2-3 (continued)

Agent	Specimen	Culture	Other	Serology
Fungi (cont.)				
P carinii	Respiratory secretions	No	DFA; toluidine blue, calcofluor, silver stains [16,17]	Yes: IFA
P marneffei	Blood or any other site	Yes: with smears of tissue	Endemic: Thailand, China, and other countries in Far East	Being developed, as are methods for amp
S schenckii	Skin; rarely blood or other sites	Yes: smears are insensitive, however		Not widely used
Yeast	Any site	Yes: with stains		Cand-Tec [70] antigen for *C albicans* with questionable specificity for invasive disease
Parasites				
Cryptosporidia	Stool; other	No	O&P with acid-fast stain; antigen detection in stool	N/A
Cyclospora	Stool	No	Acid-fast stain	N/A
E histolytica	Stool; liver abscess	Not usually used	O&P exam; antigen detection in stool	Yes: IHA, EIA
Echinococcus sp	Surgical specimen	No	Exam for "hydatid sand" in surgical specimens	Yes: IHA
Giardia lamblia	Stool; string test	No	O&P exam; antigen detection in stool	N/A
Hookworm	Stool	No	O&P for eggs	N/A
Leishmania sp	Blood; nodes	Yes: not widely available	Exam of tissue for trophozoites	Yes: IFA
Microsporidia	Stool; other sites	No	O&P exam with modified trichome stain	N/A
Plasmodium sp	Blood smears	No	Exam for ring forms and gametocytes	Yes: IFA
Schistosoma sp	Stool	No	Exam for eggs	Yes: IFA
Strongyloides sp	Stool; other sites	Not widely used	O&P for larvae	Yes: IHA
T canis	Stool; tissue	No	O&P for eggs	Yes: EIA
T gondii	Blood; CSF; nodes; tissue	Yes: tissue culture; not widely available	Giemsa and other stains; amp	Yes: IFA, EIA IgG and IgM
Taenia sp	Stool	No	Exam for eggs	
Trichinella sp	Muscle biopsy	No	Exam for cysts	Yes: bentonite flocculation
Trichomonas vaginalis	Vaginal discharge	Yes: but not widely used	Wet mount for motility; probe	N/A
Trypanosoma sp	Blood; other	No	Exam for trophozoites	Yes: CF, IHA
Viruses				
Arbovirus	Brain biopsy; blood	Rarely done		Preferred: IFA, CF, HI, EIA, IgM and IgG
Adenovirus	Any	Yes: shell vial and conventional	Antigen detection in respiratory specimens	Yes: CF, EIA
	Stool		Antigen detection 40/41	
LCM	CSF; throat; urine; serum	Yes	Biosafety level 4	
CMV	Any	Yes: shell vial and conventional	Antigen detection; probes; amp	Yes: CF, IHA, EIA, IFA

Table 2-3 (continued)

Agent	Specimen	Culture	Other	Serology
Viruses (cont.)				
EBV	Blood	No		Yes: heterophile agg; IgM and IgG VCA, EBNA, EA
Hepatitis A	Blood	No		Yes: RIA or EIA, IgM, anti-HAV
Hepatitis B	Blood	No	Amp [75]	Yes: RIA or EIA
Hepatitis C	Blood	No	Amp [49]	EIA, Western blot
Hepatitis D	Blood	No		RIA
Hepatitis E	Blood	No		EIA, Western blot
HIV [48]	Blood	Yes but lengthy incubation; may be preferred in neonates	Amp; p24 antigenemia	EIA with Western blot for confirmation
HSV	CSF	No	Amp preferred method [22]	
	Any other site	Yes: shell vial or conventional	Antigen detection; ELVIS	Available but not specific for diagnosis
Calicivirus, Norwalk virus, astrovirus: gastroenteritis	Stool	No	EM	
Measles	Nasopharynx; throat; other	Not widely used	Direct IFA	Yes: HI, EIA, IgM by IFA, EIA, RIA, CF
Mumps	Blood	No		Yes: IFA, EIA, HAI
Rubella	Throat; tissue; urine	Not widely done		Preferred: EIA, HI, IFA, CF
HPV [50]	Genital	No	Probe; in situ; amp	
Rabies	Brain biopsy	Not routine	Direct IFA	IFA, RFFIT: diagnosis and immune status
Influenza A and B	Respiratory secretions	Yes	Direct antigen detection	Yes: CF, HAI
Parainfluenza I, II, III	Respiratory secretions	Yes	Direct antigen detection	Yes: HAI, CF, EIA
	Lesion; vesicle [15]	Yes	DFA	Yes
	NP aspirates	Yes	Direct antigen preferred	N/A

Abbreviations: Agg = agglutination; Amp = amplification; CF = complement fixation; *DFA* = direct fluorescence antibody; EIA = enzyme immunoassay; ID = immunodiffusion; IFA = indirect immunofluorescence; *IHA* = inhibition hemagglutination assay; LGV = lymphogranuloma venereum; MIF = microimmunofluorescence; N/A = not applicable or not available; *O&P* = ova and parasites; * = research only.

from the wells or tubes that remain visually negative are plated onto the surface of agar plates and incubated overnight. The next day, colonies are counted to determine which of the visually negative wells actually contains organisms. The well in which no growth occurs after agar plating is considered the MBC. If a drug is "cidal," the MIC and MBC are within one to two dilutions. If the drug is inhibitory and not cidal, then there will be a more than two-well dilution difference between the MIC and MBC.

There are methods that have been developed and standardized for the susceptibility testing of *Mycobacterium tuberculosis* and yeast organisms. For molds and other species of *Mycobacterium* species, some laboratories may perform susceptibility assays that they have developed in house or as a part of NCCLS evaluation studies. The NCCLS is working on a protocol for the susceptibility testing of molds. Currently, viral susceptibility testing is in the research stage but will probably be available for clinical use in the future.

Summary of Diagnostic Methods for Parasites, Fungi, Mycobacteria, and Viral Agents

PARASITES

- Stool needs to be submitted fresh or preserved in formalin or PVA. If fresh, should be sent to lab in less than 2 hours.
- Specimens are examined microscopically by wet mount; iodine preparations and trichrome-stained preparations are used to visualize trophozoites and cysts (if present).
- In addition, there are antigen assays available for *Giardia*, *Cryptosporidium* sp, and *Entamoeba histolytica*.
- For *Microsporidia*, a modified trichrome called the *Weber stain*, is used and observations are made under oil immersion.
- For *Cyclospora*, *Cryptosporidium* sp and *Isospora* belli an acid-fast stain is preferable.
- For *Plasmodium* or *Babesia microtii*, blood is sent to the lab, and thick and thin smears are prepared and stained with trichrome stain. Ring forms in red blood cells and presence of gametes is diagnostic.
- For leishmaniasis, direct observation of tissue sections, skin snips or biopsy specimens, or culture, and serology should be considered to aid in the diagnosis.
- For microfilaria (*Wuchereria bancrofti*, *Brugia malayi*, and loa loa); blood smears are used to see microfilaria; for *W bancrofti* and *B malayi*—nocturnal, and for loa loa, diurnal.
- For *Onchocerca*, presence of microfilaria in skin snips is diagnostic.
- *Toxoplasma gondii* is usually diagnosed serologically; however, clusters of tachyzoites and, in some cases, cysts can be seen in stained tissue sections. Amplification methods are becoming more the standard for diagnosis.
- For trichinosis, detection of spiral larvae in muscle tissue in conjunction with serologic testing is confirmatory.

FUNGI

- Culture and direct stains by means of calcofluor white or Congo red are standard; amplification is available in research labs; serology may be helpful in making some diagnoses.
- For dimorphic fungi, *H capsulatum*, *B dermatitidis*, *Coccidioides immitis*, *P brasiliensis*, *Sporothrix schenckii*, and *Penicillium marneffei*, after isolation in culture, demonstration of the yeast form as a conversion from mold is necessary. Exoantigen or probe tests of the mold form of the organism are needed for definitive identification.
- *Histoplasma capsulatum*: Lung, sputum, BAL, lymph nodes, blood, bone marrow, or CSF culture requires up to six weeks for isolation and use of specific media; probe is available for culture confirmation. Requires special request from the lab for isolation of organism from blood.
- *Blastomyces dermatitidis*: Lung, sputum, BAL, skin, bone, or CSF culture is standard; rarely blood culture, but if needed, special request of the lab is required. Requires up to two to three weeks for isolation of organism. Probe is available for culture confirmation.
- *Coccidioides immitis*: Lung, sputum, BAL, CSF, skin, or rarely, blood culture is done. Requires only four to five days for isolation. This organism is a potential hazard in the lab, so alert the lab if suspected. Probe available for culture confirmation.
- Brasiliensis: Same as for *B dermatitidis*.
- *Sporothrix schenckii*: Skin; lymph nodes; less likely from respiratory or other more systemic sites; no probe because conversion is easy and takes only a short period of time. Requires only about three to four days for isolation. Mold is dematiaceous (black).
- *Penicillium marneffei*: Any tissue; blood, bone marrow; looks like *H capsulatum* in tissue and peripheral blood. Conversion from mold (with red diffusible pigment) to yeast-like form is necessary for confirmation.
- *Aspergillus* species: These can be isolated from any site; may be the pathogen or a contaminate/saprophyte.
- *Candida* and other yeast: Usually easily isolated; any specimen; may be the etiology or part of the normal flora.
- Dermatophytes: Usually isolated from specimens of hair, skin or nails; may require up to three to four weeks for isolation. A genus level identification is adequate.
- Dematiaceous molds: May be soil contaminants in lab or saprophytes in patients or may

be responsible for clinical disease. Usually require more than 48 hours for isolation. Many genera and species isolated in human disease; may need reference lab for definitive identification.

MYCOBACTERIA

M tuberculosis: Culture and AFB smear of specimens from respiratory tract, tissue, or body fluids. All specimens from nonsterile sites should first be decontaminated and concentrated. Labs should use a broth culture supplemented with agar cultures for rapid detection and identification: Requires about 10–15 days in broth culture; longer in agar. Once isolated, cultures should be identified by probes, high-performance liquid chromatography (HPLC), or sequencing for rapid identification. Susceptibility testing of all isolated is required. Two amplification assays are available for direct specimen processing but should be performed only on respiratory samples that are smear positive. To meet CDC guidelines, labs should strive to perform AFB smears within 24 hours, isolate and identify *M tuberculosis* within 21 days, and perform susceptibilities within 30 days. With use of probes, the identification of *M tuberculosis* will be reported as a complex including *M tuberculosis*, *M bovis*, *M microtii*, and *M africanum* [64].

MOTT (*Mycobacterium* SPECIES OTHER THAN *M tuberculosis*)

Any specimen sent to the lab should be processed as for *M tuberculosis*. *M avium-intracellulare* (MAI) is usually isolated within the first five to seven days, and others in varying amounts of time. Rapidly growing *Mycobacterium* species may require variable amounts of time for primary isolation, but upon transferring the isolates in the lab, less than five to seven days are required. Identification of MAI, *M gordonae*, and *M kansasii* can be done with genetic probes. The other species require HPLC, sequencing, or conventional biochemical means of identification. Susceptibility testing is not standardized, although many labs will provide either MIC or Kirby-Bauer testing if requested [64].

VIRUSES

Many viruses can be cultured in the lab. For culturing of these viruses, specimens should be transported to the lab in an appropriate container/tube that also contains appropriate viral transport media and antibiotics. A conventional culture is processed in tubes and incubated for 30 days. Alternatively, a more rapid shell vial technique, requiring 48 hours, may be employed for some viruses. For some of the viral agents that are responsible for gastroenteritis, such as calicivirus, astrovirus and Norwalk virus, an electron microscopic exam may be provided; for others, antigen-detection methods can be used on stool specimens. Amplification and probe technology is more and more widely employed for viral diagnosis. Phoning the lab with requests often enables the lab to search for reference labs that do perform the assay if it does not.

References

1. Doern GV, Vautour R, Gaudet M, et al. Clinical impact of rapid in vitro susceptibility testing and bacterial identification. *J Clin Microbiol* 1994;32:1757–62.
2. McLaughlin J. The implementation of cost-effective, clinically relevant diagnostic microbiology policies: the approach. *Clin Microbiol Newsl* 1995;17:70–71.
3. Thomson RB, Peterson LR. The role of the clinical microbiology laboratory in the diagnosis of infections. In: Noskin LA (ed), *Management of Infectious Complications in Cancer Patients.* Boston: Kluwer Academic Publishers, 1998.
4. Wilson ML. Clinically relevant, cost-effective clinical microbiology: strategies to decrease unnecessary testing. *Am J Clin Pathol* 1997; 107:154–67.
5. Dunne WM, Nolte FS, Wilson ML. *Blood Cultures III in Cumitech 1B.* Washington, DC: ASM Press: American Society for Microbiology, April 1997.
6. Reimer L, Wilson M, Weinstein M. Update on detection of bacteremia and fungemia. *Clin Microbiol Rev* 1997;10:144–65.
7. Wilson ML. General principles in specimen collection and transport. *Clin Infect Dis* 1996;22:766–77.

7a. Koneman EW, Allen SD, Janda WM, et al. (eds). *Color Atlas and Textbook of Diagnostic Microbiology*, 5th Ed. Philadelphia: Lippincott, 1997.

8. Miller JM. *A Guide to Specimen Management in Clinical Microbiology.* Washington, DC: American Society for Microbiology, 1996.
9. Bartlett JG, Ryan KJ, Smith TF, et al. *Cumitech 7A. Laboratory Diagnosis of Lower Respiratory Tract Infec-*

tions. Washington, DC: ASM Press: American Society for Microbiology, 1987.

10. Gleaves CA, Hodinka RL, Johnston SLG, et al. *Cumitech 15A. Laboratory Diagnosis of Viral Infections.* Washington, DC: ASM Press: American Society for Microbiology, 1994.

10a. Wilson ML. Clinically relevant, cost-effective clinical microbiology. Strategies to decrease unnecessary testing. *Am J Clin Pathol* 1997;107:154–67.

11. Lennette EH, Lennette DA, Lennette ET (eds). *Diagnostic Procedures for Viral, Rickettsial, and Chlamydial Infections,* 7th Ed. Washington, DC: American Public Health Association, 1995.

12. Minnich LL, Smith TF, Ray GC. *Cumitech 24: Rapid Detection of Viruses by Immunofluorescence.* Washington, DC: ASM Press: American Society for Microbiology, 1994.

13. Murray P, Washington JA. Microscopic and bacteriologic analysis of expectorated sputum. *Mayo Clinic Proc* 1975;50:339–44.

14. Fluornoy DJM, Beal LM, Smith MD. What constitutes an adequate sputum specimen? *Lab Med* 1994;25:456–9.

15. Kahn F, Jones J. Diagnosing bacterial respiratory infection by bronchoalveolar lavage. *J Infect Dis* 1987; 155:862–9.

16. Eisen D, Ross BC, Fairbairn J, et al. Comparison of *Pneumocystis carinii* detection by Toluidine blue O staining, direct immunofluorescence and DNA amplification in sputum specimens from HIV-positive patients. *Pathology* 1994;26:198–200.

17. Fraser JL, Lilly C, Israel E, et al. Diagnostic yield of bronchoalveolar lavage and bronchoscopic lung biopsy for detection of *Pneumocystis carinii. Mayo Clin Proc* 1996;71:1025–9.

18. Gray LD, Fedorko DP. Laboratory diagnosis of bacterial meningitis. *Clin Microbiol Rev* 1992;5:130–45.

19. Kiska DL, Jones MC, Mangum ME, et al. Quality assurance study of bacterial antigen testing of cerebrospinal fluid. *J Clin Microbiol* 1995;33:1141–4.

20. Perkins MD, Mirrett S, Reller LB. Rapid bacterial antigen detection is not clinically useful. *J Clin Microbiol* 1995;33:1486–90.

21. Temset A, Roux P, Poirot JL, et al. Evaluation of a monoclonal antibody-based latex agglutination for diagnosis of cryptococcosis: comparison with two tests using polyclonal antibodies. *J Clin Microbiol* 1992; 30:2544–50.

22. Lakeman FD, Whitley RJ. Diagnosis of herpes simplex encephalitis: application of PCR to cerebrospinal fluid from brain-biopsied patients and correlation with disease. *J Infect Dis* 1995;171:857–63.

23. Baron EJ, Cassell GH, Duffy LB, et al. *Cumitech 17A. Laboratory Diagnosis of Female Genital Tract Infections.* Washington, DC: ASM Press: American Society for Microbiology, 1993.

24. Hook EW, Smith K, Mullen C, et al. Diagnosis of genitourinary *Chlamydia trachomatis* infections by using Ligase Chain Reaction on patient-obtained vaginal swabs. *J Clin Microbiol* 1997;35:2129–32.

25. Briselden A, Hillier SL. Evaluation of ARRIRM VP: microbial identification test for *Gardnerella vaginalis* and *Trichomonas vaginalis. J Clin Microbiol* 1994; 32:148–52.

26. Alles AJ, Waldron MA, Sierra LS. Prospective comparison of direct immunofluorescence and conventional staining methods for detection of *Giardia* and *Cryptosporidium* spp. in human fecal specimens. *J Clin Microbiol* 1995;33:1632–4.

27. Aldeen WE, Hale D, Robeson AJ, et al. Evaluation of a commercially available ELISA assay for detection of *Giardia lamblia* in fecal specimens. *Diagn Microbiol Infect Dis* 1995;21:1137–42.

28. Kehl KS, Ciricello H, Havens PL. Comparison of four different methods for detection of *Cryptosporidium* sp. *J Clin Microbiol* 1995;33:416–8.

29. Fan K, Morris A, Reller B. Application of rejection criteria for stool cultures for bacterial enteric pathogens. *J Clin Microbiol* 1993;31:2233–5.

30. Siegel DL, Edelstein PH, Nachamkin I. Inappropriate testing for diarrheal diseases in the hospital. *JAMA* 1990;263:1027–9.

31. Yannelli B, Gurvich I, Schoch PE, et al. Yield of stool cultures, ova and parasite tests, and *Clostridium difficile* determinations in nosocomial diarrhea. *Am J Infect Control* 1988;16:246–9.

32. Peterson LC, Kelly PJ. The role of the clinical laboratory in the management of *C difficile*-associated diarrhea. *Infect Dis Clin North Am* 1993;7:277–93.

33. Ahlwalia GS, Scott-Taylor TH, Klesco B, et al. Comparison of detection methods for adenovirus from enteric clinical specimens. *Diagn Microbiol Infect Dis* 1994;18:161–6.

34. Sanders RC, Campbell AD, Jenkins AF. Routine detection of human rotavirus by latex agglutination: comparison with latex agglutination, electron microscopy and polyacrylamide gel electrophoresis. *J Virol Methods* 1986;13:285–90.

35. Stager CE, Fraire AE, Kim H, et al. Modification of the Fungi-Fluor and the Genetic Systems fluorescent antibody methods for detection of *Pneumocystis carinii* in bronchoalveolar lavage specimens. *Arch Pathol Lab Med* 1995;119:142–7.

36. Hall GS. Probe technology for the clinical microbiology laboratory. *Arch Pathol Lab Med* 1993;117:578–83.

37. Hall GS. Identifying *M tuberculosis. Advance Lab Admin.* 1995; May: 27–34.

38. Tenover FC, Unger ER. *Nucleic Acid Probes for Detection and Identification of Infectious Agents.* In: Persing DH, Smith TF, Tenover FC, et al. (eds)., *Diagnostic Molecular Microbiology: Principles and Applications.*

Washington, DC: ASM Press: American Society for Microbiology, 1993.

39. Iwen PC, Walker RA, Warren KL, et al. Evaluation of nucleic acid based test (PACE 2C) for simultaneous detection of *Chlamydia trachomatis* and *Neisseria gonorrhoeae* in endocervical specimens. *J Clin Microbiol* 1995;33:2587–91.
40. Pokorski SJ, Vetter EA, Wollan PC, et al. Comparison of Gen-Probe group A streptococcus direct test with culture for diagnosing streptococcal pharyngitis. *J Clin Microbiol* 1994;32:1440–3.
41. Persing DH. Polymerase chain reaction: trenches to benches. *J Clin Microbiol* 1991;29:1281–5.
42. Wolcott MJ. Advances in nucleic acid based detection methods. *Clin Microbiol Rev* 1992;5:370–86.
43. Goessens WHF, Mouton JW, vanderMeijden WI, et al. Comparison of three commercially available amplification assays, AMP CT, LCx, and COBAS AMPLICOR, for detection of *Chlamydia trachomatis* in first-void urine. *J Clin Microbiol* 1997;35:2628–33.
44. Eing BR, Becker A, Sohns A, et al.. Comparison of Roche Cobas Amplicor *Mycobacterium tuberculosis* assay with in-house PCR and culture for detection of *M tuberculosis. J Clin Microbiol* 1998;36:2023–9.
45. Gamboa F, Fernandez G, Padilla E, et al. Comparative evaluation of initial and new versions of the Gen-Probe amplified *Mycobacterium tuberculosis* direct test for direct detection of *Mycobacterium tuberculosis* in respiratory specimens. *J Clin Microbiol* 1998;36:684–9.
46. Reischl U, Lehn N, Wolf H, et al. Clinical evaluation of the automated COBAS AMPLICOR MTB assay for testing respiratory and nonrespiratory specimens. *J Clin Microbiol* 1998;36:2853–60.
47. Doern GV. Diagnostic mycobacteriology: where are we today? *J Clin Microbiol* 1996;34:1873–6.
48. Yen-Lieberman B. Rapid and alternative specimen source testing for HIV-1 antibodies. *Clin Microbiol Newsl* 1998;20:133–7.
49. Alte HJ, Sanchez-Pescador R, Urdea MS, et al. Evaluation of branched DNA signal amplification for the detection of hepatitis C virus RNA. *J Viral Hepatitis* 1995;2:121–32.
50. Cox JT, Lorincz AT, Schiffman MH, et al. Human papillomavirus testing by hybrid capture appears to be useful in triaging women with a cytologic diagnosis of atypical squamous cells of undetermined significance. *Am J Obstet Gynecol* 1995;172:946–54.
51. Rose N, deMacario E, Folds JD, et al (eds). *Manual of Clinical Laboratory Immunology*, 5th Ed. Washington, DC: ASM Press: American Society for Microbiology, 1997.
52. Gaydos CA, Roblin PM, Hammerschlag MR, et al. Diagnostic utility of PCR-enzyme immunoassay, culture, and serology for detection of *Chlamydia pneumoniae* in symptomatic and asymptomatic patients. *J Clin Microbiol* 1994;32:903–5.
53. Raoult D, Fournier PE, Drancourt M, et al. Diagnosis of 22 new cases of *Bartonella* endocarditis. *Ann Intern Med* 1996;125:646–52.
54. Bakken JS, Krueth J, Wilson-Nordskog C, et al. Clinical and laboratory characteristics of human granulocytic ehrlichiosis. *JAMA* 1996; 275:199–205.
55. Magnarelli LA. Current status of laboratory diagnosis for lyme disease. National Clinical Conference on Lyme Disease. *Am J Med* 1995;98:10S–14S.
56. Kwon-Chung KJ, Bennett J (eds). *Medical Mycology*, 3rd Ed. Philadelphia: Lea & Febiger, 1992.
57. Garcia LS, Bruckner DA. *Diagnostic Medical Parasitology*, 2nd Ed. Washington, DC: ASM Press, American Society for Microbiology, 1993.
58. Guichon A, Inzana TJ, Scimeca JM, et al. Cumitech 28. *Laboratory Diagnosis of Zoonotic Infections: Chlamydia, Fungal, Viral, and Parasitic Infections Obtained From Companion and Laboratory Animals.* Washington, DC: ASM Press: American Society for Microbiology, Feb 1996.
59. Kashuba ADM, Balows CH. *Legionella* urinary antigen testing: potential impact on diagnosis and antibiotic therapy. *DMID* 1996;24:129–39.
60. Durkin MM, Connolly PA, Wheat LJ. Comparison of radioimmunoassay and enzyme-linked immunoassay for detection of *Histoplasma capsulatum* var. *capsulatum* antigen. *J Clin Microbiol* 1997;35:2252–5.
61. Wheat LJ, Kohler RB, Tewardi RP, et al. Significance of *Histoplasma* antigen in the cerebrospinal fluid of patients with meningitis. *Arch Intern Med* 1989;149:302–4.
62. National Committee on Clinical Laboratory Standards. *Methods for Dilution Antimicrobial Susceptibility Tests for Bacteria That Grow Aerobically.* Approved Standard M7-A4. Villanova, PA: NCCLS, 1997.
63. Neumann MA, Sahm DF, Thornsberry C, et al. *Cumitech 6A. New Developments in Antimicrobial Agent Susceptibility Testing: A Practical Guide.* Washington, DC: ASM Press: American Society for Microbiology, February 1991.
64. Cernoch PL, Enns RK, Saubolle MA, et al. *Cumitech 16A. Laboratory Diagnosis of the Mycobacterioses.* Washington, DC: ASM Press: American Society for Microbiology, Oct 1994.
65. Baker DM, Cooper RM, Rhodes C, et al. Superiority of conventional culture techniques over rapid detection of group A streptococcus by optical immunoassay. *Diag Microbiol Infect Dis* 1995;21:61–4.
66. Dale JC, Vetter EA, Contezac JM, et al. Evaluation of two rapid antigen assays, BioStar Strep A OIA and Pacific Biotech CARDS O.S., and culture for detection of group A streptococci in throat swabs. *J Clin Microbiol* 1994;32:2698–701.
67. Phillips P, Dowd A, Jewesson P, et al. Nonvalue of antigen detection immunoassays for diagnosis of candidemia. *J Clin Microbiol* 1990;28:2320–6.

68. Haque R, Neville LM, Hahn P, et al. Rapid diagnosis of *Entamoeba* infection using *Entamoeba* and *Entamoeba histolytica* stool antigen detection kits. *J Clin Microbiol* 1995;33:2558–61.

69. Veal N, Payan C, Fray D, et al. Novel DNA assay for cytomegalovirus detection: comparison with conventional culture and pp65 antigenemia assay. *J Clin Microbiol* 1996;34:3097–100.

70. Takamoto S, Grandien M, Ishida MA, et al. Comparison of ELISA, indirect immunofluorescence assay and virus isolation for detection of respiratory syncytial virus in nasopharyngeal secretions. *J Clin Microbiol* 1991;29:470–4.

71. Dominquez A, Taber LH, Couch RB. Comparison of rapid diagnostic techniques for respiratory syncytial and influenza A virus respiratory infections in young children. *J Clin Microbiol* 1993;31:2286–90.

72. Salomon HE, Grandien M, Avila MM, et al. Comparison of three techniques for detection of respiratory viruses in nasopharyngeal aspirates from children with lower respiratory tract infections. *J Med Virol* 1989;28:159–62.

73. Reina J, Munar M, Blanco I. Evaluation of a direct immunofluorescence assay, dot-blot enzyme immunoassay, and shell vial culture in the diagnosis of lower respiratory tract infections caused by influenza A virus. *Diag Microbiol Infect Dis* 1996;25:143–5.

3 / Epidemiology and Etiology of Occupational Infectious Diseases

Daymon Evans

Background and History

The central premise of epidemiology is that injuries and illnesses are not randomly distributed. It is the science that estimates the frequency and distribution of injury and illness from the accurate knowledge of the frequency and distribution of risk factors. Epidemiology is the formal study and treatment of populations rather than the linear clinical care of individual patients. It is from the care of the individual that one learns the art of medicine, but it is only from the study of groups that we all find and share the science of medicine. Epidemiology studies the associations, causation, and ultimately the methods of control and prevention of injury and illness and their effectiveness.

The early advancement of medical science depended on the astute individual clinician who was stimulated by a single case, formed a hypothesis of causation, and began a mission of scientific proof. The Henle-Koch postulates formed the basis of the scientific method, and epidemiology was nearly synonymous with communicable disease until the middle of the twentieth century. Epidemiology expanded to other areas such as chronic disease, the behavioral sciences, injuries, and most recently to clinical pathways and outcome analysis. Epidemiology and biostatistics are being used more and more to justify or discredit treatment methods.

Today there are formal systems of surveillance to look for outbreaks, epidemics, or new associations. But infectious disease remains the number one cause of death in humans. New infectious agents and diseases are being discovered, most often by a clinician or basic scientist pursuing a premonition. Many familiar chronic and degenerative diseases are now suspected or proved to have microbiotic or immunologic causation. It was only 12 years between the isolation of a strange spiral bacteria from gastric mucosa and the *NIH Consensus Statement on* Helicobacter pylori *in Peptic Ulcer Disease* [1]. A possible association between such infectious agents as cytomegalovirus or chlamydia and coronary artery occlusion is currently being debated, as there have been conflicting studies. The postulates of infectious disease have renewed importance.

Most occupational and environmental medicine practices in the United States spend more time and effort preventing infectious disease than treating it. This textbook is intended to expand that pattern. It is assumed that the reader has some knowledge of the basic concepts of infectious disease, epidemiology, and cell structure. A review of key definitions that are central to this chapter's and following chapters' topics are presented early in the chapter. Definitions and concepts relative to the epidemiology of infectious disease, totaling over 250, are presented in bold throughout the chapter. The first set of 49 definitions are presented in reference to communicable *human* disease, although most have wider applications.

Definitions

Epidemiology: "The study of the distribution and determinants of health-related states and events in populations, and the application of this study to control health problems" [2]. It can be further subdivided into:

Descriptive epidemiology: Represents the majority of epidemiologic studies such as surveys and cross-sectional studies. It is concerned with describing communicable disease with respect to demographic fields such as age, sex, race, occupation, or area of residence. It studies populations "as is" or with "hands-off." It is less accurate than experimental, because it may imply a cause and effect (an **association**) rather than scientifically proving a cause and effect.

Experimental epidemiology: The scientific, or "**control study,**" experimentally isolates the factor to be prospectively studied as the main difference in the two groups. The study and control groups are intentionally matched for all factors except that which is to be studied. It is little used in communicable disease, except for clinical trials of antibiotics or vaccines. Withholding available treatment for infections is usually unethical, so the control group is often those receiving the traditional or standard treatment for the infectious disease.

"Shoe leather" epidemiology: A term to describe the hard and menial work of epidemiologic investigation—a reference to John Snow's wearing out his shoes collecting door-to-door information in his epic cholera study. Major U.S. field assignments are often performed by officers or fellows of the Epidemiologic Intelligence Serve (EIS), who use the "sole with a hole" emblem.

Infectious agent: Any living or biologic entity (virus, bacteria, rickettsia, fungus, or multicellular organism) that may cause an infection or illness in a higher life form. This chapter and textbook discuss those agents that may cause human infection.

Host: A human or other animal or insect that is physically supporting or sustaining an infectious agent under natural conditions. A host may or may not be ill or affected by the agent. A **definitive (primary) host** is one in which a parasite attains its sexual or mature stage, while an **intermediate (secondary) host** supports or sustains a larval or asexual stage.

Environment: Any part of the universe existing outside of a living or biologic entity.

Population: A specified and well-defined group of people, such as residents of a geographic area or employees of a company. This is the usual denominator of epidemiologic study and statistics and represents those who are at some risk of the disease under study.

Rate: The number of cases of an infection (a numerator) occurring in a given population (a denominator) over a specified period of time. Unlike a quotient or percentage, it must always specify a unit of time.

Prevalence: The number of cases of an infectious disease (both new and old) existing or active in, or over, a period of time. If a period of time is not specified, then it may be a **point prevalence**, or the number or percent infected at a point in time. **Lifetime prevalence** is the percentage of persons who will have a given condition at some time in their life. *Example*: Fifteen percent (15%) of the human population will have herpes zoster at some time in their life [3].

Seroprevalence: The percent of a population that has evidence of antibodies to an infectious agent at a point in time, implying a past exposure. A very useful statistic in investigating epidemics or clusters of infectious disease in a given area or group. *Example*: In the United States, there is a seroprevalence of 33% for hepatitis A IgM antibody in adults [4]. One of every three adults has evidence of having been exposed to (and recovered from) hepatitis A (HAV).

Incidence: The number of new cases of an infectious disease that occur over a given period of time. The number of persons exposed or at risk who do contract or develop the infectious disease, divided by those exposed or at risk who could contract or develop that infectious disease. This is usually presented as a percentage, over a given period of time (**incident rate**).

Case definition: As with many other diseases, the specific criteria needed to make the diagnosis of the specific infection. This varies from agent to agent and may require specific symptoms, examination findings, laboratory diagnosis, or a combination thereof. The most recent Centers for Disease Control and Prevention (CDC) revision of case definitions for infectious disease was in 1997 [5].

Historical controls: Comparing the outcome of an infectious disease to that recorded in the past. This could be the same as the natural history of the disease before treatment or prevention was available. *Example:* Historical controls show that nearly 50% of active pulmonary tuberculosis cases died from their disease before twentieth-century controls and treatments.

Epidemic: The incidence of an infectious disease in a specified population over and above that expected from previous experience. Generally found by **surveillance**, the formal and organized tracking of an infectious disease's statistics over time. Only two cases can be considered an **outbreak** or epidemic if no cases occurred in that population in the past. An **epizootic** is an epidemic in animals, and an **epornitic** in birds. **Plague** is an older term synonymous with an epidemic or pandemic but is also specific for diseases caused by *Yersinia pestis.*

Pandemic: An outbreak or epidemic that crosses continents and become global. This includes the class-1 diseases plague, yellow fever, and cholera but has more recently occurred with rubella, influenza, and HIV.

Epidemic curve: The plotting of the number of new cases of an infectious disease (Y axis) over a period of time (X axis). The epidemic curve can aid in the identification of the infectious agent from determining epidemics (peaks), incubation periods (steepness), and secondary cases (second spikes). Figure 3-1 shows a fictitious epidemic curve.

Endemic: The steady and constant presence (or prevalence) of an infectious agent in a given geographic area or host population. An infectious state that is never cleared from a population and is not typically occurring in epidemics. **Holoendemic** means that most of the population is affected, and **hyperendemic** means than many are infected. *Example*: Plague is endemic in some rodent populations in the western United States.

Attack rate: An incident rate or a ratio of those who become infected with a specific infectious

Figure 3-1
Sample epidemic curve plotting the number of new cases versus time. The initial peak suggests an incubation period of about three to four days, and a second peak suggests secondary cases.

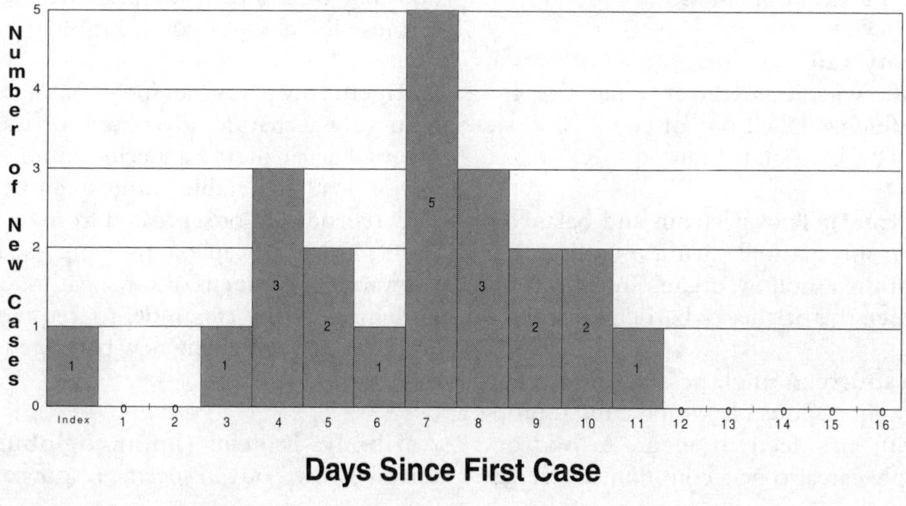

agent, calculated from the number who were exposed to that agent. *Example*: Adults living in a home with children during an influenza epidemic have an attack rate of 33% in an average year [6].

Infection: The state of having microorganisms (or parasites) entering, living, and reproducing on the physical person. It is not synonymous with disease, which means that the infection is causing symptoms (**apparent illness**). In some cases, an infection is short-lived and causes no symptoms (**inapparent illness**) or persists and causes no symptoms (colonization). *Example*: Hepatitis A infection causes apparent illness in only 30% of children under the age of 6 (therefore, 70% inapparent illness), but 70% of older children or adults have apparent illness [7].

Incubation period: The period of time from being invaded (infected) with the agent until the time that clinical manifestations occur. The time during which the agent multiplies or propagates within the infected organism until the time it causes illness. The epidemic curve in Figure 3-1 shows a peak number of persons becoming ill between three and five days after the first, suggesting an incubation period in this range.

Communicable (or infective) period: Over the course of an infection and illness, the period of time that the person is capable of passing the illness to another. Depending on the infectious agent, it may include periods of time before, during, or after clinical illness.

Case fatality rate: The percentage of persons infected who will die as a direct result. *Example*: Spanish influenza killed one of every 10 ill victims for a 10% case fatality rate.

Flora (normal): The spectrum and balance of microorganisms naturally living on a body surface or within a hollow organ. Infections can develop when this balance or barrier is disrupted.

Common source: A single person (**index case**), place, or thing responsible for infecting multiple victims with an infectious agent. A food or a water supply can also be a common source. *Example*: The potato salad served at the Smiths' family reunion in Fairfield, New Jersey, on the afternoon of June 26 was the common source for the food poisoning cases.

Reservoir: The natural habitat of an infectious agent. The substrate (person, animal, plant, insect, water, or soil) where it best survives in either an actively reproducing or dormant state. *Example*: The only reservoir for measles is the human being. When no humans are infected, the disease (rubeola) will be eradicated!

Infestation: The state of having a parasitic organism (generally an arthropod) living on the physical surface of the body. Such a person is **infested**.

Immune: The state of being unable to contract a specific infectious disease because one has acquired adequate host defense mechanisms with dedicated killing cells or antibodies. Usually this is through previous exposure (by infection or immunization), followed by an adequate host immune response. Immunity is not always complete, and an overwhelming dose of infectious agents (**inoculum**) could still cause some illness.

Inoculum: The amount of infectious agent that successfully invades or exposes a host. **Inoculation** is the process of exposing or introducing a host to an infectious agent. An **infective dose** is the number of organisms necessary to cause infection or a measurable host response. An inoculum may be less than the infective dose needed to cause infection or colonization.

Antigen: Any part of an infectious agent (a protein, polysaccharide, glycolipid, or transplanted tissue) that can induce a specific immune response in the host. If a stable antigen can be synthetically reproduced or separated from its infectious agent, it may be capable of being used as an active vaccine. Antigens of some pathogens such as influenza or HIV can undergo frequent changes and produce essentially new pathogens and new diseases.

Antibody: Proteins (**immunoglobulins**) produced by the body in specific response to microbial antigens, which may be efficient in binding to antigen to prevent or fight diseases. In response to some diseases, the human body can produce antibodies that do not seem to be entirely competent in fighting or eradicating the disease. *Examples*: Human immunodeficiency virus (HIV) and hepatitis C virus (HCV).

Vehicle (of infection): Any mode of transportation for an infectious agent from its reservoir to a person or an inanimate object, including fomites. Food or water can be vehicles.

Fomites: Inanimate objects that serve as surfaces for the spread of infectious agents. *Examples*: Door handles, drinking glasses, toys, and medical instruments.

Vector: Any animate object that serves as a carrier of an infectious agent. A **mechanical vector** passively carries the agent somewhere on its body, such as the leg of a fly. A **biologic vector** includes arthropods (insects), which may also serve a role in the replication cycle of the agent.

Cohort: Any human who may have in common the sharing of a risk and who may be the subject of study for the effect of that risk. Co-workers may be cohorts by virtue of working for the same employer, sharing a workplace risk, or being subjects of a workplace study.

Birth cohorts: All of those persons born in a given year. Children in the same grade in school are from approximately the same birth cohort. In seroepidemiology, birth cohorts are individuals born at points in time that may define natural exposure to circulating diseases. *Example*: It is published in some guidelines that persons born before 1957 may be assumed to be immune to the wild rubella and rubeola viruses that were in widespread circulation before 1957 [8].

Nosocomial infection: Infection related to or having been acquired while in a health care institution and unrelated to patients' original diagnoses.

Latent infection: Any infection that can remain asymptomatic in the host for long periods of times but with the potential to reactivate. *Examples*: tuberculosis, syphilis, HIV, and many herpesviruses.

Latent period (latency): Classically, the period between the time of invasion and infection until the time of infectivity. However, more recently with HIV, it has come to be used synonymously with *incubation period*. That is, HIV is both latent and infectious at the same time. Asymptomatic diseases with long latency (but high infectivity) can be the most difficult to control.

Carrier: A person or animal that harbors an infective and infectious agent without apparent illness themselves. A carrier can be a short-lived or a **transient carrier** or can become a long-term **chronic carrier**. A person can be a carrier before clinical illness (**incubatory carrier**) or after clinical recovery (**convalescent carrier**).

Susceptible: A person's state of being at risk for infection with an agent because the individual lacks resistance or immunity to that agent.

Susceptible pool: That group of persons in a population who are not immune to a specific infectious agent and therefore are susceptible to infection if exposed. In theory, an epidemic ends when the susceptible pool is exhausted or a high percentage of the population has developed immunity.

Herd immunity: The immunity of a population to a specific infectious agent. Theoretically there is a percent of immunity (**herd immunity threshold**) at which an epidemic ceases to propagate. This threshold is specific to each disease and is based both on its ability to reproduce and its infectivity [9]. Many mathematical models of vaccine efficacy are based on a target herd immunity.

Seroepidemiology: The use of laboratory studies of infection (antigens) and immunity (antibodies) to study patterns of human infections. **Serosurveys** are a form of observational epidemiology that studies the inapparent infection rates, dormancy, latency, herd immunity, and susceptibility of a natural population. Seroepidemiology is both expensive and time consuming but provides the most valuable information in investigating epidemics. Seroepidemiology takes the form of experimental seroepidemiology in highly structured **vaccine efficacy trials**.

Virulence: The degree to which an infectious agent can cause clinical illness, either by its ability to damage tissue and/or its ability to invade a host. It is best measured by the **case-fatality rate**.

Shedding: The process of a host excreting, exhaling, defecating, or sloughing into the environment infectious agents that are capable of infecting others. Shedding entails an active port of exit.

Isolation: The process of separating or restricting the movement of an infectious and ill person from those who are well and susceptible. Isolation is imposed for the anticipated duration of the communicable period.

Quarantine: The process of separating a well but exposed person from those who are well and susceptible but not yet exposed, for the duration of the anticipated communicable period. Quarantine is mainly of historic significance, although some quarantine commitment laws still exist.

Zoonosis: An infection transmitted from vertebrate animals (e.g., rabies and brucellosis) to humans under natural conditions.

Conventions of Reporting and Surveillance

The **International Classification of Disease (ICD)** is a system of cataloging diagnoses that periodically is updated by a committee of the World Health Organization (WHO). Originally used for epidemiologic surveillance, it is now used for financial coding as well. The ninth (ICD-9) is the system used in the United States at this time, but a major revision (ICD-10) was written and ratified in 1990. All editions have listed infectious and parasitic diseases first (e.g., in ICD-9, cholera is 001 and typhoid is 002). There are 21 chapters in ICD-10; Chapter 1 is Infectious and Parasitics Diseases (A00 to B99).

Communicable diseases are also classified as **reportable** or **not reportable**. The status of each disease is determined by the local state, and each licensed physician is responsible for knowing what is reportable and what is not reportable in their area and for making individual **case reports**. All states have strict laws of confidentiality governing their public health officers. States then create **collective reports** for their own analysis, which they pass on to the CDC. International communicable disease surveillance is done by the **World Health Organization (WHO)**. WHO also classifies diseases into five levels of surveillance and reporting [10], which are summarized in Table 3-1.

Much of the reporting of infectious disease in the United States was inconsistent before 1990. At that time, the CDC and the **Council of State and Territorial Epidemiologists (CSTE)** established a policy that requires state health departments to report cases of selected diseases (Table 3-2) to the CDC's **National Notifiable Disease Surveillance System (NNDSS)**. They also wrote specific criteria for diagnosing each communicable disease (the case definition). This document was updated in 1997 [5]. Table 3-3 contains the

Table 3-1
WHO's Five Levels of Disease Reporting

Class 1: Case Report Universally Required by International Health Regulations, under Surveillance by WHO. *Examples:*
- 1A: Plague, cholera, yellow fever
- 1B: Louse typhus, paralytic poliomyelitis, malaria

Class 2: Case Report Regularly Required Wherever the Disease Occurs. *Examples:*
- 2A: Typhoid fever, diphtheria
- 2B: Brucellosis, leprosy

Class 3: Selectively Reportable in Recognized Endemic Areas. *Examples:*
- 3A: Scrub typhus
- 3B: Coccidioidomycosis
- 3C: Schistosomiasis

Class 4: Obligatory Report of Epidemics—No Case Report Required. *Examples:* Epidemics of food poisonings or keratoconjunctivitis

Class 5: Official Report Not Ordinarily Justifiable. *Example:*
- Common respiratory illness

Table 3-2
Infectious Diseases Designated as Notifiable at the National Level, United States, 1997

Acquired immunodeficiency syndrome (AIDS)	Malaria
Anthrax	Measles
Botulism	Meningococcal disease
Brucellosis	Mumps
Chancroid	Pertussis
Chlamydia trachomatis, genital	Plague
Cholera	Poliomyelitis, paralytic
Coccidioidomycosis	Psittacosis
Cryptosporidiosis	Rabies, animal
Diphtheria	Rocky Mountain spotted fever
Encephalitis, California group	Rubella
Encephalitis, eastern equine	Congenital rubella
Encephalitis, St. Louis	Salmonellosis
Encephalitis, western equine	Shigellosis
Escherichia coli 0157:H7	Streptococcal disease, invasive group A
Gonorrhea	*Streptococcal pneumoniae*, drug-resistant
Haemophilus influenzae, invasive	Streptococcal toxic shock
Hansen's disease (leprosy), invasive	Syphilis
Hantavirus pulmonary syndrome	Syphilis, congenital
Hemolytic uremic syndrome, postdiarrheal	Tetanus
Hepatitis A	Toxic-shock syndrome
Hepatitis B	Trichinosis
Hepatitis C (non-A, non-B)	Tuberculosis
HIV infections, pediatric	Typhoid fever
Legionellosis	Yellow fever
Lyme disease	

From Centers for Disease Control and Prevention. Case definitions for infectious conditions under public health surveillance. *MMWR* 1997;46(RR-10):2.

Table 3-3
Infectious Diseases and Conditions That Are Not Nationally Notifiable but for Which Case Definitions May Be Useful for Surveillance[a]

Amebiasis	*Granuloma inguinal*
Aseptic meningitis	Leptospirosis
Bacterial meningitis, other	Listeriosis
Campylobacter infection	*Lymphogranuloma venereum*
Cyclospora infection	Mucopurulent cervicitis
Dengue fever	Nongonococcal urethritis
Ehrlichiosis	Pelvic inflammatory disease
Genital herpes	Rheumatic fever
Genital warts	Tularemia
Giardiasis	Varicella (chickenpox)

[a] Not a complete list of such diseases.
From Centers for Disease Control and Prevention. Case definitions for infectious conditions under public health surveillance. *MMWR* 1997;46(RR-10):4.

list of infectious diseases that are not nationally notifiable but for which case definitions may be useful for surveillance.

The Epidemiologic Triangle (or Triad)

For an infection to occur, a specific combination of events must occur. There must be an infectious **agent** capable of infecting a human being. The agent must be present in sufficient quantity in the **environment** to cause entry, invasion, and infection of a susceptible human **host**. This triad is called the **epidemiologic triangle or triad** (Figure 3-2) and serves as the model and outline for the rest of this chapter. We may think of the agent-environment-host triad as the three points on the corner of the triangle, and the concept of **transmission** as the three lines connecting the triangle. The transmission is completed by the existence of a **port of entry**, a **port of exit**, and a reservoir for the agent.

This model can also serve as the model for control. That is, a completed triangle is negative, and any and all factors that prevent the triangle from forming are positive. The individual factors of the agent, environment, or host can be studied individually for factors that may remove a corner and thus break the triangle. The sides can be studied for methods of breaking the triangle by blocking transmission. Infection control and preventive medicine must search for the weakest, most practical, and most economical part of the triangle to attack.

THE AGENT

Agents of concern in this text are various infectious microbial organisms or entities with the ability to cause harm to humans. The most basic instinct of infectious agents, as for all living entities, is to survive and propagate their own kind. They are not homicidal by nature, as causing rapid death to their human host serves them no purpose. The most successful viruses are those that can reach the point of being a persistent and latent infection in most humans on Earth (or **holoendemic**). Thus, herpes simplex 1 and varicella viruses are far more successful than rabies or Ebola. Some attributes of infectious agents that can increase their success and survival are listed in Table 3-4.

Agents may come in different varieties of the same species and symptomatically present as different diseases. These are called *subtypes*, *strains*, *serotypes*, or *serovars* (serologic variant), depending on the agent. Some agents may have only one pathologic form (e.g., rubella), while others may have dozens (e.g., shigella, *Escherichia coli*, cholera, adenovirus), hundreds (e.g., rhinovirus), or even thousands (e.g., influenza, salmonella).

THE HOST AND HOST FACTORS

The term *host* in this textbook implies the human unless otherwise specified, that is, when the infectious agent may have other hosts in their life cycle. Humans have a great range of factors that can influence their efficiency as a host. Called **host factors**, these include:

Figure 3-2
Epidemiologic triangle displaying the interplay between the host, environment, and agent that produces infection.

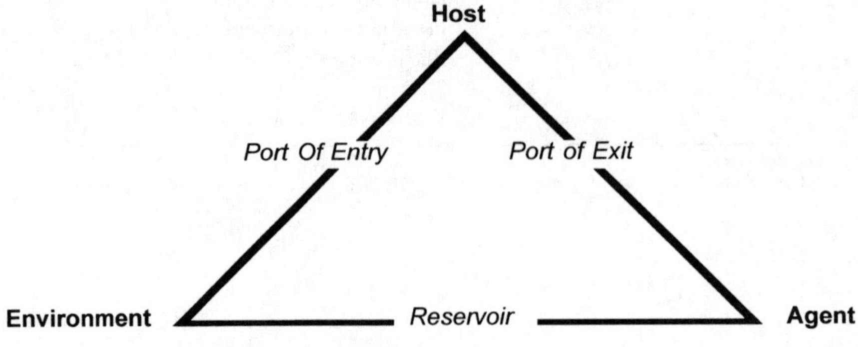

Table 3-4
Attributes of Infectious Agents Associated with Their Success

Agent must be stable and resistant to physical factors in the environment; is even more successful if it can adapt to changes in the environment.
Agent must exist in sufficient quantity in the environment to cause infection.
Agent must find the proper *vector*, or medium, to use to infect the host.
Agent must have the ability to invade and infect through a host portal of entry.
Agent must be resistant to host-defense factors once it has invaded a host and is more successful if it can actively develop resistance to host defenses.
Agent must have the ability to egress or shed from the host through a portal of exit.

Age

Young children and adults are very different when it comes to susceptibility and response to infectious diseases. We focus on adults in this text, but an understanding of this difference is essential. A history of childhood diseases is very important, especially for those entering the health care field. A fairly reliable clinical history of varicella during childhood is nearly as sensitive as laboratory confirmation. Many infections are asymptomatic (subclinical) in children but symptomatic (clinical) in adults. Examples include poliovirus, Epstein-Barr virus (mononucleosis), mumps, varicella, *Neisseria meningitidis,* and some types of influenza. Children in their preschool years have maximally efficient immune systems and can form lifelong immunity to all the diseases mentioned above. One study showed that, because of exposure to a similar strain when they were children [11], people over the age of 75 (a birth cohort) had better immunity to the Hong Kong influenza strain during an outbreak than those ages 65 to 75. The elderly may not be more susceptible to infectious agents in general but are more susceptible to complications and morbidity and mortality from infectious agents.

Socioeconomic Factors

As mentioned, many of the more highly communicable diseases are less severe in childhood. Conditions associated with lower socioeconomic class or poverty (crowding, poor hygiene and sanitation, lack of available medical care) seem to protect individuals raised in these conditions from more severe morbidity if an infectious disease is contracted in adulthood. This is most true of the highly endemic or prevalent human diseases that are spread by fecal-oral or direct transmission. However, poor nutrition or poor general health may predispose one to the complications of infection if host defenses are less than optimum. Children living in substandard conditions are more susceptible to a few diseases, such as pulmonary tuberculosis.

Genetics

Like age, inheritance is a biologic factor that cannot be altered. Genetic traits influence susceptibility to certain infections and may determine not only the clinical outcome but whether the person becomes chronically ill (e.g., hepatitis B or C). Genetics may be a factor in most, if not all, infectious diseases and helps to explain the great variations in human host response. Variations in the human leukocyte antigen (HLA) seem to correlate with both susceptibility and resistance to certain diseases.

Gender

Only a few infectious diseases seem to have a predilection for one gender over the other. Overall, males have slightly more infectious disease risk and this may be due in part to gender differences of occupation, forms of recreation, or risk-taking behaviors.

Geography

The area of residence is extremely important in individual infectious disease susceptibility. There is tremendous variation in the endemic infectious diseases from continent to continent. One may become exposed and resistant to diseases endemic in the soil of one's homeland but remain susceptible to soil pathogens in another area. In the United States, the best examples of this are cases of histoplasmosis in the Midwest and Ohio Valley and cases of coccidioidomycosis in the Southwest. Adults moving from one area to the other may be more susceptible to developing clinical illness soon after their move and may need to be taken into consideration in their pre-employment history.

Immunity

Vaccines can make a host resistant to certain diseases, but we still lack vaccines for many diseases such as the rickettsiae and most bacteria.

Environment

The environment of the Earth's biosphere is extremely delicate and is "colonized" by billions of living organisms, including humans. Each organism has evolved in its own habitat or a place where and time when the conditions of temperature, moisture, season, sunlight, and substrate availability is maximum for its survival. Many organisms have evolved life cycles that include other organisms. Humans have a comparatively wide range of habitats, as we can assure our survival almost anywhere on Earth with our technology (e.g., plumbing, energy, clothing, communication). But most important in our technology is our knowledge of the environments into which we trek or seek to reside and how we can protect ourselves from the biologic hazards we may expect to find in those environments.

Microbiologists and virologists are the primary resource experts on infectious agents, and clinicians the experts on the host and host responses. Safety, public health, and preventive medicine professionals are the resource experts on the forms of infectious agents in the environment and factors that influence them. Certainly this includes occupational and environmental health professionals. Our occupations and technology take us into environments we would not otherwise visit—that is, deep in the earth, high in the sky, or under the seas. It may be that our technology has in fact created some of the "new" infections such as legionella. We may become the new and **accidental host** when we have changed the environment or a biologic reservoir in some way. Humans may be accidental hosts for some of the most dangerous infectious agents such as Ebola virus, *Hantavirus*, rabies, and the plague.

Causality and the Postulates: A Historical Perspective

A **postulate** is an unproven assertion or assumption, a statement or formula offered as the basis of a theory [12]. The postulates for the causation of infectious disease seem simple and logical today, but their hypotheses were a major contribution to the medicine of the early nineteenth century, written by Jako Henle (1809–1885) in 1840 but further modified by his student Robert Koch (1843–1910) and published in 1890 [13]. Henle and Koch were aware that many diseases may be caused by microbes or bacteria, which they called *parasites*. Their joint hypotheses, known as the *Henle-Koch postulates*, state that:

1. The agent must be shown to be present in every case of the disease by isolation in pure culture.
2. The agent must not be found in cases of other diseases.
3. Once isolated, the agent must be capable of reproducing the disease in experimental animals.
4. The agent must be recovered from the experimental disease produced.

Henle and Koch considered #1 and #2 to be essential, and #3 and #4 to be further confirmation. The pure postulates may be difficult to adhere to in their entirety, because they did not consider that:

1. Isolation is not always possible, depending on the disease and lab techniques available (e.g., there is still no culture technique for hepatitis B).
2. Some individuals may be or have been infected but are/were not ill (inapparent infection).
3. An animal laboratory model does not exist for all human diseases. Some diseases are specific to humans, and therefore:
4. There is no experimental disease to study.

Rivers questioned the rigidity of the postulates in the presidential address to the American Immunological Society in 1937 [14]. The field of virology was exploding with new knowledge at that time and viral culture techniques were being perfected. His postulates for the viruses state that:

1. A specific virus must be found to be associated with a disease with "a degree of regularity."
2. The virus in the ill person must be proved to be the cause of the disease, not an incidental or accidental finding.
3. Infection is produced with a "degree of regularity" in susceptible hosts by means of inoculating them with material (otherwise uncontaminated) from ill individuals.

However, many other questions remained unanswered in the field of virology. It was found that antibodies to nonpathogenic viruses were often present, some viral infections cleared without stimulating the infected host's production of antibodies, and on occasion one could be infected (or reinfected) with a virus to which they already had antibodies. Answers to the remaining questions are still elusive, especially since viruses or their specific antibodies are being increasingly suspected of contributing to causation of cancers and other chronic illnesses. Many variations of postulates for causation have been published beyond the topic of infectious disease. Dr. Alfred S. Evans has written many of the more modern postulates, including the 1973 criteria we now associate with the **"paired sera"** diagnosis of acute viral illness [15].

1. Specific antibody to the virus is absent in the susceptible person.
2. Specific antibody appears during illness. Examples are transient specific IgM antibody, persistent IgG antibody, and local IgA at the site of viral multiplication.
3. Specific antibody production is accompanied by the presence of viruses in the infected tissues.
4. Absence of specific IgG indicates susceptibility.
5. Presence of specific IgG indicates immunity.
6. No other virus produces these specific antibodies.
7. Induced production (immunization) of specific antibody prevents disease.

Evans reviewed the history of postulates and the principles of causation in a book published shortly before his death [16]. The concepts of postulates eventually extended far beyond infectious disease. The most up-to-date set of concepts of epidemiologic causation are attributed to British biostatistician Austin Hill (1897–1991) [17]. Hill's criteria for observations that contribute to a valid association are listed in Table 3-5.

In 1964, the United States Surgeon General's Advisory Committee accepted Hill's criteria #1, #2, #3, #5, and #7 as the five criteria that should be fulfilled to establish a causal relationship. This was the same year they released the Surgeon General's report on the association of tobacco and lung cancer.

Correlates to Other Risks in the Workplace

Hill's criteria for the proof of causation should be very familiar to those trained in occupational and environmental medicine or other preventive medicine specialties. Rendering opinions within a scientific basis is the second point of the American College of Occupational and Environmental Medicine's Code of Ethical Conduct [18].

THE HEALTHY WORKER EFFECT

The **healthy worker effect (HWE)** states that, in general, employed persons enjoy a higher level of health than the general public, such that comparisons of workers to the general public are invalid. The concept is somewhat controversial, but most good occupational studies nevertheless use only employed populations for comparison. Some HWEs may be attributable to infectious diseases, since those with genetic or congenital vulnerability to infections may not obtain nor sustain employment. In some cases, the vulnerable may not stay in an occupation that causes them frequent illness. Industries such as health care may conduct screening for vaccine-preventable disease immunity on preplacement examination, and safety training (i.e., bloodborne pathogen training) should begin immediately. Studies have shown that the most dangerous time for injury to workers is their first year on a new job or work-

Table 3-5
Hill's Criteria for a Valid Association

1. **Consistency:** The association is consistent when results are replicated in other studies, or by different methods, or in other locations by other scientists. Also known as *reproducibility.*
2. **Strength:** The association must be of sufficient "size" or magnitude (***relative risk***) when measured by the *appropriate* tests of statistical significance. Also known as *biostatistic analysis.*
3. **Specificity:** A single risk or cause produces a specific effect. A nonspecific or a variable response to a specific exposure points away from causation.
4. **Dose-response relationship:** An increasing level of exposure or risk (in volume or duration) increases the effect.
5. **Temporal relationship:** Exposure must precede outcome. This is the only absolutely essential criterion. If a risk was not present before or during the time of the effect, it has the most perfect alibi.
6. **Biologic plausibility:** The association agrees with existing knowledge of pathobiologic processes. Also can be called *sensibility.*
7. **Coherence:** The association is compatible with existing theories and knowledge, which may include evidence from previous animal studies. The association must not contradict the principles of science nor the laws of physics.
8. **Experimental evidence:** Experiments or studies designed to interfere or block the risk or exposure will "break" the causation or association: the basic premises of prevention.

ing for a new employer [19]. This is true for both genders and all age groups. No studies have specifically focused on infections acquired during the first year of employment, but certainly there is a learning curve in many occupations and professions that is a factor in contracting infection (e.g., health care workers and the handling of sharp instruments).

INJURY CONTROL

In the epidemiologic triad for injury, the host is the human, and the agent is energy (mechanical, electrical, chemical, radiation, or thermal). The environment is those areas where both the agent (energy) and the host (the human body) are found in potential conflict.

The classic **Haddon matrix** (Table 3-6) and model for injury [20] was initially used to study the control of motor vehicle injury [21], in which the agent is kinetic energy. But the matrix model has been expanded to other forms of injury prevention. Haddon's "pre-injury" may correlate with the presence of an agent in the environment (the reservoir), creating exposure and a risk of "injury," or with the agent's invasion of the host, and "post-injury" may correlate with the individualized response of the host to the infection or infestation.

The great successes in controlling or eradicating some infectious diseases have been due as much to public sanitation (removing the agent from the environment), improved personal hygiene (removing the risk of transmission through a port of entry) and improved nutrition (improving host response), as they have been due to vaccines or antibiotics (improving host response). Infection or infestation with a pathogenic microorganism may be analogous to an "injury" and may necessitate medical care. Thus, the Haddon matrix can be modified as a model of control for biologic hazards as well.

INDUSTRIAL HYGIENE, TOXICOLOGY

The classic "four-controls" approach of industrial hygiene (substitution, engineering, administrative, and personal protection) is finding in-

Table 3-6
Haddon Matrix

Phases	Human (Host)	Vehicle (Agent)	Environment
Pre-injury	Alcohol intoxication	Utility vehicle instability	Visibility of hazards
Injury	Resistance to energy insult	Sharp/pointed edges and surfaces	Flammable materials
Postinjury	Hemorrhage	Rapidity of energy reduction (decelerate)	EMS response time/quality

creasing utility in infection control. In most cases, substitution is not relevant with respect to infectious agents. No techniques have been developed for substituting drug-sensitive for drug-resistant organisms. But the other controls concepts of engineering, administrative, and personal protection establish an excellent **"hierarchy of controls"** for infectious agents. The CDC's 1993 Draft Guidelines for Preventing the Transmission of Tuberculosis in Health Care Facilities utilized the model for the industrial hygiene hierarchy of controls [22]. The Occupational Health and Safety Administration (OSHA) quickly made the guidelines enforceable under the General Duty clause [23]. These guidelines introduced a new concept to infection control—that tuberculosis is not an infectious disease that can be occupational, but rather an occupational disease that can be infectious [24]. Hospitals and the health care industry had been willing to accept that infection control "guidelines" would still allow some occasional worker illness. OSHA was not as lenient in dealing with occupationally acquired fatal infections. Federally mandated infection control was a new and costly concept to health care.

Industrial hygiene focuses on protecting the worker from specific *known* risks by utilizing controls and protection specific to that risk. But protection of workers from communicable diseases usually needs to be more generalized, that is, based on the assumption that there are multiple unknown pathogens in the work environment. For example, **"Universal Precautions"** assume that every patient is infected with every bloodborne pathogen. Imposing Universal Precautions may involve administrative controls, engineering or barrier controls, worker education, protective tasks such as hand washing, and the utilization of protective equipment. Control of communicable diseases may often require an extensive medical history, a physical exam, laboratory evaluation for immunity, and immunization or postexposure prophylaxis. The occupational health clinician responsible for workers exposed to communicable diseases must assume many of the tasks assumed by other safety or industrial hygiene professionals in other industries. Roles analogous to the industrial hygienist's in industry may be performed by hospital epidemiologists or infection control practitioners and infection control committees in the health care work environment. They utilize many of the same principles (if not the same hardware) as the industrial hygienist, including routine surveillance and monitoring for nosocomial infections, cumulative reporting of cross-infection between patients and staff, and specific criteria for outbreak analysis. These are not just voluntary activities; they are mandated by accrediting agencies such as the Joint Commission on the Accreditation of Healthcare Organization (JCAHO) and local hospital licensing agencies.

But unlike most other workplace risks, workers with communicable illnesses can bring the risk *to* the workplace or take it *from* the workplace. A worker may also acquire disease from (or infect) not only their co-workers but also their customers and clients. Determining the work relatedness of an infection can prove more difficult than tracking a specific toxic chemical from a known point of origin.

The classic industrial hygiene approach familiar to safety and occupational health practitioners can easily be applied to communicable disease. In both cases, the emphasis and preferred solution is total removal or eradication of the risk from the work environment. However, this is rarely possible with infectious agents. If the reservoir for the diseases is only the human, then the human body becomes both the host and the environment for the agent. Such diseases may be the most amenable to eradication if a safe and efficacious vaccine can be developed and widely applied (e.g., smallpox). The agent is eradicated by removing the availability of the reservoir, i.e., the susceptibles.

For the occupational physician, the important principles of toxicology have some application in managing patients with infectious diseases. Practitioners who are familiar with chemical and toxic hazards should not be uncomfortable evaluating workers with infectious disease. Many of the same concepts apply to both (Table 3-7).

MATERIAL SAFETY DATA SHEETS

The Laboratory Centre for Disease Control, a Division of the Health Canada–Health Protection Branch has prepared Material Safety Data

Table 3-7
Comparison of Concepts of Toxicology and Communicable Disease

Toxicology Concept	ID Correlate	Similarities/Dissimilarities
Toxicity of agent	Virulence	Host response may be individualized, especially with IA. Best treatment is avoidance.
Dose	Dose	Question of dose-response relationship. A "threshold" of illness for TA, "infective dose" for IA.
Route of entry	Route of entry	Much the same for both agents. Controls with barriers, behavior, personal protection.
Exposure duration	Exposure duration	Both increase chances of illness; IA might stimulate immunity, and TA stimulate allergy.
Exposure frequency	Exposure frequency	Both increase chances of illness, but IA might stimulate immunity, and TA stimulate allergy.
Absorption	Invasion	May target specific organs and physiology. TA may have more predictable consequences than IA.
Distribution	Systemic/hematogenous	Both may cause generalized multi-organ pathology. TAs decline in concentration, but IAs multiply and increase in concentration.
Metabolism	Host response/immunity	TA metabolites may also be toxic and harmful; IA-antibody complexes may be harmful or stimulate autoantibodies.
Excretion	Shedding	TA excretion of metabolites less likely to be harmful to others than IAs, which are attempting survival by propagation (infectious).

Abbreviations: *TA* = toxic agent; *IA* = infectious agent.

Sheets (MSDSs) for infectious agents. The format is similar to chemical hazard MSDSs and was created for laboratory workers who may be exposed to infectious agents in much higher concentration and in different forms than the general public. The format is shown in Figure 3-3 and a list of infectious agents is given in Figure 3-4. The agency attaches the following disclaimer:

> Please note that although the information, opinions and recommendations contained in these Material Safety Data Sheets are compiled from sources believed to be reliable, we accept no responsibility for the accuracy, sufficiency, or reliability or for any loss or injury resulting from the use of the information. Newly discovered hazards are frequent and this information may not be completely up to date.

These MSDSs provide an excellent reference for quick answers to questions such as what it takes to inactivate an organism, survivability in the environment, and worker hazards and controls. Traditional infectious disease textbooks tend to hide such information in context or choose not to mention what is not known (e.g., the infective dose for most agents).

The American Public Health Association publishes *Control of Communicable Diseases Manual* (A. S. Benenson, editor) every five years [10]. It is an economical pocket reference that presents most of the known human infectious diseases in a standard format: name and synonyms, ICD-9 and 10 codes, identification, infectious agent, occurrence, reservoir, mode of transmission, incubation period, period of communicability, susceptibility and resistance, and methods of control. The methods of control section is further subdivided into preventive measures, control of patient contact and the immediate environment,

Figure 3-3
Format for Health Canada's material safety data sheets (MSDSs), showing 32 categories of information under nine headings.

MSDS Sheets for Infectious Agents on the Internet

Health Canada; Health Protection Branch
Laboratory Centre for Disease Control
Format
http//www.hc-sc.gc.ca/hpb/lcdc/biosafty/msds/index.html

Section **I-Infectious Agent**
Name:
Synonym or Cross Reference:
Characteristics:

Section **II-Health Hazard**
Pathogenicity:
Epidemiology:
Host Range:
Infectious Dose:
Mode of Transmission:
Incubation Period:
Communicability:

Section **III-Dissemination**
Reservoir:
Zoonosis:
Vectors:

Section **IV-Viability**
Drug Susceptibility:
Susceptibility to Disinfectants:
Physical Inactivation:

Section **V-Medical**
Surveillance:
First Aid/Treatment:
Immunization:
Prophylaxis:

Section **VI-Laboratory Hazards**
Laboratory-Acquired Infections:
Sources/Specimens:
Primary Hazards:
Special Hazards:

Section **VII-Precautions**
Containment Requirements:
Protective Clothing:
Other Precautions:

Section **VIII-Handling**
Spills:
Disposal:
Storage:

Section **IX-Miscellaneous**

epidemic measures, disaster implications, and international measures.

Agents of Infectious Disease

The infectious agents responsible for most of the occupational infections in Western civilization are no larger than a single cell. This section presents a basic review of the major classes of infectious agents. The classification and nonclinical characteristics of microbes are massive disciplines that do not always have relevance to the needs of the busy clinician. Information on the size, shape, taxonomy, and metabolism of infectious agents are not covered in detail. Chapter 2 discusses the principles of laboratory study and diagnosis of the various infectious agents.

This section also reviews attributes of the infectious agents and their products that enable them to cause disease and some of their attributes that enable them to actively develop resistance to treatment.

AGENTS OF OCCUPATIONAL INFECTIOUS DISEASE

Viruses

A virus is among the simplest of all biologic entities but represents the largest class of human pathogens. It is arguable whether viruses meet the full definition of *life form*. They are obligated to infect and reproduce within another organism to complete their life cycle. Specifically, they are obligated to invade the cells of another organism, defining them as **obligate intracellular**

Figure 3-4
One hundred seventy-one (171) agents with MSDSs on the Internet.

Infectious Agents with MSDS Data
Health Canada; Health Protection Branch
Laboratory Centre for Disease Control
http//www.hc-sc.gc.ca/hpb/lcdc/biosafty/msds/index.html

Actinobacillus spp.
Actinomyces spp.
Adenovirus (types 1,2,3,4,5,7)
Adenovirus (types 40 & 41)
Aerococcus spp.
Aeromonas hydrophila
Ancylostoma duodenale
Angiostrongylus cantonensis
Ascaris lumbricoides
Ascaris spp.
Aspergillus spp.
Bacillus anthracis
Bacillus cereus
Bacteroides spp.
Balantidium coli
Bartonella bacilliformis
Blastomyces dermatitidis
Bluetongue virus
Bordetella bronchiseptica
Bordetella pertussis
Borrelia burgdorferi
Branhamella catarrhalis
Brucella spp. (abortus, canis, melitensis, suis)
Brugia spp.
Burkholderia (Pseudomonas) mallei
Burkholderia (Pseudomonas) pseudomallei
California serogroup
Campylobacter fetus subsp. fetus
Campylobacter jejuni, coli,fetus subsp. jejuni
Candida albicans
Capnocytophaga spp.
Chlamydia psittaci
Chlamydia trachomatis
Citrobacter spp.
Clonorchis sinensis
Clostridium botulinum
Clostridium difficile
Clostridium perfringens
Clostridium tetani
Clostridium spp. (others)
Coccidioides immitis
Colorado tick fever virus
Corynebacterium diphtheriae
Coxiella burnetii
Coxsackievirus
Creutzfeldt-Jakob agent, Kuru agent
Crimean-Congo hemorrhagic fever virus
Cryptococcus neoformans
Cryptosporidium parvum
Cytomegalovirus
Dengue virus (1, 2, 3, 4)
Diphtheroids
Eastern (Western) equine encephalitis virus
Ebola virus
Echinococcus granulosus
Echinococcus multilocularis
Echovirus
Edwardsiella tarda
Entamoeba histolytica
Enterobacter spp.
Enterovirus 70
Epidermophyton floccosum, Microsporum spp. Trichophyton
Epstein-Barr virus
Escherichia coli, enterohemorrhagic
Escherichia coli, enteroinvasive
Escherichia coli, enteropathogenic
Escherichia coli, enterotoxigenic
Fasciola hepatica
Francisella tularensis
Fusobacterium spp
Gemella haemolysans
Giardia lamblia
Haemophilus ducreyi
Haemophilus influenzae
Hantavirus
Hepatitis A virus
Hepatitis B virus
Hepatitis C virus
Hepatitis D virus
Hepatitis E virus
Herpes simplex virus
Herpesvirus simiae
Histoplasma capsulatum
Human coronavirus
Human immunodeficiency virus
Human papillomavirus
Human rotavirus
Human T-lymphotrophic virus
Influenza virus
Machupo virus
Klebsiella spp.
Kyasanur Forest disease virus
Lactobacillus spp.
Legionella pneumophila
Leishmania spp.
Leptospira interrogans
Listeria monocytogenes
Lymphocytic choriomeningitis virus
Marburg virus
Measles virus
Micrococcus spp.
Moraxella spp.
Mycobacterium spp. (except bovis,tuberculosis, avium leprae)
Mycobacterium tuberculosis, M. bovis
Mycoplasma hominis, orale, salivarium, fermentans
Mycoplasma pneumoniae
Naegleria fowleri
Necator americanus
Neisseria gonorrhoeae
Neisseria meningitidis
Neisseria spp. (others)
Nocardia spp.
Norwalk virus
Omsk hemorrhagic fever virus
Onchocerca volvulus
Opisthorchis spp.
Parvovirus B19
Pasteurella spp.
Peptococcus spp.
Peptostreptococcus spp.
Plesiomonas shigelloides
Powassan encephalitis virus
Proteus spp.
Pseudomonas spp. (except malle pseudomallei)
Rabies virus
Respiratory syncytial virus
Rhinovirus
Rickettsia akari
Rickettsia prowazekii, R. canada
Rickettsia rickettsii
Ross river / O'Nyong-Nyong virus
Rubella virus
Salmonella choleraesuis
Salmonella paratyphi
Salmonella typhi
Salmonella spp. (others)
Schistosoma spp.
Scrapie agent
Serratia spp.
Shigella spp.
Sindbis virus
Sporothrix schenckii
St. Louis & Murray Valley encephalitis virus
Staphylococcus aureus
Streptobacillus moniliformis
Streptococcus agalactiae
Streptococcus faecalis
Streptococcus pneumoniae
Streptococcus pyogenes
Streptococcus salivarius
Taenia saginata
Taenia solium
Toxocara canis, T. cati
Toxoplasma gondii
Treponema pallidum
Trichinella spp.
Trichomonas vaginalis
Trichuris trichiura
Trypanosoma brucei
Ureaplasma urealyticum
Vaccinia virus
Varicella-zoster virus
Venezuelan equine encephalitis
Vesicular stomatitis virus
Vibrio cholerae, serovar 01
Vibrio parahaemolyticus
Wuchereria bancrofti
Yellow fever virus
Yersinia enterocolitica
Yersinia pseudotuberculosis
Yersinia pestis

parasites. Viruses have limited survival in the free environment and can remain infectious only from minutes to a few weeks at most (e.g., hepatitis B).

Morphology. Viruses have the common characteristics listed in Table 3-8. When a viral agent does have an envelope, it is composed of lipids, proteins, and glycoproteins acquired from the host cell when the virus buds off. The envelope (if present) will protect the virus in the extracellular environment. The outer part of the virus (the capsid or the envelope) contains the structural key to penetrate target cells that have the appropriate receptors for that virus. Part of this ability may be derived from the parts of the envelope that it acquired from a similar cell on its birth. Viruses have been known to infect almost every part of other life forms, including plants, mycoplasmas, fungi, and even bacteria (**bacteriophages**).

Subclassifications. There is only a slight tendency for viruses of specific taxonomic classifications to behave in clinically similar manners. Viruses can be classified in several ways. All contain either DNA or RNA of either single (**ss**) or double strands (**ds**) for their genetic core. They may also be classified by size, shape, and the presence or absence of an envelope (see Figure 3-5).

Pathogenic DNA viruses are usually double stranded and may be recognized and accepted into the host cell's DNA. Once incorporated, their replication occurs in the nucleus. They can use the cell's RNA polymerases for the creation of their progeny. RNA viruses are usually single stranded (except for reoviruses and birnaviruses) and must encode for some of their own enzymes. Replication is usually in the cell cytoplasm.

Table 3-8
Common Characteristics of Viruses

1. A size between 20–300 nm.
2. The structure of:
   a. A genetic *core* of DNA or RNA (but not both), which codes their genetic makeup, or *genome*.
   b. A protein coat enclosing their DNA/RNA (*capsid*).
   c. The core/capsid complex, called a *nucleocapsid*, which in some cases represents the entirety of the virion.
3. May or may not have a surrounding envelope.
4. They infect only:
   a. Specific ranges or types of host cells.
   b. Specific species of higher life forms than them.
   c. Cells that have specific *receptors* on their surface that make them vulnerable to the virus.

Entry and Invasion. Viruses have been known to infect humans by all portals of entry. They must penetrate either already broken skin or by the bite of an arthropod or other multicellular organism, or enter through the mucous membranes or epithelium of a body orifice or cavity. Some viruses have adapted multiple methods of entry into the body (e.g., HBV and varicella). **Parenteral** exposure (directly into the bloodstream) is the most efficient port of entry (i.e., **bloodborne pathogens**), but the respiratory route is also efficient and is the most difficult of the natural routes of infection to control.

Once the pathogenic virus obtains entry, it targets specific cells that have the appropriate receptors to allow intracellular invasion. Some examples of specific target cells, their receptors, and invading viruses are listed in Table 3-9.

Once the cell is penetrated, several steps occur:

1. Uncoating of the viral genome (DNA or RNA).
2. Expression of the virus genome.
3. Replication of the viral genome, by using the cell's stock of nucleic acids and often their polymerase enzymes as well.
4. Assembly of **progeny** (children or offspring) viruses.
5. Egress from the infected cell, often by lysis or killing the cell.

Clinical Characteristics. Some viruses enter, invade, and predominantly remain within the same organ system. Examples include the viral gastroenteritis caused by the rota- and Norwalk viruses in the epithelia of the intestines. In most cases, the release of progeny means lysis or killing the host cell, often producing pathologic or clinical (**cytopathogenic**) consequences. The clinical course of a viral infection depends on:

1. Virulence of the infecting virus.
2. Infective dose.
3. Port of entry.
4. Type of cells and tissues infected.

Figure 3-5
Names, shapes, and relative sizes of some vertebrate-animal viruses. (From Murphy FA, Fauguet DHL, Bishop SA, et al. Sixth report of the International Committee on Taxonomy of Viruses. Wein: Springer-Verlag, 1995, with permission.)

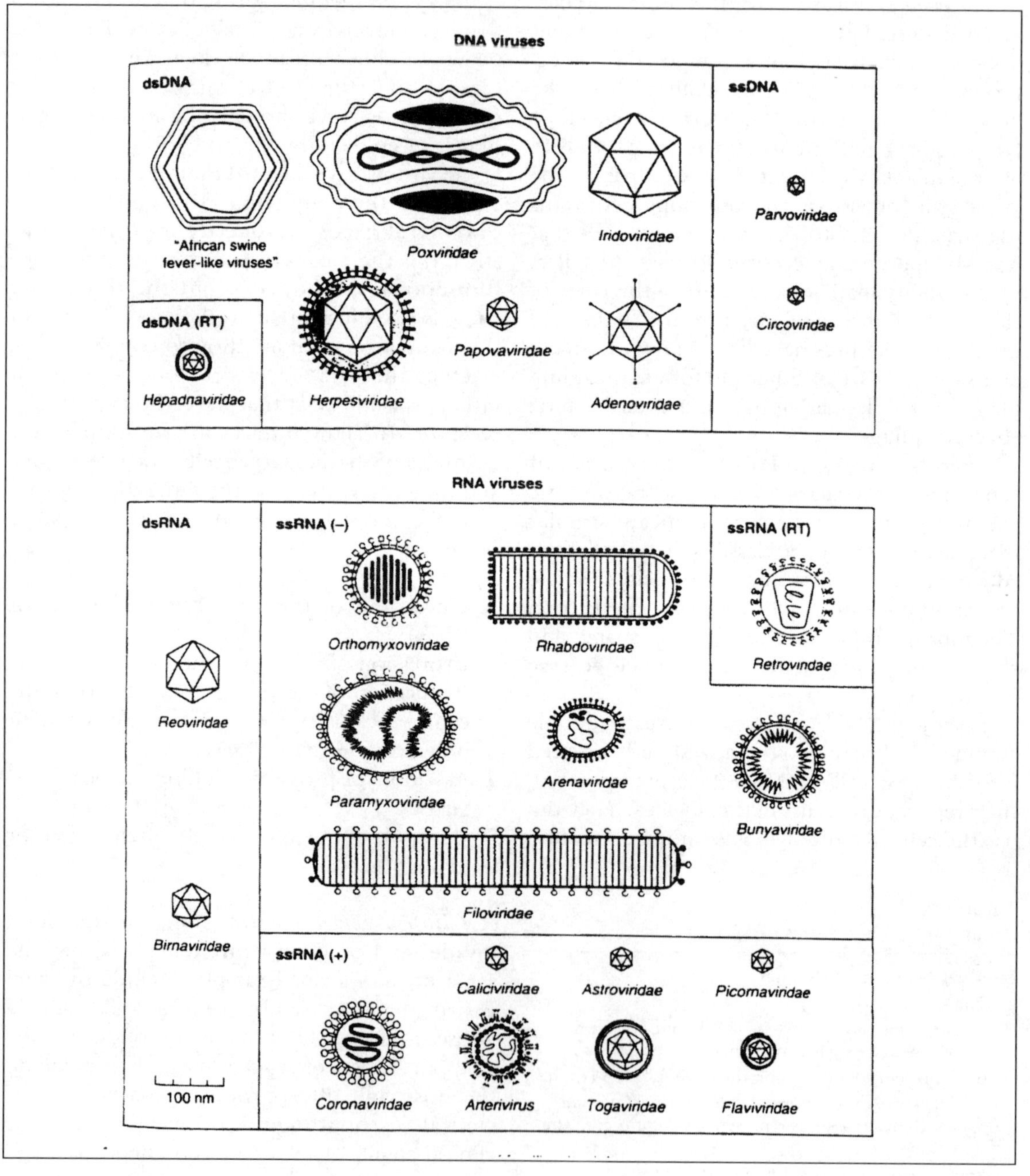

Table 3-9
Example of Viral Cell Receptors

Cells	Receptors	Infecting Virus
T4 lymphocytes	CD4	HIV
Skin/membranes	Cell-surface heparin sulfate	Herpes simplex
Oropharynx	CR2	Epstein-Barr

5. Rate of viral spread and replication.
6. Site from which the virus is shed into the environment.
7. Nature and magnitude of the immune and host defense responses.

Each point is addressed in this chapter and in the chapters on specific viral pathogens. Viral infectivity is partially dependent on the human host's genome. The small variation in human genotypes may explain why some persons are more susceptible to some types of viruses than others. Epstein-Barr virus, for instance, is fatal to the majority of persons with a specific X-linked defect. There is also variation in the degree of clinical illness, which may be a result of genetics, general health, and the level of pre-existing immunity to the causative agent or a closely related virus.

Clinical Outcomes. Viruses are difficult to treat, since they reside within the cell during their pathogenic state. The development of drugs that selectively destroy the virus without damage to the protoplasm or genetic material proves difficult.

The exact mechanism by which a virus kills its host cell is not known. Death or impairment of host cell function is responsible for most of the pathophysiology of viruses, along with consequences of the host immune responses, which are discussed later. In some cases, the infected host cells and organs are at increased risk for neoplasms. For instance, chronic hepatitis B infection increases the lifetime risk for developing primary liver cancer by a relative risk of 200.

However, not all viruses must kill the host cell to replicate. A virus may infect a cell that does not possess all of the factors it needs for replication. If the block occurs early in a replication cycle, the virus genome may be diluted by cell division to the point of viral extinction, and the host may be able to develop immunity to subsequent invasion. If the block occurs later in the replication cycle, the cell may be lysed but without releasing infectious progeny. Some DNA viruses have evolved the ability to survive in cells that are nonpermissive of viral replication, which may explain latent infection by such classes as the herpesviruses. They may still become active and infectious when conditions change in the cells.

The fate of a virus within the human body is variable. It may fall victim to an efficient immune system and meet with early eradication. Some viruses cause an active infection that leads to death (e.g., rabies) or a slowly progressive chronic illness by selectively damaging cells of a vital organ (e.g., hepatitis B, hepatitis C, slow viruses). Other viruses may remain in a latent form throughout a normal human life span (e.g., varicella and most of the herpes class of viruses). Specific antibodies may develop into latent infection but be inefficient in eradicating the disease. Nevertheless, these antibodies can be used as biologic markers or screening tests for diagnosis (e.g., hepatitis C, HIV).

Occupational Considerations. Since viruses have limited survivability in the inanimate environment, the risk of occupational viral infection risks are higher for those working in health care or in other jobs with closer contact with infectious humans (including co-workers) or animals. The great exception is the arboviruses, which are harbored by mosquitos and ticks: Those who may be working outdoors in endemic areas, at specific times of the day or night, and in specific seasons and weather conditions have a higher rate of exposure and risk for arboviruses.

Treatment of Viral Infections. RNA viruses must code for their own **RNA polymerase** (called *transcriptases/replicases*). This genome may be specific for that virus. If drugs can be developed that selectively inhibit that genome or enzyme, then viral replication may be inhibited without affecting the function of the host cells. This is the basis for the first generation of antiretroviral (HIV) drugs known as *nucleoside* *analogs* and *non-nucleoside reverse transcriptase inhibitors.* RNA viruses often also need to code for their own proteases, the enzymes that cleave larger chains of polyproteins to yield the smaller proteins needed to assemble progeny. The proteases inhibitors have been the latest generation of anti-HIV drugs.

Prevention and Prophylaxis. Despite the advances in antiviral drug therapy, the drug treatment of viral diseases is still in its infancy. Amantadine and rimantadine may help prevent or reduce the clinical illness of influenza A (Chapter 11), ribavirin may treat respiratory syncytial virus in children, and acyclovir and its precursor drugs may reduce the clinical illness from the herpesviruses.

Prevention by immunization remains the most reliable method of virus control (Chapter 5). But many viruses undergo rapid genetic variation (e.g., HIV, influenza), and this makes elusive the development of an efficacious vaccine. Other viruses (e.g., adenovirus) have so many pathogenic subtypes that developing a broadly protective vaccine is difficult.

Bacteria

Bacteria is a very broad term for single-cell organisms that may or may not cause human disease (be or not be pathogenic). They are classified as lower protists, or prokaryotic bacteria. Bacteria are present throughout the biosphere and are highly adapted to specific environments. Only pathogenic bacteria are discussed in this book. Unlike viruses, most bacteria can survive outside of hosts. Some common characteristics of human pathogenic bacteria and exceptions are listed in Table 3-10.

Classification. Bacteria are classified in many different ways, not all of which are of great clinical significance. These include:

SHAPE. Bacteria are classified by their shape as:

- **Cocci:** round, spherical, or ovoid in shape. They may be found singularly or in groups or clusters.
- **Baccilli:** basically rod shaped, with square, round, or club-shaped ends.
- **Spirilla:** corkscrew or comma shaped (vibrio and spirochetes).
- **Diplococci:** cocci occurring in pairs.

STAINING. The bacteria with semirigid cell walls are further described by their reaction to the standard **Gram's stain**. Gram-positive organisms stain a purple-black due to the peptidoglycan and teichoic acid in their cell walls. Gram-negative organisms stain pinkish due to their thinner layer of peptidoglycan yet thicker and more numerous layers of protein and poly-saccharides in their cell wall. All *Spirilla* stain gram negative.

Two thirds of cocci are gram positive, and bacilli are about evenly split between gram

Table 3-10
Characteristics of Pathogenic Human Bacteria

Single-cell organisms:	Exceptions:
Have DNA for their genetic material	—
Do not have a membrane around nucleus	—
Reproduce by asexual splitting (or binary fission)	—
Have semirigid cell walls	*Mycoplasma* (no true walls)
	Treponema (thin walls)
	Borrelia (thin walls)
	Leptospira (thin walls)
Are free living	*Rickettsia* (cell parasite)
	Coxiella (cell parasite)
	Chlamydia (cell parasite)

positive and gram negative. Mycobacteria cannot be demonstrated by gram staining and are instead stained with acid-fast preparations. All **mycobacteria**, including human tuberculosis, are acid-fast positive. They lack cell walls but have thick cholesterol-based membranes and are very resistant to most physical forces.

Pathogenic gram-negative bacteria have **pyrogenic**, fever-inducing, properties. This is due to **endotoxins**, complex phospholipid-polysaccharide macromolecules in the cell wall. Gram-negative bacteria (*Neisseria meningitidis, Yersinia pestis, Salmonella typhi*) may be among the most virulent of bacteria and be responsible for sepsis in about one fourth of those who develop gram-negative infection in the blood (**bacteremia**). Other gram-negative bacteria that cause sepsis include *Escherichia coli, Klebsiella, Enterobacter, Serratia, Proteus, Pseudomonas aeruginosa*, and *Haemophilus influenzae*.

The incidence of gram-positive bacteriemia and sepsis are increasing, mainly due to the use of medical catheters, shunts, and prosthesis, which disrupt the natural mucocutaneous barriers and introduce bacteria into the bloodstream (Figure 3-6). Shock and acute respiratory syndromes are less common with gram-positive organisms (e.g., staphylococci, enterococci, and streptococci) than with gram-negative. Many other stains have been used for bacteria, both for clinical indications as well as for classification.

Figure 3-6
Disruptions of the epithelial surfaces that may result in infection. These include surgery, burns, catheters, and trauma. (From Meakins JL. Host defenses. In: Howard RJ, Simmons RL (eds), *Surgical Infectious Disease*, 2nd Ed. New York: Appleton-Century-Crofts, 1988. Chap 11, p 154, with permission.)

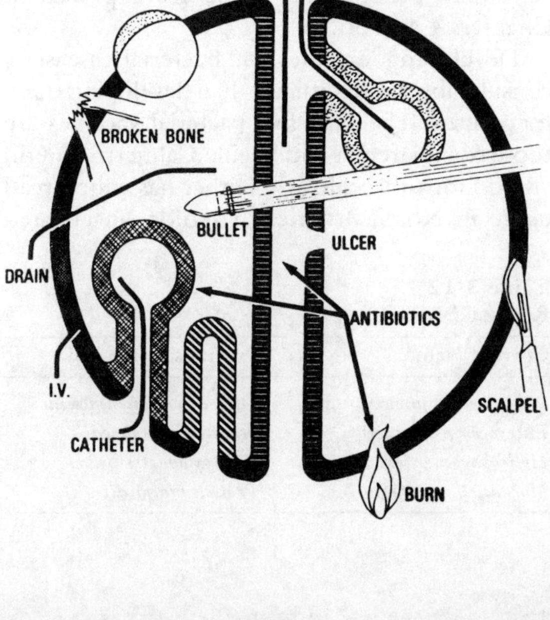

BIOCHEMICAL ACTIVITY. Most bacteria can be grown in laboratories, under a great variety of conditions and using various media. This has led to a classification of bacteria as negative or positive to lactose, sorbitol, catalase, or coagulase. Bacteria can also be classified as alpha- or beta-hemolytic on blood agar. Laboratory methods of bacteriology are discussed in Chapter 2.

GROWTH PATTERN. Bacteria are also described by their growth patterns in various atmospheres, using these definitions:

- **Strict (or obligate) aerobic:** Will not grow in the absence of oxygen.
- **Strict (or obligate) anaerobic:** Will not grow in the presence of oxygen.
- **Facultative anaerobe:** Will use oxygen if present but can also grow without oxygen.
- **Microaerophilic:** Requires oxygen concentration of 2–10% (instead of the atmospheric 20%). These bacteria may also require higher than atmospheric concentration of carbon dioxide.

Anaerobic Infections. Anaerobic bacterial infections are usually due to indigenous (flora) organisms that are normally found on the low-oxygen tension surfaces such as the gingival crevices of the oral cavity, the distal ileum and colon, and the endocervix and vagina. Anaerobic bacteria outnumber aerobic bacteria in the normal human colon about 500:1 and are also predominant in the mouth. The study of anaerobes did not begin until the 1970s because of the difficulty in obtaining cultures. Some of the most significant anaerobic organisms are listed in Table 3-11. Facultative anaerobes include Enterobacteriaceae, staphylococci, and streptococci.

Subclassifications. Several pathogenic groups of organisms do not meet the classic concept of bacteria but are generally classified with them clinically, since they produce diseases similar to

Table 3-11
Some Significant Anaerobic Organisms

Group	Organisms
Gram-positive cocci	*Peptostreptococcus*, *Peptococcus*
Gram-positive bacilli	*Clostridium perfringens* and *Clostridium tetani* (spore formers), *Lactobacillus*, *Actinomyces*
Gram-negative cocci	*Veillonella*
Gram-negative bacilli	*Bacteroides fragilis* and *Bacteroides bivivus*

bacteria and are generally sensitive to the same antibiotics as free-living bacteria. They are discussed in Chapters 12 and 28.

CHLAMYDIA. Chlamydia are obligate intracellular parasites that can infect mammals, humans, and domesticated avian species. They are responsible for the most prevalent human sexually transmitted disease (STD) but can also cause blindness and respiratory infections. *Chlamydia psittaci* can be aerosolized and is responsible for the occupational disease known as *psittacosis*. They are susceptible to antibiotics (see Chapter 12) and are treatable once recognized.

RICKETTSIA. Like viruses, rickettsia are obligate intracellular parasites, but they are also like bacteria because they divide by binary fission, are gram negative, are coccobacillary in shape, contain both RNA and DNA, have their own metabolism by electron transport, and utilize the Krebs cycle. The four subclasses are *Rickettsia*, *Coxiella*, *Ehrlichia*, and *Rochalimaea*. They are mostly distributed by arthropod vectors of ticks and lice and are a risk for outdoor workers. They were named for Dr. H. T. Ricketts, who died from occupational typhus contracted through his research. Rickettsia require a high level of precautions when handled in laboratories (see Chapter 33), because some types such as *Coxiella burnetii* and *Rickettsia rickettsii* (Rocky Mountain spotted fever) can also be inhaled by aerosol.

Nomenclature. The nomenclature for microorganisms is constantly changing (by the International Commission on Microbial Taxonomy) and may confuse clinicians who have learned different names during their training. The reasons for name changes are rarely clinically relevant but are done for taxonomic reasons. Some examples are listed in Table 3-12.

Clinical Outcomes. Bacteria are the only major class of microorganisms that seems to have a vital purpose in survival. We cannot live without bacteria, which are involved in the digestion of food, preparation of food, production of essential vitamins, and debriding the sloughing tissues of our skin and mucous membranes. A specific bacteria can be either a friend or a foe if it invades outside of its habitat on our body.

Occupational Considerations. Bacteria are found in almost every square inch of land, water, and sea. Unlike viruses, most bacteria species on Earth can live independent from higher life forms. They are highly adapted to their environment, their hosts, and often both. Many occupations expose humans to bacteria for which they do not have immunity, through environmental exposure or by physical trauma and disruption of the flora planes (Figure 3-6). Consideration of specific occupational environments and their controls is discussed in Chapter 4, Occupations at Risk. Chapter 33 on laboratory workers is especially important in the handling of all infectious agents, as is Chapter 34 on health care workers.

Prevention and Prophylaxis. Many zoonoses are bacterial or rickettsial in origin: anthrax, brucellosis, leptospirosis, Q fever, bubonic plague, Rocky Mountain spotted fever, salmonellosis, and tularemia. Precautions to be taken vary with professions; these are explored in Chapters 4 and 36.

Developing vaccines for bacterial disease is considerably more difficult than developing them for viruses. The only live bacterial vaccines are those for tularemia and bacille Calmette-Guérin (BCG) for tuberculosis. Neither has widespread usage in North America. **Toxoids** (inactivated

Table 3-12
Renamed Bacteria

Current Name	Previous Name
Streptococcus pneumoniae	*Diplococcus pneumoniae*
Enterococcus faecalis	*Streptococcus faecalis*
Helicobacter pylori	*Campylobacter pylori*
Morganella morgagni	*Proteus morganii*

toxin antigen vaccines) are given for diphtheria and tetanus, and both require frequent re-immunizations as adults. Oral vaccines have been developed for diseases naturally inoculated by ingestion (e.g., polio). Most other bacterial vaccines are made from nonviable (dead) cellular components.

Treatment of Bacterial Diseases. Most known bacterial diseases have some available, effective antibiotic or antimicrobial therapy. But drug resistance has been an emerging problem (Chapter 38) in the treatment of hospitalized patients and is now becoming a problem with treatment of outpatients. Workers in hospitals and extended care facilities may be developing colon colonization by resistant species such as vancomycin-resistant enterococcus (VRE) [25]. Although no morbidity or mortality have surfaced in these workers, they could at some point in later life become septic because of infection with this very-difficult-to-treat pathogen.

Fungi

Fungi are eukaryotic, or possess both plant and animal characteristics. **Yeasts** are defined as the spherical organisms that reproduce by budding (like bacteria), and the **molds** have branches (**hyphae**) and grow seeds (**spores** or **conidia**), behaving more like plants when they grow into masses (**mycelium**). Some are **dimorphic**, switching between molds and yeasts, depending on the environment and substrate availability. Fungi are present in most parts of the biosphere, living on environmental surfaces and in the soil, contaminating the air with their spores. Thousands of species are known, but only about 100 are pathogenic in humans. Fungi are responsible for causing both human allergic reactions (rhinitis, pneumonitis, and asthma), infections, and toxicity (**mycotoxicoses**). Even dead, or nonviable, parts of fungi can cause allergic reactions and are occasionally implicated in sick-building syndromes.

Most fungal infections are superficial infections of the skin or nails (**dermatophytosis**). Both are more common in occupations in which bathing facilities may be shared, such as military barracks or athletic gymnasiums. Deep fungal infections of the lung or systemic fungal infections are called ***mycoses***. Some human mycoses have a dimorphic form and can switch between being a yeast in tissue and a mold in the environment. Persons who work in occupations in which there is disturbance of the soil or the creation of dust are at risk for infection with aerosolized pathogenic fungi. Histoplasmosis and coccidioidomycosis may result from the inhalation of soil or dust contaminated by bird droppings. Deeper, systemic mycoses occasionally occur in healthy persons but are even more common in immunocompromised individuals. Environmental fungal infections are of great concern as nosocomial infections. Poorly controlled hospital renovation projects have resulted in lawsuits filed by transplant and other immunocompromised patients infected with aspergillus.

Fungi also produce mycotoxins, which have been suspected of being mutagenic, carcinogenic, and teratogenic. Aspergillus mycotoxins, known as ***aflatoxins***, have direct organ-toxic effects as well. The USDA controls conditions under which corn or peanuts must be stored.

Fungemia is the presence of fungi in the bloodstream, which is becoming a more common problem. *Candida* fungemia is the most common and usually occurs in those who are immunosuppressed and in whom mortality is usually high. Fungemia may also originate from the GI tract in those who have *Candida* overgrowth from antibiotic treatment. Phagocytic neutrophils and T lymphocytes are the body's major defense, and infection is more common if there are inadequate host defenses (neutropenia or cellular immunosuppression).

Parasites

All pathogens discussed in this text are human parasites. But the biomedical disciplines define *parasitology* as the study of the parasitic protozoan, helminthic, and arthropod species, and all of these organisms have multiple life-cycle stages and infective forms that can survive outside of the body of the human. Most parasitic infections are more significant in immunosuppressed hosts. They are all in the subkingdom Protozoa and classified under three phyla: Apicomplexa (the sporozoan), Sarcomastigophora (flagellates and amoebas), and Ciliophora (the ciliates).

Flagellates. Flagellates have one or more whip-like tails (**flagella**) or an undulating membrane (e.g., trypanosomes).

INTESTINAL AND URINARY FLAGELLATES. *Giardia.* Giardia has four sets of flagella and a double nuclei. They encyst on passing into the colon and may cause illness, depending on the infective dose and the health of the host. There is a high inapparent:apparent illness ratio. They are transmitted by fecally contaminated food or water and are treated at 90% efficacy with metronidazole (Flagyl).

Trichomonas. This parasite has several sets of flagella and an undulating membrane. It is sexually transmitted from the genitourinary tract but may survive short periods on personal fomites. It also has a high inapparent:apparent illness ratio and may be treated with several drugs, including metronidazole.

BLOOD FLAGELLATES. *Trypanosoma.* This group of pathogens has an elongated shape and flagella. All pathogenic forms have an intermediate insect host vector. Diseases caused by Trypanosoma include African sleeping sickness and Chagas' disease. Trypanosoma may be bloodborne and thus transmitted by transfusions. The pathogen's habitats are dependent on the mosquito species in tropical climates. The disease is hard to treat and may become chronic and have cardiac complications.

Leishmania. This infection is spread by the bite of sandflies and can cause cutaneous ulcers. It is also a bloodborne pathogen and was found in some U.S. troops upon their donation of blood after returning from the Gulf War.

Amebas. Amebas are large, amorphous moving cells, that feed by **phagocytosis** (surrounding and engulfing their meals). An active ameba forms inactive cysts and inter-mediate precysts. Cysts are found only in the colon or formed stool of humans and some primates and are very sensitive to drying. Amebic infections have a large inapparent:apparent ratio. As many as 5% of U.S. adults harbor *Entamoeba histolytica* without knowing it. Several therapies, including metronidazole, are available. The disease can cause liver abscesses.

Blood Sporozoans. The plasmodia are ameboid intracellular parasites of vertebrates and are spread by the bite of the female Anopheles mosquito. They are responsible for various forms of malaria (Chapter 25).

Cryptosporidium. Not to be confused with cryptococcosis (torulosis), which is a deep mycosis, cryptosporidiosis is caused by *Cryptosporidium parvum*, a protozoa that is spread by the fecal-oral route between humans and many domestic and wild animals in contaminated food or water. It is a **"predictive" disease for AIDS** [26] and an occupational risk for farmers, animal handlers, and day care workers. Also a coccidian protozoan like the cryptosporidium, *Toxoplasma gondii* requires the domestic cat for full completion of its life cycle. Many other animals carry infective stages of the protozoan, which may encyst in their muscle or brain tissue for life. Humans are infected by the fecal-oral route from soil contaminated with cat feces. *Toxoplasma* encephalitis is also a predictive disease of AIDS [26].

Worms. The worms are know as ***helminth*** and are multicellular parasites. There are three types of worms: nematodes (roundworms), trematodes (flukes and flatworms), and cestodes (tapeworms).

NEMATODES. Nematodes are an extremely successful phylum that infect almost every species of plant, insect, and invertebrate in the land, sea, and air. These worms cause a wide range of diseases and conditions, which are largely treatable. Infection is usually by ingestion of undercooked contaminated food or vegetables or exposure to contaminated water. The infection has a high inapparent:apparent illness ratio. The current estimated global prevalence of some nematode infections [27] is shown in Table 3-13.

TREMATODES. The flatworms have a very wide variety of life cycles and hosts. The typical flatworms are hermaphroditic, invade by ingestion, and live in the colon. However, the schistosomes have separate sexes and invade through the skin from contaminated water to live in the blood vessels. End-organ damage is common, and flatworms may serve a role in bladder or colon carcinogenesis. Trematodes are more prevalent in tropical climates.

CESTODES. Human cestodal infections include the *Taenia* (taeniasis) species of pork and beef tapeworm. Infection is contracted by eating

Table 3-13
Global Prevalence of Some Nematode Infections

Nematode	Common Name	Number Infected
Ascaris lumbricoides	Giant roundworm	1 billion
Ancylostoma duodenale or *Necator americanum*	Hookworm	800 million
Wuchereria bancrofti	Filarial worm	hundred millions
Enterobius vermicularis	Pinworm	hundred millions

the poorly cooked meat of pigs or cattle that have grazed in human fecally contaminated soil. Humans are the definitive hosts, and swine and cattle are intermediate hosts. Humans are the exclusive hosts for *Mymenolepium nana*, dwarf tapeworms, however. The broad, or fish, tapeworm (*Diphyllobothrium latum*) is the largest of the cestodes, often reaching 30 feet in length. Infection is contracted by eating poorly cooked or raw fresh water fish. Symptoms may include malnutrition and pernicious anemia. This helminth has been found in the colder climates of Alaska and Canada.

ATTRIBUTES OF MICROORGANISMS THAT ENABLE THEM TO CAUSE DISEASE

Toxigenicity

Exotoxins. Exotoxins are antigenic proteins excreted into the environment by bacteria cells (more often gram positive than gram negative) that have toxic clinical effects on specific human biologic functions or tissues. Exotoxins derive their name from the fact that they are toxic substances that have been excreted or exited the living bacterial cell. They are found either outside the cells, in the environment, or in bacterial spores. Since they are antigenic proteins, the body can form antibodies, or **antitoxins**, to most exotoxins. Exotoxins do not generally cause fever. Exotoxins may either cause illness by "**intoxication**" (poisoning) of humans who have either ingested or contacted the exotoxin of a bacteria living outside the human body or by infection when the bacteria is excreting exotoxin within the body (i.e., the intestine or a wound). Exotoxins are toxic to a wide range of cells and tissues that are specific to each exotoxin (Table 3-14).

Clostridium botulinum is an organism that lives in the soil and produces the exotoxin responsible for botulism. Botulism is an intoxication and is the most virulent exotoxin known. It is capable of causing death with ingestion of a few thousandths of one milligram of the exotoxin.

Clostridium perfringens lives in the colon of about 35% of humans and in the urogenital tract of some females. It or *Clostridium septicum* or *Clostridium novyi* may be responsible for gas gangrene. Infection with this exotoxin may be contracted from exposure to contaminated soil or from fecal contamination by injury or perforation of the gastrointestinal or female genital track (for example, by abortion).

Clostridium tetani also is present in the intestinal flora of humans and domestic animals, and its spores are widely distributed in the soil in crowded or poverty stricken areas. It is responsible for tetanus, a disease that can be prevented with "toxoid" vaccines made from inactivated toxin. Tetanus killed over 50,000 Axis troops in World War II, while Allied troops were spared because they had been immunized.

Staphylococcus can produce a toxin called *toxic shock syndrome toxin-1 (TSST-1)* when *Staphylocococus aureus* strains colonize mucous membranes. This phenomenon was discovered in the early 1980s in association with the use of super-absorbent tampons. TSST-1 is also a "**superantigen**," which means it stimulates lymphocytes to produce large amounts of IL-1 and TNF. Toxic shock syndromes have also occurred after influenza infections (Chapter 11).

Enterotoxin. An enterotoxin is any substance specifically toxic to the cells of the intestinal mucosa. An enterotoxin is a form of exotoxin. Bacterial enterotoxins are responsible for most infectious diarrhea syndromes and may cause

Table 3-14
Diseases and Exotoxins of the Clostridia and Their Target Tissues

Species and Disease	Exotoxins
C botulinum (botulism)	At least six neurotoxins that cause paralysis
C perfringens, etc. (gas gangrene)	Alpha through zeta exotoxins, which have actions of damaging: cells (necrolysis) heart muscle (cardiotoxin) collagen (collagenase) structural protein (proteolytic) fatty tissue (lipase) blood (hemolytic) erythrocytes (lecithinase)
C tetani (tetanus)	Neuromuscular contraction (tetanospasmin)
C diphtheriae (diphtheria)	Cardiac and CNS (diphtheria toxin)

illness by either infection or intoxication. Examples of enterotoxin intoxication include botulism and staphylococcal and clostridial food poisoning. Enterotoxin infections include *Salmonella enteritidis*, cholera, and bacillary dysentery (*Shigella*).

The *Escherichia coli* syndromes of enterotoxigenic (ETEC), enterohemorrhagic (EHEC), and enteroaggregative (EAggEC) disease are due to enterotoxins, while enteroinvasive (EIEC) and enteropathogenic (EPEC) are not. Salmonella has over 2,000 serotypes, and many may cause inapparent illnesses. People probably develop progressive immunity to salmonella types over a lifetime. Enteric forms of salmonella infection such as typhoid fever (*Salmonella typhi*) are rare in the United States. The gastroenteritis form is much more common but may require a 10,000 organism inoculum to cause infection. Most salmonella enterotoxins are heat sensitive and are destroyed by cooking, but a few are heat resistant.

Shigellosis may occur with a "dose" of as few as 10 bacilli. Both shigella (dysentery) and *Vibrio cholerae* (cholera) produce enterotoxins (Shiga's and choleragen, respectively) that have cytotoxic, neurotoxic, and enterotoxic (inducing fluid secretion) effects.

Species of *Staphylococcus aureus* may produce a **staphylococcal enterotoxin** while growing in foods not properly refrigerated. There are at least six types, but all are absorbed in the gut and stimulate neural receptors to cause vomiting within a few hours. No other ingested biologic toxin works as quickly. A common-source food poisoning that causes vomiting within a few hours usually proves to be *S aureus*, although other nonbiologic toxins must be included in the differential diagnosis. Inoculation of the food is often caused by a food worker with an infection on the hand or fingers. Food workers should be restricted from handling open food when they have infections of the upper body.

Most of the enterotoxins are heat sensitive (except some *Salmonella*) and can be destroyed by a temperature of 140°F (60°C). Exotoxins rarely produce fever.

Endotoxin. Endotoxins are complex phospholipid-polysaccharide macromolecules (LPS) in the cell wall of gram-negative bacteria which may have virulent properties. The toxin is not released but remains a part of the cell wall of either the living cells or its debris.

Endotoxins derive their name from the fact that they can have toxic effects while remaining part of the wall of the bacterium. They are free only if the cell is destroyed. Endotoxins do not stimulate antibody or antitoxin formation, do not have receptor cells, and are not destroyed by heat or disinfectants. There is variation in the structure and function of the cell wall, and these differences may be important both in virulence and classification of these bacteria. Endotoxins are **pyrogenic**, that is, they produce fever. The fever is caused by monocytes' producing **endogenous pyrogen** in reaction to the endotoxin effects on the thermoregulatory center in the hypothalamus.

The **lipopolysaccharide (LPS)** portion of the endotoxin is the most important in determining host tissue reaction. An **O-specific LPS** determines the serologic specificity, and the "lipid-A" portion is responsible for the toxic effect.

GRAM-NEGATIVE SHOCK. Endotoxin can induce tissue inflammation, fever, and shock in those infected; that is known as ***gram-negative sepsis.*** The lipopolysaccharides of the endotoxin can enter the bloodstream after the death of the cell. This may stimulate the complement system via the alternative pathway (discussed later) and result in the appearance of active effector molecules and inflammatory mediators such as the tumor necrosis factor, cachectin, interleukin 1, interferon, and cytokines. These can activate vascular endothelium and cause vasodilation and increased blood vessel permeability, which may result in a reduction in blood volume and hypovolemic shock. The **tumor necrosis factor (TNF)** is identical to lymphotoxin produced by activated T cells [28]. Lymphotoxin precipitates the following sequence of events: inflammation, cytotoxicity, cachexia, organ failure, shock, and death. These same biochemicals are also found in some types of cancer. Antibodies can attach to cachectic TH and lymphotoxin, which can inhibit some of the antibody response. Corticosteroids may also help block reaction to this cascade, which is possibly why they are effective treatment for some gram-negative shock victims. These agents may be beneficial in small amounts and, when absorbed from the intestinal flora, may serve to stimulate the human immune system during maturation.

CLINICAL EFFECTS. Other oxygen radicals stimulated by endotoxin may cause alveolar damage and acute respiratory distress syndrome. Endotoxins may also be responsible for stimulating the biochemical reaction that results in the invasiveness of *Haemophilus influenzae, Neisseria meningitis,* and other bacteria, causing a break in the blood-brain barrier and resulting in meningitis and shock. Endotoxin has also been shown to act on macrophages, enhancing their ability to produce oxygen radicals, which have been implicated as mediators of inflammatory tissue damage. Macrophages may stimulate the production and release of collagenase. Endotoxins have been implicated in the destruction of gum tissue in periodontal disease. Gram-negative organisms are the predominant oral flora in those with periodontitis. Endotoxins also may be the agent responsible for **byssinosis**, an occupational illness that can result from the inhalation of the products of gram-negative bacteria contaminating cotton or other vegetable fibers.

Virus-Induced Proliferation of *Host Cells.* Some DNA viruses have the ability to stimulate division of their host cells, an indirect means of increasing their own progeny. Viral antigens with these properties are called ***oncogenes.*** They increase the rate of growth of a tissue line or increase the life of individual cells and thus may cause malignancies as a result of latently infected cells. Viruses believed to function as oncogenes include Epstein-Barr, papillomaviruses, and hepatitis B (HBV).

Extracellular Enzymes. Many bacteria produce enzymes that degrade tissue in their vicinity. **Hyaluronidase** hydrolyzes hyaluronic acid from the connective tissue and is produced by many staphylococci, streptococci, and anaerobes; it facilitates their ability to form **abscesses**. Staphylococcus aureus can produce **coagulase**, which coagulates plasma and forms a fibrin mass around the lesion which helps protect bacterial abscesses. Many streptococci produce the enzyme **fibrinolysin** (also known as **streptokinase**), which facilitates their growth in coagulated tissue. This enzyme has been synthesized and used to reverse clots in patients with myocardial infarction. Dozens of other tissue-destructive enzymes are known to be produced by bacteria, and some may be considered exotoxins, as described above.

Many organisms that invade through the epithelium have the ability to actually cleave the protective secretory IgA antibodies. These are called ***IgA1 proteases*** and are produced by *N gonorrhoeae*, *S pneumoniae*, *H influenzae*, and *N meningitidis.*

Invasiveness (Infectivity)

The invasiveness of bacteria is partially determined by **adherence**. Adherence can be determined by several factors, including:

1. Surface hydrophobicity. The more hydrophobic the bacterial surface, the greater the adherence to the host cell.
2. Net surface charge. Both bacteria and host cells tend to be negatively charged, so bacteria gain an advantage if they can move toward being positively charged. Charge can depend on the anions and cations and pH of the local environment.
3. Binding molecules on the bacteria (**ligands**) and their ability to adhere to host cell receptors.
4. Presence of **pili** or **fimbriae**. These hair-like appendages on bacterial walls may facilitate attachment to host cells receptors such as epithelial cells (e.g., *E coli* to bowel epithelia, and group A streptococcus to buccal epithelia).

Host cells are not always passive, however, as they may be enticed to phagocytize the bacteria after the bacteria have adequately adhered to them. This saves the bacteria the trouble of actively invading. The bacteria is contained in a "Trojan Horse" vacuole membrane, which later dissolves. This phenomenon has been seen in vitro with the following bacteria:

1. *Shigella* species, *Yersinia enterocolitica*, and *Listeria monocytogenes* adhere to, and are phagocytized by, macrophages in the epithelium of the intestine.
2. *Legionella pneumophila* adheres to, and is engulfed by, pulmonary macrophages.
3. *Neisseria gonorrhoeae* adheres to microvilli of fallopian epithelial cells, are engulfed, and then multiply intracellularly.

METHODS OF RESISTANCE OF THE INFECTIOUS AGENT

All antibiotics work on bacteria either by disrupting their normal biochemical mechanisms or by disrupting the formation of their cell wall. Disruption of biochemical activities involves inhibiting bacteria's synthesis of nucleic acid and/or proteins, disrupting their plasma membrane, or inhibiting their normal enzyme activity in cellular metabolism. As humans have no cells with walls, cell-wall-disrupting drugs—penicillin, cephalosporins, and their synthetic relatives—have been among the most efficacious and least toxic antimicrobials. Some naturally occurring antimicrobial agents, such as the bacitracin from *Bacillus licheniformins*, have been found and commercially synthesized.

Genetic Antimicrobial Resistance

Bacteria and viruses are both **clonal**, since they are haploid and produce offspring that are exact replicas of themselves. A clonal line with improved virulence or survivability may gain a competitive advantage over other microorganisms, even of the same species.

Infectious agents may be resistant to antibiotics or disinfectants because of their own constitutional structure or genome or because of resistance they acquire during exposure. Bacteria may develop resistance by the chance mutation and development of enzymes that inactivate antimicrobials. Examples include:

1. Enzyme inactivation of aminoglycosides by acetylation, phosphorylation, or adenylation.
2. Beta-lactamases that cleave penicillins and cephalosporins.
3. Acetylases that acetylate chloramphenicol.

But often the resistance itself seems to be contagious, more than can be explained by chance single-sequence mutations. Three mechanisms of the moving of larger DNA sequences between infectious agents are known to occur: transformation, transduction, and plasmid transfer.

Transformation. Transformation is a rather inefficient and random event in which an isolated and free DNA fragment is incorporated into the chromosome of a closely related agent. Drug resistance can be transformed into another agent if this sequence codes for resistance.

Transduction. In transduction, the DNA fragment enters the recipient cells by a **bacteriophage**. A bacteriophage is a virus that infects specific bacteria as their host. This mechanism is more efficient than transformation, as larger homologous segments may be moved and it may induce multidrug resistance.

Plasmid ("R" Factor) Transfer. The most efficient and "sexiest" of resistance transfer is through the plasmids. Many bacteria have nonchromosomal "extra" genetic material not essential to their survival. A physical mating may occur between two widely different bacterial cells, wherein rather large fragments of extrachromosomal DNA is inserted through a hollow **pilus** connecting the mating cells. This DNA is called a **plasmid**, or an **"R" (residence) factor**. This process was first identified during dysentery epidemics in Japan in the 1950s, when *Shigella* species developed antimicrobial resistance factors identical to those of *E coli* strains from the colons of the same patients. But resistance is not always categorical; it may fall along a continuum.

Biochemical Antimicrobial Resistance

The methods of genetic transfers of resistance factors are better understood than the biochemical mechanisms of this resistance. But several changes in bacterial cells are known to be associated with resistance.

Enzymatic Inactivation of the Antibiotic. Several antibiotics are subject to inactivation by cleaving enzymes produced by bacteria. These include the penicillins and cephalosporins, which are inactivated by **beta-lactamases** into penicilloic and cephalosporic acids, respectively. Aminoglycosides and chloramphenicol are also known to be inactivated by specific bacterial enzymes.

Alterations in Target Site/Permeability. Many pathogenic bacteria are known to alter the coding for their cell-wall antibiotic receptor sites. This includes many of the pathogens of concern in the hospital environment, such as **methicillin-resistant *Staphylococcus aureus* (MRSA)** and penicillin-resistant *Streptococcus pneumoniae.* Bacteria may also change the permeability of their cell walls to antibiotics, especially the gram-negative bacteria, which have a cell membrane outside of their wall. This may be responsible for their resistance to tetracycline and sulfa drugs.

Unblocked Metabolic Pathways. Many antibiotics work by blocking critical metabolic pathways. Plasmids, or R factors, may code for changes in bacterial enzymes, which are either less sensitive to blocking or are able to bypass the block through an alternative pathway.

Viral Drug Resistance. The development of antiviral therapeutic agents lags decades behind that of antibacterial agents. Nevertheless, viruses seem to have developed resistance to antiviral drugs just like bacteria to antibacterial drugs. Influenza's resistance to amantadine and rimantadine can develop in a matter of days or even hours, and resistance of HIV to anti-retroviral drugs has been seen. Less is known about antiviral-drug resistance, which may be due simply to antigenic changes.

The Antibiogram

Health care organizations must track drug sensitivities of microorganisms cultured within their facilities and share these results, in written form, with prescribing physicians and clinical pharmacists. This document is called the ***antibiogram.*** An example of an annual antibiogram for three hospitals is shown in Table 3-15. The document can show the pattern of emergence of resistance over time. Antibiograms serve several purposes. They may help the clinician prescribe more effective drugs to seriously ill patients between the time of their presentation and obtaining culture results and sensitivity results. Antibiograms can also be used to control costs by serving as guideposts to the use of the least expensive but effective drugs. Hospitals can use antibiograms to establish clinical pathways and to control the development of new drug resistances. Matching antibiogram patterns of sensitivity may also have epidemiologic utility, as they may point toward a common source during a nosocomial outbreak.

The Host and Host Response

HOST RESPONSE TO INVASION

The Biologic Gradient

A host's clinical responses to invasion by infectious agents may vary greatly, ranging from rapid tissue destruction and death of the host to no clinical, or apparent, effect. Advances in microbiology and serology have led to the **"iceberg concept"** of infectious disease (Figure 3-7). The base of the iceberg is the majority of host exposures, which will not result in attachment or invasion. A smaller number may result in the development of immunity, as detected by laboratory studies, and an even smaller number result in infection with no clinical symptoms. Only those infections with clinical symptoms appear above

Table 3-15
Antibiogram from Community Hospital

PERCENT SENSITIVITY INFORMATION FOR THE TOP ISOLATES* 1/97-12/97 ICU

Community Hospital East (ICU)

	ORGANISMS	# ISOLATES	AMK	GEN	TOB	CFZ	CTN	CXM	CTX	CTZ	AMP	A/S	PEN	PIP	AZT	CIP	I/C	TET	T/S	ERY	CLN	VAN
GRAM NEG.	Pseudomonas aeruginosa	66	96	85	100					80				91	71	65	76					
	Escherichia coli	44	100	100	100	96	100	93	98	97	61	58		71		100	100		93			
	Klebsiella pneumoniae	38	100	100	100		100	100	100	100	0	78		83		100	97		97			
	Enterobacter cloacae	22	100	100	100		20	8	36	33	0	8		48		100	100		100			
	Stenotrophomonas maltophilia	14	42	38	46					15				15		46	0		60			
	Klebsiella oxytoca	12	100	100	100		100	100	100	100	0			100		80	100		100			
	Serratia marcesens	12	100	100	100		100	0	100	100	8	25		100		75	100		100			
	Proteus mirabilis	11	100	100	100		100	100	100	100	82	90		90		90	100		73			
	Morganella morganii	8	100	100	100		100	19	100	100	0	20		100		63	88		63			
	Enterobacter aerogenes	5	100	100	100	0	60	50	80	80	0	67		100		100	100		100			
GRAM POS.	Staphylococcus aureus (MSSA)	69				95					5	95	11			96		100	100	77	97	100
	Enterococcus species	59									75		66					26				86
	Staphylococcus epidermidis	51				25					0	21	2			45		63	59	31	55	100
	Staphylococcus aureus (MRSA)	42				0					0	0	0			7		82	73	12	29	100

Community Hospital North (ICU)

	ORGANISMS	# ISOLATES	AMK	GEN	TOB	CFZ	CTN	CXM	CTX	CTZ	AMP	A/S	PEN	PIP	AZT	CIP	I/C	TET	T/S	ERY	CLN	VAN
GRAM NEG.	Escherichia coli	27	100	100	100		100	89	100	95	85	81		86		100	100		100			
	Pseudomonas aeruginosa	20	100	95	100					85				90	53	45	85					
	Klebsiella pneumoniae	14	100	100	100		100	100	100	100	0	60		93		86	100		86			
	Proteus mirabilis	5	100	100	100			100	100	100	100	100		100		100	100		100			
	Enterobacter cloacae	5	100	100	100		40	10	80	80	0			80		100	100		100			
GRAM POS.	Staphylococcus aureus (MSSA)	29				100					0	100	0			90		91	100	76	100	100
	Staphylococcus epidermidis	15				30					10	20	7			27		93	60	33	53	100
	Enterococcus species	12									92		92					58				100
	Staphylococcus aureus (MRSA)	9				0					0	0	0			0		78	33	22	22	100

Community Hospital South (ICU)

	ORGANISMS	# ISOLATES	AMK	GEN	TOB	CFZ	CTN	CXM	CTX	CTZ	AMP	A/S	PEN	PIP	AZT	CIP	I/C	TET	T/S	ERY	CLN	VAN
GRAM NEG.	Escherichia coli	26	100	96	100	100		98	100	100	77	79		74	100	100	100		92			
	Pseudomonas aeruginosa	10	100	90	100					100				100	78	70	100					
	Klebsiella pneumoniae	10	100	100	100	100	100	100	100	100	10	67		100	100	100	100		90			
GRAM POS.	Enterococcus species	18									94		89					6				94
	Staphylococcus epidermidis	11				13						27	9			18		82	36	27	73	100
	Staphylococcus aureus (MSSA)	8				100						100	0			100		86	100	100	100	100
	Staphylococcus aureus (MRSA)	6				0					0	0	0			0		100	100	67	83	100

BOXES CONTAINING NO NUMBERS INDICATES THE ANTIBIOTIC WAS NOT TESTED FOR THAT PATHOGEN

*Sensitivities reported for antibiotics where at least half the isolates were tested

ABBREVIATIONS

AMK=AMIKACIN
AMP=AMPICILLIN
A/S=AMPICILLIN/SULB.
AZT=AZTREONAM
CFZ=CEFAZOLIN
CIP=CIPROFLOXACIN
CLN=CLINDAMYCIN
CTN=CEFOTETAN
CTX=CEFTRIAXONE
CTZ=CEFTAZIDIME
CXM=CEFUROXIME
ERY=ERYTHROMYCIN
GEN=GENTAMICIN
I/C=IMIPENEM/CILASTATIN
PEN=PENICILLIN
PIP=PIPERACILLIN
TZP =PIPERACILLIN/TAZOBAC.
TET=TETRACYCLINE
TOB=TOBRAMYCIN
T/S=TRIMETHOPRIM/SULFA.
VAN=VANCOMYCIN

Figure 3-7
The "iceberg concept" of host responses to infectious agents. Most intrusions of infectious agents into the host do not result in clinical symptoms. (Modified from Evans AS, Kaslow RA (eds), *Infections of Humans: Epidemiology and Control,* 4th Ed. New York: Plenum, 1997. P 26.)

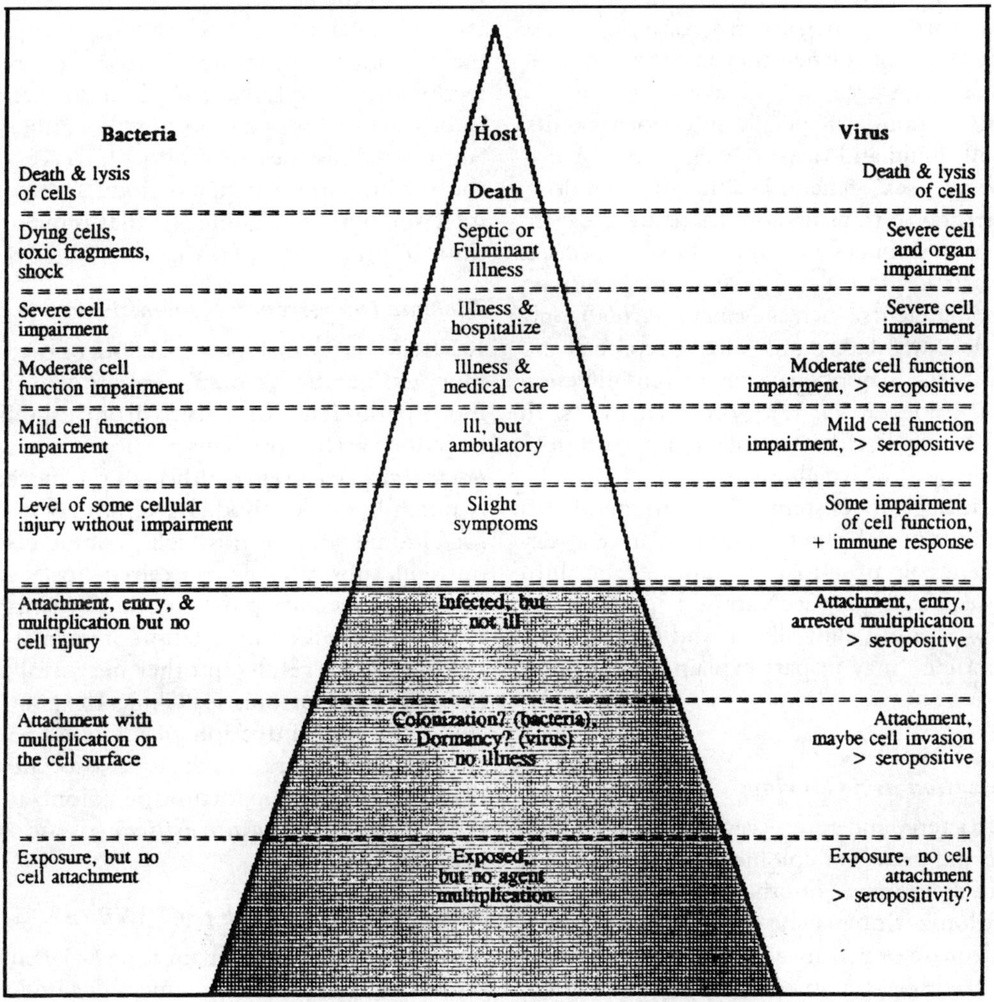

the waterline, and the very peak represents fatal host infections.

Clinical infections can be called ***apparent,*** while asymptomatic infections can be called *sub-clinical,* or ***inapparent.*** Inapparent infection can be diagnosed only by laboratory studies that detect the presence of persistent antibodies or isolate the agent. The **inapparent:apparent ratio** (subclinical:clinical ratio) is considerably wider for viruses than for other infectious agents. The ratio for human rabies is 0:100, while paralysis from wild poliomyelitis virus may be over 1,000:1. Other examples are measles, 1:99, influenza, 1.5:1, and rubella, 2:1. Because of the limits of serology testing, less is known about ratios for bacterial, fungal, and parasitic infections.

Inapparent:apparent ratios can also vary greatly depending on the age of the human host at the time of exposure. Most viral diseases have less morbidity in those who are young at the time of exposure. Hepatitis A has a ratio of 20:1 at age 5, 11:1 at 5–9, 7:1 at 10–15, and 2–3:1 after age 15. Many of the herpes viruses (e.g., Epstein-Barr, cytomegalovirus, varicella) cause more severe illness when they infect susceptible adults. There is great individual variation in how humans respond to specific infectious agents, especially fungi and viruses. Even when correcting for age, sex, general health, infective dose, and method of transmission, there are great individual differences in human host responses. This variation is called the ***biologic gradient.*** With some agents (such as *N meningitides*), only rarely does an infected individual become ill and succumb; the majority have inapparent infection or even colonization. With other agents (such as HIV), it is rare that an infected person does not have progressive illness.

These differences stem from both mendelian and multifactorial genetics and may have a very significant role in human evolution. One third of all people who were exposed to the great plagues were not clinically ill, and this "surviving genome" may in part explain why plagues have not recurred.

Colonization and Carriage

Some bacteria and fungi seem well adapted to adhere and grow in "colonies" on human skin, mucous membranes, or other epithelial surfaces. This **colonization** may be due to a combination of inadequate or permissive host immunity and/or properties of the infectious agent that allow them to attach to lectins (adhesins) on the epithelial cell surfaces. Some bacteria have appendages called ***pili*** or ***fimbriae*** that allow them to attach to specific epithelial cells. These bacteria may only colonize for a short period of time, depending on seasons, host conditions, or host behaviors. If a host is infected with an agent that it can communicate to others, the term ***carriage*** is used. Carriage can exist before (**incubatory carrier**) or after (**convalescent carrier**) illness. In some cases, the host may never be symptomatic from carriage of the agent (**healthy carrier**). The host may be either a **transient carrier**, or an indefinite, **chronic carrier**.

While bacteria and fungi tend to colonize humans, some viral infections (e.g., varicella, poliomyelitis, herpes simplex, cytomegalovirus) can remain subclinical (**latent**, or **dormant**) for the lifetime of the host. Infections with some mycobacteria species (e.g., tuberculosis) may also remain latent (inapparent). Disease (apparent infection) may be reactivated by immune deficiency or other stressors or factors not fully understood. Among the diseases most difficult to control are those with a long latency period (time between infection and clinical illness) that remain infectious to others (e.g., HIV).

Biologic Interference: Normal Flora

Resident, or normal, bacterial flora of the skin or mucous membrane may competitively inhibit more pathogenic organisms from establishing infections in the host. This phenomenon is called ***bacterial interference***, although the mechanism is not fully understood. Bacteria may compete for binding sites on host cells, compete for the nutrient substrates from expired host cells, or produce substances toxic to other organisms.

The suppression or deletion of normal bacterial flora often results in other microbial agents becoming opportunistic. Clinical examples include the **superinfection** of *Candida* vaginitis after oral antibiotics, or antibiotic-associated colitis caused by the opportunistic colonization of the colon by *Clostridium difficile* (**pseudomembranous colitis**).

Invasive Flora: Attack from Within

Not all normal flora remain forever harmless to their host. Many can cause infections under conditions of immunosuppression of the host or in situations in which a disruption of anatomic planes introduces the infectious agent into other tissues (Figure 3-6), for instance, disruption by penetrating wounds or surgery. Examples include peptostreptococcus' establishing vegetation on heart valves (infective endocarditis) after tooth extraction. Penetrating injuries of the bowel were nearly universally fatal before the advent of antibiotics. Anaerobic bacteria may compromise up to 30% of the mass of normal feces but an even higher percentage if there is peristaltic stasis or ileus. An increase in bacterial mass (as high as 10^{11} organisms per gram), along with inflammation of the bowel, may cause bacteremia and sepsis. The most serious new nosocomial infection has been **vancomycin-resistant enterococcus (VRE)**. Hospitalized patients may become colonized with VRE, although the organism may be clinically apparent only when it invades an organ or vascular space other than the bowels or GI tract. The mode of transmission is most often the unwashed hands of health care workers. It is reasonable to expect that a high percentage of hospital workers are being colonized with VRE.

Host immunosuppression may also cause normal flora to become opportunistic. This suggests that flora organisms are at least partially policed by a healthy host's immune system.

HOST RESISTANCE: THE NONSPECIFIC (INNATE) IMMUNE SYSTEM

Nonspecific (innate) immunity is the combination of inborn and natural host factors that serves to prevent the establishment of foreign invaders, including infectious agents. Innate immunity comprises barriers such as skin and mucous membranes and nonspecific physiologic and immune responses by white blood cells (**leukocytes**), blood proteins, and scavenger cells in the tissues. The host reactions of fever and inflammation are also functions of innate immunity.

Skin

The skin is the largest organ of the body and the most important barrier to infectious agents. It is constantly growing and shedding the outer cornified epithelium (epidermis), which contains most of the indigenous bacteria. The skin's normal bacterial flora does not seem to be essential for survival, as animals have been raised experimentally in microbe-free environments. Skin varies in its properties of thickness, rate of growth and flora, depending on the part of the body it covers.

Traumatic skin breaks such as abrasions, lacerations, or bites cause susceptibility to infections and may represent a large proportion of work-related infections. "Natural" breaks in the skin barrier occur at the hair follicles and at sweat and sebaceous glands. These glandular secretions have an acidic pH and a high content of long-chain fatty acids with antimicrobial activity to pathogenic organisms such as fungi. Prepubescent children have more susceptibility to ringworm and other dermatophytes before the sebaceous glands are fully developed. Lipophilic and anaerobic bacteria such as *Propionibacterium acnes* live deep in the sebaceous glands and are not exposed to surface controls. These organisms are frequently found in blood cultures, CSF cultures, bone marrow aspirates, and any other procedures that involve puncturing the skin and underlying sebaceous glands and are deemed contaminants.

Sweat glands also secrete **lysozyme (muramidase)**, an enzyme that can dissolve the bacterial cell walls of some gram-positive organisms. Normal flora of the skin (Table 3-16) have evolved the ability to colonize the skin and to inhibit more pathogenic bacteria in the competition for substrates living on the skin (bacteriologic interference). For instance, some gram-positive organisms have enzymes that break down complex lipids produced by sebaceous glands to unsaturated fatty acids, with antimicrobial activity against gram-negative organisms or fungi. It is the fatty acids of the skin that cause odor, and commercial deodorants are selectively gram-positive bacteriocidal. These products may shift the floral toward gram-negative predominance and toward gram-negative infections. The more serious bacterial infection of the skin (e.g., gangrene, necrotizing fasciitis) often represent combinations of aerobic and anaerobic organisms and may be very difficult to culture.

The skin is quite resistant to viruses but may be contaminated with viral pathogens at times. True viral or rickettsial colonization of the skin is not believed to occur. Viruses that can penetrate small abrasions in the skin include poxviruses, papillomavirus, herpes simplex, and possibly other herpesviruses. The bites of arthropod vectors transmit arboviruses and rickettsial infection. The bites of vertebrates transmit rabies and herpes B (Simian) infections. Manmade punctures of the skin (IV drug use, transfusion, needlestick) may be the mode of transmission for many viral **bloodborne** infections.

Since the outermost layer of the skin is devoid of blood vessels or nerves, very few viruses cause local infection; exceptions are molluscum contagiosum, papillomaviruses, and rarely herpes simplex). Most viral lesions of the skin are

Table 3-16
Normal Flora of the Skin[a]

Infectious Agent	Incidence	Comments
Staphylococcus epidermidis	+++	Coagulase-negative
Propionibacterium acnes (corynebacteria)	+++	Anaerobic near sebaceous glands
Diphtheroids	++	Aerobic corynebacteria
Clostridium perfringens	++	Especially groin and legs Gas gangrene
Lactobacilli	++	
Staphylococcus aureus (*S albus*)	+	Coagulase-positive nostrils, perianal area
Moraxella species	+	
Streptococcus pyogenes (Gr A)	+	
Candida albicans	Rare	
Other *Candida* spp	+	
Enterobacteriaceae	Rare	
Mycobacterium species	Rare	

[a] Predominantly gram-positive cocci and rods, with some gram-negative bacteria in moist areas of skin (under clothing, groin). Many transient organisms can also reside temporarily.
Key: +++ = most humans; ++ = many humans; + = some humans at times.

from hematogenous spread and are from other ports of entry, such as respiratory. Cutaneous manifestations of viral infections are called ***exanthems***. Exanthematous diseases have a great range of severity, prevalence, and patterns of lesion morphology and distribution. These include the "usual" childhood disease of rubeola, rubella, varicella, roseola, and erythema infectiosum. With the possible exception of varicella, exanthems are generally not infectious. Skin lesions serve as portals of exit (are infectious) for only very few viral skin infections, including poxviruses, herpes simplex, and herpes zoster. But even with acute varicella, the viruses in oropharyngeal secretions may be more important than skin in disease transmission.

Skin lesions of rickettsial infections (i.e., Rocky Mountain spotted fever, rickettsial pox, typhus, trench fever) are due to vasculitis in the blood vessels of the skin; they are not portals of exit and are not infectious.

Nose and Nasopharynx

Normal flora of the nose and nasopharynx (Table 3-17) may be highly variable, even in the same individual over periods of time. The rim of the nares has a transitional zone with facial skin and a predominance of *Staphylococcus epidermidis*. But the nose and nasopharynx also contain a large number of anaerobic diphtheroids, which rarely causes host infection. Cultures of the posterior nares or nasopharynx pose special problems because of contamination from the outer area. The area is very difficult to culture, requiring special swabs and techniques. This area is also important as an origin of infections of the sinuses or the middle ear. Outbreaks of nosocomial methicillin-resistant *Staphylococcus aureus* have been attributed to nasal-colonized health care workers. The membranes of the nose and nasopharynx have their own lysozymes and secretory IgA.

Respiratory System

The respiratory system is one of the most efficient routes of entry for infectious agents, just as it is for chemical hazards. Nasal hairs provide some filtration, but their primary function is to produce turbulence of inspired air to trap particles on mucous membranes of the respiratory tree. The nasal and sinus turbinates present a large surface area of mucous membranes that are lined with special ciliated epithelial cells. Trapped particles are moved along the surface by the cilia (the **mucociliary elevator**), toward the oropharynx. There, the trapped agents are periodically swallowed and digested. The smaller particles may

Table 3-17
Normal Flora of the Nose and Nasopharynx

Infectious Agent	Incidence	Comments
Staphylococcus epidermidis	+++	At margins of nares
Staphylococcus aureus	+++	At margins of nares
Haemophilus parainfluenzae	++	Rarely pathologic; lack LPS in walls
Diphtheroids (anaerobic corynebacteria)	++	Rarely pathologic species
Haemophilus influenzae	++	May cause otitis media
Branhamella catarrhalis	++	
Group A *Streptococcus pyogenes*	+	
Streptococcus pneumoniae	+	Rarely pathologic; lack LPS in walls
Enterobacteriaceae	+	
Moraxella nonliquefaciens	+	
Neisseria meningitidis	+	
Alpha-nonhemolytic streptococcus	Rare	

Key: +++ = most humans; ++ = many humans; + = some humans at times.

get past the nasopharynx or oropharynx but then may be caught by the mucociliary elevator of the lower pharynx or tracheal tree and moved to the oropharynx for swallowing.

The mucous membranes of the respiratory tract have more than just mechanical defenses. The cells have lysozymes and mucopolysaccharide inhibitors and phagocytic cells. The secretions also contain specific antibodies (IgA) to prevent bacteria adherence and viral penetrance and to aid in phagocytosis. The resident flora of the respiratory tree may also suppress pathogens by bacterial interference.

The smallest of infectious agents (some viruses, spores, and infective nuclei) of approximately 5–6 μm or less may reach the alveoli. There, they may be phagocytized by alveolar macrophages, but they may also cross the alveoli to cause infection by entering the lymphatic system or blood vessels. A few bacteria and many viruses invade the respiratory epithelial cells or alveolar macrophages directly and may cause clinical illness (Table 3-18).

Other viral agents that have routes of entry through the respirator epithelial cells include varicella, rubella, mumps, measles (rubeola), arenavirus, and hantavirus. Many bacterial infections of the lower lungs (Table 3-19) may be associated with oropharyngeal flora (Table 3-20).

Factors of general health and behavior have great influence on host responses of the respiratory system. Smoking damages the mucociliary function and alveolar host defenses. Acute and chronic alcoholism may be associated with colonization of the upper airway by aerobic gram-negative bacilli. Chronic use of alcohol may diminish the gag reflex and impair tracheobronchial ciliary function. All of these factors are associated with increased risk for aspiration pneumonia. Stomach acids can further damage the bronchial system and increase the risk for pneumonia due to infection of the lungs by gastrointestinal (GI) flora.

Table 3-18
Some Viruses Responsible for Respiratory Illnesses

Viruses responsible for the upper respiratory infections
Adenovirus, common cold
Rhinovirus, common cold
Coronavirus, common cold
Myxovirus, parainfluenza and respiratory syncytial
Orthomyxovirus, influenza
Viruses responsible for mononucleosis syndromes
Epstein-Barr (human gamma herpesvirus 4)
Cytomegalovirus (human beta herpesvirus 5)
Roseola infantum (human herpesvirus 6)
Human immunodeficiency virus (seroconversion illness)
Viruses responsible for sore throats (oropharyngitis)
Adenovirus
Herpes simplex, type 1
Enteroviruses (coxsackieviruses, echoviruses)
Orthomyxovirus, influenza
Myxovirus, parainfluenza and respiratory syncytial

Table 3-19
Lower Respiratory Bacterial Infections

Disease	Pathogens
Empyema	Group A streptococcus, *Streptococcus pneumoniae*
Bronchiectasis	*Pseudomonas aeruginosa*, other aerobic and anaerobic bacteria
Lung abscesses	Many bacteria
Aspiration pneumonia	Many aerobic and anaerobic bacteria

General poor health or debilitation increases the prevalence of gram-negative organisms in the GI and respiratory systems and the risk of aspiration and decreases the ability to initiate protective cough responses. The use of antacids and H_2 blockers, administered through a nasogastric tube, to prevent stress-related gastric ulcers may lower pH and contribute to pathogens' colonizing the pharynx and infecting the lungs.

Mouth and Oropharynx

The mucosa of the oropharynx and mouth have the widest range of flora of the human body (Tables 3-20, 3-21). They are sterile at birth but are contaminated by passage through the birth canal and by exposure to the mother and other humans. The various alpha and nonhemolytic streptococcal species (formerly called *viridans*) are established as the predominant organism of the flora within a few hours of birth and remain so throughout life. Various aerobic and anaerobic staphylococcus, gram-negative diplococci such as *Neisseria*, *Moraxella catarrhalis*, diphtheroids, and *Lactobacillus* are added soon afterward. After the teeth erupt, various spirochetes and fungi (*Candida* and *Actinomyces*) colonize the mouth and tonsillar tissues. Some of these organisms may be implicated in sinus, ear, or lung infections. Many of the throat flora are known to be antagonistic to group A streptococcus, yet up to 9% of people remain colonized with pyogenic forms. The mouth and oropharynx may develop a predominance of gram-negative organisms during periods of very serious illness, which can have positive associations with multiple antibiotics and length of hospital stay. This may contribute to gram-negative sepsis in the critically ill.

Several viral groups can cause lesions of the mouth or oropharynx, including herpes simplex virus and coxsackie group A types 1–24. Fungal infections of the mouth and upper respiratory systems are usually caused by normal flora in immunosuppressed individuals.

Table 3-20
Normal Flora of the Oropharynx

Infectious Agent	Incidence	Comments
Streptococcus (alpha-nonhemolytic)	+++	
Other *Streptococcus* spp	+++	*S viridans*
Branhamella catarrhalis sinusitis	+++	May cause pneumonia or otitis
Aerobic *Corynebacterium*	+++	Diphtheroids
Staphylococcus aureus	++	
Streptococcus epidermitis	++	
Streptococcus pneumoniae	++	
Bacteroides spp	++	
Haemophilus influenzae	++	
Haemophilus parainfluenzae	++	
Neisseria meningitidis	+	
Aerobic streptococci	+	
Anaerobic micrococci	+	
Pyogenic group A streptococcus	+	Up to 9% of adults
Campylobacter sputorum	+	
Gram-negative bacteria	Rare	Causes serious illness

Key: +++ = most humans; ++ = many humans; + = some humans at times.

Table 3-21
Normal Flora of the Mouth and Surface of Teeth

Infectious Agent	Prevalence	Comments
Streptococcus (alpha-nonhemolytic)	100%	Also known as *S viridans*
Anaerobic micrococci	100%	On caries
Veillonella alcalescens (anaerobic)	100%	On caries
Staphylococcus epidermidis	+++	Coagulase-negative
Lactobacillus spp	+++	
Fusobacterium nucleatum	++	
Enterobacteriaceae	++	
Bacteroides spp	++	
Peptostreptococcus	++	May cause endocarditis
Treponema spp	++	On caries
Staphylococcus aureus	+	Coagulase-positive
Candida albicans	+	Opportunistic in the immunosuppressed
Mycobacterium spp	+	

Key: +++ = most humans; ++ = many humans; + = some humans at times.

Teeth

The flora of the mouth may have great individual variation, depending on the presence of teeth and the presence of caries. Much of this variation involves the streptococcal species. *Streptococcus sanguis* and *Streptococcus mutans* colonize the tooth surface, while *Streptococcus salivarius* attaches to gingival and buccal epithelium. The combined presence of certain bacteria contributes to the formation of plaque, which results in a lower oxidation reduction potential at the level of the tooth surface. This may stimulate the growth of strict anaerobes, such as various bacteroides species and *Veillonella alcalescens.* There is also a high association of *Streptococcus mutans* with dental caries. *S mutans* produces glucans (carbohydrate polymers) and results in a strong acidic demineralizing ("**cariogenic**") force on the enamel. Those with extensive active caries have a higher number of both anaerobic bacteria and oral treponemes. They are at higher risk of anaerobic pulmonary infections after aspiration of oral secretions. Extractions or adequate dental care can reduce this risk and greatly change the mouth flora. Human bites are frequent occupational injuries in law enforcement and mental health workers, and any of these factors can increase the likelihood of anaerobic infections from human bites.

Stomach and Small Intestines

The major defense of the lower gastrointestinal track is the low pH. Bile and pancreatic secretions of the duodenum also have strong antimicrobial properties. Very few microorganisms survive in this environment even for short periods of time (Table 3-22). Susceptible organisms survive the stomach only if there is a rapid transit or if the pH is above normal. Neonates, those taking antacid medications, and those who have had surgical gastrectomy have lower acidity (**achlorhydria**) and may have different flora of the stomach and upper intestine. Achlorhydria may increase exposure to some infectious agents.

With achlorhydria, the flora is more like the flora of the mouth and oropharynx and may include anaerobic and gram-negative aerobic bacteria. The bile and pancreatic ducts are normally sterile, but infection with *Salmonella* species (including typhi), *Enterococcus*, *Bacteroides*, or *Clostridia* species is then more likely.

Distally in the small intestine, there is an increase in the number of colon-type organisms, including anaerobic bacteria and enterococci. Any disruption of the normal small or large intestine motility (e.g., surgery, obstruction, or ileus) may produce an overgrowth of facultative anaerobes of the small intestine, with clinical consequences.

Table 3-22
Normal Flora of the Stomach and Small Intestine

Infectious Agent	Incidence	Comments
Stomach, if pH 2–3	Near sterile	↑ with pH
Jejunum		↑ with pH
Enterococci	+	
Lactobacilli	+	
Diphtheroids	+	
Anaerobics	Rare	
Ileum		↑ with pH
Enterobacteria	+	
Anaerobic gram-negative bacteria	+	
Candida albicans	++	Opportunistic in immunosuppressed

Key: +++ = most humans; ++ = many humans; + = some humans at times.

Large Intestine

Like the mouth and oropharynx, the colon is sterile at birth but soon harbors the largest microbial population of the body (Table 3-23). There are up to 10^{11} organisms per gram—even higher if colon motility is decreased below normal. Children who are breast-fed seem to have a predominance of lactobacilli, but the flora pattern rapidly changes after weaning.

The flora of adult colon are predominantly anaerobic (99%) and represent over 100 species. There is also a great range of virulence of the species, which does not correlate with their prevalence in fecal flora. Facultative aerobic bacteria such as *Escherichia coli* represent 0.06% of fecal organisms but are frequent causes of clinical infection from fecal contamination of the urinary tract or surgical wounds. Variations in the virulence of the many *Bacteroides* species are related to the great variance in the toxicity of capsular polysaccharides.

The gram-positive spore-forming bacilli (e.g., *Clostridium perfringens*, *C difficile*, *C tetani*) are present in the colon of about half of humans and is responsible for the global spore contamination of soil and water. Bacterial interference is very complex in the colon, but it is known that *Shigella*, *Salmonella*, and *Cholera* pathogens are inhibited by the short-chain fatty organic acids produced by anaerobes. Specific IgA in intestinal mucosa may prevent many infections, including cholera.

The flora load of the intestine increases with conditions that slow motility. Likewise, the flora load is greatly reduced by diarrhea, which may be stimulated by many infectious agents or their enterotoxins or by intoxication from the ingestion of exotoxins. Diarrhea may be either a toxin reaction, a defense mechanism to rid the body of harmful agents, or both. In children, diarrhea is the world's leading cause of death from infectious disease. Most clinical protocols involve treating the dehydration and malnutrition associated with diarrhea, rather than trying to suppress the diarrhea itself.

Other Host Defenses

The host defenses described are by no means complete. Because of the theme of occupation-related disease in this text, the genitourinary, maternal-neonate-placental, and sexually transmitted aspects of host defenses are not presented.

Phagocytosis. In addition to all of the nonspecific host responses discussed thus far, a major part of nonspecific immunity is the defense offered by cells dedicated to ingesting and destroying foreign matter, including infectious agents. These cells are collectively called phagocytes.

DEFINITION OF PHAGOCYTE. A cell possessing the ability to ingest bacteria, other infectious or foreign agents, and other cells. Phagocytosis is the process of engulfing foreign material. Phagocytes include several different types of cells, all of which have their origin in bone marrow precursor cells (Figure 3-8). Phagocytes receive signals from foreign microorganisms, from antibodies, or from parts of the

Table 3-23
Normal Flora of the Large Intestine

Flora	Incidence
Bacteria	
Anaerobic gram-negative:	
Bacteroides	
fragilis	100%
oralis	100%
melaninogenicus	100%
Fusobacterium spp	100%
Anaerobic gram-positive:	
Clostridium	
perfringens	++
innocuum	++
tetani	+
septicum	+
ramosum	+
difficile	3%
Lactobacilli	+++
Bifidobacterium bifidum	+++
Eubacterium limosum	+++
Peptostreptococci	++
Peptococci	+
Facultative gram-negative aerobic:	
Enterococci	100%
Escherichia coli	100%
Klebsiella	++
Enterobacter spp	++
Proteus spp	+
Salmonella (2000+)	+
Pseudomonas aeruginosa	+
Shigella	Rare
Salmonella typhi	Very rare
Gram-positive aerobic:	
Enterococci	100%
Staphylococcus aureus (with nasal)	++
Streptococci (non-A)	+
Fungi	
Candida albicans	++

Key: +++ = most humans; ++ = many humans; + some humans at times.

complement system. These "opsins" prepare the microbe to be a target for a phagocyte.

TYPES OF PHAGOCYTES. *Monocytes and Macrophages.* Monocytes circulate in blood and become larger (macrophages) when they move into tissue or organs. These long-lived cells then become a stationary part of the body's reticuloendothelial system. The kidneys, spleen, peritoneum, lungs (alveolar macrophages), liver (Kupffer cells), and brain (microglial cells) all have specialized macrophages. As part of the reticuloendothelial system, the tissue macrophages are also the local housekeepers and assist in ridding the body of older cells and cellular debris. Other parts of the reticuloendothelial system performs the same function throughout the body, filtering the blood and lymphatic system of microorganism and other organic debris. The tissue-bound macrophages also can work in concert with the T cells of the acquired immune system, to which they are closely related (Figure 3-8). T cells and tissue macrophages communicate chemically by cytokines.

Granulomas are the scar tissue structures that may form due to long-term phagocytosis to some infectious or foreign agents. Granulomatous meningitis may result from tuberculosis or cryptococcus. Granulomas can also be seen in the lungs, due to tuberculosis or other infectious disease as well as chronic workplace exposures to some synthetic fibers.

Leukocytes. Leukocytes are the white blood cells that constitute the plasma of circulating blood. Their primary function is one of immunity. Lymphocytes are primarily involved in acquired immunity, while the granulocytes are involved primarily with nonspecific immunity. Leukocytes work together as a team in the face of adversity.

Granulocytes. These are circulating mature white blood cells that appear as granules on staining (neutrophils, basophils, and eosinophils) and are involved in functioning of the immune system.

Neutrophils (**polymorphonuclear leukocytes, PMNs**). These are mature circulating phagocytic granulocytes that stain neutral. The cytoplasmic granules contain biochemicals that degrade and digest ingested cellular matter.

Eosinophils. These are mature circulating granulocytes that stain acidic and contain cytoplasmic granules that can "degranulate" into immunoactive substances.

Basophils. These are mature circulating granulocytes that stain basic and contain cytoplasmic granules that can degranulate into immunoactive substances. **Mast cells** are twins of basophils and are found in the lungs, skin, tongue, and linings of the nose and intestinal tract; they are responsible for the symptoms of allergy.

Figure 3-8
The development pathways of immunoactive cells, from a common stem cell. (From Benjamini E, Sunshie G, Leskowitz S. *Immunology, A Short Course*, 3rd Ed. New York: Wiley-Liss, 1996. P 21, with permission.

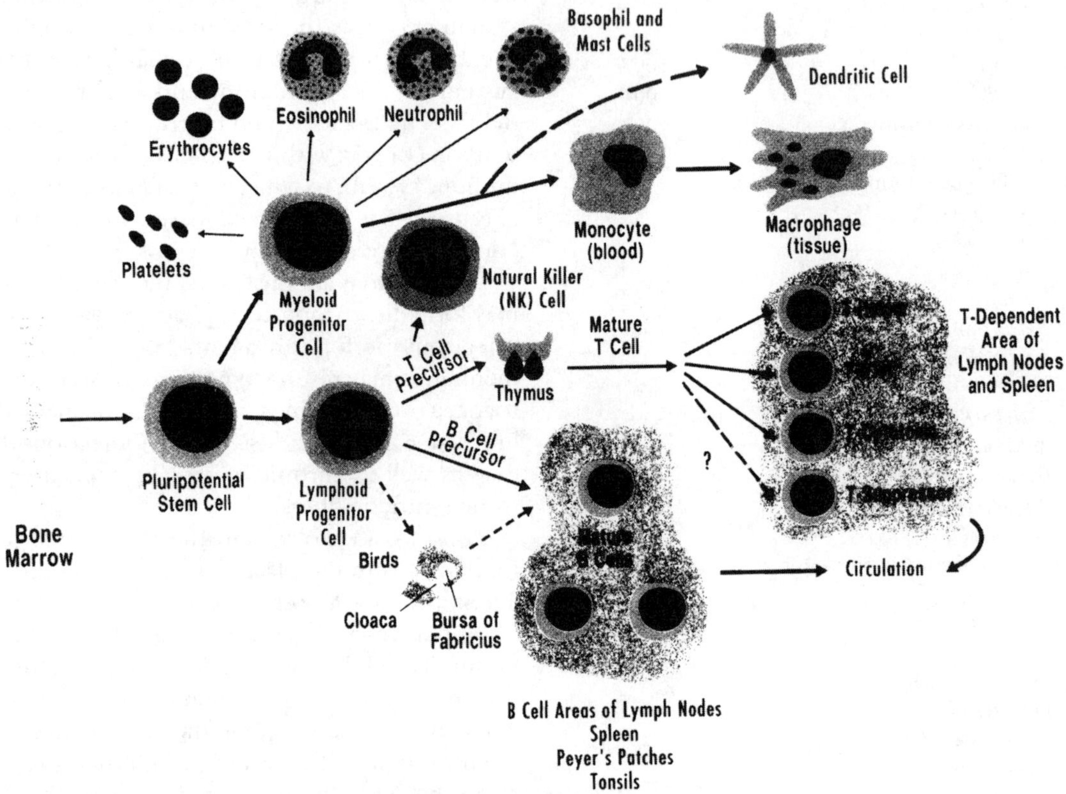

Granular leukocytes are part of the nonspecific or innate immune system and have shorter lives than the tissue macrophages. Neutrophils adhere to the infectious agent and phagocytize them, forming **phagosomes**. Neutrophiles then discharge their hydrolytic and other antimicrobial agents (**degranulation**) into the cell now called a **phagolysosome**. These agents may include hydrogen peroxide, peroxidase, chlorine, oxygen radicals, cathepsin, lysozyme, lactic acid, and acid hydrolase. Some individuals may have a deficiency in fighting catalase-producing organisms and thus have chronic *Staphylococcus aureus*, fungi, and aerobic gram-negative bacterial infections.

NATURAL KILLER CELLS (NK CELLS). Unlike the T lymphocyte cells, which have specific target cells, NK lymphocytes may have a wider range of nonspecific target cells. They do not kill by phagocytosis, but rather by releasing very potent biochemicals in the vicinity of, and in response to, a target cell. This is also called *extracellular killing*. The NK cells respond to soluble mediators such as **interferon** and the **interleukins**. These are manufactured by various leukocytes, fibroblasts, activated T lymphocytes, and even infected cells themselves. All are a call for the NK cells. This system may also play a large roll in the natural control of cancer cells.

THE INFLAMMATORY RESPONSE

Inflammation is a very nonspecific protective response to a wide variety of noxious stimuli, including infectious agents. Inflammation can also be a response to mechanical, thermal, or chemical trauma. Overreaction of the inflammatory response may be a large component of allergic, hypersensitivity, and autoimmune conditions. Specific types of responses depend on the stimulus.

The complement system may be triggered by **C-reactive proteins** in response to specific infectious agents or antigen-antibody complexes. This trigger may come from the acquired (or memory mediated) immune system and will result in inflammation in the area "requested." Explanations of the complement and acquired immune system follow.

Direct tissue injury releases the **kinin system**, a complex system of local smooth muscle, nerve, membrane, clotting, and tissue reactions that stimulate healing, inflammation, and perceptions of pain. The trigger is the activation of the **Hageman factor**, or factor VII of the clotting cascade.

Cytokines are released by activated tissue macrophages, and **monokines** by monocytes. Cytokines can induce coagulation, stimulate other phagocytes and leukocytes to enter the area and bind to vascular endothelial cells, and increase vascular permeability. Macrophages enter the area a few hours later to destroy antigens and help defend the area.

The study of these complex biochemical and tissue reactions have helped to explain the historical and physical findings of inflammation, which are:

pain	*dolor*
heat	*calor*
redness	*rubor*
swelling	*tumor*
and loss of function	

The inflammation system may be overly efficient. In many cases, inflammation remains in a tissue or joint much longer than physiologically necessary, and inflammation becomes the chief complaint. The standard treatments (ice, elevation, and nonsteroidal or even steroidal anti-inflammatory medications) offer some symptomatic relief, but there is little evidence that they modify or improve the body's reaction.

THE FEBRILE RESPONSE

Fever is generally associated with the presence of, and reaction to, infectious agents, although some drug reactions (e.g., neuroleptic malignant syndrome), hot environmental conditions, or overexertion may also cause fever. The thermostat for controlling body temperature is located in the anterior hypothalamus. This mechanism is driven by endocrine and metabolic controls, the selective control of blood flow to tissues, and sweating or shivering.

The cause of fever in the face of an infectious agent is due to cytokines produced by macrophages, the same process which initiates local inflammatory response. Several cytokines have been found to cause febrile responses: interleukin-1 (IL-1), macrophage inflammatory protein-1 (MIP-1), and the tumor necrosis factor (TNF). These same cytokines have other roles, such as improving the efficiency of T lymphocytes, stimulating fibrinogen, and increasing normal erythrocytes aggregation (the reason for elevated sedimentation rates in persons with fever).

Animal studies have shown that antibody production and T-cell proliferation are more efficient at higher body temperatures than at normal body temperature. Known harmful effects of prolonged high fever include cerebral cortex damage, stress on the heart and great vessels, and negative nitrogen balance. But the suppression of fever by medication (aspirin or acetaminophen) has not been shown to adversely affect the outcome of infections. These drugs do alleviate symptoms and make febrile patients more comfortable, however.

ACQUIRED (ADAPTIVE OR SPECIFIC) IMMUNITY

Acquired, or adaptive, immunity is that acquired after exposure to a specific antigen of an infectious agent. The average adult may have acquired immunity for as many as 10^6 to 10^8 antigens. If all of this immunity were innate, the human would need about 50 sets of chromosomes instead of the bequeathed 23.

Acquired immunity is mediated by either lymphoid tissues or specific antibodies. Acquired immunity can be either active or passive. **Passive immunity** is tantamount to "borrowing" the antibodies of another human for a temporary period. Maternal antibodies are passive immunity but are not discussed in this chapter. **Passive immunotherapy** is the administration of human blood products after exposure to a specific infectious agent or toxin. It may be thought of as an available "antidote" or "antitoxin." Passive immunization is discussed in Chapter 5. The remainder of this chapter discusses **active immunity**; the "immunization" that is acquired from the natural exposure to one of the Earth's thousands of infectious agents.

Role of the Lymphatic System

Most of the immune system's assets are derived from **stem cells**, multipurpose precursor cells derived from the bone marrow (Figure 3-8). These cells are the first stage of all circulating blood cells. **Erythroid cells** develop into red cells, **myeloid** into granulocytes, and **lymphoid** into the lymphocytes.

Some of the lymphoid cells are now known to develop in the fetal liver before migrating to the bone marrow. These cells were originally called *bursal cells* because they were found to originate from a bursae in birds. The human **B cells** are now known to function from bone marrow, a **primary lymphoid organ** (which conveniently starts with a *B*). They are the antibody-producing cells that mediate our **humoral immunity** (or "B" for blood). They are transported by the blood to **secondary lymphoid organs**, where they remain.

Some of the lymphoid cells migrate into the thymus gland and mature into **T lymphocytes** (*T* for thymus). The thymus is a gland in the upper thorax (also a *T*) that atrophies after puberty. It is also a primary lymphoepithelial organ. After migrating to the thymus gland, T lymphocytes then move to secondary lymphoid organs, where they are stored indefinitely.

The secondary lymphoid organs are the spleen, lymph nodes, appendix, tonsils, some small patches in the small bowel (**Peyer's patches**), and very small patches in other mucous membranes. The lymphatic system is both an anatomic and physiologic entity that is not discussed in detail in this text. These glands and nodes have complex anatomies and physiologies, as they maintain the red and white blood cells and foreign antigens and filter them from the blood. Lymphocytes are strategically located along lymphatic vessels.

Humoral Immunity

It is in these secondary lymphoid organs that B lymphocytes respond to specific antigens by making specific antibodies. For the purpose of this text, antigens are infectious agents but may also be other "foreign" or nonhost antigens such as toxins, cancerous cells, transplanted tissues or organs, or free allergens.

The B-cell lymphocytes secrete soluble antibodies into both vascular and extravascular body fluids, which is defined as **humoral immunity**. They work only on extracellular antigens and cannot attack intracellular antigens (in **target cells**). Each lymphocyte is programmed for a specific antibody. When a B cell encounters its triggering antigen, it gives rise to many large cells known as **plasma cells**. The plasma cells then manufactures specific antibodies for circulation in the bloodstream.

Each antibody is an **immunoglobulin**, a protein with a globular structure and a specific immune function. They fall into one of several structural and functional classes (Ig "X"). Each immunoglobulin has a basic structure of four polypeptide chains and two identical heavy (**H**) chains and two identical (**L**) chains. There are some fundamental differences and some consistent similarities between the immunoglobulins of different species, which can be utilized in some laboratory studies (Chapter 2). Immunoglobulin chemistry has developed into a scientific disciple that has produced several Nobel Prize winners. The immunoglobulin classes (isotopes) are named after the heavy chain.

IgA Immunoglobulin Antibodies. These are the major antibodies of external secretions and concentrates in body fluids, tears, saliva, and secretions of the respiratory, digestive, and genitourinary tract. They establish the guarding or "surface" immunity at the port-of-entry sites of infectious agents. They are also the major immunoglobulin of mothers' milk and may help to protect and establish the proper gastrointestinal flora in infants. Quantitatively, they are the largest class of human antibodies.

IgG Immunoglobulin Antibodies. These are the major antibodies of the "internal" body fluids (blood, lymph, cerebrospinal, and peritoneal fluid). They coat the infectious agents once they are recognized and stimulate their uptake and actions by other parts of the immune system. They provide the more long-term immunity, and their presence in laboratory studies can usually be interpreted as past exposure. They are the only antibodies that pass through the placenta and are responsible for all passive immunity.

IgM Immunoglobulin Antibodies. These are directly effective in killing bacterial cells and are manufactured acutely in response to new infectious agents. Their presence in laboratory studies can usually be interpreted as recent exposure. They are the largest of the antibodies and do not cross the placenta or blood-brain barrier. Children may be more susceptible to gram-negative infections because of their lack of IgM.

IgE Immunoglobulin Antibodies. These provide incomplete protection against parasites but are also responsible for most of the symptoms of allergic reactions due to their ability to degranulate mast cells. They have the smallest concentration but the most dramatic actions.

IgD Immunoglobulin Antibodies. These are found in the more mature B cells but are very unstable. Their true function is unknown.

Cellular Immunity

It is the T lymphocytes that control **cell-mediated immunity**, the immunity that combats intracellular antigens. It may be the more recently evolved part of the immune system. Humoral immunity and antibodies can function only outside of cells. Like B cells, T cells have receptors for antigens. However, they do not produce antibodies but rather secrete **cytokines**, specifically **lymphokines**. These agents can:

- Bind to target cells.
- Stimulate and mobilize other immune system cells or "direct traffic" for the:
  - Destruction of target cells.
  - Arousal of **phagocytes** (monocytes and macrophage).

Immature T lymphocytes can develop into one of two types of mature lymphocytes. They can become mature **helper T lymphocytes** (with CD4 receptors), which regulate cellular immune response. It is this binding site that is vulnerable to the HIV virus and these lymphocytes that are destroyed during the latent period. The other T cells are the **cytotoxic T lymphocytes** (with CD8 receptors) programmed to destroy **target cells** that are infected (or cancerous).

The Complement System

The complement system is an important part of both the humoral immune response and inflammatory reactions. It is a system of at least 28 circulating or membrane proteins that work to "complement" the actions of antibodies. It also helps to clear the body of antibody-coated antigens (**antigen-antibody complexes**). Complement is primarily responsible for the inflammatory response previously described.

Activation of the first protein by an antibody-antigen complex starts a cascade of activation of the C1–C9 proteins in the **classical complement pathway**. Components C3 or beyond trigger the release of physiologically active substances at the site of the reaction. This results is a cylindric complex's insertion into the cell wall and eventual destruction of the target cell. Some of the proteins of the cascade (C4a, C3a, and C5a) may stimulate anaphylaxis (**anaphylatoxins**) that induces tissue mast cells and serum basophils to degranulate and release histamine. Histamine increases capillary permeability and the smooth muscle contraction responsible for anaphylactic allergic reactions, vascular dilation, and damage to the endothelium caused by neutrophil adhesion. Complement can also cause **opsonization**, the preparation of the microbe to be phagocytized by macrophages.

The **alternative complement pathway** is a more primitive (evolutionarily older) system that is activated by the LPS (lipopolysaccharides of the bacterial cell wall) of endotoxin. The cells of some yeast also trigger the alternative pathway, as can some venoms from poisonous reptiles. The alternative pathway begins at C3 but may work with the classic pathway to amplify both the antibody-dependent and antibody-independent activity starting at C3.

Components of the complement systems are manufactured by liver hepatocytes, epithelial cells of the gastrointestinal tract, blood monocytes, and tissue macrophages. Components are encoded on at least eight chromosomes (1, 4, 6, 9, 11, 12, 19, and X). Genetic defects have been found for most of the components of the complement system. Individuals with a heterozygous defect of a single allele have half as much of that component and may be susceptible to some infections. Homozygous defects in the complement system are very rare. Specific genetic defects in one or more of the complement proteins may be responsible for individual susceptibility to specific infections. The complement system may also have played a role in genetic selection and evolution in the face of epidemics. At least one deficit seems responsible for vulnerability to *Neisseria* species. Meningococcal infections (*N meningitides*), can become "invasive" or septic in a small percentage of the population, while most individuals develop inapparent infection and immunity or asymptomatic colonization (see Chapter 23).

ABNORMALITIES OF IMMUNITY

Allergy

Allergic or hypersensitivity reactions are also mediated by the immune system and are defined as an exaggerated or overreactive response to a seemingly harmless antigen (renamed an **allergen**). They are divided into four classes:

- Type I: The **sensitization phase** is the production of specific IgE to an allergen, which binds to the basophils or mast cells (**sensitized**). They are triggered to degranulate on re-exposure to the antigen (**activation phase**). They release histamine, leukotrienes, heparin, and substances that activate other leukocytes. In the **effector phase**, these substances can produce an **anaphylactic reaction**, with an influx of eosinophils, increases in vascular permeability, and constriction of smooth muscles. Local cutaneous reactions at the site of the allergen can cause reactions within minutes (**wheel and flare**). If the allergen is systemically distributed, a life-threatening **systemic anaphylaxis** can occur. This type of immunity likely has its origins in providing protection from parasites.
- Type II: When a specific IgM or IgG antibody binds to a cellular surface allergen (target cell), it may trigger an activation of the complement cascade and result in cellular destruction. This is the **cytotoxic reaction**. These reactions may be seen with blood transfusion ABO group incompatibility, Rh factor incompatibility, and drug reactions. Drugs that cause agranulocytosis or hemolytic anemia are usually phagocytic or cytotoxic (type II) reactions. Many autoimmune diseases may be chronic cytotoxic reactions.
- Type III: These are the **immune complex reactions**, a triggering of the complement cascade with antigen-antibody (allergen-antibody) complexes. Granulocytes are attracted to the local area and degranulate, causing lytic reactions within a few hours. Local reactions have historically been called the ***Arthus reaction*** and may be the pathogenesis of some venom reactions. Systemic reactions have been called ***serum sickness.*** Type III pulmonary reactions are responsible for many occupational pulmonary diseases.
- Type IV: These reactions are mediated by the T lymphocytes, not antibodies. Type IV reaction has been called ***delayed hypersensitivity, or cell-mediated immunity.*** It has also been called the ***tuberculin reaction,*** as it is responsible for PPD and other positive skin tests showing local induration or redness. The allergen-activated T-lymphocytes release cytokines. Cytokines attract monocyte and macrophages, which are not specific for this allergen. Type IV reactions are delayed 24–48 hours. **Contact sensitivity** is a form of delayed hypersensitivity, in which the target cells and organ is the skin. Naturally occurring oils (such as the urushiol of poison ivy) or industrial oils can penetrate skin because of their lipophilic properties.

Autoimmunity

For reasons that are poorly understood, the immune system may malfunction and develop immune reactions to its own tissues. Antibodies become **autoantibodies**. Autoantibodies have been implicated as the cause of hemolytic anemias, Graves' disease, and myasthenia gravis. Dozens of other conditions are suspected of being autoimmune. Suspected T-cell-mediated autoimmune diseases include type I diabetes mellitus, Hashimoto's thyroiditis, and multiple sclerosis.

Most of these diseases have **multifactorial** causes, combinations of multiple genetic (**polygenic**) factors and environmental conditions. Environmental conditions may include exposure to infectious agents or occupational risks, although proof is lacking at this time.

Immune Complex Diseases

Immune complexes (antigen-antibody complexes) from infections may fail to be cleared at times and may be due to abnormalities in complement receptors. Complexes become trapped and cause direct damage to the kidney (e.g., poststreptococcal glomerulonephritis), the liver (viral hepatitis), skin, joints, or blood vessels. Systemic lupus erythematosus (SLE) is mediated by immune complexes and may cause target-organ damage in the joints, heart, kidneys, liver, or central nervous system. No infectious agent has yet been found to stimulate the production of the antinuclear antibodies of SLE.

Immunodeficiency

The **primary immune deficiency disorders** are those that are hereditary or develop as primary diseases. Much of what we know of the normal immune system comes from studying the illnesses and infections of those with specific deficits. These disorders are rare—on the order of 1 in 10,000 persons. Their approximate prevalences by percentage are listed in Table 3-24.

The B-cell disorders are called ***hypogammaglobulinemias***, but excess disorders (**monoclonal gammopathies**) and B-cell cancers also occur. Those with T-cell deficits may also develop malignancies. Excesses in the complement system can also occur if one of the inhibitor enzymes is absent. The absence of C1 esterase is one cause of persistent angioneurotic edema.

Table 3-24
Primary Immune Deficiency Disorders, by Percent

Disorder	Percent (%)
B-cell antibody mediated	50
Both B- and T-cell mediated	20
Phagocytes and/or killer cells	18
T-cell mediated	10
Complement cascade	2

Secondary immune deficiency disorders are much more common and are the result of malignancies of leukocytes (leukemias) due to medical chemotherapy or deliberate immunosuppression such as that performed with transplantation. The immune system may also fail in the face of overwhelming bacterial infections and sepsis, which usually results in death.

The Environment and Reservoirs of Infectious Agents

THE ENVIRONMENT

There will always be infectious agents in the environment, and for most diseases, there will remain susceptible hosts. The triangle is complete only when the human host is invaded through a **portal of entry**. For human-to-human diseases transmitted directly or indirectly through the environment, the **portal of exit** is just as important in the life cycle and survival of the agent. The portal of exit of an infectious agent from its host is its portal of entry into the environment, the port of exit from the environment is its portal of entry to the host.

For many agents the human is not the natural host, and is infected by "accident." This is especially true for workers who, in the course of their duties, interrupt the environment and the triangle of other natural cycles. Diseases that occur by "accident" include anthrax, brucellosis, leptospirosis, Q fever, plague, Rocky Mountain spotted fever, salmonella, tularemia, and dozens of others. Workers may utilize technology to enter new environments or environmental conditions and thus be exposed to new biohazard challenges to human host defenses. Workers may also, in the course their duties, travel to foreign environments and be exposed to infectious agents to which they are susceptible.

Exposure to the Environment

The width and breadth of one's exposure to infectious agents is positively related to the width and breadth of one's exposure to the environment and to their behavior patterns in that environment (Figure 3-9). Risk can be reduced by an awareness of the environmental hazards and the use of vaccination, chemoprophylaxis, personal protective equipment, engineering, and education on safe behavior. Each is discussed in the other chapters of this text.

The relative number and the danger of infectious agents in our environment is increasing for several reasons:

1. As the last wilderness areas of the Earth are invaded by working humans utilizing technology in the search for resources, we may be unearthing the reservoir of some virulent infectious agents for which we have not evolved innate resistance or other defense mechanisms. This may be the case for the Hantaan, HIV, and Ebola viruses.
2. New forms of infectious agents, such as the drug-resistant strains of bacteria found in hospitals, may arise from our technology. Legionellosis may be a disease that has arisen from our heating, cooling, and air-conditioning technology. Natural human *Legionella* infection from the disturbance of natural or nonmanmade environments has yet to be proved.
3. Because of the increasing prevalence of immunosuppressed persons in our society, dozens of bacteria, virus, fungi, and parasite species once considered to be harmless have been added to the list of pathogens. A dozen of these agents were included in the 1987 CDC definition of the AIDS diagnosis (**"AIDS Predicting Illness"**) [26].

Figure 3-9
Only a small portion of all potentially infectious agents are pathogenic to humans. These agents may be of inanimate, invertebrate, vertebrate, or human origin.

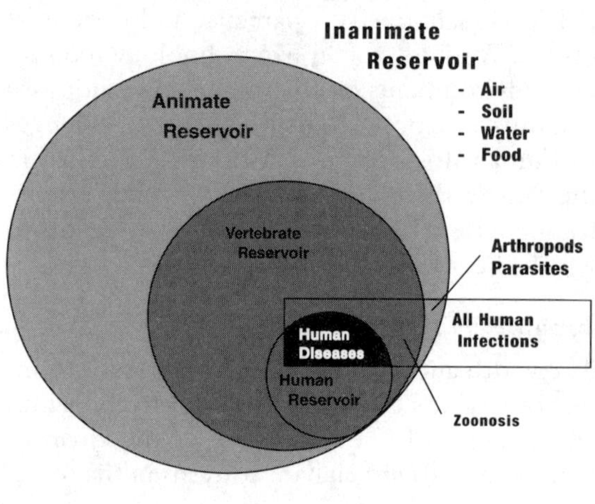

Infectivity from the Environmental Reservoir

For an infectious agent to cause human infection from the environment or reservoir, it must:

1. Be stable and resistant to the physical factors and stressors of that environment. The more it can adapt to changes in its environment, the wider its range and longer it may survive.
2. Have a port of entry into the human host.
3. Exist and enter in sufficient quantity to cause infection (**the infective dose**).
4. Have a means of reproduction to replace the natural death or loss of viability of infectious agents in the environment or the host.

Ecology of Microbes in the Environment

The total number of microorganisms in the biosphere is nearly constant. Knowledge of the growth patterns, nutritional needs, and optimal environmental conditions for various infectious agents comes from observational studies of their growth in the laboratory. The growth patterns of bacteria and some fungi in specific substrates is a principal means of identifying them in the clinical microbiology laboratory (Chapter 2). The growth equations, curves, and mathematical models of microbial growth on media in the laboratory are of little use in the study of disease in the host or their persistence in the environment.

The interrelationships between the bacteria, fungi, and viruses in the natural environment is still poorly understood. Attempts to make objects sterile or to alter their flora patterns in the natural environment by and large have failed. Any void of microbial life is eventually filled by another microbe, and even later, the original "extinct" microbe may return to the original balance of flora.

Viruses are inert in the extracellular environment. They may survive and remain infective for short periods but they do not reproduce. Viruses are known to infect all higher life forms, even down to single-cell mycoplasmas, bacteria, and algae. Neither the origins of viruses nor their true function in nature are known. But because of their reaction of pilfering and plundering genetic material, they may be the secret of Darwinian evolution. Besides sabotaging and, in rarer cases, "improving" the genome of various species, viruses may cause human epidemics that reduce the population but "improve" the human genome through the survivors. It is known that as many as 5% of persons living with the HIV virus do not seem to progress to clinical disease (AIDS). These individuals may be infected with a less virulent strain, or it is possible that they possess some genetic advantage inherited from ancestors that survived a similar virus.

THE RESERVOIRS

Both Benenson [10] and Last [2] give the same word-for-word definition for a reservoir of infectious agents: "Any person, animal, arthropod, plant, soil, or substance (or combination of these) in which an infectious agent normally lives and multiplies, on which it depends primarily for survival, and where it reproduces itself in such a manner that it can be transmitted to a susceptible host." Last adds, "the natural habitat of the infectious agent."

The known natural prevalence of a potentially infectious agent in a reservoir is called *endemicity*. For occupational and environmental health professionals, this should be considered a "risk." The presence of a potentially infectious agent in the reservoir should be approached no differently than the kinetic injury of a punch press, the carcinogenic property of vinyl chloride gas, or the consequences of a maturing cataract in an airline pilot. One must assess the risks of the environment (reservoir) and take appropriate preventive action. Evaluating and estimating which potentially infectious agents have reservoirs or infective forms in the work environment should be a routine part of any job risk evaluation. Even the physical proximity of workers to one another may help predict the incidence and prevalence of upper respiratory infection (see Chapter 11 on influenza and Chapter 14 on other upper respiratory infections).

All human infectious agents are derived from at least one of three reservoirs: humans, other living creatures, or the environment.

The Human Host as the Reservoir

Many infectious agents are exclusively human and have little or no survivability outside of the human host (Table 3-25). For these agents, the environment is removed from the equation. The human body *is* the environment, and the agent persists only as long as a single human is infected and infectious and another human remains susceptible. The agent may travel through a life cycle from human host to human host with no carrier, colonization, or dormant state. Such an agent would require very efficient routes of entry and exit and adequate infectivity to "leap frog" from one susceptible human to another (e.g., measles, mumps, rubella). The infected human's portal of exit is the susceptible human's portal of entry. Most of the **sexually transmitted diseases (STDs)** are human-specific (e.g., HIV, herpes simplex, syphilis, gonorrhea, genital chlamydia, trichomoniasis). Some infectious agents may frequently change their antigenic properties and therefore make the previously infected susceptible again (e.g., influenza).

The agent may be able to establish a long latent period of communicability and even inapparent infection (e.g., HIV, HCV, HBV). The agent may be able to establish lifelong infections with infectivity only during periods of exacerbations (e.g., varicella, herpes simplex, Epstein-Barr, cytomegalovirus). The agent may be able to colonize the healthy person and cause infections only under certain conditions such as trauma or immunosuppression (e.g., actinomycosis, *Candida albicans* infection, *M tuberculosis* infection).

The colonization of human organs or surfaces and all types of human carriers (healthy or asymptomatic, incubatory or convalescent, temporary or transient, and active or chronic) should be considered reservoirs that represent risk to susceptible humans.

The Animate Reservoir

Insects (arthropods) or animals may serve as a reservoir for about half of the known human pathogenic infectious agents of significance. Humans, animals, and arthropod hosts may inject, excrete, exhale, defecate, or slough infectious agents into the environment that are capable of infecting others. This process may also

Table 3-25
Human-Specific Infectious Agents (No Significant Animal or Environmental Reservoir)

Disease	Agent	Transmission	Vac[a]	Erad[b]	Problems
AIDS/HIV	Virus	Parenteral Sexual	No	No	Long latency Unstable antigen Attacks immune system
Actinomycosis	Bacteria	Oral	No	No	Endogenous flora
Candidiasis	Fungus	Oral	No	No	Endogenous flora
Chancroid	Bacteria	Sexual	No	No	Tracing contacts difficult
Coxsackievirus	Virus	Sexual Oral/MM[c]	No	No	Many forms, difficult diagnosis
Cytomegalovirus	Virus	Oral/MM[c]	No	No	Lifelong latency Reactivation?
Diphtheria	Bacteria	Direct	Yes	Yes	Adult immunity decay
Epstein-Barr virus	Virus	Direct/MM	No	No	Many chronic carriers
Genital chlamydia	Chlamydia	Sexual	No	No	Male carriage/high inapparent illness rate
Gonorrhea	Bacteria	Sexual	No	No	High inapparent illness rate
Granuloma inguinal	Bacteria	Sexual	No	No	Rare in U.S.
Haemophilus influenzae B	Bacteria	Droplet/MM[c]	Yes	Yes	Variation in host response
Helicobacter pylori	Bacteria	Direct?	No	No	Unknown mode of transmission
Hepatitis B	Virus	Sexual Parenteral	Yes	Yes	Chronic carriers
Hepatitis C	Virus	Parenteral	No	No	High prevalence High inapparent illness rate
Herpes simplex	Virus	Direct/MM[c] Sexual	No No	No No	High prevalence Exacerbations
Influenza	Virus	Airborne Direct/MM[c]	Yes	No	Many antigenic forms Highly prevalent Global circulation

Lymphogranuloma venereum	Chlamydia	Sexual	No	No	High inapparent illness rate, especially in females Long latency and incubation
Measles	Virus	Airborne	Yes	Possible	Highly contagious
Mumps	Virus	Droplet/MM[c]	Yes	Yes	Unimmunized children
Mycoplasma	Bacterilike	Droplet/MM[c]	No	No	High inapparent illness rate
Neisseria meningitides	Bacteria	Direct/MM[c]	Yes	No	High inapparent illness rate, floral
Pertussis	Bacteria	Droplet/MM[c]	Yes	Yes	Fail immunity as adults
Parvovirus-19 (Fifth's disease)	Virus	Direct	No	No	High inapparent illness rate
Rhinitis	Virus	Airborne Direct/MM[c]	No	No	Many serovars
Rubella	Virus	Airborne	Yes	Yes	One serovar!!
Streptococcus pneumoniae	Bacteria	Droplet/MM[c]	Yes	No	Many carriers, high inapparent illness rate
Smallpox	Virus	Airborne	Yes	GONE!	Security of culture stock and global populace susceptibility
Varicella	Virus	Droplet Contact Oral/MM[c]	Yes	No	Lifelong latency

[a] Vaccine available?
[b] Potential for eradication within a generation?
[c] Mucous membrane contact or secretions.

be called ***shedding***. The environment may also be contaminated by the infectious agents remaining in the body of dead plants and animals.

Diseases spread by vertebrate animal hosts to humans are called ***zoonoses***. Vertebrate animal vectors can be wild, livestock, or pets. Workers who handle any of these classes of vertebrates (live or dead) should take the appropriate methods of protections and prevention (Chapters 4 and 36).

Many human infectious diseases occur in predictable seasonal patterns (e.g., arbovirus encephalitis in warmer months, upper respiratory viruses in cold months). Seasonal patterns suggest that the source of infection is related to seasonal life cycles of plants or animals, seasonal environmental conditions, or seasonal human recreational or occupational behaviors that increase exposure. The reservoir remains unknown for only a few infectious agents (e.g., Ebola virus, Kawasaki agent).

The arboviruses were named for their association with arthropods (i.e., mosquitoes, mites, ticks, and flies). By definition, arboviruses propagate in arthropods. Arthropods are infected by biting infected vertebrates (especially small mammals and birds) during a period of viremia. Horses were once considered to be the reservoirs for some of the encephalitis viral diseases found in the United States, and thus named *equine*. Horses, as well as humans, may be affected, but they are not the reservoir. Nor are the living arthropods the true reservoir, as most live only part of the year. They may pass the infection to their offspring vertically or through the **transovarian route**. The virus may also live through the winter in birds or small mammals, a reservoir method known as **overwintering**.

The reservoir of the seasonal respiratory viruses has also been a mystery as to where they reside during the "off-season." For influenza, it is believed that the opposite hemisphere serves as the reservoir, as mutating influenza strains constantly circle the Earth. Animals are suspected reservoirs for several diseases. The section on "Swine Flu, the story continues . . ." in Chapter 11 describes the dramatic 80-year-long suspicion and investigation of a possible dormant domestic animal reservoir for the agent responsible for the twentieth century's most deadly epidemic.

The Inanimate Reservoir

The presence of infectious agents in or on inanimate objects in the environment is termed ***contamination***. It differs from **pollution**, the presence of noxious or toxic chemical or noninfectious agents in or on inanimate objects of the environment. Inanimate reservoirs include food and water (the human substrates). Essentially all food and water contains bacteria and fungus or their spores and may contain some viruses and parasites as well. The oral and gastrointestinal host defenses have been discussed previously. Some organisms are capable of actual multiplication within the environment of soil, plants, food, or milk. An organism will grow in the presence of the proper and sufficient nutrients and substrates. Climatic conditions also affect the relative balance of microorganisms in the biosphere.

Physical Factors in the Inanimate Reservoir

TEMPERATURE AND SEASONS. The Law of "Brownian motion" states that molecular motion increases with temperature and slows with cooling. Living creatures are much the same, becoming more active in warmer weather. Most infectious agents of concern to humans are **mesophilic**, or survive best at or just below human body temperatures. **Thermophilic** (heat loving) or **psychrophilic** (cold loving) agents are less frequently pathogenic. Human behavioral patterns change with the temperature. Recreational activity in the warmer climates increases the risk of exposure to pathogens from swimming in natural bodies of water and sewage, the risk of skin wounds and infection, and the bites of arthropod vectors.

In colder climates, humans tend to gather inside and thus share seasonal increases in the communicable respiratory infections (Chapters 11, 13, and 14). Many animals and insects that serve as hosts have life cycles that are dependent on the seasons and cause human seasonal epidemics of diseases (e.g., viral encephalitis from mosquito-borne arboviruses). Occupational infectious diseases contracted from crops peak with harvesting (e.g., sporotrichosis) and diseases contracted from domestic livestock occur in seasonal slaughters or shearing (e.g., Orf with the shearing of sheep).

HUMIDITY, WATER, AND FLOODING. Periods of draught, high humidity, or flood can change the growth pattern of bacteria and especially fungi. "El Nino" is an episodic variance of weather of warm winds blowing easterly rather than the usual westerly direction across the Pacific. Although disputed among climatologists, it may be responsible for widening the extremes of weather patterns, which could affect natural disease patterns through the changes in humidity and as a consequence of weather-related disasters.

The lack of moisture in an environment is a powerful stimulus for some microorganisms to initiate species-preservation defenses. Many fungi make spores or conidia, which can survive desiccation in the soil yet remain viable and virulent. Other spore-forming organisms and diseases are the clostridia (botulism, tetanus, gas gangrene, pseudomembranous colitis) and bacillus (anthrax, food poisoning). Bacterial endospores are the most resistant of all living entities, requiring sterilization of surgical instruments and the boiling and/or canning of preserved foods. Endospores for *Clostridium tetani* have survived in a viable state in soil for two years, and those for *Clostridium perfringens* have survived in frozen meat for one year. Drought may also increase the amount of dust in the air and serve as a vehicle for infection. Starvation from drought may lower host immunity and defenses and stimulate the occurrence of an epidemic.

Flooding is the natural disaster with the greatest impact on infectious diseases. Sanitation systems fail when clean water mixes with contaminated sewage water in reservoirs and wells. Food stocks, crops, and building structures may also be contaminated with dozens of infectious agents transmitted by the fecal-oral route. In addition, fungi thrive on the wet wood and environmental surfaces of homes and other structures. Cleanup procedures should adhere to flood-disaster guidelines for decontamination, disinfection, and disease prophylaxis [29].

LIGHT AND RADIATION. Bacteria have varying degrees of sensitivity to ultraviolet (UV), or direct, sunlight. But the spores of the bacillus and clostridia are highly resistant to light and drying. UV radiation is defined as that part of the electromagnetic spectrum of wavelengths from 100 to 400 nm (UV-A is 320–400 nm; UV-B is 290–320 nm; and UV-C is 100–290 nm). Commercial units admitting a wavelength of 253.7 nm have been used to control *Mycobacterium tuberculosis* in the venting or upper room air in health care facilities. Tubercles have remained viable in sputum for 6–8 months if kept in a cool dry location. Relative humidity has been noted to have an adverse effect on UV germicidal irradiation [30].

UV light, x-ray, and high-energy particles can all inactivate viruses. Lethal dosage varies by the type of virus. Infectivity is the most radiosensitive property of viruses, since their entire genetic content is needed for their successful replication. Damage to any part of the genome prevents replication, although some pathogenicity may still be expressed in the host cell.

GEOLOGIC BOUNDARIES (AND TRAVEL). Natural habitats are separated by natural geologic boundaries of oceans, rivers, or mountain ranges. Plants, animals, and infectious agents have adapted to local conditions and may not be able to survive outside of a geographic location or to cross a natural boundary. This is best exemplified by the hundreds of species of arbovirus, each confined to a specific reservoir area by the geologic requirements of their arthropod host. Island isolation may protect a population from a disease (for example, rabies is eradicated in Scandinavia) but could make it vulnerable to disease for which it has no acquired immunity. If an infectious agent is taken out of its natural habitat, it may find a sustaining reservoir devoid of natural enemies. Even humans seem to have some geographic and ethnic differences in disease susceptibility. For instance some native Africans seem to have a natural resistance to some forms of malaria indigenous to their native area. The geographic high prevalence of this genetic trait may be a result of the natural selection of this population to survive in this malaria-endemic area.

The speed of modern air travel negates the natural boundaries. A traveler can spread an infectious agent across the globe in a matter of hours—well less than the incubation period for most infectious diseases. The worker who is to travel to a foreign area requires both an assessment of the local reservoirs and his or her own susceptibility. Likewise, a traveler may become an index case to a native population with no acquired immunity. The usual childhood diseases of the European conquerors may have triggered high mortality epidemics in the adults of Native American tribes in North America. The principles of travel medicine are covered in Chapters 5 and 27–31.

Divisions of the Inanimate Reservoir. THE ATMOSPHERE. The atmosphere is contaminated with many infectious agents, but none are known to multiply while airborne. Winds and dust disseminate the spores of fungi and bacteria, which constantly settle on surfaces. Almost any type of sterile media dish will grow colonies if the lid is removed at room air. Contaminants from air may be responsible for the contamination of some foods and medical equipment in the health care environment. Droplet and droplet nuclei (defined later) will contaminate the air near animal and human sources. Only a few viable infectious agents are known to travel great distances in the air between hosts. These include tuberculosis, rubeola (red measles), and *Coxiella burnetii* (Q fever). Many airborne infectious agents can contaminate dust.

SOIL (AND DUST) RESERVOIRS. The soil is the largest and most important inanimate infectious agent reservoir (for **geophilic species**) and the most important inanimate source of occupational infections. The soil reservoir is dynamic. It seeds infectious agents into the air through dust or digging and into the bodies of water (including groundwater) by rain and gravity. It constantly receives agents falling from the atmosphere from gravity or precipitation, from overflowing bodies of water, and from the excretory system of higher life forms. It also receives and processes the remains of dead plants and animals. But the soil is also nature's filtering agent for infectious disease, greatly reducing the contamination of water as it seeps from the surface to the more pure groundwater.

Tens of thousands of fungi and bacterial species perform the useful function of breaking down and recycling decaying organic matter. The term ***saprophytes*** was originally defined as "plants" that live on decaying organic matter. But since bacteria and fungi are no longer classified as plants, the term ***saprobe*** has been used for any microorganism living on decaying organic matter from the soil in the inanimate reservoir.

Many soil microorganisms have a useful purpose. Some bacteria species grow in the nodules of the roots of legume plants and perform "**nitrogen fixation**," an anaerobic process performed below ground. This process converts nitrogen gas from the air into a usable form for plants and animals and is an essential function of the biosphere and food chain.

The soil (and water) also serves as the "toilet" for all creatures. Hundreds of infectious agents have adapted their life cycle to the "soil–GI tract" cycle of higher organisms. The soil is a reservoir of infectious agents "hibernating" in soil substrates in various inactive spore or cyst forms, which lie in wait to be ingested or inhaled. Only a few examples are discussed in this chapter.

Gram-Positive Soil Pathogens. Aerococcus species (viridans) are soil saprobes found throughout the biosphere. These organisms are opportunistic in immunocompromised individuals if they are ingested or in healthy individuals with trauma. They live in both fresh and saltwater and are responsible for a disease fatal to lobsters. In addition, they are airborne contaminants and are responsible for the greenish color that reliably forms on pickled or cooked meats (e.g., cold cut ham slices).

The *Nocardia* species, which cause nocardiosis, are transmitted by the inhalation of contaminated dust and can cause abscesses of the brain or other organs. These are saprobes of decaying vegetation and pose a risk to farmers in Mexico and tropical parts of Africa and Asia.

Several gram-positive cocci (peptococcus, peptostreptococcus) found in normal oral flora can survive in the soil. Newborns may be colonized early. These organisms can also cause wound infections after soil-contaminated trauma. *Staphylococcus aureus* is another gram-positive cocci that can cause food poisoning by the ingestion of an enterotoxin or wound infections from broken skin. *S aureus* is a saprobe that can live in an animal carcass for 42 days or survive or grow in meat products for up to 60 days. The streptococcal species are not believed to cause infections from soil exposure, although some have been found to live in soil for weeks to months.

Bacillus Species. Bacillus species form spores that can remain viable in the soil for many years and can also contaminate from dust. *Bacillus anthracis* causes anthrax, or woolsorter's disease. Almost all domestic and grazing mammals can be infected with *B anthracis* and contaminate the soil in populated or agricultural areas. Besides ingestion, the organism can infect by inhalation of contaminated dust or direct contamination of skin or wounds. It may also be spread mechanically by biting flies. Anthrax is among the most deadly diseases and could be used in biologic warfare or bioterrorism. The U.S. military began immunizing some troops for anthrax in 1998.

Bacillus cereus is a food poisoning by a toxin. Food is probably infected from floating spores landing on food kept at ambient temperature, but it may also directly contaminate crop foods such as rice. Spores may survive boiling up to 10 minutes.

Clostridia Species. Clostridia are colon bacteria that also form spores that can survive for long periods in the soil and require long boiling to inactivate in food. About 2–3% of humans are colonized with *Clostridium difficile*, which can overgrow in antibiotic or cancer chemotherapy–associated colitis. *C difficile* is an important nosocomial fecal-oral transmitted pathogen. *Clostridium perfringens* is also found in the GI tract of healthy persons and that of livestock, fish, or poultry. It can cause an enterotoxin poison in food contaminated by soil or feces or in inadequately cooked meat. Only 10 organisms per gram can be infective. Tetanus is caused by *Clostridium tetani*, a potent exotoxin. Spores are concentrated in animals feces and the soil in populated or agricultural areas.

Gram-Negative Soil Pathogens. It is the gram-negative bacteria that are primarily responsible for the decomposition of plant products. Workers exposed to plant or vegetable products, especially in dry environments, are at risk for illness from the inhalation of endotoxins. Symptoms may include a dry cough, tightness in the chest, headache, chills, malaise, and fever. Symptoms may peak a few hours after exposure ("**Monday fever**"), but chronic pulmonary damage and disease may occur with long-term exposure. Bacteremia does not seem to occur by inhalation. The effects may be due to a combination of toxicity and allergenicity to organic plant dusts. *Byssinosis*, or *brown lung*, has been the name given to occupational cotton-dust reaction. This syndrome and the spectrum of illnesses attributable to endotoxin inhalation is yet to be well named, however.

Aeromonas hydrophilia is a gram-negative rod that survives in soil and in both fresh and saltwater; it forms both spores and exotoxins and is a common pathogen found in both marine and freshwater animals and amphibians. In humans, *A hydrophilia* can cause wound infections and many other organ infections and sepsis. The human incidence is dramatically increasing and is most often misdiagnosed as coliforms.

Yersinia enterocolitica produces a very heat-stable enterotoxin that causes an enteric lymphadenitis mimicking appendicitis. The organism is spread by fecal-oral contaminated food or water. It can survive in water for 20 days and in soil for up to two years. *Yersinia pestis* (plague) is a "forgotten" saprobe that can survive in a human body up to nine months after death. A human carcass is probably not directly infectious to humans but may infect rodents and their arthropod vectors and thus sustain an epidemic.

Coxiella burnetii, the rickettsia that causes Q fever, has been shown to survive in dust up to 120 days. Viable organisms have been shown to travel a half-mile downwind from sites infected by domestic livestock. The rickettsia are very resistant to physical inactivation and require biosafety level 3 (described later) when their cultures are handled.

Viral Soil Pathogens. Viruses rarely survive in dry environments and generally do not cause human infections through exposure to soil or dust. Some exceptions may be the rare Hanta, Machupo, or lymphocytic choriomeningitis viral infections from the very recent contamination of dust by rodent excreta.

Fungal Soil Pathogens. Many fungi are soil saprobes (or saprophytes) and live on plant vegetation, wood, or other organic matter in the soil for months to years. Most are not pathogenic to humans. Fungal spores also contaminate some types of wood and may be responsible for some of the extrinsic allergic alveolitis from sawdust (**aeroallergens**) that afflicts woodworkers. The *Aspergillus* species (**farmers' lung**) are associated with the decay of grains, hay, and plant material. They are distributed throughout nature and are dangerous to immunosuppressed persons. Toxins from aspergillus (aflatoxins) have been associated with primary hepatocellular cancer in Africa and Asia.

Coccidioides immitis is responsible for valley and desert fever (coccidioidomycosis), which is caused by its endospores, found in the soil around rodent burrows in the southwestern United States and in Central and South America. Cryptococcosis occurs mainly in immunosuppressed individuals and is due to a yeast saprobe of pigeon droppings. The various **dermatophytosis** (skin infections) caused by fungi (*Epidermophyton*, *Microsporum*, or *Trichophyton* species) can remain infective for years in fomites contaminated with desquamated epithelium from humans or animals.

Histoplasmosis (*Histoplasma capsulatum*) is a saprobic endemic mold found in the soil around the world but most concentrated in the eastern and midwestern United States river valleys. The majority of the population in these areas have positive skin tests confirming past exposure. *H capsulatum* spores can remain viable for long periods in almost any soil but are most concentrated in soil contaminated by bird or bat excreta. This pathogen is further discussed in Chapter 13. Sporotrichosis (*Sporothrix schenckii*) is a soil saprobe that not only causes pulmonary disease but also wound infections. High-risk professions include farmers and gardeners.

Parasitic Soil Pathogens. Ascaris lumbricoides (roundworm) eggs can remain viable in favorable soil conditions for many years. An infection that occurs only in humans, it is a pure example of the agent-host-environment model with a fecal-oral route of transmission and a soil reservoir. Symptoms also positively correlate with the volume of ingested eggs (**worm load**). The eggs of various tapeworms (*Echinococcus* or *Taenia*) species may survive for months in the soil under a wide range of temperatures and conditions. *Giardia lamblia* (giardiasis) is a protozoan with a cyst that can survive for long periods in food, water, or soil. It is transmitted by the fecal-oral route.

Leptospirosis, or Swineherd's disease (*Leptospira interrogans*), is a generalized illness caused by a spirochete that contaminates the soil from the urine of a wide range of domestic, pet, and wild animals. It can remain infective in soil for weeks. A wide range of occupations, including farmers, pickers, veterinarians, miners, and lab workers who handle infected dogs or rodents, have been infected.

The incidence of toxocariasis (*T canis, T cati*) is increasing worldwide. The pathogen is a nematode with eggs that can live for months in the soil. It is transmitted by the fecal-oral route through contact with soil contaminated with pet dog or cat feces. It is the cause of visceral larva and ocular larva migrans. Toxoplasmosis (*Toxoplasma gondii*) can also be transmitted by the fecal-oral route through contact with soil contaminated with cat feces.

WATER RESERVOIRS. Bacteria, fungi, and algae contaminate water and are active in the decay and recycling of organic mater. Fortunately, most of these organisms are inactivated by commercial water-treatment methods. However, protozoa and helminths also contaminate bodies of water and are harder to inactivate. Giardiasis and cryptosporidiosis have been responsible for some very large outbreaks in municipal water supplies. Some viruses are present in water even after treatment, including polio and other enteroviruses.

Water is not homogeneous in its temperature nor flora but exists in levels called ***thermal stratification***. Seasonal changes "turn over" strata and can change the microbial content at the surface. Bodies of water differ in their oxygen content. Methane is produced by bacteria at the lower levels of bodies of water with heavy organic contamination (**biologic oxygen demand**).

Drinking Water. In the United States, 90% of drinking water is from ground sources. But 36% of tap water samples contain one or more bacterial contaminants that exceed the regulation limits. Treated drinking water should have about 0.4 ppm of available chlorine.

Bacteria is removed from water in drinking supplies by several methods. Chlorine combines with ammonia nitrogen to form chlorine compounds that have biocidal properties. Chlorination should occur after most of the organic sediment has been removed. The mixing of high levels of chlorine and hydrocarbons are suspected of making **chloramines**, which have germicidal but possible carcinogenic properties. In water treatment, anaerobic microbes may be killed by aeration and/or the use of ozone to oxidize the water. Ultraviolet light and/or chlorine dioxide may be used in commercial water-treatment facilities.

WATER AND OTHER RESERVOIRS. Some of the waterborne infectious agents also infect soil and have been already discussed. These include gram-positive agents (*Aerococcus, C difficile*) and gram-negative agents (*Aeromonas hydrophilia* in fresh and saltwater, *Enterobacter* species, and *Yersinia enterocolitica*).

Gram-Positive Bacterial Waterborne Pathogens. *Listeria monocytogenes* is gram-positive bacillus with the rare ability to survive and actually grow in cold water near the freezing point. It also survives well in soil, water, mud, food, feces, and the tissue of many wild and domestic animals. It is opportunistic in the immunosuppressed, the very elderly, very young, and pregnant women. It crosses the placenta and can cause serious neonatal infections or stillbirth. Up to 5% of humans are colon carriers. *Listeria* can be a serious threat after flooding. Few other waterborne infections are associated with gram-positive bacteria.

Gram-Negative Bacterial Waterborne Pathogens. Enterotoxigenic *Escherichia coli* is one form of **traveler's diarrhea**, a disease usually caused by ingestion of at least 100,000,000 food-borne or waterborne organisms. It is more common in underdeveloped countries and more pathogenic to visitors exposed to the toxins for the first time.

Legionella pneumophila has its reservoir in water, including treated drinking water. It may survive for months in tap and even distilled water. It is not infective by ingestion, but from aerosol transmission with rapid drying of contaminated water in air conditioning or evaporation units. It might also aerosolize from hot showers and cause nosocomial pneumonia. It requires a higher level of chlorination to control.

Typhoid fever is a human disease that can infect by the ingestion of food or water contaminated with *Salmonella typhi*. Besides fecal contamination, it may also infect through urine. A single chronic carrier may contaminate a water source or any food that he or she handles. The best known carrier was "**Typhoid Mary**," a cook in New York City responsible for typhoid epidemics [31]. This moniker is used to describe any unknowing index case of any disease.

There are over 2,000 serotypes of other *Salmonella* species, causing millions of cases of food- or waterborne infections in the United States each year. Both animal and plant foods have been implicated in *Salmonella* infections, but most often it is caused by contamination of poultry products. Pet reptiles have also been implicated. Up to 5% of children and 1% of adults may excrete organisms for over one year, making direct human-to-human fecal-oral transmission possible.

Shigella species are also spread by food and water through fecal-oral transmission. Humans are the only significant host and may become ill from less than 200 organisms. *Shigella* remains viable in water for only a few days, so human carriers may be the more important reservoir. Also known as **bacillary dysentery**, it is endemic in some tropical areas and is another travel-related enteritis.

Vibrio cholerae is the prototype human enteric disease associated with human feces-contaminated water. It is disease #001 in all 10 ICD classifications and has been responsible for many pandemics throughout history. It has a 50% mortality if untreated but less than 1% if treated. Cholera is a frequent consequence of flood or war, most recently occurring in Iraq after the Gulf War.

Viral Waterborne Pathogens. More and more viruses are being recognized as waterborne agents. Hepatitis A was among the first recognized and can survive in water and sewage for very long periods. *Rotavirus* is the world's leading cause of gastroenteritis in children and can survive for a month in water as cold as 4° C (40° F). Norwalk virus is a waterborne pathogen that causes gastroenteritis. It can live in water supplies, but the reasons for outbreaks remain a mystery.

Coxsackieviruses cause a range of human conditions and are primarily spread by direct human-to-human contact, but the virus can be isolated and remain viable in stool specimens for several weeks. It may have some waterborne spread. The echoviruses are enteric cytopathogens and can survive weeks in the environment; their transmission is believed to be directly through the fecal-oral route.

Fungal Food- and Waterborne Pathogens. Water and food are both contaminated with various forms of fungal species, but disease caused by their ingestion has not been described. Fungi seem very sensitive to digestive enzymes and gastric pH. *Candida* species can cause thrush, monilia, and lesions in the gastrointestinal organs in immunocompromised hosts. But *Candida* is in the normal flora and infection is probably endogenous in origin.

Parasitic Waterborne Pathogens. Some of these parasites were discussed in the section on soil parasites, including *Cryptosporidium*, the tapeworms, *Giardia*, leptospirosis, and toxoplasmosis.

Balantidium coli (balantidial dysentery) is a ciliated protozoa found in water contaminated by human or swine feces. It is relatively rare but has caused epidemics. *Entamoeba histolytica* is the prototype amoebic infection, occurring only in humans and often because of an asymptomatic **cyst passer** index case. It has a fecal-oral mode of spread from food or water, and individual reinfection is rare. It is another form of dysentery that may be associated with travel. *Naegleria fowleri* is an ameba that invades the brain and meninges through the nasal mucosa. It is associated with swimming in contaminated pools, hot tubs, or stagnant natural bodies of water.

One Asian trematode (*Fasciola hepatica*, or sheep liver fluke) is acquired by eating undercooked water plants contaminated by human, pig, or dog feces. But the most prevalent waterborne parasites are the *Schistosoma* trematodes (blood flukes). These trematodes directly penetrate the skin of humans who work or wade in water contaminated by animal excrement. They are found around the world in warmer climates and may infect hundreds of millions of humans while bathing or working. Some nonhuman species can penetrate the skin to cause **"swimmer's itch,"** although they do not mature further. In the United States, these have been found on beaches, including those of the Great Lakes. The skin irritation resulting from *Schistosoma* infection is often confused with **"seabather's itch,"** caused by jellyfish larvae.

FOOD-BORNE INFECTIOUS AGENTS. *Food poisoning* is a general term that means contamination of food by any of the infectious agents or their toxins or by chemicals, metal, or radionucleotides.

Bacterial Food-Borne Infections. Bacteria with specific metabolic properties are used in food processing. Examples include butter, cheese, yogurt, buttermilk, pickles, sauerkraut, olives, wine, and beer. *Actinobactor* is used in the production of vinegar. *Lactobacillus* has been cultured from 100-year-old cheese and is an essential colonic flora bacteria. The GI tract of humans and ruminants (cattle and sheep) can synthesize vitamin K and most of the B-complex vitamins.

Most all human foods are also "enjoyed" by bacteria. Commercial food processing and packaging attempts to inhibit the growth of bacteria in food. Most bacterial food contaminants grow best near room temperature. Specific food controls are covered later.

Because of the lack of direct relevance to occupational infections, milk is not discussed. It is the best single food media for infectious agents and is worthy of chapter status in most other textbooks on infectious disease.

Some food-borne infectious agents are discussed under soil or water, including *Aerococcus* species, *B cereus*, *C perfringens*, *Listerella*, *Salmonella*, *Shigella*, and *Y enterocolitica*.

Gram-Positive Food-Borne Infections. Staphylococcus aureus is an important organism in occupational medicine. Commercial food handlers with suspected staphylococcus wound infections of the upper body should be removed from the handling or preparation of open food until their wounds are treated or healed. Likewise health care workers with noninfected open wounds of the hand(s) or arm(s) should be relieved from work in patient care areas. Methicillin-resistant *Staphylococcus aureus* (MRSA) can infect and colonize health care workers. Other than the enterotoxin of *Staphylococcus*, gram-positive bacteria do not generally cause food-borne disease in healthy individuals with intact immune defenses.

Gram-Negative Food-Borne Infections. Immunosuppressed persons may become ill from *Citrobacter* species and develop severe diarrhea or septicemia. They may also become ill from various *Proteus* species (*P mirabilis* or *P vulgaris*) found in food. Hospital patients seem to be susceptible to *Proteus* urinary tract infections, bacteremia, or pneumonia after antimicrobial therapy. The oral reintroduction of a normal intestinal floral organism seems to present a risk of invasion of other organs in these patients.

E coli, either the enterotoxigenic (ETEC) or enterohemorrhagic (EHEC) form, can cause infection. The first causes a watery diarrhea, and the second a bloody diarrhea. Serotype O157:H7 is an ETEC that causes severe illness and is increasing in incidence.

Viral Food-Borne Infections. Norwalk virus has been linked with institutional epidemics in camps, schools, nursing homes, and even cruise ships. Contamination of raw shellfish and vegetables is the common mode of its spread. While *Rotavirus* seems to occur more in children, Norwalk is more common in adults. Both have been called by other names, including ***epidemic viral gastroenteritis.***

Fungal Food-Borne Infections. Mycotoxins are toxic metabolites of molds (fungi) that contaminate food. They may be produced by *Aspergillus*, *Fusarium*, and even *Penicillium* molds. The mycotoxins of most concern are the aflatoxins, the most powerful biologic carcinogens known. They may be found in grains, nuts, and some dairy products if cattle are fed mold-contaminated foods. Aflatoxins can form from the wet storage of seeds and grain. Storage of these is now under strict FDA regulations.

Parasitic Food-Borne Infections. Most of the parasites that infect food have previously been discussed under soil and water, including *Ascaris*, *Cryptosporidium parvum*, the *Echinococcus* tapeworms, *Entamoeba histolytica*, *Fasciola hepatica*, *Giardia*, *Leptospira*, and *Taenia* tapeworms.

Opisthorchis species are trematode liver flukes that encyst in fish and may cause human infection if fish is improperly cooked. Symptoms may include biliary tree inflammation and obstruction and cholangiocarcinoma. These species are endemic in some parts of Southeast Asia and in eastern Europe and the former Soviet republics. The cysts may be killed by freezing and thawing of fish.

The *Trichinella* species are nematodes that cause trichinellosis (trichinosis), a disease acquired from the ingestion of the raw or undercooked flesh of pork or other mammals. Symptoms stem from massive invasion of muscle and can vary from inapparent to fatal if cardiac and neurologic complications develop. Eosinophilia is a consistent finding. Gamma radiation or one month of deep freezing may be necessary to kill the cysts. Toxoplasmosis (an obligate intracellular sporozoan) is a similar disease acquired from cysts in undercooked pork, mutton, or beef. The definitive host is cats, but many other domestic animals may serve as intermediate hosts. It has a high association with immune suppression and is an AIDS predicting disease [26] in the form of an associated encephalitis.

Other Food-Associated Infectious Agents. The agent for **scrapie** is the most recently discovered infectious organism. It has been called a ***prion*** and is a filterable self-replicating agent that may cause slowly progressive neurologic diseases. Scrapie may be contracted by the ingestion of infected animal tissues, although this has not been proved to occur in humans at the present time. This infection and the causative organism are covered in more detail in Chapter 22.

THE NOSOCOMIAL RESERVOIR. Hospital and health care facilities are worthy of a section heading equal to that of food, water, or soil. These facilities are "meeting places" for the most virulent, infective, and drug-resistant infectious agents shed from the most ill hosts, into the environment or onto environmental surfaces and medical equipment and instruments, exposing the most susceptible of human people (the very young, the very old, the immunosuppressed, and those with broken skin or other compromised defenses).

Many gram-negative organisms are nosocomial threats. Over two thirds of all cases of *Klebsiella* pneumonia are acquired during hospitalization. The organism has been found to grow in bronchodilator solutions, surviving for several days. Other gram-negative water bacteria such as *Pseudomonas aeruginosa*, some nontuberculous mycobacteria such as *Avium*, and *Legionella* can live and multiply in a hospital's warm water supply. *Legionella* can aerosolize from hot showers and be responsible for nosocomial pneumonias. *Pseudomonas* has also been found to grow in the water in vaporizing respiratory equipment. *Enterobacter* species are gram-negative rods with a history of nosocomial fecal-oral spread. These organisms caused a nationwide epidemic of septicemia from IV solutions in 1971. *Enterobacter* species may survive in the water reservoirs of medical equipment (e.g., nebulizers, incubators) for 21 days.

Mechanical-vector arthropods have also been found in hospitals. *Streptococcus pyogenes* (responsible for many infections, including impetigo, erysipelas, puerperal fever, strep throat, and necrotizing fasciitis) has been cultured from the legs of flies caught in hospitals. Most hospitals are required to have double sets of entry and exit doors and sealed windows to protect patients and workers from insect vectors.

The Transmission of Infectious Agents: The Triad Completed

MODELS OF TRANSMISSION

Some models of infection have added a fourth component to the agent-host-environment model—the **vehicle**. The definition for *vehicle of infection transmission* is "the mode of transmission of an infectious agent from its reservoir to a susceptible host. This can be person-to-person, food, vector-borne, etc." [2].

The four-component model conceives of transmission as one in a blend of four nouns. The triangular model uses three nouns connected by the action verb *transmission*. The triangular-model concept is preferred for this text on occupational infections because much of infectious disease transmission is related to human behavior and tasks and much of it can be prevented by teaching, learning, and training, all verbs denoting *control*.

TYPES OF TRANSMISSION

An infectious agent must be transmitted, either directly or indirectly, from one place to another. A standard system of nomenclature for classifying transmission has been accepted. The practical interpretation of this nomenclature comprises favorite questions on tests and board exams. Standard terms and new definitions not yet covered in the text are presented in bold, and examples of some of the more common diseases are given, although not all are directly relevant to the workplace. Unless otherwise specified, all hosts are human. The section after that on the types of transmission reviews the portals of entry and exit and is followed by a section on means of controlling transmission.

Direct Transmission

Direct transmission means the transference of infectious agents directly and rather immediately into the portal of entry of a susceptible host. There is **no vehicle, vector, nor "floating" to the host**, either actively or passively. For most diseases, direct contact means that between humans or their "gravity-sensitive" body fluids. Examples of direct transmission are listed in Table 3-26.

Droplet Spread. Examples of bacteria transmitted by droplets (the vehicle) are group A beta-hemolytic streptococcus, *Mycoplasma pneumoniae*, *Streptococcus pneumoniae*, pneumonic plague, and *Neisseria meningitidis*. Examples of viruses spread by droplets are *Rubella*, adeno-, rhino-, corona-, and coxsackieviruses, mumps, parvovirus, Epstein-Barr virus, and CMV and other herpesviruses.

Droplet spread is the transmission by the "gravity-sensitive" or "falling" body-fluid projectiles from coughing, sneezing, singing, spitting, or talking. Various texts list this distance as anywhere from 3 feet (1 meter) [2] to 6 feet [32]. In droplet spread, the portal of entry is the mucous membrane surfaces of the lungs, nose, mouth, throat, or conjunctiva. Not all infectious agents with this respiratory-nasal-oral portal of exit must be considered direct transmission, however. An infectious agent that can be spread by "floating" a greater distance is considered to be *indirectly* transmitted.

Indirect Transmission

Indirect transmission occurs when an infectious agent is removed from its reservoir and carried to the susceptible host over a distance of at least several feet and up to many miles. The type of

Table 3-26
Examples of Direct Transmission

Skin to skin	
• By touching or embracing (staphylococcus, enterococcus, scabies, pediculosis)	
Percutaneous	
• By biting (rabies, cat scratch, hepatitis B, encephalitis)	
• Wound contamination with an environmental contaminating infectious agent (tetanus, sporotrichosis, *Staphylococcus aureus*, aeromonas)	
Mucous membrane to mucous membrane	
• By sexual intercourse (syphilis, gonorrhea, chlamydia, HIV, HBV)	
• By kissing (Epstein-Barr virus, CMV, mycoplasma)	
Maternal-fetal	
• *Transplacental transmission* is the passage of an infectious agent from mother to unborn fetus across the placenta. Examples of agents with this route of transmission are rubella, HIV, and cytomegalovirus. This route is also called *vertical transmission*, although vertical transmission may also include infection of the infant by agents that colonize the birth canal (e.g., *Listeria*, HIV, Group B *Streptococcus*).	

indirect transmission is further defined by the mechanism of that transmission.

Vehicle (Vehicle-Borne) Spread. This is the contact of an infectious agent and a susceptible host through contact with *contaminated inanimate objects.* Commonly used objects or articles such as environmental surfaces, clothing, bedding, toys, or money can serve as fomites (vehicles). Infection by ingestion (of food or water) is also a form of indirect transmission. The transmission of a bloodborne pathogen by transfusion, needlestick, or tissue transplantation are all considered indirect; the respective vehicles in these examples are the blood unit, the needle, and the tissue specimen.

The infectious agent may contaminate only the vehicle (e.g., Epstein-Barr virus in saliva on a child's toy), or it may actually live and multiply in the vehicle (e.g., *Staphylococcus aureus* in a jar of unrefrigerated mayonnaise).

Vector (Vector-Borne) Spread. This is defined as the indirect transmission of an infectious agent to a susceptible host by an animate or living entity. These are generally small species that move intentionally in the cycle of their own survival but infect incidentally. The vectors can be further subdivided.

MECHANICAL VECTORS. Mechanical vectors move the agents to the host via their own contaminated body organs or surfaces. An insect, such as a fly, that carries on its legs infectious bacteria (e.g., Streptococcus pyogenes) as it moves from a fecal meal to a human wound is an example of mechanical vectorization. Fleas, cockroaches, and flies have been shown to be mechanical vectors for the transmission of Pasteurella to open wounds and Salmonella and Shigella to food. These insects may also carry the infectious agent in their GI tract. Mechanical vectors are not a natural part of the life cycle of infectious agents; the vector just happens to be "contaminated," or "colonized," with the agent, which causes it no harm.

BIOLOGIC VECTORS. These are the classic insect (arthropod) vectors that serve a role in the life cycle of the infectious agent. The agent passes through one or more life cycles in the arthropod before it can become infective to man by its bite. For example, the female Anopheles mosquito spreads malaria to humans, and the Plasmodium parasite that causes malaria needs the mosquito as part of its life cycle. The agent may or may not cause harm to the arthropod.

Biologic-vector transmission is further divided into **transovarial transmission**, the passing of the infection "vertically" from a female arthropod to her offspring, and **transstadial transmission**, the continuation of the infection in the arthropod host as it moves from one life-cycle stage to another (i.e., from a nymph to an adult).

Airborne Spread. This is the movement of infectious agents into the susceptible host by the air. Infectious agents in this class can be inhaled directly into the alveoli of the lungs, past the mechanical host defenses of the nose and throat. Airborne indirect transmission is further divided into two vehicle classes.

DUST. Dust is any organic or inorganic material capable of floating in the air for any distance. The dust particle itself is the vehicle and may carry spores or exotoxins. Exposure to infections from dust is a risk in any profession exposed to wind, dryness, or the mechanical disturbance of soil (Chapters 4, 10, 13, 15, 16). It may also be a risk to laboratory workers (Chapter 33).

DROPLET NUCLEI. Droplet nuclei are the smallest of infective vehicles, generally less than 5 μm in size. They can be produced naturally by the evaporation of droplet body fluids from infected hosts and float long distances to cause infections. They are the most difficult diseases to prevent but fortunately are relatively few in number. They include tuberculosis (and other Mycobacterium), influenza (orthomyxoviruses), rubeola (measles), and varicella (chickenpox). Droplet nuclei may also be produced unnaturally by mechanical devices in laboratories or abattoirs (slaughter-houses). Note that some diseases that cause infection by droplet nuclei can also cause disease by direct droplets. For example, influenza can infect not only indirectly by droplet nuclei, but also closer by the direct droplets dispersed in the air by a sneeze or cough.

IMPORTANCE OF THE TRANSMISSION CLASSES

These classifications of transmission may seem rather didactic and confusing, but they are important to understand in order to understand methods of controls. They are not just rigid definitions left unchanged out of respect for the original writer. Knowing the differences in the definitions of the transmission classes and why spread of airborne droplets is direct and that of airborne droplet nuclei is indirect will help to understand and classify controls. In the hospital isolation system, the former can be prevented by wearing a simple surgical mask near the patient's bedside in the regular semi-private room, while the latter requires the wearing of a high-efficiency particulate-air (HEPA) respirator everywhere in a negative ventilated private room with the door closed.

Transmission systems should not be confused with the portal-of-entry and portal-of-exit concepts discussed next. These are entirely different but equally important. For instance *fecal-oral* describes routes of entry and exit, not the method of transmission. Fecal-oral transmission can be direct, in cases of oral-anal sexual transmission, or indirect, in cases of food or water contamination. Although an organism may be the same agent, transmitted by the same portal of entry, and same port of exit, one cannot *control transmission* without knowing the *type of transmission*. Safe sex practices will not prevent hepatitis A food poisoning nor will safe food-handling prevent sexual transmission of hepatitis A.

If it is learned how an agent is transmitted, its transmission may be prevented or blocked years before its identity is known. Thanks to John Snow's work on discovering the mechanism of transmission of cholera, it could be prevented a century before its etiology was identified. The risk factors for AIDS transmission were identified a few months after the disease's existence was recognized and several years before the infectious agent was isolated or named. Perhaps the best examples for this text are, however, the dozen or more infectious diseases that were named after occupations, implying that the risk factors of transmission were known years or even centuries before the respective agents were named.

Infectious agents do not always have a single port of entry, exit, or method of transmission. The most successful (i.e., difficult to control) infectious agents have more than one method of transmission. The varicella-zoster virus (VZV), for instance, can be transmitted directly by contact with vesicular fluid (zoster) or by airborne droplet (varicella). However, it can also be spread indirectly by droplet nuclei from respiratory secretions (varicella) or by fomites (varicella or zoster). Note that this agent produces two separate disease forms, infects for life, and can randomly reactivate. The weakness of the virus is that it infects only humans, has no other reservoir, and survives only a few minutes outside the human body. But despite there now being an effective vaccine, the disease may still take a century to eradicate. It will not be eradicated until the last human with latent VZV dies, and/or all humans on Earth have immunity.

PORTALS OF ENTRY

For infection to occur, there must be a portal of entry into a susceptible host. Often, the portal of entry and the portal of exit are in the same organ system and are also the organs affected. For example, if an individual releases an agent into the air by coughing, another may acquire it by inhaling, and the respiratory tree and lung suffer the pathogenicity of the agent. But many infections are far from being this simple.

The Respiratory System as a Port of Entry

As with the chemical and toxic occupational and environmental risks, the respiratory route is the most important and efficient natural means of entry for harmful agents. Infections contracted by the respiratory route are the most difficult to control, since humans obligatorily take "sample specimens" of their immediate atmosphere (air) 12–20 times a minute in breathing. Most of the great pandemics in history (the Plague, Spanish influenza, leprosy) have been primarily acquired by the respiratory route. Most of the "usual" childhood illness (e.g., measles, rubella, varicella, mumps) are also acquired by inspiration or by direct contamination of the upper respiratory system from the respiratory secretions of cohorts. More than any other pathogens, respiratory-acquired infections do not spare the healthy.

The mechanical and immunologic host defenses of the respiratory system were previously described in this chapter, and controls are discussed later. Infectious agents are transmitted to the respiratory system in one of the following ways:

- Directly by gravity-influenced droplets from a human or other vertebrate in the immediate vicinity.
- Indirectly by dust (a vehicle) from a source of any distance.
- Indirectly by a floating droplet nuclei from a human or other vertebrate beyond the immediate inspiration zone.

Bacterial agents known to cause infection from some distance include tuberculosis, Q fever, and legionella; viral agents include influenza, rubeola, and rubella. Outbreaks of all these agents have been reported in the workplace or in military units.

But not all human-specific diseases acquired by inspiration have the respiratory system as the portal of exit. The poxviruses (e.g., varicella, vaccinia, monkeypox) for instance can be aerosolized from vesicles. And some animal respiratory secretions can aerosolize to cause infection in animal researchers. This recently occurred in two laboratory workers doing research on swine influenza [33].

Gastrointestinal System as a Port of Entry

The term ***fecal-oral spread*** is not synonymous with a gastrointestinal portal of entry. It implies a gastrointestinal exit *and* an oral route of entry as a means of transmission of an agent. Fecal-oral spread may be direct or indirect from mechanical vectors or on vehicles such as food, water, or fomites. Orally acquired bacterial infections may also be called ***enteric fevers***; these are covered in Chapter 18. Some enteric fevers may be a humans-only disease transmitted by the fecal-oral route and spread predominantly by the hands of humans (e.g., shigella), or by water (e.g., cholera, typhoid). However, others may be transmitted by ingestion of food contaminated by the infected feces of domestic animal hosts (e.g., *Yersinia enterocolitica*, *Salmonella*, or *Campylobacter*).

Most fecal-oral viral infections are classified in the genus *Enterovirus* (echovirus) or *Reovirus* (rotavirus). A large percentage of these are subclinical and inapparent, especially in adults. Norwalk virus occurs infrequently as an epidemic of adult diarrheal illness contracted by ingestion of feces-contaminated food or water. Hepatitis A virus (HAV) is a fecal-oral agent that infects food more often than water.

Not all orally acquired infections are of fecal origin. Many viruses and bacteria may be acquired orally, nasally, by direct droplet, or in some combination. This includes most of the herpes class of viruses (cytomegalovirus, Epstein-Barr virus, herpes simplex, influenza, rhinovirus) as well as bacteria such as group A beta-hemolytic streptococcus, diphtheria, and mycoplasma.

Skin as a Port of Entry

The skin is very important as a portal of entry, especially for occupationally acquired infections. The normal flora and host defenses of the skin were discussed previously. Work-related skin infections include not only those associated with the trauma of cuts and abrasions, but also those associated with occupationally acquired contact dermatitis or other rashes, which may serve as a source of wound infections or a route for bloodborne pathogens or other serious exposures. Skin and wound infections are of special consequences in health care workers, not only because of the possible exposure to body fluids and drug-resistant organisms, but also because of the cost of restricting caregivers from working.

A full discussion of all infections that gain entry through the skin or wounds is beyond the scope of this chapter. Some of the more common agents of wound infections are discussed in the previous section on the inanimate reservoir and soil.

Percutaneous Entry. Percutaneous infections are those acquired by penetration of the skin, including trauma (cuts or abrasions), penetration by instruments (needlesticks), or bites of animals or arthropods. Needlesticks are covered in more detail in Chapters 4, 24, and 34. Blood transfusions may also serve as an indirect percutaneous source of infectious agents. Besides the more common pathogens of HIV, HBV, and HCV, rare transfusion-related bloodborne pathogens include cytomegalovirus, arboviruses, HTLV-1, babesiosis, Epstein-Barr virus, Creutzfeldt-Jakob disease, brucellosis, leptospirosis, malaria, *Borrelia*, and syphilis. These infections could legally be considered work-related health problems that fall under workers' compensation if they occur as complications of a transfusion given in the course of treating a work-related injury.

ARTHROPOD BITES. The arboviruses are defined as viruses that replicate in both vertebrates and arthropods (mosquitoes, ticks, midges, or sandflies) during their life cycle and transmit disease between vertebrates by arthropod bites. Thousands of arboviruses have been identified and recorded by the *International Catalogue of Arboviruses* [34], and some are listed in Table 3-27. Some of these arboviral diseases are covered in more detail in the chapter on travel-related viral infections (Chapter 27).

Table 3-27
Major Classes of Arboviruses and Their Disease

Togaviridae family, alphavirus genus (horses, birds)
Eastern equine encephalitis (mosquitoes)
Western equine encephalitis (mosquitoes)
Venezuelan equine encephalitis (mosquitoes)
Flaviviridae family (birds, groundhogs, monkeys)
St. Louis encephalitis (mosquitoes)
Japanese B encephalitis (mosquitoes)
Powassan encephalitis (ticks)
Dengue fever (mosquitoes)
Reoviridae, orbivirus genus
Colorado tick fever (ticks)
Bunyaviridae family
California encephalitis (mosquitoes)
LaCrosse encephalitis (mosquitoes)
Jamestown Canyon encephalitis (mosquitoes)
Rhabdoviridae family, vesiculoviruses (domestic animals)
Vesicular stomatitis (sandflies, mosquitoes, blackflies)

Rickettsia akari (rickettsialpox) is spread by the bites of ticks and has as its reservoir house mice and rats. *Rickettsia rickettsii* (Rocky Mountain spotted fever) has as its reservoir dogs, rodents, and other small mammals. Lyme disease (*Borrelia burgdorferi*, Chapter 26) is the most recently recognized of the tick-borne diseases and can have a chronic course. Animal hosts vary according to the stage of the *Ixodid* ticks. The malarial parasites, which are spread by mosquitoes, are covered in Chapter 25.

ANIMAL BITES. Wound infections are the most common complications of animal bites and are covered in parts of Chapters 4 and 36. Rabies is covered in Chapter 20. *Pasteurella* species of bacteria can cause localized infections and osteomyelitis from cat or dog bites, especially in colder weather. *Streptobacillus moniliformis* can cause a serious systemic illness and multiple organ abscesses after rat bites and may have a mortality up to 7%; in the United States, most cases are related to laboratory rat bites. Both *Pasteurella* and *S moniliformis* are very sensitive to penicillin and its derivatives. *Herpesvirus simiae* is a close relative of herpes simplex and has its reservoir in the mouths of macaque and other Old World monkeys. Thirty-one cases have been reported, with a 68% fatality rate. Most deaths have been occupationally related. In laboratories, this virus should be handled only under biosafety level 4.

PORTALS OF EXIT

To survive, infectious organisms must have a portal of exit from a host, either directly into another susceptible host or into the environment to await indirect entry into a susceptible host. Surprisingly few infectious diseases enter, exit, and cause disease all in the same organ systems. Examples include some respiratory diseases (tuberculosis, influenza, and rhinoviruses) and some of the diarrheal illnesses spread by the fecal-oral route. There are five classic portals of exit from a human or animal reservoir, but for occupational infectious diseases, one might add a unique sixth.

Bleeding wounds may be considered a portal of exit for those exposed to human blood in the course of their employment.

Respiratory Portal of Exit

Factors influencing the efficiency of the human respiratory system as a portal of exit include:

- Intensity and propulsion of discharge of secretions from the system. This can range from drainage and direct contact or contamination of fomites, to coughing, to the most efficient means, sneezing.
- Size of the droplets being exited, which generally range from 1 to 20 μm. The size of the droplets can also be influenced positively by ambient humidity and negatively by ambient temperature.
- Wind currents in the local area.
- Concentration of viable and infective units. Infective doses by inhalation can be as low as 7 virions for an adenovirus [35], 10 bacilli for *M tuberculosis*, and 1,300 bacteria for anthrax.

It is well established that many respiratory viruses (e.g., influenza, respiratory syncytial virus, and rhinoviruses) can be spread by direct contact of mucous membranes with hands and other fomites. There may be nearly 2 million particles extruded from a sneeze, compared to under 100,000 from a cough [36]. But more infective particles may be released in a cough because of the deeper origin in the lungs [37].

Many studies of the infectivity of respiratory viruses have been conducted by Knight's group [37] and include mathematical theories and models of the infectivity of viruses in zero gravity [35]. Knight and colleagues have also theorized that some respiratory diseases may be more infectious in space travel, since larger drops float longer and further. All U.S. space modules, starting with Apollo, have used HEPA air filters. Table 3-28 summarizes the behavior of spherical objects in still air.

Gastrointestinal Portal of Exit

Very few infectious organisms are known to be spread by vomiting. However, bloody vomitus should be considered a bloodborne pathogen risk, especially in patients with hepatitis B. Oral secretions may transmit many viruses, as discussed previously, including most of the "usual" childhood illnesses and the herpes family of viruses. Respiratory and oral secretions may be mixed, especially in ill children. Rabies can exit the body via saliva and be infective by a bite.

Many fecally excreted infectious agents can persist in the soil and water for long periods; and examples are given in Table 3-29.

Skin as a Portal of Exit

Organisms in superficial lesions such as the lesions of impetigo, syphilis, and chickenpox can be dislodged easily. Other organisms (e.g., plasmodia, HBV) exit the body via the percutaneous route through breaks in the skin, insect bites, and needles.

Genitourinary Tract as a Portal of Exit

The sexually transmitted diseases are not discussed but serve as an important portal of exit (and entry) for many diseases that may also be acquired occupationally, including HIV, HBV, and HSV. A careful sexual history and possibly a genitourinary examination may be needed for the differential diagnosis of a work-related illness.

Table 3-28
Behavior of Spherical Infectious Particles (in Still Air)

Diameter	To Fall 3 Meters	Transmission
100 μm	10 seconds	Very direct only
40 μm	1 minute	Direct only
20 μm	4 minutes	Direct
10 μm	17 minutes	Some indirect?
≥6 μm	May float	Caught by nasal hair
0.6–6.0 μm	Floats	Into lungs

Table 3-29
Fecally Excreted Infectious Agents and Their Environmental Survival

Bacteria
- *Bacillus cereus* spores may survive for years in environment of soil or water, including surviving cooking.
- *Clostridium* spores may survive in soil for months to years and in meat for 330 days.
- *Aeromonas*, *Listeria*, and *Salmonella* have long survival in water or soil.
- *Citrobacter* species and cholera survive well in water.
- *Escherichia coli* (enterotoxigenic) survives 84 days in soil or stool.
- *Yersinia enterocolitica* can survive in soil for 540 days, water for 20 days, and cold seawater for up to 105 days.
- *Salmonella typhi* can survive in ashes for 130 days, dust up to 30 days, and feces for 60 days. One human carrier can expel billions of infectious units and infect many others.

Viruses
- Echoviruses (enteroviruses) may survive pH as low as 3, and can survive in stool for three weeks at room temperature.
- Hepatitis A (an RNA picornavirus) can survive long periods in water and sewage.
- Rotavirus can live for months in water near freezing.
- Norwalk virus' survival conditions are unknown.

Parasites
- *Ascaris* (roundworm) and *Toxocara* eggs can live months in soil.
- *Balantidium* protozoan cysts can survive months and possibly years in soil.
- *Cryptosporidium parvum* oocysts and *Giardia* and *Amoeba* cysts can survive several months in moisture or water.
- Almost all tapeworm cysts can live months in the environment.

Salmonella typhi is shed from human urine and can contaminate food or water, causing typhoid fever.

A few zoonotic diseases are known to be shed from urine. *Leptospira* species can be shed from the urine of animals for up to 11 months after initial infection and from the urine of infected humans for up to one month. Rodent-urine contamination of the soil and dust may be a method of transmission of Lassa fever and Hantaan, Junin, and Machupo viral infections.

Principles of Controlling Occupational Infectious Disease

This chapter has described the concepts of the agent, host, and environment triad and their linkage by transmission. This section addresses the principles of control of occupational infectious disease risks at these four levels, utilizing the classic industrial hygiene (IH) approach of *recognition*, *evaluation*, and *control.*

For most workplace risks, the goals are to quantitatively contain the risk at a safe level. For infectious agents, the goal is to prevent or at least control exposure of the susceptible worker host to a less-than-infective dose of an infectious agent. Despite the great advances made in the treatment of infectious disease during the last century, such treatment remains a large part of clinical medicine.

The tools and methods to control or prevent infectious diseases at the level of the infectious agent, the susceptible host, or the environment are rather limited. All infectious agents from the environment cannot be eliminated, nor should they be. Nor can all workers be rendered immune to all infectious agents. The weak link is transmission. The spread of cholera was controlled a century before the agent was identified because the method of transmission was learned (fecal-oral) and the reservoir (contaminated water) identified by John Snow. Avoiding the drinking of potentially human-feces contaminated water controlled the disease, and this behavior also controlled dozens of other diseases, with identical reservoirs for transmission.

The first steps in the classic IH evaluation of a health hazard is to acquire knowledge of the existence of the threatening agent, then knowledge of the workplace process. In evaluating infectious diseases, knowledge of the workplace and the work process and its environment often precede the evaluation of risks for specific infectious agents, which must in turn first be known to control them at the source, pathway, and/or at the worker. The classic IH method may, however, be translated to evaluation of risks for transmission of occupational infectious agents:

Classic Industrial Hygiene Evaluation	*Evaluation of Occupational Infectious Agents*
"Control" at the:	"Transmission" at the:
Source	"Agent"
Pathway	"Environment"
Worker	"Host"

IH professionals can obtain area or personal samples for many nonbiologic hazards. But the culturing or isolating of all possible infectious agents in a work environment is rarely practical. Workers in only a few occupations may be constantly exposed to a single known infectious agent, for example, laboratory, food, or pharmaceutical workers who handle or utilize a potentially infectious agent as an inherent part of their job. Most workers who are exposed to infectious agents are exposed to a variety of agents in a less predictable, random pattern. Examples include hospital workers and those who work in the wilderness. Their protection and job precautions may be "generalized" and relate to behavioral patterns (e.g., washing hands, using insect repellents) but may also be agent specific (e.g., HBV vaccination, rabies vaccination).

The hierarchy of classic industrial hygiene controls, in order of importance, is:

1. **Substitution** (of the agent).
2. **Engineering controls**.
3. **Administrative controls**.
4. **Personal protection controls**.

Since infectious agents are rarely of value to the workplace, **avoidance** or **eradication** of them can "substitute" for classic IH substitution. Most methods of control involve more than one level, or "**integrated controls**." For instance, the control program for tuberculosis in a health care facility may involve the use of negative-pressure rooms and ultraviolet lighting (engineering controls); require that all employees screen patients for tuberculosis symptoms and risk factors at the time of entry into the health care system (administrative controls); require that medical staff have special training in the recognition of tuberculosis (administrative controls); and require that staff be trained to use N-95 respirators when in contact with potential tuberculosis patients (personal protection). No one level of control alone will suffice.

CONTROLLING THE AGENT

Substitution

The use of the concept of substitution for infectious agents has limited applications. Live, attenuated vaccines are a form of substitution of a less virulent agent (antigen) to stimulate immunity (Chapter 5). The less virulent oral poliovirus (an enterovirus) vaccine may "substitute" for the wild virus found in municipal sewage [38]. When the wild virus has been completely substituted in the environment and in the human host, it will be eradicated. The rare cases occurring presently are due to mutation of the vaccine virus "back" to a pathogenic or paralytic strain.

The ability to use a true in-vivo substitution of one less virulent infectious agent for another may be less difficult than attempting eradication, especially for organisms that are normal residents of human flora. In the early antibiotic era, there were outbreaks of the penicillin-resistant *S aureus 80/81* phagotype, transmitted from mothers to infants in newborn nurseries, and later from infant to infant. After this, newborns were deliberately colonized with *S aureus 502A*, a less virulent organism that inhibited the virulent form by bacterial interference.

Eradication (Extinction) of an Infectious Agent

The complete extinction of a human infectious agent from the planet is the ultimate goal of infection control, since only a few seem to serve an otherwise essential role in the biosphere. Smallpox was eradicated in 1979. Eradication of wild poliomyelitis before 2000 is a current goal; the remaining hurdles are cultural and political rather than technical. Very few other infectious agent extinctions are expected in our lifetime. Some factors that may contribute to the possibility of eradication of a human infectious disease and agent are presented in Table 3-30.

Table 3-30
Factors Contributing to Eradication of an Infectious Agent

- The disease exists only in humans (Table 3-25), with no animal or insect hosts or vectors, and no environmental survival (reservoir). That is, the entire reservoir is approachable and treatable if the agent is only transmitted directly human to human.
- The disease has a very low inapparent:apparent ratio: Cases are not missed and do not have "silent" symptoms.
- The disease has a rather distinct clinical presentation, narrow differential diagnosis, and therefore a reliable clinical diagnosis and accurate case reporting. An example is the characteristic clinical course and presentation of mumps (parotitis).
- The incubation and communicable period is short, with little to no carriage, colonization, or latency states. Measles, with its short incubation and infective period, is easier to eradicate than varicella-zoster virus or latent tuberculosis, both of which may persist for life and become reactivated.
- A highly efficacious vaccination or other highly reliable prevention exists and is widely delivered. The susceptible population is reduced ("herd immunity"), or the susceptibles are so isolated and remote from the active cases that the infectious agent is routed to a dead end.
- The disease has only a single serotype or strain. Rubella has only one form, while influenza and salmonella have thousands.
- The cost of eradication should also be cost effective. Rubella would not have been worthy of vaccine research or been on the International Task Force for Disease Eradication list had it not been for the discovery of the costly congenital rubella syndrome (CRS). Rubella is otherwise a mild disease of rare clinical consequence.

The most difficult diseases to eradicate are those with a wide and well-protected "endemic" reservoir. Human rabies is rare in most parts of the world, and adequate vaccines are available for both humans and animals, but vaccination of all wild animals in the global reservoir is impossible. The best hope is, at least, eradication of "urban rabies."

Eradicating the Agent Within the Host. Treatment, or chemotherapy, for illness of human infectious disease represents a large portion of general clinical practice. The many classes and mechanisms of action of antimicrobials is beyond the scope of this chapter. The development of new classes of antimicrobial agents barely keeps pace with the development of resistance. Antiviral resistance is now seen with amantadine and rimantadine for influenza (Chapter 11) and antiretroviral medications for HIV (Chapter 24). Many parasites have also developed resistance to previously effective treatments.

There may at rare times be indications for treating asymptomatic workers, especially those in health care, or groups of workers colonized with bacteria that pose a risk to their patients or clients. Health care personnel who were carriers of group A streptococcus (GAS) have infrequently been linked to sporadic outbreaks of surgical site, postpartum, or burn wound infections [39–45] and food-borne transmission of GAS-caused pharyngitis [46]. Investigations of nosocomial infections have shown a link between methicillin-resistant *Staphylococcus aureus* and health care workers [47–54]. However, CDC guidelines do not advise "routine" culturing of specimens from health care workers unless they have been linked epidemiologically to infected patients [8]—that is, not unless they have been common caregivers to two or more patients who have been positive for the condition. Epidemics of diseases among workers at non-health care facilities have also been reported. One recent study reported 165 of 232 workers at a textile plant who tested PPD-positive after exposure to an undiagnosed co-worker with active pulmonary tuberculosis [55].

Eradicating the Agent in the Environment. Complete eradication of an infectious agent in inanimate reservoirs (air, soil, water) is rarely possible. Even eliminating an infectious agent in animate reservoirs is challenging.

However, one major reservoir of very serious infectious agents is approachable by controls, that is, health care facilities and their patient care equipment. Here, the goal is eradication of infectious agents, or at least reducing the **bioburden** of agents to a level below the infective doses. The eradication or reduction of infectious agents in the health care environment has developed into a field of study generally termed *Sterilization and Disinfection.*

STERILIZATION AND DISINFECTION. Research in this field has contributed most of the available information on the physical and chemical sensitivities of all infectious agents and life forms. The research for new technology and products is very competitive and driven by commercial interests. Three major problems have evolved, and these have only recently been addressed.

1. *Terminology.* A confusing vocabulary has developed in the field [56]. The public, health professionals, and even manufacturers have deviated from the true dictionary definitions. Different classification systems have also evolved.
2. *Regulations.* Several agencies have been involved in the regulation and testing of germicides, leading to conflicts, inconsistencies, and gaps in control.
3. *Safety issues.* Both patients and health care workers may suffer harmful effects from the chemicals and hardware used in sterilization and disinfection. Some germicidal agents have been found to damage delicate instruments, or the instruments' lumina have not been adequately drained and have caused injury to patients [57].

TERMINOLOGY AND CLASSIFICATION: GERMICIDAL TERMS

Cleaning: In the health care environment, the removal of *visible* dirt, debris, soil, or any organic or inorganic material from the surface of objects. It is a very crude but major reduction of the bioburden and potential substrates. It *must* precede all disinfection or sterilization procedures, as effectiveness is inversely related to the amount of initial debris.

Bioburden: The sum total of the number and range of biologic contamination on, or in, an inanimate object. This is analogous to the flora count on an animate surface.

Antibacterials: Germicidal chemicals that may counteract, inhibit and, to some limited degree, destroy some bacteria. These include many over-the-counter products for household cleaning, dishwashing, and bathing. The sale of such products greatly increased throughout the 1990s.

Antiseptics: The relatively mild antimicrobial germicides used to reduce microbes on the skin or living tissues. Applies only to those agents meant for direct contact on *biologic surfaces,* as opposed to environmental surfaces (disinfection).

Disinfectants: Germicidal agents used to destroy or inhibit the growth of most pathogenic bacteria and some viruses on environmental or *nonbiologic surfaces.* Some bacteria (mycobacteria and endospores) and some viruses may survive some disinfectants.

Disinfection: Any process that reduces pathogenic infectious agents. Does not imply the complete destruction of all pathogenic infectious agents.

Spores: A small dormant or inactive single-cell reproductive body produced by some bacteria, fungi, or lower plants as a means of surviving adverse conditions. **Endospore** is the inner layer of the wall of a bacterial spore. Spores are the most difficult of all infectious agents to kill (Figure 3-10).

Bacteriostat(ic): Chemical products intended to retard or inhibit the *growth* of bacteria, including bacteriostatic chemical polymers used in the manufacturing of building materials surfaces (such as restaurants or hospitals) or medical products.

Bacteriocide: Germicide used to *kill* pathogenic bacteria, rather that just inhibit or retard their growth.

Sterilization: The highest level (gold standard) of germicidal processes; the killing or inactivating of all living entities and their by-products, including endospores.

Figure 3-10
Levels of infectious agent survival from categories of germicidal agents, from the most resistant to the least resistant. Sterility implies the absence of all infectious agents, including bacterial spores. This survival order is approximately the same to heat, light, salinity, and pH.

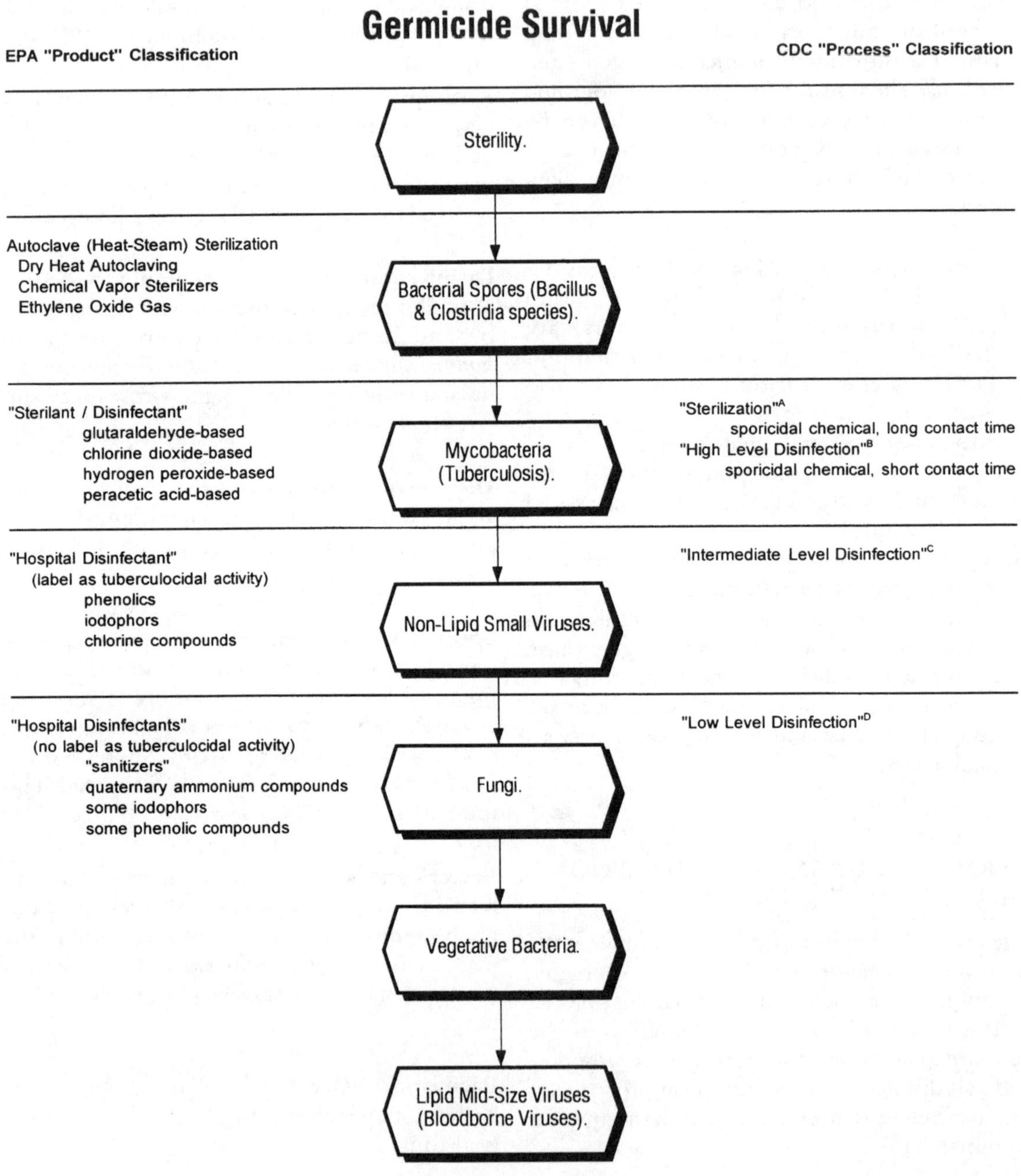

A Appropriate only for critical or semi-critical instruments that are damaged by heat and can not be autoclaved (i.e., laparoscopes). Not capable of being biologically monitored and requires cumbersome post exposure manipulation such as rinsing, drying, and wiping with sterile towels. Less than true sterilization.

B Appropriate only for semi-critical instruments that are damaged by heat and cannot be cleaned by autoclaving (i.e., colonoscopes). Requires washing with sterile water before next use.

C Appropriate for between-patient processing of certain noncritical instruments or devices or for environmental surfaces, such as spills of blood or microbial cultures.

D Appropriate for between patient processing of certain noncritical instruments/devices or for routine cleaning and housekeeping.

Sterility Assurance Level: The probability of a microorganism surviving on an object of less than 1 in 1 million (10^6). Used as a definition for level of sterilization.

Decontamination: A less desirable term (than *sterility assurance level*), which implies only that some effort was used to make an object reasonably free of microorganisms and thus reduce the risk of disease transmission. The word alone does not imply the degree to which that risk has been reduced, however.

CLASSIFICATION SYSTEMS FOR GERMICIDAL PROCESSES

One of the standard systems for classifying inanimate surfaces in the hospital environment was developed by Spaulding in 1972 [58] and involves three germicidal levels.

1. **Critical.** Instruments or devices that are to contact normally sterile body cavities (including vascular) must be sterilized.
2. **Semi-critical.** Instruments or devices that touch mucous membranes may be either sterilized or disinfected.
3. **Noncritical.** Instruments or devices that touch skin or the patient only indirectly can be cleaned and then disinfected with an intermediate-level disinfectant, sanitized with a low-level disinfectant, or simply cleaned with soap and water.

Spaulding also classified the chemical germicidal agents by "activity" level.

1. **High-level disinfection.** Kills vegetative microorganisms but not necessarily a high number of bacterial spores when it is used for contact times of 10–30 minutes. They are capable of sterilization only with contact times of 6–10 hours. These qualify for the current EPA designation "sterilant/disinfectants" and include the glutaraldehyde-, chlorine dioxide-, hydrogen peroxide-, or peracetic acid-based products.
2. **Intermediate-level disinfection.** Kills vegetative bacteria, including *M tuberculosis*, all fungi, and most viruses. These are the iodophors, phenolics, and chlorine (bleach) compounds. A 1:10 dilution of household bleach (sodium hypochlorite) will inactivate HBV and HIV in a blood spill.
3. Low-level disinfection. Kills all vegetative bacteria, with the exception of M tuberculosis, some fungi, and a few viruses. Does not kill spores. These are EPA registered as "hospital disinfectants" or "sanitizers" and include the quaternary ammonium compounds, some iodophors, and some phenolics.

REGULATION OF CHEMICAL GERMICIDES

In the United States, two different agencies regulate chemical germicides: the Environmental Protection Agency (EPA) and the Food and Drug Admin-istration (FDA). Agents formulated as sterilants or disinfectants had been regulated by the EPA, but both agencies recently agreed that agents used on specific medical devices fall under the purview of the FDA. The FDA also regulates all sterilization devices, such as autoclaves and dry heat ovens, and any products to be used in direct contact with human tissues. The FDA also oversees manufacturers' recommendations and the compatibility of device and germicide. The agency still oversees the manufacturing and testing of sanitizers, disinfectants, hospital disinfectants, and sterilant/disinfectants ("sporicides"), including testing for potency, stability, and toxicity to humans. The CDC does not have regulatory powers but only makes recommendations for infection control for each infectious agent or process category. OSHA has the responsibility for assuring worker safety and controlling exposure to germicides and germi-cidal processes.

METHODS OF STERILIZATION

Infectious agents can be classified by the temperatures needed to inactivate them, which comprise a spectrum, from the bacterial endospores (*Bacillus* and *Clostridia*), which require high temperatures and are the hardest to kill, to the medium-size lipid viruses, which can be killed at lower temperatures (Figure 3-10). Fortunately, HIV and the other blood-borne viruses are at the lowest level on the spectrum, and relatively few virulent organisms are at the highest.

Although the other methods of sterilization seem to follow the same kill chart, heat remains at least three orders of magnitude superior to the best liquid-chemical sterilization process. Monitoring is done with a "**spore test**," using harmless spore-forming organisms such as *Bacillus stearothermophilus*. Quality is also controlled with heat-change tapes and slow-change chemical indicator strips. Steam under pressure is the gold standard. Methods of sterilization for medical instruments include:

- **Autoclaving:** Temperature of 250°F (121°C), at 15–20 lb per square inch of pressure, for 30 minutes. The timer should not be set until the necessary temperature and pressure are reached. Errors include overloading, overcrowding, leaving organic debris, using nonporous wrapping, and failure in settings. Other errors may include autoclaving materials such as plastic. Serious steam burns can occur with malfunctioning units but are otherwise safe for workers.
- **Dry heat:** Most autoclaves can be converted to dry heat sterilization, which is more suitable for powders, oils, and some fine instruments used in dental offices. Dry heat sterilization must reach 325°F (163°C) for one hour. Instruments must cool before being used.
- **Chemical vapor sterilizers:** These have the advantages of leaving cutting instruments free of corrosion, of being faster, and of requiring no cooling time. Chemical vapor sterilization requires 270°F (132°C) for 20 minutes at 25 lb per square inch. These sterilizers are more expensive, and noxious gases may develop if the proper sterilizing bags are not used or certain metals are sterilized. Excellent ventilation is required.
- **Ethylene oxide:** This gas is the first choice for sterilizing fine heat-sensitive instruments. It has a broad killing spectrum but requires many hours of contact. It is also explosive over a 3% concentration and can cause burns if traces are left on gloves or clothing. It is also very toxic, possibly carcinogenic, and falls under a full OSHA standard.
- **Chemical sterilants:** Chemical sterilants fall into two classes: the chlorine compounds and the glutaraldehydes. They should be used in closed units and in excellent ventilation. Goggles and gloves should be worn, and instruments should be well cleaned before contacting the chemicals. These solutions can disinfect in a few minutes, but it usually takes 6–10 hours for sterilization. More dilute solutions are used for disinfection.

Only one chlorine compound (Exospor) is accepted as a sterilant. It contains sodium chlorite, which releases nascent oxygen upon contact with cell surfaces and leaves harmless residues. It is a noxious chemical that also damages many metal surfaces on instruments. The glutaraldehydes are used in acidic, neutral, and alkaline forms. Two percent (2%) alkaline is the most widely used. All chemical sterilants should be used according to FDA-approved manufacturers' recommendations.

CONTROLLING THE ENVIRONMENT (RESERVOIR)

The success of attempting to control the environment or reservoir of infectious agents is generally limited to controlling that environment in the near proximity of the susceptible host and their ports of entry. Means of controlling infectious agents by removing them near their source of origins is known as ***source-control techniques***. The appropriate safety and industrial hygiene techniques depend on the nature of the work, risks associated with infectious agents, and the nature of the source of the infectious agents. Appropriate techniques may include regular culturing of a reservoir for harmful infectious agents (e.g., hospital hot-water systems for levels of *Legionella* and *Mycobacterium avium*).

Controlling the Airborne Environment

Outdoors. Control of infectious agents in the air is impossible. Dust can be locally and partially controlled by the spraying of water or oil. Three percent (3%) formaldehyde can be used in some areas of suspected heavy contamination by *Histoplasma capsulatum* or *Coccidioides immitis* fungus. This concentration requires an EPA permit. Those doing the work should wear particulate respirator masks and should ideally be native to the area. A one percent (1%) hypochlorite spray can be used for suspected viral dust contamination, such as *Hantavirus.*

Indoors. Attempts to completely sterilize indoor air by filtration, propylene glycol, and UV light have all met with failure. There are limits on the infection control afforded by ventilation [59]. The best controls generally involve controlling directions of indoor airflow. The size and viability of bioaerosols may depend on their electric charge, moisture content, hygroscopicity, density, cell composition, and shape. Naturally occurring viable bioaerosols (droplets or droplets nuclei from coughing or sneezing) have been discussed.

Source-control techniques have had some success in health care facilities. **Negative-pressure ventilation** is achieved by having the exhaust-air velocity exceed intake in an area that contains and encloses the source. No air should escape the enclosure (e.g., patient's room), and directional flow can be measured with smoke tubes as a quality control. Exhaust air is passed through a **HEPA filter**, defined as one capable of filtering out 99.97% of particles 0.3 μm or less in diameter. If HEPA filters are not used, then the exhausted air should be discharged well above the re-entry zone. High-power UV lighting (with eye protection) and laminar air flow is used in surgical suites with some success for high-risk cases, such as total joint replacements.

General ventilation can be one of two types. **Single-pass ventilation** systems take 100% of exhausted air out of the structure and obtain 100% of intake fresh air from outside the structure. This is the desirable system for infection control but is expensive because the fresh air must be controlled to the proper temperature and humidity. Most structures use **recirculated ventilation**, in which only a portion of the exhausted air is replaced by fresh.

Viable bioaerosols of infectious agents not naturally infectious by bioaerosols could theoretically be produced by laboratory spills or centrifuge accidents. The infectivity of such agents would also depend on the method of aerosol generation, the nature of liquid that surrounds the microorganism, and the size or weight of the organism itself. Laboratory safety protocols for most infectious agents call for allowing 30 minutes for aerosols to settle before beginning cleanup.

Another concern is the possibility of aerosolized bloodborne or tissue-borne pathogens generated by laser plumes or by high-speed high-energy surgical "power" tools. This was a concern for hepatitis B patients even before HIV was described, but studies showed that high-speed dental drills did not produce particles small enough for inspiration [60]. Note that HBV infections have been spread by direct splatter of infected body fluid onto mucous membranes; however, transmission by aerosolization has not been reported. Experimental studies have shown that aerosols produced by surgical instruments can culture HIV [61]. Other experimental studies have shown that surgical drills have produced inspirable particles of bone or tendon of 5 μm or less, laser plumes have produced particles between 0.3–100 μm, and electrocautery has produced particles of 0.7 μm [62–64]. It is unlikely that a paper mask would offer protection from particles this small, but several serosurveys of dentists and orthopedic surgeons [65] who regularly use these instruments show no increased risk of HIV infection in these groups. No cases of HIV transmission from aerosolized tissue or blood have been confirmed. The source-control devices being utilized perform suctioning near the aerosolization of plumes by **smoke evacuators**. These consist of a vacuum pump, HEPA filter, hose, and an inlet nozzle. A **capture velocity** of 100–150 feet per minute, with the inlet nozzle held within 2 inches of the surgical site [66,67] is recommended.

Control of the Water and Soil Environment

Water is a dynamic resource cycling between bodies of fresh water, the ground, the sea, and evaporation into the atmosphere and precipitation from the atmosphere. This is called the ***hydrologic cycle.*** Water can be contaminated at any point in the cycle but is most likely to be contaminated by the lower atmosphere during precipitation and on contact with (and runoff from) the soil. The least contaminated water is that found in **groundwater**, the zone of saturation deep in the soil and earth. The upper portion of this zone is the **wa-**

ter table, which must be penetrated by wells in order to use groundwater sources. Thus, the purest and most contaminated and polluted water on Earth may be separated only by a relatively thin layer of soil. This layer is nature's water filter, which **percolates** or **recharges** groundwater. It is at the mercy of man and civilization and is violated by septic tanks and wells. The outermost layer of soil, which can generate dust, is called the ***surficial level***.

Preschool-age children usually eat a certain amount of soil and dust, purposefully or during play. This averages a few hundred milligrams per day, more in children with nutritional deficiencies or pica. Gardening, some turf sports, and many occupations pose a risk for swallowing or inhaling dust and soil. Pollutants such as metals and organic toxins may be of greater concern than microorganisms. Soil, of course, is a major route of entry of infectious agents for many animals and grazing livestock.

Night soil is the historic polite name for human excreta, which may contaminant soil or spill into wells or other water sources. The protection of water involves both the treatment of drinking water and the control and containment of human garbage and fecal waste (**sewage**).

The reader is referred to other sources [68,69] for in depth discussion of water treatment, sanitation technology, and regulations. Chlorination and other treatments of drinking water have been the most important technologies in reducing infectious disease in the last century. The time-tested yardstick of fecal contamination of drinking water is the **coliform determination**, or culturing of those organisms most frequently found in the colon of human and other warm-blooded animals. Coliform bacteria serve as the **indicator organisms** of fecal contamination. High coliform counts on cultures signify inadequate treatment of water or point contamination after treatment. Various enteric viruses (HAV, polio, coxsackie) as well as echo-, reo-, rota-, and Norwalk viruses may contaminate water. Standard or economical tests for quality control of viral contamination have not been developed, nor do tests exist for the protozoans of concern (*Giardia lamblia*, *Cryptosporidium*, and *Cyclospora*), which were responsible for very large outbreaks in the 1990s.

The 1989 Surface Water Treatment Rules (ESWTR) established stricter baseline filtration, disinfection, and pathogen-removal requirements for surface water in response to *Giardia* and viral infections. It also created a schedule of new contaminants and pollutants to be regulated over the turn of the millennium. ESWTR did not specifically cover groundwater drinking sources nor adequately address *Cryptosporidium* or more heavily contaminated water. We have entered a new era of conflict between the microbial rules for drinking water and concern with the **microbial and disinfection by-products (M-DBP)**. These include trihalomethanes such as chloroform, haloacetic acids, bromates, chlorite, and other by-products of water treatment that may be toxic and/or carcinogenic. The EPA has formed a **Regulatory Negotiation Committee** (the "**Reg Neg**") to address the conflicts between microbial control and M-DBP [70]. A schedule for data collection, public comment, and rule promulgation deadlines began in November 1998.

The majority of U.S. citizens obtain water from wells or groundwater sources. More recent EPA amendments (1996, section 1428) to the Safe Drinking Water Acts call for the establishment of state-regulated **Wellhead Protection Programs**. At this writing, 44 states have approved programs [70].

The greatest single threat to the water supply is flooding because of the resultant mixing of sewage with drinking water supplies. For rescue agency workers or contractors working in post-flood areas, it may also pose the greatest occupational threat from water contamination.

In an emergency, any water suspected of being contaminated with bacteria may be treated with any of the following treatments:

1. Vigorous boiling for 20 minutes.
2. Chlorine tablet, 1 per quart.
3. Chlorine bleach, 2 drops per quart, then letting water stand for 30 minutes.
4. Iodine tablets, 1 per quart, letting water stand for 30 minutes.
5. Tincture of iodine, 2% USP, 5 drops per quart, letting water stand for 30 minutes (water should be cool).

Note that the above processes are for the treatment of water contamination by infectious agents. They will not reduce chemical or metal pollutants. More information on waterborne infections is presented in Chapters 8, 18, 27–30, and 35.

Control of Food Vehicles

It is important for occupational and environmental health clinicians to be familiar with infection controls for food processing and preparation for the following reasons.

1. Although few domestic cases of food poisonings are adjudicated as workers' compensation, they may be covered by workers' comp if a worker travels in the course of employment. The clinician should be familiar with principles of protection from food-borne contaminants and have the knowledge to serve as a resource for employers and workers.
2. Infectious-agent poisonings may be considered in the differential diagnosis for the evaluation of acute illness in workers.
3. Agriculture and food services is the largest industry in the United States and most other nations. Occupational physicians should have a basic understanding of food workers' roles and be members of the team needed to deliver safe produce and food products.

The protection of food from contamination by infectious agents should be practiced at every stage in the planting, growth, harvesting, processing, packaging, distributing, displaying, and preparing of food. The surface of foods can be contaminated by soil, insects, rodents, and aerosols from coughing or sneezing and by the hands or body fluids of food handlers. Almost all diseases caused by the ingestion of soil or water can also contaminate food. Milk is the food vehicle that has been most difficult to control and thus has been progressively regulated for well over a century. Milk and dairy products should be considered body fluids, and a superb culture media. About two dozen diseases, including brucellosis, tuberculosis and Q fever, have been associated with diseased cattle or milk. Milk is also very susceptible to contamination after pasteurization. Mastitis of cows has been caused by various streptococcus, staphylococcus, *Pasteurella* species, and *Listeria monocytogenes.* Traces of antibiotics used to treat mastitis may become milk pollutants or allergens. *Campylobacter* and various *Salmonella* species are found in high concentration in cattle, pigs, chickens, and in the agricultural environment. Controlling these agents so that livestock, milk, and dairy products are not infected has proved difficult and sometimes impossible.

All foods contain some bacteria, although most are not pathogenic. Bacteria is used in the processing of many foods, including *Lactobacillus* for sauerkraut, *Acetobacter* for vinegar, and various yeasts for bread and beer, but many pathogenic bacteria can grow in foods at or around room temperatures. Even refrigerated foods eventually spoil, due to the psychophilic organisms that can grow at 32–40°F (0–5°C).

The solute content of food can also affect growth. For instance, the microbial cells must compete with solutes such as sodium chloride for the **available water (a_w)** in food. With the exception of *Staphylococcus aureus*, bacteria are rather poor competitors, whereas molds are excellent. Table 3-31 shows the decrease in water activity with salinity. Most infectious agents have a specific range of a_w that will support its growth. Greater solute content may not kill a bacteria, only inhibit or halt its growth. Processed foods such as canned soup tend to be very high in salt content and may require the addition of water before preparation.

However, temperature and a_w have an inverse relationship, since more heat is required to inhibit bacteria as the a_w becomes lowered. But the pH also affects growth. The interplay between

Table 3-31
Salinity and Water Activity in Food (Available Water)

Percent NaCl	Water Activity (a_w)
0.9	0.99+
1.7	0.99
3.5	0.98
7.0	0.96
10.0	0.94
13.0	0.92
16.0	0.90
22.0	0.86

these factors can be used in food preservation technology. *Clostridium botulinum* will not grow in a food with a pH below 5.0 *and* an a_w of less than 0.935, although it would grow without the two in combination. This is called the ***hurdle effect*** and is a basic concept of food processing. It requires experimentation to determine the properties of each food and the processing needed to inhibit microbial growth in it and preserve its quality.

The use of disinfectants and sanitizers on food-preparation surfaces is also important and is similar to the medical disinfection and sterilization technology previously described. The personal hygiene and training of food workers is just as important, however.

An in-depth discussion of food protection technology is available in other texts [68,71]. There are also many excellent food-safety resources available on the Internet, including the *Bad Bug Book* (Figure 3-11) published by the FDA and available at *http://vm.cfsan.fda.gove/~mow/intro.html.* This website lists the most prevalent infectious agents in food and gives a detailed description of each. The table on the onset, duration, and symptoms of food-borne illness is an excellent tool to use for the differential diagnosis of suspected food-borne illness (Figure 3-12). Other useful technical information is available through the U.S. Department of Agriculture, Food Safety and Inspection Service, at *http://www.fsis.usda.gov.*

Recent well-publicized adverse food events, such as deaths from *E coli* 0:157, *Salmonella* content in chickens, and the "new" pathogenic protozoa *Cyclospora cayetanensis* found in imported strawberries, have all heightened public interest in food safety. One example of a conjoint public and private food-safety campaign is the Fight BAC!™ program by the program Partnership for Food Safety Education (Figures 3-13 and 3-14).

Training programs and certifications for food-service professionals will expand in the future. The **Hazard Analysis Critical Control Points (HACCP)** program has expanded, and training information and data is available at *http://nal.usda.gov;fnic/foodborne/foodborn.htm.* There is very little controversy concerning the principles of food-poisoning prevention at the consumer level. The 10 basic principles are presented in Table 3-32. Employer- or company-sponsored picnics or "pitch-ins" may reduce liability and other losses due to food poisoning by posting warnings about this problem before such events.

Global Food Status. According to the Food and Agriculture Organization (FAO) of the United Nations, 25% of all global food pro-duction is lost to insect infestation, rodents, bacteria, molds, and premature germination. Food-borne bacteria are responsible for 9,000 deaths and up to 80 million cases of diarrheal illness in the United States alone. Data is less accurate globally, but diarrhea is the leading cause of infant death. The inability of nations to satisfy each other's food quarantine and health regulations is often a barrier to trade. Food laws are often misused for political agendas.

Food Irradiation. The irradiation of food was first performed in 1905, but perfected in the 1940s and 50s. Health and safety officials from 39 countries have approved the irradiation of some 40 types of foods. This technology holds great promise in addressing many long-standing and global food problems. The people of the United States are far behind most nations in their

Table 3-32
Ten Principles of Food Poisoning Prevention

1. Keep hot foods hot, and cold foods cold. Refrigerated food should be well below 40°F (5°C) and cooked food above 165°F (74°C).
2. Do grocery shopping trips last, on the way home. Pick cold and frozen foods last. Most groceries now have these items last in the market loop aisles.
3. Keep thermometers visible; and set at under 40° F (5° C) in the refrigerator and under 0° F (–18°C) in the freezer.
4. Thaw meat in the refrigerator or in water-tight bags in water, and never let it sit out (unrefrigerated) more than two hours.
5. Refrigerate leftovers immediately. Reheat them to high temperatures.
6. Keep ice chests cold on picnics and camping trips. Both have high associations with food poisonings.
7. Pay special attention to creams, custards, mayonnaise, pudding, yogurt, or any daily products left sitting out or open.
8. Cutting boards and counter tops in contact with raw foods should be cleaned with bleach and hot water to avoid cross-contamination.
9. Wash hands before and after eating or preparing meals.
10. When in doubt, throw it out!

Figure 3-11
The FDA's "Bad Bug Book" homepage on the Internet. Each underlined agent is a hypertext link to more information on that agent. (Available at *http://vm.cfsan.fda.gov/~mow/intro.html.*)

The *"Bad Bug Book"*

This handbook provides basic facts regarding foodborne pathogenic microorganisms and natural toxins. Some technical terms have been linked to the National Library of Medicine's Entrez glossary. Recent articles from Morbidity and Mortality Weekly Reports have been added to selected chapters to update the handbook with information on later outbreaks or incidents of foodborne disease. At the end of selected chapters on pathogenic microorganisms, hypertext links are included to relevant Entrez abstracts and GenBank genetic loci. A more complete description of the handbook may be found in the Preface.

PATHOGENIC BACTERIA

- Salmonella spp.
- Clostridium botulinum
- Staphylococcus aureus
- Campylobacter jejuni
- Yersinia enterocolitica and Yersinia pseudotuberculosis
- Listeria monocytogenes
- Vibrio cholerae O1
- Vibrio cholerae non-O1
- Vibrio parahaemolyticus and other vibrios
- Vibrio vulnificus
- Clostridium perfringens
- Bacillus cereus
- Aeromonas hydrophila and other spp.
- Plesiomonas shigelloides
- Shigella spp.
- Miscellaneous enterics
- Streptococcus

Enterovirulent Escherichia coli Group (EEC Group)

- Escherichia coli - enterotoxigenic (ETEC)
- Escherichia coli - enteropathogenic (EPEC)
- Escherichia coli O157:H7 enterohemorrhagic (EHEC)
- Escherichia coli - enteroinvasive (EIEC)

PARASITIC PROTOZOA and WORMS

- Giardia lamblia
- Entamoeba histolytica
- Cryptosporidium parvum
- Cyclospora cayetanensis Updated!
- Anisakis sp. and related worms
- Diphyllobothrium spp.
- Nanophyetus spp.
- Eustrongylides sp.
- Acanthamoeba and other free-living amoebae
- Ascaris lumbricoides and Trichuris trichiura

VIRUSES

- Hepatitis A virus
- Hepatitis E virus
- Rotavirus
- Norwalk virus group
- Other viral agents

NATURAL TOXINS

- Ciguatera poisoning
- Shellfish toxins (PSP, DSP, NSP, ASP)
- Scombroid
- Tetrodotoxin (Pufferfish)
- Mushroom toxins
- Aflatoxins
- Pyrrolizidine alkaloids
- Phytohaemagglutinin (Red kidney bean poisoning)
- Grayanotoxin (Honey intoxication)

APPENDICES

- Infective dose
- Epidemiology summary table
- Factors affecting microbial growth in foods

Home

Hypertext last edited: 1998-APR-06 by mow@cfsan.fda.gov

Figure 3-12
Onset duration, and symptoms of food-born illness from the FDA's "Bag Bug Book" website on the Internet. Useful in the differential diagnosis of food-related illness. (Available at *http://vm.cfsan.fda.gov/!mow/app2.html.)*

Onset, Duration, and Symptoms of Foodborne Illness

Approximate onset time to symptoms	Predominant symptoms	Associated organism or toxin
Upper gastrointestinal tract symptoms (nausea, vomiting) occur first or predominate		
Less than 1 h	Nausea, vomiting, unusual taste, burning of mouth.	Metallic salts
1-2 h	Nausea, vomiting, cyanosis, headache, dizziness, dyspnea, trembling, weakness, loss of consciousness.	Nitrites
1-6 h mean 2-4 h	Nausea, vomiting, retching, diarrhea, abdominal pain, prostration.	*Staphylococcus aureus* and its enterotoxins
8-16 h (2-4 h emesis possible)	Vomiting, abdominal cramps, diarrhea, nausea.	*Bacillus cereus*
6-24 h	Nausea, vomiting, diarrhea, thirst, dilation of pupils, collapse, coma.	Amanita species mushrooms
Sore throat and respiratory symptoms occur		
12-72 h	Sore throat, fever, nausea, vomiting, rhinorrhea, sometimes a rash.	*Streptococcus pyogenes*
2-5 days	Inflamed throat and nose, spreading grayish exudate, fever, chills, sore throat, malaise, difficulty in swallowing, edema of cervical lymph node.	*Corynebacterium diphtheriae*
Lower gastrointestinal tract symptoms (abdominal cramps, diarrhea) occur first or predominate		
2-36 h, mean 6-12 h	Abdominal cramps, diarrhea, putrefactive diarrhea associated with *C. perfringens*, sometimes nausea and vomiting.	*Clostridium perfringens, Bacillus cereus, Streptococcus faecalis, S. faecium*
12-74 h, mean 18-36 h	Abdominal cramps, diarrhea, vomiting, fever, chills, malaise, nausea, headache, possible. Sometimes bloody or mucoid diarrhea, cutaneous lesions associated with V. vulnificus. Yersinia enterocolitica mimics flu and acute appendicitis.	*Salmonella* species (including *arizonae*), *Shigella*, enteropathogenic *Escherichia coli*, other *Enterobacteriacae Vibrio parahaemolyticus, Yersinia enterocolitica, Pseudomonas aeruginosa* (?),*Aeromonas hydrophila, Plesiomonas shigelloides, Campylobacter jejuni, Vibrio cholerae* (O1 and non-O1) *V.vulnificus, V. fluvialis*
3-5 days	Diarrhea, fever, vomiting abdominal pain, respiratory symptoms.	Enteric viruses
1-6 weeks	Mucoid diarrhea (fatty stools) abdominal pain, weight loss.	*Giardia lamblia*
1 to several weeks	Abdominal pain, diarrhea, constipation, headache, drowsiness, ulcers, variable -- often asymptomatic.	*Entamoeba histolytica*
3-6 months	Nervousness, insomnia, hunger pains, anorexia, weight loss, abdominal pain, sometimes gastroenteritis.	*Taenia saginata, T. solium*
Neurological symptoms (visual disturbances, vertigo, tingling, paralysis) occur		
Less than 1 h	*** SEE GASTROINTESTINAL AND/OR NEUROLOGIC SYMPTOMS (Shellfish Toxins) (this Appendix)	Shellfish toxin
	Gastroenteritis, nervousness, blurred vision, chest pain, cyanosis, twitching, convulsions.	Organic phosphate
	Excessive salivation, perspiration, gastroenteritis, irregular pulse, pupils constricted, asthmatic breathing.	Muscaria-type mushrooms
	Tingling and numbness, dizziness, pallor, gastro- hemmorrhage, and desquamation of skin, fixed eyes, loss of reflexes, twitching, paralysis.	Tetradon (tetrodotoxin) toxin
1-6 h	Tingling and numbness, gastroenteritis, dizziness, dry mouth, muscular aches, dilated pupils, blurred vision, paralysis.	Ciguatera toxin
	Nausea, vomiting, tingling, dizziness,	Chlorinated hydrocarbons

	weakness, anorexia, weight loss, confusion.	
2 h to 6 days, usually 12-36 h	Vertigo, double or blurred vision, loss of reflex to light, difficulty in swallowing. speaking, and breathing, dry mouth, weakness, respiratory paralysis.	*Clostridium botulinum* and its neurotoxins
More than 72 h	Numbness, weakness of legs, spastic paralysis, impairment of vision, blindness, coma.	Organic mercury
	Gastroenteritis, leg pain, ungainly high-stepping gait, foot and wrist drop.	Triorthocresyl phosphate
Allergic symptoms (facial flushing, itching) occur		
Less than 1 h	Headache, dizziness, nausea, vomiting, peppery taste, burning of throat, facial swelling and flushing, stomach pain, itching of skin.	Histamine (scombroid)
	Numbness around mouth, tingling sensation, flushing, dizziness, headache, nausea.	Monosodium glutamate
	Flushing, sensation of warmth, itching, abdominal pain, puffing of face and knees.	Nicotinic acid
Generalized infection symptoms (fever, chills, malaise, prostration, aches, swollen lymph nodes) occur		
4-28 days, mean 9 days	Gastroenteritis, fever, edema about eyes, perspiration, muscular pain, chills, prostration, labored breathing.	*Trichinella spiralis*
7-28 days, mean 14 days	Malaise, headache, fever, cough, nausea, vomiting, constipation, abdominal pain, chills, rose spots, bloody stools.	*Salmonella typhi*
10-13 days	Fever, headache, myalgia, rash.	*Toxoplasma gondii*
10-50 days, mean 25-30 days	Fever, malaise, lassitude, anorexia, nausea, abdominal pain, jaundice.	Etiological agent not yet isolated -- probably viral
Varying periods (depends on specific illness)	Fever, chills, head- or joint ache, prostration, malaise, swollen lymph nodes, and other specific symptoms of disease in question.	*Bacillus anthracis, Brucella melitensis, B. abortus, B. suis, Coxiella burnetii, Francisella tularensis, Listeria monocytogenes, Mycobacterium tuberculosis, Mycobacterium* species, *Pasteurella multocid*, *Streptobacillus moniliformis, Campylobacter jejuni, Leptospira* species.
Gastrointestinal and/or Neurologic Symptoms - (Shellfish Toxins)		
0.5 to 2 h	Tingling, burning, numbness, drowsiness, incoherent speech, respiratory paralysis	Paralytic Shellfish Poisoning (PSP) (saxitoxins)
2-5 min to 3-4 h	Reversal of hot and cold sensation, tingling; numbness of lips, tongue & throat; muscle aches, dizziness, diarrhea, vomiting	Neurotoxic Shellfish Poisonir (NSP) (brevetoxins)
30 min to 2-3 h	Nausea, vomiting, diarrhea, abdominal pain, chills, fever	Diarrheic Shellfish Poisoning (DSP) (dinophysis toxin, okadaic acid, pectenotoxin, yessotoxin)
24 h (gastrointestinal) to 48 h (neurologic)	Vomiting, diarrhea, abdominal pain, confusion, memory loss, disorientation, seizure, coma	Amnesic Shellfish Poisoning (ASP) (domoic acid)

January

mow@cfsan.fda.gov

Figure 3-13
Four general principles for the consumer to avoid cross-contamination of food. (From: Fight-Bac™ Campaign of the Partnership for Food Safety Education.)

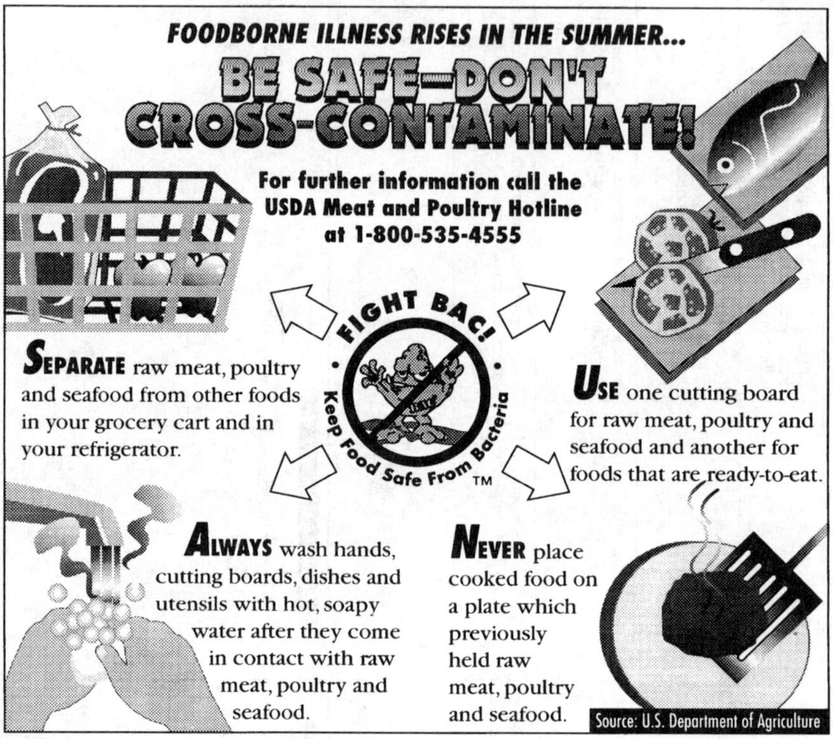
FOODBORNE ILLNESS RISES IN THE SUMMER...
BE SAFE—DON'T CROSS-CONTAMINATE!
For further information call the USDA Meat and Poultry Hotline at 1-800-535-4555
FIGHT BAC!
Keep Food Safe From Bacteria
TM
SEPARATE raw meat, poultry and seafood from other foods in your grocery cart and in your refrigerator.
USE one cutting board for raw meat, poultry and seafood and another for foods that are ready-to-eat.
ALWAYS wash hands, cutting boards, dishes and utensils with hot, soapy water after they come in contact with raw meat, poultry and seafood.
NEVER place cooked food on a plate which previously held raw meat, poultry and seafood.
Source: U.S. Department of Agriculture

acceptance of irradiated products because of myths and fears regarding nuclear technology. The first international acceptance was the 1983 **Codex Alimentarius Commission** issued by a joint expert committee of the FAO, the World Health Organization, and the International Atomic Energy Agency [72]. The Codex declared that irradiation up to 10 kiloGrays (1,000 rads) posed no toxologic, nutritional, or microbiologic hazards and that no further testing was needed.

Most irradiation of food employs gamma rays and the cobalt-60 radioisotope. Cobalt-60 is produced by neutron bombardment of cobalt-59 and then is double encapsulated into "pencils" for use at irradiation plants. It has a half-life of only 5.3 years. No other source of radiation has proved as economical, safe, or effective. The food is passed by conveyor belts through the energy field; dosage, belt speed, and energy are specific for each food. The food receives energy but does not itself become radioactive. The main purpose of food irradiation is to kill bacteria that may be in a growth cycle. DNA is far more sensitive to radiation energy than nutrients such as nucleoproteins, carbohydrates, fats, enzymes, and vitamins. Even damage of only a few percent of bacterial DNA will stop its replication. Irradiation with dosages of up to 10 kGy is called ***radurization*** or ***radicidation*** and is the upper limit currently approved. This dosage is sufficient to kill *Salmonella*, *Campylobacter*, *Bacillus cereus*, *Staphylococcus aureus*, fungi, and protozoa cysts. *Clostridium botulinum* may survive, but the number of organisms is reduced and the pathogen becomes more sensitive to heat, pH, and salt. Complete sterilization using much higher doses is called ***radappertization***.

Irradiation of food produces **radiolytic products**. These are mostly natural metabolites such as acetaldehyde, carbon dioxide, glucose, peroxide, and formic acid. They are also naturally present in foods and may be generated by heat processing or cooking. Irradiation causes the formation of unstable and reactive free radicals but in less volume than that resulting from toasting, frying, and freeze drying [73]. In any case, the free radicals are inactivated by liquids such as saliva. No mutagenic effects have been found in animals fed heavily irradiated food.

Food irradiation is not meant to substitute for **good manufacturing practices (GMPs)**. Food is still subject to surface contamination after treatment, and irradiation cannot make spoiled or bad food into good food. Furthermore, radiation does not kill all preformed bacterial toxins nor all viruses.

For most foods, the color and odor produced by bacteria are the warnings of spoilage. However, studies by European and Scandinavian countries have shown no increased risk of food spoilage after bacteria has been irradiated. Note that pasteurization, freezing, and preservatives used in food processing also destroy some bacteria. Although the shelf life of produce may be prolonged, the look and smell of spoilage is the same in irradiated food as that in nonirradiated food. Other theoretic advantages of food irradiation are less dependence on insecticides, fumigants, preservatives, or other pollutants of food and lower energy costs for refrigeration. In reality, however, these methods of control are still used in conjunction with irradiation.

Control of the Animate Reservoir

ARTHROPOD CONTROL. The largest attempts to control animate vectors of infectious agents (viruses, parasites, and rickettsia) in their natural environment has involved arthropods. Although some good control of arthropod-transmitted diseases has occurred, manmade changes in the environment or wars often promote their resurgence. Arthropods that are associated with human diseases include fleas, flies, lice, mites, roaches, mosquitoes, and ticks. Flies and roaches can mechanically transmit infectious organisms, especially enteric fecal-oral pathogens such as typhoid, shigella, and cholera.

Most of the science of controlling arthropods is related to their ranges, climactic requirements and preferences, geologic boundaries, and seasons. Routine surveillance and surveys of mosquito populations are conducted in most areas by trained and licensed public employees or contractors. Studies of larval samples from artificial or still bodies of water are also conducted. Various traps are available for capturing adult mosquitoes. Arthropod **vector abundance** is measured several ways, such as the number of mosquitoes caught per **light-trap night**. Measured overabundance of a specific vector species may predict human outbreaks of the disease it causes.

Larvicides, fogging units, or mists are used in specific areas of **harborage** of mosquitoes, and these efforts are increased when populations and thus the risk for transmission of infection increases. However, these **chemical controls** are the least preferred because of environmental concerns and the development of resistance to the chemicals.

Other controls have included **biologic controls**, such as introducing arthropod parasites, natural insect predators, and minnow fish to eat larva. Building reservoirs and ditches that maintain some movement of water (**mechanical control**) to prevent stagnation is the best single prevention, as larvae must have still water to complete their life cycle. Migrating birds play a role in distributing viruses associated with mosquitoes and encephalitis. Only a few species of birds suffer illness from mosquito bites and viremia. Trying to control the arboviruses in their wild primary host would prove most difficult.

Human vaccines have been developed for only a few of the arthropod-vector diseases, but horses are routinely immunized for Venezuela (VEE), eastern (EEE), and western (WEE) equine encephalitis. The majority of arthropod-borne viral infections do not have vaccines nor effective therapies. Other forms of control and preventions of arthropod-associated infections are covered in the chapters of the text on malaria (Chapter 25), meningitis (Chapter 23), and travel (Chapters 27–31).

RODENT CONTROL. **Murine rodents** are those that live and feed in the fringes of the human habitat—the house mouse, roof rat, and Norway rat. Wild rodents are the principal hosts of many tick (larval and nymphal stages) diseases, including some forms of tick-borne encephalitis and other illnesses (Kayasnur Forest, Crimean-Congo hemorrhagic fever, Powassan, and Colorado tick fever). Adult ticks more often bite large animals, including humans. Rodents can

Figure 3-14
Front and back side of brochure on the four simple steps to food safety.
(From: Fight-Bac™ Campaign of the Partnership for Food Safety Education.)

Be a BAC Fighter

Although an invisible enemy may be in your kitchen, you have four powerful tools to *Fight BAC!*™ washing hands and surfaces often, avoiding cross-contamination, cooking to proper temperatures, and refrigerating promptly. So, be a BAC Fighter and make the meals and snacks from your kitchen as safe as possible.

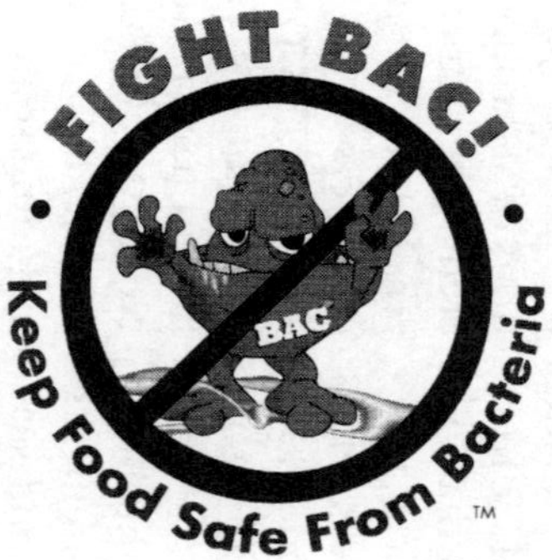
FIGHT BAC!
Keep Food Safe From Bacteria
BAC
TM

For More Information About Safe Food Handling and Preparation

USDA's Meat and Poultry Hotline
1-800-535-4555

FDA's Food Information and Seafood Hotline
1-800-332-4010

Partnership for Food Safety Education Web Site
www.fightbac.org

Or contact your local cooperative extension office.

Apply the Heat...and *Fight BAC!*™

Cooking food to the proper temperature kills harmful bacteria. So *Fight BAC!*™ by thoroughly cooking your food as follows:

Raw Food	Internal Temperature
Ground Products	
Hamburger	160°F
Beef, veal, lamb, pork	160°F
Chicken, turkey	165°F
Beef, Veal, Lamb	
Roasts & Steaks	
medium-rare	145°F
medium	160°F
well-done	170°F
Pork	
Chops, roasts, ribs	
medium	160°F
well-done	170°F
Ham, fresh	160°F
Sausage, fresh	160°F
Poultry	
Chicken, whole & pieces	180°F
Duck	180°F
Turkey (*unstuffed*)	180°F
Whole	180°F
Breast	170°F
Dark meat	180°F
Stuffing (cooked separately)	165°F
Eggs	
Fried, poached	*Yolk & white are firm*
Casseroles	160°F
Sauces, custards	160°F

This chart has been adapted for home use and is consistent with consumer guidelines from the U.S. Department of Agriculture (USDA) and U.S. Food & Drug Administration (FDA).

PARTNERSHIP FOR FOOD SAFETY EDUCATION ™

Fight BAC!™

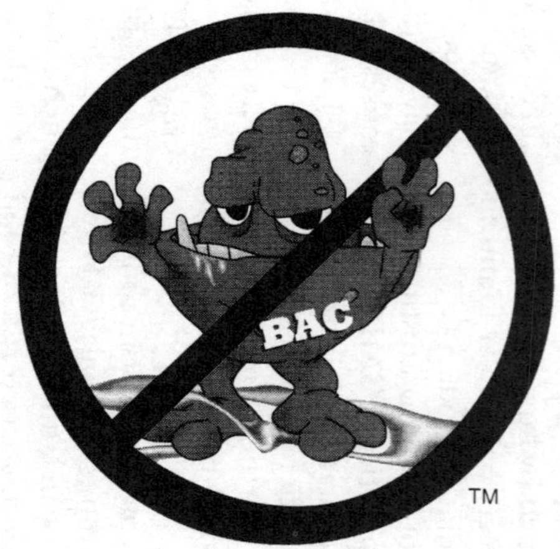
BAC
TM

Four Simple Steps to Food Safety

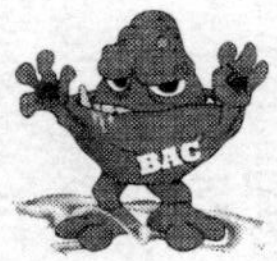

Right now, there may be an invisible enemy ready to strike. He's called BAC (bacteria) and he can make you and those you care about sick. In fact, even though you can't see BAC — or smell him, or feel him — he and millions more like him may have already invaded the food you eat.

But you have the power to *Fight BAC!*™ and to keep your food safe from harmful bacteria. It's as easy as following these four simple steps:

Clean: Wash hands and surfaces often

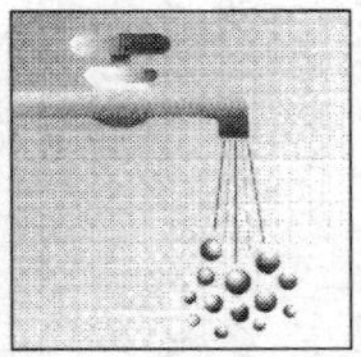

Bacteria can spread throughout the kitchen and get onto cutting boards, utensils, sponges and counter tops. Here's how to *Fight BAC!*™:

- Wash your hands with hot soapy water before handling food and after using the bathroom, changing diapers and handling pets.
- Wash your cutting boards, dishes, utensils and counter tops with hot soapy water after preparing each food item and before you go on to the next food.
- Use plastic or other non-porous cutting boards. These boards should be run through the dishwasher — or washed in hot soapy water — after use.
- Consider using paper towels to clean up kitchen surfaces. If you use cloth towels, wash them often in the hot cycle of your washing machine.

Separate: Don't cross-contaminate

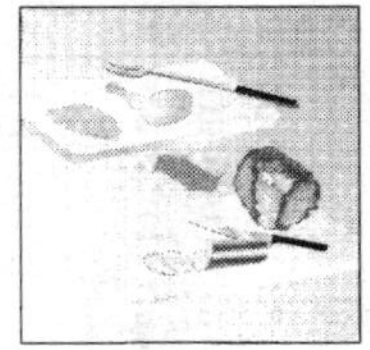

Cross-contamination is the scientific word for how bacteria can be spread from one food product to another. This is especially true when handling raw meat, poultry and seafood, so keep these foods and their juices away from ready-to-eat foods. Here's how to *Fight BAC!*™:

- Separate raw meat, poultry and seafood from other foods in your grocery shopping cart and in your refrigerator.
- If possible, use a different cutting board for raw meat products.
- Always wash hands, cutting boards, dishes and utensils with hot soapy water after they come in contact with raw meat, poultry and seafood.
- Never place cooked food on a plate which previously held raw meat, poultry and seafood.

Cook: Cook to proper temperatures

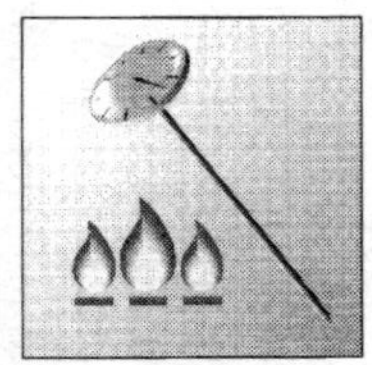

Food safety experts agree that foods are properly cooked when they are heated for a long enough time and at a high enough temperature to kill the harmful bacteria that cause foodborne illness. The best way to *Fight BAC!*™ is to:

- Use a clean thermometer, which measures the internal temperature of cooked foods, to make sure meat, poultry, casseroles and other foods are cooked all the way through.
- Cook roasts and steaks to at least 145°F. Whole poultry should be cooked to 180°F for doneness.
- Cook ground beef, where bacteria can spread during processing, to at least 160°F. Information from the Centers for Disease Control and Prevention (CDC) link eating undercooked, pink ground beef with a higher risk of illness. If a thermometer is not available, do not eat ground beef that is still pink inside.
- Cook eggs until the yolk and white are firm. Don't use recipes in which eggs remain raw or only partially cooked.
- Fish should be opaque and flake easily with a fork.
- When cooking in a microwave oven, make sure there are no cold spots in food where bacteria can survive . For best results, cover food, stir and rotate for even cooking. If there is no turntable, rotate the dish by hand once or twice during cooking.
- Bring sauces, soups and gravy to a boil when reheating. Heat other leftovers thoroughly to at least 165°F.

Chill: Refrigerate promptly

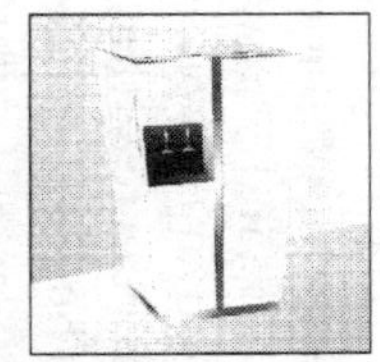

Refrigerate foods quickly because cold temperatures keep harmful bacteria from growing and multiplying. So, set your refrigerator no higher than 40°F and the freezer unit at 0°F. Check these temperatures occasionally with an appliance thermometer. Then, *Fight BAC!*™ by following these steps:

- Refrigerate or freeze perishables, prepared foods and leftovers within two hours or sooner.
- Never defrost food at room temperature. Thaw food in the refrigerator, under cold running water or in the microwave. Marinate foods in the refrigerator.
- Divide large amounts of leftovers into small, shallow containers for quick cooling in the refrigerator.
- Don't pack the refrigerator. Cool air must circulate to keep food safe.

serve as reservoirs for *Hantavirus* and *Leptospires*, transmitting infection through their dried urine and feces. Fortunately, rodents have a rather limited. local range and predictable environment. Methods of rodent control include isolation, substitution, treatment, shielding, and prevention. Prevention involves the removal of food sources, places of harborage, and adequate maintenance. It often involves training of humans to control rodents' food stores and wastes, including pet foods. Structural integrity and the removal of debris or supplies that may serve as harborage areas for rodents should be part of the eradication process and the ongoing preventive maintenance. Community and local resident education is essential to ongoing prevention in residential areas.

The safest rodent poisons are the anticoagulants. They take several days to work, and the rodents do not learn to associate the bait with illness. Some rodenticides are too toxic to be used inside. In areas where the presence of *Hantavirus* is suspected, cleanup should be done with personal protective equipment (PPE), including HEPA-filter respirators, disposable coveralls, and shoe covers. All PPE should be decontaminated or destroyed after use.

ZOONOSIS CONTROL. Most animals on Earth have their own pathogenic infectious agents. Relatively few can also infect humans. One disease—brucellosis—can serve as an excellent, nearly ideal, model for the control of zoonotic diseases. Brucellosis (also known as *Mediterranean*, *Malta*, or *undulant fever*) is a complex of diseases caused by small gram-negative rods that infect a wide range of domestic and wild mammals. Besides the wide range of animals, it can infect a wide range of tissues and organs through a wide range of portals of entry, portals of exit, and modes of transmission. The differential diagnosis for *Brucella* is further complicated by its relatively long and variable incubation period, range of symptoms, and spontaneous relapses and remissions. Doubtless, thousands of human cases remain undiagnosed and treated around the world.

Brucella species include *B abortus* (cattle), *B suis* (swine), *B canis* (cats and dogs), and *B melitensis* (sheep and goats). Besides animal-to-animal sexual and other routes of transmission, the pathogen is transmitted between domestic and wild animals (cattle, caribou, dogs, and coyotes). Humans may be infected by handling infected tissues, aborted fetuses and placentas, blood, urine, discharges, and other body fluids as well as by ingestion of contaminated milk or cheese. There is a high association of the infection with occupations that involve handling animals or animal products and with hunting, in which dead game is handled. The bacteriologist Alice Evans, who did most of the pioneering studies of the disease, was occupationally infected and suffered brucellosis relapses for 20 years. Humans can contract the infection by ingestion, mucous membrane or sexual organ contact, the blood-borne route, and by minor percutaneous injuries. Hundreds of clinical laboratory workers were occupationally infected before the use of biologic safety cabinets was introduced, suggesting aerosol transmission as well. Completing brucellosis's claim to being the "perfect" zoonotic disease is the fact that it can remain viable and infectious in the environment (soil) up to 125 days and in carcasses for 135 days.

Brucellosis also serves as a superb model for infection control at the agent, host, environment, and transmission levels. Where research, regulation, and other intervention efforts have been implemented, the disease has become rare. Less than 100 cases occur in the United States each year. Some of the methods and principles of control for brucellosis are presented in Table 3-33. Brucellosis should rank high in the differential diagnosis for any fever of unknown origin in a worker with occupational risks for the disease.

Levels of Control for Zoonotic Diseases. Most nations have their own restrictions and quarantine laws for handling animal species. Many have specific holding areas and mandatory inspections. Regulations may be imposed to protect local livestock, pets, and native species from infectious agents. All municipalities in the United States have rabies vaccination laws for pets (Chapter 20).

HIGH-TECHNOLOGY APPLICATIONS FOR ANIMATE RESERVOIR CONTROL. The National Aeronautics and Space Administration (NASA) and the National Institute of Allergy and Infectious Diseases (NIAID) are cooperatively funding research grants for the development of remote sensing and geographic information

Table 3-33
Brucellosis as an Example of Integrated Controls

1. Eradication of the agent
   - By antibiotics (tetracycline, streptomycin, rifampin) at the level of the human host or the animal host after definitive or presumed diagnosis.
   - By laws requiring pasteurization, of the animal body fluid known as milk.
2. Eradication of the host(s):
   - By slaughtering the infected host herd (swine or cattle).
3. Control of the environment
   - By establishing and enforcing aggressive control laws, the disease is eliminated from the host and eventually from the environment (i.e., placental or body fluid contamination of the pasture's soil is eliminated after a four-month quarantine of the unused pasture). This may be done by fencing (a barrier or a containment).
   - By totally eliminating the disease from the environment through the use of administrative controls and regulation (e.g., those of the Scandinavian countries).
4. Control of transmission
   - By immunizing domestic animals and thus making them nonsusceptible if exposed to soil, wild animals, or infected cohorts. An adequate vaccine does not exist for humans.
   - By use of personal protective equipment (e.g., long-arm rubber gloves while delivering cattle).
   - By education. Training animal and agricultural workers on the risks for the disease and how to prevent transmission. Also by basic training of physicians and veterinarians about the disease and how to recognize cases.

system (RS/GIS) technologies to control infectious diseases [75]. The purpose is to predict future disease outbreaks and identify areas where specific control programs should be concentrated.

A study conducted by Notre Dame and the University of Kentucky is using aerial multi-spectral videography to detect electromagnetic radiation from ground objects in the Ohio Valley. Known tire dumps and their infrared "fingerprint" are used to detect the location of other tire dumps from aerial studies. This technology can also be used to estimate the size of dumps, which can be up to 50,000,000 tires in size. Water remaining in tires serves as a breeding ground for mosquitoes. Tire dumps will pose several risks for clean-up workers when they are eventually abated.

University of Maryland researchers are using satellites to study ocean height, temperature, and phytoplankton and zooplankton blooms in the Indian Ocean shores off India and Bangladesh. These blooms can harbor cholera, and measurable variables of the blooms have been correlating with outbreaks. Other RS/GIS grantees include [75]:

- Yale grantees' study of specific vegetation and landscape patterns in residential Westchester County, New York, the major hot spot of tick-borne Lyme disease.
- Studies of hantavirus host (rodent) habitats in the Southwest.
- Studies of Brazilian environmental factors that correlate with leishmaniasis and schistosomiasis.
- Studies of the distribution of helminthic diseases in China.
- Studies of the epidemiology of malaria in Mali.

CONTROLLING HOST RESPONSE

Controlling the human host response to infectious disease is the domain of clinical medicine. Unfortunately, infectious disease still represents a large proportion of the practice of medicine. Specific antimicrobial treatment and prophylaxis is discussed in other chapters, and immunizations are covered in Chapter 5.

Wellness and Susceptibility

Two of the most rapidly expanding fields of interest and knowledge in clinical medicine are the human immune system and the effects of physical activity. The 1996 release of the Surgeon General's Report on Physical Activity and Health summarizes, by organ system, the positive relationship between activity and health [76]. The effects of various forms of stress on the human immune system are unrefutable. A Medline search for review articles associating stress with immunity published just in the English language since 1990 retrieves 50 reviews. These reviews average over 98 references each. Some of the more interesting are listed as recommended readings. Every known part of the human immune-system response is significantly affected by stress. The veterinary literature confirms the same associations in animals studies. The improved life span of AIDS patients may in part be due to increased social acceptance of the disease.

This is not surprising to experienced corporate-based occupational health practitioners. Workplace stressors such as mandatory overtime, layoffs, management changes, mergers, and even the rumors of these things impact absenteeism and illness due to infectious diseases. These adverse health effects are too often dismissed as "blue flu," "mass psychogenic illness," or well-disguised job actions. The association between workplace stress and immunity has been inadequately studied.

The better studies of the relationship between stressors and infectious diseases have come from college health services. A large serial study of one class of cadets attending the U.S. Military Academy at West Point correlated many factors with the risk of development of clinically apparent infectious mononucleosis in cadets first infected with Epstein-Barr viruses [77]. Illness was significantly predicted to occur in cadets who had overachieving fathers, strong personal motivation and commitment to, and identification with, a military career, coupled with a relatively poor academic performance. The study corrected for all other socioeconomic and demographic data.

CONTROLLING TRANSMISSION: INTERRUPTION

The bugs are many; your doors and windows are few.
—Daymon Evans (*I just made it up*)

Despite the thousands of known infectious agents, contaminating almost every square inch of the Earth, and with essentially every multicellular organism on life serving as a host, humans can be protected by adherence to a few basic principles. Transmission is the weakest point in the epidemiologic triad and is broken by any blockage of the portal of entry, the portal of exit, or another break in the transmission of viable infectious agents into a susceptible host or from an infecting host. Controlling the agent within the host or environment is much more difficult than controlling the transmission.

Transporting Infectious Agents

Several agencies regulate the movement of infectious agents and vectors of human disease. These include the Public Health Service Foreign Quarantine regulations and the Department of Transportation. The U.S. Department of Agriculture regulates the importation and interstate shipment of animal pathogens and prohibits the importation, possession, or use of certain exotic animal disease agents that pose a serious disease threat to domestic livestock and poultry. Figure 3-15 shows the required packing and labeling of etiologic agents [78].

Models of Transmission Control

This chapter presents two models for preventing transmission of infection, although both are covered elsewhere in the text. These models reflect the principles of **containment** and **isolation**, as demonstrated and practiced by **laboratory biosafety levels (BSL)** [79] and the CDC's **hospital isolation categories** [80]. Both sets of principles govern the safety of workers as well as the general public.

Containment (Biosafety). The best model for the containment (rather than destruction) of infectious agents is the microbiology laboratory and shipping laws regarding infectious agents. **Primary containment** is the protection of personnel and their immediate environment from exposure to infectious agents. **Secondary containment** is the protection of the environment external to the laboratory. The three elements of laboratory containment of infectious agents are (1) laboratory practice and technique, (2) safety equipment, and (3) facility designs. Each is covered in detail in Chapter 33 on laboratory workers.

Biosafety is defined as the application of specific safety protocols to the handling of biologic risks, both specimens of infectious agents and animals that may be infected. The full force of biosafety levels include a combination of engineering controls, administrative controls, work practices and procedures and, on occasion, medical interventions.

All infectious agents are classified by risk into **biosafety levels** 1 through 4 (BSL 1–4) for microbiologic and biomedical laboratories. Four categories of risk also are used for the handling of animals (ABSL 1–4) [81]. The principal piece of safety equipment in the laboratory is the **biologic safety cabinet (BSC)**; the cabinet serves

Figure 3-15
Proper biosafety packaging and labeling of an etiologic agent for transport. (Available at *http://www.cdc.gov/od/ohs/biosfty/bmbl/fig4.gif.*)

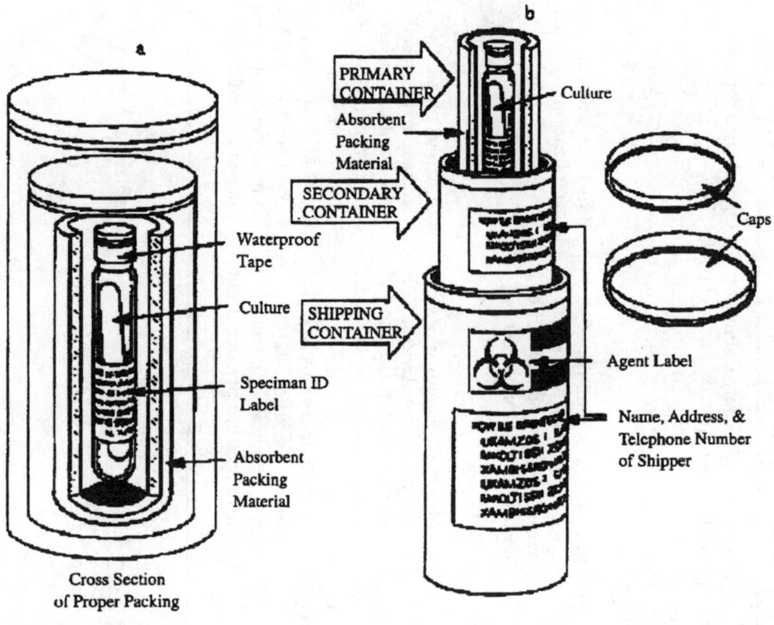

as an excellent model for the prevention of all types of transmission. These cabinets are the ultimate invention for local source-control, or containment, techniques. These techniques include:

- *Air transmission* by the use of controlled directional flow away from workers' respiratory portals of entry and through HEPA filtration to be exhausted outside, BSCs utilize negative pressure as local source control.
- *Direct transmission* by the use of solid and see-through barriers that prevent exposure of workers' skin or mucous membranes to splashes or aerosolization. The surfaces are nonporous and can be easily cleaned. Direct transmission also requires various levels of personal protective equipment (e.g., gloves, goggles, gowns).

BSCs are governed by regular inspection and maintenance schedules. Class-1 BSCs provide a basic barrier as well as splash protection and air flow in the front and out of the top. Class-1 BSCs are not intended to protect the specimen or product. Levels 2, 3, and 4 are intended to protect the product/specimen and contain several subclasses, which are differentiated by design and air flow pattern. Class 3 is gas-sealed or air-tight and exhausts externally through at least two HEPA filters.

Standard safe-laboratory practices and behavior are learned in training, which helps to prevent accidental transmission by the oral, mucous membrane, or percutaneous routes. Protocols also exist for the disposal of cultures and other laboratory wastes in the secondary containment program. The levels of biosafety for infectious agents are presented in Table 3-34 and are covered in more detail in Chapter 33. Only some viruses currently fall under BSL-4; these are listed in Table 3-35.

Isolation and Quarantine. Isolation and quarantine are not synonymous. **Quarantine** is the restriction of the activities or habitat of well persons or animals (i.e., contacts) who have been exposed to a communicable agent. Quarantine should be for no longer than the maximum known period of incubation or infectivity of the specific pathogen. The purpose of quarantine is to protect the well and susceptible.

There are quarantine laws for immigrants and imported animals in most countries. Authority

Table 3-34
Summary of Biosafety Levels (BSLs)

	Biosafety Levels (BSLs) for Infectious Agents			
BSL	**Agents**	**Practices**	**Safety Equipment (Primary Barriers)**	**Facilities (Secondary Barriers)**
1	Not known to cause disease in healthy adults	Standard microbiologic practices (SMP): Wash hands before/after; no eat, drink, smoke, or cosmetics; no mouth pipetting; clean surfaces; splash spill precautions; biohazard disposal.	None. Biologic Safety Cabinet (BSC) not required.	Open Bench top sink.
2	Associated with human disease, a hazard of auto-inoculation, ingestion, or mucous membrane exposure	SMP plus "Limited Access, Biohazard" signage, sharps precautions, biosafety manual (BSM) defining needed water decontamination or medical surveillance.	BSC 1 or 2, containment of all devices with potential splash or aerosolizing capacity. PPEs of lab coats, gloves, face protection.	BSL 1 plus autoclave or other sterilization available.
3	Indigenous or exotic agents with potential for aerosol transmission; disease may have serious or lethal consequences	BSL 2 plus "Controlled Access"; decontamination of all waste and clothing before laundering; baseline serology on worker.	BSC 1 or 2, all manipulations done with containment devices. PPE: protective lab clothing, gloves, respiratory protection as needed.	BSL 2 plus physical separation from access corridors; self-closing double doors; exhausted air (not recirculated). Negative airflow into laboratory.
4	Dangerous/exotic agents that pose high risk of life-threatening disease. Aerosol-transmitted lab infections or related agents with unknown risk of transmission.	BSL 3 plus clothing change before entering; shower on exit. All material decontaminated on exit from facility.	All primary barriers plus all procedures in a BSC 3, or ½ with full-body air-supplied positive-pressure personnel suit.	BSL 3 plus separate building, or isolated zone. Dedicated supply/exhaust vacuum and decontaminated systems.

Vertebrate Animal Biosafety Levels (ABLSs) for Infectious Agents

BSL	Agents	Practices	Safety Equipment (Primary Barriers)	Facilities (Secondary Barriers)
1	Not known to cause disease in healthy human adults	Standard animal care and management practices, including appropriate medical surveillance programs.	As required for normal care of each species.	Standard animal facility nonrecirculation of exhausted air; directional air flow recommended.
2	Associated with human disease. Hazard: ingestion, percutaneous and mucous membrane exposure	ABSL-1 practices, limited access; biohazard warning signs; sharps precautions; biosafety manual; decontamination of all infectious wastes and of animal cages prior to washing.	ABSL-1 equipment, primary barriers; containment equipment appropriate for animal species; PPE: lab coats, gloves, face and respiratory protection as required.	ABSL-1 facility plus autoclave available; hand-washing sink available in the animal room.
3	Indigenous or exotic agents with potential for aerosol transmission; disease may have serious health effects	ABSL-2 practices, controlled access; decontamination of clothing before laundering; cages decontaminated before bedding removed; disinfectant foot bath as needed.	ABSL-2 equipment, containment equipment for housing animals and cage dumping, class $\frac{1}{2}$ BSCs for procedures (inoculation, necropsy) that may >infectious aerosols. PPEs: appropriate respiratory protection.	ABSL-2, facility, physical separation from access corridors; self-closing double doors, access sealed penetration; sealed windows autoclave available in facility.
4	Dangerous/exotic agents that pose high risk of life-threatening disease; aerosol transmission, or related agents with unknown risk of transmission	ABSL-3 practices, entrance through change room where personal clothing removed and lab clothing on. Shower on exiting, all water decontaminated before removal from facility.	ABSL-3 equipment, maximum containment equipment (i.e., class 3 BSC or partial containment equipment with combination with full-body air-supplied positive pressure suit used for all procedures and activities.	ABSL-3 facility, separate building or isolated zone; dedicated supply/exhaust zone; vacuum and decontamination systems. Floor drains with traps and disinfectant. Windows sealed.

Table 3-35
Infectious Agents Requiring Biosafety Level-4 Containment

Bacteria
None
Fungi
None
Parasites
None
Viruses
Arenaviridae
Lassa, Junin, Machupo, Sabia, Guanarto
Bunyaviridae[a]
Genus *Nairovirus*: Crimean-Congo hemorrhagic fever
Filoviridae
Ebola
Marburg
Flaviviridae[a]
Tick-borne encephalitis complex
Russian spring-summer encephalitis
Kyasanur Forest
Omsk hemorrhagic fever
Herpesviridae
Alphaherpesviridae
Herpes simplex virus
Herpes B (monkey, simian)
Poxviridae
Orthopoxivirus
Variola
Monkeypox

[a] Arthropod-borne viruses.

to place U.S. citizens in strict or complete quarantine is left to the states. Forty-two states permit the involuntary commitment of tuberculosis patients to treatment facilities [82]. U.S. citizens are very rarely involuntarily confined. However, workers may be the subjects of "modified quarantine" from their workplace to protect patients in health care facilities. Terms such as "furlough," "reassignment," or "leave of absence" are used as synonyms for "modified quarantine" in these guidelines. An example is the removal of a health care worker with known or possible susceptibility to varicella from days 10 to 21 after an exposure or removal of a food service worker with hepatitis A (HAV) until one week after jaundice has subsided [8]. With the varicella and HAV vaccines now available, such removal should occur less frequently.

HISTORY OF HOSPITAL ISOLATION. The first recommendations for hospital isolation precautions were published in 1877 and ultimately resulted in special infectious disease hospitals. But nosocomial infections continued to occur because patients were not segregated by disease. By 1910, some aseptic practices were developed and the "cubicle," or multi-bed wards, were built to replace single open rooms in hospitals. This crude isolation system was called *barrier nursing*. It was not until the 1950s and '60s that infectious disease hospitals and tuberculosis sanitoriums closed. Acute care hospitals began developing isolation wards and rooms.

The first official manual of isolation precautions was published by the CDC in 1970 [83] and was revised for the first time in 1975 [84]. There were seven categories based on the existing knowledge of transmission. These were Strict Isolation, Respiratory Isolation, Protective ("reverse") Isolation, Enteric Precautions, Wound and Skin Precautions, Discharge Precautions, and Blood Precautions. Color-coded stickers and signage were made for each category. However, the system did not protect against the development of nosocomial infections, nor was the effectiveness of the system empirically studied.

The next guidelines, written by interdisciplinary panels of experts, were published in 1983 [85]. They allowed hospital infection control committees to have some flexibility and clinicians to customize precautions to the specific disease and the patient. Protective Isolation was deleted because of lack of efficacy. Blood Precautions were expanded to include other "body fluids." There were four categories of Isolation (Strict, Contact, Respiratory, and Tuberculosis/AFB) and three categories of Precautions (Enteric, Drainage/Secretion, and Blood and Body Fluid). Many questions and controversies persisted regarding diseases such as measles, rubella, respiratory syncytial virus, and influenza. All of these were inadequately isolated by the respiratory precautions.

Many addenda and other guidelines were published for specific diseases, including HIV "**Universal Precautions (UP)**" (1985), hemorrhagic fever precautions (1988), parvovirus B-19 precautions (1989), and tuberculosis precautions (1990, 1993, 1994). Some nongovernment-affiliated experts initiated a **Body Substance Isolation (BSI)** system that was adopted by many hospitals. It had the advantages of both ease and implementation but the disadvantage of being weak on precautions for airborne diseases, and it did not recommend routine hand washing if gloves had been worn. Thus, the OSHA Bloodborne Pathogen standard was implemented in 1991 [86], but confusion and conflict continued over the use of UP versus BSI. Hand washing (Table 3-36) is basic to all isolation principles.

PRESENT ISOLATION SYSTEMS. The most recent guidelines [80] have simplified the UP and BSI principles into a single level called ***Standard Precautions (SP)***. SP simultaneously reduces the risk of both bloodborne and other pathogens. All of the other previous categories of isolation and precautions are collapsed into a single set of **Transmission-Based Precautions**. The three major types of hospital transmission (airborne, droplet, and contact) are recognized as more important than specific diagnoses or infectious body substances (Table 3-37). These precautions are consistent with the most recent thinking—that the mode of transmission is indeed the weak link in the epidemiologic triad.

But besides the airborne, droplet, and contact modes of transmission, one must not forget the common-vehicle and vector-borne modes of transmission. These modes of transmission are not generally considered nosocomial, as they are covered by the "business-as-usual" or "institutional infrastructure" of general housekeeping as well as insect and other vermin control. Common-source controls include the safe handling of food and water and the disinfection and sterilization of surfaces and equipment. These things are taken for granted by clinicians in U.S. hospitals. However, with the increasing prevalence of immunosuppressed patients and drug resistance in U.S. hospitals, they may be the subject of increasing clinician scrutiny and control in the future.

Table 3-36
Principles of Hand Washing in Health Care

1. Hands should be washed before and after gloving.
2. Gloves should never be substituted for hand washing.
3. Disposable gloves must not be reused.
4. Nonlatex and powder-free alternatives should be available for workers (and patients) with sensitivities to latex and/or powder.
5. Fingernails should be kept short to avoid soiling and to prevent glove tearing.
6. Petroleum-based lotions and hand treatments should not be used, since they threaten the integrity of latex.
7. Hands should be dried completely, either by hand blowers or papers towels that are beyond the splash range of other hand washers.

Table 3-37
1996 CDC Isolation Categories for Hospitals: Examples by Disease

Standard Precautions (body fluids)
- Use for the care of all patients, with all other categories

Airborne Precautions
- Measles
- Varicella (includes disseminated varicella-zoster virus)
- Tuberculosis (includes special N-95 respirators)

Droplet Precautions
- Invasive *Haemophilus influenzae*, type B (meningitis, pneumonia, epiglottitis, sepsis)
- Invasive *Neisseria meningitides* (meningitis, pneumonia, sepsis)
- Diphtheria
- Mycoplasma pneumonia
- Pneumonic plague
- Group A streptococcus (pharyngitis, pneumonia, scarlet fever)
- Adenovirus
- Influenza
- Mumps
- Parvovirus B19 (Fifth's disease)
- Rubella

Contact Precautions
- GI, respiratory, skin, or wound infection or colonization with a multidrug-resistant bacteria judged to be of clinical or epidemiologic significance, i.e., vancomycin-resistant enterococcus (VRE) or methicillin-resistant *Staphylococcus aureus* (MRSA)
- *Clostridium difficile*
- Diapered or incontinent patients; *Escherichia coli* 0157:H7, shigella, hepatitis A, or rotavirus

1996 Transmission-Based Precautions. Standard Precautions synthesize the major features of UP and BSI and apply them to all patients who receive care in hospitals, regardless of their diagnosis or presumed infection status. SP applies to:

- Blood.
- All body fluids, secretions, and excretions except sweat, regardless of whether or not they contain visible blood.
- Nonintact skin.
- Mucous membranes.

Standard Precautions are included within all of the other Transmission-Based Precautions [80]

Figure 3-16
Four categories of "transmission-based" hospital isolations, per the 1996 CDC Recommendations. (Adapted from Centers for Disease Control. Guidelines for isolation precautions in hospitals. Hospital Infection Control Practices Advisory Committee (HICPAC). *Infect Control Hosp Epidemiol* 1996;17:24–52.)

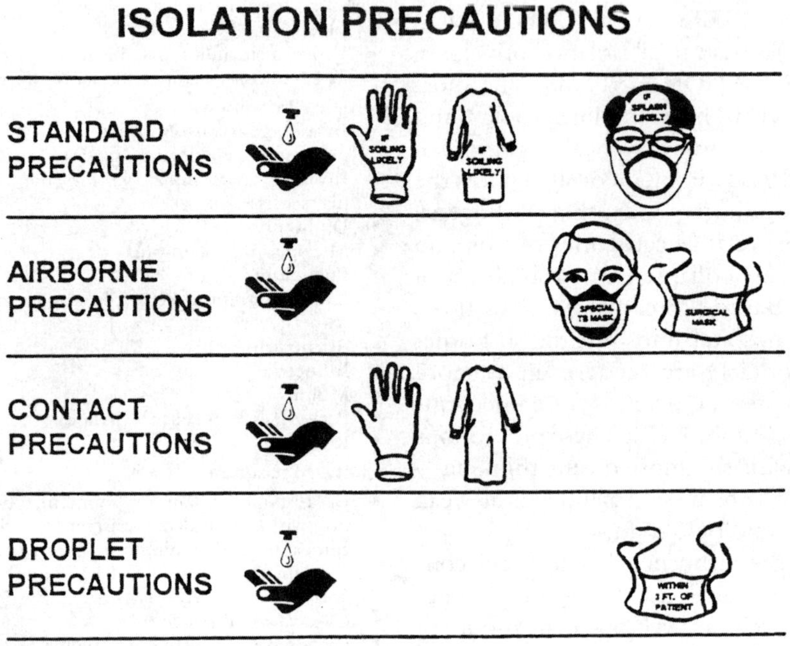

(Figure 3-16). These precautions are designed for patients proved or suspected to be infected with highly transmissible or epidemiologically important pathogens for which additional precautions, beyond SP, are needed to interrupt transmission in hospital.

Airborne Precautions ("A"). These are designed to reduce transmission of infectious disease spread by droplet nuclei (5 μm or less in size) that may remain suspended in air for long periods of time and may be infective for some distance. It should be used in combination with special air handling such as negative pressure and with personal protection.

Droplet Precautions ("D"). These are designed to reduce transmission of infections diseases spread by droplet nuclei (over 5 μm in size) through coughing, sneezing, or talking or during the performance of procedures on the airway from a distance of about 3 feet or less. One becomes infected by droplet nuclei from an infected individual coming into contact with respiratory surfaces or the mucous membranes of the mouth or eyes.

Contact Precautions ("C"). These are designed to reduce the risk of transmission of epidemiologically important microorganisms by direct skin-to-skin contact and physical transfer of microorganisms to a susceptible host from a colonized or infected person. They also protect against indirect transmission from the intermediate or inanimate objects.

Some diseases, such as *Varicella* (A and C), may require more than one form of isolation. A complete list of recommended precautions and their duration is found in Appendix A of reference 80; it is too extensive for publication in this chapter. This document also lists 97 references to the literature. Table 3-37 lists isolation categories by example, and Table 3-38 lists recommended categories of isolation based on clinical syndromes pending confirmation.

Table 3-38
Clinical Syndromes Warranting Additional Precautions To Prevent Transmission of Epidemiologically Important Pathogens Pending Confirmation of Diagnosis

Clinical Syndrome	Potential Pathogen	Precautions
Diarrhea		
Incontinence or diaper	Enteric pathogens	C
Adult, recent antibiotic use	*Clostridium difficile*	C
Meningitis	*Neisseria meningitides*	D
Rash or exanthems		
Petechial/fever	*Neisseria meningitides*	D
Vesicular	Varicella	A, C
Mac-pap, coryza, fever	Measles (rubeola)	A
Respiratory infections		
Cough/fever/upper lobes/HIV-/any lobes/HIV+	Tuberculosis	A
Paroxysmal or severe cough	Pertussis (epidemic)	D
Infant or child, croup	Respiratory syncytial virus or parainfluenza	C
Multidrug resistance risk		
Previous history of resistant organisms	Resistant agent?	C
Skin, GI, or wound nosocomial infection	Resistant agent?	C
Skin or wound abscess or drain not coverable	*Staphylococcus aureus,* or group A streptococcus	C

Abbreviations: *A* = airborne; *D* = droplet; *C* = contact.

Gloving

There are three indications for gloving in the health care environment [80]:

1. To provide a protective barrier and prevent gross contamination of the hands when touching blood, body fluids, secretions, excretions, mucous membranes, and nonintact skin. Gloving in these situations protects the worker and is mandated by OSHA [86].
2. To reduce the likelihood that microorganisms present on the hands of personnel will be transmitted to patients during invasive or other patient-care procedures that involve touching a patient's mucous membranes or nonintact skin. This protects the patient.
3. To reduce the likelihood that the hands of personnel contaminated with microorganisms from a patient or a fomite can transmit these microorganisms to another patient. In this situation, gloves must be changed between patient contacts and hands washed after gloves are removed. This protects other patients but also serves to protect the worker.

Wearing gloves does not replace the need for hand washing, because gloves may have small, inapparent defects or may be torn during use. Gloves can also become contaminated during removal and are therefore to be used only once.

Hand Washing

Hand washing (see Table 3-36) is the single most important procedure for preventing nosocomial infections [87,88]. It is just as important in preventing the spread of infection in childcare and food industries. Multiple agencies and organizations, including OSHA, CDC, FDA, the Association of Operating Room Nurses (AORN), and the Association for Practitioners of Infection Control and Epidemiology (APIC), have published guidelines on hand-washing techniques. Hand washing is included in all categories of hospital isolation in the CDC guidelines.

OSHA 29 CFR 1910.1030, sections (d)(2)(III–IV) do not address hand-washing agents or technique. They do address the availability of hand-washing facilities and recommended frequency as well as "alternative" methods of hand washing such as antiseptic towelettes if workers subsequently wash hands with soap and water as soon as feasible. This is to cover field workers in emergency medical services, law enforcement, and mobile blood collection units. All fixed health care facilities must have hand-washing facilities available. Passing through stairs or doors and thus making environmental contamination possible is a violation of section (d)(2)(III). OSHA also requires adequate training in hand washing.

Hand washing serves two main purposes:

1. Removal of gross contamination by organic and inorganic debris by the friction of rubbing the hands together, and the "degreasing" properties of soap and lather.
2. Removal of some microorganisms from the skin, depending on the soap or hand-washing solution.

Bar soap should be kept on a draining rack to prevent contamination. Fresh soap products should not be added to old dispensers; disposable dispensers are recommended. Lotions should be in small personal containers, as *Pseudomonas aeruginosa* has been associated with infections in refillable lotion containers.

CDC and APIC guidelines for general patient care call for application of non-antimicrobial soap followed by vigorous rubbing together of lathered hands for 10–15 seconds. Antimicrobial soaps *should* be used in caring for newborns, the immunosuppressed, and in performing invasive procedures. Preoperative hand washing should be done for 120 seconds, or 20 seconds if using an alcohol-based product. General hand-washing recommendations for health care workers are listed in Table 3-36. Hot water has traditionally been recommended but may increase drying and be associated with the development of rashes and dermatitis in health care workers or others who wash frequently. When harsh soaps are required, such as in hospital units, workers should wet their hands before applying soap to avoid skin contact with undiluted, full strength soap and the possible resultant irritation.

In non-food and non-health-care workers, hand washing is part of general personal hygiene (see below). Hands should be washed before preparing food for consumption by others. They should also be washed after defecating or urinating and after handling items that may be contaminated.

Commercial training programs and products are available to teach hand-washing techniques. Glo-Germ [89] is a commercial company that makes a fluorescent dye that is applied and then blacklighted after hand washing for quality control.

General Personal Hygiene

No topic can serve as a better conclusion to this large and complex chapter than the topic of personal hygiene. *Personal hygiene* is defined as those protective measures and behaviors under the responsibility of the individual that maintains his or her own health and prevents the spread of disease. Personal hygiene is most important for preventing direct transmission. Workers in health care, food, and some manufacturing industries may work under more specific guidelines, regulations, or employer policies. Regardless of the industry or regulations, all employers should have either written policies or at least a "company culture" that includes the principles listed in Table 3-39.

Table 3-39
Principles of Personal Hygiene

1. Wash hands in soap and water immediately after urinating, defecating, or touching any mucous membranes. This is especially important before eating, drinking, or preparing food for others or after handling fomites such as money or tickets.
2. Keep hands and any unclean personal articles (e.g., toothbrush, hairbrush, nail clippers) away from the mouth, nose, eyes, ears, genitalia, and wounds of others.
3. Keep fingernails trimmed and clean.
4. Avoid using common unclean eating utensils, drinking cups, linen, handkerchiefs, combs, or brushes of others.
5. Avoid exposing others to spray from the nose or mouth when coughing, sneezing, laughing, or talking.
6. Keep body and clothing clean and nonoffensive to others.

References

1. NIH Consensus Statement, *Helicobacter pylori in Peptic Ulcer Disease.* Bethesda MA: National Institutes of Health, Feb 7–9, 1994.
2. Last JM (ed). *A Dictionary of Epidemiology*, 3rd Ed. New York. Oxford University Press, 1995. Pp 55–6.
3. Hope-Simpson RE. The nature of herpes zoster: a long-term study and a new hypothesis. *Proc R Soc Lond* 1965;58:9–20.
4. *Third National Health and Nutrition Examination Survey (NHANES III).* DHHS 94-1308. Hyattsville, MD: U.S. Department of Health and Human Services, National Center for Health Statistics, 1994.
5. Koo D, Wharton M. Case definitions for infectious conditions under public health surveillance. *MMWR* 1997;46(RR-10):1–56.
6. Glezen WP, Couch RB. Influenza viruses. In: Evans AS, Kaslow RA (eds), *Viral Infections of Humans: Epidemiology and Control*, 4th Ed. New York: Plenum, 1997. P 482.
7. Centers for Disease Control and Prevention. Prevention of hepatitis A through active or passive immunization. Recommendations of the Advisory Committee on Immunization Practices. *MMWR* 1996;45(RR-15):1.
8. Centers for Disease Control and Prevention. Draft guidelines for infection control in health care personnel. *Federal Register* 1997;62(173):47275–327.
9. Fine PEM. Herd immunity: history, theory, practice. *Epidemiol Rev* 1993;15:265–302.
10. Benenson AS (ed). *Control of Communicable Diseases Manual*, 16th Ed. Washington, DC: American Public Health Association 1995. Pp xxiv–v. (Also available on CD ROM.)
11. Houseworth WJ, Spoon MM. The age distribution of excess mortality during A2 Hong Kong influenza epidemics compared with earlier A2 outbreaks. *Am J Epidemiol* 1974;94:348–50.
12. *Stedman's Pocket Medical Dictionary* (abridged from 24th Ed). Baltimore, MD: Williams & Wilkins, 1987. P 602.
13. Koch R. Uber bacteriologische Forschung. *Int Med Cong (Berl)* 1891;1:35.
14. Rivers T. Viruses and Koch's postulates, *J Bacteriol* 1937;33:1–12.
15. Evans AS. Causation and disease: the Heenle-Koch postulates revisited. *Yale J Biol Med* 1976;49:175–95.
16. Evans AS. *Causation and Disease. A Chronological Journey.* New York: Plenum Press, 1993.
17. Hill AB. The environment and disease: association or causation? *Proc R Soc Med* 1965;58:295–300.
18. Code of Ethical Conduct, American College of Occupational and Environmental Medicine. Washington, DC. Adopted by ACOEM Board of Directors, October 15, 1993.
19. Suskind F. Another look at the link between work injuries and job experience. *Month Labor Rev* 1982; 105:38.
20. Haddon W Jr. The changing approach to the epidemiology, prevention, and amelioration of trauma. The transition to approach etiology rather than descriptively based. *Am J Public Health* 1968;58:1431–8.
21. Haddon W Jr. A logical framework for categorizing highway safety phenomena and activity. *J Trauma* 1972;12:193–207.
22. Centers for Disease Control. Draft guidelines for preventing the transmission of tuberculosis in health-care settings, second edition. *Federal Register*, October 12, 1993;58:52809–54.
23. Memorandum for Regional Administrators (letter) Re: Enforcement Policy and Procedure for Occupational Exposure to Tuberculosis. Roger A. Clark, Director of Compliance Programs, Occupational Health and Safety Administration. Washington, DC, October 8, 1993.
24. Gerberding JL. Occupational infectious diseases or infectious occupational diseases? Bridging the views on tuberculosis control. (Editorial.) *Infect Control Hosp Epidemiol* 1993;14:12, 686–8.
25. Recommendations for preventing the spread of vancomycin resistance. Recommendations of the Hospital Infection Control Practices Advisory Committee (HICPAC). *MMWR* 1995;44:RR–12.
26. Revision of the CDC surveillance case definition for acquired human immune insufficiency virus. Conference of State and Territorial Epidemiologists, Center for Disease Control, Atlanta. *MMWR* 1987;36(suppl 1):1s.
27. Brooks GF, Butel JS, Morse SA. *Jawetz, Melnick, and Adelberg's Medical Microbiology*, 21st Ed. Stamford, CT: Appleton & Lange, 1998.
28. Urbaschek B, Urbaschek R. Introduction and summary. Perspective on bacterial pathogenesis and host defense, *Rev Infect Dis* 1987;9:(suppl 5):S431–6.
29. *Prevention Guidelines: A Guide to Action* (Topic 43, weather): Flood: a prevention guide to promote your personal health and Safety. Atlanta: CDC Office of Public Affairs, 1994. Pp 1150–6.
30. Riley RI, Kaufman JE. Effect of relative humidity on the inactivation of airborne *Serratia marcescens* by ultraviolet radiation. *Appl Microbiol* 1972;23:1113–20.
31. Soper GA. The curious career of Typhoid Mary. *Bull NY Acad Med* 1939;15:698–712.
32. Cassens BJ. *Preventive Medicine and Public Health*, 2nd Ed. Philadelphia: Harwal Publishing, 1992. P 6.
33. Wentworth DE, McGregor MW, Macklin MD, et al. Transmission of swine influenza virus to humans after exposure to experimentally infected pigs. *J Infect Dis* 1997;175:7–14.
34. Karabatsos N (ed). *International Catalogue of Arboviruses.* San Antonio: American Society of Tropical Medicine and Hygiene, Subcommittee on Information Exchange, 1985.

35. Knight V, Couch RB, Landahl HD. The effect of the lack of gravity on airborne infection during space flight. *JAMA* 1970;214:513–8.
36. Gerone PJ, Couch RB, Keefer GV, et al. Assessment of experimental and natural viral aerosols. *Bacteriol Rev* 1966;30:576–88.
37. Knight V (ed). *Viral and Mycoplasma Infections of the Respiratory Tract.* Philadelphia: Lea and Febiger, 1973.
38. Kelly S, Winsser J, Winkelstein W Jr. Poliomyelitis and other enteric viruses in sewage. *Am J Public Health* 1957;47:72–7.
39. Mastro TD, Farley TA, Elliott JA, et al. An outbreak of surgical-wound infections due to group A streptococcus carried on the scalp. *N Engl J Med* 1990;323:968–72.
40. Viglionese A, Nottebart VF, Bodman HA, et al. Recurrent group A streptococcal carriage in a health care worker associated with widely separated nosocomial outbreaks. *Am J Med* 1991;91:329S–33S.
41. Paul SM, Genese C, Spitalny K. Postoperative group A B-hemolytic streptococcus outbreak with the pathogen traced to a member of a healthcare worker's household. *Infect Control Hosp Epidemiol* 1990;11:643–6.
42. Ridgeway EJ, Allen KD. Clustering of group A streptococcal infections on a burns unit: important lessons in outbreak management. *J Hosp Infect* 1993;25:173–82.
43. Berkelman RL, Martin D, Graham DR, et al. Streptococcal wound infections caused by a vaginal carrier. *JAMA* 1982;247:2680–2.
44. Schaffner W, Lefkowitz LB Jr, Goodman JS, et al. Hospital outbreak of infections with group A streptococci traced to an asymptomatic anal carrier. *N Engl J Med* 1969;280:1224–5.
45. Richman DD, Breton SJ, Goldmann DA. Scarlet fever and group A streptococcal surgical wound infection traced to an anal carrier. *J Pediatr* 1977;90:387–90.
46. Decker MD, Lavely GB, Hutcheson RHJ, et al. Food-borne streptococcal pharyngitis in a hospital pediatrics clinics. *JAMA* 1986;253:679–81.
47. Boyce JM, Opal SM, Byone-Potter G, et al. Spread of methicillin-resistant *Staphylococcus aureus* in a hospital after exposure to a health care worker with chronic sinusitis. *Clin Infect Dis* 1993;17:496–504.
48. Sherertz RJ, Reagan DR, Hampton KD, et al. A cloud adult: the *Staphylococcus aureus*–virus interaction revisited. *Ann Intern Med* 1996;124:539–47.
49. Belani A, Sherertz RJ, Sullivan ML, et al. Outbreak of staphylococcal infection in two hospital nurseries traced to a single nasal carrier. *Infect Control* 1986;7:487–90.
50. Kreiswirth BN, Kravitz GR, Schlievert PM, et al. Nosocomial transmission of a strain of *Staphylococcus aureus* causing toxic shock syndrome. *Ann Intern Med* 1986;195:704–7.
51. Boyce JM. Methicillin-resistant *Staphylococcus aureus* in hospitals and long-term care facilities: microbiology, epidemiology, and preventive measures. *Infect Control Hosp Epidemiol* 1992;13:725–37.
52. Boyce JM, Landry M, Deetz TR, et al. Epidemiologic studies of an outbreak of nosocomial methicillin-resistant *Staphylococcus aureus* infections. *Infect Control* 1981;2:110–6.
53. Walsh TJ, Standiford HD, et al. Randomized double-blinded trial of rifampin with either novobiocin or trimethoprim-sulfamethoxazole against methicillin-resistant *Staphylococcus aureus* colonization: prevention of antimicrobial resistance and effect of host factors on outcome. *Antimicrob Agents Chemother* 1993;37:1334–42.
54. Mulligan ME, Murray-Leisure KA, Ribner BS, et al. Methicillin-resistant *Staphylococcus aureus*: a consensus review of the microbiology, pathogenesis, and epidemiology with implications for prevention and management. *Am J Med* 1993;94:313–28.
55. Valway SE. An outbreak involving extensive transmission of a virulent strain of mycobacterium tuberculosis. *N Engl J Med* 1998;338:633–9.
56. Glaser ZR. A dictionary for central sterilization. *Infect Control Steril Technol* 1998;4(4):14–46.
57. Durante L. Investigation of an outbreak of bloody diarrhea association with an endoscopic cleaning solution and demonstration of lesions in an animal model. *Am J Med* 1992;92(5):476–80.
58. Spaulding EH. Chemical disinfection and antisepsis in the hospital. *J Hosp Res* 1972;9:5–31.
59. Nardell EA, Keegan J, Cheny SA, et al. Airborne infection: theoretical limits of protection achievable by building ventilation. *Am Rev Respir Dis* 1991;144:302–6.
60. Petersen NJ. An assessment of the airborne route in hepatitis B transmission. *Ann NY Acad Sci* 1980;353:157–66.
61. Johnson GK, Robinson WS. Human immunodeficiency virus-1 in the vapors of surgical power instruments. *J Med Virol* 1991;33:47–50.
62. Jewett DL, Heinshohn PA, Bennett C, et al. Blood-containing aerosols generated by surgical techniques. A possible infectious hazard. *Am Ind Assoc J* 1992;53:228–31.
63. Heinsohn PA, Jewett DL. Exposure to blood-containing aerosols in the operating room: a preliminary study. *Am Ind Hyg Assoc J* 1993;54:446–53.
64. Heinsohn PA, Jewett DL, Balzer L, et al. Aerosols created by some surgical power tools: particle-size distribution and qualitative hemoglobin content. *Appl Occup Environ Hyg* 1991;6:773–6.
65. Tokars J, Chamberland ME, Schable CA, et al. A survey of occupational blood contact and HIV infections among orthopedic surgeons. *JAMA* 1991;268:489–94.
66. Evaluation of a smoke evacuator used for laser surgery. *Lasers Surg Med* 1989;9:276–81.
67. NIOSH Health Hazard Evaluation and Technical Assistance reports, HETA 85-126-1932 (1989) and HETA 88-101-2008 (1990). Also at *http://www. cdc.gov/niosh/hc11.html*.

68. Koren H, Bisesi M. *Handbook of Environmental Health and Safety*, 3rd Ed. Boca Raton, FL: Lewis (CRC) Publishers, 1996. Volume 2, Chaps 3–7, pp 233–608; Volume 1, Chap 2, pp 107–201.

69. Okun DA. Water quality management. In: Last JM, Wallace RB (eds), *Maxcy-Rosenau-Last Public Health and Preventive Medicine*, 13th Ed. Norwalk, CT: Appleton & Lange, 1992. Pp 618–48.

70. Environmental Protection Agency, Office of Ground Water and Drinking Water. Regulatory Negotiation Committee. Website updates at *http://www.epa.gov/OGWDW/sdwa/mdbp*.

71. Frank JF, Barnhart HM. Food and dairy sanitation. In Last JM, Wallace RB (eds), *Maxcy-Rosenau-Last Public Health and Preventive Medicine*, 13th Ed. Norwalk, CT: Appleton & Lange, 1992. Pp 589–618.

72. *The Microbiologic Safety of Irradiated Food*, Codex Alimentarius, CX/FX/83/9. Rome, 1983.

73. Merritt C. Radiolytic products—are they safe? *Safety Factors Influencing the Acceptance of Food Irradiation Technology.* Vienna, International Atomic Energy Commission. TECDOC-490, 1989.

74. Irradiation in the production, processing, and handling of food, U.S. Food and Drug Administration, final rule. *Federal Register* 1989;55(85):18538–44.

75. *Satellites Help Scientists Focus on Emerging Diseases.* (Factsheet.) Bethesda, MD: Office of Communications, National Institute of Allergy and Infectious Diseases, National Institutes for Health, 1998. Available at *http://www.naiaid.nih.gov/factsheets/emergdis.htm*.

76. *Physical Activity and Health: A Report of the Surgeon General.* Atlanta, GA: U.S. Department of Health and Human Services, Centers for Disease Control and Prevention, National Center for Chronic Disease Prevention and Health Promotion, 1996.

77. Kasl SV, Evans AS, Niederman JC. Psychosocial risk factors in the development of infectious mononucleosis. *Psychosom Med* 1979;41:445–66.

78. Figure 4, Packing and Labeling of Etiologic Agents, graphic. U.S. Government. Available at *http://www.cdc.gov/od/biosfty/bmbl/fig4.gif*.

79. Richmond JY, McKinney RW. *Biosafety in Microbiological and Biomedical Laboratories*, 3rd Ed. Washington, DC: U.S. Department of Health and Human Services, 1993.

80. Centers for Disease Control and Prevention. Guideline for isolation precautions in hospitals. Hospital Infection Control Practices Advisory Committee (HICPAC). *Infect Control Hosp Epidemiol* 1996;17:53–80 or *Am J Infect Control* 1996;24:24–52. Available at *http://www.cdc.gov/ncidod/hip/isolat/isolat.htm*.

81. *Guide for the Care and Use of Laboratory Animals.* HEW (NIH) 86-23, Rev 1985 and Laboratory Animal Welfare Regulations 9 CFR Subchapter A, Parts 1,2,3, 1985.

82. Tuberculosis control laws—United States, 1993. Recommendations of the Advisory Council for the Elimination of Tuberculosis. *MMWR* 1993;42:(RR-15).

83. National Communicable Disease Center. *Isolation Techniques for Use in Hospitals.* (PHS #2054.) Washington, DC: NCDC, 1970.

84. Centers for Disease Control. *Isolation Techniques for Use in Hospitals*, 2nd Ed. (HHS #80-8314.) Washington, DC: CDC, 1975.

85. Garner JS, Simmon BP. *CDC Guideline for Isolation Precautions in Hospitals.* (HHS #83-8314.) Atlanta: U.S. Department of Health and Human Services, 1983. Also in *Infect Control* 1983;4:245–325 and *Am J Infect Control* 1984;12:103–63.

86. Occupational exposure to bloodborne pathogens; final rule. Department of Labor, Occupational Safety & Health Administration. *Federal Register* 56(235): 64175–82, 1991.

87. Centers for Disease Control. Guidelines for Handwashing and Hospital Environmental Control, 1985. *MMWR* 1987;36(2S suppl).

88. Hart PD. Current recommendations for handwashing compliance in the clinical setting. *Infect Control Steril Technol* 1996;2(3):1.

89. Glo-Germ®, P.O. Box 537, Moad, Utah 84532. 1-800-842-6622; *http:\www.glogerm.com*.

Recommended Reading and Resources

IMMUNOLOGY

Benjamini E, Sunshie G, Leskowitz S. *Immunology: A Short Course*, 3rd Ed. New York: Wiley-Liss, 1996.

Primer on allergic and immunologic diseases. *N Engl J Med* (Special Ed). 1997;278(22):1799–2034.

BASIC MICROBIOLOGY

Brooks GF, Butel JS, Morse SA. *Jawetz, Melnick, and Adelberg's Medical Microbiology*, 21st Ed. Stamford, CT: Appleton & Lange, 1998.

ENVIRONMENTAL HEALTH AND CONTROLS

Koren H, Bisesi M. *Handbook of Environmental Health and Safety* (Two Vols), 3rd Ed. Boca Raton, FL: Lewis (CRC), 1996.

EPIDEMIOLOGY AND CONTROL BY DISEASES

Benenson AS (ed). *Control of Communicable Diseases Manual*, 16th Ed. Washington, DC: American Public Health Association 1995. (Also available on CD-ROM.)

"DEFINITIVE" TEXTBOOKS OF INFECTION EPIDEMIOLOGY

Evans AS, Brachman PS. *Bacterial Infections of Humans: Epidemiology and Control*, 3rd Ed. New York: Plenum, 1998.

Evans AS, Kaslow RA. *Viral Infections of Humans: Epidemiology and Control*, 4th Ed. New York: Plenum, 1997.

HEALTH CARE WORKERS

Charney C, Schirmer J. *Essentials of Modern Hospital Safety.* Chesea, MI: Lewis, 1990.

Charney C, Schirmer J. *Essentials of Modern Hospital Safety*, Vol 2. Chesea, MI: Lewis, 1993.

Levy RM. *Employees at Risk: Protecting the Health of the Health Care Worker.* New York: Van Nostrand Reinhold, 1991.

BLOODBORNE PATHOGEN TRAINER AND CONTINUING MEDICAL EDUCATION

Favero MS, Bolyard EA. *Physician Update, Bloodborne Pathogens.* Tampa, FL: Medical Group Learning Systems, 1996. Section 4, Microbiologic Consideration; Disinfection and Sterilization Strategies and Potential for Airborne Transmission of Bloodborne Pathogens. (3 CME Cat-1 Credits, 1-800-547-0308.)

STRESS AND IMMUNITY

Abraham E. Effects of stress on cytokine production. *Methods Achiev Exp Pathol* 1991;14:45–62.

Anderson JL. The immune system and major depression. *Adv Neuroimmunol* 1996;6(2):119–29.

Ballieux RE. Bidirectional communication between the brain and the immune system. *Eur J Clin Invest* 1992;22(suppl 1):6–9.

Bonneau RH, Kiecolt-Glaser R. Stress-induced modulation of the immune response. *Ann NY Acad Sci* 1990;594:253–69.

Khansari DN, Murgo AJ, Faith RE. Effects of stress on the immune system. *Immunol Today* 1990;11(5):170–5.

Nelson RJ, Demas GE. Seasonal changes in immune function. *Q Rev Biol* 1996;71(4):511–48.

Rabin BS, Ganguli R, Lysle DT, et al. Interaction between the brain and immune system. *Immunol Ser* 1990;52:125–54.

Smith JA, Pyne DB. Exercise, training and neutrophil function. *Exerc Immunol Rev* 1997;3:96–116.

Sternberg EM, Chroousos GP, Wilder RL, et al. The stress response and the regulation of inflammatory disease. *Ann Intern Med* 1992;117(10):854–66.

4 / Occupations at Risk

Geoffrey A. Kelafant

Until recently, infectious disease has played a significant role in the health of individuals, populations, and even the course of history. Improvements in hygiene and technology have greatly reduced the burden of suffering in many developed areas. Despite these advances, much of the world is still at risk from infectious diseases, which have significant morbidity and mortality.

As the world shrinks, the possibility of being confronted with unfamiliar diseases increases. Infected individuals can travel farther and faster than ever before. The classic definition of occupational disease blurs in cases of work-related infectious disease, as the occupational risk becomes merely being present in an area and not just working in a particular job. Since some of these diseases are virtually unknown to many health care practitioners, it is crucial to maintain a high index of suspicion in order to recognize infections when they occur.

Diseases Affecting Those Who Work With People

HEALTH CARE WORKERS, PERSONAL CARE WORKERS, AND DAY CARE WORKERS

In some countries, health care workers face the greatest risk of acquiring occupational infectious disease. In the United States, more health care workers die from hepatitis B sequelae every year than the combined total of firefighters and policemen killed in the line of duty. After decades of confusion, it has become clear that health care workers are at significant risk from tuberculosis infection as well. Concern for health care workers has involved health care facilities and systems in the regulatory milieu as never before. Entire industries have been created over the last 10 years to address this single problem.

Health care workers may acquire diseases via airborne, fecal-oral, bloodborne/percutaneous, or direct contact routes. Although in theory a huge number of diseases may be spread to health care workers (and from health care workers), the most commonly cited are found in Table 4-1. Diseases known to have been contracted from percutaneous injuries in laboratory and research facilities are listed in Table 4-2.

PUBLIC SAFETY AND EMERGENCY RESPONSE WORKERS

Public safety and emergency response workers face risks similar to those faced by health care workers. In addition, depending on the particular job, they may also be at risk for zoonotic disease (from animal bites or contact), waterborne disease (in divers, rescue personnel), arthropod-borne disease, and soil-borne disease. Because of the diverse and sometimes odd nature of the tasks these workers are often asked to perform, persistent or unusual infections require a thorough investigation. Zoonotic, waterborne, arthropod-borne, and soil-borne disease are discussed elsewhere in this chapter.

Diseases Affecting Those Who Work with Animals

Although advances in hygiene and technology have made zoonotic diseases a curiosity in some countries, there remain dozens of diseases that can spread from animals to man (Table 4-3). Numerous occupations (Tables 4-4 and 4-5) in-

Table 4-1
Infectious Diseases Affecting Health Care Workers and Routes of Transmission

Airborne	Fecal-Oral	Percutaneous/Bloodborne	Direct Contact
Adenovirus	Hepatitis A	AIDS/HIV	Herpetic whitlow
Influenza	Norwalk virus	Crimean hemorrhagic fever	Tinea corporis
Measles	Polio	Ebola virus	Warts
Meningococcal disease	Salmonellosis	Hepatitis B	
Mumps	Shigellosis	Hepatitis C	
Parvovirus B19		Lassa fever	
Pertussis		Marburg virus	
Respiratory syncytial virus			
Rubella			
Tuberculosis			
Varicella			

volve extensive contact with animals, animal tissues, animal waste, and animal products. Ticks, fleas, and mites may be closely associated with some animal species. These diseases may be acquired via airborne spread, the fecal-oral route, contact with blood, secretions, or fluids, or direct contact or bites. Some are spread via multiple routes.

Diseases Affecting Those Who Work Outdoors

Numerous occupations involve outdoor work (Table 4-6). The two potential exposures presenting the greatest risk to outdoor workers are soil-borne and arthropod-borne disease (Table 4-7). Soil organisms, predominantly fungi, may cause infection through inhalation or direct inoculation through the skin. Arthropod-borne disease, which may be viral, rickettsial, protozoal or bacterial, is acquired through contact with mosquitoes, ticks, fleas, and mites. The spectrum of arthropod-borne disease is staggering, with well over 200 arboviral infections alone.

Diseases Affecting Those Who Work Around Water

Diseases are easily transmitted by water. Some occupations, such as diving or working with sewage or biohazardous waste, entail significant exposure to water. Additionally, agricultural work and construction work may involve exposure to water. Many diseases, especially those that are transmitted via the fecal-oral route, may be acquired during work activities involving water exposure (Table 4-8). Other diseases may involve only the skin.

Diseases Affecting Travelers

Travel-related occupational infectious disease is a relativistic field: It depends on the observer's

Table 4-2
Diseases Acquired Percutaneously

Blastomycosis
Brucellosis
Cryptococcosis
Creutzfeldt-Jakob disease
Diphtheria
Ebola virus
Gonorrhea
Herpes simplex
Herpes B virus
Japanese encephalitis
Leptospirosis
Malaria
Mycoplasmosis
Rocky Mountain spotted fever
Scrub typhus
Sporotrichosis
Staphylococcal disease
Streptococcal disease
Syphilis
Toxoplasmosis
Tuberculosis
Yellow fever

frame of reference. Many of the diseases mentioned in this book may be of concern to a traveling worker, depending on point of origin, destination, and the type of work performed. Some are vaccine preventable and some have chemoprophylaxis and or treatment available. Table 4-9 lists vaccine preventable diseases: Please note that availability and effectiveness of vaccines varies widely.

Diseases Affecting Those Who Work Indoors

Many building-related illnesses are respiratory in nature, usually presenting as asthma or hypersensitivity pneumonitis, and do not represent true infections. Infectious organisms (bacteria, fungi, viruses, and protozoa) may reside in heating, cooling, and ventilation systems or be introduced

Table 4-3
Occupational Zoonotic Disease by Animal

Animal Group	Diseases
Amphibians	*Edwardsiella tarda* Salmonellosis Sparganosis
Armadillos, sloths, anteaters	Leprosy
Bats	Duvenhage virus Histoplasmosis Kasokero virus *Lyssavirus* Mokola virus Rabies Salmonellosis Yuli virus
Birds	Campylobacteriosis Cryptococcosis Erysipeloid Histoplasmosis Newcastle disease Ornithosis *Pasteurella multocida* Salmonellosis Tuberculosis Yersiniosis
Camels, llamas	Brucellosis Campylobacteriosis Plague Q fever Salmonellosis
Cats	Campylobacteriosis *Capnocytophaga* Cat-scratch disease Cutaneous larval migrans Dermatophytosis Leptospirosis Plague Q fever Salmonellosis Strongyloidiasis Toxoplasmosis Visceral larval migrans Yersiniosis
Cattle	Anthrax Brucellosis Campylobacteriosis Cowpox Dermatophilosis Leptospirosis Milker's nodules *Mycobacterium bovis* Pseudocowpox Q fever Salmonellosis Streptococcosis Yersiniosis
Dogs	American trypanosomiasis Blastomycosis Brucellosis Campylobacteriosis Capnocytophaga Cat-scratch disease Cutaneous larval migrans Dermatophytosis Echinococcosis Ehrlichiosis Giardiasis Leptospirosis Lyme disease Pasteurellosis Plague Q fever Rabies Rocky Mountain spotted fever Salmonellosis Strongyloidiasis Trichostrongylosis Visceral larval migrans Yersiniosis
Fish	Cholera Erysipeloid Nanophyetiasis Salmonellosis Vibriosis

Table 4-3 (continued)

Animal Group	Diseases
Horses	Anthrax Brucellosis Cryptosporidiosis Dermatophilosis Eastern equine encephalitis Equine *Morbillivirus* Glanders Leptospirosis Salmonellosis Venezuelan equine encephalitis Western equine encephalitis Yersiniosis
Lizards	Salmonellosis
Marsupials	Anthrax Dermatophytosis Leptospirosis Melioidosis *Mycobacterium bovis* Pasteurellosis Q fever Salmonellosis Scabies
Pigs	Anthrax Brucellosis Influenza Leptospirosis *Pasteurella multocida* Salmonellosis Streptococcosis Yersiniosis
Primates	Amebiasis Ascariasis Campylobacteriosis Cestodiasis Dengue Dermatophilosis Giardiasis Hepatitis A Herpes B virus Leprosy Marburg virus Measles Monkeypox Salmonellosis Shigellosis Strongyloidiasis Tanapox Trichostrongylosis Tuberculosis Yaba virus
Rabbits, hares	Campylobacteriosis Dermatomycosis Dermatophilosis Leptospirosis Plague Q fever Salmonellosis Tularemia Yersiniosis
Raccoons	*Edwardsiella tarda* Rabies Salmonellosis
Rodents	American trypanosomiasis Babesiosis Cestodiasis Colorado tick fever Dermatophytosis Hantavirus Leptospirosis Listeriosis Lyme disease Lymphocytic choriomeningitis Murine typhus Plague Powassan encephalitis Rabies Rat-bite fever Relapsing fever Rickettsialpox Rocky Mountain spotted fever Salmonellosis Scrub typhus Yersiniosis
Seals, sea lions, walruses	Erysipeloid Influenza A Seal finger
Sheep, goats	Anthrax Brucellosis Campylobacteriosis Cryptosporidiosis Dermatomycosis Dermatophilosis Leptospirosis Orf Plague Q fever Salmonellosis Yersiniosis
Snakes	*Aeromonas hydrophila* *Edwardsiella tarda* *Escherichia coli* Mesocestoidiasis *Morganella morganii* *Mycobacterium ulcerans* *Proteus vulgaris* *Providencia* Q fever Salmonellosis Sparganosis
Turtles, tortoises, terrapins	Campylobacteriosis *Edwardsiella tarda* Salmonellosis
Whales, dolphins, porpoises	Erysipeloid *Mycobacterium marinum* Seal finger

Table 4-4
Occupational Groups at Risk for Zoonotic Disease

Agricultural workers	Pest control workers
Animal handlers	Primate handlers
Animal husbandry workers	Ranchers
Butchers	Research laboratory workers
Cannery workers	Sewer workers
Cattle breeders	Sheepherders
Dairy farmers	Slaughterhouse workers
Fishermen	Stockyard workers
Forestry workers	Trappers
Hunters	Travelers
Livestock handlers	Veterinarians
Meat and poultry workers	Weavers
Miners	Zookeepers
Packing house workers	

Table 4-6
Outdoor Workers at Risk

Agricultural workers	Hunters
Construction workers	Lumberjacks
Excavators	Miners
Foresters	Travelers
Geologists	

Table 4-5
Occupations at Risk and Specific Zoonotic Diseases

Occupations	Diseases
Bird handlers	Cryptococcosis Histoplasmosis Newcastle disease Ornithosis Pasteurellosis Tuberculosis
Butchers, slaughterhouse workers	Anthrax Brucellosis Leptospirosis Listeriosis Q fever Streptococcosis Tuberculosis (cutaneous) Tularemia
Fisherman	Erysipeloid Nanophyetiasis Swimming pool granuloma
Livestock handlers	Anthrax Brucellosis Cryptosporidiosis Dermatophilosis Dermatophytosis Leptospirosis Listeriosis Q fever Streptococcosis *Salmonella* (cutaneous) Tuberculosis
Pest control workers	Hantavirus Leptospirosis
Poultry workers	Cryptococcosis Erysipeloid Newcastle disease Ornithosis Pasteurellosis
Primate handlers	Giardiasis Hepatitis A Herpes B virus Marburg virus Measles Monkeypox Shigellosis Tuberculosis Yabapox
Sheep handlers	Anthrax Brucellosis Dermatophilosis Echinococcosis Orf Q fever
Veterinarians, animal handlers	Anthrax Brucellosis Cat-scratch disease Erysipeloid Leptospirosis Listeriosis Milker's nodules Newcastle disease Q fever Rabies *Salmonella* (cutaneous) Toxoplasmosis Tuberculosis (cutaneous) Tularemia

Table 4-7
Diseases Affecting Those Who Work Outdoors

Arthropod-borne Diseases	Soil-borne Diseases	Other Diseases
Viral	Blastomycosis	Amebiasis
California encephalitis	Chromomycosis	Hantavirus
Colorado tick fever	Coccidioidomycosis	
Crimean-Congo hemorrhagic fever	Cryptococcosis	
Dengue	Cutaneous larval migrans	
Eastern equine encephalitis	Maduromycosis	
Japanese encephalitis	Melioidosis	
La Crosse encephalitis	Mycetoma	
Powassan encephalitis	Nocardiosis	
Rift Valley fever	Paracoccidioidomycosis	
Russian spring-summer encephalitis	Sporotrichosis	
Sandfly fever	Strongylodiasis	
St. Louis encephalitis	Tetanus	
Venezuelan equine encephalitis		
Western equine encephalitis		
Many others		
Rickettsial		
Ehrlichiosis		
Louse-borne typhus		
Murine typhus		
Rickettsialpox		
Rocky Mountain spotted fever		
Scrub typhus		
Trench fever		
Bacterial		
Lyme disease		
Plague		
Relapsing fever		
Tularemia		
Protozoal		
African trypanosomiasis (Sleeping sickness)		
American trypanosomiasis (Chagas' disease)		
Babesiosis		
Malaria		

Table 4-8
Diseases Affecting Those Who Work Around Water

Amebiasis	Polio
Amebic meningoencephalitis	Schistosomal dermatitis
Cholera	Schistosomiasis
Escherichia coli	Shigellosis
Erysipeloid	Swimming pool granuloma
Hepatitis A	Typhoid
Leptospirosis	Vibriosis
Nanophyetiasis	Other diseases spread by fecal contamination

Table 4-9
Vaccine-Preventable Diseases

Cholera
Diphtheria
Hepatitis A
Hepatitis B
Influenza
Japanese encephalitis
Lyme disease
Malaria
Measles
Meningococcal disease
Mumps
Pertussis
Plague
Pneumococcal disease
Polio
Rabies
Rubella
Tetanus
Tick-borne encephalitis
Typhoid
Typhus
Varicella
Yellow fever

Table 4-10
Organisms Affecting Those Who Work Indoors

Aspergillus
Histoplama capsulatum
Influenza
Legionella pneumophila
Mycobacterium tuberculosis
Naegleria fowleri

Table 4-11
Diseases Affecting Those Who Work Around Food

Anthrax
Brucellosis
Erysipeloid
Leptospirosis
Listeriosis
Milker's nodules
Nanophyetiasis
Ornithosis
Q fever
Streptococcosis
Tuberculosis (cutaneous)
Tularemia

into the indoor environment via water, carpets, plants, animals, birds, pillows, bedding, dust, wet or damp materials, outside air, and humans. Organisms implicated in infectious building-related illness are listed in Table 4-10.

Diseases Affecting Those in Food Production

Although many disease outbreaks associated with food involve consumers of contaminated food products and not workers, there are occupational infectious disease risks associated with employment in the food industry (Table 4-11). Most of these diseases are associated with the processing of raw food product, mainly affecting those who slaughter and butcher livestock and poultry.

Bibliography

Calisher CH. Medically important arboviruses of the United States and Canada. *Clin Microbiol Rev* 1994;7:89–116.

Casey KR. Atypical pneumonia and environmental factors. *Clin Chest Med* 1991;12:285–302.

Centers for Disease Control and Prevention. *Epidemiology and Prevention of Vaccine-Preventable Diseases*, 5th Ed. Atlanta: CDC, 1999.

Centers for Disease Control and Prevention. *Health Information for International Travel 1996–97.* Atlanta: CDC, 1999.

Centers for Disease Control and Prevention. Immunization of health care workers: recommendations of the Advisory Committee on Immunization Practices (ACIP) and the Hospital Infection Control Practices Advisory Committee (HICPAC). *MMWR* 1997;46:RR-18.

Cohen R. Occupational infections. In: LaDou J (ed), *Occupational Medicine.* East Norwalk, CT: Appleton & Lange, 1990.

Fang G, Araujo V, Guerrant RL. Enteric infections associated with exposure to animals or animal products. *Infect Dis Clin N Am* 1991;5(3):681–701.

Ferson MJ. Infections in day care. *Curr Opin Pediatr* 1993;5:35–40.

Fox JG, Lipman NS. Infections transmitted by large and small laboratory animals. *Infect Dis Clin N Am* 1991;5:131–61.

Garibaldi R, Janis B. Occupational infections. In: Rom WN (ed), *Environmental and Occupational Medicine*, 2nd Ed. Boston: Little Brown, 1992.

Gerberding JL, Holmes KK. Microbial agents and infectious diseases. In: Rosenstock LR, Cullen MR (eds), *Textbook of*

Clinical Occupational and Environmental Medicine, Philadelphia: Saunders, 1994.

Kelafant GA (ed). *Guidelines for Employee Health Services in Health Care Facilities* (hypertext document). Chicago: American College of Occupational and Environmental Medicine, Medical Center Occupational Health Section, 1998. Available at *http://www.occenvmed.net/ehsg.*

Kligman EW, Peate WF, Cordes DH. Occupational infections in farm workers. In: Cordes DH, Rea DF (eds), Health hazards of farming. *Occup Med State Art Rev* 1991;6(3): 429–46.

Lanphear BP. Transmission and control of bloodborne viral hepatitis in health care workers. In: McDiarmid MA, Kessler ER (eds), The health care worker. *Occup Med State Art Rev* 1997;12(4):717–30.

Madkour, MM. Occupation-related infectious arthritis. *Bailliere's Clin Rheumatol* 1989;3:157–92.

Seltzer JM. Biologic contaminants. In: Seltzer JM (ed), Effects of the indoor environment on health. *Occup Med State Art Rev* 1995;10;1:1–26.

Sepkowitz KA. Occupationally acquired infections in health care workers. (Parts I and II). *Ann Intern Med* 1996;125: 826–35, 125:917–28.

Snashall D. Occupational infections. *Br Med J* 1996;313: 551–4.

Udasin IG. Biologic agents. In: Brooks SM, Gochfeld M, Herzstein J (eds), *Environmental Medicine*. St. Louis: Mosby, 1995.

University of Maryland Farm Safety Database. *Occupational Diseases* (hypertext document), 1997. Available at *http://www.inform.umd.edu/EdRes/Topic/AgrEnv/ndd/occsafe/INFECTIOUS_DISEASES.html.*

Internet Sources

Centers for Disease Control and Prevention. Access to information on hospital occupational health, immunizations, travel medicine, and infectious diseases. Also provides access to an electronic version of the *Morbidity and Mortality Weekly Report*. Available at *http://www.cdc.gov/.*

National Library of Medicine. Free Medline searches; links to a wide variety of medical topics. Available at *http://www.nlm.nih.gov/.*

Occupational and Environmental Medicine Resources. Access to the Guidelines for Employee Health Services in Health Care Facilities (Medical Center Occupational Health Section of the American College of Occupational and Environmental Medicine); home page for the Medical Center Occupational Health Section; information on the Medical Center Occupational Health Mailing List and archives of the list; links to hundreds of general medical as well as occupational and environmental medicine resources. Available at *http://www.occenvmed.net/.*

Duke University Occupational and Environmental Medicine. Access to information on the Occupational and Environmental Medicine Mailing List and archives of the list; compilation of recent government (e.g., CDC, NIOSH, EPA) documents pertinent to occupational and environmental medicine; links to many occupational and environmental medicine resources. Available at *http://152.3.65.120/oem/.*

5 / Vaccine-Preventable Diseases in Occupational Medicine

Ellen R. Kessler and Diane Dickerson

Employers have both a legal and ethical duty to provide a safe work environment for their employees and those who visit their workplaces. They also have a major business interest in supporting employees' health and welfare, maximizing their satisfaction and productivity, and preventing needless corporate financial burdens due to absenteeism. Because of these imperatives, employers have an obligation to protect the work force from occupationally acquired infections and diseases by making available an ongoing employment-based immunization program.

This chapter addresses current immunization guidelines for the prevention of accidentally acquired infections and suggests strategies for increasing compliance with these guidelines. Subsequent chapters address exposure prevention and postexposure prophylaxis for work-related infectious diseases for which there are no available immunizations. Later chapters also provide more detailed information regarding the signs and symptoms and the epidemiology of diseases that can be prevented through comprehensive workplace immunization programs.

There has always been an obvious need for infectious disease prevention programs within health care facilities, and more recently there is a growing awareness of similar needs among other industries. Employers' ever-expanding responsibility and opportunity to protect their employees from occupationally acquired diseases are evidenced by the increased numbers of employees traveling to foreign countries and the development of newly engineered vaccines such as the hepatitis A vaccine. Unfortunately, the effectiveness and cost-efficiency of adult immunization programs as tool for preventing disease are often overlooked. The underutilization of vaccines capable of preventing diseases and decreasing their morbidity and mortality remains a reality. The case of an unfortunate cardiovascular surgical resident who had not been immunized against hepatitis B and, despite adherence to infection control practices, contracted the disease and then transmitted the infection to 19 patients is a stark reminder of this underutilization [1].

Fortunately, there are nationwide campaigns in progress to ensure compliance with childhood vaccination programs and there is increasing participation of medical insurance providers in offering preventive services, including immunizations. However, the hesitancy of much of the adult population to participate in immunization programs warrants close attention and points up the need for more concentrated efforts to increase compliance. Reasons (or rationales) for noncompliance include:

- Denial of need for protection.
- Resistance or lack of interest.
- Inconvenience, time, and pain associated with vaccine administration.
- Misunderstandings regarding the need, effectiveness, and safety of vaccines.
- Indications for vaccinations and administration schedules vary according to age, medical conditions, and work environments.
- Inconvenience and costs associated with vaccine availability.

To overcome these obstacles, employers and occupational health professionals must directly address employees' misconceptions and concerns. This requires active physician support and an in-depth understanding of the importance and efficacy of the vaccines appropriate for specific work environments. It also requires ongoing educational efforts to inform potential vaccine recipients of the importance of acquiring immunity to certain vaccine-preventable diseases. Continuous highlighting of other workplace hazard controls, such as the observance of administrative and workplace health and safety procedures and the use of appropriate personal protective equipment, is also warranted and should be an integral component of the employee education process. For many companies, computerized tracking systems are instrumental in evaluating the progress of their immunization efforts as well as identifying specific departments or employee groups that require more targeted educational programs or other strategies to improve compliance.

Recommended Vaccines for Adults

The United States Public Health Service Advisory Committee on Immunization Practices (ACIP) regularly publishes the most recent recommendations regarding specific immunizations for adults and children in the *Morbidity and Mortality Weekly Report*. Discussion of every available vaccine is beyond the scope of this chapter; however, immunization recommendations for certain occupational groups, including travelers to foreign countries, is addressed in this chapter. Tables 5-1, 5-2, and 5-3 outline the most commonly used vaccines for adults in occupational settings.

INFLUENZA VACCINE

Outbreaks of influenza type A or B virus typically peak in the winter and cause community-wide epidemics every one to three years. Each year, the virus undergoes an antigenic drift that precludes complete natural or vaccinated immunity from the previous year. In some years, there is a total antigenic shift in which the virus is entirely dissimilar from previous years and subsequently is responsible for pandemic or worldwide epidemics.

Influenza outbreaks occur explosively, and one person can infect many others. An epidemic usually peaks between two to three weeks following the first reported cases in a community and continues for approximately five to six weeks. School-age children typically have the highest attack rate (50%), but theirs is generally a mild illness of fever and upper respiratory tract infection.

Mortality rates are significant for residents of long-term care facilities, for those who have underlying medical conditions, such as cardiac and pulmonary disease, and for newborns and the elderly.

The inactivated virus vaccine, which is composed of two A subtypes and one B subtype of the influenza virus, is the mainstay for prevention of the spread of disease. Viral subtypes that have been identified from the previous year go into the formulation of the vaccine for the upcoming year. Ongoing clinical trials are investigating more effective and convenient methods of prevention, such as intranasal administration of vaccine.

Many occupational health services provide annual influenza vaccination programs for their employees. In some industries, such as health care, a vaccination program is an imperative because the employees have direct contact with populations at risk for complications of influenza. In other settings, the employer recognizes that there is an easily attainable reduction in costs related to absenteeism during the flu season when the vaccine is both encouraged and provided, especially if vaccination is available at the worksite.

TETANUS TOXOID

Tetanus is an often fatal disease characterized by severe muscle spasms that typically occur in the neck and trunk muscles. These manifestations are caused by an exotoxin produced by the *Clostridium tetani*, an anaerobic or microaerophilic bacillus that proliferates at the site of injured tissue—typically a crush or puncture wound. The disease is most likely to occur in rural settings, where there is a greater exposure to animals and contaminated soil. Employee populations most at risk are those in agriculture and forestry industries.

Essentially all working-age individuals who were born in or have resided in the United States received the completed series of tetanus as a pre-

Table 5-1
Immunizing Agents and Immunization Schedules for Health Care Workers (HCWs)[a]

Generic Name	Primary Schedules and Booster(s)	Indications	Major Precautions and Contraindications	Special Considerations
Immunizing Agents Strongly Recommended for Health Care Workers				
Hepatitis B (HB) recombinant vaccine	Two doses IM 4 weeks apart; third dose 5 months after second; booster doses not necessary.	*Pre-exposure:* HCWs at risk for exposure to blood or body fluids. *Postexposure:* See Table 5-2.	On the basis of limited data, no risk of adverse effects to developing fetuses is apparent. Pregnancy should not be considered a contraindication to vaccination of women. Previous anaphylactic reaction to common baker's yeast is a contraindication to vaccination.	The vaccine produces neither therapeutic nor adverse effects on HBV-infected persons. Prevaccination serologic screening is not indicated for persons being vaccinated because of occupational risk. HCWs who have contact with patients or blood should be tested 1–2 months after vaccination to determine serologic response.
Hepatitis B immune globulin (HBIG)	0.06 mL/kg IM as soon as possible after exposure. A second dose of HBIG should be administered 1 month later if the HB vaccine series has not been started.	*Postexposure prophylaxis* (Table 5-2): For persons exposed to blood or body fluids containing HBsAg and who are not immune to HBV infection, 0.06 mL/kg IM as soon as possible (but no later than 7 days after exposure).		
Influenza vaccine (inactivated whole-virus and split-virus vaccines)	Annual vaccination with current vaccine. Administered IM.	HCWs who have contact with patients at high risk for influenza or its complications; HCWs who work in chronic care facilities; HCWs with high-risk medical conditions or who are aged ≥ 65 years.	History of anaphylactic hypersensitivity to egg ingestion.	No evidence exists of risk to mother or fetus when the vaccine is administered to a pregnant woman with an underlying high-risk condition. Influenza vaccination is recommended during second and third trimesters of pregnancy because of increased risk for hospitalization.
Measles live-virus vaccine	One dose SC; second dose at least 1 month later.	HCWs[b] born during or after 1957 who do not have documentation of having received 2 doses of live vaccine on or after the first birthday or a history of physician-diagnosed measles or serologic evidence of immunity. Vaccination should be considered	Pregnancy; immunocompromised persons,[c] including HIV-infected persons who have evidence of severe immunosuppression; anaphylaxis after gelatin ingestion or administration of neomycin; recent administration of globulin.	MMR is the vaccine of choice if recipients are likely to be susceptible to rubella and/or mumps as well as to measles. Persons vaccinated during 1963–1967 with a killed measles vaccine alone, killed vaccine followed by live vaccine, or with a vaccine of unknown

(continued)

Table 5-1 (continued)

Generic Name	Primary Schedules and Booster(s)	Indications	Major Precautions and Contraindications	Special Considerations
Measles live-virus vaccine (cont.)		for all HCWs who lack proof of immunity, including those born before 1957.		type should be revaccinated with 2 doses of live measles virus vaccine.
Mumps live-virus vaccine	One dose SC, no booster.	HCWs[b] believed to be susceptible can be vaccinated. Adults born before 1957 can be considered immune.	Pregnancy; immunocompromised persons[c]; history of anaphylactic reaction after gelatin ingestion or administration of neomycin.	MMR is the vaccine of choice if recipients are likely to be susceptible to measles and rubella as well as to mumps.
Rubella live-virus vaccine	One dose SC; no booster.	Indicated for HCWs,[b] both men and women, who do not have documentation of having received live vaccine on or after their first birthday or laboratory evidence of immunity. Adults born before 1957, *except women who can become pregnant*, can be considered immune.	Pregnancy, immunocompromised persons[b]; history of anaphylactic reaction after administration of neomycin.	The risk for rubella vaccine-associated malformations in the offspring of women pregnant when vaccinated or who become pregnant within 3 months after vaccination is negligible. Such women should be counseled regarding the theoretical basis of concern for the fetus. MMR is the vaccine of choice if recipients are likely to be susceptible to measles or mumps, as well as to rubella.
Varicella-zoster live-virus vaccine	Two 0.5 mL doses SC 4–8 weeks apart if ≥ 13 years of age.	Indicated for HCWs[b] who do not have either a reliable history of varicella or serologic evidence of immunity.	Pregnancy, immunocompromised persons,[c] history of anaphylactic reaction following receipt of neomycin or gelatin. Avoid salicylate use for 6 weeks after vaccination.	Vaccine is available from the manufacturer for certain patients with acute lymphocytic leukemia (ALL) in remission. Because 71%–93% of persons without a history of varicella are immune, serologic testing before vaccination is likely to be cost effective.
Varicella-zoster immune globulin (VZIG)	Persons < 50 kg: 125μg/10 kg IM; person ≤ 50 kg: 625 μg.	Persons known or likely to be susceptible (particularly those at high risk for complications, e.g., pregnant women) who have close and prolonged exposure to a contact case or to an infectious hospital staff worker or patient.		Serologic testing may help in assessing whether to administer VZIG. If use of VZIG prevents varicella disease, patient should be vaccinated subsequently.

(continued)

Table 5-1 (continued)

Generic Name	Primary Schedules and Booster(s)	Indications	Major Precautions and Contraindications	Special Considerations
BCG Vaccination				
Bacille Calmette-Guérin (BCG) vaccine (tuberculosis)	One percutaneous dose of 0.3 mL; no booster dose recommended.	Should be considered only for HCWs in areas where multidrug-resistant tuberculosis is prevalent, a strong likelihood of infection exists; and where comprehensive infection control precautions have failed to prevent TB transmission to HCWs.	Should not be administered to immunocompromised persons,[c] pregnant women.	In the United States, tuberculosis-control efforts are directed toward early identification, treatment of cases, and preventive therapy with isoniazid.
Other Immunobiologics That Are or May Be Indicated for Health Care Workers				
Immune globulin (hepatitis A)	Postexposure: One IM dose of 0.02 mL/kg administered ≤ 2 weeks after exposure.	Indicated for HCWs exposed to feces of infectious patients.	Contraindicated in persons with IgA deficiency; do not administer within 2 weeks after MMR vaccine, or 3 weeks after varicella vaccine. Delay administration of MMR vaccine for ≥ 3 months and varicella ≥ 5 months after administration of IG.	Administer in large muscle mass (deltoid, gluteal).
Hepatitis A vaccine	Two doses of vaccine either 6–12 months apart (HAVRIX) or 6 months apart (VAQTA).	Not routinely indicated for HCWs in the United States. Persons who work with HAV-infected primates or with HAV in a research laboratory setting should be vaccinated.	History of anaphylactic hypersensitivity to alum or, for HAVRIX, the preservative 2-phenoxyethanol. The safety of the vaccine in pregnant women has not been determined; the risk associated with vaccination should be weighed against the risk for hepatitis A women who may be at high risk for exposure to HAV.	
Meningococcal polysaccharide vaccine (tetravalent A, C, W1356, and Y)	One dose in volume and by route specified by manufacturer; need for boosters unknown.	Not routinely indicated for HCWs in the United States.	The safety of the vaccine in pregnant women has not been evaluated; it should not be administered during pregnancy unless the risk for infection is high.	

(continued)

Table 5-1 (continued)

Generic Name	Primary Schedules and Booster(s)	Indications	Major Precautions and Contraindications	Special Considerations
Typhoid vaccine, IM, SC, and oral	IM vaccine: One 0.5 mL dose, booster 0.5 mL every 2 years. SC vaccine: two 0.5 mL doses, ≥ 4 weeks apart, booster 0.5 mL SC or 0.1 ID every 3 years if exposure continues. Oral vaccine: Four doses on alternative days. The manufacturer recommends revaccination with the entire four-dose series every 5 years.	Workers in microbiology laboratories who frequently work with *Salmonella typhi*.	Severe local or systemic reaction to a previous dose. Ty21a (oral) vaccine should not be administered to immunocompromised persons[c] or to persons receiving antimicrobial agents.	Vaccination should not be considered an alternative to the use of proper procedures when handling specimens and cultures in the laboratory.
Vaccinia vaccine (smallpox)	One dose administered with a bifurcated needle; boosters administered every 10 years.	Laboratory workers who directly handle cultures with vaccinia, recombinant vaccinia viruses, or orthodox viruses that infect humans.	The vaccine is contraindicated in pregnancy, in persons with eczema or a history of eczema, and in immunocompromised persons[c] and their household contacts.	Vaccination may be considered for HCWs who have direct contact with contaminated dressings or other infectious material from volunteers in clinical studies involving recombinant vaccinia virus.
Other Vaccine-Preventable Diseases				
Tetanus and diphtheria (toxoids [Td])	Two IM doses 4 weeks apart; third dose 6–12 months after second dose; booster every 10 years.	All adults.	Except in the first trimester, pregnancy is not a precaution. History of a neurologic reaction or immediate hypersensitivity reaction after a previous dose. History of severe local (Arthus-type) reaction after a previous dose. Such persons should not receive further routine or emergency doses of Td for 10 years.	Tetanus prophylaxis in wound management.[d]

(continued)

Table 5-1 (continued)

Generic Name	Primary Schedules and Booster(s)	Indications	Major Precautions and Contraindications	Special Considerations
Pneumococcal polysaccharide vaccine (23 valent)	One dose, 0.5 mL, IM or SC; revaccination recommended for those at highest risk ≥ 5 years after the first dose.	Adults who are at increased risk of pneumococcal disease and its complications because of underlying health conditions; older adults, especially those age ≥ 65 who are healthy.	The safety of vaccine in pregnant women has not been evaluated; it should not be administered during pregnancy unless the risk for infection is high. Previous recipients of any type of pneumococcal polysaccharide vaccine who are at highest risk for fatal infection or antibody loss may be revaccinated ≥ 5 years after the first dose.	

[a] Persons who provide health care to patients or work in institutions that provide patient care, e.g., physicians, nurses, emergency medical personnel, dental professionals and students, medical and nursing students, laboratory technicians, hospital volunteers, and administrative and support staff in health-care institutions.
[b] All HCWs (i.e., medical or nonmedical, paid or volunteer, full time or part time, student or non-student, with or without patient-care responsibilities) who work in health care institutions (e.g., inpatient and outpatient, public and private) should be immune to measles, rubella, and varicella.
[c] Persons immunocompromised because of immune deficiency diseases, HIV infection, leukemia, lymphoma or generalized malignancy or immunosuppressed as a result of therapy with corticosteroids, alkylating drugs, antimetabolites, or radiation.
[d] Refer to CDC UPDATE ON ADULT IMMUNIZATION: Recommendations of the Advisory Committee on Immunization Procedures (ACIP), *MMWR* 1991;40(No RR-12):1–94.
Abbreviations: *IM* = intramuscular; *HBV* = hepatitis B virus; *HBsAg* = hepatitis B surface antigen; *SC* = subcutaneous; *HCW* = health care workers; *HIV* = human immunodeficiency virus; *MMR* = measles, rubella vaccine.
Adapted from Centers for Disease Control. Immunization of health-care workers: recommendations of the Advisory Committee on Immunization Practices (ACIP) and the Hospital Infection Control Practices Advisory Committee (HICPAC). *MMWR* 1997;46(No RR-18):1–34.

requisite for enrollment into school. However, it is essential that previously vaccinated employees receive booster vaccinations with the tetanus and diptheria vaccine (Td) at least every 10 years. Therefore, it is important to determine the Td vaccination status of all employees, particularly foreign-born individuals from rural areas of Africa, Asia, and South America, where immunization programs may not be routine.

MEASLES MUMPS AND RUBELLA VACCINE (MMR)

In the United States, the incidence of measles declined considerably after the introduction of the live, attenuated MMR vaccine in 1963. In 1983, only 1,493 cases were recorded; however, this trend dramatically reversed in the years 1989–1991, with a peak of 27,786 recorded cases in 1990. After this brief period, the downward trend resumed, and in 1997 only 135 cases were documented, which is the lowest annual incidence ever recorded [2].

Worldwide, measles infection continues to be problematic: Each year, there are an estimated 36.5 million cases and 1 million deaths caused by the disease, most of them in Africa. Since 1997, most of the recorded cases in the United States have been imported from Germany, Italy, Brazil, China, France, Pakistan, and the Philippines.

Health care workers and other employees who may have contact with measles carriers should be required to show evidence of immunity. This is particularly true for individuals who travel to countries where measles is poorly controlled. ACIP defines immunity as physician documentation of infection, serologic evidence of immunity, or documentation of two doses of the MMR vaccine administered after 16 months of age. Individuals born before 1957 are considered to have natural immunity; however, serologic sampling of hospital workers has indicated that approximately 5% of those born before 1957 were not immune to measles. Because nearly 30% of all health care workers who acquired measles at work between 1985 and 1989 were born before 1957 [3,4], the ACIP recommends that consideration be given to vaccinating an individual if there is reason to believe the person, regardless of age, is not immune.

In both children and adults, rubella virus presents as a mild febrile disease accompanied by a maculopapular rash. However, rubella can cause intrauterine death or devastating congenital abnormalities in the developing fetus. A single dose of live, attenuated rubella vaccine as part of the MMR will elicit an adequate antibody response in nearly 99% of susceptible individuals. In the United States, two doses of MMR are recommended as part of the childhood vaccination program. Medical personnel and all women of childbearing age who are likely to come in contact with individuals who have rubella or with patients in prenatal clinics should have serologic proof of immunization or physician-written documentation of at least one rubella immunization at the time of, or after, the first birthday.

PNEUMOCOCCAL VACCINE

In the United States, pneumococcal infections are responsible for approximately 40,000 deaths per year—that is, for more deaths than any other vaccine-preventable infection [5]. Individuals at risk who should be vaccinated include those age 65 or older and individuals with chronic diseases such as cardiovascular disease, pulmonary disease (excluding asthma), diabetes mellitus, chronic liver disease, alcoholism, and asplenism.

The Americans with Disabilities Act (ADA) of 1990 laid the foundation for more individuals with chronic illnesses to enter the work force. In addition, individuals age 65 or older remaining

Table 5-2
Recommended Postexposure Prophylaxis for Percutaneous or Permucosal Exposure to Hepatitis B Virus, United States

Vaccination and Antibody Response Status of Exposed Person	MBsAg[a] Positive	Treatment When Source Is HBsAg Negative	Source Not Tested or Status Unknown
Unvaccinated	HBIG[b] × 1; initiate HB vaccine series[c]	Initiate HB vaccine series.	Initiate HB vaccine series.
Previously vaccinated:			
Known responder ±	No treatment.	No treatment.	No treatment.
Known nonresponder	HBIG × 2 or HBIG × 1 and initiate revaccination	No treatment.	If known high-risk source, treat as if source were HBsAg positive.
Antibody response unknown	Test exposed person for anti-HBs[e] 1. If adequate,[d] no treatment. 2. If inadequate,[d] HBIG × 1 and vaccine booster.	No treatment.	Test exposed person for anti-HBs: 1. If adequate,[d] no treatment. 2. If inadequate,[d] initiate revaccination.

[a] Hepatitis B surface antigen.
[b] Hepatitis B immune globulin; dose 0.06 mL/kg intramuscularly.
[c] Hepatitis B vaccine.
[d] *Responder* is defined as a person with adequate levels of serum antibody to hepatitis B surface antigen (i.e., anti-HBs ≥ 10 IU/mL; *inadequate response to vaccination* is defined as serum anti-HBs < 10 mIU/mL.
[e] Antibody to hepatitis B surface antigen.
Adapted from Centers for Disease Control. Immunization of health-care workers: recommendations of the Advisory Committee on Immunization Practices (ACIP) and the Hospital Infection Control Practices Advisory Committee (HICPAC). *MMWR* 1997;46(No RR-18):1–34.

Table 5-3
Vaccines for Foreign Travelers

Vaccine or Toxoid	Indications	Schedule	Major Contraindications	Comments
Hepatitis B		See Table 5-2.		
Hepatitis A		See Table 5-1.		
Poliovirus	a. Health care workers and laboratory workers who may be in close contact with patients excreting wild poliovirus or who handle specimens from such patients. b. Members of community with current disease by wild polioviruses. c. Travelers to developing countries outside the Americas.	*Unimmunized adults:* IPV. Two doses at 4–8 week intervals, third dose 6–12 months after second (can be as soon as 2 months). Dose: 0.5 mL SC. *Partially immunized adults:* Complete primary series with either vaccine. IPV schedule shown above; OPV schedule is two doses 6–8 weeks apart, and third dose 6–12 months after second (can be given as early as 6–8 weeks after second if need urgent). No need to repeat doses if schedule is interrupted. Booster: OPV: None. IPV: None.	IPV: a. Pregnancy. b. Anaphylactic allergy to neomycin or streptomycin. *OPV:* a. Vaccine recipient or household contact is immunodeficient or immunosuppressed (including HIV infection). b. Pregnancy is relative contraindication; OPV may be used if immediate protection is needed. c. Anaphylactic allergy to neomycin or streptomycin. Malignancy. Chemotherapy. Radiation therapy.	In episode of potential exposure to wild poliovirus, adults who had only three doses of OPV or IPV previously may be given one more dose of either preparation.
Japanese encephalitis		Two or three doses given one week apart.	Pregnancy. Severe illness. Previous serious reaction to vaccine.	
Plague[a]	First dose (1 mL IM); second dose (0.2 mL IM) four weeks later; dose (0.2 mL IM) 3–6 months after dose two.			
Yellow fever[a]	One dose (0.5 mL SC).			
Meningococcal polysaccharide (tetravalent A, C, W135, and y)		See Table 5-1.		
Typhoid IM, SC, and oral		See Table 5-1.		
Rabies	Travelers planning to be more than 30 days in an area of the world where rabies is a constant threat.		Known reaction.[b] Neomycin allergy.[b] Thimerosal allergy.[b]	

(continued)

Table 5-3 (continued)

Vaccine or Toxoid	Indications	Schedule	Major Contraindications	Comments
Rabies, human diploid cell (HDCV)		Three doses (0.1 mL ID) on days 0,7, and 21 or 28.		Boost after two years or test serum for antibody level. Must not use chloroquine for malaria prophylaxis until three weeks after completion of third ID dose of vaccine.
Rabies, human diploid cell or rabies vaccine absorbed (RVA)		Three doses (1 mL IM in deltoid area) on days 0,7, and 28.		Boost after two years or test serum for antibody level.

[a] See manufacturer's package insert for recommendations on dosage.
[b] Not major contraindication.
Abbreviations: *ID* = intradermal; *IPV* = inactivated poliovirus vaccine; *OPV* = oral poliovaccine; *PO* = orally; *SC* = subcutaneously.

in, or returning to, the workplace is a growing trend. While the employee's primary care provider is generally responsible for providing the pneumococcal vaccine, the occupational health center may play an invaluable role by identifying employees at risk and directing them to their primary care provider or their company's occupational health service for appropriate vaccination.

VARICELLA VACCINE

Varicella (chickenpox) and herpes zoster (shingles) are clinical manifestations of the varicella-zoster virus (VZV). Varicella, the primary infection, is extremely contagious but is generally regarded as a benign, self-limited infection of childhood. However, varicella can be life-threatening for premature infants, individuals who are immunocompromised, and patients with chronic lung or skin afflictions. Any person over the age of 13 who has active infection may also suffer serious and sometimes fatal complications.

Approximately 9% of individuals older than age 15 are considered to be nonimmune, but a higher percent is found among people raised in the tropics or subtropics. Herpes zoster, the localized reactivation of the primary infection, occurs in all age groups but most commonly in the elderly.

In the workplace setting, VZV vaccine is underutilized. This is particularly true among health care workers who do not have a positive history of immunity to the disease. VZV vaccine has proved to be safe in healthy nonpregnant individuals and can reduce the costs of a hospital VZV-control program [6]. Concerns have been raised regarding the risk of transmission of virus following vaccination, particularly if the individual develops a varicella-like rash following immunization. To date, the benefits have far outweighed the theoretical risks; thus, susceptible health care workers should receive the vaccine. Nonimmune employees who are likely to travel to countries where VZV is prevalent or have exposures to nonimmunized children, as in a childcare setting, should consider vaccination.

HEPATITIS B VACCINE

Hepatitis B vaccine, which was first made available in 1976, has been a significant factor in the decline of transmission of hepatitis B virus (HBV) among health care workers. At one university hospital, the incidence of clinical HBV decreased from 82 cases per 100,000 between 1980 and 1984 to 0 cases between 1985 and 1989 [7].

Although hepatitis B vaccine—a highly purified viral antigen manufactured initially from pooled donor serum and later genetically engineered—has proved to be safe, the rate of acceptance among health care workers is strikingly inadequate. Many health care workers and other employees who come in contact with blood and other potentially infectious material (OPIM), believe they are not at risk for contracting the disease. Although the Occupational Safety and Health Administration (OSHA) Bloodborne Pathogen Standard mandates that employers offer potentially exposed employees the vaccine series at no cost, aggressive immunization campaigns are often lacking.

Prevaccination serologic screening for prior infection is not warranted for individuals receiving the vaccine series. Postvaccination testing for antibodies may be advisable if the individual is likely to have ongoing risk of injuries from sharp instruments or needlesticks. Knowledge of the individual's antibody response after completion of the hepatitis series aids in the determination of the need for immediate postexposure prophylaxis in the event of an accident.

In a significant percentage of individuals, antibodies to HBV following vaccine gradually decrease over time. However, studies have shown that despite waning antibody titers to HBV, vaccine-induced immunity persists and will probably prevent clinical hepatitis or viremia [8]. Therefore, booster doses may be unnecessary. ACIP continues to assess the need for booster doses as more data become available (see Table 5-2) [9].

HEPATITIS A VACCINE

In response to the recent FDA approval of two hepatitis A vaccines, ACIP has published recommendations for the prevention of hepatitis A virus (HAV) [10]. In most pre-exposure settings, the vaccine can be used instead of immune globulin (IG). In postexposure settings, IG is generally recommended.

Employees who travel to, or work in, countries that have high or intermediate HAV endemicity should be vaccinated before departure. HAV is superior to IG for individuals ages 2 or older who plan frequent travel or who reside for long periods of time in high-risk areas. U.S. travelers to other countries in North America (except Mexico and Central America), western Europe, Japan, Australia, or New Zealand are not considered to be at greater risk than those who travel within the United States.

Employees who work with HAV-infected primates or with HAV in a research laboratory are the only occupational groups shown to be at increased risk for HAV infection because of occupational exposure. Although outbreaks of hepatitis A have been documented in other work settings, such as food handling, health care centers, sewage treatment facilities, and child care centers, pre-exposure immunization is not routinely recommended.

POLIOVIRUS VACCINE

In the United States, control of poliomyelitis has essentially been achieved because of the success of the polio vaccination program that began in the 1950s. Since 1980, fewer than 150 cases of paralytic paralysis have been reported, most of which were associated with vaccination; a handful of cases have been due to importation of the wild poliovirus into the United States. Prevention of epidemics due to imported virus can be sustained only by ongoing early childhood vaccination programs. Routine vaccination of adults who reside in the United States is not recommended because of the low probability of exposure and the high probability of immunity in the adult population.

Adults should receive the poliovirus vaccine only if they have a high risk of exposure to the virus. All health care workers and laboratory workers who are in close contact with patients excreting wild poliovirus or who handle specimens from those patients should receive the vaccine. Travelers to developing countries outside the Americas are also candidates for vaccination against polio. In order to reduce the risk of vaccine-associated paralytic paralysis (VAPP), ACIP recommends the use of inactivated poliovirus vaccine (IPV) instead of oral poliovirus vaccine (OPV) in unvaccinated adults. Adults who have previously been immunized and are receiving a booster dose are not considered to be at risk for VAPP; either OPV or IPV is recommended for them.

LYME DISEASE VACCINE

Lyme disease is a tick-borne infection caused by the spirochete *Borrelia burgdorferi*. It is the most common tick-borne disease in the United States. An average of 12,500 cases were reported to the CDC during 1993–1997 [11]. The disease primarily occurs in the northeastern, mid-Atlantic, upper north central regions of the United States as well as in the northwestern regions of California. The transmission of the spirochete from the tick occurs after 24–48 hours of attachment to the individual. Transmission peaks from April through July, when the nymphal stages of the tick vectors of Lyme disease, *Ixodes scapularis* and *I pacificus*, are actively seeking hosts.

Approximately 85% of individuals with symptomatic Lyme disease have the typical erythema migrans rash. If untreated, the infection can cause arthritis or neurologic symptoms such as radiculoneuropathy or encephalopathy. Antibiotics are usually effective in eradicating the disease completely.

Recently, two Lyme disease vaccines, LYMErix and ImuLyme have been developed; they use recombinant *B burgdorferi* lipidated outer-surface protein A (rOspA) as an immunogen. To date, only LYMErix has been approved by the Food and Drug Administration (FDA) for use in the United States. When vaccinated, the individual is protected by the production of OspA antibodies, which kill the Lyme spirochetes in the gut of the vector tick between time of attachment and transmission to the host.

LYMErix has been approved for individuals ages 15–70 and is administered as a three-dose regimen given over a 12-month period. The protective efficacy of the vaccine has been shown to be 75% after the third dose; however, the duration of protection is unknown. Antibody titers have been shown to decrease over time, and it is likely that booster doses will be necessary.

Recommendations for the Lyme disease vaccine target individuals who are at risk for exposure to infected ticks. The vaccine is recommended for individuals who live, work, or recreate in regions of high or moderate risk for Lyme disease and are likely to have frequent or prolonged contact with infected ticks. The vaccine may be considered for those who are exposed to tick-infested areas, but the exposure is not considered to be frequent or prolonged. The vaccine is not recommended for persons who have minimal or no exposure to the tick-infested areas. The vaccine is also not recommended for individuals in geographic regions with the lowest incidence of the disease. The decision to vaccinate short-term travelers to highly endemic areas should be considered if frequent or prolonged exposure is anticipated.

RABIES VACCINE

Rabies is a fatal viral disease of the central nervous system that can infect most mammals. The most susceptible animals are bats, raccoons, skunks, coyotes, foxes, wolves and unvaccinated dogs, cats, and livestock. Occupational groups such as veterinarians, veterinary technicians, animal control officers, wildlife workers and other animal handlers who are frequently exposed to these animals, are at particular risk of viral transmission, and exposures may be inapparent. Laboratory workers who work with the live rabies virus, spelunkers (cave explorers), certain construction workers, and travelers to foreign countries where canine rabies is a problem should also be considered at risk for exposure to rabies. All of these workers should undergo the three-dose pre-exposure series with the rabies vaccine. This is particularly necessary if the individual is working in a remote area where the vaccine is not readily available. If a rabies exposure takes place, postexposure immunization with two doses of the vaccine is still necessary, even if the exposed individual has received the pre-exposure series.

The newer rabies vaccines have proved to be safe and better tolerated than the earlier formulations. Most of the symptoms (i.e., fever, rash, muscle aches) have been due to preservatives in the vaccine; the most recently approved preservative-free vaccine may significantly decrease these side effects.

Vaccines for Health Care and Laboratory Workers

Health care and laboratory workers are exposed to a variety of infections in the occupational setting. Most of these exposures are in some manner representative of exposures from the community that these workers serve. However, because of the increased diversity of communities, the types of infectious disease exposures have become more varied. In addition, laboratory workers are more likely to encounter a greater variety of infectious agents when handling cultures or infected animals for research purposes.

To support employer immunization programs, the Centers for Disease Control and Prevention (CDC) has published three vaccine-preventable disease categories to serve as guidelines for the use of vaccines [12].

1. Diseases for which active immunization is strongly recommended because of their special risks for health care workers: hepatitis B, influenza, measles, mumps, rubella, and varicella.
2. Diseases for which active and/or passive immunizations may be indicated in certain circumstances: tuberculosis, hepatitis A, meningococcal disease, pertussis, typhoid fever, and vaccinia.
3. Diseases for which immunization of all adults is recommended: diphtheria, tetanus, and pneumococcal disease.

It cannot be overemphasized that sound preventive measures such as standard precautions, thorough hand-washing, and the use of personal protective equipment are the most important methods for reducing the risk of transmitting nosocomial infections to other patients and health care workers. Vaccines that are safe and effective in reducing nosocomial infections must be promoted and made easily available to all employees, including those working night and weekend shifts. Extended clinic hours and on-site vaccination programs help to increase employee participation in employers' vaccination campaigns, especially at certain times such as during the annual influenza season.

Vaccines for Travelers to Foreign Countries and Endemic Areas

It has become more commonplace for employees in both the public and private sector to have work duties that require either frequent travel or a temporary assignment outside the United States. In addition, international agencies recruit health care workers to volunteer their time to reconstruction efforts in countries devastated by war, natural disaster, or poverty. The possibility of exposure to malaria, yellow fever, typhoid, polio, hepatitis A, meningitis, and other infectious diseases must be evaluated prior to travel abroad. Not infrequently, these assignments occur unexpectedly and preclude adequate time for optimal vaccination. For workers whose jobs entail travel, particularly in certain endemic areas, all possible health and safety measures must be taken, which necessitates having the most current information on infectious disease outbreaks in a particular area. The CDC's Traveler's Health Hotline (404-332-4559 [phone]; 404-332-4565 [fax]; *http://www.cdc.gov/travel/travel.html* [website]), as well as most travelers clinics, may be instrumental in providing necessary information on recommended immunizations and schedules. Table 5-3 categorizes the most frequently required immunizations for individuals who travel abroad.

Future Vaccines

Several new and promising vaccines are in development, undergoing clinical trials, or awaiting approval for licensing. For instance, a U.S. Food and Drug Administration advisory panel has recommended the approval of two vaccines for the prevention of Lyme disease in people ages 15 and over. Other vaccines that hold considerable promise include malaria vaccine, respiratory syncytial virus (RSV) vaccine, rotavirus vaccine, and *Streptococcus pneumonia* vaccine. In addition, major research has been launched to develop new tuberculosis vaccines [13].

Role of Employers and Occupational Health Professionals

Over the past decade, significant progress has been made in dealing with work-related infectious disease exposure and prevention. Legislative directives, most notably OSHA's Bloodborne Pathogen Standard, broke new ground on the prevention front by mandating employer responsibility for at-risk employees. Compliance with this standard resulted in hepatitis B vaccination campaigns. Unfortunately, employees' acceptance of this and other safety-proven vaccines has sometimes been disappointing, and the occurrence of preventable work-related infectious diseases continue to be of concern. Employers, particularly in the health care industry, have generally assumed responsibility for providing the appropriate immunizations according to recommended guidelines, but this becomes an increasingly difficult task when, for example, hospitals merge to become complex hospital systems, and outpatient services and physician practices are purchased by these systems.

Besides employers, occupational health professionals also play a major role in influencing employees and increasing their understanding and acceptance of preventive procedures such as vaccines. Providing employees with immunization programs not only supports workers' health and safety, but also saves dollars for the organization over the long term—namely, through decreases in lost workdays, and thus increased productivity, as well as decreases in workers' compensation costs. However, in order to realize the long-term gains, employers must be willing to bear the costs associated with the administration of vaccines as well as with ongoing employee education and efforts to gain increased employee acceptance of them.

References

1. Harpaz R, Von Seidlein L, Averhoff FM, et al. Transmission of hepatitis B virus to multiple patients from a surgeon without evidence of inadequate infection control. *N Engl J Med* 1996;334:594–95.
2. Advances in global measles control and elimination. *MMWR* 1998;47(No RR-11):5.
3. Braunstein H, Thomas S, Ito R. Immunity to measles in a large population of varying age. *Am J Dis Child* 1990;144:296–8.
4. Smith E, Welch W, Berhow M, et al. Measles susceptibility of hospital employees as determined by ELISA. *Clin Res* 1990;38:183A.
5. Prevention of pneumococcal disease: recommendations of the Advisory Committee on Immunization Practices (ACIP). *MMWR* 1997;46(No RR-8):3.
6. Nettleman M, Schmid M. Controlling varicella in the healthcare setting: the cost effectiveness of using varicella vaccine in healthcare workers. *Infect Control Hosp Epidemiol* 1997;18:504–8.
7. Lamphear BP, Linneman CC Jr, Cannon CG, et al. Decline of clinical hepatitis B in workers at a general hospital: relation to increasing vaccine-induced immunity. *Clin Infect Dis* 1993;11:10–14.
8. Hadler SC, Margolis HS. Hepatitis B immunization: vaccine types, efficacy and indications for immunization. In: Remington JS, Swartz MN (eds), *Current Topics in Infectious Diseases.* Boston: Blackwell Scientific, 1992. Pp 282–308.
9. Centers for Disease Control. Hepatitis B virus: a comprehensive strategy for eliminating transmission in the United States through childhood immunization: recommendations of the Advisory Committee on Immunization Practices (ACIP). *MMWR* 1991; 40(No RR-13):1–25.
10. Centers for Disease Control. Prevention of hepatitis A through active or passive immunization: recommendations of the Advisory Committee on Immunization Practices (ACIP). *MMWR* 1996;45(No RR-15):11–23.
11. Centers for Disease Control and Prevention. Recommendations for the use of Lyme disease vaccine: recommendations of the Advisory Committee on Immunization Practices (ACIP). *MMWR* 1999;48(No RR07):1–14.
12. Centers for Disease Control and Prevention. Immunization of health-care workers: recommendations of the Advisory Committee on Immunization Practices (ACIP) and the Hospital Infection Control Practices Advisory Committee (HICPAC). *MMWR* 1997;46(No RR-18): 1–34.
13. Centers for Disease Control and Prevention. Development of new vaccines for tuberculosis: recommendations of the Advisory Council for the Elimination of Tuberculosis (ACET). *MMWR* 1998;47(No RR-13):1–6.

6 / Legal Challenges

Susan O. Cassidy

Managing employees with health problems is an increasingly complex legal challenge. Prior to 1990, workers' compensation and state disability laws determined employers' duties and workers' benefits. The explosion of laws providing new protections and benefits for workers has led to confusing and often conflicting duties for employers. The primary reasons for this confusion are the diversity of purpose and the lack of common goals of the various legislation.

Workers' compensation provides compensation for lost wages (indemnity costs), medical expenses, and financial compensation for permanent impairment, but only if an individual has a work-related injury or illness. Under the workers' compensation system, workers injured or made ill as a result of their job are generally entitled to specified benefits without regard to the duration or permanency of the impairment.

The Americans with Disabilities Act (ADA) legislated the integration of disabled individuals back into the workplace and into society. The ADA does not provide financial benefits, but rather seeks to level the playing field for impaired individuals whose disability is substantial and of significant duration. Under the ADA, workplace accommodations are required if they will enable a qualified individual with a disability to perform the essential functions of his or her job.

The Family Medical Leave Act (FMLA) provides covered individuals with unpaid time away from work to recuperate or care for an ill family member. Unlike workers' compensation, the ADA and FMLA apply to specified disabled or medically ill individuals, regardless of whether or not their illness or injury is job related. While certain short-term illnesses may be covered under workers' compensation and the FMLA, they are expressly excluded from ADA protections.

Managing the exposure and communicability issues associated with infectious disease in the workplace adds substantially to the complexity of the legally mandated employer duties. The potential for significant effects on business productivity and for exposure to huge financial losses makes it imperative that employers and health care professionals have a firm grasp of the areas of conflict and overlap and of the scope of employee protections under these laws. Further complicating this complex interplay of medicine and employment protections are privacy and confidentiality concerns as well as the laws regulating the collection and release of medical information. In addition to the federal laws that address medical record requirements for specified medical conditions, there is a patchwork of state statutory and case law that differs across state borders.

Workers' Compensation

HISTORICAL OVERVIEW

Common law imposed employer duties such as the provision of a safe place to work, safe tools, and equipment and the need to give adequate warnings when a servant (employee) could not appreciate a danger. Further, employers were expected to train fellow servants to minimize workplace accidents and injuries [1]. Common law permitted an injured employee to bring legal action against their employer for breach of these duties, but the remedies for injury or death were inadequate due to the "unholy trinity" of common law defenses. These three employer defenses—fellow-servant doctrine, contributory negligence, and assumption of risk—left many workers without recourse or compensation for work-related injuries or illnesses. In this way, courts, reflecting societal desires to encourage and support continued industrial growth and expansion, shielded employers from much of the financial burden for worker injury. Many of these same defenses continue to exist in one form or another in the current American tort system.

Fellow Servant Doctrine

In the absence of an express written contract, a master was not liable to an employee for the injuries caused by the negligence of a fellow servant. Such negligence was a risk incident to employment and was assumed by the employee. It was believed that this would lead to co-workers being careful and watchful of each other. The harshness of this doctrine was mitigated by several well-recognized exceptions—situations in which fellow servants did not have a common master, those in which servants were not engaged in the same enterprise, and those wherein injury was caused by the negligence of a vice principal acting as the employer's agent or supervisor [2].

Contributory Negligence

Under common law, employees had a duty to exercise reasonable care for their own safety. Where an employee failed to exercise reasonable care or take prudent safety precautions, the individual was barred from recovery from the employer under a contributory negligence defense. This defense was weakened with the enactment of statutes expressly imposing worker safety requirements for certain categories of employees and creating comparative negligence defenses.

Assumption of Risk

Under common law, employees were deemed to have voluntarily assumed certain risks incident to working. Such risks included those that a mature worker was presumed to know even if the individual worker did not have actual knowledge, and also included extraordinary or substantial risks of which the worker had actual knowledge. In contrast to the contributory negligence defense, grounded in tort theories of duty and breach of such duty, assumption of risk theory was contractual in nature. Consequently, the presence or absence of fault had little role in raising or mitigating an assumption of the risk defense. However, even when an employee could prove that he did not assume the risk of the danger that caused his injury, he could be barred from recovery if the employer could show contributory negligence [3].

In the nineteenth century, rising industrial injury and death rates prompted enactment of employer liability legislation. The fellow servant doctrine defense was eroded in 1855, when the state of Georgia enacted provisions for railroad worker protections for workers injured by the negligence of a fellow worker. By the early 1900s, almost every other jurisdiction in the United States had enacted statutes providing similar protections [4]. In 1908, Congress passed legislation that covered interstate railroad workers, and later seamen, under an employer's liability act system. These protections soon proved inadequate, as workers continued to have the burden of invoking the legal system to obtain recovery from employers for workplace injuries.

European counties were struggling with their own forms of compensation for injured workers. Both the German and British systems of compensation greatly influenced the ultimate form of workers' compensation in the United States. In 1884, Germany enacted the first workers' compensation act when it passed legislation establishing a compulsory system of accident insurance for employees in manufacturing, mining, and transportation industries [5]. Great Britain enacted. The Workmen's Compensation Act of 1897, which served as the template for the legislation passed in the United States in the early 1900s [6]. The British act set forth limitations on the scope of coverage, "arising out of and in the course of employment" [7]. This enduring phrase is still found in state workers' compensation statutes throughout the United States. While the Workmen's Compensation Act of 1897 provided coverage for hazardous jobs, it did not contain insurance provisions, leaving that burden on employers as a cost of doing business.

While it is beyond the scope of this chapter to cover all employee protection legislation, it is important to recognize that once legislative rule-making began in this arena, many laws providing protections to certain worker groups were passed. Such early legislation included the Federal Employees' Compensation Act, the Federal Employers' Liability Act, the Jones Act, the LongShore and Harbor Workers' Compensation Act, the Federal Coal Mine Health and Safety Act of 1969, and the Federal Black Lung Benefits Legislation.

GENERAL PROVISIONS

While the provisions and policies of workers' compensation statutes have evolved over the intervening years, general themes continue to characterize this system of legal recovery for work-related illness and injury. The elective nature of workers' compensation coverage gave way to presumptive coverage, wherein a worker was presumed to be covered by their employer unless coverage was contractually waived, and finally to the compulsory coverage system used in a majority of states. Constitutional objections to such state action have been overcome by amending state constitutions to grant the state the necessary legislative power to enact workers' compensation laws [8].

Generally, a "covered employer" is an employer with at least one employee. Covered employees are those incurring an injury that arises out of, and in the course of, the employment relationship. In most states, an employee with a preexisting condition aggravated or accelerated by the workplace is also covered under workers' compensation. In addition to compulsory coverage, a key component of all workers' compensation systems is the exclusive coverage provision. Exclusivity provisions enable an ill or injured worker or their dependents legal recovery regardless of fault; they also provide for financial compensation to the worker and ensure the coverage of the costs of medical treatment without the necessity of bringing suit against the employer. The price for these employee protections was employer protection from negligence suits brought by their employees. Much controversy and uneasiness continues to surround exclusivity provisions. Employee advocates argue that such provisions eviscerate the due process rights of injured individuals by limiting recovery to modest compensation for injuries and illness without the ability to sue to recover for employer negligence. Under this no-fault system, employers have lost the right to assert contributory negligence, assumption of risk, and fellow servant defenses but can limit their financial exposure and get fixed costs by insuring the liability. Despite no-fault provisions, certain employee actions—for example, self-inflicted injuries and intoxication—can preclude financial recovery. Workers' compensation systems operate by spreading the cost of workplace illness and injuries across society, as the costs to employers are then incorporated into the price of products and cost of services.

BENEFITS

Employee benefits under workers' compensation vary by state and are based on a wage-loss rationale, a medical-loss rationale, or a combined scheme. A wage-loss approach compensates an individual who suffers a loss of wages or diminished earning capacity, while a medical-loss approach provides for compensation for a medical loss—for example, loss of vision or an extremity—without regard to loss of wages or diminished earning capacity [9]. Regardless of the approach, the system generally provides only modest compensation to the injured or ill worker, and the standardized schedule of awards in some states results in inadequate and inequitable remedies for some individuals.

THIRD-PARTY LIABILITY

While workers are generally barred from bringing suit against their employer and must accept workers' compensation as their sole remedy if they sustain a work-related illness or injury, they are not prohibited from seeking legal redress from third parties. Increasingly, affected employees are initiating suit against co-workers, including physicians employed by the company. While co-workers may have immunity for nonintentional acts under state workers' compensation statutes or under case law, a few states permit actions to be brought against anyone other than the employer. In these states, a worker or their dependents may bring legal action against a co-worker whose negligence results in injury or loss of life [10].

Affected employees are not prohibited from suing employers and others for property damage. In addition, employees may sue the involved third party if injury is the result of negligent inspection or performance by company vendors. Employers and their insurers have also been successfully sued by employees who can demonstrate bad faith in the processing or administration of a workers' compensation claim [11]. Such actions create an opportunity for large monetary awards for relatively minor injuries.

Claimants have also utilized product liability statutes when injury has occurred as the result of a specific product or instrument. Courts have increasingly embraced strict liability in many product liability suits against product manufacturers, opening the door for substantial monetary awards. Dual capacity liability may be claimed, in addition to the workers' compensation claim if a worker is injured while using a product manufactured by his employer. Private physicians treating employees for workers' compensation claims are liable for medical malpractice under the usual tort statutes of duty and breach of that duty with resultant harm. Physicians who are employed by the company may escape liability for negligence under co-worker immunity provisions of the workers' compensation statutes, but it could be argued that they are independent contractors and therefore subject to tort liability as third party.

INTENTIONAL TORTS

Workers' compensation immunity does not extend to employers' intentional torts against workers. Employers have been successfully sued for intentional infliction of emotional distress [12], retaliation and discrimination [13], and sexual assault [14]. Increasingly, courts are permitting claims of intentional torts to be filed as part of workers' compensation claims. In such instances, employees have received enhanced awards without the necessity of separate tort actions against their employers. Additionally, employers may face criminal liability if serious injury or death has resulted from an employer's failure to remediate a known hazard, or in instances in which an employer knew or should have known of employee exposure to highly hazardous materials or operations.

Most states permit discharged employees to sue for retaliatory discharge if there is evidence that an employee was fired for filing a workers' compensation claim. In addition, workers' compensation legislation does not pre-empt federal law, thus permitting claims for age, gender, or disability discrimination or other federal discrimination claims to be brought against employers. Furthermore, state actions, including but not limited to harassment, libel, slander, and false imprisonment, are not barred by workers' compensation laws.

COVERAGE

Workers' compensation coverage hinges on employee status, employment relatedness, and the medical condition at issue. Compensation is available only if there is a reasonable nexus between the injury and the job. States have enacted specific exclusions, such as commuting to and from work and employer recreational activities, as well as specific inclusions and criteria, such as cardiac injury. As a general rule, coverage is available if the accident occurs on company premises, during travel between company sites, or during travel required as part of the job. Home offices are also considered company premises for purposes of workers' compensation coverage if the employee regularly performs work for the company there. Most state workers' compensation laws require claimants to demonstrate that they sustained their injuries or illnesses *during the course of their employment* and that their *condition arose out of their employment* [15]. The course of employment inquiry considers time, location, and circumstances of the incident, while the "arising out of" inquiry involves evaluation of the underlying cause of the claimant's injuries.

In the area of work-related infectious diseases, courts have generally limited coverage to workers who can demonstrate that their employment exposed them to increased risk of infection compared to that of the general public [16]. Historically, such workers have been health care workers exposed to infected patients, corrections and law enforcement officers, and workers who, by the nature of their jobs, are required to work in unsanitary conditions. Unlike accidents or acute injuries when infectious diseases are involved, it is more difficult to prove causality for purposes of workers' compensation. Reasons for this include the long latency period of many infectious diseases prior to the development of clinical symptoms and/or signs, the prevalence of certain infections in the community, and the lack of specific markers to track the source of infection. When infections suddenly develop due to sudden exposure to infectious agents in the workplace, there is generally little difficulty demonstrating work relatedness. However, some states permit claimants legal recovery under workers' compensation if they can prove that their job placed them at increased risk for their illness. In a Connecticut case, a dental hygienist was awarded workers' compensation after the court concluded that "it is more likely than not that Claimant's infection with hepatitis arose out of and in the course of her employment" [17]. To be compensable, a disease is not required to be one that arises solely out of the particular kind of employment in which the employee is engaged, nor must it be due to causes in excess of the ordinary hazards of that particular type of employment [18] .

Further, it is now not always necessary to actually contract an illness or disease to recover under workers' compensation. In *Doe v Stamford* [19] the state's highest court recently held that a police officer who, during the course of restraining a prisoner, was exposed to but had not contracted a potentially fatal contagious disease, was entitled to recover the reasonable expenses that he incurred for medically appropriate testing and treatment. The claimant police officer was exposed to HIV and tuberculosis during two separate incidents three months apart. The HIV exposure was the result of his thumb, which had an open wound, coming into contact with medical pads contaminated with bodily fluids from a criminal suspect who was HIV positive. The tuberculosis exposure resulted from repeated close physical contact with another criminal suspect who, it was later learned, had active disease [20]. The court held that these exposures constituted compensable "injuries" within the definitional boundaries of the state's workers' compensation act.

Confidentiality and Release of Medical Information

Expanded collection of individual health data has led to renewed public concern about and awareness of the uses and potential misuses of personal health information. Computerized recording of medical data and technologic advances in diagnostic testing and genome identification and mapping have left workers increasingly concerned that employers' knowledge and access to such data may negatively impact their employment status. It is against this backdrop that heightened care must be exercised in the collection and release of medical information, regardless of the setting or payment system.

It has been generally recognized that workers seeking payment for medical expenses and wage replacement waive confidentiality of the medical information related to the work-related injury or medical condition. While specific laws governing medical records vary by state, there has been an increasing tendency to narrow the scope of the medical information available to payers without express release by the claimant. Several states limit this access to the treating physician or curtail the content and scope of discussions between employers and their agents and the claimant's physician. Further, the ADA sets forth confidentiality requirements for the protection and release of employee medical information. The ADA's express intention to provide protection of employee medical data must be considered when releasing any type of employee medical data. Even where state laws purport to give greater freedom to release medical information, they are not a defense to a wrongful disclosure claim under federal legislation such as the ADA. While states are free to require greater protections for employee medical information, they cannot provide less protection than outlined in the ADA or other laws. This aspect of the preemption of state laws by federal laws, such as the ADA, has not received the attention it deserves, particularly in regard to the use and disclosure of medical information in the workers' compensation setting. Currently, it is not uncommon for employee medical information related to a workplace incident, including symptoms and diagnosis, to be freely shared with numerous individuals within the company or insurance environment. EEOC Enforcement Guidance documents provide clarification regarding employer confidentiality duties [21].

> An employer must keep any medical information on applicants or employees confidential, with the following limited exceptions:
>
> - Supervisors and managers may be told about necessary restrictions on the work or duties of the employee and about necessary accommodations;
> - First-aid and safety personnel may be told if the disability might require emergency treatment;
> - Government officials investigating compliance with the ADA must be given relevant information on request;
> - Employers may give information to state workers' compensation offices, state second injury funds or workers' compensation insurance carriers in accordance with state workers' compensation laws;
> - Employers may use the information for insurance purposes. For example, an employer may submit medical information to the company's health insurance carrier if the information is needed to administer a health insurance plan in accordance with § 501(c) of the ADA.

EEOC guidelines on release and disclosure of medical information clearly specifies that such information is lawfully disclosed within the company only on a strict *need-to-know basis* and stipulates that employee medical information must be kept separate from personnel records. This applies to workers' compensation information, such as diagnosis or symptoms, as well as to non-work-related medical conditions. Documents containing medical information that need to be put into the personnel file, must have all medical information removed prior to placement in that file [22].

While many state workers' compensation forms signed by claimants authorize release of medical information and records to the payer and the state, it has become increasingly important for health care professionals to obtain a signed, specific release prior to disclosing any medical information to anyone besides the claimant. Such medical releases should clearly specify to whom the information is to be released, the scope of the medical information being released, and the duration of the authorized release interval. Further, each page of information should be stamped "not authorized for re-disclosure."

Special care must be exercised not to exceed the scope of the release, and if sensitive medical information such as substance abuse, psychiatric information or HIV/AIDS data is involved, it is imperative that specific federal and state laws regarding the process and procedures for lawful release are followed. Many states have specific laws regarding HIV/AIDS testing and information release—for example, New York State requires that a special state form be utilized to lawfully release such information. Connecticut, while not requiring a special form, has a statute prescribed paragraph that must be included on the medical release form. As of July 1998, 32 states have enacted HIV/AIDS reporting requirements for revealing the identities of individuals so diagnosed. Such reporting requirements have rigid confidentiality and release protections.

In the workers' compensation setting, and in general, even if lawful consent can be obtained, it is prudent not to release or discuss any medical information that is not relevant to the narrow scope of issues at hand. Physicians have been successfully sued for release of HIV data that they received during the course of treating a workers' compensation injury. A New York court ruled that a physician who had released medical records, which included HIV status, had violated the law because she had not utilized the state-required consent form. In this case, the physician treating the claimant for a workers' compensation injury had released the medical records to the Pennsylvania workers' compensation board pursuant to a subpoena [23]. When releasing medical information relevant to the workers' compensation claim to anyone, including the employer or the state, specific consent by the claimant for the release should be obtained. If an overriding public health consideration or a demand for medical information pursuant to a subpoena arises, it is prudent to obtain legal advice to frame the issues, ensure that the most conservative approach is taken, and provide for a defensible position in the event of future legal scrutiny.

The Family and Medical Leave Act

In addition to workers' compensation benefits, employees with occupationally related infectious diseases are also likely to be entitled to unpaid FMLA leave [24]. The FMLA was enacted to provide workers with time to recuperate from a health condition or, in certain circumstances, to provide care for others. An employee receives up to 12 weeks of unpaid leave per 12-month period in any of the following circumstances:

- Child care following the birth of a child or placement of a child for adoption or foster care.
- The employee's need to care for a spouse, child, or parent who has a serious health condition.
- A serious health condition that makes the employee unable to perform the essential functions of his or her position.

Serious health condition is defined as:

- Inpatient care or any period of incapacity or any subsequent treatment in connection with such inpatient care.
- Absence from work plus treatment by a health care provider.
- Pregnancy.
- A chronic condition requiring treatment.
- Permanent or long-term condition requiring supervision.
- Multiple treatments for a nonchronic condition.

It is likely that most employees who contract an occupationally related infectious disease will be entitled to FMLA leave, as well as paid time off, for the time they are rendered unable to work due to their illness. Exceptions to FMLA entitlement occur when an employee has not been employed long enough to be eligible or has previously exhausted their FMLA benefits within the same benefits year. FMLA leave can run concurrently with paid time off under workers' compensation, the employer's sick-days program, or short-term disability, provided the employer notifies the employee that the paid time off is also being counted against the 12 weeks that the individual may be entitled to under the FMLA.

Americans with Disabilities Act (ADA)

In 1990, Congress passed landmark legislation to address inequities faced by individuals with disabilities. In the employment sector, this federal law trumps state legislation, including workers' compensation laws. While states are free to provide greater protections to its citizens under workers' compensation statutes, they cannot enact laws that violate or narrow protections provided under the ADA. Individuals with an illness or injury may be covered by one, both, or neither law. In addition, FMLA and state disability laws may come into play and must be reconciled with the rights, duties, and benefits of workers' compensation and the ADA.

Title I of the ADA prohibits employers from discriminating against qualified individuals because of disability in all aspects of employment [25]. This contrasts with workers' compensation law, which provides a scheme for prompt and fair settlement of employees' claims (for lost wages, lost earning capacity, and medical expenses) against employers for occupational injury and illness. An employee with an occupational injury or illness generally has a "disability" for workers' compensation purposes, but may not have a "disability" for purposes of the ADA [26]. Further, ADA proscriptions temper or invalidate states' worker exclusion laws. In its guidance document, the EEOC expressly addresses the apparent conflict of the ADA with state health and safety laws, which permit or require an employer to exclude individuals with certain disabilities from employment. The ADA does not allow such exclusion except where the employer can demonstrate that the individual is a "direct threat" [27]. Further, even if an individual poses a "direct threat" to himself/herself or other employees, the employer has a duty to investigate whether the threat can be reduced or eliminated by reasonable accommodation. If an employer cannot show that an individual is a direct threat or that reasonable accommodation is not possible, exclusion of an employee based on a state law is not a defense to a claim of ADA discrimination by a covered individual.

Return-to-Work Issues

FULL-DUTY REQUIREMENTS

In addition to invalidating state exclusionary laws, the ADA impacts "return to full-duty requirements." Many workers' compensation schemes permit an employer to require that an injured employee be able to return to "full duty" before returning to work. If an employer uses the term *full duty* to apply to job functions that are "marginal" in nature, it is in violation of the ADA if the individual can perform the *essential* functions of the job with or without reasonable accommodation. Unlike workers' compensation systems, in which the treating physician releases an individual to return to work, under the ADA the employer bears the ultimate legal responsibility for deciding whether an employee with a disability-related occupational injury or illness is ready to return to work [28].

DIRECT-THREAT ANALYSIS

Under the ADA, the return-to-work decision about an employee who has a communicable or potentially communicable disease should trigger a direct-threat analysis. The provisions of the ADA come into play if an individual with such a condition desires to return to work in a setting that causes the employer concern about the individual's medical condition relative to the safety of that individual or co-workers. Under the ADA, the direct-threat standard must be satisfied before an employer can lawfully prevent a covered individual from returning to his or her job. It is important to remember that not all workers with an occupationally related infectious disease are covered by the ADA. Those with self-limited infections of short duration, regardless of their severity, may not be covered unless the employer causes protections to attach by "regarding the individual as disabled" [29].

EEOC regulations define *direct threat* as one that presents a significant risk of substantial harm to the health or safety of the individual worker or other workers and that cannot be eliminated or reduced by reasonable accommodation. An individualized assessment of the worker's present ability to perform the essential functions of the job is required. The standard must be applied uniformly and reasonable medical judgment based on current medical knowledge and/or the best available objective evidence with respect to the infectious disease must be utilized. Further, the specific behavior or condition that would pose a threat must be identified. If a significant risk of substantial harm is identified, then reasonable accommodations that may reduce or eliminate the risk must be considered. ADA regulations, as promulgated by the EEOC, define the factors to be considered when assessing whether an individual presents a direct threat. These factors are [30]:

- Duration of the risk.
- Nature and severity of the potential harm.
- Likelihood that the potential harm will occur.
- Imminence of the potential harm.

A direct-threat analysis should also include a determination of the likelihood and imminence of the danger. Similar to the concerns and issues raised if an individual has a mental condition, factors such as failure of prior treatment, treatment noncompliance, and evaluation of recent and past behavior are relevant to the assessment of likelihood of harm. For example, in the infectious disease setting, a health care worker's failure or refusal to use Universal Precautions or other protective equipment is a crucial piece of the behavioral assessment of that worker. As noted above, even if an employee, by nature of his/her medical condition does not meet the "disability" impairment threshold for ADA protection, the individual can become covered under the provisions of the ADA if the employer reacts to and treats the person as if such an impairment existed. This is an important consideration in the infectious disease setting, in which the risks of disease transmission (to co-workers, customers, and patients) must be balanced against the rights of the affected individual to be in the workplace as long as he/she can perform his/her job.

Prior to enactment of the ADA and the plethora of HIV and AIDS cases in which legal action was taken by individuals seeking disability protections and financial remuneration, perhaps the best known case involving infectious disease and employment rights was *School Board of Nassau County v Arline*. This case was brought under Section 504 of the 1973 Rehabilitation Act after a school teacher who had been treated for tuberculosis was denied the right to return to her teaching job despite her lack of contiguousness with other people at work. In *Arline*, the

U.S. Supreme Court ruled that a teacher with reactivation of tuberculosis was protected under Section 504 of the Rehabilitation Act and that the relevant inquiry was whether or not she was "otherwise qualified." To answer this, the court held that an individualized inquiry as to whether or not she posed a threat of infection to the students must be conducted. Based on the public health authorities' contention that she had been treated and did not pose a threat of infection, she was reinstated in her job. In *Arline*, the American Medical Association (AMA) submitted an amicus brief that articulated the standards for conducting the appropriate inquiry as to threat of infection [31]. The AMA's position, largely adopted by the court, focused on facts based on the state of medical knowledge, and reasonable medical judgments drawn from these facts, concerning:

- Nature of the risk (how the disease is transmitted).
- Duration of the risk (how long the carrier is infectious).
- Severity of the risk (the potential harm to third parties).
- Probability that the disease will be transmitted and will cause varying degrees of harm.

The court then touched on the employer's duty to reasonably accommodate workers when appropriate [32].

The majority of the infectious disease cases under the ADA have involved HIV-positive individuals (with or without AIDS) alleging denial of employment due to their disease status. These cases provide a template for the standards and assessment process required in managing the employment status of employees with infectious diseases. A recent U.S. Supreme Court decision broadened the scope of ADA protection for HIV-positive individuals, ruling that HIV-positive status alone invokes ADA protections [33]. This effectively negates the need for an HIV-positive individual to be substantially impaired in one or more major life activities in order to be considered disabled under the ADA.

Direct threat and safety concerns have been successfully raised by employers, with courts declining to follow the EEOC's interpretation of the direct threat standard. In *Doe v University of Maryland*, the court upheld the right of the hospital to exclude an HIV-positive neurosurgery resident from its training program because the individual presented an appreciable risk of catastrophic harm [34]. Courts have also upheld hospitals' rights to reassign HIV-positive individuals to other jobs if they present appreciable risk of catastrophic harm in their present jobs. In a Texas case, the court ruled that it was permissible for the employer to reassign an HIV-positive surgical technician [35]. In another case in which a surgical technician was suspected of being HIV-positive, a Michigan court ruled that while infrequent, there was some contact (hands in direct contact or in the immediate vicinity of an incision) that was essential to the success of a surgical procedure and that this was an essential job function. The hospital was not required to restructure the essential functions of the job by providing another person in the operating room [36].

Decisions about employees' ability to work should be based on sound scientific knowledge as to the nature of the infectious agent, its infectivity and invasiveness, the mode of transmission, the host status, and the susceptibility of co-workers and others working near or in close contact to the affected individual. Currently, aside from the Bloodborne Pathogen Standard and the general duty clause, there is little OSHA or state statutory guidance regulating the return to work of an individual being treated or recently treated for an infectious disease. The proposed OSHA tuberculosis standard does, however, provide some clarification regarding employer duties in the infectious disease setting [37]. Medical removal protection requirements provide for employees with suspected or confirmed infectious tuberculosis to be kept out of the workplace until they are determined to be noninfectious. The proposed standard outlines benefit and wage provisions as well as job modification guidance and employee/employer notification requirements.

In managing an employee with an infectious disease, the initial step is evaluating the individual's present ability to perform essential job duties. Attention to the physical and emotional job demands should be evaluated and documented. If there is no issue regarding the employee's ability to perform the essential job tasks, the inquiry should then focus, if appropriate, on the safety of others in the workplace. This involves an evaluation of the affected individual's proximity to co-workers and customers/clients and an assessment of contaguousness. As previously stated, current scientific medical literature and accepted sources should be consulted. Prior to exclusion of an infected individual from returning to work, public health officials should be contacted for their input. All steps in the evaluation process should be carefully documented: specifically, the nature of the infectious disease in question, the status of the affected employee, including their compliance with treatment and job-required protective equipment, and the type of work they perform. Care should be taken not to generalize based on the virulence of the infectious agent, as disease stage, ease of transmission, and co-worker/patient/customer issues and job requirements are also important factors to consider in the individualized assessment. If it is established that there are legitimate reasons for concern about the individual's presence in the workplace relative to safety, attention must then shift to consideration of available means to mitigate or reduce the likelihood of harm. This may include modification or change of job duties or even reassignment of the individual to a vacant position.

In *Bragdon v Abbott*, a recent case involving an HIV-positive claimant who, under the ADA, brought legal action against a dentist who refused to treat the individual in his office, the U.S. Supreme Court held that the patient's disease status must be assessed to determine whether or not it poses a significant threat to the health and safety of others and, if a health risk was shown to exist, whether or not it could be eliminated by safety procedures. In *Bragdon*, this objective inquiry was held to be required under the ADA to justify the dentist's refusal to treat the patient in his office. This type of individualized assessment will be required when evaluating employees with infectious diseases if they desire to return to work.

Historically, the causality issues associated with infectious diseases have resulted in many exposures and infections being handled outside the workers' compensation system. Articles in the legal and public health literature have highlighted the difficulty of proving causation of infectious disease by work-related factors if the disease is prevalent in the community [31]. Additionally, for ease of management or financial reasons, many workplace incidents and exposures have been handled on-site at the company's premises, or through the employer's group health plan. Prior to prophylaxis after HIV exposure and other expensive testing and treatments, many workplace needlestick exposures were handled in the hospital's employee health department. Given the inconsistent reporting and causation issues surrounding work-related infectious diseases, it is likely that their true magnitude has been unappreciated.

There is a strong likelihood that infectious diseases will become a greater issue in the workers' compensation arena, presenting special workplace safety concerns and ADA compliance challenges. Technologic advances in molecular epidemiologic analysis, improved diagnostic testing, the advent of new infections, better identification of common disease agents, and the resurgence of infections once thought to be controlled or eradicated, will lead to an increased number of workplace infectious disease challenges. In addition, employee protection laws, such as the ADA, which have paved the way for individuals with chronic diseases to remain in the workplace, will further compound the challenges. These laws will drive demographic changes in the health status of the "typical" American worker. Changes in employee medical benefit, retirement, and disability plans will also lead to an increased number of individuals with medical conditions remaining at work. Such changes will lead to a greater number of employees who are immunocompromised by virtue of age, organ transplantation status, steroid use, cancer or other chronic diseases, working along side a greater number of employees with acute and chronic infections. Further, there will be an increase in the number of employees who are chronic infectious disease carriers or have acute but undiagnosed infectious disease, e.g., hepatitis or HIV [31].

The increased globalization of U.S. businesses has resulted in an explosion in employee travel on company business to remote places where food preparation, water safety, and general sanitation are frequently substandard and constitute significant health hazards from infectious disease. While most companies comply with the immunization requirements for foreign country entry, few adequately prepare their employees for the challenges they will encounter. Further, the ADA has significantly limited companies in denying overseas work assignments based on the presence of significant medical conditions in the employee or their dependents. Employees with complex and serious medical conditions may now accept an overseas assignment despite the absence of adequate medical resources or exposure concerns present in the foreign country.

The availability of vaccines and immunizations for diseases such as hepatitis B has led to increased employer responsibilities in preventing work-related infectious disease. While OSHA requires employers to provide HBV vaccine for all employees who are at risk of infection, employers should consider providing other immunizations at no cost to employees [31]. This has both public health and employer productivity benefits. If an employee has not had a childhood infectious disease nor immunization for that disease, contracting the disease secondary to a workplace exposure not only results in costs and morbidity for the individual employee, but also opens the door to a widespread workplace outbreak of the disease. Additionally, the company may incur third-party liability for dependents of the employee who become infected, particularly if they suffer serious sequlae.

The resurgence of multidrug-resistant tuberculosis has led OSHA to develop the proposed occupational tuberculosis standard, which contains requirements for medical surveillance for the disease. While still in the proposal stage, these OSHA standards will be legally mandated when the rule is finalized.

The role of occupational medicine professionals in the management of infectious disease issues in the workplace will continue to expand. In addition to medical treatment issues, the direct-threat standard will shape and guide decision-making in striking the delicate balance between an infected individual's right to be in the workplace and the employer's duty to protect the safety and well-being of co-workers and others. The ADA provides a clearly articulated legal mandate stating that the direct-threat standard requires an individualized assessment based on current, objective scientific evidence about the medical condition and consideration of reasonable accommodations that may mitigate any threat to workplace safety and health. While pre-employment medical examinations became extinct after enactment of the ADA, the need for occupational medicine physicians with strong clinical, public health, and legal knowledge has never been greater.

References

1. Hood JB, Hardy BA, Lewis HS. *Workers' Compensation and Employee Protection Laws.* St. Paul, MN: West Publishing, 1990. P 1.
2. Ibid. P 2.
3. Ibid. P 4.
4. Ibid. P 5.
5. Ibid. P 7.
6. Ibid.
7. Ibid.
8. Ibid. P 27.
9. Ibid. P 29.
10. Ibid. P 35.
11. *Simkins v Great West Cas. Co.,* 831 F2d 792 (8th Cir 1987).
12. *Childers v Chesapeake & Potomac Tele. Co.* (1989).
13. *Smolarek v Chrysler Corp.* (1989).
14. *Paroline v Unisys Corp.* (1989).
15. Rothstein MA, Craver CB, Schroeder EP, et al. *Employment Law.* St. Paul, MN: 1994.
16. Rothstein MA, Craver CB, Schroeder EP, et al. *Employment Law.* St. Paul, MN: 1994.
17. *Hansen v Gordon,* 221 Conn 29 (1992).
18. Ibid. P 36.
19. 241 Conn 692 (1997).
20. Ibid. P 694.
21. Equal Employment Opportunity Commission. *ADA Enforcement Guidance: Pre- employment Disability-Related Questions and Medical Examinations.* Washington, DC: EEOC, Oct 15, 1995.
22. 42 USC §12201(c) ; 29 CFR 1630 app. §1630.14(b); 29 CFR. 1630 app. §1630. P 3.
23. *Doe v Roe,* 190 A2d 463, 599 NYS2d 350 (1993).
24. 29 USCA §§2601–54.
25. 42 USC §12112(a); 29 CFR §1630.4.
26. Equal Employment Opportunity Commission. *ADA Enforcement Guidance: Workers' Compensation and the*

ADA. Washington, DC: EEOC, Sept 3, 1996. No 915.002. P 7.

27. Equal Employment Opportunity Commission. *ADA Enforcement Guidance: Workers' Compensation and the ADA*. Washington, DC: EEOC, Sept 3, 1996. No.915.002. P 9.
28. Equal Employment Opportunity Commission. ADA Enforcement Guidance: Workers' Compensation and the ADA. Washington, DC: EEOC, Sept 3, 1996. No.915.002. P 14.
29. 42 USC 12102–13 (1994).
30. Ibid.
31. Richards EP, Rathbun KC. *Law and the Physician: A Practical Guide*. Boston: Little, Brown, 1993. Chap 23.
32. *School Board of Nassua County v Arline,* 107 SCt 1123 (1987).
33. *Bragdon v Abbott,* 8 AD Cases 239, US, No 97-156, 6/25/98.
34. 50 F3d 1261 (4th Cir 1995).
35. *Bradley v University of Texas M.D. Anderson Cancer Ctr.,* 3 F3d 922, 925 (5th Cir 1993).
36. *Mauro v Borgess Medical Ctr.,* 886 F Supp 1349 (WD Mich 1995).
37. Occupational Exposure Rule for Tuberculosis Standard (g)5(i), (ii), (iii), (iv).

7 / Medical Surveillance of Workers

Timothy J. Key, Freddy G. McMurry, and Victor S. Roth

Fundamentals of Medical Surveillance

A medical surveillance program should be part of a company's occupational health services. The employer has a clear ethical and legal responsibility to provide these services for its workers. It is important to understand the general principles that are the foundation for medical surveillance. Medical surveillance for infectious diseases is only part of most surveillance programs. In some, it is a very limited part, but it plays a larger role in others. Two types of surveillance programs in which it plays a larger role are highlighted in this chapter: programs for animal handlers and those for health care workers.

Merriam-Webster's Online defines *surveillance* as a "close watch kept over someone or something"; the word is derived from the French term *vieller*, which means "to watch." The surveillance process implies an observational process and incorporates many epidemiologic principles and terms. The occupational medicine provider must be familiar with biostatistical methods and must be comfortable applying epidemiologic principles. Many excellent biostatistical and epidemiologic reviews for workplace applications are available [1–3]. To develop a sound medical surveillance program, an understanding of the prevention triad is necessary. Primary prevention is institution of measures aimed at preventing the occurrence of disease. This involves (in order of preference), material substitution, engineering controls, administrative controls, and personal protective equipment [4]. This sequence of measures attempts to eliminate or control exposure. If the hazard cannot be eliminated or controlled, then attempts are made at limiting exposure through work practices or protective equipment. Personal protective equipment is the least desirable of these four control strategies since failure at this level results in immediate exposure of the worker to the hazard. Secondary prevention is detection of disease at a subclinical stage or at such an early stage that it is reversible or its progression can be stopped. Strictly defined, medical surveillance falls under secondary prevention. Tertiary prevention is the medical treatment of disease once it is clinically present and not reversible.

The fundamental goal of any medical surveillance program is early detection of workplace disease at a reversible stage. Although medical surveillance programs are classified as secondary prevention, they should function as complements to primary prevention efforts. Workplace professionals such as industrial hygienists, safety professionals, and occupational medicine specialists generally perform primary prevention efforts. A well-designed medical surveillance program has occupational medical professionals who actively participate in implementing primary prevention controls in the workplace in conjunction with other occupational health and safety professionals. In general, the activities of the industrial hygiene, safety, and occupational medicine professionals are the driving force behind the medical surveillance program.

Fundamentals of Medical Surveillance Programs

REASONS FOR MEDICAL SURVEILLANCE PROGRAMS

The most common reasons for employers to establish surveillance programs are concern for the health and fitness of employees and the need to comply with governmental regulations [5]. Many employers are beginning to realize that good employee health promotes good business and productivity [6]. Unfortunately, economic constraints make it difficult for some employers to implement an occupational health program, thus resulting in more hazardous workplaces [7]. Quality medical surveillance programs have many benefits [8]. A medical surveillance program should be complementary to the existing industrial hygiene, safety, and occupational health programs. The occupational medicine provider who serves as director of the surveillance program can alleviate the job demands placed on the industrial hygienist and other health and safety professionals. Regulatory compliance issues can be addressed as a team, drawing on the expertise of diverse health and safety professionals.

BARRIERS TO ESTABLISHING PROGRAMS

There may be barriers to establishing a medical surveillance program [8]. A major obstacle is the existence of an institutional, or corporate, culture that de-emphasizes safety. This could be the result of either employer or employee attitudes, or both. For a safety culture to exist, top management must "buy into" and champion safety. Usually, employees will either rise or fall to the safety performance level expected and rewarded. The success or failure of a medical surveillance program depends on the support of top management. The employer must emphasize to employees the reasons for surveillance and allow them adequate time to participate in the surveillance program. Employees' mistrust of the employer's motives render many surveillance programs ineffective. It should be clearly stated that the medical surveillance program is not intended to identify employees for punitive reasons or to find cause for their dismissal. In some hazardous workplaces, lower ranking employees are more likely to be injured and are less likely to be enrolled in a medical surveillance program than higher ranking employees [9]. Employers should have a job-protection policy that incorporates work accommodations or job transfer for those employees discovered to have a medical condition by medical surveillance. If employees have the opinion that the surveillance program is simply a method to terminate workers, they will not participate.

PROGRAM COMPONENTS

A medical surveillance program benefits from use of a computer tracking system, of which there are many commercially available software packages. The system will provide a database of surveillance activities [10–13] and can assist in identification and timely scheduling of needed examinations. It can also serve as a communication tool between medical and other health and safety professionals and management. Epidemiologic analysis of the database can assist in identification of workplace problems. Early identification of workplace trends allows for more effective preventive measures and gives added value to the provision of medical surveillance services. Maintenance of the database by a knowledgeable individual is crucial; a poorly maintained database will miss individuals needing examinations and fail to identify problems. Understandably, advice based on a faulty database will be of poor quality and useless. In addition, poor advice could have adverse financial consequences for the occupational medical service unit and others involved in the surveillance program.

The confidentiality of workplace information has undergone an unprecedented assault from advances in information technology. The construction of comprehensive databases on workplace information, made possible by computer technology, has been a two-edged sword. On the positive side, relational databases have made the query for useful workplace information possible. Aggregation of occupational health data needs to take place for information to be useful and applicable, as the data should be used in decisions about programs [14]. On the negative side, unscrupulous use of this technology can violate the rights of workers. Confidentiality must be protected and not compromised because of technology or surveillance issues.

Training employees about good work practices has proved to be an effective tool for workplace safety. The goal of any training program is employees' acquisition of the knowledge and attitudes to perform safe work practices. Appropriate training is a regulatory requirement when hazardous work is being done. The Hazard Communication Standard, 29 CFR 1910.1200, imparts to employees a "right-to-know" about workplace hazards and entitles them to training that will protect them from the hazard [5,15,16]. The training program should be generated and supervised by the departments involved in the actual training. The occupational medicine services unit should be involved as an information resource and actively participate when needed. Sometimes an occupational medicine provider may be able to give added weight to a safety issue, encouraging the employee to take notice. The occupational medicine provider must be aware of adult learning models and adapt any presentations or discussions to the workers' needs and capabilities. Workers with cognitive disabilities may be present in the workplace; these employees will have difficulty learning and applying, on the job, new material and skills learned. Employers have a legal obligation under the Americans with Disabilities Act (ADA) to provide reasonable accommodations in all employment aspects, including training.

Medical evaluations are important to the medical surveillance program. The preplacement medical examination or periodic examination is probably the best time for the occupational medicine provider to discuss with the employee ways to reduce exposure risks. Evaluations for injuries or illnesses are a time to discuss workplace practices and retrain employees on basic safety issues. Any injury or illness event should prompt an incident evaluation and job-safety analysis. This may include a walk-through of the workplace by the occupational medicine professional. This allows the occupational medical service unit to learn more about the workplace and interact more with the employees at the actual worksite.

ETHICAL, LEGAL, AND REGULATORY ISSUES

The confidentiality of workplace information has undergone an unprecedented assault from information technology and employers' demands of access to medical information. Likewise, the continued advances in genetic technology and its expected role in disease prevention will have a significant impact on the workplace [17]. The ethical and legal questions raised by these workplace confidentiality issues will continue to evolve through debate in the professional arena and in the courtroom [18–22, 23–27].

The American College of Occupational and Environmental Medicine's (ACOEM) *Code of Ethical Conduct* (points 5 and 6) sets a standard for professional ethical conduct regarding confidentiality. Point 5 states "keep confidential all individual medical information, releasing such information only when required by law or overriding public health considerations, or to other physicians according to accepted medical practice, or to others at the request of the individual." Point 6 states "recognize that employers may be entitled to counsel about an individual's medical work fitness, but not to diagnoses or specific details, except in compliance with laws and regulations." ACOEM's position paper Confidentiality of Medical Information in the Workplace addresses the changing legal issues and the ethical challenges [23]. The Association of Occupational and Environmental Clinics (AOEC) has created a Patient Bill of Rights that also addresses these issues [24].

The Americans with Disabilities Act (ADA) has reshaped the legal landscape of the workplace and the duties of the occupational health professional. The ADA prohibits discrimination against the disabled individual seeking employment. Although simple in its intent, it has proved difficult in its interpretation. The inherent ambiguity of the ADA definitions of "disability," "qualified individual," "reasonable accommodations," "direct threat," and "undue hardship" requires case-by-case analysis when applying the law. The following discussion highlights basic aspects of the ADA concerning medical surveillance and is not intended to be all-inclusive. Comprehensive reviews of the ADA are available, and the provider of medical surveillance must be knowledgeable in its interpretation for workplace screening [25–28]. The U.S. Equal Employment Opportunity Commission and the U.S. Department of Justice have excellent Internet sites at *www.eeoc.gov* and *www.usdoj.gov*, respectively. The medical surveillance process impacts the entire employment process and is subject to the ADA.

Knowledge of the ADA and its protections is essential if the occupational medicine provider is to appropriately make decisions regarding job placement. Individuals with physical and mental impairments will apply for positions and must be carefully evaluated for the presence of disability, as defined by the ADA, and the need for reasonable accommodations. To quality for ADA protection, a disabled person must be qualified for the job. An employer has no legal obligation to hire unqualified people but is obligated to provide reasonable work accommodations for a disabled individual who is otherwise qualified to perform the job. Reasonable accommodation entails an employer's provision of flexibility in job structure or work environment or of special equipment without imposing undue hardship on the employer. Key terms here are *reasonable accommodation* and *undue hardship*. These are both relative terms with the clear implication that many factors must be included in the decision. The decision about what constitutes reasonable accommodation depends on the individual needs of the disabled person. It is helpful for the occupational medicine provider to have a current job description from the employer, including essential functions of the job for which the individual is applying.

The ADA covers all aspects of the employment process. A job applicant is protected from having to divulge any medical information or submit to any medical examination prior to being offered a job. The employer may not ask any question to which the answer may reveal information about the existence of a disability. However, the employer is allowed to ask the applicant if essential job functions can be performed with or without reasonable accommodations. The ADA requires that if an employment entrance examination is performed, it be required for all new employees in the same job category.

The ADA has had a major impact on the periodic examination of current employees. If the periodic examination is mandatory for employment, it must be job-specific in its scope. Employees may voluntarily participate in periodic medical surveillance examinations offered by their employer. Still, only job-related information may be released to the employer.

The Occupational Safety and Health Act General Duty Provision mandates employers provide "safe and healthful working conditions" [29,30]. The Occupational Safety and Health Administration (OSHA) Strategic Plan for 1997 through 2002 has three goals [31,32]. The first is to improve workplace safety and health for all workers, as evidenced by fewer hazards, reduced exposures, and fewer injuries, illnesses, and fatalities. The second is to change workplace culture to increase employer and worker awareness of, commitment to, and involvement in safety and health. The third is to secure public confidence through excellence in the development and delivery of OSHA's programs and services. OSHA promulgates health standards that may pertain to a specific workplace or apply broadly to all workplaces. The National Institute of Occupational Safety and Health (NIOSH) may be asked to provide the technical information for standards. OSHA is ultimately responsible for implementation and enforcement of the standard. There may be local guidelines and regulations by governing local bodies/organizations, which may impact occupational health and safety issues. Occupational medicine providers must know what role they will play in workplace surveillance and be able to interact with these local organizations effectively.

RELATIONSHIP TO HAZARD EVALUATION

The need for medical surveillance is a function of exposure. If no potential for exposure to hazardous agents existed in the workplace, there would be no need for medical surveillance. Proper exposure assessment is a prerequisite for planning and implementing an appropriate medical surveillance program [8,33]. Exposure assessment is typically a function of industrial hygiene, safety and health, and occupational medicine professionals. These safety and health professionals function as a team to anticipate, recognize, evaluate, and control hazards. The occupational medicine provider should be involved in this process. Communication between professionals is essential in achieving the goal of prevention of occupational illness and injury.

One fundamental industrial hygiene principle to understand is the difference between the terms *toxic* and *hazardous*. The toxicity of an agent is a function of the capability of that agent to cause harm. Determination of hazard is a probability assessment of the likelihood that harm will occur. Many toxic substances are present in the workplace. In many cases, these toxic agents are not hazards to the worker because proper industrial hygiene and safety procedures render the potential for causing injury or illness to the worker nonexistent. Hazard types are broadly classified as physical, chemical, biologic, and ergonomic.

Risk assessment as a process has taken on increasing importance due to an increasingly complicated workplace environment. Biologic research continues to expand in scope and present new types of exposure risks. Likewise, increasing productivity demands placed on workers and poorly designed work processes have presented new and increased hazards to the worker. Risk is a probability determination of an adverse outcome. A formal risk assessment process is the characterization of the probability of an adverse health effect from exposure to an agent. The risk assessment process is systematic and scientific in its approach [34]. The process at its most basic level is a risk-benefit analysis. Sequential steps detailed by the National Academy of Science include hazard identification, dose-response assessment, exposure assessment, and risk characterization [35].

Hazard identification is typically the initial step in the process. During this step, agents undergo a toxicity assessment. Available literature must be reviewed to gather evidence on known toxicity. Some sources of information include current toxicologic and medical research articles on the agent, standard toxicologic and medical reference books, and the Material Safety Data Sheet (MSDS). The Hazard Communication Standard, 29 CFR 1910.1200, requires that the manufacturer of that chemical agent must supply a current MSDS of a chemical.

Next, an estimate of dose-response should be obtained. The dose-response estimate is needed when deciding on an allowable exposure level for the agent. As Paracelsus, the father of toxicology, said in the 1500s, "the dose determines that a thing is not a poison" and having an idea of how much dose of an agent is required before an adverse response occurs is important in the surveillance process. Dose-response estimations and occupational exposure limits are often inexact or poorly known for many agents [41,42].

Exposure assessment is critical to effective risk assessment. It is exposure to a toxic agent in sufficient amounts that makes the agent hazardous to the worker. Unfortunately, accurate exposure assessment is frequently very difficult to obtain. Ideally, a quantitative exposure amount could be calculated for all workers and then compared to a well-defined dose-response curve allowing exact risk characterization. Realistically, quantitative calculations often have a wide margin of error and often the exposure estimate is simply a qualitative, yes-no determination as to whether exposure has occurred. Constraints in exposure estimation, coupled with limitations in detailing dose-response curves, make risk characterization difficult. Typically, the industrial hygiene or safety professional performs the exposure estimate, but the occupational medicine provider must be aware of the inherent limitations of the process. Some strategies have been developed for more effective exposure assessment [10,36–42]. In many cases, some type of surrogate for exposure has to be defined. The use of a job-exposure matrix attempts to use many factors, such as work duration, job description or occupational titles, to make a quantitative estimate of exposure. In some industries, biologic monitoring is done to augment environmental monitoring [43–46]. Biologic monitoring involves taking a specimen from the employee, such as urine or blood, and measuring it for the presence of a chemical or its metabolite to assess exposure. For biologic monitoring to be useful, the exposure of interest must be capable of leading to, or resulting in, some sort of cumulative toxin or biochemical process that can be quantitatively measured and extrapolated to an exposure estimate.

The final step is risk characterization, at which time all available information is used to define and analyze the potential risk to the worker plus estimate the severity of the adverse outcome. Once the risk has been characterized, the issue of risk management and risk communication becomes important. Risk management consists of institutional policy decisions to control risk. Risk management involves all aspects of the employer-employee relationship. Typical examples are:

- Provisions in the institutional policy and procedure manual.
- Institutional financial protection.
- Additional employee training.
- Implementation of engineering controls.
- Substitution of less toxic materials.
- Personal protective equipment.
- Occupational health services.

Risk communication is conveying information about the elements of risk inherent in the workplace and work process to all involved parties. Timely and accurate risk communication is essential in preservation of the institutional good-citizen image [47].

The risk assessment process should drive the medical surveillance process. Some might argue that if the risk assessment and risk management processes work correctly, there would be no need for medical surveillance. Medical surveillance is a method of monitoring or measuring the controls put in place to manage risk. As pointed out previously, there are some inherent limitations in the risk assessment process. Without medical surveillance, some workers, especially the most susceptible, would succumb to occupational illnesses or injuries. In these cases, the medical surveillance process may be able to spur the risk assessment process, limiting and controlling institutional risk. For example, if during the periodic medical examinations, workers reported high rates of symptoms or exhibited signs of illnesses or if biomarkers were present, this would be communicated to the safety and occupational personnel so that an exposure assessment would be done. The medical surveillance process provides needed redundancy to ensure worker safety [48].

Activities of Occupational Health Professionals

The occupational medicine provider must be proficient at performing an occupational medical history and a focused physical examination plus obtaining information pertinent to the workplace. Standard occupational medicine textbooks can be used to formulate a working guideline for incorporation into the medical surveillance program. An exposure history template was developed by the Agency for Toxic Substances and Disease Registry (ATSDR) and National Institute for Occupational Safety and Health (NIOSH). This template, which is comprehensive, is available from ATSDR [49].

As in any type of medical encounter, the history obtained from the employee provides the most important information for decision making in occupational medicine. It is important to understand exactly what the employee does in his job, how he does it, what materials are used, and the current workplace environment. Likewise, it is important to know the employee's past job history and workplace exposures plus any leisure activities or hobbies that could have an impact on health. This is greatly facilitated by having the employer furnish a current job description, but the job description does not replace direct history obtained from the employee. Many times an employee does multiple tasks outside his or her job description, and it may be these tasks are causing or could potentially cause problems. In addition, the employee may need additional training or protective equipment to safely perform additional tasks not covered in the job description.

To facilitate the interview process, most occupational medicine providers formulate a health questionnaire covering general medical plus specific occupational information. The questionnaire is typically a combination of check-off type questions, a listing of specific items, and then descriptive elaboration by the employee. Typically, the employee fills out the questionnaire prior to the interview and reviews it with the medical professional during the interview and examination. The length of the interview and examination is directly proportional to the complexity of the situation. Young healthy employees with no symptoms or signs of disease and a very brief work history can be evaluated quickly, while employees with symptoms or signs of disease or with a complex work-exposure history can be very time consuming.

In the medical surveillance process, the occupational medicine provider's initial encounter with a worker is typically the preplacement examination. At this point in the employment process, the individual has been offered a job on the condition that he/she undergo a medical examination. Up to this point, the employee has not had to provide any medical information to the employer, as governed by the ADA. The employer has deemed the applicant qualified for the job, and the medical examination is done to assess if the applicant can perform the essential functions of the job with or without reasonable accommodations. The applicant is required to provide a complete medical history to allow for this determination but is provided confidentiality in its disclosure.

Essentially, the preplacement examination is a risk assessment process during which the medical professional is attempting to determine if the individual can safely work, based on knowledge of the individual and knowledge of the workplace. Such issues as employee susceptibility and direct threat come into consideration. Certainly, some medical conditions present a direct threat to the individual and their co-workers. The ADA defines *direct threat* as a reasonable probability of substantial harm to self or others. For example, an individual with a well-controlled seizure disorder cannot be considered a direct threat even though it is possible that he could have a seizure on the job. The ADA does not allow speculation on all possibilities but only what is a reasonable possibility.

Current employees may voluntarily participate in periodic medical surveillance examinations that may be comprehensive in nature, similar to the preplacement examination. In institutions in which periodic examinations are mandatory for continued employment, they must be job specific in scope. Any periodic examination participant is entitled to medical information confidentiality and ADA protection. The employer is only entitled to job-related information.

Episodic examinations will be driven by the occurrence of symptoms and injuries. These unanticipated patient interactions should be seen as a chance to measure how well the occupational safety and medical surveillance programs are functioning. They present an opportunity for the occupational medicine provider to learn more about the workplace, that is, to become informed of work process changes and new workplace hazards. Episodic examinations serve as a two-pronged relationship builder through (1) providing care for the employees and (2) working with the other occupational health professionals in the provision of a safe workplace.

An employer may offer an exit examination to an employee leaving the institution. In general, exit examinations are not well received by employees. Once the decision has been made to change jobs, most employees will not schedule an exit examination, unless some overriding health concern exists.

This has been an overview of medical surveillance in general. The next two sections deal with the medical surveillance of two specific groups of workers—animal handlers and health care workers—specifically surveillance for infectious diseases. These two groups of workers certainly have the greatest exposure risk to infectious diseases when compared with other classifications of workers.

Medical Surveillance of Animal Handlers with an Emphasis on Infectious Diseases

OVERVIEW

Medical surveillance plays an important role in the protection of the health and safety of animal handlers. The surveillance is exposure driven through environmental monitoring performed by the workplace health and safety professionals. In an animal care facility, the institutional veterinary staff is usually the principal source of exposure information. Medical surveillance needs vary between institutions, and it is critical for occupational health professionals to work closely with the animal care facility professionals to ensure that an effective program exists. Animal care facilities operate in a very emotional public environment. Maintaining a good institutional-citizen image to the public is critical. Likewise, possessing an internal institutional culture with an emphasis on high standards for occupational safety and health is important. Animal care facilities are not immune to the same type of restructuring and cost-benefit analysis performed in the private corporate setting. Institutional characteristics, in particular financial resources, are important determinants of the very existence of workplace medical surveillance. The monetary value of medical surveillance to the animal care facility can be difficult to account for in the budgetary process. It is crucial that the occupational health professional involved in the program have a clear understanding of the institution's surveillance requirements. This must be coupled with sensitivity for the budgetary constraints faced by the animal facility managers. Medical surveillance programs should be provided for all personnel involved in care and research use of animals [14]. It is estimated that there are over 90,000 animal handlers in the United States [4].

Occupational health programs for animal handlers require cooperative participation of all representatives of activities related to animal research [14]. Effective programs rely on strong administrative support and interactions among several institutional groups and programs. These groups and programs are generally considered to be the research programs, the animal care and use program, the environmental health and safety program, occupational health services, and administration. Investigators and their staffs represent the research program. Veterinarians represent the animal care program and the institutional animal care and use committee. The environmental health and safety program is represented by the industrial hygienist and other safety professionals working directly with the animal care facility program. The occupational health program is represented by the occupational health professional. The administration is represented by human resources, finance departments, facility-maintenance personnel, and the institution's operating administrators. Day-to-day responsibility for safety in this environment resides with the laboratory supervisors and the animal care facility supervisors.

The purpose of a medical surveillance program for animal handlers is to monitor the effectiveness of engineering controls, work practices, and use of personal protective equipment [50]. The scope and duties of a medical surveillance program depend on the needs of the animal care center. Services provided should be based on an adequate risk assessment of the animal care facility. This assessment should consider:

- Animal handler's contact with animals.
- Exposure intensity of the contact.
- Exposure frequency of that contact.
- Physical and biologic hazards presented by the animals and their husbandry activities.
- Hazardous nature of the agents and protocols used in the research.
- Individual susceptibilities of the animal handlers.
- Occupational history of the animal handlers and the experience of other animal handlers in other settings [14].

Assessment of risk involves evaluating the worksite for work activities that create higher risks of occupational injury and illness. An example would be animal handlers' direct handling of macaques leading to potential herpes B virus exposures. Another example is handling and removing soiled litter from cages with increased exposure to specific agents [14]. Setting up appropriate controls is based on identification of persons at high risk, which is done through interaction with environmental health and safety staff as well as during the preplacement medical evaluations, periodic medical evaluations, and episodic medical evaluations. It is important for all involved in administering the program that adverse health outcomes are quickly recognized and evaluated to determine whether the control program has failed [14].

It is essential for the facility to have a policy statement regarding animal handler selection, medical evaluations and medical surveillance, and relocation and dismissal plans. During preplacement medical evaluation, animal handlers need to be informed about hazards that will be encountered in their jobs and about safe work practices. Information about reporting procedures and the medical surveillance program must also be covered at this time [50].

Confusion over interpretations of broad regulatory requirements or contractual obligations by funding agencies has led to some institutions' developing broad, expensive programs that have lacked relevancy to the needs of animal handlers [14]. Generally, focused programs will better serve their needs. A narrowly focused animal care program will require a narrowly focused surveillance program. A comprehensive animal care program may appear to require a comprehensive surveillance program but may only need a focused surveillance program specific to the needs of animal handlers. The majority of comprehensive animal research centers are located or associated with academic centers that have access to an academic occupational medicine service capable of meeting all its needs and requirements and serving as a resource for specific issues and questions. If this is not the case, access to a primary care service or occupational medicine service, with an interest and willingness to assume the duties and responsibilities, is required.

Primary contacts/persons from both the occupational medical service unit and animal care program should be designated to facilitate communication. The contact person from the occupational medical service unit should develop a working knowledge of the exposures and risks involved at the animal care facility, especially in the area of zoonoses. This individual must be willing to make worksite visits and be capable of developing a medical surveillance program based on the exposure risk assessment.

REGULATIONS THAT AFFECT PROGRAMS

Animal care and research facilities are subject to numerous regulations. These regulations can be federal, state, local, and institutional. The focus is generally on the federal regulations. Federal regulations are Occupational Safety and Health Administration (OSHA) standards and guidelines, Centers for Disease Control and Prevention (CDC) recommendations, and National Institutes of Health (NIH) guidelines.

There are several OSHA standards that may apply, based on activity. The "general duty" clause of the original Occupational Safety and Health Act of 1970 requires employers to provide a safe and healthy workplace. The OSHA Bloodborne Pathogens Standard (29 CFR 1910.1031) requires the employer to provide hepatitis vaccination if there is a risk of exposure. The OSHA Occupational Exposure to Hazardous Chemicals in Laboratories Standard (29 CFR 1910.1450) requires medical surveillance if exposures routinely occur above the action level. Other OSHA standards that could apply are the OSHA Hazard Communication Standard (29 CFR 1910. 1200), the OSHA Ethylene Oxide Standard (29 CFR 1910.1047), and the OSHA Formaldehyde Standard (29 CFR 1910.1048).

CDC guidelines are applicable if institutions receive federal funding. *The Public Health Service Policy on Humane Care and Use of Laboratory Animals* and the *Biosafety in Microbiological and Biomedical Biotechnical Laboratories* guidelines require that institutions provide occupational health services to animal handlers [51,52]. The *Biosafety in Microbiological and Biomedical Laboratories* is being revised at this time. The current edition was published in 1993. It is directed at research programs involving experimentally or naturally infected vertebrates and has recommendations regarding serum banking that are no longer believed to be necessary, as other approaches are now used. The guidelines recommend limiting access of individuals who would be highly susceptible or who would likely have more complicated courses of illness if infected. It is now recommended that serum banking of a baseline sample be secured for specific agents under Biosafety level 2. This applies if a substantial risk of infection exists and there is a reliable method to measure immunologic response to the specific infectious agent. Biosafety level 3 agents require serum banking if the previously mentioned criteria are met. Immunizations should be given when safe and effective vaccines exist and there is a clearly identified risk for employees. Such vaccines as hepatitis B, yellow fever, rabies, polio, and diphtheria/tetanus would be considered applicable. It is also recommended that a TB surveillance program be in place [14].

The NIH Guidelines for Research Involving Recombinant DNA Molecules requires occupational health services for employees working with viable recombinant DNA containing microorganisms that need Biosafety level 3 or greater. One of the requirements is a record of agents handled by the individuals involved. Another requirement is the maintenance of serial serum samples for monitoring of serologic changes [14].

HAZARDS AND RISK ASSESSMENT

Medical surveillance is a means of measuring the effectiveness of risk assessment and control of hazards and risk of exposure. One needs to understand what the hazards are in an animal handler facility and use appropriate methods to assess risk of exposure [53]. Animal handlers may encounter any of the following type of hazards: physical hazards, chemical hazards, or biologic hazards [14,58]. Physical hazards can be classified as animal bites, scratches, and kicks and may result in exposure to infectious agents. Biologic hazards can be divided into zoonotic infections, allergens, and research protocol infections. All of these hazards are potentially present in animal care and research facilities. Risk assessment efforts should be directed at detecting these hazards [14,40,54–62].

The occupational health professional must be familiar with all workplace hazards and be comfortable interfacing with the animal care professional about the workplace assessment. Substantial contact with an animal is not a sufficient indicator of risk. A determination should be based on the nature of hazards associated with the care and use of research animals and the intensity and frequency of employee exposure to these hazards [14].

Safety procedures can minimize the potential risks of exposure to zoonotic infections. These procedures include [4]:

- Purchase of pathogen-free animals if possible.
- Use of a holding facility for quarantine of newly acquired animals and animals suspected of being infected; in such a facility the animals can be evaluated for pathogens and treated appropriately.
- Vaccination of animal handlers.
- Use of specialized containment caging or chemical restraint and protective clothing.

The risk of animal handlers' acquiring a zoonotic disease has declined, especially for those handling small animals. The major reason is that, currently, these animals are more often bred in barrier facilities [4]. Large animals still pose considerable risk because they are frequently obtained from the wild or from facilities that are not true barrier facilities [4]. Animals used as models in infectious disease studies pose a threat regardless of where they were bred [4,14]. Transmission of zoonotic agents to animal handlers is either by direct contact with infected animals or indirectly by exposure to contaminated equipment or supplies [4]. Aerosolization of infectious agents is considered the main way most zoonotic diseases are transmitted [4]. Bites, scratches, and exposure to contaminated equipment, resulting in direct inoculation, are other means of transmission [4,14].

Animal handlers need to be continually reminded of the importance of reporting all wounds and accidents. This enables the occupational medicine services unit to initiate appropriate follow-up measures. Animal handlers need to be educated about the importance of reporting any gastrointestinal, respiratory, or dermal conditions with symptoms that are similar to those occurring in animals they are tending. This helps surveillance program personnel to decide if control measures are working correctly and effectively. The following is a brief overview of some zoonoses that may affect animal handlers. They are presented according to general animal groupings. The groupings are rodents and rabbits, carnivores, ungulates, and nonhuman primates.

Rabbits and Rodents

Zoonotic diseases associated with modern rodent- and rabbit-research holding facilities are infrequent. However, there are reports of cases of lymphocytic choriomeningitis virus, Korean hemorrhagic fever caused by Hantavirus, leptospirosis, the tapeworm *Hymenolepis nana*, and ringworm that were purportedly acquired in laboratory facilities. Most infections acquired by animal handlers from rodents and rabbits are via direct contact with the animals or the animals' excretions or indirectly via aerosolized contaminants. Proper handling of rabbits and rodents is the most effective measure of preventing bites and scratches from these species [63].

Carnivores

Dogs, cats, and ferrets are the most common carnivores used in laboratory settings, and rabies is the most important zoonotic disease associated with carnivores. This is because carnivores are not likely to have come from barrier breeding facilities. Bites and scratches are the most common source of zoonotic disease transmission to animal handlers [63].

Ungulates

Ungulates such as sheep and goats present little risk for transmission of zoonotic disease to humans because these animals being are kept in herds and thus good husbandry conditions usually exist. Potential exposure is from direct contact or indirectly through aerosolized contaminants. Improper handling can result in kicks, butts, bites, or being stepped on, which potentially may result in exposures. Q fever is a concern in certain research projects involving ungulate parturition products or materials contaminated by these products [63].

Nonhuman Primates

The two infectious agents that present major risks for transmission of zoonotic infection from nonhuman primates to humans are simian immunodeficiency virus (SIV) and herpes B virus [64–66]. The morbidity of human SIV infections has not been clearly defined [11]. The morbidity of herpes B virus is very clear: Although it causes minimal adverse effects in macaques, in humans in can cause rapidly progressive encephalomyelitis, with a fatality rate approaching 70%.

The best approach to either of these infections and other potential zoonoses transmitted by nonhuman primates is prevention of exposure. Education about the risks of exposure is very important. Animal handlers should receive instruction about protocols and procedures involved in handling nonhuman primates. They need to be able to demonstrate the steps to be taken in the event of an injury or potential exposure. The use of restraint cages and chemical restraint should be encouraged whenever any interaction is planned with nonhuman primates. Protective equipment such as gloves, face shields, and arm protectors should be used [53]. This is especially important in handling macaques. When nonhuman primates have been experimentally inoculated with SIV or similar types of viruses, Biosafety level 2 practices should be followed [64].

CONTROL METHODS

It is generally accepted that engineering controls should be considered the best approach to reducing exposure risks, although it is understood that constraints may be present that require other approaches. Using administrative or work practice controls is the next best approach. The final and least acceptable method is personal protective equipment. Animal care facilities are no exception to this approach to controlling hazards and exposures. Engineering controls are generally considered to be the best barriers to exposure to animals [14]. These barriers may consist singly or in combination of such items as fume hoods, biologic safety cabinets, special caging, and room ventilation. Administration and work practices consist of measures to reduce the number of employees exposed and reduce contacts with animals. For the protection of individual animal handlers, efforts are directed at reducing exposures by percutaneous, ingestion, and inhalation [14]. These measures should apply to tasks of handling, transporting, and restraining animals as well as to housekeeping, waste disposal, and cage cleaning. It is important also to address issues of personal hygiene to reduce the risk of exposure and provide facilities that make it easy to maintain a high standard of personal cleanliness [53]. Hand washing is very important in preventing the spread of infectious contaminants [63]. Eating, drinking, smoking, and applying cosmetics should not be permitted in laboratories or animal containment areas [14,53,63]. Two principles should be followed in regard to protective measures [63]. One, protective measures are meant to reduce exposures, based on knowledge of risks involved in caring for animals. Two, good hygiene helps reduce risk of contamination. Personal protective equipment consists of equipment such as gloves, shoe covers, protective clothing, face shields, earplugs, and respirators. Animal handlers should be given the appropriate personal protective equipment based on potential exposure to hazardous agents [53]. This equipment protects the individual wearing it against splashes and splatters and should not be presumed to offer protection against needlesticks or bites [63].

The most important preventive strategy is education. Animal handlers must be trained in the use of control measures [14,53,63] and in proper handling of animals to avoid bites and scratches. It is also important to educate handlers on proper disposal methods for animal bedding and waste products and other contaminated body materials as well as on Universal Precautions and other good personal hygiene measures. They also need to understand the importance of immediately reporting accidents and adverse incidents [14,63]. Training should be done at least annually and must be appropriate to animal handlers' education level, experience in the facility, and language skills [14,53,63].

TYPES OF MEDICAL EVALUATIONS

An important part of an animal handler's medical surveillance program is the medical evaluation. There are basically three types of medical evaluation: preplacement, periodic, and episodic evaluations. These evaluations should be used to gather information about animal handlers and as educational times for the animal handlers. The term *evaluation* is more appropriate because the term *examination* implies physical examination. The encounter should be to find out information about the health of the animal worker, and for the most part, this can be done by questionnaires and focused interviews. A decision to conduct further evaluation should be based on information elicited during the history taking. The educational portion of the evaluations involves explaining health exposure risks, the reporting mechanisms for accidents and injuries, and how the medical surveillance program functions to protect the animal handler.

Preplacement Evaluation

The preplacement evaluation is used to establish a baseline of health information before an individual starts on the job and has any exposures at the worksite. It is a time to identify pre-existing conditions that can affect an individual's capacity to perform the essential functions of a position. This time can be used to discuss medical conditions that might alter an individual's risk profile, such as active tuberculosis or pregnancy, and to address the needs for reasonable accommodations. From an educational standpoint, it is time to educate animal handlers about potential risks, the use of personal protective equipment, and the medical symptoms that should prompt the individual to obtain an occupational health evaluation [14,58,69].

Periodic Evaluation. The periodic medical evaluation is the main component of a medical surveillance program. This evaluation needs to be designed to verify the success of the occupational health and safety program in reducing exposure risk. Components of the evaluation need to focus on the individual animal handler's risk of exposure. Careful inquiry must be made in regard to symptoms that may be early warnings of potential disease. These symptoms may prompt measures to prevent progression of the disease process. Physical examinations need not be a routine part of the periodic evaluation unless warranted by a change in health status [14]. The best use of the occupational health professional's time is taking a careful history, based on knowledge of the animal handler's exposure risk. This knowledge is gained by the health professional's visiting the worksite. Time should also be devoted to informing the animal handler of workplace hazards and inquiring about warning signals of illness.

Episodic Evaluation

Episodic health evaluations are evaluations of work-related injuries or medical follow-up of early warning symptoms of illness and persistent symptoms [14]. Animal handlers should be encouraged to report all suspected work-related injuries and illnesses as soon as possible [67]. All accidental exposure incidents need to be evaluated to determine if they warrant medical evaluation.

A special type of episodic evaluation is when a female handler becomes pregnant. An evaluation by the occupational health professional, with input from her personal physician, will ensure proper medical surveillance and work assignment changes, thus helping to reduce the exposure risk for the animal handler and her fetus [63].

There should be a regular systematic review of these examinations by the animal care facility managers, the environmental health and safety professionals, and the occupational health professional. Changes in the program examinations should be based on changes in exposures for the animal handlers. Work force changes should be accounted for as well. The injury and illness experience needs to be looked at to determine changes in the surveillance program. Last, new guidelines may require changes in surveillance procedures.

ISSUE OF SERUM BANKING

Serum banking is typically for the purpose of giving an institution the ability to compare serum obtained after a worker's acute illness or exposure with prior samples from the same individual. It has often been a standard component of animal handler surveillance programs. It is actually more useful from a medicolegal standpoint than for the benefit of the animal handler in almost all instances. Guidelines from the late 1980s and early 1990s called for routine serum banking [14,64,65]. More recent guidelines recommend serum banking in very limited cases in which serologic monitoring can follow the progression of a potential infection or disease state. These guidelines also recommend testing of the obtained serum specimen along with its banking. In general, serum banking should be used only if there is a clear reason for obtaining the samples and there is a plan to analyze the data as part of a risk-assessment strategy.

There are issues that need to be addressed by a policy statement concerning serum banking, and a program should be implemented to address chain-of-custody issues. Just as it is important to maintain an appropriate chain of custody for urine drug screens, it is also important for serum banking. The policy statement should make clear that there must be no tampering with or misplacing or mislabeling of specimens as well as address issues of confidentiality and identification of specimens. There should be identifiers that identify the specimens but do not reveal the donor to the casual observer. The specimens have to be handled appropriately before being stored so that the specimen does not deteriorate sooner than anticipated. The specimens must be retained in a storage unit that will maintain the correct temperature level. The unit must have a back-up energy source so that if a power outage occurs, the specimens are not ruined. Deterioration of the specimens over time due to natural processes and the freezing process itself need to be addressed. The policy statement must cover all of these issues. The institution will also have to consider the cost of maintaining the specimens in a secure manner. Finally, animal handlers should give informed consent regarding the collection, storage, and use of such specimens. They should also be given the opportunity to decline participation without punitive action by the employer.

IMMUNIZATIONS AND SEROLOGIC TESTING

Animal handlers should be offered immunizations known to be safe and effective. Recommendation for immunization vary according to risk and hazard assessments. This information will come from the institutional veterinarians and the occupational health and safety professionals. Hepatitis B vaccination also should be offered, based on the requirements of the OSHA Bloodborne Pathogen Standard (29 CFR 1910.1030). In general, all animal handlers should have current tetanus and diphtheria immunization status. Other vaccinations offered might include those for yellow fever, rabies, and polio.

Rabies should be offered to all animal handlers involved with animals potentially infected with rabies. It should be provided to those who capture or destroy wild animals on site. Those who inspect sites where rabies virus is used should also be considered for vaccination. Periodic serologic monitoring should be offered.

Serologic testing for toxoplasmosis should be obtained for immunocompromised animal handlers or females capable of childbearing who anticipate exposure to cats or their feces. If titers are not interpreted as protective, then the animal handler should be counseled regarding potential health risks to themselves or fetus. The supervisor needs to make the decision about providing job reassignments for these animal handlers [67].

GENERAL GUIDELINES FOR A PROGRAM

Medical surveillance for animal handlers has changed dramatically over the last decade. Formerly, most programs relied heavily on serum banking as the cornerstone of their programs. They attempted to be all-encompassing in their design, but unfortunately, they often accomplished nothing more than looking good "on paper" when accrediting groups inspected animal care facilities. In recent years, the emphasis has changed to a more focused and simple approach. Serum banking is used sparingly, and comprehensive annual examinations are not routinely performed anymore. More cooperation exists between research personnel, animal care facility personnel, occupational health and safety professionals, and the occupational health professionals [14]. This has led to more practical and often long-term cost-effective medical surveillance programs for animal handlers. Emphasis is placed on risk assessment and control of hazardous exposures rather than a standard, comprehensive evaluation of individual animal handlers that has little relevance to their specific risks. The National Institute of Health (NIH) and the National Institute of Environmental Health Sciences (NIEHS) have programs that are based on this tailored approach [63,67]. The program at our institution, the University of Alabama, is modeled after these programs, although our institution does not follow exactly the same approaches as those of the NIH and the NIEHS because of financial constraints and the particular needs of our animal resource program. The following is a presentation of a model program that draws from parts of all three programs.

There must be a written policy statement about the medical surveillance program for animal handlers. The purpose of an animal handlers' medical surveillance program needs to be stated. In essence, it is to protect the health of the worker. The clinical interactions are used to provide appropriate immunizations, to review good work practices, and to educate the animal handlers in regard to risk assessment and exposure reduction. The program is available not only to the animal handlers of the animal care facility [14,53,63,67], but also to all that come in contact with animals on a routine basis. The animal handlers' surveillance program is divided into three categories:

1. Small animals, mainly rodents and rabbits.
2. Large animals, mainly cats, dogs, and livestock.
3. Nonhuman primates, namely, marmosets, monkeys, and apes.

Preplacement Evaluation

A preplacement evaluation is offered to all participants [63,67]. It should consist of an occupational and personal medical history, safety and health counseling, tuberculin skin testing, and appropriate immunizations. Additional requirements are based on that initial evaluation. A focused examination may be required, based on the results of the occupational or personal medical history. Other special diagnostic tests are performed as indicated by an individual animal handler's medical or occupational history or job assignment.

The occupational and personal medical histories are used to determine if reasonable accommodations are necessary for the individual. The occupational and environmental portion of the history covers information about past experiences with animals and with which type of animals; it also includes past work history and questions regarding adverse incidents in past employment. The counseling part of the evaluation should be an integral part of the occupational history and should include (1) a description of the job and the essential functions of the job, the different types of animals the worker will have contact with and the hazards and risks associated with them, and any other potential work hazards and risks. At this time and during orientation, the animal handler receives instructions regarding Universal Precautions and the availability of the occupational health service unit for evaluation of injuries and accidents and issues of occupational health risk.

At the preplacement evaluation, the animal handler is given appropriate immunizations based on the animal contact they will have and in compliance with federal, state, and local regulations.

The animal handler is started in a tuberculosis surveillance program. Those who will be working with large animals are offered additional services [63,67]. Rabies immunization and serologic monitoring should be offered to those who would be considered at high risk of exposure to rabies. There should be serologic testing for toxoplasmosis for those who would be at risk [67], namely, immunocompromised workers and any females with childbearing potential who will be exposed to cats or cat feces. If an animal handler fits in one of these categories and lacks immunity to toxoplasmosis, the individual is counseled in regard to susceptibility to infection and associated risk. The person's supervisor should be notified of the need for job reassignment of the worker.

If there is a high risk of exposure to Q fever, counseling should be offered [67]. Animal handlers that will have direct involvement with *Coxiella burnetii* or handle products of parturition or other contaminated materials from sheep, goats, cattle, or cats are considered at risk. They should be advised of signs and symptoms to look for and the importance of early treatment. Animal handlers with medical conditions that could be adversely affected by Q fever infection are advised of the potential risk and may be advised to avoid work in those areas of high risk of exposure.

Additional services should be offered to those involved in work with nonhuman primates [67]. All animal handlers are enrolled in the tuberculosis surveillance program. At this time, it is emphasized that tuberculosis has devastating consequences for nonhuman primates and may cause the loss of the whole colony. It is stressed that it is important that the animal handler not infect the nonhuman primates. Rubeola screening is offered at preplacement because the animal handler must have evidence of immunity to rubeola or be vaccinated. Rubeola is a common infection in nonhuman primate colonies. Hepatitis A and B vaccinations are offered if animal handlers will be working with experimentally infected nonhuman primates. Rabies immunization is offered to animal handlers who will be working with quarantined nonhuman primates. Animal handlers can voluntarily enroll in a retrovirus exposure surveillance program. Additionally, animal handlers working with nonhuman primates are given instruction on appropriate measures to take in the event of injuries and potential exposures to herpes B virus from macaques and to simian immunodeficiency virus from other monkeys and apes, whether they are naturally or experimentally infected.

Periodic Evaluation

Periodic evaluations are usually given annually. An occupational history is conducted to detect early signs and symptoms of disease. Further medical evaluation is based on the findings of the history; at this time, tuberculin skin testing or other means of evaluating a worker's tuberculosis status is performed. Those working with nonhuman primates may need to have more frequent surveillance in the tuberculosis program. Immunization status is reviewed and updated as necessary. Those who received rabies immunization starting two years after the series was completed require serologic testing to determine their immune status.

SUMMARY

A medical surveillance plan for animal handlers should provide for the safety and good health of all those who work with animals. The program needs to focus on the specific needs of the animal handlers, based on an adequate health risk assessment of the specific animal care facility. The occupational medicine service unit should be involved in policy and procedure issues that have an impact on the health of the animal handlers. The occupational health professional should have a good working knowledge of the facility and the hazards and risks involved. There should be regular interaction between the animal care facility managers, the environmental health and safety professionals, and the occupational health professional. There should be a computerized data collection system that will augment the surveillance program; it should be used to review and aggregate information about the control methods and the surveillance program. The program should not add unnecessary items that will eventually dilute the services rendered to the animal handlers.

Medical Surveillance of Health Care Workers with an Emphasis on Infectious Diseases

OVERVIEW

It is well recognized that health care workers are frequently exposed to a variety of occupational insults that can result in serious acute or chronic adverse health effects [68]. Although occupational exposure to infectious disease is not a risk that solely affects health care workers, this group clearly has more intensity of such exposures and a far greater variety of exposures to potentially virulent infectious agents than most other occupational work groups. For these reasons alone, it is imperative that a well-organized surveillance program be in place in health care facilities. Those who run such facilities must also recognize that OSHA regulations mandate some infectious disease surveillance. However, the overriding incentive for infectious disease surveillance of health care workers should be that these programs benefit health care–facility employees as well as the patient populations they serve, many of whom have compromised health.

Surveillance programs for infectious diseases are already in place in most health care facilities. The remainder of this section details well-recognized infectious disease surveillance protocols as well as touches on other possible surveillance protocols that may be adapted, depending on the potential for exposure that may exist in an individual facility.

Surveillance programs should always coexist with primary and secondary prevention. Primary prevention of an infectious disease is action taken to prevent initiation of the disease process. These activities remove or reduce risk factors [69]. Such measures include Universal Precautions (e.g., for bloodborne pathogens), personal protective equipment (e.g., respirators, gowns, gloves), engineering controls (e.g., ventilation, ultraviolet lighting), and preexposure vaccination. Secondary prevention of infectious disease involves intervention early in a disease process, when that process may be reversible or when the disease progression may be limited. For infectious diseases, secondary prevention may involve medical treatment such as medication, surgery, or postexposure vaccination [2].

Other chapters in this text cover specific infectious diseases, including surveillance for these diseases, in greater detail. The examples in this section cover the important elements that should be included in employee surveillance programs for most health care facilities.

SPECIFIC INFECTIOUS DISEASE SURVEILLANCE IN HEALTH CARE WORKERS

Hepatitis

Hepatitis B. Occupational exposure to hepatitis B was a major impetus for OSHA's Bloodborne Pathogen Standard, which became effective March 6, 1992, and applies to all persons occupationally exposed to blood or other potentially infectious materials. According to the standard, exposure determination is based on the definition of occupational exposure without regard to personal protective clothing or equipment. Reviewing job classifications within the work environment and listing exposures into two groups are steps in making the exposure determination. The first group includes job classifications in which all of the employees have occupational exposure, such as operating room scrub nurses. In such cases, it is not necessary to list specific work tasks. The second group includes those job classifications in which some of the employees have occupational exposure, such as workers in a hospital laundry where some of the workers are assigned the task of handling contaminated laundry, while others are not.

Surveillance for hepatitis B, either preplacement or postexposure, is based on blood tests for hepatitis B antibodies and hepatitis B antigen. These blood tests also help to determine whether or not an employee is a chronic carrier of the disease, carries the protective antibody, or needs to be vaccinated for the disease.

For those health care workers covered under OSHA's Bloodborne Pathogen Standard (see above), a series of three hepatitis B vaccines should be initiated at the time of the preplacement exam, provided that there is no previous history of hepatitis B or previous administration of hepatitis B vaccine. If there is a history of previous disease or previous vaccine administration, then blood testing for the presence of hepatitis B antibodies should be performed to determine whether immunity is present. Employers are not required to offer hepatitis B vaccination (1) to employees who have previously completed the hepatitis B vaccination series, (2) when immunity is confirmed by antibody testing, or (3) if the vaccine is contraindicated for medical reasons. Employee participation in a prescreening program is not required in order to obtain a hepatitis B vaccination series.

For prevaccination surveillance testing, when immunity or prior history of disease status is uncertain, one should consider performing blood testing for the hepatitis B surface antigen (HBsAg) and the antibody to hepatitis B surface antigen (anti-HBs). The hepatitis B surface antigen (HBsAg) is positive in chronic carriers. The antibody to hepatitis B surface antigen (anti-HBs) indicates immunity following disease recovery or following a successful immunization series.

If necessary, postvaccination surveillance for immunity (anti-HBs) should be performed at least 1–6 months after completion of the vaccine series. If such results indicate a nonresponder, 15–25% achieve an adequate antibody response after one additional dose and 30–50% after three additional doses [70].

A recombinant vaccine that carries no risk of bloodborne pathogen transmission eventually replaced the initial plasma-derived formulation of the hepatitis B vaccine. The standard schedule for immunization involves three injections in the deltoid muscle at 0, 1, and 6 months. The three-dose series confers a protective antibody response in more than 90% of healthy young adults, but response rates decline with age and may be as low as 50% in the elderly. Response is also lower in those with renal failure, diabetes mellitus, chronic hepatic disease, HIV infection, obesity, and in those who smoke. The response rate is slightly better in women than in men [71].

The anti-HBs (hepatitis B surface antibody) is the major protective mechanism in individuals who have had an episode of hepatitis B or have had the series of hepatitis B vaccinations. Its presence usually indicates lifelong immunity [72].

The employer must make the hepatitis B vaccine and vaccination series available to all employees who have occupational exposure as well as provide a postexposure evaluation and follow-up to all employees who experience an exposure incident. The vaccine and vaccinations, as well as all medical evaluations and follow-up, must be made available by the employer at no cost to the employee.

If a health care employee has a parenteral (e.g., needlestick or cut) or mucous membrane (e.g., splash to eye or mouth) exposure to the blood or other body fluid of a patient potentially infected with hepatitis B, the following procedural measures are recommended:

- The employee's hepatitis B history and vaccination status should be established and blood drawn for HBsAg and anti-HBs.
- If the patient is known to be HBsAg positive and is not known to be immune, the employee is immediately given hepatitis B immune globulin (HBIG) at a dose of 0.06 mL/kg. Employees who received HBIG within the last three months do not need another injection.
- If the hepatitis B surface antigen (HBsAg) status of the patient is unknown, a blood sample is drawn from the patient and sent to the laboratory for HBsAg testing.
- After results of the above are known, the following should be implemented:
  - If the health care employee's anti-HBs status is positive, indicating immunity, no further steps are taken.
  - If the patient's status is HBsAg negative and the health care employee's HBCoreAg and anti-HBs are also negative, the employee is offered the hepatitis B vaccine.
  - If the patient's HBsAg is positive, but the employee's HBCoreAg and anti-HBs are both negative, HBIG (0.06 mL/kg) is given along with the first dose of hepatitis B vaccine. HBIG must be given within seven days after exposure but preferably should be given within 24–48 hours. The vaccination series should be completed according to the recommended schedule (at 0, 1, and 6 months).

Hepatitis C. If the possibility of a health care worker's contracting hepatitis C following a parenteral or mucous membrane exposure is of concern, the following procedural measures are recommended:

- The health care employee's hepatitis C history should be established and blood drawn for anti-HCV.
- If the hepatitis C status of the patient is unknown, the blood should be drawn from the patient and sent for testing of the antibody level to hepatitis C (anti-HCV).
- If the source is found to be infected (anti-HCV positive) and the health care employee is anti-HCV negative, then the employee should be informed of the need for medical follow-up. Serologic monitoring for anti-HCV is repeated at 1 and at 6 months. Counseling should be made available to the employee.

There is no known effective immunoprophylaxis or chemoprophylaxis for hepatitis C. The Centers for Disease Control and Prevention (CDC) no longer considers the use of immune serum globulin an appropriate option.

Hepatitis A. Routine administration of hepatitis A vaccine, even in health care personnel, is not recommended. Consequently, regular surveillance of health care workers for hepatitis A is usually not standard procedure. Adherence to well-recognized precautions against transmission via the fecal-oral route is the best preventive measure. Vaccination of personnel in highly endemic areas or after exposure to hepatitis A has not been adequately studied. On the other hand, administration of immune globulin within 2 weeks following a known hepatitis exposure is quite effective in preventing infection and may be advisable in outbreak situations.

Hepatitis D and E. Infection with hepatitis D virus occurs only in persons with coexisting acute or chronic hepatitis B infection. In this population, high-risk individuals include people from Mediterranean countries, individuals with hemophilia, and parenteral drug users. An antibody assay for hepatitis D is available.

Hepatitis E, which is rare in the United States, is a designation for an epidemic form of hepatitis that is apparently transmitted by the fecal-oral route. It is a diagnosis of exclusion. The role of passive immunization for either hepatitis D or E is unclear.

Tuberculosis

Health care workers, including home health nurses, staff in long-term care facilities, and emergency medical technicians should be included in a tuberculosis (TB) screening and prevention program [73,74]. Such a program should include tuberculin skin testing for all health care workers upon employment and at intervals determined by their future risk of exposure in that facility.

Mantoux tuberculin skin testing is the standard method used for TB screening. This test is administered by intradermal injection of 0.1 mL of purified protein derivative (PPD) containing 5 tuberculin units (TU), into either the volar or dorsal surface of the forearm. A disposable tuberculin syringe, with the needle bevel facing up should be used. If this procedure is done correctly, it should produce a discrete, pale elevation of the skin (wheal), 6–10 mm in diameter.

Two-step TB skin testing is used to distinguish boosted reactions from those reactions due to new infections. If the skin test reaction to an initial (first) test is read as negative, a second test should be done 1–3 weeks later. A positive reaction to this second test is most likely a boosted reaction and not a new infection. Using the result of the second test in the two-step method, a person should either be classified as previously infected (but not a new converter), if the test is positive, or uninfected, if the second test is negative. In the latter case (two-step negative persons), a positive reaction to any subsequent test is likely to represent a new infection with *M tuberculosis* (new converter). Two-step TB skin testing is recommended for the initial (preplacement) skin testing of health care workers, who will be retested periodically (annually).

A trained health care worker should interpret the tuberculin skin test within 48–72 hours after the injection. A positive reaction may still be read up to one week following the injection. However, if a patient who fails to return within 72 hours has a negative test, tuberculin testing should be repeated.

Measurement of the area of induration (palpable swelling) is the way a test is interpreted, not the erythema around the site of injection (Table 7-1). The appropriate cut-off measurement for a health care worker should be similar to the measurement limits used for persons not in health care occupations. The difference is that determination of what constitutes a positive tuberculin skin test for health care workers is also dependent on the prevalence of TB in the health care facility. In facilities with little if any exposure to TB, 15-mm induration may be an appropriate cut-off for persons with no other risk factors. On the other hand, for workers in facilities that regularly care for TB patients, 10-mm induration may be an appropriate cut-off.

Varicella

Varicella vaccine was granted U.S. licensure in 1995. Vaccination is desirable for persons who lack a reliable history of varicella. Special efforts should be made to assess an individual health care worker's immunity to varicella by obtaining either a reliable history of disease or through surveillance by measurement of serum antibody titers. Those who are susceptible—for example, health care workers serving immunocompromised patients—should receive varicella vaccine. The occurrence of varicella in pregnant women is very rare, since 90% of females of childbearing age are immune. However, a fetal varicella syndrome, characterized by multiple congenital malformations, has been described [75]. Therefore, it is advisable to weigh the risks and benefits of administering varicella vaccine to a nonimmune female health care worker of childbearing age.

Although historical information may be an important factor in predicting immunity, recent studies have shown that 2–5% of all health care workers are susceptible to varicella [76,77]. Additionally, this study found that historical information was ineffective in predicting immune status for measles, rubella, mumps, and varicella.

Human Immunodeficiency Virus

Surveillance data suggest that most health care workers with acquired immunodeficiency syndrome (AIDS), acquired the human immunodeficiency virus (HIV) infection through a nonoccupational route [78]. However, as increasing numbers of patients with AIDS are hospitalized, the risk of exposure to HIV can be expected to increase further. Thus, preventing transmission of HIV to health care workers will require efforts to reduce the incidence and dosage of exposure to blood and body fluids through the use of Universal Precautions [79].

If, despite ongoing efforts to prevent HIV exposure, exposure takes place, in addition to appropriate medical treatment, surveillance of the exposed employee for the disease needs to begin immediately. Baseline testing of the health care worker to establish HIV antibody status at the time of exposure should be performed. If the source patient is seronegative and has no clinical evidence of AIDS or symptoms of HIV infection, further follow-up is usually not necessary. If the source person has recently engaged in behavior associated with contracting HIV infection, baseline and follow-up antibody titer measurements should be obtained at 6 weeks, 12 weeks, and 6 months postexposure [80]. It is unclear whether an extended follow-up period (e.g., 12 months) is indicated in certain cases. A recent study showed a mean seroconversion time frame of 46 days following exposure, with a median of 65 days [81].

Mumps

An effective vaccination program for those that are susceptible is the best approach to preven-

Table 7-1
Classification of Positive Tuberculin Skin Tests in Health Care Workers

5-mm Induration	10-mm Induration	15-mm Induration
Known or suspected HIV	Medical conditions, excluding HIV	No known risk factors for TB
Close contacts of persons with infectious TB	IV drug users with known negative HIV	

tion of occupational transmission of mumps. Personnel should be considered immune if they have (1) documented physician-diagnosed mumps, (2) documentation of receipt of one dose of live mumps vaccine on or after their first birthday, or (3) serologic evidence of immunity. Persons born prior to 1957 may be considered immune from naturally acquired infection [82].

Rubella

Serologic screening of personnel for immunity to rubella need not be done before vaccinating against rubella, unless the medical facility considers it cost effective or the person getting the vaccination requests it [14]. Rubella vaccination should be required for health care workers who work in a facility where exposure and consequent transmission to patients could have life-threatening consequences. This would include those who care for immunocompromised, pediatric, or obstetric patients. For the same reason, special consideration should be given to susceptible female health care workers of childbearing age who are at risk of exposure to rubella (such as those that work with pediatric patients). However, vaccination for rubella carries its own risk for this latter group, and women should be counseled to avoid pregnancy for a period of 30 days following the administration of vaccine.

References

1. Lewitt MH. Epidemiology and biostatistics. *Occup Med State Art Rev* 1997;12:587–99.
2. Pottinger JM, Herwaldt LA, Perl TM. Basics of surveillance—an overview. *Infect Control Hosp Epidemiol* 1997;18:513–27.
3. Schenker MB. Biostatistics and epidemiology. In: LaDou J (ed), *Occupational and Environmental Medicine*. Stamford, CT: Appleton & Lange, 1997. Pp 783–804.
4. Fox J, Lipman N. Infections transmitted by large and small laboratory animals. *Infect Dis Clin North Am* 1991;5:131–59.
5. Colligan MJ, Sinclair RC. The training ethic and the ethics of training. *Occup Med State Art Rev* 1994; 9:127–34.
6. McCunney RJ, Anstadt G, Burton WN, et al. Advantage of a healthy work force. *J Occup Environ Med* 1997; 39:611–13.
7. Boden LI, Cabral H. Company characteristics and workplace medical testing. *Am J Public Health* 1995; 85:1070–75.
8. Robinson ST. Role of industrial hygiene in medical surveillance. *Occup Med State Art Rev* 1990;5:469–78.
9. Abatemarco DJ, Delnevo CD, Rosen M, et al. Medical surveillance practices of blue-collar and white-collar hazardous waste workers. *J Occup Environ Med* 1995;37: 578–82.
10. Burdorf A, Sorock GS, Herrick RF, et al. Advancing epidemiological studies of occupational injury—approaches and future directions. *Am J Ind Med* 1997;32:180–3.
11. Leigh JP, Miller TR. Job-related diseases and occupations within a large workers' compensation data set. *Am J Ind Med* 1998;33:197–211.
12. Maizlish N. Designing prevention-oriented software for workplace health and safety. *Am J Ind Med* 1997;31:64–74.
13. Sorock GS, Smith GS, Reeve GR, et al. Three perspectives on work-related injury surveillance systems. *Am J Ind Med* 1997;32:116–28.
14. National Research Council. Occupational health and safety in the care and use of research animals. Washington, DC: National Academy Press, 1997.
15. Baram M. Generic strategies for protecting worker health and safety. *Occup Med State Art Rev* 1996;11:69–77.
16. Joseph AJ. Right-to-know training of workers with IQ less than 70: a pilot study. *Am J Ind Med* 1997;32:417–20.
17. Khoury MJ, Genetics Working Group. From genes to public health: the applications of genetic technology in disease prevention. *Am J Public Health* 1996;86:1717–22.
18. McCunney RJ. Preserving confidentially in occupational medical practice. *Am Fam Physician* 1996;53:1751–6.
19. Rischitelli, DG. The confidentiality of medical information in the workplace. *J Occup Environ Med* 1995; 37:583–93.
20. Rothstein MA. A proposed revision of the ACOEM code of ethics. *J Occup Environ Med* 1997;39:616–22.
21. Rothstein MA. Legal and ethical aspects of medical screening. *Occup Med State Art Rev* 1996;11:31–9.
22. Tilton SH. Right to privacy and confidentiality of medical records. *Occup Med State Art Rev* 1996;11:17–29.
23. American College of Occupational and Environmental Medicine. Position paper on the confidentiality of medical information in the workplace. *J Occup Environ Med* 1995;37:594–6.
24. Association of Occupational and Environmental Clinics. Patient Bill of Rights. 1987. Available at *http://occ-env-med.mcduke.edu/oem/aoec.html.library*.
25. Langer CS. Title I of the Americans with Disabilities Act. *Occup Med State Art Rev* 1996;11:5–16.
26. Stillman NG, Donmoyer KT. Occupational health issues under employment law. *Occup Med State Art Rev* 1996;11:41–55.

27. U.S. Department of Justice. Americans with Disabilities Act Home Page. Available at *http://www.usdoj.gov/crt/ada/adahom1.html.*

28. U.S. Equal Employment Opportunity Commission. The ADA: Your Responsibilities as an Employer. Available at *http://www.eeoc.gov/facts/ada17.html.*

29. Jones DL. Occupational health services and OSHA compliance. *Occup Med State Art Rev* 1996;11:57–68.

30. Occupational Safety and Health Administration. *All About OSHA*. OSHA 2056, 1994.

31. Antti-Poika M. Implementation of a quality system for the examination of occupational diseases. *Occup Med* 1995;45:298–304.

32. Occupational Safety and Health Administration. OSHA Strategic Plan FY1997–FY2002, 1997. Washington, DC: OSHA, 1997.

33. Manno M. Risk assessment. *Toxicol Lett* 1995;77:45–7.

34. Bell JG, Bishop C, Gann M, et al. A systematic approach to health surveillance in the workplace. *Occup Med* 1995;45:305–10.

35. National Academy of Science. Risk assessment in the federal government: managing the process. Washington, DC: National Academy Press, 1983.

36. Hansson SO. Critical effects and exposure limits. *Risk Anal* 1997;17:227–36.

37. Jarvholm B. Relative risk and excess rate models in exposure-response analysis. *Am J Ind Med* 1997;31:399–402.

38. Anderson JTL, Astrakianakis G, Band PR. Standardizing job titles for exposure assessment in the pulp and paper industry. *Appl Occup Environ Hyg* 1997;12:611–4.

39. Cordes DH, Rea DF. Work-site risk assessment. *Prim Care* 1994;21:267–74.

40. Crook B. Review: methods of monitoring for process microorganisms in biotechnology. *Ann Occup Hyg* 1996;40:245–60.

41. Goldberg M, Levin SM, Doucette JT, et al. A task-based approach to assessing lead exposure among ironworkers engaged in bridge rehabilitation. *Am J Ind Med* 1997;31:310–8.

42. Tornero-Velez R, Symanski E, Kromhout H, et al. Compliance versus risk in assessing occupational exposures. *Risk Anal* 1997;17:279–92.

43. Lowery LK. Role of biomarkers of exposure in the assessment of health risks. *Toxicol Lett* 1995;77:31–8.

44. Murthy LI, Halperin WE. Medical screening and biological monitoring. *J Occup Environ Med* 1995;37:170–84.

45. Schulte PA. Opportunities for the development and use of biomarkers. *Toxicol Lett* 1995;77:25–9.

46. Zober A, Will W. Biological monitoring and risk assessment in occupational settings. *Int Arch Occup Environ Health* 1996;68:389–93.

47. Jardine CG, Hrudey SE. Mixed messages in risk communication. *Risk Anal* 1997;17:489–98.

48. Matte TD, Fine L, Meinhardt TJ, et al. Guidelines for medical screening in the workplace. *Occup Med State Art Rev* 1990;5:439–56.

49. Agency for Toxic Substances and Disease Registry. *Taking an Exposure History. Case Studies in Environmental Medicine:* 26. Atlanta, GA: U.S. Department of Health and Human Services, 1992.

50. Hunskaar S, Fosse R. Allergy to laboratory mice and rats: a review of its prevention, management and treatment. *Lab Anim* 1993;27:206–21.

51. National Institutes of Health. *Public Health Service Policy on Humane Care and Use of Laboratory Animals.* Rockville, MD: Department of Health and Human Services, 1996.

52. U.S. Department of Health and Human Services. *Biosafety in Microbiological and Biotechnical Laboratories.* Publication No. (CDC) 93-8395. Washington, DC: U.S. Government Printing OIffice, 1993.

53. National Research Council. *Guide for the Care and Use of Laboratory Animals.* Washington, DC: National Academy Press, 1996.

54. Culver J. Preventing transmission of blood-borne pathogens: a compelling argument for effective device-selection strategies. *Am J Infect Control* 1997;25:430–3.

55. Hathon L. Engineering controls for abating airborne biologic, chemical and physical contaminants in healthcare workplaces. *Occup Med State Art Rev* 1997;12:635–9.

56. Kacergis JB, Jones RB, Reeb CK. Air quality in an animal facility: particulates, ammonia, and volatile organic compounds. *Am Ind Hyg Assoc J* 1996;57:634–40.

57. Khuder SA, Arthur T, Bisesi MS, et al. Prevalence of infectious diseases and associated symptoms in wastewater treatment workers. *Am J Ind Med* 1998;33:571–7.

58. LaMontagne AD, Mangione TW, Christiani DC, et al. Medical surveillance for ethylene oxide exposure: practices and clinical findings in Massachusetts hospitals. *J Occup Environ Med* 1996;38:144–54.

59. LaMontagne AD, Rudd RE, Mangione TW, et al. Determinants of the provision of ethylene oxide medical surveillance in Massachusetts's hospitals. *J Occup Environ Med* 1996;38:155–68.

60. Plaut M, Zimmerman EM, Goldstein RA. Health hazards to humans associated with domestic pets. *Annu Rev Public Health* 1996;17:221–45.

61. Society for Healthcare Epidemiology of America position paper: management of healthcare workers infected with hepatitis B virus, hepatitis C virus, human immunodeficiency virus, or other bloodborne pathogens. *Infect Control Hosp Epidemiol* 1997;18:349–63.

62. Stave GM. Control of biological hazards. *Occup Med State Art Rev* 1996;11:79–85.

63. National Institutes of Health. Health and Safety Manual: *http://www.niehs.nih.gov/odhsb/manual/lftfrm.html.*

64. Centers for Disease Control and Prevention. Perspectives in disease prevention and health promotion guide-

lines to prevent simian immunodeficiency virus infection in laboratory workers and animal handlers. *MMWR* 1988;37:693–4, 699–704.

65. Holmes G, Chapman L, Stewart J, et al. Guidelines for the prevention and treatment of B-virus infections in exposed persons. *Clin Infect Dis* 1995;20:421–5.
66. National Institutes of Health. *Protection of NIH Personnel Who Work with Non-Human Primates.* Manual 3044-2. Washington, DC: NIH, 1993.
67. National Institutes of Health. Animal Exposure Surveillance Program: *http://oacu.od.nih.gov/exposure/aesp.html.*
68. Rogers B. Health hazards in nursing and health care: an overview. *Am J Infect Control* 1997;25:248–61.
69. Matte TD, Fine L, Meinhardt TJ, et al. Guidelines for medical screening in the workplace. *Occup Med: State Art Rev* July–September 1990;5(3).
70. American Academy of Family Physicians: *Recommendations for Hepatitis B Pre-exposure Vaccination and Post-exposure Prophylaxis.* Reprint # 529. Kansas City, MO: AAFP, August 1992.
71. Reynolds EE, Baron RB, Perez-Stable EJ. *Who needs Hepatitis and Varicella vaccines? Fam Prac Recert* April 1997;19(4):33–51.
72. Aach R, Hirschman SZ, Holland PV. The ABCs of viral hepatitis. *Patient Care* August 15, 1992.
73. Centers for Disease Control. *Core Curriculum on Tuberculosis*, 3rd Ed, Atlanta: CDC, 1994.
74. Holmes SJ. Review of Recommendations of the Advisory Committee on Immunization Practices, Centers for Disease Control and Prevention, on varicella. *J Infect Dis* 1996;174(Suppl 3):S342–4.
75. Connan L, Ayoubi J, Icart J, et al. Intra-uterine fetal death following maternal varicella infection. *Eur J Obstet Gynecol Reprod Biol* 1996;68(1–2):205–7.
76. Sepkowitz K. Occupationally acquired infections in healthcare workers. *Ann Intern Med* 1996;125:826–34.
77. Oliveira J, da Cuhna S, Corte-Real R, et al. The prevalence of measles, rubella, mumps and chickenpox antibodies in a population of health care workers. *Acta Med Port* 1995;8(4):206–14.
78. Chamberland ME, Conley LJ, Bush TJ, et al. Healthcare workers with AIDS. National surveillance update. *JAMA* 1991;266(24):3459–62.
79. Lamphear BP. Trends and patterns in the transmission of bloodborne pathogens to health care workers. *Epidemiol Rev* 1994:16(2):437–50.
80. Centers for Disease Control and Prevention. Public Health Service guidelines for the management of healthcare worker exposures to HIV and recommendations for postexposure prophylaxis. *MMWR* 1998;45:1–39.
81. Busch MP, Satten GA. Time course of viremia and antibody seroconversion following human immunodeficiency virus exposure. *Am J Med* 1997;102(Suppl 5B): 117–24.
82. Bolyard EA, Tablan OC, Williams WW, et al. Guidelines for infection control in health care personnel. 1998. *Am J Infect Control* 1998;19:407–63.

8 / Employee Education and Training

Peter P. Greaney

Training

Employee training and education are forms of primary prevention and are integral components of effective health and safety programs. In fact, training is a required element in many standards set forth by the Occupational Safety and Health Administration (OSHA). More than 100 occupational safety and health standards require that workers be provided with some type of training to protect them from work-related hazards. These standards not only specify certain content that the training must include and certain administrative requirements, such as training duration and frequency, but also require that the employer demonstrate the effectiveness of the education program in transferring the necessary skills and knowledge.

Effective training requires more than merely subjecting employees to prepackaged programs or scripted material on health and safety. Training programs that actively engage workers will be most effective in achieving improvements in workplace safety. They often work best if participants have the opportunity to listen, look at visuals, ask questions, and participate in problem solving, planning, and practice with equipment. Hands-on exercises are the most effective training method [1], and class size should be kept as small as possible in order to maximize the opportunity for participation in activities that reinforce information retention. Training must be conducted during working hours and at no cost to the employee. The training should be conducted at the time of the initial assignment of an employee and periodically thereafter.

Training needs to be individualized to the exposures of the specific workplace and the required practices of the employees in that workplace. For example, in training a correctional officer on prevention of tuberculosis exposure, if the individual will not be involved with the actual medical care of the patient, then the information on isolation rooms and personal protective equipment should be limited. In this situation, more emphasis should be placed on administrative procedures and policies regarding actions to take when prisoners exhibit symptoms of tuberculosis, have active diseases, or are taking anti-tuberculosis medications. Other considerations when designing training programs are worker demographics and educational level and the training environment.

Some people compare training employees on occupational risks and hazards to the medical practice of obtaining patients' informed consent [2]. All jobs have inherent risks that must be fully understood and agreed to by the employee. The problem arises, however, from the variation in the employer's perception of risk and the employee's. Employers will typically underestimate risk, and those with less information will have a tendency to overestimate it [2]. The goal of effective training and education, therefore, should be to strike a balance between these biases.

An employer has the ethical and the moral responsibility to conduct training that is properly conceived and properly conducted in order to avoid harm to employees as well as to the organization [3].

Work Practices for Infection Control

Since employees may be a major source of contamination from, and transmission and distribution of, infectious diseases, training on the desired work practices to prevent exposure to infections is essential.

Infection control practices involve the training of employees to perform certain activities in specified manners, thus reducing or avoiding exposures. For example, employees may be instructed to wash their hands regularly, wear certain protective equipment, or keep certain items refrigerated. Universal Precautions are an example of work practices designed to protect health care workers from occupational exposure to HIV and other bloodborne pathogens. These precautions entail the use of appropriate types of barrier protection such as gloves, masks, gowns, or goggles whenever contact with blood or nonintact tissue is probable [4].

It is the responsibility of the employer to ensure that employees are properly informed of the potential health hazards and are provided training on how to minimize or reduce these hazards. Recommendations for employers in protecting workers from disease caused by exposure to bloodborne pathogens have been published in the Department of Labor and Department of Health and Human Services Joint Advisory Notice [5]. In developing programs to protect workers, employers should follow these steps [5]:

1. Classification of work activity.
2. Development of standard operating procedures.
3. Provision of training and education.
4. Development of procedures to ensure and monitor compliance.
5. Workplace redesign.

Infection control work practices should be based on knowledge and analysis of the work activities and work system as a whole [6]. The analysis should include evaluation of what the worker does in terms of activities or functions, how the work is done, and results of the work and worker characteristics. The risk of exposure to infectious agents will vary, depending on the job activity of the worker, which in turn will vary, depending on the occupation or job category. It is therefore important to have a thorough understanding of the particular risks inherent in a given occupation so that targeted training and education programs can be developed [7]. OSHA's bloodborne pathogen standard, 29 CFR 1910.1030, for example, requires that employees be provided training on the modes of transmission of bloodborne pathogens, the methods for recognizing job tasks and other activities that may involve exposure to blood and other potentially infectious materials, and the use and limitations of methods that will prevent or reduce exposure, including appropriate engineering controls, work practices, and personal protective equipment [8]. In a laboratory setting, the most important element of prevention is strict adherence to standard microbiologic practices and techniques. Persons working with infectious agents or other potentially infectious materials must be aware of the potential hazards and must be properly trained in how to handle these materials [9].

Each workplace with potentially infectious material should develop or adopt a detailed operations manual. This operations manual should include standard operating procedures (SOP) for all activities having the potential for exposure. The operations manual should identify specific hazards that will or may be encountered and should specify practices and procedures designed to minimize or eliminate the hazards. Once these SOP are developed, both an initial and periodic worker education program should be provided to all potentially exposed workers. No worker should engage in such tasks or activities before receiving training pertinent to SOP work practices and required protective equipment.

Enforcing proper work practices is the responsibility of the director or supervisor. Employers should monitor compliance with SOP and monitor the workplace to ensure that required work practices are observed by employees and that protective clothing and equipment are provided and properly used.

The employer should maintain records documenting SOP and work practices. In addition, complete training records, indicating the dates of training sessions, the content of those training sessions, the names of all persons conducting training and the names of all those receiving training, should be kept.

Control of work practices implies control over the behavior of individual workers. Behavioral health and safety programs began to gain popularity in the late 1980s. These programs are based on behavior modification through observation, feedback, and positive reinforcement. An effective behavior modification program requires supervision, motivation, and education of employees. It also requires commitment from all levels of management within an organization. One study found that employees' work behavior positively correlated with their perceptions of management's commitment to them [10].

Work practices controls take on greater importance when engineering controls are either not feasible or inadequate and when there is the potential for significant exposure to infectious agents when an employee is outside of controlled spaces. In many cases, work practice controls are required to complement engineering controls. The ability to influence work practices implies control over the behavior of individual workers on the job. Close supervision of workers is needed in order to enforce compliance with proper work practices.

Personal Protective Equipment

Following a 1987 directive to form the Occupational Safety and Health Administration (OSHA), the Centers for Disease Control issued guidelines recommending the use of protective gloves, protective clothing, and special procedures. Following that directive, OSHA issued the final bloodborne pathogens standard, "Occupational Exposure to Bloodborne Pathogens; Final Rule," which requires health care institutions to protect their employees from all occupational exposures to bloodborne pathogens [11].

Personal protective equipment (PPE) controls exposure by isolating the employee from the emission source. PPE is used to supplement engineering controls and work practices and is indicated whenever hazards cannot be totally eliminated through the use of engineering controls. In cases in which engineering controls are not practical or possible, PPE may form the primary barrier between the employee and infectious materials.

Respirators are a common type of PPE; they are used when protection from an inhaled contaminant is required. Respirators can range from a simple surgical mask to HEPA filter masks, depending on the agent and potential for exposure. Surgical masks serve mainly to protect the patient, animal, or product from exposure to the worker's exhaled organisms. HEPA filter masks have been shown to be effective in protecting health care workers from exposure to infectious particles, particularly *Mycobacterium tuberculosis* [12]. Training for respirator use must include a fit test, a written medical history questionnaire, and medical clearance.

Other forms of personal protective equipment include gloves, coats, gowns, shoe covers, boots, face shields, safety glasses, and goggles.

The proper choice of PPE depends on the type of work and the potential route of exposure. For example, the protective clothing required for performing tasks with an associated risk of bite or laceration consists of leather or steel-mesh reinforced hand and arm wear.

The PPE standard, 29 CFR 1910.132–137, includes requirements for eye and face protection, respiratory protection, occupational head protection, occupational foot protection, and electrical protective devices. It also requires that employees are trained to know when and why PPE is necessary, what type of PPE is necessary, how it is to be worn, the limitations of the PPE, and the proper care, maintenance, useful life, and disposal of the PPE. In addition, the employer must document that the employee has received and understood the required training through written certification that contains the name of each employee, the date(s) of training, and the subject of the certification [13].

Engineering Controls

Implementation of engineering controls is the preferred method for effective and reliable control of prolonged or highly infectious potential. Engineering controls are intended to contain biohazards at their source, reduce their airborne concentration, and limit their movement throughout the worksite. Controls include safety equipment such as enclosed containers, cabinets, sharps disposal containers, and ventilation hoods designed to remove or minimize exposures to hazardous biologic materials. Engineering controls act at the source of the emission and eliminate or reduce employee exposure without reliance on self-protective action by the employee. Although PPE provides a cheaper alternative to engineering controls, it does not eliminate the source of the exposure, often fails to provide the degree of protection required, and may create additional hazards by interfering with the user's vision, hearing, and mobility. Employees should be properly trained on the proper use of the engineering controls as well as its proper maintenance.

Personal Hygiene

Often overlooked is the great importance of personal hygiene, which includes personal habits, the use of protective clothing, provision and use of shower facilities, and cleaning of protective clothing so that biologic contaminants are not transferred to others.

A food handler, for example, is an obvious potential source for the dissemination of potentially infectious material, but workers in other settings such as the research laboratory, animal facilities, health care centers, and meat and poultry processing facilities are other significant sources of dissemination.

It is important that, when at work, employees follow strict habits of personal hygiene such as regular hand washing with soap and water. This should be done after eating, drinking, smoking, and using the toilet. Employees should keep their fingernails trimmed and clean and their hair clean and neat [14].

Clothing can be a potential source of infectious contamination. Employees should be instructed to keep their clothes neat and clean. If special protective clothing is available, it is recommended that employees wear it at work instead of street clothes. If protective clothing is provided, employees should not be allowed to wear work clothing home, as it may be another source of contamination.

Training Essentials

Training is an essential element in all preventive strategies and should include information on:

- Potential hazardous exposures.
- Bloodborne pathogens, including hepatitis A, B, and C as well as HIV.
- Methods of protection: engineering, work practice, and universal precautions.
- Statistics related to these pathogens.
- Immunization: what it does and does not do.
- Instructions on routine clean-up techniques, working in a safe manner, and cleanup of contamination.
- Housekeeping issues.

References

1. Wallerstien N, Rubenstein H. *Teaching About Job Hazards: A Guide For Workers and Their Providers.* Washington, DC: American-Public Health Association, 1993.
2. Dutton DB. Medical risks, disclosure, and liability: slouching toward informed consent. *Science Technol Human Values* 1987;12:48–59.
3. Colligan MJ, Sinclair RC. The training ethic and the ethics of training. *Occup Med* 1994;9(2):127–34.
4. Centers for Disease Control. Update: universal precautions for prevention of transmission of human immunodeficiency virus, hepatitis B virus, and other bloodborne pathogens in healthcare settings. *MMWR* 1988;37:377–88.
5. U.S. Department of Labor, U.S. Department of Health and Human Services. Joint Advisory Notice: protection against occupational exposure to hepatitis B virus (HBV) and human immunodeficiency virus (HIV). *Federal Register* 1987;52:41818–24.
6. DeJoy DM, Gershon RR, Murphy LR, et al. A work-systems analysis of compliance with universal precautions among health care workers. *Health Educ Q* 1996;23(2):159–74.
7. Bin Zakaria M, Lerche NW, Chomel BB, et al. Accidental injuries associated with nonhuman primate exposure at two regional primate research centers (USA), 1988–1993. *Lab Anim Sci* 1996;46(3):298–304.
8. 29 CFR 1910.1030.
9. *Biosafety in Microbiological and Biomedical Laboratories,* 3rd Ed. Washington, DC: U.S. Department of Health and Human Services Public Health Service, Centers for Disease Control and Prevention and National Institutes of Health. 1993.
10. Shore LM, Wayne SJ. Commitment and employee behavior: comparison of affective commitment and continuance commitment with perceived organizational support. *J Appl Psychol* 1993;78(5):774–80.
11. OSHA's bloodborne pathogens standard: analysis and recommendations. *Health Devices* 1993;22(2):35–92.
12. Nicas M. Respiratory protection and the risk of *Mycobacterium tuberculosis* infection. *Am J Ind Med* 1995;27:317–33.
13. 29 CFR 1910.132.
14. *Food and Drug Administration Food Service Sanitation Manual.* DHEW Publication No (FDA) 78-2081. Washington, DC: U.S. Government Printing Office, 1976.

II / Diseases

9 / Occupational Tuberculosis

John D. Meyer

Tuberculosis (TB), the "White Plague" of the nineteenth and early twentieth centuries, exhibited a progressive decline with the introduction of public health measures at the turn of the century and subsequently with the development of antimicrobial therapy in the 1940s and 50s. More recently, an upsurge in the incidence of TB in the United States has followed the AIDS epidemic beginning in the 1980s. Other factors that combined to produce this increase were relaxation of traditional public health measures aimed at diagnosis and treatment of infection, and alterations in the social fabric, including increased immigration from endemic areas and burgeoning homeless shelter and prison populations. The rise of multidrug-resistant TB, exacerbated by increases in HIV infection and difficulty in tracking infected homeless individuals, has accentuated the risk of serious illness, or even death, in those developing active TB. Although evidence now points to a decline in infection rates after a decade of increase, this is no cause for relaxation of preventive and control efforts.

The rise in the incidence of TB has placed a substantial segment of the working population at risk for acquiring this infection. The Occupational Safety and Health Administration (OSHA) estimates that over 5 million workers are exposed to TB in the course of their work; for this reason, OSHA has proposed a regulatory standard to protect these individuals in the course of their employment [1]. This chapter outlines the epidemiology of occupational exposure to TB and surveillance measures, and reviews prevention and control strategies to mitigate exposure and subsequent infection.

Pathogenesis and Transmission

Tuberculosis (TB) results from infection with *Mycobacterium tuberculosis (M tuberculosis)*, an obligately aerobic thick-walled bacterium. High concentrations of lipid in the thick wall make the bacterium resistant to decolorization with acid alcohol, and hence the mycobacteria (along with related bacteria such as *Nocardia* and *Corynebacterium*) are termed *acid-fast. Mycobacterium tuberculosis* has a length of 1–4 μm and a thickness of 0.3–0.6 μm. Patients with active pulmonary or laryngeal tuberculosis expel organisms into ambient air through coughing, sneezing, or speaking. Larger droplets then settle onto nearby surfaces and, although laden with bacilli, are generally noninfectious. Smaller droplets, 1–5 μm in diameter, termed *droplet nuclei*, desiccate and remain suspended in the air, able to travel substantial distances indoors and stay airborne for several hours. These particles, containing one to three active TB bacilli, are small enough to bypass upper respiratory defenses and filtration at the level of the bronchioles and may be inhaled deep into the lungs. Once in the alveolar space, they are ingested by macrophages, which attempt to contain them by nonspecific cellular immune mechanisms. The organisms may multiply intracellularly if not destroyed by macrophages, and a logarithmic increase in bacilli may appear during the first to third week following infection. Cell-mediated immune mechanisms (type IV, or delayed-type hypersensitivity) are activated after the third week in the previously uninfected host. Increased bacterial destruction via lymphokine-activated macrophages combines with increased macrophage death to form a granulomatous tubercle with a necrotic or caseating center, a pathologic hallmark of TB.

Depending on host resistance factors, tuberculosis infection may be successfully contained at this stage, or it may spread and become disseminated throughout the lungs and the rest of the body. If successfully contained, caseous or granulomatous foci may be replaced by fibrous or calcified tissue. The Ghon focus, a single, small peripheral nodule seen on radiographs and often accompanied by ipsilateral calcified hilar nodes, is an example of contained primary tuberculosis. Primary tuberculous infection can spread when containment mechanisms fail and TB bacilli multiply in liquefied gaseous material. Cavity formation occurs when delayed-type hypersensitivity (DTH) reactions of the host lead to destruction of bronchial and hilar structures and cavitation. Coughing and other maneuvers spread the organisms throughout the lungs and create satellite foci of infection. Hematogenous dissemination to other sites throughout the body may occur.

The DTH reaction is the basis for the most common method of diagnosing tuberculosis infection. Purified protein derivative of tuberculin (PPD), an extract of the bacterial cell wall, stimulates a cell-mediated immune response when injected intradermally in subjects who have sustained primary tuberculous infection. This inflammatory response produces an area of induration, the extent of which is used to assess the likelihood of reactivation and the need for preventive therapy. In individuals with primary tuberculosis infection, the PPD reaction becomes positive four to 12 weeks following exposure and initiation of infection. This time delay should be borne in mind when investigating tuberculosis outbreaks or exposure to active cases of TB. Guidelines for the reading of PPD skin testing are discussed later in this chapter.

Latent TB infection may occur in an untreated person at any point in the individual's lifetime. Pulmonary tuberculosis demonstrates a predilection for reactivation in the apical and posterior upper lobes of the lung, reflecting the high partial pressure of oxygen available there for mycobacterial growth. The reactivated TB may be arrested, resulting in evidence of fibrocalcific scarring on radiographs, or the infection may progress, resulting in pulmonary infiltrates, effusions, cavitation, empyema, and fibrosis as well as miliary dissemination to other tissues.

The risk of TB reactivation is greatest in the first years after primary infection. Five to 15% of immunocompetent individuals develop active TB within two years after the initial infection. The incidence of reactivation of latent disease then declines to a low level for the remainder of exposed individuals' lives unless the immune mechanisms holding the infection in check are disrupted. The cumulative lifetime risk of tuberculosis reactivation has been estimated at 10%. This reflects both the high initial incidence of the infection, coupled with ongoing sporadic cases of reactivation among individuals with remotely acquired infection [2].

Reactivation of TB depends on many factors related to the host's immune response to infection, which determines whether the infecting organisms will be contained or will multiply and disseminate. Host factors that appear to determine the competence of the immune response include age, nutritional status, and concomitant illnesses such as acquired immune deficiency syndrome (AIDS), diabetes mellitus, renal insufficiency, lymphoreticular malignancies, and silicosis. Chemotherapeutic agents and corticosteroids compromise the immune system and may also lead to reactivation of TB. The greatest risk of reactivation occurs in individuals with HIV infection at a rate as high as 10% per year. Additionally, although susceptibility to infection with *M tuberculosis* is not increased in people with HIV infection, they develop active TB upon initial infection at a higher rate and in a shorter period of time (as quickly as one month after exposure) than do immunocompetent individuals. Manifestations of tuberculosis in HIV-infected patients may differ significantly from typical presentations, and involvement outside the lungs is more common.

Epidemiology of Occupational Tuberculosis

Recognition of TB as an occupational hazard of health care personnel lagged behind the improvements in public health measures aimed at its control. Standard texts from the 1920s and 1930s maintained that there was no danger from workers' breathing the expired air of consumptive patients or being coughed upon by TB patients [3]. Pioneering studies by Heimbeck in Oslo in the 1920s demonstrated 95% tuberculin test conversion in nursing students by the time of graduation; furthermore, 22% of these initially negative nurses developed clinical tuberculosis, compared to 1.5% of 200 initially tuberculin positive nurses [3]. Despite similar compelling data, the recognition and control of TB as an occupational hazard made little progress. With the advent of antituberculous therapy and continued success in identification, isolation, diagnosis, and treatment of patients, occupationally acquired TB became less frequent but, paradoxically, more conspicuous in the general trend toward reduced incidence of the disease.

In the interval between the development of antituberculous therapy and the onset of the AIDS epidemic, few studies attempted to quantify TB risk, either in specific occupational settings or in the general population. A 1973–74 study of employees of the Board of Education of New York City found an overall 12% tuberculin reactivity in 61,000 employees; differences in prevalence within this cohort were related to ethnic group, socioeconomic status, age, and sex [4]. Berman and colleagues analyzed results of a five-year (1971–76) tuberculin screening program in a Baltimore hospital [5]. The study calculated an annual risk for TB infection of 1.4%, although the authors attributed the higher-than-expected conversion rate to a booster effect and to exposure in the community. Other studies during this period found conversion rates of 0.11–4.5%, depending on such factors as location and patient population. Screening and treatment programs during this era became underfunded, and public health measures atrophied, despite evidence that tuberculin reactivity was prevalent in as much as one fourth of some segments of the population.

The increase in TB as a concomitant opportunistic infection in patients with HIV paralleled the worldwide AIDS epidemic in the 1980s. Risks to health care workers of TB infection became disproportionately skewed toward areas and institutions that provided care to the homeless, indigent, and inner-city populations. Additionally, with the rise in cases of multidrug-resistant (MDR) tuberculosis, the perception of increased risk of severe illness and even death from TB became more widespread. Evidence for the increased risk to health care workers was drawn both from prevalence data on skin test conversions and from incidence data on new skin test conversions in outbreaks of TB in facilities. Postexposure rates of employee PPD conversions have been noted to range from 4% to 77%, with most reported incidence rates from 15% to 30% [6]. Eight cases of active MDR-TB developed in health care workers in New York and Miami hospitals in the period 1990–91. Epidemiologic evidence linked these cases to nosocomial transmission from infected patients [7].

Annual PPD conversion rates have in general increased in the 1980s and 1990s when compared with rates before the AIDS epidemic. Routine exposure to patients in some hospitals has resulted in conversion rates of 5–10% per year [8]. In an attempt to quantify risk for its proposed standard, OSHA has calculated estimates of relative risk for TB skin test conversion ranging from 1.47 to 9.0, based on results from a 1994 Washington State hospital survey, a statewide survey in North Carolina, and data from 1989 to 1991 at Jackson Memorial Hospital in Miami [1]. Higher risks of PPD conversion (14.5% over four years) were found in employees who worked on wards where patients with culture-confirmed TB were cared for, as opposed to 1.4% in those who did not work around these patients [9]. Furthermore, risk was not limited to those with direct patient contact; it was also increased in other workers, such as clerks, on the same wards. Health care tasks that increase the likelihood of contact with airborne bacilli also carry higher risk. Pulmonary fellows converted at an 11% rate during their two-year training period; this incidence compares to a 2.4% conversion rate in infectious disease fellows, who would have cared for a similar patient population, indicating that respiratory aerosol generation by patients was an important determinant of infectivity [10].

Data on occupational risk outside of hospital-based health care are considerably more sparse.

Increased numbers of individuals with TB are isolated or cared for in settings such as prisons, homeless shelters, medical laboratories, hospices, and home health care services. Populations in correctional facilities, where high-risk individuals are overrepresented, have TB case rates that are estimated to be three to 11 times higher than in the general population. A two-year employee-screening program in New York State prisons found a PPD conversion rate of 1.9%. Relative risks for conversion were 1.64 in guards and 2.39 in medical employees in facilities with known TB cases [11]. Occupational exposure was estimated to account for 33% of new tuberculosis infections in this study.

Facilities for chronic and long-term care present another setting where workers may be exposed to infection. Facilities for the elderly continue to house a cohort of individuals for whom chemoprophylaxis of tuberculous infection had not yet been instituted and who thus present a risk for reactivation. Positive PPD rates among residents range from 10% to as high as 40%. In addition, by virtue of age and illness, the uninfected may be particularly susceptible to primary infection from fellow residents. Large-scale screening studies of workers in these facilities do not exist; a smaller study from Canada [12] found a 15.7% rate of positive tuberculin testing in 286 staff from a hospital and two chronic care facilities, paralleling a 14% rate among residents. A high rate of positive reactions (39.5%) was found among staff in elderly and mental health care services in a New Zealand hospital, implying that exposure may be much higher than had been suspected [13].

A five-fold risk for active tuberculosis in laboratory workers was noted in a large 1971 survey study in the UK [14]. Technicians in "morbid anatomy" departments (those working with tissue) were at the greatest risk for development of disease. Little current data exists on PPD conversion rates or transmission of TB in laboratories. Tuberculosis of the skin from primary inoculation, termed *prosector's wart*, is a well-known phenomenon in pathologists and related technical personnel [15]. Cutaneous inoculation tuberculosis in laboratory personnel as a result of injuries by sharp instruments has been described [16].

The relationship of silicosis to the development of active tuberculosis infection has been well known for the last century and is the subject of an extensive literature. Active tuberculosis has been found to develop in as many as 25% of workers with silicosis; these workers have at least a threefold higher risk of death from TB infection. Work in silica-exposed occupations, such as quarrying, pottery, stone carving, and ship building and repair, is associated with higher incidence of tuberculosis [17]. Because of the high rate of disease in these individuals, some authorities have suggested prolonged, even life-long, chemoprophylaxis for silicotic workers who exhibit PPD conversion [18].

Diagnosis of Tuberculosis

Diagnosis of *Mycobacterium tuberculosis* infection is based on the tuberculin PPD skin test. Immunocompetent individuals with active TB infection and healthy subjects with past primary tuberculosis but no evidence of active disease will react to the application of this test. The preferred method for the test consists of intracutaneous injection of 0.1 mL of 5 tuberculin units (5TU) of a standardized PPD preparation sufficient to result in a small wheal on the forearm or other injection site. The test is read 48 and 72 hours following injection and should be interpreted by personnel with adequate training and experience. A positive result is based on the extent of induration at the injection site; redness or erythema may be present in many individuals and may extend well beyond the injection site, but should not be measured or considered as positive.

The Centers for Disease Control and Prevention (CDC) have established guidelines for the interpretation of the test, based on the likelihood of the degree of induration predicting the presence of infection. Since the predictive value of a positive test depends on the prevalence of a condition in the population, a much higher positive threshold is set for use of the test in populations expected to have a low risk of exposure or development of infection. The CDC classification [19], shown in Table 9-1, outlines the criteria for a positive test.

Table 9-1
CDC's Criteria for a Positive PPD Skin Test

Skin Test Result	Groups
5-mm induration	• HIV-infected persons • Recent close contacts of persons with active TB • Persons with abnormal radiographs indicative of fibrotic change from inactive TB
10-mm induration	• Injecting drug users known to be HIV seronegative • Persons with medical conditions increasing the risk of progression to active TB: silicosis, chronic renal failure, diabetes mellitus, high-dose steroid or immunosuppressive therapy, hematologic malignancies, ≥10% body weight • Children <4 years old • Persons from areas of high prevalence of TB (Asia, Africa, Caribbean, Latin America) • Persons from indigent or medically underserved populations • Residents of long-term care facilities • Persons from high-risk populations in community, as determined by local public health authorities
15-mm induration	• Persons not meeting any of the above criteria

PPD conversions in health care workers should be interpreted according to the above guidelines. Two additional points, however, should be kept in mind in this interpretation. The first is that individual risk factors outside of the work environment must be considered in the interpretation. For example, a worker who is receiving therapy that may be severely immunosuppressive or who has HIV infection will be considered to be in a higher risk group for reactivation, and therefore a skin test of 5- to 9-mm induration may represent a positive test. The second point is that in health care settings where tuberculosis is treated, close contact with infectious patients places workers at increased risk. In these workers, a skin test result of 10-mm induration is probably sufficient to indicate a positive result, even in the absence of other risk factors. By contrast, if a facility presents a low or minimal risk for TB exposure, a cutoff point of 15 mm may be used to judge a result positive if the individual has no other risk factors. In general, in facilities that treat tuberculosis patients, an increase in skin-test induration of 10 mm or more in a two-year period indicates a skin test conversion; for facilities in which the risk of exposure is minimal, a cutoff point of 15 mm or more may be used [19].

Reaction to PPD skin testing may gradually wane, and if many years have passed since initial TB infection, an individual may have a negative reaction to skin testing. This reduction in cell-mediated hypersensitivity may be reversed by repeated administration of the tuberculin skin test, a phenomenon termed *boosting*, which can be used to determine whether an individual has sustained a remote primary tuberculous infection. A two-step testing protocol has been recommended to avoid misinterpretation of the boosting phenomenon in subjects, including health care workers, who may need repeated testing [19]. An initial negative PPD is followed by placement of a second 5TU skin test one to three weeks later. If this second test is judged to be positive, the result likely represents previous primary TB infection rather than a new conversion, and the individual should be evaluated accordingly. If the second test remains negative, a subsequent test with a positive result indicates a newly converted case. Interpretation of the result is again dependent on individual risk factors and the risk of exposure to tuberculosis. In elderly populations, the booster phenomenon may not be present until three or more tests have been performed, and therefore an increase of 15 mm following a previous negative test is used as the criterion for a true skin test conversion.

Bacille Calmette-Guérin, or BCG, is used in many parts of the world to immunize individuals, primarily as a control measure in regions where tuberculosis incidence is high. The protection afforded by BCG vaccination is variable and may relate to host, environmental, and bacterial virulence factors. Reactivity to a tuberculin skin test develops soon after vaccination; postvaccination skin test results may range from 3- to 19-mm induration. The size of skin test reactions does not correlate with the degree of protection against TB that may be afforded by BCG [20]. Additionally, there is poor correlation between the size of tuberculin skin test reactions and protection against developing active tuberculosis. BCG vaccination may complicate the diagnosis of tuberculosis infection, because the PPD reaction that results cannot be distinguished from that produced by mycobacterial infection. Decreases in tuberculin reactivity due to BCG vaccine wane over time, however, and after 10 years may be minimal or absent. The following guidelines may be used in determining the probability of *M tuberculosis* infection in an individual exhibiting induration on PPD skin testing:

- Larger reaction size, generally 15mm or greater.
- History of close contact with a case of active tuberculosis.
- Country of origin or residence in an area with a high prevalence of tuberculous disease.
- Longer time interval since BCG administration [19,21].

Thus, an adult health care worker who was immunized with BCG as a child in a country with a high TB prevalence could be considered to have evidence of TB infection with a PPD reaction of 10 mm or greater. It is essential to consider the other factors noted above that put the individual at increased risk for active tuberculosis infection, and a history of BCG vaccination should neither preclude participation in PPD screening nor lead the interpreter to conclude reflexively that BCG administration is the sole cause of an indurated skin test.

Subjects who, because of immunosuppressive illness, may be anergic should be tested with other companion antigens at the time of PPD testing. Mumps, *Candida*, and tetanus toxoid antigens may be administered in addition to PPD; if 3-mm induration is evidenced on any skin test (including the PPD), the individual may be considered not anergic, and PPD results interpreted accordingly. Individuals with HIV infection who are not anergic should be assessed according to CDC guidelines, which describe reactions of 5mm or greater as a positive result. Evaluation for preventive therapy in those who do not exhibit a response to skin-testing antigens should be made on the basis of additional clinical and epidemiologic information, such as evidence of exposure to another individual with active TB.

For subjects who exhibit a positive PPD test, radiography is used to determine whether evidence of active or prior pulmonary tuberculosis infection is present. Additionally, any patient with symptoms indicative or suggestive of TB infection should have radiography performed. A posterior-anterior (PA) view is the standard radiographic procedure; additional views, such as apical lordotic views, may be needed, depending on the PA view or clinical evidence.

The classic finding of healed primary TB is the Ghon complex, described above. However, other findings, such as multiple fibrotic or calcific foci, may be seen in cases of old, healed tuberculosis. The presence of these lesions is not necessary for the diagnosis of past primary TB infection, and in many cases there may be no abnormalities. A normal chest radiograph in an otherwise asymptomatic healthy-appearing individual with a positive PPD excludes the possibility of active pulmonary tuberculosis.

Patchy or nodular infiltrates in the apical or subapical upper lobes or the superior segments of the lower lobes are characteristic of active pulmonary tuberculosis, although radiographic abnormalities may occur throughout the lungs. Cavitation, adenopathy, empyema, and pleural effusion may also be seen in active cases. Miliary spread of the disease appears as multiple nodular densities throughout the lung fields. Abnormalities on chest radiography may indicate TB, particularly when characteristic findings appear along with a positive skin test, but such abnormalities should not be considered diagnostic of the disease in the absence of bacteriologic evidence.

Presentation of pulmonary tuberculosis in HIV-infected patients may be atypical and can reflect the level of immune response to infection.

Infiltrates in any zone of the lungs may be seen, usually in conjunction with prominent hilar and mediastinal adenopathy. Miliary disease may also be seen. Extrapulmonary disease is more frequent in HIV-infected persons and should always be considered when clinical evidence points to tuberculosis infection and chest radiographs remain normal.

Culture of a sputum specimen and its examination after staining for acid-fast bacilli (AFB) are the major procedures for the diagnosis of pulmonary tuberculosis. The specimen should be obtained after instruction and supervision by a health care worker to avoid mistakenly culturing saliva and nasal mucus. Sputum production may be induced with saline aerosols if the patient is unable to spontaneously produce any. Failure to demonstrate AFB on a smear does not exclude the diagnosis of TB; only 60% of patients with a positive culture have a positive AFB smear. A positive culture for *M tuberculosis* makes the definitive diagnosis of TB. Since cultures may take from four to eight weeks to yield a positive identification, however, therapy may be instituted for a provisional diagnosis of TB on the basis of clinical signs, symptoms, radiographic findings, and AFB smear results. Drug susceptibility testing is essential for all positive initial cultures, and the results should be used to guide modifications in antibacterial therapy. To assess effectiveness of, and response to, therapy as well as the infectiousness of the patient, follow-up sputum examination and culture should be obtained at least monthly until cultures become negative.

Preventive Therapy

Individuals who experience a recent PPD skin test conversion should be considered for preventive therapy with isoniazid (INH). The decision to treat with INH may be complex and should balance the risks of reactivation of tuberculosis and development of active infection with those of the hepatic toxicity of INH. Prophylaxis with isoniazid has been demonstrated to reduce the risk of active tuberculosis by as much as 90% in adults if a full course is given. The highest priority should be assigned to treating individuals with positive skin tests, regardless of age, if they [19]:

- Are known or suspected of having HIV infection, or are known injecting drug users.
- Have close contacts with a person with infectious tuberculosis.
- Have a medical condition that increases the risk of active tuberculosis (e.g., diabetes, silicosis, or immunosuppressive drug therapy).
- Have chest radiographic findings indicative of previous TB but have received inadequate or no treatment.
- Are known recent converters, whose skin test has changed from negative to positive within the past two years.

In addition, preventive therapy may be indicated for significant skin test reactions (as measured against the CDC guidelines noted above) in individuals in high-incidence groups. These include those born in foreign countries with high TB endemicity, medically underserved or indigent populations, and residents of long-term care or custodial facilities. Preventive therapy for health care workers and others with occupational exposure should be strongly considered if the skin test reaction is 10 mm or greater and the worker is under age 35, particularly if TB is prevalent in the work facility [19].

Strategies for prophylaxis of individuals with PPD conversion who are over age 35 remain problematic. Elevations of serum transaminase activity and clinical hepatitis occur more frequently in those over 35; several deaths have been reported from isoniazid-associated hepatitis. Since daily alcohol users, pregnant women, patients with chronic liver disease, and injecting drug users are all at increased risk for the development of INH-associated hepatitis, the decision to treat these individuals should be made with care. Many investigators have recommended against the use of INH in low-risk reactors, based on the toxicity of the drug and a lack of cost effectiveness of treatment [22]. More recent studies have indicated a benefit to monitored INH therapy, which includes intermittent liver function testing and practitioner visits, for low-risk converters. Potential benefits of therapy in higher risk converters were consequently felt to be much greater and to outweigh the risks of the medication [23]. The decision to treat a converter over age 35 should therefore be based on a careful assessment of the risk of reactivation and should include a plan by which liver function can be monitored (generally monthly) and the individual undergoing treatment can be assessed for signs of drug toxicity.

The recommended course of INH therapy for adults is 300 mg once daily for a six- to 12-month period. Individuals with HIV infection and those with silicosis should receive a full 12-month course; more prolonged, even lifelong, therapy in silicosis has been recommended by some [18]. From 10% to 20% of individuals taking INH develop asymptomatic transaminase elevations; many of these elevations resolve even if the drug is continued. Elevations of three to five times the upper limits of normal or symptomatic adverse reactions should lead the clinician to strongly consider halting therapy. Peripheral neuropathy may develop as a side effect of INH therapy and can be generally ameliorated by concomitant pyridoxine (50 mg once daily) administration. Individuals with existing peripheral neuropathy or with conditions such as diabetes that may predispose to its development should be carefully evaluated and monitored while undergoing prophylactic therapy.

Discussion of therapy for active tuberculosis is beyond the scope of this text. Practitioners should seek consultation with a physician who has expertise in the management of tuberculosis, in particular if multidrug-resistant TB is suspected.

Prevention and Control Strategies

ENGINEERING AND PROTECTIVE EQUIPMENT

Primary prevention strategies include rapid identification of patients with active tuberculosis and prompt isolation until they are determined to be noninfectious. Engineering controls, including negative pressure isolation rooms, increased room ventilation, local exhaust ventilation, high-efficiency particulate air (HEPA) filtration, and ultraviolet (UV) radiation are appropriate mechanisms for reducing the concentration of airborne droplet nuclei, limiting their dispersal throughout an institution and thus decreasing the potential for inhalation of pathogenic bacilli. Increased ventilation to a patient or isolation room reduces airborne particle concentration through dilution. Six air changes per hour to an isolation room will reduce the concentration of droplet nuclei by 99.75% under ideal conditions. This represents the recommended standard for TB isolation rooms. Additional mixing factors, based on ventilation characteristics of the room and the amount of "dead space," which mixes more slowly, can be used to calculate necessary additional ventilation to the room. Additionally, the fact that figures used for dilutional ventilation represent mean clearance of particles from the entire room should be kept in mind. Workers involved in patient care are not protected in the immediate breathing zone of a patient actively aerosolizing viable mycobacteria.

Negative pressure airflow, which results from maintenance of a pressure gradient between the interior of a hospital room and the surrounding work area, is an effective strategy for limiting the spread of airborne pathogens in hospitals and related facilities. Combined with appropriate ventilation controls, these systems reduce the risk of transmission to workers in adjacent areas. Negative-pressure mechanisms, however, are delicate and susceptible to a variety of disturbances, particularly in large facilities, where a variety of influences can disrupt them. Reversal of normal pressure patterns can result from such simple maneuvers as opening the door to the room, thus obviating the protective effect of airflow into the room. Maintenance and inspection of pressure systems must be frequent and systematic; lax maintenance of systems is more likely than poor original design to cause failure of protective mechanisms. Once again, negative-pressure systems do not control potentially high concentrations of infective droplets in the breathing zone of the tuberculosis patient. Finally, some authorities draw attention to occasional overemphasis on room ventilation and stationary engineering controls, pointing out that these do little to reduce nosocomial TB spread from patients in whom active TB has not yet been diagnosed and who have not yet been isolated [24].

HEPA filtration of room or confined-area air has been considered as an adjunct to other ventilatory controls, particularly in situations in which ventilation is substandard or circulated air must, for engineering reasons, be recirculated back into the room. HEPA filters designed to capture particles 0.3 μm in diameter with an efficiency of 99.97% will be effective in removing the 1- to 5-μm droplet nuclei, the sizes at which pathogenic bacteria are inhaled. Disadvantages of HEPA filtration include the filters' resistance to entrainment of air through them, with consequent costs in energy and potential for leakage around the filter, the need for periodic maintenance and replacement, without which effectiveness is considerably reduced, and the failure of local or free-standing units to capture particulates in the vicinity. OSHA, in its proposed TB standard, intends to mandate the use of HEPA filtration in cases in which air from isolation rooms cannot be exhausted away from employees, intake vents, and the public, or must be recirculated within the building [1].

Ultraviolet germicidal irradiation, or UVGI, has been suggested for use as a bacteriocide in several settings within the hospital, including isolation rooms, air-system ductwork, and recirculating room air cleaners. There remain differences of opinion regarding the efficacy of UVGI in reducing the airborne burden of *M tuberculosis*. Claims have been made that irradiation results in reduction of viable organisms equivalent to over 20 air changes per hour [24]. By contrast, other investigators have estimated the result of bacterial inactivation by UVGI at only 1.6 air changes per hour and have thus not considered it an appropriate method of reducing bacterial aerosols in areas where they may be constantly generated [25]. The CDC recommends the use of UVGI as a supplemental air-cleaning mechanism in isolation and treatment rooms and in waiting rooms, emergency facilities, and other areas where undiagnosed patients with active TB may be found [19]. It is not recommended as a stand-alone substitute for HEPA filtration of air that must be recirculated or for negative pressure in isolation rooms.

Personal protective equipment, in the form of mask respirators, must be used when engineering controls cannot fully mitigate the hazards of contact with patients with active tuberculosis, or when circumstances prevent the use of these controls. In particular, the areas where respiratory protection is needed include isolation rooms, where the worker is exposed to high local concentrations of droplet nuclei, procedure areas where generation of aerosols with high infective potential is likely, and enclosed areas where engineering controls are not feasible, such as ambulances and other forms of transport. Respiratory protective devices must meet standards and performance guidelines developed by NIOSH. These criteria are:

1. Filtration efficiency of 95% or greater for particles of 1 μm at flow rates of 50 L per minute.
2. Ability to be reliably quantitatively or qualitatively fitted such that fit testing results in leakage in no more than 10% of cases.
3. Ability to fit faces differing in size and other characteristics.
4. Ability to check for facepiece fit [19,26].

HEPA filter negative-pressure respirators, which filter particles of 0.3 μm, with 99.97% efficiency, have been considered effective under these guidelines. Additionally, under more recent NIOSH criteria, N-95 respirators, which meet particle removal efficiency standards of 95% for 0.3 μm particles, will meet criteria for use in TB prevention guidelines. The use of HEPA filter masks has been problematic because of evidence that particles leak around face seals in 10–20% of subjects, thereby reducing their protective effect. Cost and discomfort of the masks may hinder their widespread acceptance.

The common surgical mask lacks effective filtration for small particles and is of little use to the worker exposed to aerosols generated by a patient with TB. However, such a mask can be useful for temporary, short periods in patients who may present a risk within the facility, for example, those being transported for tests or procedures or those who have not yet been admitted to an isolation room. These masks will stop expulsion of most respiratory droplets and reduce the generation of droplet nuclei. Masks should be changed if wet with secretions or sputum, as forceful coughing may then expel particles from the mask. In addition, they are uncomfortable and stigmatizing for the patient, and they should not be used as a prolonged substitute for effective isolation procedures.

In accordance with the OSHA respirator standard, individuals should undergo determination of medical fitness to wear a respiratory protective device. Although infrequent, some medical conditions may result in the inability to wear a respirator mask; individuals with such conditions should be kept from known or direct exposure to patients with active tuberculosis (e.g., direct patient contact or attendance at high-risk procedures). A related issue is the need for greater protection in performing procedures, such as bronchoscopy or chest physiotherapy, which result in the generation of large volumes of potentially infectious particulates. Positive-pressure or powered HEPA filter respirators may be more effective choices for individuals who perform these procedures regularly. Although data regarding the utility and efficacy of respiratory protection in the prevention of TB in institutions are sparse, both the CDC recommendations for health care facilities and the proposed OSHA standard are firm in their stance regarding respirators, and individuals responsible for safety and health in these facilities must familiarize themselves with procedures for a respiratory protection program.

SCREENING AND SURVEILLANCE

Secondary prevention, the early diagnosis of disease (while the individual is in a stage amenable to therapeutic intervention), is achieved by systematic screening of exposed workers through PPD skin testing, with subsequent evaluation and prophylactic treatment of positive reactors. The fundamental principles of PPD testing are outlined above. Their application to workers exposed to tuberculosis is discussed here.

Any facility that houses or cares for persons with suspected or confirmed tuberculosis should develop a risk assessment that determines the job tasks and individuals having potential exposure to *M tuberculosis* along with the nature and frequency of exposure. This exposure assessment will in turn mandate which workers should be included in a surveillance program and determine the frequency of testing. Each employee determined to have occupational exposure, as defined by the employer in the exposure control plan, should participate in a medical surveillance program that systematically and periodically tests for infection with tuberculosis. In addition, provisions for appropriate medical evaluation and follow-up should be made for employees who sustain an "exposure incident," although they may not have been included in the exposure determination or may not have been reasonably anticipated to have exposure.

An initial two-step protocol for PPD skin testing should be performed on hire, or on initiation of a surveillance program, for all employees not known to be previously positive or who cannot document a negative skin test in the past 12 months. Individuals who exhibit the booster phenomenon (an initial negative test followed by a second, positive PPD), indicative of past tuberculosis infection with subsequent waning of cell-mediated immune response, can be excluded from subsequent testing. Individuals with a boosted reaction should be evaluated by a physician for possible prophylactic treatment. Health care facilities and other worksites should gain complete, reliable information on baseline skin test status of employees prior to initial assignment in jobs with occupational exposure. BCG vaccination should not be considered a contraindication to PPD testing, as noted above; it is important to remember that these individuals may also exhibit a boosted reaction on two-step testing. The interpretation of positive tests under the guidelines noted above must be performed by medical professionals skilled and practiced in their interpretation. The employee should not, and should not be expected to, read and interpret her own test results.

Periodic retesting should be performed at least annually for those employees with exposure. The CDC recommends that frequency of PPD testing be based on a risk assessment of the health care facility, which is in turn related to the number of cases of infectious tuberculosis present and the potential for transmission to workers. These recommendations vary for different facilities; testing as frequently as every three months is suggested for workers in facilities with the highest risk, defined as areas with an elevated rate of skin test conversions, evidence of a cluster of conversions, or evidence of transmission between patients or from patients to workers [19]. At the very least, employers should provide TB skin testing every six months for employees who enter AFB isolation rooms, perform or are present during high-hazard procedures, transport suspected or confirmed infectious patients in enclosed vehicles, or work in intake areas of facilities where six or more confirmed cases per year of infectious TB have been encountered. These workers are considered to be exposed more intensely and frequently. Other workers, with lower risks of exposure, should be retested yearly. Under the proposed OSHA standard, employers are exempted from periodic retesting if they can demonstrate that their facilities, if located in counties with sufficiently low or negative yearly rates of TB, do not provide medical services to TB patients and have not had a case of infectious TB in the past 12 months. These facilities should, however, be aware of changes in the local incidence of TB and of suspected exposures occurring at the worksite.

Individuals in health care and other exposed work settings who have a PPD conversion should have chest radiography performed to exclude the possibility of active tuberculosis. In the absence of radiographic evidence and clinical signs and symptoms of tuberculosis, evaluation for prophylactic treatment with isoniazid is warranted. PPD conversion after known exposure to multidrug-resistant TB presents an additional challenge in the treatment of primary tuberculosis. If the source of exposure is known or strongly suspected to have multidrug-resistant TB, a careful assessment of the exposed worker's health and immunologic status is mandated. Individuals at greater risk of developing active tuberculosis include HIV-infected subjects, others with immunosuppression from other medical conditions or therapies, the very young, and the elderly. All these should be considered for multiple-drug prophylactic therapy. This usually consists of the addition of rifampin to the prophylactic regimen but should be tailored to known susceptibilities of the isolate or to the pattern of drug resistance in the specific setting. If conversion after multidrug-resistant TB exposure is suspected, consultation with a specialist with expertise in the treatment of tuberculosis is advisable.

A PPD conversion in the workplace may be a sentinel event, indicating that other workers or patients have had similar exposures. A history of contacts and possible exposures should be elicited from the individual with a newly converted skin test. If this history indicates that exposure took place within the facility, contacts of the suspected source should be identified and tested. A similar protocol should be followed in identifying contacts of a suspected or confirmed case of a worker with active TB within a facility; patients and co-workers must be identified and tested for evidence of TB infection [19]. If exposure is recent, sufficient time to convert to a positive skin test may not have elapsed, and any identified contacts who are skin-test negative should have repeat PPD testing in three months. If additional positive tests are found on follow-up, they are grounds for assessing current controls and preventive measures against the spread of TB within the facility. A similar challenge may occur if probable sources cannot be identified within the facility. The period within which the worker was likely to have become infected can be estimated, based on previous negative skin test results, which range from 10 weeks before the last negative PPD to two weeks before skin test conversion. Hospital records during this time, including those from the laboratory and the infection control service, should be examined to determine possible sources of infection. Additional screening within the new converter's occupational group or area co-workers may be necessary to determine the likelihood of transmission from a common source. If there is evidence of such transmission, evaluation of procedures for TB control in the facility are in order. Since this type of investigation requires extensive work, it is necessary to keep accurate and current records of the PPD status of workers who may sustain TB exposures.

Workers who exhibit PPD conversion but have no symptoms or signs of active tuberculosis may continue work at their current job without restriction, whether or not they are taking INH. They should be advised to report any signs or symptoms of active tuberculosis, including productive cough, fever, chills, night sweats, and weight loss. Prompt assessment for the possibility of active TB infection is indicated if these symptoms develop in a skin test converter. Workers who cannot take isoniazid, or must have it discontinued before completing a full course, should be made aware of the potential for development of active TB infection.

Individuals with active pulmonary or laryngeal tuberculosis may transmit the infection to patients and co-workers. These workers should be excluded from the workplace until they have been demonstrated to be noninfectious through appropriate treatment. Adequate and continuing therapy, resolution of cough, and three consecutive negative AFB smears should be documented before an excluded individual is allowed to return to work. Special care must be taken to ensure that an infected individual continues to comply with treatment, that treatment remains adequate (based on laboratory tests of sensitivity), and that sputum and other secretions remain negative for AFB. Patients who discontinue treatment before they are considered cured should be evaluated promptly. If evidence indicates that they may continue to be, or have reverted to being infectious, they should once again be excluded from work until the above criteria have been met. Individuals with tuberculosis at sites other than the larynx or lung are generally considered noninfectious with respect to the workplace, and need not be excluded if concurrent respiratory tract TB has been excluded [19]. However, for individuals with cutaneous tuberculosis, caution should be exercised to ensure that exposure via direct contact with actively infected lesions will not occur.

The Future

Although tuberculosis's threat to health is not nearly as menacing as it was in the nineteenth century, reports of its demise have proved greatly exaggerated. Newly emerging diseases and therapies have led to its resurgence at a time when public health efforts aimed at its control are becoming moribund for lack of funds. The threat of drug resistance in an organism notorious for its imperviousness to eradication has added a further concern. Control of the threat of tuberculosis has now come under the purview of both the CDC and, with the promulgation of a proposed standard, the Occupational Health and Safety Administration. Regulation may now address what should have been assumed as prevention and control. Under proposed standards, health care facilities and other employers whose workers may come into contact with infectious tuberculosis will be required to define their population at risk, obtain knowledge regarding those employees' exposure status, institute appropriate and ongoing surveillance measures, and maintain effective controls and measures for the reduction of exposure among their personnel. Although evidence of the efficacy and cost-effectiveness of engineering controls and personal protective equipment may not be complete [5], the failure to rapidly recognize and take adequate control measures for exposure appears to be the single most important factor in nosocomial transmission of tuberculosis infection. Current guidelines and proposed standards, while imperfect, provide a framework by which exposure reduction and surveillance can be instituted for the protection of exposed employees. From a public health perspective, exposure reduction additionally benefits those who may not fall under the immediate protection of health and safety standards but whose work may inadvertently put them at risk. Ongoing vigilance is needed to reduce the burden that a new resurgence of an old disease has placed on workers who are responsible for patient care and human services.

References

1. U.S. Department of Labor, Occupational Safety and Health Administration. Occupational exposure to tuberculosis; proposed rule. *Federal Register* 1997;62 (201):54159–308.
2. Comstock GW. Frost revisited: the modern epidemiology of tuberculosis. *Am J Epidemiol* 1975;101:363–82.
3. Sepkowitz KA. Tuberculosis and the health care worker: a historical perspective. *Ann Intern Med* 1994;120: 71–9.
4. Reichman LB, O'Day R. Tuberculous infection in a large urban population. *Am Rev Respir Dis* 1978;117:705–12.
5. Berman J, Levin ML, Orr ST, et al. Tuberculosis risk for hospital employees: analysis of a five-year tuberculin skin testing program. *Am J Public Health* 1981; 71:1217–22.
6. Bowden KM, McDiarmid MA. Occupationally acquired tuberculosis: what's known. *J Occup Med* 1994;36: 320–5.

7. Centers for Disease Control. Nosocomial transmission of multidrug-resistant tuberculosis among HIV infected persons—Florida and New York, 1988–1991. *MMWR* 1991;40:585–91.
8. Markowitz SB. Epidemiology of tuberculosis among health care workers. *Occup Med State Art Rev* 1994;9: 589–608.
9. Boudreau AY, Baron SL, Steenland NK, et al. Occupational risk of *Mycobacterium tuberculosis* infection in hospital workers. *Am J Ind Med* 1997;32:528–34.
10. Malasky C, Jordan T, Potulski F, et al. Occupational tuberculous infections among pulmonary physicians in training. *Am Rev Respir Dis* 1990;142:505–7.
11. Steenland K, Levine AJ, Seiber K, et al. Incidence of tuberculosis infection among New York State prison employees. *Am J Public Health* 1997;87:2012–7.
12. Langille DB, Sweet LE. Tuberculin skin testing in a hospital and two chronic care facilities in Prince Edward Island. *Can J Infect Control* 1995;10:41–4.
13. Lawson J, Caygill J. Results from a Mantoux screening programme of staff in the care of elderly and mental health fields at Wakari Hospital, Dunedin. *N Z Med J* 1995;108:222–4.
14. Harrington JM, Shannon HS. Incidence of tuberculosis, hepatitis, brucellosis, and shigellosis in British medical laboratory workers. *Br Med J* 1976;Mar 27;1(6012): 759–62.
15. Goette DK, Jacobson KW, Doty RD. Primary inoculation tuberculosis of the skin: prosector's paronychia. *Arch Dermatol* 1978;114:567–9.
16. Sharma VK, Kumar B, Radotra BD, et al. Cutaneous inoculation tuberculosis in laboratory personnel. *Int J Dermatol* 1990;29:293–4.
17. Rosenman KD, Hall N. Occupational risk factors for developing tuberculosis. *Am J Ind Med* 1996;30:148–54.
18. Morgan E. Silicosis and tuberculosis. *Chest* 1979; 75:202–3.
19. Centers for Disease Control and Prevention. Guidelines for preventing the transmission of *Mycobacterium tuberculosis* in health-care facilities, 1994. *MMWR* 1994;43:RR-13.
20. Schein MF, Heubner RE. Tuberculin skin testing. In: Rossman MD, MacGregor RR (eds), Tuberculosis: *Clinical Management and New Challenges.* New York: McGraw-Hill, 1995. Pp 73–88.
21. Snider DE. Bacille Calmette-Guérin vaccinations and tuberculin skin tests. *JAMA* 1985;253:3438–9.
22. Moulding, T. Preventive treatment of tuberculosis: a clinician's perspective. In: Rossman MD, MacGregor RR (eds), *Tuberculosis: Clinical Management and New Challenges.* New York: McGraw-Hill, 1995. Pp 89–105.
23. Salpeter SR, Sanders GD, Salpeter EE, et al. Monitored isoniazid prophylaxis for low-risk tuberculin reactors older than 35 years of age: a risk-benefit and cost-effectiveness analysis. *Ann Intern Med* 1997;127:1051–61.
24. Nardell EA, Riley RL. Precautions to prevent transmission. In: Rossman MD, MacGregor RR (eds), *Tuberculosis: Clinical Management and New Challenges.* New York: McGraw-Hill, 1995. Pp 57–72.
25. Macher JM, Alevantis LE, Chang Y-L, et al. Effect of ultraviolet germicidal lamps on airborne microorganisms in an outpatient waiting room. *Appl Occup Environ Hyg* 1992;7:505–13.
26. Hodous TK, Coffey CC. The role of respiratory protective devices in the control of tuberculosis. *Occup Med State Art Rev* 1994;9:631–57.

10 / Occupational Legionellosis

Stephen F. Wintermeyer

Legionnaires' disease is a disease first identified after an outbreak of pneumonia that affected attendees at an American Legion Convention in Philadelphia in 1976. In December 1977, just 16 months after the outbreak, scientists from the Centers for Disease Control (CDC) published a description of the epidemic [1] and of work pointing to a previously unidentified bacteria as the pathogenic agent [2]. The organism was later named *Legionella pneumophila*. Subsequently, many similar organisms have been identified, and a new taxonomic family, the Legionellaceae, has been created. There are presently 40 species in the Legionellaceae family; approximately 18 have been shown to cause pneumonia in humans [3,4].

Legionnaires' disease, with pneumonia as its primary feature, is the most common disease caused by *Legionella* species. There is also a second, less important, clinical form of legionella infection known as *Pontiac fever* [5,6], which is an acute, self-limited illness that spontaneously resolves, resulting in full recovery. The term *legionellosis* will be used in this chapter as a synonym for *legionnaires' disease*.

After years of being regarded as an uncommon pathogen, *Legionella* has been shown to be an important cause of community-acquired pneumonia [7,8]. Legionnaires' disease can occur both in epidemic and sporadic forms.

Legionella lives in water and has been found in many different sites. It is transmitted primarily by inhalation of aerosols containing the pathogen and can best be thought of as an organism transmitted by aerosolization of contaminated water sources (both indoor and outdoor). Methods of protection should focus on environmental controls, not specific occupational controls.

Epidemiology

INCIDENCE AND PREVALENCE

Legionella has consistently been shown to be one of the three or four most common causes of community-acquired pneumonia [9]. In a large American study, it was shown to cause 6.7% of cases of community-acquired pneumonia, the third highest percentage for a specific organism [10]. Pneumonia caused by legionella tends to be more severe than other types of community-acquired pneumonia. Not surprisingly, the percentage of legionella pneumonias among community-acquired pneumonia cases resulting in admission to a hospital intensive care unit (ICU) is higher than the percentage among cases of community-acquired pneumonia. Torres and colleagues [11] found legionella to cause 14% of severe cases of community-acquired pneumonia in their study, a total exceeded only by *Streptococcus pneumoniae.*

The true incidence of legionellosis in the United States is unclear. The reported number of cases of legionellosis in the United States in 1994 was 1,535 [12]. Comparing this to a predicted incidence of 268,000 (6.7% times 4,000,000, the number of community-acquired cases of pneumonia that occurs in the United States annually), it is clear that there is a large discrepancy. The explanation for the discrepancy is threefold:

1. Possible overestimate of legionella cases.
2. Underdiagnosis of legionella cases.
3. Underreporting of legionella cases.

It is unclear how much of each factor is involved. Since legionellosis is not a chronic disease, prevalence is not a parameter of concern.

RISK FACTORS FOR TRANSMISSION

Water is the natural habitat of legionella. This fact must always be kept in mind when discussing transmission of legionella. Legionella organisms have been found in a variety of water reservoirs, including hospitals' potable water [13–16], residential potable water [17–19], aerosol equipment cleansed by tap water [20], a decorative fountain [21], a hotel potable water system [22], an ice machine [23], lakes and rivers [24], a whirlpool [25], a grocery mist machine [26], a cooling tower [27], a nursing home [28], and industrial plants [29].

The role of legionella colonization of water reservoirs in causing the disease is well established. The actual role that colonization of cooling towers plays has been challenged [30], but this is a specific issue and does not change the acceptance of water colonization as fundamental to the pathogenesis of legionella infection.

The reason that legionella is found in many water supplies is quite simple: It is well adapted to live in these environments. In fact, it is best to view legionella as an organism well adapted to living in water and as filling a niche that is a fundamental part of that environment. Several important adaptations by *pneumophila* include the following:

- Non-legionellaceae microbiota in natural samples for the multiplication of *L pneumophila* [31].
- Predilection for warmer temperature (≥ 35° C) [24,32].
- Utilization of sediment for nutrition [32].
- Predilection to grow on surfaces [33].
- Ability to live in amoeba [34,35].

These multiple adaptations need to be kept in mind when attempting to understand the transmission of legionella in order to prevent its transmission.

Aerosolization of water contaminated by legionella and then directly inhaled into the lungs is considered the most common method of transmission [6,9,30]. However, there may be other methods of transmission as well. Transmission of legionella to hospitalized patients via respiratory equipment filled with contaminated water has been documented [36]. Woo and colleagues [37] have discussed in detail how legionella may be transmitted by respiratory equipment and aerosol-generating devices. Aspiration is another possible mode of transmission. Johnson and colleagues [38] showed that 30% of nosocomial pneumonia in head and neck surgical patients was due to legionella. Given that such patients are very prone to aspiration, the study was felt to be circumstantial evidence that legionella can be transmitted by aspiration. Graman and associates [23] demonstrated a case of nosocomial legionella pneumonia associated with legionella contamination of an ice machine in an ICU; microaspiration was the presumed method of transmission. It should be noted that data clearly demonstrating oropharyngeal colonization by *L pneumophila* have been lacking. Finally, legionella can be transmitted by direct inoculation of a wound by contaminated tap water. Lowry and colleagues [39] demonstrated three cases of sternal wound infection with legionella occurring after the wounds were contaminated with legionella during bathing or dressing changes using tap water.

It is important to emphasize that there has been no documented cases of person-to-person transmission of legionnaires' disease. Fifteen years ago, Yu and co-workers [40] concluded that person-to-person transmission of *L pneumophila* did not occur. There has been no evidence to refute this conclusion since. Obviously, lack of person-to-person transmission eliminates a major problem in controlling legionella and differentiates it from varicella, tuberculosis, and pertussis among other contagious diseases. It also clearly changes the risk of contracting the disease. One does not need to worry about exposures to other humans, including co-workers, only about exposure to contaminated water.

As might be expected for an organism that is not transmitted by a person-to-person route, the attack rate for legionella is only 2–4%. The attack rate in the 1976 Philadelphia outbreak was 4% [1]. A study of health care workers during an outbreak of nosocomial legionnaires' disease in 1984 revealed an attack rate of 2.4% [41].

As with any infectious disease, host factors play a role in the development of legionellosis. Advanced age and an underlying debilitating condition, such as chronic obstructive pulmonary disease, diabetes, cigarette smoking or alcohol abuse, have been shown to be risk factors for legionellosis [6,10,18]. In addition, diseases and therapy resulting in an immunocompromised state, such as organ transplantation, are important risk factors [6,42].

Occupational Risk Factors

As noted previously, legionellosis should be considered more a disease that is transmitted from an environmental source than an occupational disease. It has been made clear from studies of epidemics of legionnaires' disease that the important feature has been exposure to a contaminated water source, not the occupation of the victims or nonvictims of the epidemic.

With this in mind, one can postulate what occupations may be at increased risk for legionellosis over the general population. Occupations taking people into close contact with water that is not decontaminated come to mind. For natural waters, such occupations as park rangers, fishing tour guides, and canoe guides come to mind; for manmade water sources, plumbers, heating, ventilation, air conditioning (HVAC) workers, and construction workers. The data in the literature are clearly lacking: Only health care workers [41], industrial plant workers [29], and a remodeling laborer [19] have been discussed. To clearly identify specific occupations at risk, two things are needed. One is much improved accuracy in diagnosing legionellosis among physicians caring for patients with pneumonia. The second would be a case control study of legionella patients, looking at their occupations. Unfortunately, neither is likely to occur soon.

Prevention and Control

ADMINISTRATIVE CONTROLS

Administrative controls, at best, can play only a limited role in preventing occupational and environmental legionella infections. The reason is simply that the reservoir for legionella infection is water. Prohibiting people from using water is not practical.

One situation in which administrative controls might be useful is in cleaning respiratory therapy equipment. Such equipment, cleaned by tap water, can be a source of legionella infection [37]. Instituting a policy by which only sterile water is used to clean and rinse respiratory therapy equipment is a reasonable policy that could succeed in practice. Another administrative control that could be useful is a policy of washing wounds only with sterile water, not tap water, which has been shown to be a source of legionella wound infections [39]. Again, this administrative control is reasonable, since it involves changing behavior for only one specific activity, and its rationale is easy for health care providers to understand.

Other potential administrative polices are not likely to succeed. It is not practical to prohibit individuals from drinking tap water, using ice from ice machines or taking showers, even though all are water sources associated with legionella infection [15,23,43]. It is also not practical to prohibit individuals with risk factors for legionella, such as diabetes [44], immunocompromised states [10] and smoking [18], from working near water. Although such individuals have an increased risk for legionella relative to the general population, prohibiting them from working around potential sources of legionella would not be practical. There are too many potential exposure sites. In addition, prohibiting work for individuals who do not pose a threat to others, even if they are at greater risk themselves, is a very difficult position to defend legally.

SAFE WORK PRACTICES AND ENGINEERING CONTROLS

When discussing safe work practices and engineering controls for legionella, one must always keep in mind that legionella is an organism that is well adapted to live in various water reservoirs and will typically do so, unless specific actions are taking place to eliminate it. Empirical support for this postulate include the following:

- The organism's ability to live in water for long periods of time [45].
- Its isolation from many different sites when sought after [13,24,46,47].
- Its positive relationship with other organisms, such as bacteria [31] and amoeba [34].
- Its ability to flourish in hot water tanks (≤ 60°C) [48].

Safe work practices—i.e., administrative controls—have a limited role in preventing legionella, as discussed above. Engineering controls have a much more fundamental role. These can best be divided into active disinfective measures and design, operation, and maintenance measures [49].

Active disinfection measures include copper-silver ionization, thermal eradication, chlorination, instantaneous steam heating, ultraviolet irradiation, and ozonation [49,50]. Copper-silver ionization has been shown to be effective in keeping legionella numbers in water systems at acceptably low levels [49]. The system works by producing copper and silver ions, which are released into hot water going through the system. These positively charged ions bind to negatively charged sites on the bacteria, which disrupts the bacterial cell membrane and thus alter permeability, leading to the death of the organism. One drawback to this system is that it only works on those parts of the plumbing system that are regularly in use.

A second method of disinfection is thermal eradication, or heat and flush [49]. In this method, hot water tank temperatures are first elevated to 70°C (158°F). Next, this hot water is used to flush all faucets and shower heads to kill legionella colonizing these distal sites. When it reaches the distal outlets, the water temperature must be at least 60°C. Flushing should occur for at least 20–30 minutes. Recolonization can be reduced by maintaining the water temperature at 60°C. This technique has the advantage of not requiring any special equipment and thus is particularly useful in terminating an outbreak [49,51]. Unfortunately, this technique is time consuming and labor intensive, which makes it expensive. The hot temperatures can also make scalding a hazard [52].

Chlorination is a third active disinfection measure [49,50] that has been shown to be effective in controlling legionella [50]. Its main advantage is that it provides disinfection of an entire system rather than only a specific area. However, the technique has several disadvantages, which make it less than optimal. Relatively high levels of chlorine (3 ppm) are needed [50], because the organism is very tolerant to chlorine [53]. Corrosion of pipes is also a major problem. The formation of halogenated organic compounds, which are potential carcinogens, is a theoretical disadvantage [50].

A fourth active disinfection measure is instantaneous steam heating [49]. In this method, water is heated to a very high temperature (≥ 88° C), then mixed with an appropriate volume of cold water to achieve the desired temperature. A major advantage of this technique is that it alleviates the need for hot water storage tanks, which are well-known sites for growth of legionella [32].

A fifth method of active disinfection is ultraviolet (UV) irradiation [49,54]. UV light has been shown to be very effective in killing *L pneumophila* [54]. This method of disinfection works by sending water through a UV sterilizer unit on its way to a designated area. Advantages of UV sterilization include the fact that the method produces no harmful by-products and does not damage the plumbing system. One major disadvantage is that there is no residual disinfectant effect in the water; therefore, any sites of legionella colonization downstream will not be affected. A second disadvantage is that UV light loses some of its effectiveness at high water temperatures.

A final method of active disinfection is ozonation [50], since ozone is effective in killing *L pneumophila* [54]. An advantage of ozonation is that it kills bacteria and viruses instantaneously. A major disadvantage is that an onsite ozone generator is necessary because of the relatively short half-life of ozone. The need for on-site generator(s) increases the cost considerably. At present, ozonation is not a recommended method of active disinfection.

In addition to the active disinfection techniques discussed above, engineering controls for legionella include design, operation, and maintenance measures [49]. These measures are effective by eliminating conditions under which legionella flourishes.

One useful measure is the removal of aerators on faucets. Such aerators accumulate sediment in which legionella grows well [33]. Another measure eliminates sludge, which can accumulate in the bottom of hot water storage tanks. Placement of an accessible drain valve at the lowest point facilitates removal of the sludge, a primary area for possible growth of legionella. The number of infrequently used spurs in the system should be minimized and their length minimized. The longer these sections are, the more stagnant the water and the greater the potential for growth of legionella. The storage temperature of hot water should be 60° ± 2.5°C. Legionella are rapidly killed at this temperature. Higher temperatures are not necessary and increase the risk of scalding [52]. The hot-water temperature at outlets such as sinks and baths should be 50–60°C. The cold water temperature at these outlets should be ≤ 20°C, as legionella growth is inhibited by temperatures less than 20°C. If a hot-water system is not in use for at least one week, the water temperature should be raised to 60°C for at least one day before the system is brought back on line. In addition to these measures, routine cleaning and maintenance is necessary. Cold-water tanks should be examined, cleaned, and disinfected on an annual basis. Hot-water tanks should be examined and drained quarterly.

To facilitate the evaluation and use of the engineering controls that have been discussed, a few key points must be mentioned [49]. The disinfection plan for buildings should be designed on a case-by-case basis. The active disinfection methods that have proved cost effective are copper-silver ionization and thermal irradiation, although the other disinfection methods may be appropriate under special circumstances. In general, it is easier to prevent colonization in a new system than to eliminate colonization that is already established. Eradication of legionella is not necessary for the desired clinical outcome. Best and colleagues [14] showed that no legionella cases occurred in their hospital if the percentage of sites contaminated with legionella was kept under 30%. One must keep in mind that the goal is to prevent cases of disease, not to eliminate legionella from every possible site where it may be. Keeping this goal in mind can help make sure that money spent on engineering controls is spent wisely.

PERSONAL PROTECTIVE EQUIPMENT AND PREVENTIVE MEASURES

Personal protective equipment does not have a role in the prevention of legionella infections. There are two reasons for this. One is the fundamental occupational medicine principle that engineering controls, if available, are better means of prevention than personal protective equipment, and as discussed above, there are a variety of effective engineering controls available to prevent legionella infection. The second reason is that the reservoir of legionella is water, and individuals may become exposed to water almost anywhere. Thus, personal protective equipment would have to be worn virtually all the time to avoid inhalation of water particles potentially contaminated with legionella. Such a plan is obviously not practicable.

Is there any scenario in which personal protective equipment would be indicated? From the practical viewpoint, no. From a theoretical point of view, yes. Given that a self-contained breathing apparatus can protect against inhalation of respirable particles (≤ 5 μm), which may contain *L pneumophila* [37], one can imagine a situation in which an individual would use personal protective equipment. For example, if a severely immunocompromised patient needed to be transferred for a test or procedure and the transfer required passing through an area of a building, such as an unused wing or tunnel, where legionella was documented to exist in the water supply, it might be reasonable to provide that patient with personal protective equipment.

As discussed above, the key preventive measures are engineering controls. Administrative controls may be helpful to a lesser extent. Personal protective equipment, however, is not helpful. Of course, one could always use a concern regarding legionella infection to try to obtain other health benefits. Since cigarette smoking is a risk factor for legionella [18,55], one might suggest to a smoker concerned about legionella that he/she stop smoking.

EMPLOYEE EDUCATION AND TRAINING

All hospital employees need to undergo infection control education and training. It is very helpful to provide information concerning legionella to these employees during their orientation. In addition, it is reasonable to provide information on legionella to other individuals who theoretically might be at increased risk of legionella infection. Such individuals include plumbers and HVAC workers.

Certain key points should be covered in such training. It should be emphasized that legionella infections are more common than previously thought and are probably highly underdiagnosed. The reservoir for legionella is water, and the organism has been found in many different types of water reservoirs. Stagnant water is particularly likely to harbor legionella. Aerosolization of stagnant water should be done only after efforts have been made to disinfect the water or it has been demonstrated to be free from legionella. Finally, such workers should know that very effective treatment is available for legionella and that person-to-person spread does not occur.

MEDICAL SURVEILLANCE

From a public health point of view, medical surveillance for legionella remains important. It is one of the three or four most common causes of community-acquired pneumonia [9], yet it probably is severely underreported. Nevertheless, legionella is a reportable disease and should remain so. Physicians should be encouraged to make a specific diagnosis when they treat a patient for community-acquired pneumonia. The urinary antigen test (see below) is a very simple, benign, and useful test in making a diagnosis. In addition to public health officials, hospital infection control practitioners need to use medical surveillance to monitor legionella infections among patients, since legionella is a known cause of nosocomial infection [56].

For the occupational medicine practitioner, a high index of suspicion for legionella is useful when treating patients with pneumonia, but a broad medical surveillance program for legionellosis is not likely to be of value. Given the widespread reservoirs of legionella, a surveillance program would have to be so broad that it could not be cost effective. A surveillance program focusing on one exposure site, such as a reservoir for a confirmed outbreak, would be reasonable on a temporary basis to ensure that no further individuals were infected from that site.

A surveillance program could be conducted using questionnaires asking about pneumonia symptoms (legionnaires' disease) and flulike symptoms (Pontiac fever). Given the short incubation times of these illnesses, the questionnaires would not need to be given longer than a month after the outbreak. Baseline serologies and follow-up serologies in three months would provide valuable, objective information. Such a surveillance program could even be conducted for a time as short as three months and then stopped. If no further cases were found in this time, it is likely the problem would not recur.

ENVIRONMENTAL MONITORING

Biologic testing plays a very important role in the prevention of legionellosis, because it is a method by which efficacy of engineering controls are monitored. Biologic testing as it relates to hospitals has been well documented [49] and is discussed here.

Biologic testing should be done at least annually. Given legionella's predilection for hot-water, all hot water tanks should be sampled. A sample of distal sites, which include faucets and shower heads, should also be tested. A minimum of 10 distal sites is recommended. For large hospitals (500 beds or more), testing two sites per 100 beds is recommended. Distal sites from units caring for patients at increased risk of acquiring legionellosis should be included.

If legionella is found in hot-water tanks and the hospital is known to have nosocomial legionella infections, disinfection of the water system should be considered. If no known cases of nosocomial legionellosis have occurred, disinfection depends on the results of testing the distal sites. If less than 30% of distal sites are positive, disinfection need not be done, and periodic biologic testing should continue. If more than 30% of distal sites are positive, disinfection should be considered. Even if testing of hot-water tanks is negative, if at least 30% of distal sites are positive, disinfection of the system should be considered.

A sterile, Dacron swab can be used to obtain samples from faucets and shower heads. To obtain a faucet sample, the swab is inserted and rotated four times around the known circumference as it is pushed further into the faucet. The swab should then be placed in transport medium or moistened by 0.5 mL of faucet water prior to being taken to laboratory. For a shower head, water is first allowed to trickle through the opening to moisten it. Next, a sterile swab is rotated four times over the entire surface of the shower head. It should then be transported to the lab in a similar fashion as described above.

To obtain samples from a hot-water tank, the first 10–50 mL are collected after the drain valve at the base of the tank is opened. After water is allowed to drain for 15–30 seconds, another 10–50 mL is collected. The first sample is from the drain pipe, while the second is from the tank.

Because legionella cannot grow on standard media, buffered charcoal-yeast extract (BYCE) agar plates with selective antibiotics and growth factors are used.

IMMUNIZATION AND PROPHYLACTIC MEASURES

Pre- and Postexposure Measures

At the present time, there is no vaccination available for any of the Legionellaceae. Work on a vaccine is being done, but even the most encouraging results [57] still have a long way to go. At this time, there is no prophylactic medical regimen advised for legionellosis. It is unlikely that a prophylactic regimen will be used in the future without improved understanding of the epidemiology of legionnaires' disease and the ability to predict when it may occur. One can theorize a benefit of empirically starting therapy on an individual with the risk factors for severe legionella infection (e.g., a patient with diabetes or in an immunocompromised state) who has been exposed to a source known to cause legionella in other individuals. However, such treatment would be appropriate only on a very limited, case-by-case basis.

In addition, there are currently no nonpharmacologic measures recommended. Legionella has a relatively low attack rate, so prophylaxis of individuals that have been exposed to a water reservoir known to contain legionella is not indicated. The organism is not transmitted person to person, so there is no need for isolation practices.

Compliance

Since there are currently no pre- or postexposure measures to use, compliance is a moot point.

METRICS TO ASSESS ADEQUACY OF PREVENTION MEASURES

As discussed above, testing for legionella in the water systems of hospitals and other buildings is fundamental for monitoring the need for, and the effects of, engineering controls. Since it has been shown empirically that hospital water systems with 30% or less of their distal sites positive for legionella do not have nosocomial infections [14], the adequacy of preventive measures has been based partially on keeping the percentage of contaminated distal sites less than 30% [49]. Of course, the truly important metric is the number of cases of legionellosis or Pontiac fever seen. The goal should be zero. What is considered acceptable may depend on the circumstances of each specific situation.

Symptoms and Signs

There are two predominant clinical manifestations of legionella infection: legionnaires' disease and Pontiac fever. Legionnaires' disease is much more significant clinically and is discussed first, followed by a discussion of Pontiac fever and then a discussion of less common types of infection.

The clinical symptoms of legionnaires' disease have been well described [1,6,9,44,58]. Pneumonia is the typical clinical syndrome, and it can vary widely in severity. As legionellosis has become more widely recognized, there is a greater appreciation of the milder presentations of the disease, not just the more severe cases. The early symptoms are nonspecific and include fever, malaise, myalgias, headache, and anorexia. The symptoms begin two to 10 days after exposure. The fever may be very high, over 40°C in some cases. Initially, cough may be nonproductive but subsequently is often productive of at least a small amount of sputum. Chest pain may occur and is sometimes pleuritic. In addition to the pulmonary symptoms, gastrointestinal and neurologic symptoms are common. Approximately 40% of individuals have gastrointestinal symptoms, particularly diarrhea. Abdominal pain, nausea, and vomiting also may occur. Neurologic symptoms range from mild headache to confusion, stupor, and photophobia.

On physical examination, the signs of legionnaires' disease are those of pneumonia and are not specific for the disease. Fever is common, with a mean temperature of 38.8°C [44]. Tachycardia (mean heart rate = 110) and tachypnea (median respiratory rate = 32) are also common [44]. Most patients have at least one sign of pneumonia, such as dullness to percussion, crepitation, or bronchial breath sounds.

Of note is that hyponatremia ($Na^+ \leq 130$) can be useful in pointing toward legionella as the cause of a community-acquired pneumonia. Chest radiography frequently reveals patchy alveolar infiltrates initially; these often progress to multilobar consolidation [59].

Pontiac fever is a self-limited, flulike illness [5,6]. Symptoms include fever, chills, headache, malaise, and myalgia that have their onset after a one- to two-day incubation period. Chest pain, chest congestion, and mild cough are common. After two to five days, symptoms resolve and there are no permanent sequelae.

Extrapulmonary legionellosis is unusual but worth mentioning. Legionella has been documented to cause sinusitis, cellulitis, pancreatitis, peritonitis, pyelonephritis, pericarditis, endocarditis, and wound infection [9,39]. In these cases of legionellosis, symptoms and signs are typical for infections involving the particular organ involved.

Differential Diagnosis

The symptoms and signs of legionnaires' disease are typical for pneumonia. Thus, in a nonhospitalized individual the differential diagnosis includes other types of community-acquired pneumonia. Common bacterial causes of community-acquired pneumonia other than legionella are *Streptococcus pneumoniae*, *Haemophilus influenzae*, *Chlamydia pneumoniae*, *Staphylococcus aureus*, a variety of other streptococcal species, and *Mycoplasma pneumoniae* [7,10,11]. Several symptoms—diarrhea, abdominal pain, and headache [10]—are more typical of legionella pneumonia than other bacterial pneumonias and are therefore suggestive of legionnaires' disease. In addition, a markedly elevated temperature (≥ 40°C) is suggestive of legionnaires' disease [10].

There are also other conditions that can mimic community-acquired bacterial pneumonia and therefore legionnaires' disease. One such condition is viral pneumonia. Chest radiography may be useful in differentiating viral pneumonia from bacterial pneumonia, since viral pneumonia tends to cause more diffuse lung abnormalities radiographically. Occasionally, an acute flare-up of sarcoidosis can mimic pneumonia. Also, acute hypersensitivity pneumonitis can present like pneumonia. The diagnosis of these latter conditions is typically made on biopsy, although the results of certain blood tests may be suggestive of the diagnosis.

In addition to being a common community-acquired pneumonia, legionellosis is also a common nosocomial pneumonia [56]. Therefore, the differential diagnosis of nosocomial legionellosis includes other types of nosocomial infection. Common non-legionella causes of nosocomial pneumonia include *Pseudomonas aeruginosa*, *Serratia marcescens*, and *Staphylococcus aureus* [56].

The symptoms and signs of Pontiac fever are typical for the flu. Other etiologies of flulike syndromes include metal fume fever and polymer fever. Since these clinical entities are self-limited, there is usually no incentive to identify a specific etiology unless the condition is recurrent. Likely, many cases of Pontiac fever go undiagnosed and are attributed to the flu.

Diagnostic Evaluation

As in working up any type of medical condition, the diagnostic evaluation of suspected legionellosis includes a detailed medical history, physical examination, and laboratory evaluation. The laboratory evaluation includes certain routine tests, followed by more specific tests as the differential diagnosis is narrowed.

The typical presentation of legionellosis is that of a community-acquired pneumonia. Therefore, in the medical history, one must ask about systemic symptoms, such as fever, and respiratory symptoms, such as cough. It is also important to ask specifically about neurologic symptoms, such as headache and confusion, and gastrointestinal symptoms, such as nausea, vomiting, diarrhea and abdominal pain, since these can be suggestive of legionellosis. In addition, one should be sure to ask about exposures. Has the individual been involved in any situations where water has been aerosolized? Does the individual do any work with old plumbing or stagnant water? Does the individual know of others who have similar symptoms? If so, a point of legionella source outbreak may have occurred.

The physical examination of an individual presenting with a history suggestive of community-acquired pneumonia should include the vital signs, complete pulmonary examination and examination of other pertinent organ systems. It is very important to measure the temperature as legionellosis tends to cause higher temperatures than other types of community-acquired pneumonia. Other physical findings are those typical for pneumonia: tachycardia, tachypnea, tactile fremitis, egophony, and crackles. Other pertinent organ systems to examine include the cardiac, gastrointestinal, and musculoskeletal systems and the extremities. These systems do not have specific findings of legionellosis but may have specific findings useful for diagnosing other diseases on the differential diagnosis.

Routine laboratory evaluation typically reveals a polymorphonuclear leukocytosis, a very nonspecific finding. A sputum Gram's stain showing many polymorphonuclear leukocytes with few organisms suggests an atypical pneumonia, such as legionellosis. Hyponatremia has been associated with legionellosis [44,58,60] and is helpful in pointing to the diagnosis but cannot be used to make the diagnosis.

The chest radiograph is useful in confirming a diagnosis of pneumonia but cannot be used to specifically diagnose legionellosis [6,9]. Typical findings of legionellosis include early unilateral alveolar infiltrates, late bilateral infiltrates, and pleural effusions [59]. Pleural effusions are present in approximately 30% of cases. In immunosuppressed patients, bilateral nodular opacities which may capitate, may occur [61].

The diagnosis of legionellosis requires specialized laboratory testing. Commonly used tests include cultures for the organism, direct fluorescent antibody testing, and urinary antigen testing [3,6,9]. These tests are discussed in detail below.

Isolation of legionella from a respiratory sample is diagnostic of legionnaires' disease, since the organism has not been found to colonize the oropharynx and only rarely found to colonize the respiratory tract. Unfortunately, legionella does not grow on routine laboratory media and samples require special handling in media. Acid washing of sputum samples reduces the growth of other organisms, which increases sensitivity. The best media for legionella growth is buffered charcoal-yeast extract (BCYE) agar. To deter the growth of other organisms, antibacterial and antifungal agents are added to the media. Dyes are added to enhance the visibility of legionella colonies. The sensitivity of sputum culture for legionella has ranged from 11% to 70% in different studies [6]. The yield tends to be better when specimens are processed immediately. Bronchoalveolar lavage (BAL) specimens are more sensitive (66%) than sputum samples [62].

The legionella urinary antigen test is extremely useful. It is rapid, inexpensive, and benign, since all it requires from the patient is a urine sample. The test has a sensitivity of 70% and a specificity close to 100% [9,16]. Another advantage of this test is that the urinary antigen remains positive for weeks despite antibiotic therapy. The major disadvantage of the urinary antigen test is that it is useful only for *L pneumophila* serogroup 1. However, this disadvantage is not so significant, because 90% of legionella infections are caused by *L pneumophila*, and of these, more than 80% are caused by serogroup 1 [3]. At this point and time, the best first step in evaluating an individual with suspected legionnaires' disease is a urinary antigen test.

Direct fluorescent antibody staining is another rapid test that can be clinically useful. This test can be done in two hours and is highly specific. However, the sensitivity is only 30–70% [63] because of the need for a large number of organisms to be present before they can be easily visualized.

Serologic tests are not useful to the individual physician caring for a patient with possible legionellosis, but they are useful for epidemiologic studies. The diagnosis of legionellosis based on antibody titers requires samples from the acute phase and convalescent phase (approximately six to eight weeks later). The diagnosis is made if there is either a fourfold increase in the antibody titer to 1:128 or more, or if there is a single convalescent titer of 1:256 or more in a patient with a history consistent with legionellosis. The specificity of serologic tests to diagnose legionellosis secondary to *L pneumophila* is estimated to be 95%. The sensitivity and specificity of serologic tests to diagnose legionellosis secondary to other legionella species have not been established.

Most cases of legionella can be diagnosed from urine or sputum samples. In the case of an individual with severe pneumonia felt to possibly be legionellosis but in whom the urine antibody test and sputum samples have been negative, a bronchoscopy with bronchoalveolar lavage may be indicated to secure the diagnosis.

Pontiac fever is diagnosed by antibody seroconversion in individuals having a clinical illness consistent with Pontiac fever. Culture and direct fluorescent antibody staining of clinical specimens have not been shown to be useful in making the diagnosis.

Treatment and Rehabilitation

Since the original description of legionnaires' disease, erythromycin has been known to be effective in treating the disease [1]. For much of the last 20 years, erythromycin has been the standard therapy for treating legionella infections. Recently, newer macrolides (azithromycin and clarithromycin) and the fluoroquinolones have become widely accepted as appropriate therapy for legionella infections.

Since legionellosis typically presents as a community-acquired pneumonia prior to a specific diagnosis being made, it is important to cover Legionellaceae when empirically treating community-acquired pneumonia. The standard empiric treatment for community-acquired pneumonia, regardless of severity or presence of co-morbid conditions, includes a macrolide [7,64]. For an outpatient with co-morbid conditions, a fluoroquinolone is added to the macrolide. For hospitalized patients, a second- or third-generation cephalosporin is added to the macrolide.

Erythromycin is still commonly used to treat legionellosis, but azithromycin will likely become the standard of care in the near future. In laboratory studies, azithromycin has been shown to be more effective against *L pneumophila* than erythromycin [65]. In clinical studies, azithromycin has been shown to be effective and well tolerated in the treatment of legionellosis [66,67]. The biggest advantage of azithromycin over erythromycin is that it can be given once per day rather than four times per day. It also causes fewer side effects. Azithromycin is now available in intravenous form, thus allowing it to be used for severely ill patients. Clarithromycin is another macrolide with greater activity against *L pneumophila* than erythromycin [68]. It is an alternative to azithromycin or erythromycin for the outpatient treatment of community-acquired pneumonia [64]. However, since it is not available in intravenous form, it cannot be used for severe cases.

The fluoroquinolones have been shown to be more effective in vitro than erythromycin [68]. Ciprofloxacin has been shown to be clinically effective in the treatment of patients with legionellosis [68,69], as has ofloxacin [68]. Levofloxacin and trovafloxacin are accepted alternatives to macrolides for the treatment of any case of adult community-acquired pneumonia [64]. Because macrolides can interact with immunosuppressive agents commonly used for transplantation patients, legionellosis in such patients should be treated with ciprofloxacin or levofloxacin [6,69]. Because of its ability to be effective when given in daily doses, levofloxacin is the better choice of the two.

Several other agents have been shown to be effective against legionella and may have a role in treatment in certain cases, such as in patients allergic to macrolides or fluoroquinolones. These include rifampin, trimethoprim-sulfamethoxazole, tetracycline, and doxycycline [1,9,64,68]. Rifampin in combination with a macrolide or a quinolone is recommended for the treatment of severe legionellosis [9,70].

No clinical trials have specifically compared the efficacy of different antibiotics against non–*L pneumophila* Legionellaceae. Given similarities in experimental data and anecdotal reports [4,68], it seems reasonable to advocate the same treatment for these organisms as has been discussed for *L pneumophila*.

In addition to antibiotic therapy, treatment of legionella often requires supportive care, particularly in severe cases. Such care may include intravenous fluids, supplemental oxygen, intubation, mechanical ventilation, and chest physiotherapy. The type and frequency of supportive modalities depends on the severity of the case and should be decided on a case-by-case basis.

Occupational Considerations

As has been emphasized throughout this chapter, it is best to think of legionellosis as an environmental disease rather than an occupational one, for a variety of water sources can serve as reservoirs for legionella. Since legionella is so widespread, no specific occupation can be considered immune to the threat.

Since certain occupations involve more contact with water, they theoretically could put workers at greater risk. Such occupations include canoe trip guides, fishing guides, plumbers, and HVAC workers. However, no study has examined the relative risks of different occupations for legionellosis.

Since legionellosis has been well documented as a nosocomial infection, it is reasonable to ask if health care workers are at higher risk for legionnaires' disease. Marrie and colleagues [41] investigated this issue and found that the risk of infection among health care workers during an outbreak of legionnaires' disease was low (2.4%). It is low primarily because legionellosis is not spread person-to-person, and individuals who are able to work full time, such as health care workers, are unlikely to be immunocompromised. The reason that nosocomial legionella infections are common is probably not due to any unique problem with the water supply of hospitals, but rather that immunosuppressed individuals, who are at increased risk of infection, are present as patients in hospitals and that there is a better job of specifically diagnosing the specific cause of pneumonia (such as legionella) in hospitalized patients compared to the general population.

What should an occupational medicine physician do if a patient is diagnosed with a community-acquired pneumonia? In addition to providing appropriate therapy, the physician should investigate whether the illness may be work related. The possibility that the pneumonia is due to legionellosis should be investigated. The legionella urine-antigen test is easy to use to diagnose legionellosis and is a good first-line test to run. If legionellosis is diagnosed, there are several subsequent steps to take to determine if the infection is work related [29]. One is to investigate whether other work related cases exist at the patient's workplace. Next, attempts can be made to isolate legionella from water reservoirs at work. If legionella is isolated, the environmental isolate should be compared to that isolated from the patient. If they match, the worksite is likely the source; if not, there is another source. Given the large number of potential reservoir sites and the many species and serotypes within the family Legionellaceae, this final matching step is critical to perform. This type of logical, step-by-step investigation should help prevent outbreaks in the future.

References

1. Fraser DW, Tsai TR, Orenstein W, et al. Legionnaires' disease: description of an epidemic of pneumonia. *N Engl J Med* 1977;297:1189–97.
2. McDade JE, Shepard CC, Fraser DW, et al. Legionnaires' disease: isolation of a bacterium and demonstration of its role in other respiratory disease. *N Engl J Med* 1977;297:1197–1203.

3. Muder RR. Legionnaires' disease. In: Gorbach SL, Bartlett JG, Blacklow NR (eds), *Infectious Diseases*, 2nd Ed. Philadelphia: Saunders, 1998. Pp 614–21.

4. Fang GD, Yu VL, Vickers RM. Disease due to Legionellaceae (other than *Legionella pneumophila*): historical, microbiological, clinical and epidemiological review. *Medicine* 1989;68:116–32.

5. Kaufmann AF, McDade JE, Patton CM, et al. Pontiac fever: isolation of the etiologic agent (*Legionella pneumophila*) and demonstration of its mode of transmission. *Am J Epidemiol* 1981;114:337–47.

6. Roig J, Domingo C, Morera J. Legionnaires' disease. *Chest* 1994;105:1817–25.

7. American Thoracic Society. Guidelines for the initial management of adults with community-acquired pneumonia: diagnosis, assessment of severity, and initial antimicrobial therapy. *Am Rev Respir Dis* 1993;148:1418–26.

8. Bartlett JG, Mundy LM. Community-acquired pneumonia. *N Engl J Med* 1995;333:1618–24.

9. Stout JE, Yu VL. Legionellosis. *N Engl J Med* 1997; 337:682–7.

10. Fang GD, Fine M, Orloff J, et al. New and emerging etiologies for community-acquired pneumonia with implications for therapy: a prospective multicenter study of 359 cases. *Medicine* 1990;69:307–16.

11. Torres A, Serra-Batlles J, Ferrer A, et al. Severe community acquired pneumonia: epidemiology and prognostic factors. *Am Rev Respir Dis* 1991;144:312–8.

12. Cases of selected notifiable diseases, United States, weeks ending December 31, 1994, and January 1, 1994 (52nd week). *MMWR* 1995;43:968.

13. Stout JE, Yu VL, Vickers RM, et al. Ubiquitousness of *Legionella pneumophila* in the water supply of a hospital with endemic Legionnaires' disease. *N Engl J Med* 1982;306:466–8.

14. Best M, Yu VL, Stout J, et al. Legionellaceae in the hospital water supply: epidemiological link with disease and the evaluation of a method for control of nosocomial legionnaires' disease and Pittsburgh pneumonia. *Lancet* 1983,2(8345):307–10.

15. Shands KN, Ho JL, Meyer RD, et al. Potable water as a source of legionnaires' disease. *JAMA* 1985;253: 1412–6.

16. Plouffe JF, Webster LR, Hackman B. Relationship between colonization of hospital buildings with *Legionella pneumophila* and hot water temperatures. *Appl Environ Microbiol* 1983;46:769–70.

17. Stout JE, Yu VL, Muraca P, et al. Potable water as a cause of sporadic cases of community-acquired legionnaires' disease. *N Engl J Med* 1992;326:151–5.

18. Straus WL, Plouffe JF, File TM, et al. Risk factors for domestic acquisition of Legionnaires' disease. *Arch Intern Med* 1996;156:1685–92.

19. Rampling A, Butt CJ, West AA, et al. Community acquired legionnaires' disease following minimal exposure to a contaminated source. *J Infect* 1997; 35: 300–2.

20. Brady MT. Nosocomial legionnaires' disease in a children's hospital. *J Pediatr* 1989;115:46–50.

21. Hlady WG, Mullen RC, Mintz CS, et al. Outbreak of legionnaires' disease linked to a decorative fountain by molecular epidemiology. *Am J Epidemiol* 1993;138: 555–62.

22. Schlech WF, Gorman GW, Payne MC, et al. Legionnaires' disease in the Caribbean: an outbreak associated with a resort hotel. *Arch Intern Med* 1985;145: 2076–9.

23. Graman PS, Quinlan GA, Rank JA. Nosocomial legionellosis traced to a contaminated ice machine. *Infect Control Hosp Epidemiol* 1997;18:637–40.

24. Fliermans CB, Cherry WB, Orrison LH, et al. Ecological distribution of *Legionella pneumophila*. *Appl Environ Microbiol* 1981; 41:9–16.

25. Mangione EJ, Remis RS, Tait KA, et al. An outbreak of Pontiac fever related to whirlpool use, Michigan 1982. *JAMA* 1985;253:535–9.

26. Mahoney FJ, Hoge DW, Farley TA. Community wide outbreak of legionnaires' disease associated with a grocery store mist machine. *J Infect Dis* 1992;165:736–9.

27. Dondero TJ, Rendtorff RC, Mallison GF, et al. An outbreak of legionnaires' disease associated with a contaminated air conditioning cooling tower. *N Engl J Med* 1980;302:365–70.

28. Brennen C, Vickers RM, Yu VL, et al. Discovery of occult legionella pneumonia in a long stay hospital: results of prospective serological survey. *Br Med J* 1987;295:306–7.

29. Muraca PW, Stout JE, Yu VL, et al. Legionnaires' disease in the work environment: implications for environmental health. *Am Ind Hyg Assoc J* 1988;49:584–90.

30. Muder RR, Yu VL, Woo AH. Mode of transmission of *Legionella pneumophila*: a critical review. *Arch Intern Med* 1986;146:1607–12.

31. Wadowsky RM, Yee RB. Effect of non-Legionellaceae bacteria on the multiplication of *Legionella pneumophila* in potable water. *Appl Environ Microbiol* 1985;49:1206–10.

32. Stout JE, Yu VL, Best MG. Ecology of *Legionella pneumophila* within water distribution systems. *Appl Environ Microbiol* 1985;49:221–8.

33. Wright JB, Ruseska I, Athar MA, et al. *Legionella pneumophila* grows adherent to surfaces in vitro and in situ. *Infect Control Hosp Epidemiol* 1989;10:408–15.

34. Wadowsky RM, Butler LJ, Cook MK, et al. Growth-supporting activity for *Legionella pneumophila* in tap water cultures and implication of hartmannellid amoeba as growth factors. *Appl Environ Microbiol* 1988;54: 2677–82.

35. Barker J, Brown MR, Collier PJ, et al. Relationship between *Legionella pneumophila* and *Acanthamoeba polyphaga*: physiologic status and susceptibility to chemi-

cal inactivation. *Appl Environ Microbiol* 1992;58:2420–5.

36. Arnow PM, Chou T, Weil D, et al. Nosocomial legionnaires' disease caused by aerosolizal tap water from respiratory devices. *J Infect Dis* 1982;146:460–7.
37. Woo AH, Goetz A, Yu VL. Transmission of legionella by respiratory equipment and aerosol generating devices. *Chest* 1992;102:1586–90.
38. Johnson JT, Yu VL, Best MG, et al. Nosocomial legionellosis in surgical patients with head and neck cancer: implications for epidemiological reservoir and mode of transmission. *Lancet* 1985;2:298–300.
39. Lowry PW, Blankenship RN, Gridley W, et al. A cluster of legionella sternal wound infections due to postoperative topical exposure to contaminated tap water. *N Engl J Med* 1991;324:109–13.
40. Yu VL, Zuravleff JJ, Gavlik L, et al. Lack of evidence for person-to-person transmission of legionnaires' disease. *J Infect Dis* 1983;147:362.
41. Marrie TJ, George J, Macdonald S, et al. Are health care workers at risk for infection during an outbreak of nosocomial legionnaires' disease? *Am J Infect Control* 1986;14:209–13.
42. Roig J, Aguilar X, Ruiz J, et al. Comparative study of *Legionella pneumophila* and other nosocomial-acquired pneumonias. *Chest* 1991;99:344–50.
43. Venezia RA, Agresta MD, Hanley EM, et al. Nosocomial legionellosis associated with aspiration of nasogastric feedings diluted in tap water. *Infect Control Hosp Epidemiol* 1994;15:529–33.
44. Kociuba KR, Buist M, Munro R, et al. Legionnaires' disease outbreak in southwestern Sydney, 1994: clinical aspects. *Med J Aust* 1994;160:274–7.
45. Skaliy P, McEachern HV. Survival of the legionnaires' disease bacterium in the water. *Ann Intern Med* 1979;90:662–3.
46. Morris GK, Patton CM, Feeley JC, et al. Isolation of the legionnaires' disease bacterium, environmental samples. *Ann Intern Med* 1979;90:664–6.
47. Alary M, Joly JR. Factors contributing to the contamination of hospital water distribution systems by legionellae. *J Infect Dis* 1992;165:565–9.
48. Vickers RM, Yu VL, Hanna SS, et al. Determinants of *Legionella pneumophila* contamination of water distribution systems: 15 hospital prospective studies. *Infect Control* 1987;8:357–63.
49. Allegheny County Health Department. *Approaches to Prevention and Control of Legionella Infection in Allegheny County Health Care Facilities.* Pittsburgh: Allegheny County Health Department, 1997.
50. Muraca PW, Yu VL, Goetz A. Disinfection of water distribution systems for *Legionella:* a review of application, procedures and methodologies *Infect Control Hosp Epidemiol* 1990;11:79–88.
51. Yu VL, Liu Z, Stout JE, et al. Legionella disinfection of water distribution systems: principles, problems, and practice. *Infect Control Hosp Epidemiol* 1993;14:567–70.
52. Mirowski GW, Frieden IJ, Miller C. Iatrogenic scald burn: a consequence of institutional infection control measures. *Pediatrics* 1996;98:963–5.
53. Kuchta JM, States SJ, McNamara AM, et al. Susceptibility of *Legionella pneumophila* to chlorine in tap water. *Appl Environ Microbiol* 1983;46:1134–9.
54. Muraca PW, Stout JE, Yu VL. Comparative assessment of chlorine, heat, ozone and UV light for killing *Legionella pneumophila* within a model plumbing system. *Appl Environ Microbiol* 1987;53:447–53.
55. Marston BJ, Lipman HB, Breimen RF. Surveillance for legionnaires' disease: risk factors for morbidity and mortality. *Arch Intern Med* 1994;154:2417–22.
56. American Thoracic Society. Hospital-acquired pneumonia in adults: diagnosis, assessment of severity, initial antimicrobial therapy, and preventative strategies. A consensus statement. *Am J Respir Crit Care Med* 1995;153:1711–25.
57. Blander SJ, Horwitz MA. Major cytoplasmic membrane protein of *Legionella pneumophila*, a genus common antigen and member of the hsp 60 family of heat shock proteins, induces protective immunity in a guinea pig model of legionnaires' disease. *J Clin Invest* 1993;91:717–23.
58. Woodhead MA, Macfarlane JT. Legionnaires' disease: a review of 79 community acquired cases in Nottingham. *Thorax* 1986;41:635–40.
59. Kroboth FJ, Yu VL, Reddy SC, et al. Clinicoradiographic correlation with the extent of legionnaires' disease. *AJR* 1983;141:263–8.
60. Yu VL, Kroboth FJ, Shonnard J, et al. Legionnaires' disease: new clinical perspective from a prospective pneumonia study. *Am J Med* 1982;73:357–61.
61. Elbright J, Tarakji E, Brown W, et al. Multiple bilateral lung cavities caused by *Legionella pneumophila*: case report and review. *Infect Dis Clin Pract* 1993;2:195–9.
62. Kohorst WR, Schonfeld SA, Macklin JE, et al. Rapid diagnosis of legionnaires' disease by bronchoalveolar lavage. *Chest* 1983;84:186–90.
63. Zuraleff JJ, Yu VL, Shonnard J, et al. Diagnosis of legionnaires' disease: An update of laboratory methods with new emphasis on isolation by culture. *JAMA* 1983;250:1981–5.
64. Gilbert GN, Moellering RC, Sande MA (eds). *The Sanford Guide to Antimicrobial Therapy.* 1999, 29th Ed. Vienna, VA: Antimicrobial Therapy, 1999. P 28.
65. Edelstein PH, Edelstein MA. In vitro activity of azithromycin against clinical isolates of *Legionella* species. *Antimicrob Agents Chemother* 1991;35:180–1.
66. Myburgh J, Nagel GJ, Petschel E. The efficacy and tolerance of a three-day course of azithromycin in the treatment of community-acquired pneumonia. *J Antimicrob Chemother* 1993,31(suppl E):163–9.
67. Kuzman I, Soldo I, Schonwald S, et al. Azithromycin

for treatment of community acquired pneumonia caused by *Legionella pneumophila*: a retrospective study. *Scand J Infect Dis* 1995;27:503–5.

68. Edelstein PH. Antimicrobial chemotherapy for legionnaires' disease: a review. *Clin Infect Dis* 1995;21(suppl 3):S265–76.

69. Hooper TL, Gould FK, Swinburn CR, et al. Ciprofloxacin: a preferred treatment for legionella infections in patients receiving cyclosporin A. *J Antimicrob Chemother* 1988;22:952–3.

70. Moffie BG, Mouton RP. Sensitivity and resistance of *Legionella pneumophila* to some antibiotics and combinations of antibiotics. *J Antimicrob Chemother* 1988; 22:457–62.

11 / Occupational Influenza

Daymon Evans

In common language, *the flu* has come to mean any generalized communicable illness of the upper respiratory or gastrointestinal systems. A wide discussion of all of the possible pathogens and illnesses that could be mislabeled *the flu* is beyond the scope of this chapter. The discussion is limited to that relatively severe and highly communicable upper respiratory infection caused by the RNA orthomyxoviruses A, B, or C. Influenza should not be confused with *Haemophilus influenzae* (*H flu*), a bacteria that can cause upper respiratory infections. When first cultured from purulent sputum during outbreaks in 1892 by Pfeifer [1] it was presumed to be the pathogen responsible for clinical influenza [2]. Its etiology as the influenza pathogen was questioned after the 1918 Pandemic, and its name was officially changed to *hemophilus influenza* in 1920 to recognize both its historical association with influenza and its dependence on blood components or the "blood-loving" nature of the bacteria [3]. The virus responsible for human influenza was first isolated in 1933 [4]. Hemophilus influenza B vaccine (Hib) is now part of the childhood immunization panel and should not be confused with influenza vaccines.

The size of this chapter is a reflection of the incidence of this disease in working populations, its dynamic epidemiologic characteristics, the challenges of surveillance, and the complexity of treatment and prevention options. Influenza and influenza-like illness (ILI) infect more workers annually than all diseases in this textbook combined and are responsible for spikes of absenteeism and financial costs to all employers. This may be the first medical textbook chapter to specifically address influenza in the workplace.

"Occupational influenza" may be an administrative nonentity, in that influenza is rarely accepted as a compensable occupational disease. Influenza is considered a normal disease of life by most workers' compensation carriers and state statutes because there is no evidence that the risk, incidence, or prevalence varies among professions or worksites. Widening the definition of occupations to include students and military personnel will include a major population of influenza victims, include classic routes of transmission, and include the study groups for much of our scientific and observational knowledge of the disease.

Influenza is a disease of great consequence to employers because of the expense of absenteeism and medical care. The direct medical costs of influenza in mid-1990 dollars are estimated to be as much as $4.6 billion in an average year, but total and direct costs of a severe influenza season are at least $12 billion [5]. Much of this cost is absorbed by employers.

Especially vulnerable are hospitals and other acute health care facilities, with their simultaneous high patient workloads and high employee absenteeism [6–9]. Both may be attributable to influenza. Management is challenged to maintain adequate staffing of in-patient units during influenza epidemics and may have to resort to the expense of contracting workers from outside agencies. Well employees may be asked to work longer shifts or overtime, and the more dedicated caregivers may report to work despite their own illness and thus contribute to the nosocomial aspects of an epidemic [10–12].

However, the employer and the worksite can serve pivotal roles in community influenza prevention, education, and intervention. Employers offering influenza vaccine and/or prophylactic antiviral prescriptions will recover their costs in most years [13–19]. A recent case control study by Campbell and Rumley [13] showed that a North Carolina textile plant saved $2.58 for each $1.00 invested in an employee vaccination program. A survey study by 3M showed that employees receiving sequential (annual) immunizations had reductions in absenteeism [19].

Practitioners of occupational and environmental medicine will frequently be asked to consult and/or attend influenza prevention efforts. This is good public health and a wise business investment. Occupational medicine practitioners (OMPs) should enthusiastically accept these offers and maintain their up-to-date knowledge on influenza epidemiology, immunization, and other prevention strategies. They should be able to serve their client companies and patients as a year-round resource for influenza control and prevention planning. When influenza infects workers, it affects their health and productivity. Some occupations may logically seem more at risk than others, but there is little evidence that infection rates vary significantly among jobs or worksites. With the majority of adults spending one fourth of their life at, or in route to or from, work, there is little doubt that employment and the workplace are major factors in human-to-human influenza transmission. Society may not accept influenza as a compensable occupational disease but cannot deny its existence as an environmental disease. It remains one of the most studied, most fascinating, least understood, and prevalent human afflictions. The workplace should not be a missed opportunity for the implementation of adult influenza immunization and education.

Epidemiology

INCIDENCE AND PREVALENCE

Influenza is the world's leading respiratory infection and is a threat to all populations. Less than half of those hospitalized with acute respiratory disease during the influenza months are over age 65 or have a chronic medical condition [20] (the classic high-risk patient), and half of all patients hospitalized by complications of influenza are employed.

Influenza may seem to come in seasonal epidemics, but in reality, it is an endemic human disease continually encircling the Earth. A strain may take one to two years to circle the globe, and 20% of the Earth's human population will have at least one influenza infection in an average year [21]. A geographic area and its population have their season at any given point in time and likely serve as the reservoir for the disease, which seemingly disappears for much of the year. A pandemic is defined as "an epidemic occurring over a very wide area, crossing international boundaries and usually affecting a large number of people" [22].

History and Influenza

Only by understanding the history of human influenza can we afford this disease the respect it deserves. Its stealth motivates us to maintain our surveillance systems and to fund further research on surveillance, prevention, and treatment.

Pre-Twentieth Century Outbreaks. A favorite exercise of medical historians is to diagnose the Great Plague of Athens, which occurred in 430 BC. Thucydides gave extensive descriptions of the clinical syndrome and the spread of this epidemic [23], which killed one third of the Greek army and precipitated the downfall of the Empire. Langmuir and colleagues have postulated that this plague was an especially virulent influenza strain with a high rate of secondary staphylococcus infection and toxic shock syndrome [24].

Influenza-like illnesses (ILIs) have been recorded throughout history [25] under many different names, such as the grip. The English term comes from sixteenth-century Italians who noted that the illness could "influence" others to have the illness and/or possibly that a winter constellation could "influence" the illness. Since the sixteenth century, at least 31 global pandemics of ILI have been recorded, averaging 4 to 5 per century [26].

The first publications on the quantitative impact of influenza can be attributed to Robert Graves [27]. He counted new graves in Dublin cemeteries starting in 1837. William Farr recorded details of the London Epidemic of 1847 and first described the concept that death rates may vary by seasons [28]. We now call this *excess mortality.* He described peaks occurring in colder months, attributable to influenza complications. Both Graves and Farr were members of the London Epidemiological Society, one of the first professional organizations to formally study disease dynamics.

The 1918 Spanish Flu Pandemic. The Great 1918 Pandemic has been the most rapid and deadly communicable epidemic of the twentieth century. Five of every 1,000 Americans died, with a final U.S. death toll estimated at 675,000. This is more American deaths than those caused by all wars in this century. As an emergency measure, public gatherings were banded in many places, and there was an international shortage of caskets during the 1918 pandemic.

The illness would begin as a typical influenza case but could rapidly develop into severe pneumonia. Fever could reach 105°F and cause dementia and hallucinations. Mahogany-colored spots would appear over the cheekbones, and cyanosis and death could occur in a few hours. The case fatality rate was about 10%. The mystery of why the disease targeted young adults was not solved for a generation.

It was called the Spanish flu because it was mistakenly believed to be the same virus responsible for an epidemic in Spain that spring. It spread along railroad lines and with the movement of troops. News of the epidemic was overshadowed by the First World War. World War I caused 8.5 million deaths, but over 20 million died in a few weeks from this influenza. In February of 1998, the Molecular Pathology Division of the Armed Forces Institute of Pathology obtained permission from the City Council of Brevig Mission, Alaska, to study the frozen remains of citizens who died in the 1918 pandemic [29]. Eighty-five percent of Mission residents died in a single week. It is hoped that the 1918 strain will finally be identified.

Subsequent Pandemics. The 1918 pandemic was most likely a strain that is now labeled influenza A (H1N1) and was likely due to a major change in the antigenic nature of the influenza virus. Other major changes in the antigens occurred with the 1957–1958 Asian flu A(H2N2), which was responsible for 70,000 deaths in the United States (Table 11-1). The most recent pandemic was the Hong Kong flu A(H3N2), responsible for 34,000 deaths during 1968 and

Table 11-1
Pathogenic Human Influenza Viruses

Type	Subtype	Prototype	U.S. Mortality	Status
A	H1N1	A/New Jersey/8/76	500,000+ in 1918 Spanish Flu; 675,000 over ensuing several years	Swine reservoir?[a] Other H1N1s circulating
	H2N2	A/Japan/305/57	70,000+ in 1957 Asian Flu	Not in circulation at present
	H3N2	A/Hong Kong/1/68	34,000 in 1968 Hong Kong Flu; maybe 400,000 since 1968[b]	The most virulent in present circulation
	H5N1	Unnamed, first found in terns 1961	0 (but 6 in Hong Kong, 1997/8 "Bird Flu"?)[c]	Chickens slaughtered. Next global threat?
B	None	B/Lee/40[d]	No data; but less than A subtypes	In circulation, but epidemics infrequent
C	None	C/Taylor/1233/47[e]	Believed to be minimal	In circulation, but clinically inapparent

[a] See discussion of swine influenza, page 11–4.
[b] See reference 64.
[c] See references 30, 31. All cases confined to Hong Kong area at present writing.
[d] First isolated by Francis in 1940. (Francis T Jr. A new type of virus from epidemic influenza. *Science* 1940;92:405–8.)
[e] First isolated by Taylor in 1947. (Taylor RM. Studies on survival of influenza virus between epidemics and antigenic variant of the virus. *Am J Public Health* 1949;39:171–8.)

1969. Gene segments for both the 1957 and 1968 subtypes were closely related to influenza viruses previously found in wild bird species. Pandemics "scares" have occurred with the swine flu in 1976, the Russian flu in 1977, and the current bird flu [30,31].

The Swine Flu. A deadly respiratory epizootic began in pigs in the midwestern United States in the early autumn of 1918. Swine veterinarian Dr. J. S. Koen believed this disease to be the same as the human Spanish influenza and named it *swine* influenza [32]. This influenza still occurs in pigs in the Midwest each autumn but is not as deadly as it was during the 1918 outbreak.

This swine virus was isolated by Shope in 1930 [33], three years before an influenza virus was isolated from a human [4]. Serologic surveys conducted by Shope in 1936 [34] showed that many humans over age 12 had antibodies to this swine virus isolate. This was confirmed by other studies and led to the assumption that the swine influenza isolate was closely related to the 1918 human pandemic strain, and possibly identical.

This offered an explanation for why the 1918 disease was so deadly to young adults. Older persons had been exposed to a similar virus that had circulated in an 1890 pandemic, and they may have had some antibody cross-protection. Further comparative human birth cohort-swine serosurveys conducted by Davenport [35] and others in the 1950s confirmed that a virus very similar to the swine influenza virus circulated from 1918 until about 1928.

Laidlaw [36] postulated that swine influenza was the surviving form of the 1918 human virus. Shope proved that swine could be infected with influenza from humans under experimental conditions [37], and later by natural conditions [38]. He found older hogs on New Jersey farms with neutralizing antibodies to a human influenza virus; these antibodies were not found in younger hogs. In the Asian flu pandemic in 1957, it was again found that some hogs were infected with human influenza [39]. The 1968 pandemic strain was also found in pigs [40] in an area where humans and swine lived in close proximity on an island. However, these researchers did not believe that influenza could be spread from swine to humans, only that swine were the secondary victims of a human disease.

In the early 1960s, there were several unconfirmed reports of swine influenzas infecting humans behind the Iron Curtain. A collaborative team from the Illinois Department of Health and the University of Illinois Veterinary College studied human sera for swine virus in 1966 [41]. They found those with direct swine contact to have a relative risk of 21for having swine influenza antibodies. There may have been human-to-human spread, since those who had contact with swine workers (but not swine) had a higher incidence of swine influenza antibodies than that of the general public who were exposed to neither. They concluded that swine influenza was not a true occupational hazard, because the infection was inapparent.

It was not until 1974 that swine influenza virus was isolated from a human, some 44 years after being isolated in hogs [42]. The victim was a 14-year-old immunosuppressed boy who did not have contact with swine until a few days before his death, when he came into contact with two pigs on a farm. Both pigs were seropositive for the strain, and both of his parents were negative. A year later, a family of six who lived on a hog farm in Wisconsin were all found to be positive, with the index case showing a positive paired sera [43]. Several more cases of illness due to swine influenza were reported from Missouri, Wisconsin, and Minnesota, but it was the outbreak among recruits at Fort Dix, New Jersey, in 1976 that sparked international attention. No contact between soldiers and swine could be identified, so it was suspected that spread was human to human. The Fort Dix epidemic created a public health panic because:

- The 230 infected recruits were young and healthy.
- Previous pandemics had began in military units.
- There was evidence of human-to-human spread.
- The swine influenza endemic in New Jersey hogs had been found 40 years earlier and had a direct linkage to the 1918 pandemic.

Because of the fear of a return of the 1918 pathogen, a massive public health initiative resulted in one fourth of the U.S. population receiving a monovalent swine influenza vaccine. An epidemic did not occur, but the rare and highly publicized vaccine complications of Guillain-Barré syndrome damaged public confidence in the influenza vaccine and the public health surveillance of influenza. Formal influenza control has yet to fully recover credibility, although a risk factor for Guillain-Barré has not been associated with subsequent vaccines [44,45].

Most recently, two workers became ill with an influenza-like illness after performing nasal swabs on pigs. The pigs were artificially infected with a swine influenza, A(H1N1), in experiments at the University of Wisconsin—Madison [46]. The two workers cultured the identical strain despite adhering to animal biosafety level 3 containment practices [47]. These workers were the eighth and ninth humans proved to have been infected with swine influenza directly from hogs [48–53]. Both survived, but the majority of patients in previously reported cases died.

Antigen Nomenclature and Clinical Correlation

An influenza virus was first isolated from chickens during a fowl plague in 1901 [32]; the pathogen is now known to be A(H7N7). Influenza B and C were isolated in 1940 and 1947, respectively. Influenza was found to grow in embryonated chicken eggs, and this led to many advances in culture technique, serologic testing, and eventually vaccine development. The influenza virus is a single-stranded RNA myxovirus and contains three sets of proteins. It is the nucleoprotein portion that distinguishes A, B, and C from one another.

Influenza C is the simplest in structure and contains only a single glycoprotein. It has been associated only with minor epidemics and less severe illness, and serosurveys confirm many inapparent infections and near 100% immunity for this type by age 5 [54]. Influenza C may be more endemic than epidemic. Influenza B, however, can cause epidemics, although much less often than the more prevalent A. In addition, influenza B usually causes less severe illness than A.

Influenza A and B each have two types of projecting glycoproteins, the hemagglutinin (H) and the neuraminidase (N). These glycoproteins are responsible for the antigenic variations in the subtypes and are the sites of antibody attachment and inhibition.

A standard system of nomenclature was developed for influenza A and underwent revisions in 1971 [55] and 1980 [56]. It is as follows:

- Type (A, B, or C).
- Host of origin (influenza A), if, and only if, it is not human.
- Geographic origin, a city or region where first found.
- Isolation (strain) number assigned sequentially.
- Year of isolation.
- If influenza A, then a description of antigenic specificity (subtype) of the surface antigens:
- *H*: hemagglutinin (one of 12 types; 1, 2, 3, and 5 pathogenic to humans).
- *N*: neuraminidase (one of nine types, 1 and 2 pathogenic to humans).

Examples: B/Beijing/184/93: a human influenza B virus first isolated in Beijing in 1993.
A/Nanchang/933/95 (H3N2): a human influenza A (H3N2) virus first isolated in Nan-chang in 1995.
A/Duck/Ukraine/1/63 (H7N2): an avian influenza A (H7N2) virus first isolated from ducks in the Ukraine in 1963.

The World Health Organization (WHO) maintains reference isolates for both human (WHO Collaborating Centres for Reference and Research on Influenza) and nonhumans (WHO Centres for the Study of Influenza Ecology in Animals). Reference matching is made on request.

An influenza A virus can undergo genetic recombinations and create newborn progeny subtypes. Genetic reassortment between two different influenza A viruses has been postulated to be the mechanism of the "antigenic shift" [57,58] when they simultaneously infect and replicate in the same victim cell. Shifts are believed to be changes of up to 50% of the nucleotide sequence and may be responsible for new pathogens and major epidemics or pandemics in a general population lacking immunity to this new subtype. The more minor changes are the antigenic drift (either influenza A or B) of less than

1% of the nucleotide sequence. Humans may have at least partial antibody protection from previously closely related infection.

Influenza A is known to be present both endemically and epidemically in many animal species (e.g., chickens, ducks, hogs, horses, mink, and seals) and could theoretically be the source for new human subtypes. Types B and C are primarily human viruses and are more antigenically stable than A. H1N1 was the primary human subtype circulating until an antigenic "double" shift to H2N2 in 1957 created the Asian Flu Pandemic (see Table 11-1). An antigenic shift to H3N2 in 1968 resulted in the Hong-Kong Flu Pandemic.

It was believed that only one subtype could circulate at a time until A(H1N1) reappeared in 1977 and subsequently co-circulated with A(H3N2). Some strains may "cycle" over a period of decades, possibly centuries. The antigenic shifts seen in this century may not represent new human pathogens. There is some serologic evidence from birth cohorts that the strain that caused a severe epidemic in 1889 and 1890 was very similar to the influenza A (Hong Kong) strain (H3N2) of 1968 [59]. During the 1968 Hong Kong Flu, persons over the age of 75 had lower morbidity and mortality than those ages 65–74 [60]. It has also been shown that 26% of persons born between 1857 and 1877 had antibodies to the A/Japan/305/7(H2N2) subtype, implying that an Asian-like flu may have circulated in the middle of the nineteenth century [61].

In December 1997 the entire chicken population of Hong Kong was slaughtered after 18 humans with chicken contact were infected with an A(H5N1) subtype [30,31]. There were six deaths including the 3-year-old boy who was the index case. Because cases have been confined to the Hong Kong area and there has not been human-to-human transmission, a "Bird Flu" epidemic has not yet occurred.

Excess Mortality

Expanding on the principle first described by Graves and Pearl and Frost [62,63] the term *excess mortality* is used to describe the death toll from the 1918 pandemic. *Excess mortality* is defined as those seasonal deaths that occur above the number predicted on the basis of a stable death rate. In the United States and other temperate areas, excess mortality occurs in the winter months and is essentially synonymous with influenza and its complications.

The excess mortality concept has undergone many statistical revisions, including the present P-I (pneumonia and influenza) index published weekly in *Morbidity and Mortality Weekly Reports.* Most of the 20,000 or so "excess" deaths in an average year in the United States are the elderly and chronically ill. Spikes occur with pandemics (Figure 11-1). The most recent influenza A subtype (H3N2) continues to circulate, and may have contributed to as many as 400,000 deaths in the United States since 1968 [64]. In the 20 flu seasons between 1972 and 1992, there were over 10,000 deaths in seven winters, over 20,000 deaths in nine winters, and over 40,000 deaths in four winters. These deaths may be only a fraction of the true deaths in which influenza was a precipitating factor.

Morbidity from influenza starts to rise at about age 40. Currently, at least 90% of influenza deaths occur in citizens over the age of 65 [65], up from 62% for the same age group in the 1970s [66]. Many fatalities occur in those with chronic cardiac, pulmonary, renal or metabolic diseases, anemia, and/or immunosuppression. Even if those with chronic illnesses survive influenza and its complications, the illness may further weaken their conditions and contribute to shortened life spans. Mortality from influenza may continue to increase as life expectancy increases for all of the high-risk populations, e.g., organ-transplant recipients, premature neonates, persons with cystic fibrosis, congestive heart failure patients, and those living with acquired immunodeficiency syndrome (AIDS).

Seasonality

In North America, the influenza season runs from December through March, but surveillance is vigilant from October through April. Epidemics typically are concentrated in a three-week period; the mode month is February [67]. In tropical areas, epidemics most often occur during the rainy season.

In localized outbreaks, epidemics can evolve rapidly, with little warning, and often end as sud-

Figure 11-1 / Monthly mortality from influenza in Massachusetts from 1887–1921 and in 90 U.S. cities from 1922–1956. (From Collins SD, *Influenza in the United States,* 1887–1957. Public Health Monograph #48. Washington, DC: Government Printing Office, 1957.)

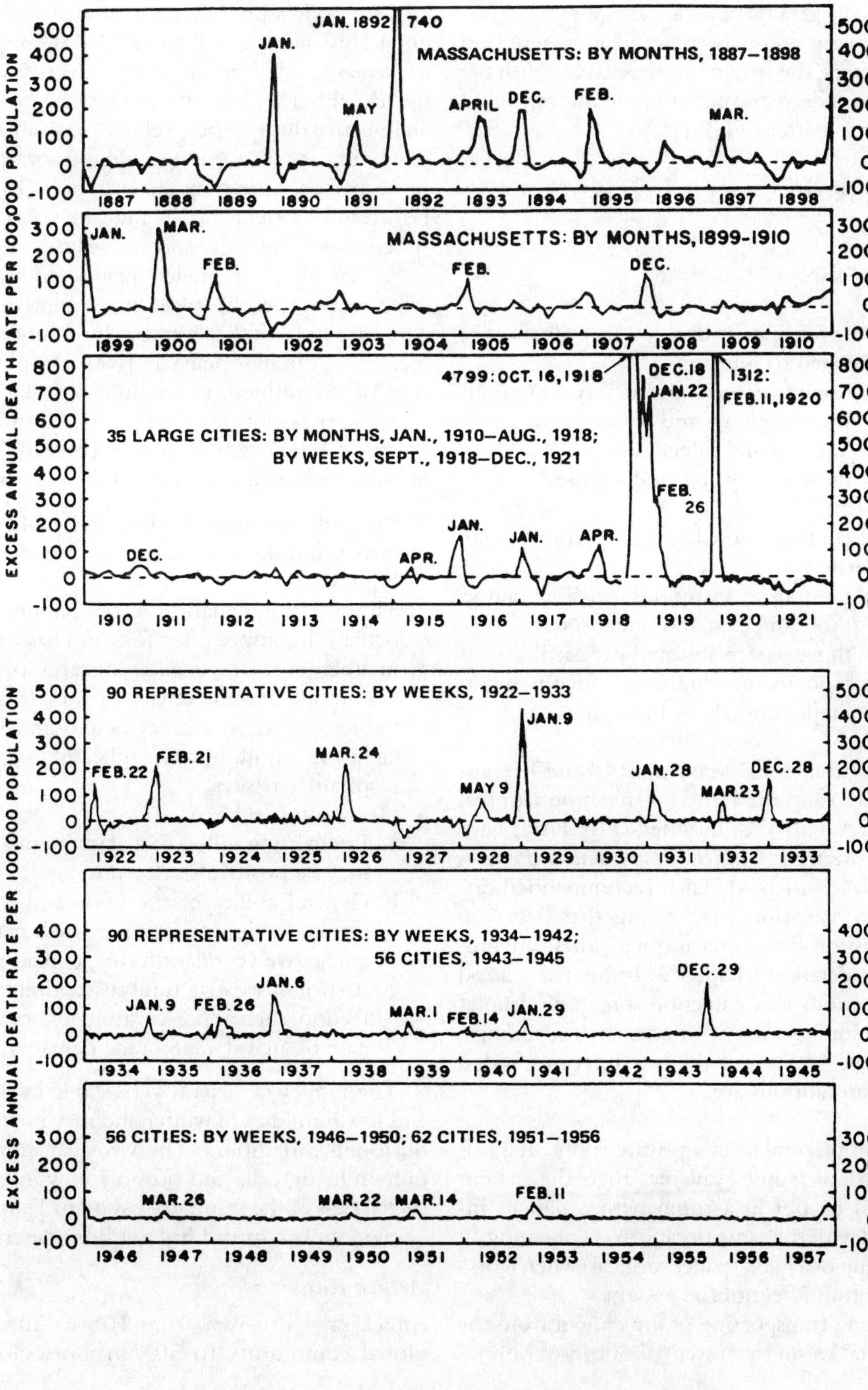

denly as they start. There are also sporadic and isolated cases, and serosurveys often confirm that subclinical, or asymptomatic, epidemics have occurred in the general population. Sporadic or isolated cases can occur anytime and anywhere, and in most cases, the origin is untraceable. With the speed of modern travel, an epidemic can jump oceans in a matter of hours.

TRANSMISSION RISK FACTORS

Infectivity

Influenza is spread by:

1. Airborne respiratory droplets (see Chapter 2) from human to human:
   With: respiratory or upper airway secretions.
   From: the coughing and sneezing of those infected and infectious.
   To: those susceptible and exposed.
   By: air.
2. Direct contact (see Chapter 2), from human to human:
   With: respiratory secretions, possibly saliva.
   From: those infected and infectious.
   To: those susceptible and exposed.
   By mucous membrane to mucous membrane, directly or by fomites.

The Centers for Disease Control and Prevention (CDC) and the Hospital Infection Control Practices Advisory Committee (HICPAC) have jointly written the *Guideline for Isolation Precautions in Hospitals* [68]. Their recommended categories of isolation were changed in 1997 to "transmission-based precautions"; these are presented in detail in Chapter 2. Influenza is listed under "serious viral infection spread by droplet transmission" (along with adenovirus, mumps, parvovirus 19, and rubella). Recommended droplet precautions are:

1. Patient placement in a private room. If a private room is not available, then the patient should be put in a room with a patient infected with the same organism ("cohorting").
2. Wearing of a mask (paper surgical) when working within 3 feet of the patient.
3. Limiting transporting of the patient from the hospital room (for essential purposes only).

The expired infective influenza nuclei is believed to be about 1–5 μm in size [69] and is therefore inspirable into the deep lower lung, past the healthy body's physiologic and anatomic barriers. (This meets the CDC-HICPAC definition of *airborne transmission.*) An infective droplet nuclei (either an infected evaporated droplet or an infective dust particle vehicle) can remain suspended in the air for longer periods of time and be dispersed widely by air currents. Other airborne microorganisms include mycobacterium tuberculosis, rubeola, and varicella.

As few as five particles may be an adequate infective dose for the lower lungs; approximately a hundredfold of that number is required for infection of the nasopharynx [69]. Deep inspiration of the influenza-contaminated expired air of another is the most efficient and infectious means of influenza transmission [69,70]. The infectivity and incubation period then depends on:

1. The dose or number of infective viral particles inspired or direct contact with mucous membranes.
2. The site of inoculation: Deep pulmonary inoculation is more infectious and has a shorter incubation than nasopharyngeal or oral.
3. The individual infectivity of the virus strain (which can have a great range) and its efficiency in invading and replicating in human respiratory tissues.
4. Host factors such as:
   a. Pre-existing full or partial immunity (which may be positively related to age).
   b. General ability of the body and immune system to fight infection, which may have a negative correlation to age in adults.
   c. Anatomic or structural susceptibility to infection, such as pre-existing pulmonary disease or airway membrane damage.

The influenza virus is very stable in the cold and low humidity of winter and may be infective on fomites for hours. The virus can reproduce only in living cells and possibly only in the epithelial cells of the respiratory system. Transfusion or bloodborne spread has not been described.

Attack Rates

Attack rates can vary from 10% to 20% in the global community to 50% in more closed or crowded communities or schools. The highest attack rate recorded is 72% aboard an unventilated aircraft [71]. Population attack rates are also influenced by the four sets of factors mentioned above, plus a fifth factor, which is the virulence or ability of an influenza strain to cause clinical disease. There is a range from predominantly inapparent infection (influenza C) to the 10% fatality rate of the 1918 pandemic. Socioeconomic class also appears to be a factor in community attack rates. Data from the comprehensive Houston observational studies have shown that small children in low-income families are at greater risk than preschool children of middle income families [72,73]. Conversely, people in the higher socioeconomic group may have higher attack rates and more severe illness as adults. Those with a more hygienic and less crowded and exposed childhood will have less immunity as adults. This principle is operational in the attack rates of many other infections, such as hepatitis A, rubella, measles, varicella-zoster virus, mumps, cytomegalovirus (CMV), mononucleosis, and many other herpesviruses. This principle of immunity related to socioeconomic status might also be relevant to adults in their workplace job categories. Those working in crowded or high person-to-person contact positions may, over time, develop better influenza immunity than those working in a more socially protected environment.

Incubation Period

The incubation period for influenza virus is one to five days. Studies have shown that nasal shedding begins one day before the onset of clinical illness [70]. This explains why isolating or cohorting the ill has always failed to prevent transmission. This relatively short incubation period accounts for both the rapid development and the rapid demise of epidemics when the susceptible pool is exhausted or was not exposed or infected.

Infective Period

The period of infectivity is usually up to five days [21] but may be as many as seven days in coughing children [74]. Maximum infectivity occurs when viral concentrations are highest in nasal and respiratory secretions, and this is simultaneous with maximum symptoms [75]. Viral concentrations can be very high and infectivity prolonged in patients with influenza pneumonia [76].

Having all ill and infectious persons remain away from the public during the time of their illness may greatly reduce community and workplace spread. Blunting of the community epidemic curve can be seen when school Christmas vacations occur just after the start of an epidemic [77–79]. There is no evidence that infective periods are prolonged in immunocompromised individuals, nor is there evidence of chronic human carriers of the influenza virus.

Places of Transmission, the Workplace

Any settings where people "mix" in enclosed areas is conducive to the transmission of influenza, especially if ventilation or air exchange is inadequate. These settings include structures such as office buildings, schools, churches, theaters, and nightclubs as well as commercial forms of transportation such as buses, aircraft, and ships and their gates, terminals, and docks. When persons from different geographic areas converge into crowded areas, a single index source can infect large numbers of people. This occurred, for example, aboard a commercial aircraft in Alaska in 1977 [71], when 72% of passengers were infected by a single coughing passenger after the plane was detained 4½ hours. The ventilation system was off during this time. The epidemic was identified because passengers were diverted to an area where all cases were seen by one physician, who initiated an investigation. Outbreaks of influenza are also common on cruise ships [80] when the travel time is shorter than the incubation period. Many outbreaks in traveling military units have been reported. Influenza vaccines should be considered for any travel medicine itinerary.

Community Spread

The first signs of an influenza outbreak classically occurs in primary schools and day care centers. The association is with immature personal and respiratory hygiene and contamination of shared fomites. Influenza A(H3N2) viruses are generally more serious infections in children than influenza A(H1N1) or B [81]. The disease is then brought home to adults by the children. Longitudinal observation studies (in Seattle, Tecumseh, and Houston) have all shown higher attack rates in adults with school-age children in the home. In an eight-year study of Houston families [82], the highest age block for infection was ages 6–10, when 39.3% of the children had influenza illness and 47.7% of the children showed serologic evidence of influenza infection each year. The percentage of attack rates dropped with increasing age, but an average of 33% of adults in families with school-age children had an influenza infection each year.

Adults then transmit influenza to their workplace [79]. That is to say, transmission is "horizontal" among students at school, then "vertical" among generations at home, then "horizontal" again among co-workers in the workplace in the latter part of an epidemic. Longini and colleagues have used data from the Seattle and Tecumseh studies to develop mathematical models to estimate the frequency of community-acquired infection and secondary attack rates [83,84].

Often, the elderly population and shut-ins are the last to be infected. Hospitalization rates rise relatively late in an epidemic season. When the P-I index curves are superimposed on influenza activity curves, it consistently shows that pneumonia mortality peaks about two weeks after the peak of influenza morbidity.

Many communities have *action levels*, a preset percentage of absenteeism during which schools or nonessential businesses may close. The early closing of schools has been a controversial means of aborting an early influenza epidemic. The flattening of the epidemic curve seen with holiday breaks has been hard to reproduce on demand. (Often, it is the high absenteeism of faculty that necessitates school closures.) High absenteeism in primary schools portends heavy absenteeism in the workplace in a matter of a few days to a week or 10 days.

Susceptibility

Susceptibility to influenza is universal. There are no humans born who are immune to influenza infection, although some may have inapparent, subclinical infections. Infection confers immunity to the infecting influenza strain and closely related strains. When a new influenza subtype emerges (i.e., an antigenic shift occurs), people of all ages and locales are susceptible, and a pandemic is possible.

Cross-Species Transmission: the Reservoir?

The origin of new human pathogenic strains has been one of the many mysteries of influenza. Influenza A has its reservoir in many wild birds and domestic farm animals and causes them both clinical and subclinical infections. There is little doubt that the major gene pool and reservoir for mammalian and avian influenza A is wild birds, but direct infection from bird-to-human is rare. Influenza A viruses become pathogenic to humans through a genetic intracellular mixing between strains. This may occur in birds or in humans, but certainly occurs in the domestic pig [85]. The pig may be the genetic "mixing bowl" for new human influenza strains.

The duck ponds on farms in Southern China are places where pigs, humans, and both wild and domestic birds share close contact. All three twentieth-century pandemics can be traced to origins in China. For this reason, the United States supports influenza research and new strain surveillance laboratories on the China mainland. This surveillance monitors animals and the humans in close contact with them, as an early warning system for the next pandemic [64]. Documented cases of transmission to or from humans remains mostly isolated and anecdotal. At this writing, there has not been a sustained human influenza epidemic that can be directly documented to have begun with animal-to-human transmission. Nor is there solid evidence that an animal species is serving as the reservoir for a recycling human influenza. It is very plausible, and even probable, that both occur, but this theory has so far escaped proof by the scientific method. It is interesting and fortunate to note that none of our more popular pet animals (cats, dogs, or parrots) have been found to carry influenza A. Nor has influenza B or C been found to be infectious to animals.

Much is written on the interspecies transmission of influenza and the potential threat of a new pandemic of animal origin. Please refer to any of the excellent reviews prepared by Webster and colleagues [86–88] for more information.

OCCUPATIONAL RISK FACTORS

Exposure to Children

All observational and community studies show that the first signs of an influenza outbreak occurs in schools and day care centers. Children may have greater susceptibility and therefore higher attack rates than adults and may also have a longer period of infectivity. The immature personal hygiene and normal behavior of children may be contributory (e.g., not covering their face when coughing or sneezing, not washing their hands, and contaminating shared toys and other fomites with their saliva or respiratory secretions). Adult day care workers, teachers, and pediatric clinic employees may be the earliest adults infected and should receive early vaccination for influenza each year.

Prolonged Face-to-Face Exposure

Prolonged one-on-one exposure to a single individual in a ventilation zone of a meter or less can increase the chances of obtaining an infective viral dose. Occupations with such contact include dentists and dental hygienists, hairdressers and barbers, manicurists, massage and physical therapists, taxi drivers, and benefit agency workers. Unfortunately, none of these professions are included in the occupations recommended for annual immunization by the CDC [89]. The risk may be even higher if contact with an infected individual or individuals occurs in enclosed or poorly ventilated areas during cold weather.

High-Volume Population Exposure

Exposure can also be related to a high volume of brief encounters with the general public or in handling fomites such as money or tickets. Workers with this type of exposure include cafeteria cashiers and other food service workers, ticket takers, receptionists, tellers, sales and counter clerks, and even politicians on handshaking campaigns. These high-risk occupations should be considered in recommending influenza vaccine or anti-influenza medications for workers.

Enclosed Areas

Perhaps the greatest risk is associated with places where large numbers of persons from wide geographic areas gather in enclosed quarters for long periods of time. This type of exposure occurs in airline work, military barracks, college or boarding school dormitories, military ships or submarines, jails and detention centers, and tour buses. Temporary or episodic gatherings in offices or other sealed energy-efficient buildings also may increase exposure risk. These occur in cafeteria lines, time clock lines, or meetings. Designated smoking areas may also be transmission points, serving as nidi of higher risk, coughing employees. A designated smoking area may still be preferred to a no-smoking policy, which often provokes workers to "meet and sneak" a smoke in poorly ventilated closets, toilet stalls, or other confined spaces.

Schools and Universities

Classroom students are particularly susceptible to all communicable respiratory or orally transmitted infections, including influenza, mycoplasma, mononucleosis, CMV, meningococcal meningitis, streptococcus, and other respiratory viruses. Student-related risk factors include:

- Younger age and therefore less acquired immunity to influenza strains.
- Crowding in classes, dorms, and lines for registrations or meals.
- Frequent social gatherings or sporting events, either as participants or spectators.
- Dancing, kissing, or more intimate sexual contact.
- Antigen "melting pot," as students from wide geographic areas converge after traveling in mass commercial transportation (buses, aircraft, trains).

University students have been readily available subjects for study through campus student health services. Studies conducted on campus students have included analysis of individual risk factors, vaccine-efficacy trails, antiviral-drug efficacy [90], seroprevalence studies [91], age-related attack rates for Russian flu [92], and pulmonary function and influenza [90] and are the first studies to show that two antigenic variants can cocirculate in a given season [93]. Most notable has been the extensive studies conducted by the late Dr. Alfred S. Evans on students at Yale, the University of Wisconsin [94], and at a university in the Philippines [95]. His studies show very little difference in campus epidemics among students in temperate climates versus those in tropical climates, but his study conducted in the Philippines did find that Philippine students very rarely have group A streptococcus, mycoplasma pneumonia, adenovirus, or Epstein-Barr infections. The symptoms of ILI are more specific for influenza contracted in a tropical environment.

Influenza is a risk for all students, but that risk may decrease with each year on campus, as one's immunity matures [94]. These serial serologic surveys show that as many as 4% of students have inapparent (subclinical) influenza infections. Taking one or more fall semester final examinations while ill is nearly a rite of passage for North American students.

The Military

Wars have been lost and empires have collapsed because of respiratory epidemics. Most military personnel, especially new recruits reporting for basic training, have the same risk factors listed above for students. Basic training is a risk epidemiologically equivalent to the freshman year. The dynamics of influenza epidemics can often be traced by troop movements [96] and is often the source of infection for civilian populations [97]. The onset of the 1986 influenza epidemic in the United States can be directly traced to a returning Navy squadron [96].

Troops have been the subject of influenza studies [98], influenza-vaccine complication studies [99], and vaccine-efficacy trials [100]. The Commission of Influenza of the Armed Forces Epidemiological Board (in the Department of Defense) monitored effectiveness of influenza vaccine and provided the most quoted statistic, "70–90 percent effective," for influenza vaccines [89]. The military is the one exception to influenza vaccinations being voluntary.

Animal Exposure

Only nine cases of documented transmission of swine influenza to humans have been reported; several cases were fatal [48–53]. At least two cases occurred despite state-of-the-art precautions in a research facility. Nonetheless, it is known that much of the Earth's domestic swine population is endemically infected with influenza A subtype H1N1. A study performed in Austria in 1994 showed that 24.5% of that country's fattening pigs, on 41% of Austrian farms, had antibodies to A(H1N1) [101]. A subsequent seroprevalence study of 137 veterinarians in Austria found that 8.8% were positive for this A(H1N1) [102]. A statistically significant number ($p \leq 0.01$) of these positive individuals were swine practitioners.

A complete review of all animal influenza studies is beyond the scope of this text. There are no practical or routine precautions recommended for influenza protection in livestock animal handlers, other than receiving the yearly influenza vaccine and the general precautions of hand washing and avoiding direct mucous membrane contact with any animal respiratory fluids. A virulent human influenza pandemic originating from a pig, chicken, or other animal remains a theoretical day-to-day threat to the human population.

The Health Care Setting

Health care workers (HCWs) in health care institutions, and health care students in training, have risks similar to those listed above for classroom students. In addition, there is the direct hands-on contact that HCWs have with the sickest, hospitalized influenza sufferers. There are many reports of nosocomial epidemics of influenza [10,11]; health care workers may be the index cases for these [12], especially in long-term or chronic care facilities where the residents have limited exposure to others [9,103–107].

Health care workers are always a top priority for immunization programs [89]. Many advisory and accrediting agencies require or strongly recommend that employers offer influenza immunizations to their employees [108]. A recent randomized vaccine study of both HCWs and residents of long-term facilities in Scotland showed reduced patient mortality (odds ratio of 0.56) if over 60% of employees were immunized [109]. Immunizations of employees produced a better clinical outcome for the residents than for the workers themselves.

Nevertheless health care workers probably do not have a higher overall rate of influenza infection than the general public. During an especially severe influenza season, this author conducted a nonscientific survey of ILI-associated absenteeism within our three-hospital network (Community Hospitals of Indianapolis). The survey covered a 30-day period from mid-December 1993 to mid-January 1994 and included absenteeism reports from 115 departments of nearly 5,000 employees. The overall influenza-like-illness rate for direct caregivers in the hospital was 40.7%. The insurance office workers located off campus and with no patient contact had an 89.5% ILI rate. But 77.8% of the ill hospital caregivers used sick days compared to only 29.4% of the insurance office workers. Our county health department had requested that direct caregivers stay at home when symptomatic. These recommendations were publicized in employee newsletters, bulletin boards, and in other highly visible places in the facilities. The higher percentage of ill clinical workers staying home may show some evidence of compliance.

Of particular interest were two urgent care centers serving similar populations and patient volumes. The North Clinic, a temporary modular building with poor ventilation had 15 employees, all of whom lost work from illness in the 30-day period. None of the 10 employees in the newer and well-ventilated East Clinic were ill during that same period.

Immunosuppressed health care workers have dual indications for immunization and should also be considered for antiviral chemoprophylaxis by their primary care physician. There has been no advantage achieved from giving two-dose immunizations to HIV-infected workers [110].

The Aerospace Environment

Very little has been published on respiratory infection in space travel, and there have been very few respiratory infections reported during space flight. Having an ILI disqualifies an astronaut from a mission, as was dramatically presented in the 1995 film *Apollo 13*.

Since the infective influenza virus is only a few microns in size, it is relatively unaffected by gravity. A biophysical model in a paper by Knight and colleagues [69] speculates that influenza may actually be less infectious in zero gravity. But respiratory disease with larger infective particles (over 20 μm) may be more infective in zero gravity than in gravity, since, at zero gravity, they are free-floating and have the potential for inoculation by in-spiration.

Prevention and Control

ADMINISTRATIVE CONTROLS

The primary preventive measure for influenza is immunization; antiviral medications are a distant secondary measure. Employers may not be able to control influenza as they might other occupational risks. But activities can be directed toward supporting employees' utilization of sick-time benefits. The following dozen suggestions represent this author's own ideas developed from 20 years of on-site and institutional medical practice. Employers may take small steps to improve morale for the working ill and possibly reduce workplace transmission or absenteeism. These may include:

- Providing boxes of tissues in widely available locations, with waste containers in very close proximity.
- Providing fresh drinking water or juices in widely available locations, with an ample supply of disposal drinking cups.
- Putting up signs reminding employees to cover their face while coughing or sneezing and to wash their hands after possible contamination with respiratory or oral secretions.
- Offering temporary or brief periods of "amnesty" from termination for those calling in sick when they have no sick-time entitlement. Employees feeling forced to work even while ill could diminish workplace productivity and promote workplace infectivity.

Administrative actions to preserve productivity may include:

- Allowing partial sick days or "sick hours" for those who need to leave because of illness.
- Relieving or reducing any procedural "hoops" for getting time-off for doctor visits for the worker or their dependent family members.

More long-range or proactive planning may include:

- Having "action levels" of absenteeism at which certain nonessential departments or work areas will close.
- Considering temporary or contingency "work-at-home" options for employees in positions in which this may be possible.
- Providing on-site day care for ill children of employees (if practical and local regulations permit).

Actions for those employers or agencies who maintain on-site occupational nursing or dispensaries may include:

- Considering extended hours to cover shift workers.
- Being well stocked with symptomatic medications and self-treatment printouts for influenza or common cold sufferers.
- Providing or arranging for discounts for antiviral medications (e.g., amantadine, rimantadine) prescribed by their own physician through benefits prescription plans or called into the dispensary (check local dispensing laws).

Ideally, employers should be able to track vacation or elective days off versus days off for illness or influenza-like illness. This is the only way to track true absenteeism due to influenza or to conduct studies on the efficacy of immunization or other steps for prevention or intervention [19]. Employers may also insist that their health insurance vendors have prevention programs and have adequate availability of primary care physicians near the worksite(s). Employers may also insist that deductibles for after-hour or urgent-care clinics be financially reasonable.

When prevention fails, the best advice is for ill employees to remain at home during times of peak symptoms. Symptoms correlate positively with infectivity. This is especially important in health care or long-term care facilities, where ill employees may infect their patients.

Once the influenza virus has invaded a worksite, influenza vaccine is not a practical solution. The immunizations may take two weeks to confer immunity, and stocks of vaccine may be exhausted by the time the epidemic begins. Neither is antiviral medications a full substitute for immunization.

SAFE WORK PRACTICES AND ENGINEERING CONTROLS

Ventilation

Controlled scientific studies of the association between ventilation and human influenza activity have not been conducted, but there have been enough episodic reports [70,96,97,111,112] of high infectivity rates in poorly ventilated areas to lend evidence to this logical and plausible assumption. The National Institute for Occupational Safety and Health (NIOSH) proposal for indoor air quality states:

> Building-related illnesses can result in serious illness and death. Indoor transmission of diseases caused by obligate pathogens (microbes that require a living host) is common in indoor environments, especially those that are overcrowded and inadequately ventilated. Diseases in this category include influenza, rhinovirus or colds, and measles.

Whenever possible, and when the task and facilities allow, workstations should be designed to allow 2–3 feet between the faces of workers and their co-workers, customers, or clients.

If the presumed 5-μm-or-less size of the infective influenza particle is correct, then influenza should technically fall under "Airborne Precautions" rather than "Droplet Precautions" under HICPAC recommendations [68]. This level of precaution calls for a private room with negative pressure of 6–12 air exchanges per hour and vented either into a high-efficiency particulate air (HEPA) filter or outdoors. The tuberculosis isolation and controls [113,114] (HEPA filtration, negative pressure rooms, N-95 respirators) could be the best "packaged process" when victims of a virulent strain receive medical care. No information is available on the effects of ultraviolet light on the influenza virus, however.

Research or laboratory workers who may be handling human respiratory secretions or other biologic hazards should do so only if wearing proper face protection or under a class II (or III) biological safety cabinet [115]. Those handling respiratory fluids from humans or other animals known to carry influenza, or material that may have been in contact with the cloaca of potentially infected avian species, are recommended to follow biosafety level 2 practices [47]. Note that these guidelines were published in 1993, before the swine-to-worker cases that were reported in 1997 despite level 3 precautions [46]. The best advice for those working with animals is, as for everyone, annual influenza immunizations and frequent hand washing after any biologic contamination.

Safe Work Practices

Appropriate safe work practices need to be specific for each workplace and its inherent tasks. For example, day care workers should wash their hands frequently after potential contamination with children's respiratory or oral secretions. Some principles apply to all workplaces, however. These are:

1. Good general housekeeping and clean, well-maintained hand-washing (and hand-drying) facilities in restrooms.
2. Trash containers should be readily available in all work areas and should be lined to minimize direct handling of trash by custodians.
3. Those who handle money or other potentially infected fomites (e.g., cashiers, ticket takers, ushers) should wash their hands before and after work and before and after meals. They should avoid hand-to-mouth or other mucous-membrane contact in the interim, between hand washings.

During influenza epidemics, employers may consider some methods of avoiding the "herding" of employees. Employers could consider staggering some daily activities, namely:

1. Staggering work times to avoid congestion at elevators, stairwells, and time clocks.
2. Staggering mealtimes to avoid cafeteria lines.

There are more formal recommendations for health care institutions to follow when dealing with their staff and with influenza patients [68,108]. Specific infection control education is also mandated by various regulations and local statutes for health care facilities. The 1994 CDC Recommendations for the Prevention of Nosocomial Influenza [68, section III-D] states:

> As much as possible during periods of influenza activity in the community, have the hospital's employee health service evaluate patient-care staff who have symptoms of febrile upper respiratory tract infection suggestive of influenza for possible removal from duties that involve direct patient contact. Use more stringent guidelines for staff working in certain patient-care areas, e.g., ICUs, Nurseries, and units with severely immunosuppressed patients.

These recommendations also suggest restricting hospital visitors who have a febrile respiratory illness.

The only absolute protection is complete isolation from other humans from late fall to early spring, yearly. The only practical protections remain vaccination, the observance of good personal hygiene by covering the face when coughing or sneezing, and politely encouraging the same behavior in symptomatic co-workers.

PERSONAL PROTECTIVE EQUIPMENT

> Obey the laws and wear the gauze. Protect your jaws from septic paws.
>
> —Rhyme propagated by the San Francisco Board of Health during the 1918 Pandemic. (Citizens could be jailed for not wearing their gauze masks.)

Personal protective equipment is not generally available nor practical for influenza control; although dental professionals, respiratory therapists, and others who are directly exposed to respiratory secretions (or who exposure their patients) should wear paper masks or face shields, or both. The plausible conclusion is that influenza transmission is probably not interrupted by wearing a regular paper surgical mask within 3 feet.

If a health care institution chooses to apply "airborne" rather than "droplet" HICPAC precautions for influenza, NIOSH-approved N-95 masks developed for tuberculosis protection could theoretically protect one from influenza. These masks filter below 1 μm, but no agency or organization has yet recommended the use of N-95 masks for influenza control, nor have studies been conducted on their effectiveness for influenza. These masks require training and fit testing and are more expensive than regular surgical paper masks. They would be routinely available only in facilities where potentially infectious tuberculosis patients may receive care (see Chapter 9).

EMPLOYEE EDUCATION AND TRAINING

Education in good personal hygiene should include covering the mouth and nose when coughing or sneezing. Employees should wash their hands if there has been mucous contamination of the hands or if they have had contact with objects possibly contaminated by the respiratory or oral secretions of others.

Many non-health-care employers are finding personal communicable disease prevention programs to be useful within their periodic training and development or health promotion programs. "Preventing Communicable Disease" is a topic appearing on training and development agendas along with timely topics on preventing workplace violence and preventing sexual harassment. Commercial products such as Glo-Germ can aid training in hand-washing techniques.

Employees should be trained to seek early and adequate treatment when they first have symptoms of infection. This may shorten the time of illness, prevent organ damage or failure, and prevent secondary bacterial infection. Non-health-care workers should also be encouraged to stay home when ill with symptoms of influenza, and such directives at times may be given from health departments. Employees should also be encouraged to "save" some sick days for when they are actually ill, so they will be less likely to report to work when ill but out of sick leave.

Most important is employee education about the value of the influenza vaccine, and a concerted effort by the employer to remove negative myths and misconceptions regarding influenza vaccines. This education should include the information that the vaccine is dead and does not and cannot cause nor spread influenza. The information should be in the language and writing style appropriate for the worker. The employer can share the "when's and where's" of local immunization efforts with their employees if unable to directly provide immunization on-site. An excellent public promotion package for the Medicare population [65] is the U.S. "Fight Flu" Program (*http://www.fightflu.hcfa*) (Figure 11-2). This web address has uncopyrighted color posters available for downloading. An excellent multipage fact sheet on influenza for the consumer is available from the National Institute of Allergy and Infectious Disease at *http://www.niaid.nih.gov/factsheets.flu.htm*.

Health care workers should be taught the importance of receiving immunizations as recommended by the CDC [68] and trained to answer questions on influenza vaccine asked by their patients. All workers in health care should be knowledgeable about influenza and be able to encourage vaccination and other precautions for their patients. It is unacceptable for physicians or other health care professionals to discourage patients from receiving influenza immunization based on their own ignorance or limited personal experiences.

MEDICAL SURVEILLANCE

International Surveillance

It is only a question of when, not if, the next pandemic will occur. International surveillance has been coordinated by the World Health Or-

Figure 11-2 / Example of a color poster available on the Internet: US "Fight Flu" Program [65].

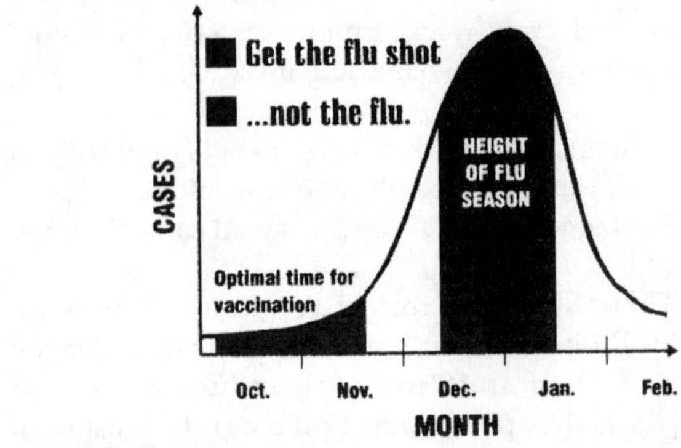

ganization since 1970 and is extensive, expensive, and truly global. An excellent source of information on influenza data should exist in the former U.S.S.R., where all clinic visits were reported to a central computerized database. This same database was used to confirm excuses for work or school absence. Unfortunately, no studies analyzing this data have been published since 1977 [116].

A comparison of new antigenic variants of influenza found in laboratory experiments performed on sera from representative populations is one method used to predict population susceptibility and severity of epidemics. Information collected from influenza epidemics in various parts of the world is used in decisions about vaccine valency. The United States supports influenza research and new-strain surveillance laboratories on the China mainland. This surveillance includes animals and humans in close contact with animals, as an early warning system for possible epidemics [64].

United States Surveillance

Surveillance in the United States is coordinated by the Centers for Disease Control and Prevention, National Center for Infectious Disease, in Atlanta. Influenza is not a reportable illness in the U.S. and is not linked to the National Notifiable Disease System (NNDSS), but local and state health departments like to know of outbreaks or clustering of influenza-like-illness, including reports from the workplace. In the United States, influenza surveillance has four levels:

1. *U.S./WHO Collaborating Laboratory Surveillance System:* Most of these 70 laboratories are within state or local health departments, and some are within universities or hospital networks. Each week of October through May, the collaborating labs report the total number of specimens received for respiratory virus testing and the number of influenza-positive isolates of A[H1N1], A[H3N2], A[non-specific], and B. All donors are typed by age groups: 1, 1–4, 5–24, 25–44, 45–64, 65 or over, or unknown. Beginning in 1998, information has been electronically submitted to the CDC. Some representative isolates are submitted to the WHO Collaborating Center for Surveillance, Epidemiology, and Control of Influenza at the CDC for complete antigenic characterization and antiviral resistance testing.
2. *Sentinel Physician Surveillance Network:* Each week from October through May, approximately 140 preselected and representative primary care providers, or "sentinel" physicians, report the number of patient visits for the week and the number of those patients who were examined for influenza-like illness, according to the above age groups. Some of the physicians collect nasal and throat swabs for virus isolation in the Collaborating Labs. This data is reported to the CDC. Sentinel physicians may also participate in other community health surveillance projects, such as lead levels.
3. *The 122 U.S. Cities Surveillance System:* Vital statistics from 122 major U.S. cities representing about half of the U.S. population are reviewed weekly. Recorded are (1) the number of death certificates filed due to all causes and (2) the number of deaths for which pneumonia was identified as the underlying cause of death and for which influenza was mentioned in any position on the certificate. This information is reported to the Epidemiology Program Office (EPO) of the CDC each week. A seasonal baseline is calculated using the proportion of pneumonia and influenza deaths observed since 1983 (the P-I Index). If that number varies by a statistically significant amount, influenza deaths are said to be above epidemic threshold (excess mortality).
4. *State and Territorial Epidemiologist's Report:* In each week of October through May the epidemiologists from each state or territory report the estimated level of influenza activity in their area as:
   - No Activity.
   - Sporadic Activity, defined as sporadically occurring cases of influenza-like illness or culture-confirmed influenza, with no outbreaks detected.
   - Regional Activity, defined as outbreaks of influenza-like illness or culture-confirmed influenza occurring in counties representing less than or equal to 50% of that state or territory's population.

- Widespread Activity, defined as outbreaks of influenza-like illness or culture-confirmed influenza occurring in counties representing over 50% of that state or territory's population.

These reports comes to EPO-CDC via the National Electronic Telecommunications Systems for Surveillance (NETSS). Methods used to make this determination vary from state to state and may include local sentinel physician networks, reports on increased visits for respiratory illness to hospital emergency rooms or outpatient clinics, school or worksite absenteeism reporting, nursing home surveillance, and reports of laboratory-diagnosed influenza.

Other Surveillance Definitions

- *Expanded reporting period:* Influenza can occur at any time of the year. Information on isolates in the summer may provide valuable information on the strain coming in the usual season.
- *Expanded sources of surveillance:* State epidemiologists or local health officials may request that other institutions or facilities assist in data collection to accommodate special needs for information.

Published Sources of Surveillance Data

A report titled *Prevention and Control of Influenza: Recommendations of the Advisory Committee on Immunization Practices (ACIP)* [89] is published by the CDC each year in late April or early May as part of the *Morbidity and Mortality Weekly Report's* "Recommendations and Reports" co-subscription. The report includes information on the trivalent vaccines being prepared for the upcoming season, updates on influenza epidemiology, recommendations for targeted groups, timing of vaccination, and the latest antiviral medication protocols for influenza. It is the best annual source for influenza information and is available over the Internet at *http://www.cdc.gov/epo/mmwr/mmwr*. A weekly "Influenza Update Summary, for the week ending mm/dd/yyyy" is posted by the CDC and can be viewed, download, or printed from the Internet at *http://www.cdc.gov/ncidod/diseases/flu/weekly.html*. The report includes a map of the 50 states shaded by their influenza activity levels (Figure 11-3).

Surveillance information is available through the CDC Voice Information Systems at 888-232-3228 or by fax document #361100 at 888-232-3299. These reports include percentages of upper respiratory illnesses that have cultured positive for influenza, the prevalent strains, and age-related trends.

Individual cases of influenza are not investigated. Exceptions are the severe or fatal cases with rare complications (e.g., encephalitis, myocarditis, rhabdomyolysis) that may suggest an especially virulent strain with specific organ pathogenicity. Other exceptions include influenza suspected to be of animal origin. These influenza A viruses that cannot be subtyped by hemagglutination inhibition testing using the standard H1N1 antisera included in the influenza reagent kit distributed by the CDC should be sent to the CDC influenza branch immediately. In any of these situations, the State Health Department and the Influenza Branch of the CDC (404-639-3591) should be contacted immediately.

Excess Mortality and the P-I Death Index

Since 1918, excess mortality has systematically been used as an index for the recognition of influenza epidemics. The method of data collection was further refined by Collins and Lehmann [117]. Figure 11-1 is from a monograph published in 1957 [118] and provides graphic evidence of influenza epidemics over a 70-year period in the state of Massachusetts and major U.S. cities. The graph is one year short of catching another pandemic.

The methodology of tracking excess mortality was refined by CDC biostatistician R. E. Serfling [119] in 1963. He used a linear regression function to represent data in a smoother sine curve and to produce advanced warning of variation and excess deaths. Excess mortality is now called the *P-I deaths* (pneumonia and influenza attributable deaths) and is a method of reporting developed by Choi and Thacker in 1981 [120]. This is the statistic reported weekly in the *Morbidity and Mortality Weekly Report*, from 122 U.S. cities of greater than 100,000 population, and on the CDC web site.

Figure 11-3 / Example of a Weekly Influenza Activity Report. (From National Centers for Infectious Disease, Centers for Disease Control and Prevention, available on the Internet at *http://www.cdc.gov/ncidod/diseases/flu/weekly.html*).

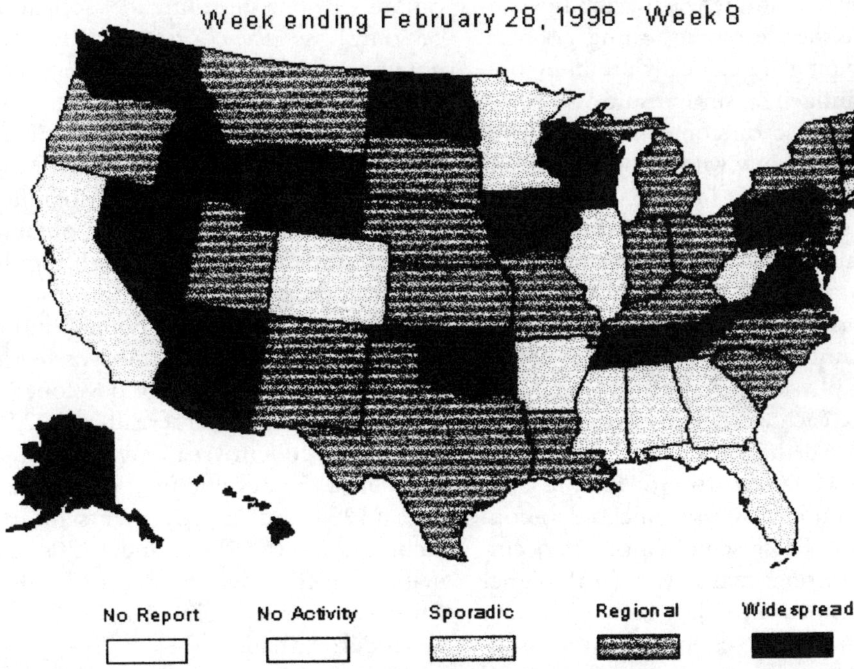

The defined *epidemic threshold* occurs when 7.2% of all deaths are attributable to pneumonia and influenza. This represents 1.645 standard deviations above the seasonal baseline. The expected seasonal baseline is projected using a robust regression procedure in which a periodic regression model is applied to observed percentages of deaths from P-I since 1983. Simonsen and colleagues have recently proposed adding a *severity index* to the equation, for more accurately comparing the severity of individual epidemics [121].

Deaths "officially" or directly attributable to influenza may only be a fraction of the deaths in which influenza was a precipitating factor. Those with pre-existing cardiac or pulmonary disease have a higher mortality from influenza, but this may not be reflected in their death certificates. Nosology protocols give a higher preference to the cardiac and pulmonary International Classification of Disease (ICD) codes. At present, at least 45,000 Americans die each year from combined influenza and pneumonia, ranking it as the sixth leading cause of death.

Family and Observational Studies

The most reliable morbidity data on influenza comes from longitudinal studies of defined and natural populations, or *observational studies.* These studies depend on the use of serosurveys to study patterns of infection and patterns of spread. It is from these studies that infectivity rates, community patterns of spread, and serosurvey data has been gathered. The largest studies have been conducted in Tecumseh, Cleveland, Seattle, and Houston. The Influenza Research Center in Houston has been the most prolific source of information on community-wide influenza.

Biologic Testing

Embryonated hen's eggs were the very first cultures used for diagnosing influenza and remain the standard culture technique. Various monkey-kidney cultures are far superior but in recent years have become too expensive for routine use. Individual clinical influenza infection is proved by a fourfold increase in influenza-specific IgM antibody titer. Neither serologic testing nor viral culturing and typing are clinically useful in individual cases of influenza, since results will be returned after the case outcome is determined. Such testing is done only within the formal surveillance systems described above or in various academic or research projects. The network of laboratories capable of conducting influenza studies is maintained by WHO and the CDC. The major coordinating reference and "indexing" labs are maintained in Atlanta and London.

The sentinel physicians report the number of patients they see each week who have symptoms that meet the case definition of ILI. These symptoms are nearly 100% sensitive for finding cases of influenza, but under 50% specific for lab-confirmed influenza. These same symptoms occurring in tropical settings may have a much higher specificity for influenza [95]. A certain number of these patients are selected for laboratory studies. Blood is returned to reference labs and cultured and/or serotyped at public expense. It is from these local reports that national trends are reported in the influenza weekly reports in the *Morbidity and Mortality Weekly Report* and on the Internet. Employer-based medical clinics have not traditionally been a part of the sentinel system, and this is one reason that scientific knowledge on influenza in the workplace is less than adequate. An on-site occupational clinic could be an epidemiologically ideal source for study, especially if the clinic is well staffed and efficient and cares for a stable work-force population, with little year-to-year change in demographic variables. A major corporation or occupational medical professional organization could be in an excellent position to initiate such observational studies or to conduct clinical trials of administrative, environmental, or behavioral control studies of influenza.

Pre- and Postexposure Influenza Vaccine

Influenza vaccine is the best method available for preventing the disease, even though it is one of the least efficacious of civilian vaccines and its efficacy and utilization varies from year to year. Influenza vaccination is not considered a routine adult or childhood immunization, but is recommended for specific populations. Antiviral medications are not a substitute for vaccination, as they can only lessen the course of the disease and cannot prevent infection. Influenza vaccines are provided free to Medicare B recipients, members of most state Medicaid plans, and members of many HMO or private insurance plans. Many health care plans restrict the availability of influenza vaccination—that is, they make it obtainable with restrict availability only through the designated primary care provider.

History of the Vaccine. Human influenza was first isolated in chicken embryos in the 1930s, and the first vaccines were developed from the allantoic fluid shortly thereafter [122]. The vaccinations frequently caused symptomatic reactions until the development of the zonal centrifuge [123] and improvements in attenuation techniques in the 1960s and 1970s. Only information on the adverse effects of influenza vaccines made available since the 1970s is applicable to modern vaccine [124].

Valency Selection Process ("the Committee"). The Food and Drug Administration's Vaccine and Related Biological Products Advisory Committee (VRBPAC) recommends three strains to U.S. vaccine product makers. Decisions are based on antigenic analyses of recently isolated influenza viruses and the antibody responses of persons vaccinated in the previous season. The vaccination strains must be selected nine to 10 months before the season, with no assurance that the selections are accurate or that antigenic drift may not occur by the time product is shipped. There are two major subtypes of influenza A in circulation: H1N1 and H3N2 (see Table 11-1). The vaccine is updated annually to include the three strains most likely to circulate (a trivalent vaccine). Usually this is one of each circulating A-subtype strain and one B-strain. One or more will change from the previous year. Although the current influenza vaccine may contain one or more of the antigens administered in previous years, annual vaccination with the current vaccine is necessary, since immunity declines in the year following a vaccination. Product remaining from the previous season should not be used. Annual changes made in the valency are reasons to retake the vaccine each year, and any similarity is not justification to avoid the vaccine. Repeated exposures to the same antigen can booster immunity [19].

Detailed information on the vaccine, the coming influenza season, and any changes in recommendations is published in the *Morbidity and Mortality Weekly Report, Recommendations and Reports* in late April or early May, and at the Internet address *http://www.cdc.gov/epo/mmwr/mmwr_rr.html.*

Influenza Vaccine Products Available in the United States. It takes months to produce, package, and distribute the vaccine each year, plus a month or more for nationwide administration. Seventy million doses are given in the United States each year. If a pandemic were to emerge, the manufacturing process could switch to a monovalent vaccine in order to maximize production, but there may not be time to produce enough vaccine to protect the entire population. The variability of the egg market and supply may also affect production during a crisis. (This is not affected by the price of tea in China, but rather by the price of eggs.)

In 1996/1997, Parke-Davis voluntarily initiated a recall of some vaccine product because of decreased potency of one component antigen, A/Nanchang/933/95(H3N2). The company discovered and reported the problem during their own postmanufacturing surveillance. This was not a product safety issue [125], but the company did drop out of the market for the following year. The vaccine is made from highly purified, egg-grown viruses that have been made noninfectious (inactivated). The methods of production may vary among manufacturers and may include both proprietary purification methods and the use of antibiotics. All contain the mercury-based preservative thimerosal that is found in many other vaccines and which in rare cases can cause localized allergic reactions.

Current U.S. Products, As of 1998.

- Fluvirin, Evans/Medina Medical Limited, 1-800-932-1950. Contains thimerosal 0.01% (1:10,000). Polymyxin, neomycin, and beta-propiolactone is used in manufacturing but cannot be detected in the final product. This is a surface antigen, or "split-virus," vaccine. The dose is 0.5 mL intramuscularly. The manufacturer states that the vaccine is contraindicated for individuals under the age of 4.
- FluShield, Wyeth-Ayerst, 1-800-358-7443. Uses no more than 5 μg of gentamicin sulfate, which is not detectable in the final product. Also contains thimerosal, 1:10,000. The manufacturing process adds the step of disrupting the lipid-containing membrane of the virus. The dose is 0.5 mL intramuscularly.
- Fluzone, Connaught Laboratories, 1-800-822-2463. Also uses thimerosal but does not use antibiotics in manufacturing. The manufacturing process also adds the step of disrupting the lipid-containing membrane of the virus. The dose is 0.5 mL intramuscularly.
- Fluogen, Parke-Davis. Not marketed in 1997/1998 [126].

Mechanism of Action. All of the influenza vaccines used in North America contain killed virus and work as a passive vaccine. All of these products are "split-virus," "subvirion," or "purified surface antigen." Whole-virus vaccines have a history of increased febrile reactions and side effects and are not recommended for children under the age of 13.

Children who have not previously been exposed to influenza have a primary antibody response to the vaccine, and for children under age 9, it is recommended they have a second dose to achieve an adequate antibody titer. The second dose should be given no sooner than 30 days after the first, but still before December. Most re-vaccinated adults and children develop high postvaccination hemagglutination-inhibition (HI) antibody titers in a booster-type immune response. These antibody titers are protective against illness caused by strains similar to those in the vaccine or the related variants that may emerge during outbreak periods [89]—that is, there may be an adequate booster reaction even if the two vaccine antigens are not exactly the same.

Elderly persons and persons with certain chronic diseases may develop lower postvaccination antibody titers than healthy young adults and may remain susceptible. If such persons develop influenza-like illness despite vaccination, the vaccine can still be effective in preventing lower respiratory tract involvement or other secondary complications. Vaccine reduces the risk of hospitalization and death.

Lasting antibodies to influenza are of the IgG class and are specifically reactive against the hemagglutinin and neuraminidase portions of the vaccine strain. Population data have shown that serum HI antibody titers correlate inversely with the occurrence of influenza virus infection [127]. Antibody titers peak at about 10–14 days after a vaccine booster and then decline over the coming months. This is the primary reason for the recommendation of annual re-vaccination.

The vaccine antigen stimulates production of antibodies only to the three strains. The vaccine will fail if infection is overwhelming or if the infecting strain is not closely related to the vaccine antigen and will not offer cross-protection from respiratory illness caused by other viruses or bacteria.

Timing: When To Immunize. Vaccine must be ordered months in advance, and supplies may be depleted before the epidemics actually start. Estimating the volume of vaccine to order should be based on past experience. Utilization may vary from year to year, depending on the extent of the epidemic, severity of symptoms, and media coverage.

Epidemics occur from October to May in North America. Activity is usually low until December, with peaks usually occurring in late November to early March, although new subtypes may circulate a month or two earlier. An unusually early report of widespread activity may be taken as a sign of a highly vulnerable population and a severe epidemic. Vaccine products are usually available sometime in September, and the ideal time for immunizing persons in the general population is mid-October to mid-November (see Figure 11-2).

Health officials may issue recommendations for earlier immunization. Vaccine can be given later, however, especially if there is reason to believe that peak activity will occur later in the season, but no opportunities should be missed to offer vaccination to high-risk patients or workers when they visit a health care provider's office or clinic.

Recently there has been a pattern of offering discount influenza vaccines in "we are the first" marketing campaigns by supermarkets, pharmacies, and shopping malls. Public immunization dates may be moving to an earlier time each year, and "herd" immunization could be falling by the time of peak activity several months later. The vaccine should be offered up to as late as April in some years (if available). Clinics doing international travel preparation should consider having extra vaccine products available for the off-season.

Who Should Be Immunized. GENERAL GUIDELINES. Influenza vaccine is strongly recommended for anyone 6 months or older who, because of age or underlying medical condition, is at increased risk for complications of influenza. Health care workers and others (including household members) in close contact with persons in high-risk groups should also be vaccinated. Vaccine may be administered to any person who wishes to reduce the chance of becoming infected with influenza and missing work or school. The following groups are at increased risk for influenza-related complications and are strongly advised to be vaccinated [89]:

- Persons 65 or older.
- Residents of nursing homes or other facilities housing persons of any age with chronic medical conditions.
- Adults and children with chronic disorders of the pulmonary or cardiovascular systems, including children with asthma.
- Adults and children who have required regular medical follow-up or hospitalization during the preceding year because of chronic metabolic diseases, including diabetes mellitus, renal dysfunction, hemoglobinopathies, or immunosuppression, including that caused by medication.
- Children and teenagers (6 months to 18 years of age) who are receiving long-term salicylate (aspirin) therapy and therefore may be at risk for developing Reye's syndrome after influenza infection.
- Women who will be in the second or third trimester of pregnancy during the influenza season.

PREGNANCY GUIDELINES. This sixth category was added during 1997 by the Advisory

Committee on Immunization Practices (ACIP). Influenza-associated excess mortality among pregnant women was reported only during the 1918–1919 and 1957–1958 pandemics. Some case reports had suggested an increased risk for serious medical complications of influenza as a result of increases in heart rate, stroke volume, and oxygen consumptions; decreases in lung capacity; and changes in immunologic function.

A recent abstract [128] of the impact of influenza during 17 interpandemic influenza seasons documented that the relative risk of hospitalization for selected cardiorespiratory conditions among pregnant women increased from 1.4 during weeks 10–14 of gestation to 4.7 during weeks 37–42. The comparison (RR = 1.0) was to women who were one to six months' postpartum. Women in their third trimester of pregnancy were hospitalized at a rate comparable to that of nonpregnant women who have high-risk medical conditions for whom influenza vaccine has traditionally been recommended. Using data from this study, it was estimated that an average of one to two hospitalizations among pregnant women could be prevented for every 1,000 pregnant women immunized.

However, pregnant women who have medical conditions that increase their risk for complications from influenza should be vaccinated before the influenza season, regardless of the stage of pregnancy. Studies of influenza immunization of more than 2,000 pregnant women have demonstrated no adverse fetal effects associated with influenza vaccine [89]. Because influenza vaccine is not a live vaccine, major systemic reactions are rare. Many experts consider influenza vaccination safe during any stage of pregnancy, but because spontaneous abortion is common in the first trimester and unnecessary exposures have traditionally been avoided during this time, some experts and obstetricians prefer delaying influenza vaccination until the second trimester to avoid coincidental association of the vaccine with early pregnancy loss. There is no contraindication of vaccine during breast-feeding [89].

GROUPS THAT CAN TRANSMIT INFLUENZA TO PERSONS AT HIGH RISK. Persons who are clinically or subclinically infected and who attend to and/or live with members of high-risk groups (e.g., the elderly, transplant recipients, or persons with AIDS) can and likely will transmit influenza virus to them. Efforts to protect these members of high-risk groups against influenza may be improved by reducing the chances of exposure to influenza from their care providers. Therefore, the following groups should be vaccinated [89]:

- Physicians, nurses, and other personnel in both hospital and outpatient-care settings.
- Employees of nursing homes and chronic care facilities who have contact with patients or residents.
- Providers of home care to persons at high risk (e.g., visiting nurses, hospice, or volunteer workers).
- Household members, including children, of persons in high-risk groups.

VACCINATIONS OF OTHER OCCUPATIONAL GROUPS. Employers may want to consider offering vaccination to workers who provide essential community services, who reside in dormitory type housing, or have the occupational risks described previously, although these groups are not generally included in the recommended groups for vaccination.

VACCINATION OF INDIVIDUALS WITH HIV/AIDS. There is no data of specific influenza risk published for HIV/AIDS patients, but you may expect them to have a worse course of illness. Vaccine is recommended for HIV-infected individuals [89]. The vaccine has produced protective antibody titers in HIV-infected persons who have minimal AIDS-related symptoms and high CD4 plus T-lymphocyte cell counts. Those with lower counts have not had protective antibody levels develop [129] nor have they responded to boosters or second doses [110].

VACCINATION OF TRAVELERS. The influenza season is reversed to April to September in the southern hemisphere. Those traveling there during these times should receive the most recent vaccine. More up-to-date information can be obtained from travel services or the WHO Influenza Website at *http//www.who.ch/programmes/emc/flu.*

Contraindications. For those with contraindications to influenza vaccine, antiviral prophylaxis with rimantadine or amantadine may be considered. Breast-feeding is not a contraindication to vaccination, as it poses no safety risk to mother or infant. Nor does breast-feeding adversely affect the immune response to vaccine [89]. Contraindications to influenza vaccine are:

- People with known allergies to eggs or egg protein products (absolute) or to thimerosal preservative (relative) should *not* receive this vaccine until consulting with their physician. But if the individual is at very high risk for influenza mortality, you may want to refer the person for allergy evaluation and desensitization protocols [130].
- Adults with acute febrile illnesses should not be vaccinated until symptoms have abated. But minor upper respiratory tract infections or allergic rhinitis is not a contraindication to the vaccination of children.
- A past history of Guillain-Barré syndrome (of any etiology) is an absolute contraindication for influenza vaccination.
- First-trimester pregnancy. Women who have medical conditions that increase their risk for complications from influenza should be vaccinated before the influenza season regardless of the stage of pregnancy.

Dosage. For all adults, the dosage of all U.S. products is 0.5 mL intramuscular, with the deltoid as the muscle of choice. All studies are based on intramuscular injections. Infants and young children should be immunized in the anterolateral aspect of the thigh. Manufacturers' recommendations should be followed for storage of vaccine products; generally they need to be refrigerated and protected from light.

Local Reactions. The most common side effect is a mild local reaction (at the vaccination site), which occurs in 10–15% of people. The reaction is usually mild, generally lasts less than 24 hours, and does not inhibit daily activities.

Systemic Reactions. Low-grade fever, malaise, myalgia, and headache may occur following vaccination. These symptoms, if they occur, usually begin six to 12 hours after injection and can persist up to two days. Systemic reactions occur in only 10–15% of children who have not been exposed to influenza virus in the past and in only about 1–2% of adults who are receiving yearly vaccines.

IMMEDIATE SENSITIVITY REACTIONS. Immediate sensitivity (allergic) reactions (e.g., hives, angioedema, allergic asthma, systemic anaphylaxis) rarely occur after influenza vaccination. These are most likely due to the traces of egg protein that remain in the product. Any individual with a history of similar reaction to dietary egg products should avoid influenza shots.

DELAYED SENSITIVITY. Delayed hypersensitivity reactions to the thimerosal used as a preservative in all influenza and many other vaccines have been reported. However, thimerosal sensitivity is not an absolute contraindication, as these reactions are confined to local reactions [131]. A past history of recurrent and significant local reactions with other immunization or purified protein derivative (PPD) tuberculin injection sites may be related to thimerosal sensitivity. A true positive PPD, with induration, should not be confused with thimerosal allergy by the patient or their providers.

Drug Interactions. There has been one study [132] showing decreased theophylline clearance (increased half-life of 122%) after influenza immunization, but this finding has been refuted by others [133–137]. Likewise, one study [138] showed an effect of influenza vaccine on warfarin efficacy, but this finding was refuted by another study [139]. Most manufacturers of vaccine do not include warnings of theophylline or warfarin interactions.

Great Britain has reported several small series in which there has been a high incidence of exacerbation of asthma after influenza vaccine [140,141]. This finding has been refuted by other studies, including the United Kingdom Committee on Safety of Medicines, which had only five reports of alleged asthma or bronchospasm exacerbations in 40,000,000 doses administered between 1963 and 1991 [142]. This controversy was reviewed by Watson in 1997 [143]. At present, no manufacturer or agency states that asthma is a contraindication to influenza immunization.

Late Complications. The most publicized and significant complication of influenza vaccination has been the Guillain-Barré syndrome (GBS) associated with the 1976/1977 monovalent influenza (swine flu) vaccine. The Nationwide Influenza Immunization Project was abruptly halted on December 16, 1976, after clusters of this complication were reported. A rapid nationwide study showed a relative risk of 4–8 times (compared to the unvaccinated) for the incidence of GBS. The excess risk for GBS was about 1 in every 100,000 immunizations [144]—two to three cases per 100,000—compared to a rate of about one to two cases per 100,000 population in the general population. Analysis of the 1976–1977 cases showed associations with ages 18–64, with most cases of GBS starting the second week after vaccination. There was also an association with having had a past history of GBS.

Surveillance of the influenza vaccinations since that time has not shown an increased relative risk for GBS associated with influenza vaccine [44,45]. Many manufacturers still list GBS as a possible complication, and most providers still list GBS on the informed consent for influenza vaccine. A past history of GBS is an absolute contraindication, however. The postulated mechanism for the inactivated influenza antigens causing GBS is molecular mimicking of myelin by viral protein in the vaccine, which triggers an autoimmune response. Theories of a persistent influenza virus gene in neural cells as a cause of chronic degenerative diseases of the central nervous system are unproved [145].

False-positive HIV and hepatitis C screening tests (ELISA) in blood donors who had received influenza vaccine with 1991 products was first reported in 1992 by blood banks in the Great Lakes area. Immunization with the 1991 product had an odds ratio of 81 for false-positive test results, which is significant at $p \leq 0.01$ [146]. Donors reverted to HIV-negative status on HIV screening tests in an average of 75 days, but false-positive results on hepatitis C screening may persist longer. Donors with false-positive test results were accepted as future donors after proof of false-positive status. If an influenza vaccine is suspected of being responsible for any transient false-positive test, it should be reported to VAERS (1-800-822-7967) [147].

Efficacy. When vaccine and epidemic strains of virus are well matched, achieving high vaccination rates among persons living in close proximity (e.g., nursing homes and other chronic care facilities) can reduce the risk for outbreaks by inducing "herd" immunity. The Commission on Influenza of the Armed Forces Epidemiological Board, U.S. Department of Defense, oversaw and measured the effectiveness of the influenza vaccine for many years. It reported an effectiveness of 70–90% for those under age 65 [35,89].

All 17- to 21-year-old recruits at Lowry Air Force in Denver were vaccinated for a period of 30 years (3,000 to 5,000 per year), which resulted in vaccine efficacy of 72–95% in 70% of the years [100]. Only the antigenic shift of 1968 and the major drift of 1972 reduced efficacy below 60%. This study also included immunizations for adenovirus, which essentially made that disease extinct at the Air Force base; the only maker of the adenovirus vaccine discontinued the product in 1996 despite its high efficacy [148].

One study of healthy working adults has shown that those who receive the vaccine have 25% fewer respiratory infections, 43% fewer sick days, and 44% fewer physician visits for respiratory illness [14]. Vaccination reduced direct medical costs by $5.99 and indirect costs by $40.86 per person vaccinated. In the elderly and those with chronic medical conditions, the efficacy may be less. Vaccine reduces hospitalization by 70% and deaths by about 85% for the elderly not in nursing homes [149]. Among elderly nursing-home residents, the vaccine can reduce the risk of hospitalization and pneumonia by about 50–60% and the risk of death by 75–80% [89].

If antigenic drift results in the circulating virus's becoming different from the vaccine virus strain, the overall efficacy of the vaccine may be reduced to near zero in preventing illness in a single season [18]. However, the vaccine is still likely to lessen the severity of the illness and prevent influenza complications and death.

Concomitant Administration of Other Vaccines. The target groups for influenza and pneumococcal vaccines have great overlap, such as those age 65 or older and those with increased susceptibility to infection (e.g., patients with HIV, splenectomy, sickle cell disease, diabetes mellitus, chronic disorders of the lungs or heart, and cirrhosis). Influenza and pneumococcal vaccines may be administered together, at different sites, without an increase in side effects. Pneumococcal vaccine is covered by Medicare when ordered by a physician. It may be given at any time of the year and is a once-in-a-lifetime vaccination for most people. Influenza vaccine can be given to children together with DTaP vaccine.

Future Directions. Currently, there has been more than 30 years' usage of "cold-adapted" live influenza vaccines in Russia and the former U.S.S.R. Their efficacy and safety appear to be comparable to inactivated vaccine used in the West [150], and some U.S. manufacturers will be conducting trials in the United States in the near future.

There has also been some research on genetic-based vaccines that has shown that a small part of the influenza virus' genetic code could be inserted into a few cells in the human body. These cells would make minute amounts of a part of the virus, which in turn would stimulate the production of high levels of protective antibodies against the virus when humans are inoculated. Other progress in research on inactivated vaccines may include increasing the dose of hemagglutinin and neuraminidase antigens, which will increase the antibody response [151].

Trials of various forms of live, attenuated intranasally administered influenza vaccine were conducted in Japan in the 1990s and are reviewed by Kuno-Sakai [152]. In the United States, a 10-site phase-three double-blind trial in children using a nasal spray vaccine made by Aviron of Mountain View, California [153] was concluded. The results affirmed the vaccine's efficacy: Only 1% of immunized children had positive culture results, versus 18% of the placebo group. This spray vaccine was the product of 20 years' research on cold-adapted influenza vaccine. The advantage of cold-adapted vaccine stems from the fact that cold-adapted influenza viruses cannot grow at the warmer temperatures found in the lower respiratory tract, but do grow well in the cooler nasal passages. This allows the vaccine to mimic a natural infection and induce both IgA mucosal as well as systemic immunity without actually causing disease. The FDA approved the vaccine for use in children in 1999, and approval for use in adults is expected soon.

Antiviral Chemotherapy and Prophylaxis for Influenza A

There are two drugs with specific indications for the treatment of influenza A viruses: amantadine and the closely related drug rimantadine hydrochloride. Neither are indicated for B, C, or parainfluenza viruses. Because these drugs do not interfere with the immunogenicity or efficacy of influenza vaccines, vaccine and antiviral medication can be given together, although medication cannot substitute for vaccination. These drugs are indicated for individuals with contraindications to immunization, for coverage in the immediate postvaccine period, when vaccine is not available (i.e., not yet delivered or supply exhausted), and to fight epidemics in high-risk situations.

History and Usage. The initial indication for amantadine chloride was for parkinsonism and other extrapyramidal diseases. In 1976, it was approved for use against type A influenza virus, for both the treatment and prophylaxis of adults and children over the age of 12 months. Rimantadine was approved in 1993 for influenza A treatment.

Available Products. Amantadine is marketed by Endo Laboratories as Symmetrel and under its generic name by Duramed, Warner-Chilcott, Novapharm, Pharmaceutical Associates, and Endo Generics [126]. It is sold both as capsules and liquids. Rimantadine is marketed as Flumadine by Forest and is available in both tablets and syrup.

Mechanism of Action. The mechanisms of action of these two drugs is unknown, but they appear to prevent the release of infectious viral nucleic acid into the host cells by interfering with the function of the transmembrane domain of some viral proteins. They may also prevent virus assembly during virus replication.

Therefore "prophylaxis" with these drugs is not true prophylaxis. They cannot prevent infection but can only significantly inhibit viral replication to the point of preventing clinical illness if the person is taking adequate doses of the drug at the time of infection. Thus, "treatment" is started after apparent infection has begun, while "prophylaxis" is treatment at the time of infection. As the dosages are the same, the two drugs are discussed simultaneously in this section with their dual indications of treatment and prophylaxis of influenza A.

When these drugs are used to arrest an influenza A epidemic in progress, the goal is to reduce the viral load and shedding from those infected, thus protecting susceptible persons. Fortunately these drugs do not seem to block or reduce antibody response or future immunity to the infecting strain. Both drugs have produced drug-resistant strains of influenza A, which appear to be equally as infectious and pathogenic as sensitive strains.

Indications: Who and Why. When prescribed for treatment, drug administration should begin as early in the clinical illness as possible. When used for prophylaxis, each of these drugs is effective only while being taken. Full susceptibility to infection returns hours after the last dose. Anti-influenza chemoprophylaxis is not a substitute for vaccination, although many of the indications for its use are the same as those for use of vaccine. These drugs can be given during the 14 days after influenza immunization to cover the period of time it takes for a full immune response to develop. This technique may be especially effective during an epidemic, both to prevent or reduce the patient's clinical illness and to protect their cohorts.

Indications for amantadine or rimantadine prophylaxis include the following persons:

- Unvaccinated individuals who have frequent contact with others at high risk (e.g., household contacts, visiting nurses, volunteer workers).
- Unvaccinated workers in hospitals, clinics, and chronic care facilities. Chemoprophylaxis should be given during the period of peak influenza activity—within the two weeks after immunization if there has been community-wide spread of the virus. Prophylaxis should be considered for all workers regardless of their vaccination status if the outbreak is caused by a variant strain of influenza A that might not be controlled by the vaccine received.
- Persons with immune deficiencies who may have an inadequate influenza vaccine response. This includes patients with advanced HIV or AIDS. There are no available data on interactions of amantadine or rimantadine with other medications the patient may be taking, such as antiretroviral medications. These patients should be monitored very closely by the prescribing physician.
- Persons for whom influenza vaccine is contraindicated and high-risk patients or workers who refuse to take influenza vaccine for whatever reason.
- Anyone who wishes to avoid influenza A illness, after consultation with the prescribing physician.

Utilization and Medical Directives (Standing Orders). Although many indications are shared by the antiviral drugs and vaccines, these drugs are not as easy or safe to dispense as vaccine. Vaccine candidates are easily screened and require essentially no follow-up, and specific physician orders or prescriptions are not needed. However, candidates for antiviral drugs require more careful history and even physical examination to screen for possible contraindications, as these drugs have relatively frequent and serious side effects. Standing orders for administration of antiviral medication to large numbers of workers may not be practical nor advisable, unless the prescriber is willing and able to be available to attend to all complications. It may be more practical and ethical for employers to make administrative or financial arrangements to have the drugs available if and only if prescribed by their own primary care physicians.

Contraindications and Precautions. Contraindications to the antiviral drugs include known hypersensitivity to any drugs in the amantadine/rimantadine class as well as pregnancy and breast feeding, unless the potential benefit justifies the potential risk to the embryo, fetus, or infant. Both amantadine and rimantadine should be used with extreme caution in those with a history of epilepsy or other seizures, especially if they are not currently taking seizure medication, and should be given with caution to depressed or potentially suicidal patients and those with a history of psychiatric illness. Death has occurred with a 2-μg overdose of amantadine (a 10-day supply or 20 pills).

Dosage. The duration of amantadine prophylaxis or treatment of influenza A should be two to three weeks at most. The drug should not be taken continuously or during an entire influenza season nor during prolonged travel. Long-term therapy is indicated only for patients with Parkinson's disease, in whom it has an entirely different set of side effects, including drug withdrawal or dose reduction syndromes such as neuroleptic malignant syndrome. The only approved indications for amantadine are short-term treatment and prophylaxis for influenza A.

The amantadine dose for healthy adults is 200 mg/day, either two 100-mg doses taken together or two 100-mg doses taken twice daily. A half dose (100 mg/day) is indicated for individuals over 65 years old and those with congestive heart failure, peripheral edema, or orthostatic hypotension. Amantadine is excreted unchanged in the urine. Peak concentration is 4 hours, and the half-life is 15 hours. Amantadine clearance is greatly reduced in adults with renal impairment, and its elimination half-life is increased two- to threefold if creatinine clearance is less than 40 mL/min/1.73 m^2. Therefore, half dosage is also recommended for patients with renal failure; even further reductions may be indicated (consult package insert for dosing details).

When amantadine is used for therapy, dosage should begin as soon as possible after symptoms begin and until 24–48 hours after symptoms resolve. Its use for postexposure prophylaxis should continue for no more than 10 days.

The recommended dose of rimantadine is also 100 mg twice daily, with halving of dosage for the same indications as amantadine. Its peak concentration is about six hours, and its half-life about 25 hours. When the drug is used for therapy, dosing should begin as soon as possible after symptoms begin and for a total of seven days.

Adverse Effects. Amantadine has been associated with a higher incidence of adverse central nervous system reactions than rimantadine. Both drugs are pregnancy category C, and embryotoxic effects have been noted in high doses in rats. Both drugs also concentrate in breast milk and should not be used by nursing mothers. Tables 11-2 and 11-3 are from Forest Pharmaceutical, makers of Flumadine (rimantadine hydrochloride) [126].

Individual Prophylaxis. When administered prophylactically to healthy adults or children before and through an epidemic period, both amantadine and rimantadine are approximately 70–90% effective in preventing illness caused by naturally occurring strains of type A influenza viruses [89]. Factors of cost, compliance, potential side effects, and the anticipated period of the peak epidemic should be considered when determining the period of prophylaxis, as the drug is effective only while being taken.

Table 11-2
Adverse Effects of Rimantadine

Adverse Effect[a]	Rimantadine (n = 1,027) (%)	Control (n = 986) (%)
Nervous System		
Insomnia	2.1	0.9
Dizziness	1.9	1.1
Headache	1.4	1.3
Nervousness	1.3	0.6
Fatigue	1.0	0.9
Gastrointestinal System		
Nausea	2.8	1.6
Vomiting	1.7	0.6
Anorexia	1.6	0.8
Dry mouth	1.5	0.6
Abdominal pain	1.4	0.8
Whole-body asthenia	1.4	0.5

[a] Serious adverse effects occurring at 0.3% or less include hallucinations, seizures, and heart failure or blocks.
From *Physicians' Desk Reference*, 52nd Ed. Montavale, NJ: Medical Economics Company, 1998.

Table 11-3
Comparison of Adverse Effects of Rimantadine and Amantadine
(Six-Week Prophylaxis Study, 200 mg a Day, in Healthy Adults)

Adverse Effect	Rimantadine (n = 145) (%)	Placebo (n = 143) (%)	Amantadine (n = 148) (%)
Insomnia	3.4	0.7	7.0
Nervousness	2.1	0.7	2.8
Impaired concentration	2.1	1.4	2.1
Dizziness	0.7	0.0	2.1
Depression	0.7	0.7	3.5
Total percentage with adverse reactions	6.9	4.1	14.7
Total percentage withdrawn from study	6.9	3.4	14.0

From *Physicians' Desk Reference*, 52nd Ed. Montavale, NJ: Medical Economics Company, 1998.

Individual Treatment. If started within 48 hours of symptoms, amantadine and rimantadine can prevent or severely limit symptomatic disease. They are not effective in preventing subclinical infection—that is, the person is still infected with influenza and will develop antibodies that may provide some protection to that and related viruses in the future. It is not known whether antiviral therapy will prevent complications of influenza A among individuals at high risk.

If drug resistance develops, it is usually to both drugs. Drug resistance is more likely to occur when these drugs are used for treatment rather than prophylaxis. Naturally occurring strains of influenza do not seem to be resistant to amantadine or rimantadine. Persons infected with influenza A and taking one of these drugs will shed sensitive virus for a few days, but then may shed resistant organisms after five to seven days. Therefore, people should stop taking these drugs as soon as possible. Preferably, they should be taken only for three to five days total, or for 24 to 48 hours after symptoms have resolved. Any virus isolated from a person receiving these drugs should be reported to the state health department, which may elect to send cultures to the CDC for antiviral sensitivity testing.

Breaking up Epidemics. When influenza outbreaks are confirmed or suspected in institutions housing persons at high risk for influenza, antiviral chemoprophylaxis should begin immediately. Contingency plans should be in place to start treatment of all consenting residents and staff. These plans should include pre-approved orders from attending physicians, or the ability to obtain prescriptions on short notice. All residents should be treated, regardless of whether they have had influenza vaccination. Treatment should continue for two weeks or until one week after the end of the outbreak. Dosage should be individually determined, based on guidelines listed above. Current CDC recommendations [89] are that only nonimmunized employees should be offered chemoprophylaxis. However, if the strain is known to be an influenza A that was not covered by the vaccine, all employees should be offered antiviral treatment.

Chemoprophylaxis may also be considered for controlling influenza A outbreaks in other facilities such as dormitories, military settings (aircraft, ship, or submarine barracks), and worksites providing critical public functions. In such cases, every effort should be made to separate those taking the drug for treatment from those taking the drug for chemoprophylaxis. This may help prevent spread of the infection and decrease the chance of prophylaxis failure due to the development of drug resistance in the facility.

Recent Advances. Research on the use of neurominidase inhibitors has recently produced two new FDA-approved type A and B anti-influenza drugs: Glaxo's inhaled powder, zanamivir (Relenza), and Roche's oral capsule, oseltamivir phosphate (Tamiflu). Both medications must be taken within two days of symptom onset: zanamivir as two inhalations (10 mg total) twice daily at two-hour intervals on the first day, and then two inhalations twice daily at 12-hour intervals for five days; oseltamivir as a 75-mg capsule twice daily for five days. These drugs can reduce the duration of illness by one to three days but are indicated only for type A and B influenza in adults. Possible side effects include nausea and/or vomiting, bronchitis, insomnia, and vertigo.

Compliance with Recommendations

Although efforts to protect the general public from exposure to influenza usually prove unsuccessful, efforts aimed at high-risk groups can be effective. Special efforts have been made to target individuals over the age of 65 because of their higher mortality from influenza, and compliance with recommendations has greatly improved. Medicare initiated reimbursement for influenza vaccine in 1993 [156], although the paperwork involved is not generally cost effective for many private influenza campaigns or employers. The official federal program that targets elderly populations partners HCFA with the National Coalition for Adult Immunization and the CDC. Companies should also make special efforts to see that their retirees are offered vaccination.

Many older people remember vaccines from the 1940s to mid-1960s that were less pure and had more side effects due to impurities. Since these vaccine side effects of fever, headache, muscle aches, and fatigue were essentially the same as those of influenza, many mistakenly assumed that the vaccine infected them with influenza. Although no influenza vaccine ever used in the United States could have been capable of transmitting influenza infection, this misconception persists and has continued to have a negative effect on utilization of influenza vaccine.

Only about 20% of those in the other groups for whom vaccination is recommended are compliant each year. Even with the massive public health campaigns for immunization with the 1976 Swine flu, only about 25% of the U.S. population was immunized. National health objectives for the year 2000 include vaccination of 60% of those at risk for severe influenza-related illness. Objectives for 2010 will be even more ambitious.

The public expects modern vaccines to be highly efficacious, and they remain relatively disappointed with influenza products. But vaccine does fail when there is circulation of an influenza virus that is dissimilar from that used in the vaccine and offers little if any protection. And it has been shown that individuals can get more than one influenza A subtype infection in a single season [157]. The Japanese have vaccinated nearly 100% of children, but epidemics persist.

Surprisingly few studies have been done on the utilization of influenza vaccines in health care workers. Doebbeling and colleagues [158] studied factors associated with utilization of influenza vaccines by hospital workers over two seasons. Among the professional nursing staff, they found positive associations with age, salary and employment time and negative associations with absenteeism. Nonprofessional support staff showed positive associations with age, female gender, salary, and length of employment. Nonprofessional staff had an association only with age. An assumption can be made that the more one knows about influenza and the more experience one has with its complications, the more likely one is to elect annual immunization.

If employers cannot offer the vaccine to employees on-site, they should provide information on the immunizations through their benefit plans or community services. Employers should also be cooperative in allowing health care providers to publicize times and places of influenza vaccinations, especially those convenient to the workplace. Table 11-4 summarizes factors that may increase utilization of influenza vaccine. The left column denotes minimal effort, service, or employer cost, while the right column moves the spectrum toward increased effort, convenience, and cost.

Metrics To Assess Adequacy of Preventive Measures

The best incentive for taking measures to prevent influenza is the dollar. Many articles have been published on the efficacy and cost-benefit analysis of influenza vaccine, although most recent studies have concentrated on immunization for the elderly [14,159–162] and Medicare [163,164], HMO, HIV-infected [165] and chronic lung disease [166] populations rather than for workers per se [13,14,167]. All studies show a positive benefit from immunization, and influenza vaccine is often used as an example of cost-benefit efficacy in methodology papers [168,169]. Fewer cost-benefit analyses of antivi-

Table 11-4
Spectrum of Factors That Impact Employees' Utilization of Influenza Vaccine

Factor	Positive Impact	Negative Impact
Education	Provided	Not provided
Educator	Knowledgeable provider	Less knowledgeable
Place	At worksite	Off worksite
Time	Organized availability	Make own arrangements
	During work time	Outside work time
	All shifts	Limited shifts
	Multiple dates	Limited dates
Ends	When vaccine gone	When scheduled times for immunization end
How	Walk-in	Appointment
	No waiting	Waiting lines
Cost	Free to employees	Employee pay/co-pay
Who	Employee and family	Employee only

ral drugs for influenza have been published. No studies have evaluated the benefits of personal protective equipment, education, or administrative controls.

Direct costs of influenza illness include physician and office fees, cost of laboratory tests, cost of prescription and nonprescription drugs, hospital charges for acute and/or extended care, and cost of supplies. But these costs may represent only 20–30% of the total cost. Indirect costs are those of absenteeism to industry, schools, and government and the economic costs of years of life lost (life insurance, burial, dependent support) for individuals who die from influenza. Costs of prevention are those of vaccine and antiviral medications, the staff and facilities to immunize or examine, medical treatment for adverse effects of vaccinations and antiviral medications, and the loss of employees' productive time going to and from the provider's facility or the pharmacy.

In light of these direct and indirect costs, why do so many individuals choose not to take the vaccine? An "individual" decision-analysis model was constructed by Dr. Stephen C. Schoenbaum of the Harvard Pilgrim Health Plan of New England in 1987 [170]. He presented two decision equations applicable to the individual, one during the preseason and one during an influenza epidemic. They are summarized in Tables 11-5 and 11-6. Table 11-7 presents a model for estimating work loss for the individual worker.

Those at high risk for morbidity or mortality from influenza have higher relative costs associated with illness than those with higher incomes. Schoenbaum's model fails to consider the occupational or social variables that may affect the individual's chances of being infected (attack rates). Employers and their contracted providers can best influence the individual equations by offering convenient low-cost vaccination (see Table 11-4).

Table 11-5
General Benefit-Cost Model of Preseason Influenza Immunization from an Individual's Perspective

Expected Benefits = Cost of having influenza
× average annual probability of an epidemic (0.33)
× average attack rate if an epidemic year (0.2–0.3)
× vaccine efficacy rate if taken (0.6–0.7)
= $0.33 \times 0.2 \times 0.6$ = 4% of the cost of having influenza *or*
$0.33 \times 0.3 \times 0.7$ = 7% of the cost of having influenza
Expected Costs = Cost of receiving the vaccine + cost of having a significant reaction

Reprinted from Schoenbaum SC. Economic impact of influenza. The individual's perspective. *Am J Med* 1987;82(6A):26–30. © 1987 with permission from Excerpta Medica Inc.

Table 11-6
Benefit-Cost Model for Protection of an Individual Against Influenza During an Epidemic

Expected Benefit = Pre-season expected benefits (from Table 11-5)
× 1/preseason probability of an epidemic
× anticipated residual occurrence rate
= pre season expected benefits × 1/0.33 × approx 1.0[a]
= 3 × (pre-season expected benefits)
= 12 – 20% of the cost of having a case of influenza

Expected Costs = Cost of receiving vaccine
+ cost of having a reaction
+ cost of receiving antiviral medication for two weeks
+ cost of reaction to antiviral medication

[a] Early in an epidemic, the residual occurrence rate is almost as high as the originally anticipated occurrence rate
Reprinted from Schoenbaum SC. Economic impact of influenza. The individual's perspective. *Am J Med* 1987;82(6A):26–30. © 1987 with permission from Excerpta Medica Inc.

Symptoms and Signs

CLINICAL EPIDEMIOLOGY

For the purpose of epidemiologic surveillance, the case definition for an *influenza-like illness* is a fever over 100° F and either a sore throat or cough [171]. This definition is highly sensitive for the diagnosis of clinically apparent influenza but has poor specificity. Onset of symptoms can be as soon as 24 hours after exposure and viral invasion but is usually 48 to 96 hours postexposure. The communicable (infective) period may

Table 11-7
Annual Work-Loss Benefit Model of Influenza Vaccine, Individual Perspective

Severe epidemic year, not vaccinated:	
Chance of illness (40% attack rate)[a]	0.40
Chance will have work absenteeism (50%)[b]	0.50
Days absent (average 4)	4.00
Average number of days absent (multiply all three above)	0.80
Mild epidemic year, not vaccinated:	
Chance of illness (20% attack rate)[a]	0.20
Chance will have work absenteeism (30%)[b]	0.30
Days absent (average 3)	3.00
Average number of days absent (multiply all three above)	0.18
Severe epidemic year, vaccinated:	
Chance of illness (40% attack rate)[a]	0.40
Divided by vaccine efficacy (40%, 60% failure)[c]	0.24
Chance will have work absenteeism (50%)[b]	0.50
Days absent (average 4)	4.00
Average number of days absent (multiply all above)	0.48
Mild epidemic year, vaccinated:	
Chance of illness (20% attack rate)[a]	0.20
Divided by vaccine efficacy (80% success, 20% failure)[c]	0.04
Chance will have work absenteeism (30%)[b]	0.30
Days absent (average 3)	3.00
Average numbers of days absent (multiply all above)	0.04

[a] Assumes that severe epidemic years have an influenza attack rate of 40%, and mild epidemic years 20%.
[b] Assumes that in severe epidemic years, there is more severe illness, with 50% of workers becoming ill and losing an average of four days, and in milder epidemic years, there is milder illness, with 30% of workers becoming ill and losing an average of three days.
[c] Assumes that vaccine is one half as effective in severe epidemic years, compared with mild epidemic years—40% versus 80%—due to antigenic drift and/or mismatching.

precede symptoms by a few hours and peaks with the peak illness and symptoms of fever, cough, and/or nasal discharge. Communicability and viral shedding ends two to three days after peak symptoms but may persist for up to seven days in children and those with primary influenza pneumonia.

The attack rate in the general public is 10–20% annually but can reach over 70% in closed or less ventilated environments, including the workplace [21,71]. The observational influenza studies performed in Cleveland [172], Seattle [173], Houston [174], and Tecumseh [175] consistently showed higher attack rates (20–50%) in adults living in households with infected children. Houston HMO studies of 1981–1983 show that the rate of physician visits for acute respiratory disease during the 10-week peak influenza season is about 12% for employed persons and their adult family members [176]. A U.S. study show that vaccinated workers average 0.31 physician visits for ILI, compared to 0.55 for unvaccinated workers [14]. Scandinavian studies show an average work absence due to influenza to be 4.9 days [167].

PREVALENCE OF SYMPTOMS

Of all healthy people infected by influenza, about 20% have inapparent illness and 30% have some respiratory symptoms without fever. However, 50% have a full-blown illness, that is, respiratory symptoms, chills and fever, sore throat, myalgia, headaches, malaise, and persistent cough [74,157,177–180]. Severity of symptoms varies from strain to strain, year to year, depending on host-related factors such as age and previous immunity.

CLINICAL COURSE

Onset of influenza symptoms is usually abrupt. The first symptoms are usually fever, sore throat and myalgia, followed closely by cough (usually nonproductive), coryza, headache, and fatigue. Easy fatigability may last a week or more, and a dry cough may be protracted, lasting two weeks or more. Temperatures can range from 100°F to 103°F and possibly higher in children. Gastrointestinal symptoms are less prevalent in adults than in children but may include loss of appetite or tussive vomiting. Constipation from decongestants, antihistamines, or antitussive medication; abdominal pain or vomiting from nonsteroidal anti-inflammatory medications; and diarrhea secondary to antibiotic prescriptions are often mistakenly blamed on the primary illness. Predominant, primary gastrointestinal symptoms generally are not attributable to influenza viruses. *Stomach flu* and *intestinal influenza* are misnomers used to describe illnesses caused by other organisms.

COMPLICATIONS

Influenza is usually a self-limited illness; healthy American adults who contract it usually lose about four calendar days from work. About 5% of adults who become ill develop significant lower respiratory tract conditions such as tracheobronchitis or pneumonitis. The pneumonitis can be either primary influenza or a secondary bacterial pathogen. Common bacteria influenza-associated pneumonias include *Streptococcal pneumoniae*, *Staphylococcus aureus*, or *Haemophilus influenzae*. If death occurs from secondary bacterial pneumonia, it usually happens within one to two weeks from the onset of pneumonia symptoms. Secondary infections of the sinus or middle ear are common after influenza.

Most influenza-related deaths occur in those with pre-existing heart or lung disease who are over 65. Rates of hospitalization of the elderly may increase two- to five-fold [89] during a major influenza epidemic. Those with weakened immune systems or heart or lung disease are more prone to succumb to pneumonia and/or pulmonary edema with hypoxia. Some have theorized that influenza can precipitate myocardial infarction due to primary myocardial invasion [181], but no association between myocardial infarction and viral antibodies has been found [182]. Myocarditis and rhabdomyolysis in association with some strains of influenza A [183] have been documented, however [184].

The majority of adults hospitalized with acute respiratory infections clinically or epidemiologically related to influenza are not in a high-risk group recommended for influenza vaccination [20]. Most are employed.

Reye's syndrome is a rare complication of influenza [185]. Hallmarks of the syndrome are encephalopathy and fatty microvesiculation of the liver associated with the use of salicylate by individuals with influenza B (more than A), especially children and young adults. The syndrome has a mortality of up to 40% and may also complicate primary varicella infection. The use of salicylates is contraindicated for individuals with all influenza-like illnesses.

Some of the more rarely reported cases of organ failure—cardiac, liver, and renal failure—have been associated with specific influenza strains, particularly new or pandemic strains. One report suggested that influenza virus may infect peripheral lymphocytes [186]. A toxic shock-like syndrome as a complication of influenza infection has also been reported.

The Asian influenza of 1957–1958 was suspected of causing viremia and contributing to a higher incidence of schizophrenia in children born of mothers infected in mid-pregnancy [188]. An association between influenza and schizophrenia would support the hypothesis of schizophrenia as a neurodevelopmental disorder. The matter is unresolved because of conflicting studies; these are well reviewed by Hayase and Tobita [145] and McGrath and Castle [188].

PATHOPHYSIOLOGY

Infection may result from as few as five influenza-infected droplet nuclei inspired into the deep lung or approximately 100 or more droplet nuclei coming into contact with the nasopharyngeal mucosa [69]. The degree and depth of tissue reaction may be positively correlated with both the infectivity and the severity of symptoms and illness associated with the specific influenza strain.

The columnar epithelium is destroyed by the replicating intracellular influenza virus, possibly stripping it down to the bare basement membrane [189]. The dead and infected epithelium is then sloughed off, and lymphocytic infiltrates can develop in the lung, causing fibrosis or pulmonary edema. The slow regeneration of the columnar epithelium may be responsible for the prolonged dry throat and cough that are characteristic of influenza. Repair of the mucosal surfaces is necessary to restore the mucociliary escalator clearance systems, which protect the lower respiratory tree and help clear damaged tissue. Influenza injury of the lung may also impair the function of pulmonary macrophages. It may be this impairment that increases the infected individual's vulnerability to other pulmonary pathogens and thus increases the chance of bacterial pneumonia.

There is no evidence to support the belief that the mammalian influenza virus can replicate anywhere other than in respiratory system cells [190]. The neuraminidase portion of the influenza virion may be the part responsible for the invasion of the very susceptible lower respiratory mucous membranes, but there are several case reports of the culturing of influenza from other body organs, including skeletal muscles, cardiac muscle, and lymphocytes. The actual pathogenesis of influenza complications such as encephalitis, myositis, myalgia, and Reye's syndrome is unknown.

IgA- or mucous-membrane-mediated immunity to specific influenza viruses may offer partial protection from closely related strains, but it is IgG immunity that seems to provide the most lasting natural immunity.

Differential Diagnosis

Because of the nature of this text, this discussion of differential diagnosis pertains only to adults. As previously mentioned, the definition of *influenza-like illness (ILI)* is any febrile illness with either a sore throat or a cough, regardless of the season in which the illness occurs. Synonyms for self-limited upper (above the epiglottis) respiratory infection are upper respiratory infections (URI), acute viral rhinitis, the common cold (or ICD-9 460, ICD-10 J00), pharyngitis, and laryngitis.

Since influenza (ICD-9 487 and ICD-10 J10,11) is not a reportable disease, clinical epidemiologic information is not collected. A definitive diagnosis can be made only by confirmatory laboratory studies. Dozens of microorganisms, with hundreds of serotypes, can cause ILI. Many more serious infections can begin with ILI symptoms, including many viral and some bacterial meningitides (Chapter 23), *Legionella*

(Chapter 10), other upper respiratory tract infections (Chapter 12), and chlamydial infections (Chapter 14).

BACTERIA

Mycoplasma *Pneumonia*

Also known as primary atypical pneumonia, *Mycoplasma* pneumonia shares many characteristics with influenza, including fever, headache, malaise, and persistent paroxysmal coughing. Like influenza, Mycoplasma pneumonia may also occur in epidemics in military units or institutions and has a higher frequency in older children and young adults. However, with Mycoplasma pneumonia, there is a much flatter epidemic curve, due to its longer incubation of six to 32 days and its communicable period of several weeks. Also, it is more likely to occur in late summer or early fall, unlike influenza, which occurs from late fall through early spring.

Streptococcus (Group A Beta-Hemolytic)

Streptococcus infection shares with influenza the symptoms of fever and sore throat but is less likely to cause significant cough. An individual with streptococcal sore throat usually presents with more positive physical findings, such as cervical lymphadenopathy, tonsillitis, and edema, redness, or petechiae of the throat or palate. Rapid tests for streptococcus may aid in the diagnosis.

Other Viral Infections

If it were practical to perform viral cultures on all adults with upper respiratory cold symptoms, only half would be positive. Overall, influenza viruses would represent about 10–15% of positive cultures, but during a mid-winter outbreak of upper respiratory illness, these viruses could account for over 50%. Corona viruses would represent another 10–15%, but the largest class represented would be the over 100 serotypes of rhinoviruses (20–40%), or even higher in the fall [21]. The clinical course for all of the viruses is essentially the same, as are their short incubation periods. But many other viruses can cause ILI if there is associated viremia. Even the initial seroconverting viremia of the human immune virus is usually described as an *influenza-like illness.*

Significant fever is almost always present with influenza, while it is less characteristic of other respiratory viruses (Figure 11-4 and Table 11-8). Cervical adenopathy, productive cough, pleuritic pain, and visible lesions of the oropharynx are more characteristic of other viruses (such as mononucleosis, coxsackievirus, CMV, or other herpesviruses) and bacterial pharyngitis. Influenza is most accurately diagnosed "epidemiologically" by the prevalence of similar illness in the community or worker cohorts. Health care practitioners should not hesitate to access up-to-date surveillance information to aid in diagnosis.

Diagnostic Evaluation

White blood cell counts are usually normal (5,000–10,000/cu mm) in persons with influenza, but there is a relative lymphocytosis [191]. Leukopenia may be present in up to 50% of cases during the acute phase of the illness. White counts over 15,000 suggest bacterial or secondary infection. Diagnostic laboratory tests should focus on secondary infection in the seriously ill, especially if there is pre-existing cardiac or pulmonary disease. Other diagnostic testing should be performed on the basis of symptoms for example, chest radiography or arterial blood gas measurement for individuals with respiratory crisis and electrocardiography or heart monitoring for persons with cardiovascular complications.

Performing specific virology studies is not clinically practical, since test results will not be available until after the illness has run its clinical course. Some surveillance utilizing the sentinel-physician system is done for epidemiologic and planning purposes, and more intensive studies may be indicated when an epidemic is suspected of having an animal origin and/or there is the threat of a major antigenic shift [30,31]. Direct immunofluorescence detection of antigen in ciliated epithelial cells from nasopharyngeal swab is now available for rapid diagnosis and is becoming the confirmation test of choice.

Influenza cannot be distinguished from other respiratory illnesses by clinical examination of the patient. Definitive diagnosis requires specific influenza testing by one of several methods. These include:

Figure 11-4 / Example of an educational poster available on the Internet. (From the National Institute of Allergy and Infectious Disease at *http://www.niaid.nih.gov/*.)

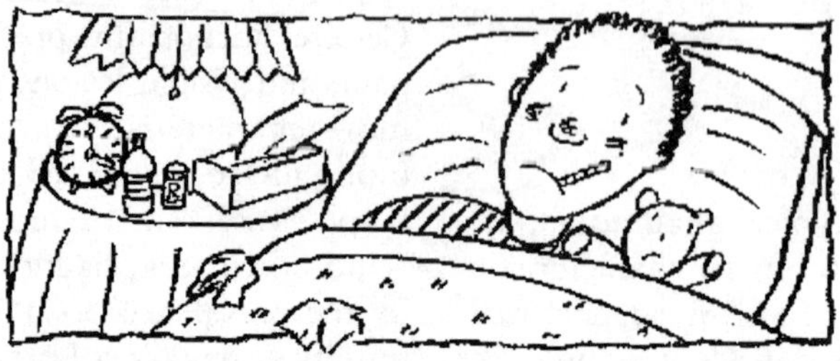

Is It a Cold or the Flu?

Symptoms	Cold	Flu
Fever	Rare	Characteristic, high (102-104°F); lasts 3-4 days
Headache	Rare	Prominent
General Aches, Pains	Slight	Usual; often severe
Fatigue, Weakness	Quite mild	Can last up to 2-3 weeks
Extreme Exhaustion	Never	Early and prominent
Stuffy Nose	Common	Sometimes
Sneezing	Usual	Sometimes
Sore Throat	Common	Sometimes
Chest Discomfort, Cough	Mild to moderate; hacking cough	Common; can become severe
Complications	Sinus congestion or earache	Bronchitis, pneumonia; can be life-threatening
Prevention	None	Annual vaccination; amantadine or rimantadine (antiviral drugs)
Treatment	Only temporary relief of symptoms	Amantadine or rimantadine within 24-48 hours after onset of symptoms

1. Virus isolation (the gold standard) either by:
   a. Standard method (which use fertilized chicken egg or tissue culture as the culture medium) performed within 72 hours of onset of illness, using one of the following specimens:
      (1) Nasal wash (can use saline).
      (2) Nasopharyngeal aspirate.
      (3) Nasal and throat swab.
      (4) Transtracheal aspirate.
      (5) Bronchoalveolar lavage.
   b. Rapid culture assay, using one of five specimens listed above.
2. Detection of viral antigens by:
   a. Enzyme immunoassay (e.g., EIA or IFA).
   b. Electron microscopy.
   c. Polymerase chain reaction (PCR).
3. Serologic testing.

VIRUS ISOLATION

Virus isolation methods have the advantage of producing virus of sufficient quantity for full antigenic characterization, which is needed for matching with vaccines. The disadvantage is that results are not available for four and a half days,

Table 11-8
Characteristics of Adult Upper Respiratory Infections: Acute and Early Symptoms

Characteristic	Influenza	Other Virus	Bacteria
Symptoms			
High fever	+++	+	++
Acute onset	+++	++	+
Swollen cervical lymph nodes	+	++	++
Oral or pharyngeal lesions	0	++	++
Productive cough	+	++	+++
Shortness of breath	0	+	++
Copious nasal discharge	++	+++	+
Conjunctivitis	+	++	++
Pleuritic chest pain	+	++	+++
Complications			
Rapid recovery	+++	+	++
Secondary sinusitis	+	++	+++
Secondary bronchitis	+	+	++
Secondary pneumonitis	++	+	++
Epidemiology			
Short incubations	++	+	–
Mid-winter epidemic	+++	++	+
Children ill first	+++	++	+
Quick epidemic curve	+++	+	0
Excess mortality	+++	0	+

on average, and are thus of little use to the clinician. The rapid culture assays detect viral antigens in cell culture; the results of these "nonstandard" cultures are available in 18 to 40 hours. State health departments should be contacted for information on local laboratory support for influenza surveillance.

ANTIGEN DETECTION ASSAYS

There are several methods for the diagnosis of influenza infection directly from clinical material. Cells from the clinical specimen can be stained using immunofluorescent antibody to detect the presence of viral antigen. Nasal washes, nasopharyngeal aspirates, nasal throat swabs, gargling fluid, transtracheal aspirates, and bronchoalveolar lavage are suitable clinical specimens. Commercially available EIAs can be used to test for the presence of viral antigens. At present, EIA test kits are available for the detection of influenza A only.

Other less frequently used methods include immunostaining, visualization of viral antigens by electron microscopy, detection of viral RNA by molecular hybridization, and reverse transcriptase polymerase chain reaction (PCR). When direct antigen-detection methods are used for the diagnoses of influenza, it is important to save an aliquot of the clinical sample for further testing, if necessary. These samples may be used for culture confirmation of direct test results and virus isolation for subtyping of influenza A isolates by a public health laboratory. Full antigenic characterization of the virus may be performed by the U.S. World Health Organization (WHO Collaborating Center for Surveillance, Epidemiology, and Control of Influenza, Influenza Branch, CDC). This characterization is necessary for the detection and tracking of antigenic variants, an essential part of the selection of optimal influenza vaccine components.

SEROLOGIC TESTING: SERODIAGNOSIS

Because most human serum contains antibodies to influenza, the diagnosis of influenza cannot be made from a single serum sample. Paired serum specimens are required for serologic diagnosis of influenza infection. The presence of a four-fold increase in specific monoclonal IgG or IgM during the disease course confirms recent infection: IgM peaks at two weeks, and IgG at four to seven weeks following infection [191]. A finding of high IgG early in the course of the illness or a stable IgG after a second serologic test indicates immunity that pre-exists the illness. A compliment fixation or hemagglutinin test showing a four-fold increase of IgG or IgM in sera compared to the level during the acute phase and convalescence a few weeks later confirm recent influenza infection.

The acute specimen should be collected within a few days of the onset of illness, and the convalescent sample should be collected approximately two to three weeks later, for IgM, or four weeks later, for IgG. Hemagglutination inhibition tests are the preferred method for serodiagnosis. A positive result is a four-fold or greater rise in titer between the acute and convalescent samples to one type of a subtype of virus. For example, starting with an initial serum dilution of 1:10, a two-fold (doubling) serum dilution would result in a concentration of 1:20. A four-fold or higher increase in titer between the acute and convalescent phase serum—that is, an increase from 1:20 to 1:80 or higher—would be considered positive. A two-fold increase between the two sera is within the margin of error for the test and should not be considered a positive finding. To assure that a rise in titer is due to infection rather than recent influenza vaccination, the vaccination history of the patient must also be taken into account.

Treatment and Rehabilitation

The 1918 pandemic occurred many years before vaccines, antiviral medication, or antibiotics were available, yet 90% of infected persons survived and acquired lifelong partial protection from A(H1N1) influenza. Influenza is usually a self-limited illness, but the severity of the illness and an individual's risk for complications may well correlate with whether and to what degree the illness is self-limited.

Rest is the best treatment, and the profound fatigue of early illness may be nature's best defense mechanism. Hydration is essential to replace body fluids lost because of fever and to assist repair of respiratory tissues damaged by viral invasion. Frequent sips and swallows of fluids may help to relieve coughing stimulated by the damaged respiratory epithelium. Hydration is needed for the proper operation of the mucociliary escalator function and for coughing to clear infected sections.

The use of prescription cough suppressive medication in influenza is controversial. Salt water or analgesic gargles may relieve coughing, and smokers should abstain from smoking. A cool-mist humidifier in the bedroom may assist rest, but the water should be changed every eight hours to prevent pseudomonas contamination. Although appetite may be suppressed, the patient should eat regular meals of nonspicy but nutritious foods. The complex carbohydrates of fruits and vegetables may help to provide energy and reduce fatigue.

Over-the-counter analgesics, decongestants, and antihistamines may afford some symptomatic relief. Acetaminophen, not aspirin, should be used for fever in children and adolescents. Amantadine or rimantadine may lessen the severity and course of influenza A if started within 48 hours of onset of symptoms. The same dose is used as that for prophylaxis (200 mg daily for healthy adults; 100 mg daily for those over age 65 and those known to have renal impairment). Antibiotics should be used only for confirmed or strongly suspected secondary bacterial infection, evidenced by a positive chest radiogram, purulent or bloody sputum, pleuritic pain, or positive Gram's stain.

Some have claimed that influenza may cause permanent impairment of pulmonary function [90], but recovery is usually complete and permanent sequelae from influenza or its treatment are very rare.

Occupational Considerations

Companies and other organizations should have business and operating contingency plans for periods of high employee absenteeism due to influenza. Every few years, this could be as high as 50% during a period of a few days. Companies should remove as many administrative, financial, and time barriers as possible for their workers to receive influenza immunizations and/or treatment (see Table 11-4) in an effort to maximize utilization of vaccination. If an employer is unable to provide on-site administration of influenza vaccine by their own or contracted nurses, then benefits managers should pressure their health plan vendors to cover prevention services such as influenza vaccine and anti-influenza chemoprophylaxis. An organization's plans should include access to health care providers near the workplace and reasonable co-payments for outpatient visits for vaccination and ILI treatment. Formal employee-sponsored health promotion or wellness programs should include credits and incentives for utilization of annual influenza immunizations. Other recommendations for administrative support are discussed on pages 233–235.

There has been a tendency in the 1990s for human resources and benefits departments to combine previous categories of days-off into a single bank of paid time-off to simplify their record keeping. This impairs the ability to study workers' illnesses in detail [19]; thus, questions such as the efficacy of influenza vaccines or other prevention programs will remain unanswered. ("No data in, no data out.")

Occupational health providers should be aware of the factors that put an individual at high risk for influenza and of recommendations for immunization and make a year-round effort to identify workers for education about, and offering of, vaccination. Providers should also be familiar with the epidemiology of influenza and the community and occupational risk factors for the disease. All occupational health practitioners should be able to provide information on the disease, its prevention, and how to implement and promote influenza prevention programs.

References

1. Pfeifer R. Vorlaufige mitt heilunger uber die erreger der influenzae. Dtsch Med Wochenschr 1892;18:28–34.
2. Pfeifer R. Die aetiologie der influenza. *Z Hyg Infektioskr* 1893;13:357–86.
3. Winslow CE, Broadhurst J, Buchanan RE, et al. The families and genera of the bacteria: final report of the committee of the Society of American Bacteriologists on Characterization and Classification of Bacterial Types. *J Bacteriol* 1920;5:191–229.
4. Smith W, Andrewes CH, Laidlaw PP. A virus obtained from influenza patients. *Lancet* 1933;2:66–8.
5. *Influenza Factsheets.* Bethesda, MD: National Coalition for Adult Immunizations. June, 1997.
6. Pachucki CT, Walsh Pappas SA, Fuller GF, et al. Influenza A among hospital personnel and patients; implications for recognition, prevention, and control. *Arch Intern Med* 1990;149:77–80.
7. Hammond GW, Cheang M. Absenteeism among hospital staff during an influenza epidemic. Implications for immunoprophylaxis. *Can Med Assoc J* 1984;131: 449–52.
8. Williams WW, Preblud SR, Reichedlderfer PS, et al. Vaccines of importance in the hospital setting. *Infect Dis Clin North Am* 1989;76:501–4.
9. Mast EE, Harmon MW, Gravenstein S, et al. Emergency and possible transmission of amantadine-resistant viruses during nursing home outbreaks of influenza (AH3N2). *Am J Epidemiol* 1991;134:986–97.
10. Balkovic ES, Goodman, A, Rose FB, et al. Nosocomial influenza A(H1N1) infection. *Am J Med Technol* 1980;46:318–20.
11. Van Voris LP, Belshe RB, Shaffer JL. Nosocomial influenza B virus infection in the elderly. *Ann Intern Med* 1982;96:153–8.
12. Centers for Disease Control. Suspected nosocomial influenza cases in an intensive care unit. *MMWR* 1988;37:3.
13. Campbell DS, Rumley MH. Cost-effectiveness of the influenza vaccine in a healthy, working-age population. *J Occup Environ Med* 1997;39(5):408–14.
14. Nichol KL, Lind A, Margolis KL, et al. The effectiveness of vaccination against influenza in healthy working adults. *N Engl J Med* 1995;333:889–93.
15. Smith JWG, Pollard R. Vaccination against influenza: a five-year study of the post office. *J Hyg (London)* 1979;83:157–70.
16. Greene CC, Beaver GT. A study of mass influenza inoculation in a large industry. *J Occup Med* 1960;2: 263–70.
17. Philipp R, Harvey K, Fletcher G, et al. Sickness absence from work and influenza immunization. *J Soc Occup Med* 1987;37:128–9.
18. Wiengarten S, Staniloff H, Ault M, et al. Do hospital employees benefit from the influenza vaccine? A placebo-controlled clinical trail. *J Gen Intern Med* 1988; 3:32–7.
19. Olsen GW, Burris JM, Burlew MM, et al. Absenteeism among employees who participated in a workplace influenza immunization program. *J Occup Environ Med* 1998;40(4):311–6.
20. Glezen WP, Decker M, Perrotta DM. Survey of underlying conditions of persons hospitalized with acute respiratory disease during influenza epidemics in Hous-

ton, 1978–1981. *Am Rev Respir Dis* 1987;136: 550–5.

21. Benenson AS (ed). *Control of Communicable Diseases Manual*, 16th Ed. Washington, DC: American Public Health Association, 1995. Pp 245–51.
22. Last JM (ed). *A Dictionary of Epidemiology*, 3rd Ed. New York: Oxford University Press, 1995. P 121.
23. Jones HS. *Thucydidis Historiae*. Exfor, Engl: Clarendon Press, 1942.
24. Langmuir AD, Worthen TD, Solomon J, et al. Thucydides syndrome; a new hypothesis for the cause of the Plague of Athens. *N Engl J Med* 1985;313(16): 1027–30.
25. Townsend JF. History of influenza epidemics. *Ann Med History* 1933;5:533–47.
26. Douglas RG. Influenza. In: Goldman L, Bennett JC (eds), *Cecil Textbook of Medicine*, 19th Ed. Philadelphia: W.B. Saunders, 1992. Chap 36, 1815.
27. Graves RJ. Influenza. In: Graves RJ, Gerhard WW (eds), *System of Clinical Medicine*. Philadelphia: E. Barrington and G.D. Hasvwell, 1848. P 462.
28. Farr W. *Tenth Annual Report of the Registrar General*. H.M.S.O., London, 1847.
29. *The American Experience: #1005, Influenza 1918, Latest Findings (Transcript)*. WGBH (PBS). Produced and Directed by Robert Kenner and hosted by David McCullough. Broadcast on Public Television, 1998.
30. Centers for Disease Control. Update: isolation of an avian influenza A (H5N1) viruses from humans—Hong Kong, 1997–1998. *MMWR* 1998;46,52,53: 1245–7.
31. World Health Organization. *Emerging and other Communicable Diseases, Fact Sheet #188, Influenza A(H5N1)*, January 9, 1998. Available at *http://www.who.ch/programmes/emc/flu/h5n1.htm*.
32. Centanni E, Savonuzzi O (cited by Stubbs EL). Fowl plague. In: Bister HE, Schwarte OH (eds), *Diseases of Poultry*, 4th Ed. Ames, IA: Iowa State University Press, 1965.
33. Shope RE. Swine influenza (a series of papers). *J Exp Med* 1931;54:349–85.
34. Shope RE. The incidence of neutralizing antibodies for swine influenza virus in the sera of human beings of different ages. *J Exp Med* 1936;63:669–84.
35. Davenport FM, Hennessy AB, Francis T. Epidemiologic and immunologic significance of age distribution of antibody to antigenic variants of influenza virus. *J Exp Med* 1953;98:641–56.
36. Laidlaw PP. Epidemic influenza: a virus disease. *Lancet* 1935;1:1118.
37. Shope RE, Francis T. The susceptibility of swine to the virus of human influenza. *J Exp Med* 1936;64:791.
38. Shope RE. Serological evidence for the occurrence of infection with human influenza virus in swine. *J Exp Med* 1938;67:739–48.
39. Kaplan MM, Payne AM. Serological survey in animals for type A influenza in relation to the 1957 pandemic. *Bull WHO* 1959;20:465–88.
40. Kundin WD. Hong Kong influenza virus infection among swine during a human epidemic in Taiwan. *Nature (London)* 1970;228:857.
41. Schnurrenberger PR, Woods GT, Marti RJ. Serologic evidence of human infection with swine virus. *Am Rev Respir Dis* 1970;102:356–61.
42. Smith TF, Burgert EO, Dowdle WR, et al. Isolation of swine influenza virus from autopsy lung tissue of man. *N Engl J Med* 1976;294:708–10.
43. O'Brien RJ, Noble GR, Easterday BC, et al. Swine-like influenza virus infection in a Wisconsin farm family. *J Infect Dis* 1977;136 (suppl):S390–6.
44. Hurwitz E, Schonberger LB, Nelson DB, et al. Guillain-Barré syndrome and 1978–79 influenza vaccine. *N Engl J Med* 1981;304:1557.
45. Kaplan JE, Katona P, Hurwitz ES, et al. Guillain-Barré syndrome in the United States, 1979–1980 and 1980–1981. Lack of association with influenza vaccination. *JAMA* 1982;248:698–700.
46. Wentworth DE, McGregor MW, Macklin MD, et al. Transmission of swine influenza virus to humans after exposure to experimentally infected pigs. *J Infect Dis* 1997;175:7–14.
47. Department of Health and Human Services. *Biosafety in Microbiological and Biomedical Laboratories*, 3rd Ed. Publication #(CDC) 93-8395. Washington, DC: U.S. Government Printing Office, 1993. Pp 44–67. Available at *http://www.cdc.gov/od/ohs/biosfty/*.
48. Top FH, Russell PK. Swine influenza at Fort Dix, IV: summary and speculation. *J Infect Dis* 1977;135 (suppl):S376–80.
49. Hinshaw VS, Bean WJ Jr, Webster RB, et al. The prevalence of influenza viruses in swine and the antigenic and genetic relatedness of influenza viruses from man and swine. *Virology* 1978;84:51–62.
50. Dasco CC, Couch RB, Six HR, et al. Sporadic occurrence of zoonotic swine influenza virus infections. *J Clin Microbiol* 1984;20:833–5.
51. Patriarca PA, Kendal AP, Xakowski PC, et al. Lack of significant person-to- person spread of swine influenza-like virus following fatal infection of an immunocompromised child. *Am J Epidemiol* 1984;119:152–8.
52. Rota PA, Rocha EP, Harmon MW, et al. Laboratory characterization of a swine influenza virus isolated from a fatal case of human influenza. *J Clin Microbiol* 1989;27:1413–6.
53. Wentworth D, Xian X, Cooley AJ, et al. An influenza A(H1N1) virus closely related to swine influenza responsible for a fatal case of human influenza. *J Virol* 1994;68:2051–8.
54. Dykes AC, Cherry JD, Nolan DE. A clinical, epidemiologic, serologic, and virologic study of influenza C virus infection. *Arch Intern Med* 1980;140:1295–8.

55. A revision of the system of nomenclature for influenza virus. *Bull WHO* 1971;45:119–124.

56. A revision of the system of nomenclature for influenza viruses: a WHO memorandum (meeting February, 1980). *Bull WHO* 1980;58(4):585–91.

57. Laver WG, Webster RG. Studies on the origin of pandemic influenza III. Evidence implicating duck and equine influenza viruses as possible progenitors of the Hong Kong strain of human influenza. *Virology* 1973;51:383–91.

58. Scholtissek C. Influenza virus genetics. *Adv Genet* 1979;20:1–36.

59. Schoenbaum SC, Coleman MT, Dowdle WR, et al. Epidemiology of influenza in the elderly: evidence of virus recycling. *Am J Epidemiol* 1976;103:166–73.

60. Houseworth WJ, Spoon MM. The age distribution of excess mortality during A2 Hong Kong influenza epidemics compared with earlier A2 outbreaks. *Am J Epidemiol* 1974;94:348–50.

61. Masurel N, Marine WM. Recycling of Asian and Hong Kong influenza A virus hemagglutinins in man. *Am J Epidemiol* 1973;97:44–9.

62. Pearl R. Influenza studies: on certain general statistical aspects of the 1918 epidemic in American cities. *Public Health Rep* 1919;34:1743–83.

63. Frost WH. The epidemiology of influenza. *Public Health Rep* 1919;34(33):1823–6.

64. Gross PA. Preparing for the next influenza pandemic: a reemerging infection. *Ann Intern Med* 1996; 124(7):682–5.

65. United States Health Care Finance Administration Program. Fight-flu campaign. Available at *http://www.medicare.gov/fightflu/fightflu.html.*

66. Glezen WP, Payne AA, Snyder DN, et al. Mortality and influenza. *J Infect Dis* 1982;146:313–21.

67. Couch RB, Kasel JA, Glezen WP, et al. Influenza: its control in persons and populations (Houston Surveillance Program). *J Infect Dis* 1986;153:431–40.

68. Hospital Infection Control Practices Advisory Committee (HICPAC). *Guidelines for Isolation Precautions in Hospitals.* Atlanta: Centers for Disease Control, 1996. Also published in: *Infect Control Hosp Epidemiol*, 1996;17:53–80, and *Am J Infect Control* 1996;24:24–52.

69. Knight V, Couch RB, Landahl HD. The effect of the lack of gravity on airborne infection during space flight. *JAMA* 1970;214:513–8.

70. Couch RB. Epidemiology of influenza—summary of influenza, Workshop IV. *J Infect Dis* 1973;128:361–86.

71. Moser MR, Bender TR, Marelolis NS, et al. An outbreak of influenza aboard a commercial airliner. *Am J Epidemiol* 1979;110:1–7.

72. Glezen WP, Frank AL, Taber LH, et al. Influenza in childhood. *Pediatr Res* 1983;17:1029–32.

73. Glezen WP, Paredes A, Taber LH. Influenza in children: relationship to other respiratory agents. *JAMA* 1980;243:1345–9.

74. Frank AL, Taber LH, Wells JM, et al. Patterns of shedding of myxoviruses and paramyxoviruses in children. *J Infect Dis* 1981;144:433–41.

75. Couch RB, Douglas RG Jr, Feson DS, et al. Correlated studies of a recombinant influenza virus vaccine. III. Protection against experimental influenza in man. *J Infect Dis* 1971;124:473–80.

76. Lefrak EA, Stevens PM, Pitha J, et al. Extracorporeal membrane oxygenation for fulminant influenza pneumonia. *Chest* 1974;66:385–8.

77. Glezen WP. Consideration of the risk of influenza in children and indications for prophylaxis. *Rev Infect Dis* 1980;2:408–20.

78. Glezen WP, Couch RB, Taber LH, et al. Epidemiological observations of influenza B virus infections in Houston, Texas, 1976–1977. *Am J Epidemiol* 1980;111:13–22.

79. Glezen WP, Couch RB. Interpandemic influenza in the Houston Area, 1974–1976. *N Engl J Med* 1978; 298:587–92.

80. Acute respiratory illness among cruise-ship passengers—Asia. *MMWR* 1988;37(4):63–6.

81. Frank AL, Taber LH, Wells JM. Comparison of infection rates and severity of illness for influenza A subtypes H1N1 and H3N2 (Houston). *J Infect Dis* 1985;151:73–80.

82. Glezen WP, Couch RB. Influenza Viruses. In: Evans AS, Kaslow RA (eds), *Viral Infections of Humans, Epidemiology and Control.* 4th Ed. New York, London. Plenum, 1997. P 482.

83. Longini IM Jr, Kiipman JS. Household and community transmission parameters from final distribution of infections in households. *Biometrics* 1982;38:115–26.

84. Longini IM Jr, Koopman JS, Montao AS, et al. Estimating household and community transmission parameters for influenza. *Am J Epidemiol* 1982;115:736–48.

85. Webster RG, Bean WJ, Gorman OT, et al. Evaluation and ecology of influenza A viruses. *Mirobiol Rev* 1992;56:152–79.

86. Webster RG. Influenza virus: transmission between species and relevance to emergency of the next human pandemic. *Arch Virol* 1997;13(suppl):105–13.

87. Webster RG, Shortridge KF, Kawaoka Y. Influenza: interspecies transmission and emergency of new pandemics. *FEMS Immunol Med Microbiol* 1997;18 (4):275–9.

88. Webster RG, Sharp GB, Claas ED. Interspecies transmission of influenza viruses. *Am J Respir Crit Care Med* 1995;152(4 pt 2):S25–30.

89. Centers for Disease Control. *Prevention and control of influenza: recommendations of the Advisory Committee on Immunization Practices. MMWR* 1997;46: RR-9.

90. Little JW, Hall WJ, Douglas RG Jr, et al. Airway hyperactivity and peripheral airway dysfunction in influenza A infection. *Am Rev Respir Dis* 1978;118:295–303.

91. Evans AS, Niederman JC, Sawyer RN, et al. Prospective studies of a group of Yale University freshmen. II. Occurrence of acute respiratory infections and rubella. *J Infect Dis* 1971;123:271–8.

92. Layd PM, Engelberg AL, Dobbs HI, et al. Outbreak of influenza A/USSR/77 at Marquette University. *J Infect Dis* 1980;142:347–52.

93. Kendal AP, Schieble J, Cooney MK, et al. Cocirculation of two influenza A(H3N2) antigenic variants detected by virus surveillance in individual communities (Berkeley and Seattle). *Am J Epidemiol* 1978;108: 308–11.

94. Evans AS, Dick EC, Nystuden K. Influenza in University of Wisconsin students. *Arch Environ Health* 1963;6:62–9.

95. Evans AS, Espiritu-Campos L. Acute respiratory diseases in students at the University of the Philippines, 1964–69. *Bull WHO* 1971;45:103–12.

96. Klontz KC, Hynes NA, Gunn RA, et al. An outbreak of influenza A. Taiwan/1/86 H1N1 infections at a naval base and its association with airplane travel. *Am J Epidemiol* 1980;129:341–8.

97. Lebiush M, Rannon L, Kark JD. An outbreak of A/USSR/90/77 H1N1 influenza in army recruits. Clinical and laboratory observations. *Mil Med* 1982;147: 43–8.

98. Evans AS. Serologic studies of acute respiratory infection in military personnel. *Yale J Biol Med* 1975; 48:201–9.

99. Roscelli JD, Bass JW, Pang L. Guillain-Barré syndrome and influenza vaccination in the U.S. Army, 1980–88. *Am J Epidemiol* 1991;133:952–5.

100. Meikejohn G. Viral respiratory disease at Lowry Air Force Base in Denver, 1952–1982. *J Infect Dis* 1983;148:775–84.

101. Nowotny N, Mostl K, Maderbacher R, et al. Serological studies in Austrian fattening pigs with respiratory disorders. *Acta Vet Hung* 1994;42:377–9.

102. Nowotny N, Armin D, Klemens F, et al. Prevalence of swine influenza and other viral, bacterial, and parasitic zoonoses in veterinarians. *J Infect Dis* 1997;76(5): 1414–5.

103. Horman JT, Stetler HC, Israel E, et al. An outbreak of influenza A in a nursing home. *Am J Public Health* 1986;124:114–9.

104. Patriarca PA, Weber JA, Parker RA, et al. Risk factors for outbreaks of influenza in nursing homes; a case-control study. *Am J Epidemiol* 1986;76:501–4.

105. Centers for Disease Control. Outbreak of influenza A in a nursing home—New York, December 1991 to January 1992. *MMWR* 1992;41:129–31.

106. Gross PA, Rodstein M, LaMontagne JR, et al. Epidemiology of acute respiratory illness during an influenza outbreak in a nursing home. *Arch Intern Med* 1988;148:559–61.

107. Catter ML, Renzullo PO, Helgerson SD, et al. Influenza outbreaks in nursing homes: how effective is influenza vaccine in the institutionalized elderly? *Infect Control Hosp Epidemiol* 1990;11:473–8.

108. Centers for Disease Control. Draft guidelines for infection control in health care personnel, 1997 (section 22, respiratory viral infections). *Federal Register* 1997;62(173)September 8:47275–327.

109. Potter J, Stott DJ, Roberts MA. Influenza vaccination of health care workers in long-term-care hospitals reduces the mortality of elderly patients. *J Infect Dis* 1997;175:1–6.

110. Miotti PG, Nelson KE, Dallabetta GA, et al. The influence of HIV infection on antibody responses to a 2-dose regimen of influenza vaccine. *JAMA* 1989;262: 779–83.

111. Cheson F, Hewitt D. Spread of influenza in a factory. *Br J So Med* 1952;6:68–75.

112. Ksaizek TG, Olson JG, Irving GS, et al. An influenza outbreak due to A/USSR/77-like (H1N1) virus aboard a U.S. Navy ship. *Am J Epidemiol* 1980;112: 487–94.

113. Centers for Disease Control. Guidelines for preventing the transmission of *Mycobacterium* tuberculosis in health-care facilities. *MMWR* 1994;43(RR-13):69–88.

114. Department of Health and Human Services and Centers for Disease Control. Guidelines for preventing the transmission of *Mycobacterium* tuberculosis in health-care facilities, Notice (Supplement #3, Engineering Controls). *Federal Register*, 1994;V59(208)October 28:54276–88.

115. Occupational Health and Safety Administration. *Technical Manual, Section V, Hospital Investigations, Health and Hazards.* Washington, DC: OSHA, 1988.

116. Baroyan OV, Rvachev LA, Ivannikow YG. *Modeling and forecasting of influenza epidemics for the territory of the USSR.* Moscow: Gameleya Institute of Epidemiology and Microbiology, 1977.

117. Collins SD, Lehmann J. Trends and epidemics of influenza and pneumonia, 1918–1951. *Public Health Rep* 1951;6:1487–505.

118. Collins SD. *Influenza in the United States, 1887–1957.* Public Health Monograph #48. Washington, DC: Government Printing Office, 1957.

119. Serfling RE. Methods for current statistical analysis of excess pneumonia-influenza deaths. *Public Health Rep* 1963;78:494–506.

120. Choi K, Thacker SB. An evaluation of influenza mortality surveillance, 1962–1979. 1. Time series forecasts of expected pneumonia and influenza deaths. *Am J Epidemiol* 1981;113:215–22.

121. Simonsen L, Clarke MJ, Williamson GD, et al. The impact of influenza epidemics on mortality: introducing a severity index. *Am J Public Health* 1997;87(12): 1944–50.

122. Salk JE. Reactions to concentrated influenza virus vaccines. *J Immunol* 1948;58:369–95.
123. Baker RS, van Frank RM. Purification of large quantities of influenza virus by density gradient centrifugation. *J Virol* 1967;1:1207–16.
124. Tyrrell DAJ, Schild GC, Dowdle WR, et al. Development and use of influenza vaccines. *Bull World Health Organ* 1981;59:165–73.
125. Poland GA. Lessons from the influenza vaccine recall of 1996/1997. *JAMA* 1997;278(12):1022–3.
126. *Physicians' Desk Reference*, 52nd Ed. Montavale, NJ: Medical Economics Company, 1998.
127. Hobson D, Curry RL, Beare AS, et al. The role of serum hemagglutination-inhibiting antibody in protection against challenge infection with influenza A and B viruses. *J Hyg (Lond)* 1972;70:767–77.
128. Neuzil KM, Reed GW, Mitchel EF, et al. Influenza morbidity increases in late pregnancy. *Abstracts of the IDSA*, 34th Annual Meeting, 1996:48.
129. Safrin S, Rush JD, Mills J. Influenza in patients with human immunodeficiency virus infection. *Chest* 1990;98:33–7.
130. Murphy KR, Strunk RC. Safe administration of influenza vaccine in asthmatic children hypersensitive to egg proteins. *J Pediatr* 1985;106:931–3.
131. Aberer W. Vaccination despite thimerosal sensitivity. *Contact Dermatitis* 1991;24:6–10.
132. Renton K. Decreased elimination of theophylline after influenza vaccination. *Can Med Assoc J* 1980;123:288.
133. Goldstein RS. Decreased elimination of theophylline after influenza vaccination. *Can Med Assoc J* 1982;126:470.
134. Britton L, Ruben FL. Serum and theophylline levels after influenza vaccination. *Can Med Assoc J* 1982;126:1375.
135. Fischer RG. Influence of trivalent influenza vaccine on serum theophylline levels. *Can Med Assoc J* 1982;124:1312.
136. San Joaquin VH, Reyes S, Marks MI. Influenza vaccination in asthmatic children on maintenance theophylline therapy. *Clin Pediatr* 1982;21:724–6.
137. Stults B, Hasisaki P. Influenza vaccination and theophylline pharmacokinetics in patients with chronic obstructive lung disease. *West J Med* 1983;139:651–4.
138. Kramer P. Effect of influenza vaccine on warfarin anticoagulation. *Clin Pharmacol Ther* 1984;35:416.
139. Lipsky GA. Influenza vaccination and warfarin anticoagulation. *Ann Intern Med* 1984;100:835–7.
140. Hassan WU, Henderson AF, Keaney NP. Influenza vaccination in asthma. *Lancet* 1992;339:194.
141. Daggett P. Influenza and asthma. *Lancet* 1992;339:367.
142. Palache AM, van der Velden JW. Influenza vaccination in asthma. *Lancet* 1992;339:741.
143. Watson JM, Cordier JF. Nicholson KG. Does influenza immunization cause exacerbations of chronic airflow obstruction or asthma? *Thorax* 1997;52(2):190–4.
144. Schonberger L, Bregman DJ, Sullivan-Bolyai JZ, et al. Guillain-Barré syndrome following vaccination in the national immunization programs, United States 1976–1977. *Am J Epidemiol* 1979;110:105–23.
145. Hayase Y, Tobita K. Influenza virus and neurological diseases. *Psychiatry Clin Neurosci* 1997;51(4):181–4.
146. Mac Kenzie WR, Davis JP, Peterson DE, et al. Multiple-false positive serologic tests for HIV, HTLV-1, and hepatitis C following influenza vaccination. *JAMA* 1992;268(8):1015–7.
147. Vaccine Adverse Event Reporting System, P.O. Box 1100, Rockville, MD 20849-1100. Toll-free phone: 1-800-822-7967.
148. Howell MR, Nang RN, Gaydos CA, et al. Prevention of adenoviral acute respiratory disease in army recruits: cost-effectiveness of a military vaccination policy. *Am J Prev Med* 1998;14(3):168–75.
149. Centers for Disease Control, *Influenza Vaccine, 1998* (Factsheet). Atlanta: CDC, 1998. Available at *http://www.cdc.gov/ncidod/diseases/flu/fluvac.htm.*
150. Kendal AP. Cold-adapted live attenuated influenza vaccines developed in Russia: can they contribute to meeting the needs for influenza control in other countries? *Eur J Epidemiol* 1997;13(5):591–609.
151. Couch RB, Ketiel WA, Cate TR. Improvement of inactivated influenza virus vaccines. *J Infect Dis* 1997;176(suppl 1):S38–44.
152. Kuno-Sakai H. Intranasal application of inactivated influenza virus vaccines. *Jpn J Clin Med* 1997;55(10):2738–45.
153. *Nasal Flu Vaccine Proves Effective in Children.* Press Release, National Institute for Allergy and Infectious Disease. 1997. Available at *http://www.niaid.nih.gov/dateline.*
154. Bamford MJ. Neuraminidase inhibitors as potential anti-influenza drugs. *J Enzyme Inhib* 1996;10(1):1–16.
155. Hayden FG, Osterhaus AD, Treaner JJ. Efficacy and safety of the neuraminidase inhibitor zanamivir in the treatment of influenza virus infections. GG167 Influenza Study Group. *N Engl J Med* 1997;337(13):874–80.
156. Centers for Disease Control. Implementation of the Medicare influenza benefit program. *MMWR* 1994;43:771–3.
157. Frank AL, Taber LH, Wells JM. Individuals infected with two subtypes of Influenza A virus in the same season. *J Infect Dis* 1983;147:120–4.
158. Doebbeling BN, Edmond MD, Davis CS, et al. Influenza vaccination of health care workers: evaluation of factors that are important in acceptance. *Prev Med* 1997;26(1):68–77.

159. Mullooly JP, Bennett MD, Hornbrook MC, et al. Influenza vaccination programs for elderly persons; cost-effectiveness in a health maintenance organization. *Ann Intern Med* 1994;121(12):947–52.

160. Fedson DS. Influenza and pneumococcal vaccination of the elderly; newer vaccines and prospects for clinical benefits at the margin. *Prev Med* 1994;23(5): 751–5.

161. Gross PA, Hermogenes AW, Sacks HS, et al. The efficacy of influenza vaccine in the elderly person. A meta-analysis and review of the literature. *Ann Intern Med* 1995;123(7):518–27.

162. Hampson AW, Irving LB. Influenza vaccination: cost-effective health care of the older adults? *J Qual Clin Prac* 1997;17(1):3–11.

163. Centers for Disease Control. Medicare influenza vaccine demonstration—selected states, 1988–1992. *JAMA* 1992;267(13):1734–5.

164. Final results: Medicare influenza vaccine demonstration—selected states, 1988–1992. *MMWR* 1993;42 (31):601–4.

165. Rose DN, Schechter CB, Sacks HS. Influenza and pneumococcal vaccination of HIV-infected patients: a policy analysis. *Am J Med* 1993;94(2):160–8.

166. Gorse GJ, Otto EE, Daughaday CC, et al. Influenza vaccination of patients with chronic lung disease. *Chest* 1997;112(5):1221–33.

167. Kumpulainen V, Makela M. Influenza vaccination among healthy employees; a cost-benefit analysis. *Scand J Infect Dis* 1997;29(2):181–5.

168. Jefferson T, Mugford M, Gray A, et al. An exercise on the feasibility of carrying out secondary economic analysis. *Health Econ* 1996;5(2):155–65.

169. Kent DL. The basics of decision analysis. *J Dent Educ* 1992;56(12):791–9.

170. Schoenbaum SC. Economic impact of influenza. The individual's perspective. *Am J Med* 1987;82(6A):26–30.

171. Wharton M, Chorba TL, Vogt RL, et al. Case Definitions for Public Health Surveillance. *MMWR* 1990;39:RR-13.

172. Jordan WS Jr, Badger GF, Dingle JA. A study of illness in a group of Cleveland families, XVI: The epidemiology of influenza, 1948–1953. *Am J Hyg* 1958;68:169–89.

173. Fox JP, Hall CE, Cooney MK, et al. Influenza virus: infection in Seattle families, 1975–1979. *Am J Epidemiol* 1982;116:212–27.

174. Taber LH, Paredes A, Glezen WP, et al. Infection with influenza A/Victoria virus in Houston families, 1976. *J Hyg (Camb)* 1981;86:303–13.

175. Monto AS, Davenport FM, Napier JA, et al. Effect of vaccination of a school-age population upon the course of an A2/Hong Kong influenza epidemic. *Bull WHO* 1969;41:537–42.

176. Glezen WP, Decker M, Joseph SW, et al. Acute respiratory disease associated with influenza epidemics in Houston, 1981–1983. *J Infect Dis* 1987;155:1119–26.

177. Frank AL, Taber LH. Variation in frequency in natural reinfection with influenza A viruses. *J Med Virol* 1983;12:17–23.

178. Frank AL, Taber LS, Glezen WP, et al. Influenza B virus infections in the community and the family. The epidemics of 1976–1977 and 1979–1980 in Houston, TX. *Am J Epidemiol* 1983;118:313–25.

179. Frank AL, Taber LH, Glezen WP, et al. Reinfection with influenza A (H3N2) virus in young children and their families. *J Infect Dis* 1979;140:829–35.

180. Frank AL, Taber LH, Porter CM. Influenza B virus reinfection. *Am J Epidemiol* 1987;125:576–86.

181. Bainton D, Jones GR, Hole D. Influenza and ischemic heart disease—a possible trigger for acute myocardial infarction. *Int J Epidemiol* 1978;7:231–9.

182. Pönka A, Jalanko H, Pönka T, et al. Viral and mycoplasmal antibodies in patients with myocardial infarction. *Ann Clin Res* 1981;13:429–32.

183. Finland M, Parker F, Barnes M. Acute myocarditis in influenza A infection. *Am J Med Sci* 1945;207:455–68.

184. Leebeek FW, Baggen MG, Mulder LJ, et al. Rhabdomyolysis associated with influenza A virus infection. *Neth J Med* 1995;46(4):189–92.

185. Corey L, Rubin RJ, Hattiwick MA, et al. A nationwide outbreak of Reye's syndrome. *Am J Med* 1976;61:615–25.

186. Wilson B, Planterose DN, Naginton J, et al. Influenza A antigens on human lymphocytes *in vitro* and probably *in vivo*. *Nature* 1976;259:582–4.

187. O'Callaghan E, Sham P, Takei N. Schizophrenia after prenatal exposure to 1957 A2 "(H2N2)" influenza epidemic. *Lancet* 1991;25;337(8752):1248–50.

188. McGrath J, Castle D. Does influenza cause schizophrenia? A five year review. *Aust NZ J Psychiatry* 1995;29(1):23–31.

189. Schiff LJ. Studies on the mechanisms of influenza virus infection in hamster trachea organ culture. *Arch Ges Virus-forsch* 1974;44:195–204.

190. Larson EW, Dominik JW, Rowberg AH, et al. Influenza virus population dynamics in the respiratory tract of experimentally infected mice. *Infect Immunol* 1976;13:438–47.

191. Wallach J. *Interpretation of Diagnostic Tests*, 6th Ed. Boston: Little Brown, 1996. P 756.

Readings on Future Pandemics and Planning

Glezen WP. Emerging infection; pandemic influenza. *Epidemiol Rev* 1996;18(1):64–76.

Hayden FG. Antivirals for pandemic influenza. *J Infect Dis* 1997;176(suppl 1):S56–61.

Kilbourne ED. Perspectives on pandemics; a research agenda. *J Infect Dis* 1997;176(suppl 1):S29–31.

Monto AS. Prospects for pandemic influenza control with currently available vaccines and antivirals. *J Infect Dis* 1997;176(suppl 1):S32–7.

Shortridge KF. The next pandemic influenza virus? *Lancet* 1995;346(8984):1210–2.

12 / Occupational Chlamydial and Rickettsial Respiratory Infections

Daniel J. Martin

Chlamydial and rickettsial agents have been found to be important pathogens in the workplace. They are nonmotile, gram-negative, obligate intracellular organisms. *Chlamydia* species have a biphasic life cycle [1], and while they are prokaryotic, they are distinct from the Eubacteria. *Chlamydia* have a spore-like extracellular elementary body (EB) that attaches to the host cell, enters via endocytosis [2], and reorganizes via growth and replication into the reticulate body (RB). Various bird species act as a reservoir for the bacteria. Eventually the organisms are released from the cell to initiate further infection. Four species of *Chlamydia* have been identified: *Chlamydia psittaci*, *Chlamydia trachomatis*, *Chlamydia pneumoniae*, and *Chlamydia pecorum*. The first three are potential human pathogens and exhibit a variety of different presentations, including respiratory infection. Clinical and serologic factors may be similar for these species, providing the physician with some diagnostic difficulty.

The family Rickettsiaceae includes two groups of the genus *Rickettsia*: the typhus group and the spotted fever group. *Rickettsia* are bacteria that utilize a cycle of mammalian reservoirs and arthropod vectors. Primarily zoonotic diseases, they tend to be fastidious and may produce endotoxin [3]. Their clinical manifestations reflect the proliferation of the organism in the endothelium of small blood vessels, resulting in characteristic rashes and vasculitic complications.

Coxiella burnetii, the agent of Q fever, and *Bartonella* are two species related to *Rickettsia*. *C burnetii* is unique among this group in that it is quite a hardy organism and has the potential of causing severe economic damage when outbreaks occur among livestock. *Bartonella* species include *Bartonella quintana*, *B henselae*, and *B elizabethae*. These organisms cause bacteremic illness and should be considered in the differential diagnosis of cases of culture-negative endocarditis. *Orientia tsutsugamushi* was formerly a member of the *Rickettsia* genus. In its endemic area, it is a relatively common arthropod-borne zoonosis that causes infection in a considerable percentage of those exposed.

This chapter focuses primarily on *Chlamydia psittaci*, the agent of psittacosis, *Chlamydia pneumoniae*, the TWAR agent, and *C burnetii*, the agent of Q fever. Mention is also made of *Chlamydia trachomatis*, *Rickettsia prowazekii*, *Rickettsia typhi*, *Rickettsia rickettsia*, *Orientia tsutsugamushi*, and *Bartonella quintana*. See Table 12-1.

Pathogens

CHLAMYDIA

In 1879, Dr. J. Ritter described seven patients who became ill after exposure to his brother's parrots in Uster, Switzerland. He termed their illness *pneumotyphus* [4]. In 1892, Morange observed similar events related to parrots and coined the term *psittacosis* (*psittakos*; Greek for "parrot") [5]. In 1907, Halberstaedter and von Prowazek examined the "mantled" intracytoplasmic organisms in tissue from patients with trachoma. They classified these organisms as Chlamydozoaceae

Table 12-1
Chlamydial and Rickettsial Infections and Their Epidemiology and Clinical Features

Disease	Organism	Vector/Reservoir	Geographic Distribution	Clinical Aspects	Diagnosis	Therapy
Psittacosis	*Chlamydia psittaci*	Birds	Worldwide	Fever, headache, tracheobronchitis or atypical pneumonia	Culture, MIF, CF titers	Tetracycline, doxycycline for 10–14 days
Trachoma	*Chlamydia trachomatis*	Humans	Worldwide	Ocular/urethritic/pneumonitic presentations; female sterility	Culture with FA, ELISA, MIF, DFA	Azithromycin 1 gm single-dose; doxycycline, ofloxacin, erythromycin for 7 days
TWAR pneumonia	*Chlamydia pneumoniae*	Humans	Worldwide/favors tropics	Upper and lower respiratory infection	IgG and IgM MIF, CF, cell culture of throat swab	Tetracycline, erythromycin, azithromycin, clarithromycin for 10–14 days
Q fever	*Coxiella burnetii*	Domestic ungulates	Worldwide (except New Zealand)	Acute form with flu-like onset, then atypical pneumonia; chronic forms include endocarditis	CF, IFA, MIF, ELISA, blood culture	Tetracycline, doxycycline, erythromycin for 2–4 weeks for acute; doxycycline, quinolone combinations for chronic, for 2–3 years or more
Epidemic typhus	*Rickettsia prowazekii*	*Pediculus humanus corporis*/humans	Worldwide	Headache, fever, chills, truncal rash with facial and palmar sparing	ELISA, MIF, tissue staining	Single-dose doxycycline, 100 mg, for epidemic; longer courses of doxycycline, chloramphenicol, or tetracycline for Brill-Zinsser disease

Murine typhus	*Rickettsia typhi*	*Xenopsylla cheopsis/ Rattus* spp.	Worldwide; parallels rodent populations	Milder than *Rickettsia prowazekii*; headache, fever, truncal rash	IFA, LA, Dip-S-Ticks	Doxycycline, chloramphenicol, tetracycline, quinolones effective
Rocky Mountain spotted fever	*Rickettsia rickettsii*	*Dermacentor andersonii*	Worldwide (various spotted fevers)	Fever, headache, wrist and ankle rash that spreads centripetally	Staining of rash biopsy, LA, IFA, CF	Tetracycline, chloramphenicol, doxycycline for 7 days
Scrub typhus	*Orientia tsutsugamushi*	Chiggers (larval *Leptotrombidium* spp.)/rodents	Eastern Asia, western Pacific	Eschar, local adenopathy, fever, headache, spreading truncal rash	IFA, IIP, Dip-S-Ticks	Tetracycline or doxycycline for 7 days (single-dose or 3-day course)
Trench fever	*Bartonella quintana*	*Pediculus humanus*	Worldwide	Variable duration of fever, bacteremia, shin pain	IFA, blood "subculture"	Erythromycin, doxycycline, tetracycline (optimum regimen)

CF = complement fixation; DFA = direct immunofluorescent antibody; ELISA = enzyme-linked immunosorbent assay; FA = fluorescent antibody; IFA = immunofluorescent antibody; IIP = indirect immunoperidase; LA = latex agglutination; MIF = microimmunofluorescence.

(*chlamys*; Greek for "mantle") [6]. Laboratory isolation and microscopic examination of the etiologic agent involved in a human outbreak of psittacosis was performed in 1930 [7]. Similar identification was taking place in British, United States, and German laboratories [8]. Subsequent reports showed that transmission could be achieved via nonpsittacine birds, such as chickens, turkeys [9], petrels [10], pigeons [11], and ducks [12]. Previously felt to be viral, these organisms were correctly classified as bacteria in 1966 [13], and the agents trachoma, psittacosis, and lymphogranuloma venereum (LGV) were grouped together under the genus *Chlamydia*. It is now apparent that virtually any bird species may act as a reservoir for *C psittaci*, and the terms *psittacosis*, or *ornithosis*, for human infection, and *avian chlamydiosis* (*AC*), for bird infection, are more properly used [14–16].

C trachomatis is the cause of ocular trachoma (serotypes A–C), genitourinary tract infections (serotypes D–K), and lymphogranuloma venereum (serotypes L1–3) [17]. Recognized in antiquity, treatments for trachoma were first described in China in the twenty-seventh century BC, and Egypt in the nineteenth century BC [18]. The characteristic cytoplasmic inclusions were first noted in tissue from an infant with trachoma in 1909 [19], were later found in the cervical and urethral cells of an infected child's parents [20], and in the urethrae of men with nongonococcal urethritis [21]. Currently, *C trachomatis* is recognized as a common sexually transmitted pathogen worldwide, making it an important public health issue.

A third chlamydial species, *C pneumoniae* (TWAR), was first isolated from the conjunctiva of a child in Taiwan in 1965 and termed *TW 183* (for "Taiwan"). The same agent was later isolated in Seattle in 1983 and was referred to as *AR 39* (for "acute respiratory") [22]. A retrospective analysis of sera stored from a 1978 springtime epidemic among young adult Finns revealed positive complement fixation (CF) titers in 78% of these pneumonias. This indicated that the organism could also cause epidemic outbreaks of respiratory disease [23]. In 1986, Grayston isolated the organism [24] and confirmed its etiologic role via use of the microimmunofluorescent antibody (MIF) test in a group of Washington University students with pneumonias and bronchitis. Combining the TW and AR prefixes, he referred to it as the *TWAR agent*. Originally considered a strain of *C psittaci*, the organism was ultimately recognized as a new species and given the name *C pneumoniae* because of its most frequently recognized manifestation [25]. Subsequent reports have illuminated the role of this organism in close-population and barracks outbreaks [26–29]. *C pneumoniae* is also a cause of bronchitis, sinusitis, and other milder forms of respiratory disease [30].

RICKETTSIA AND RELATED PATHOGENS

In 1935, an Australian medical officer named E. H. Derrick described a febrile illness that afflicted 20 employees of a Brisbane, Queensland, meat-processing plant. The puzzling disease was named *Q* (for "query") *fever* [31]. Burnett and Freeman showed that a rickettsial organism could be isolated from the blood and urine of Derrick's patients [32], and the organism was soon recovered from the Rocky Mountain wood tick in Montana by Davis and Cox [33]. The agent thus came to be known as *Coxiella burnetii*. *C burnetii*, an important occupational pathogen, has now been found in 51 nations on five continents [34], and both acute and chronic forms of infection have been described. *C burnetii* is a pleomorphic gram-negative coccobacillus, an intracellular parasite that is highly infectious to humans. It exhibits phase variation, with transformation between a phase I "virulent," and phase II "avirulent," form [35]. Within cells, it multiplies within acidic phagolysosomes, making it difficult to eradicate. While animal infection is usually subclinical, human infection can result in a variety of febrile illnesses, including pneumonitis.

Louse-born typhus (also known as *jail fever*) is another ancient disease that continues to command our attention. Epidemics were first noted in the 1400s, and 3 million deaths in Europe and the Soviet Union were attributed to typhus between 1918 and 1922 [36]. The causative organism, *Rickettsia prowazekii*, is transmitted from person to person by the human body louse, *Pediculus humanus corporis*. Transmission is aided by crowded, unsanitary conditions such as those that occur during wars or following natural disasters [37]. Recrudescence of epidemic typhus may occur years later and is called *Brill-Zinsser disease*. Murine typhus is caused by *Rickettsia typhi* and parallels the worldwide distribution of *Rattus* rats, its primary reservoir. Originally differentiated from the clinically similar typhus-like illnesses in 1926, it was eventually isolated from rats and its main vector, the flea *Xenopsylla cheopis* [38]. Transmission occurs when infected flea feces is rubbed into a pruritic bite. *Rickettsia rickettsii* is a tick-borne organism that causes a characteristic vasculitic rash on the trunk and extremities, a disease known as *Rocky Mountain spotted fever (RMSF)*. The first descriptions of the disease came from the Native American tribes of Montana [39]. The role of ticks in transmission was demonstrated when the disease was contracted by volunteers bitten by ticks removed from a patient with RMSF [39]. Similar illness is produced by other members of the spotted fever group. Organisms such as *Rickettsia conorii*, *Rickettsia australis*, and *Rickettsia akari* are also transmitted from mammals and marsupials to humans through an arthropod vector, resulting in characteristic rashes and clinical syndromes. These illnesses appear to occur within certain geographic areas, an important epidemiologic clue to their identity. Rocky Mountain spotted fever was investigated by Howard Taylor Ricketts in the Bitterroot Valley of Montana in the early 1900s, and the organism was subsequently named in recognition of his work [3,40]. The main vectors of spotted fevers are several species of ticks, and the main reservoirs of disease are mammalian vertebrates such as rodents and dogs. The Rocky Mountain wood tick, *Dermacentor andersoni*, appears to be the most important vector in cases of RMSF.

Scrub typhus is also due to an obligate intracellular organism. Formerly classified as a rickettsial infection, it is now considered to represent a distinct genus, *Orientia tsutsugamushi* [41]. The prototype strains were termed *Gilliam*, *Karp*, and *Kato*. It is now apparent that there is great heterogeneity within the species: Investigators having identified more than 40 strains in Japan alone [42]. Subsequent analysis has shown that there is an impressive degree of genotypic and immunotypic variation, even between strains recovered within a given country [43]. Scrub typhus is an illness that results when humans are infected as accidental hosts. It derives its name from the vegetation that most frequently harbors its vector, the larval stage (chigger) of trombiculid mites [44]. This illness is seen mostly in Eastern Asia and the Western Pacific, including Australia. Field troops in Vietnam were at risk [45], and other occupations are at risk as well [46,47].

Bartonella quintana (named for its supposed five-day fever), was first described as a cause of febrile outbreaks in World War I troops and was thus termed *trench fever* [48]. Affecting up to 1 million troops in Europe in World War I, the organism made an epidemic reappearance in World War II. *B quintana* is likely spread via the body louse, and its transmission and epidemics are related to conditions of poor sanitation and hygiene [49]. In England, control of the organism was achieved to a large degree by the issuance of new clothing to returning trench warfare soldiers [50]. Phylogenetic analyses have further explored the relationship of these organisms to other proteobacteria. Thus, removal of the family Bartonellaceae from the order Rickettsiales has been proposed [51]. Another important species is *Bartonella henselae*, isolated in 1986 [52]. Transmitted by cats or their fleas, *B henselae* poses a special danger to immunocompromised individuals, especially the HIV infected.

Epidemiology

INCIDENCE AND PREVALENCE

Chlamydia psittaci

Chlamydia psittaci is commonly found in birds, including companion (pet) birds and poultry. Cases occur both sporadically and in outbreaks. The latter are often associated with a commercial source, such as an abattoir (slaughterhouse). Seroprevalence studies suggest that the disease occurs much more commonly than is reported [53]. It is likely that any bird species can be host to this organism, although psittacine birds (e.g., parrots, parakeets, cockatoos) are most often infected. Outbreaks in ducks and turkeys are especially important for economic reasons. In 1978, a single infected flock of turkeys resulted in a cost of $19,000 for a Nebraska poultry-processing plant [54].

Vertical transmission has been seen and is believed to most likely be the result of exposure to the organism in the urogenital tract or, in some cases, the result of postnatal exposure. Intrauterine infection occurs in some species, such as chickens [55], while not in other species [56]. The usual route of transmission among animals is most likely inhalation of infectious aerosols, but fecal ingestion is also a potential route [57]. Sexual transmission has been noted in sheep [58]. Infected birds may be either asymptomatic, acutely, subacutely, or chronically infected. There is a 5–15% carriage rate among asymptomatic birds, which may increase to 100% when birds are subjected to the stresses of overcrowding and breeding [8,59–61]. Selected avian populations have surprisingly high rates of prevalence. Belgian commercial turkeys were antibody-positive in 50–75% [62], and testing of German turkey flocks revealed positive results on enzyme-linked immunosorbent assay (ELISA) in 20–70% of apparently healthy birds [63]. Approximately 18% of pigeons from a public park in Spain had *Chlamydia* isolated from their feces, and approximately 30% had positive antibody tests [64]. Up to 13% of free-living raptors in the Munich area had positive cloacal swabs by the ELISA method [65]. Birds may also become acutely infected after years of latent infection [66,67].

Many other species of animals have been noted to be susceptible to infection with *C psittaci*, including horses [68,69], crocodiles [70], sheep [71], cows [72], goats [73], swine [74], bears [75], dogs [76], cats [77], and koalas [78]. Transmission from these reservoirs to humans has also been noted to occur [79,80]. Orthozoonotic infection (between species) has been documented [81].

The incidence of human infection with *C psittaci* (psittacosis) is difficult to determine with certainty. Problems in diagnosis, serologic cross-reactivity with other *Chlamydia* species, and low rates of reporting, contribute to what is likely a considerable underestimate of the true incidence and prevalence of the disease. Each year, only 100–200 cases of *C psittaci* are reported to the Centers for Disease Control and Prevention (CDC) and the British (CDSC) each year [82], although seroprevalence studies suggest that a much higher rate of infection is actually occurring. Most of the reported cases involve adults 15–44 years of age [82]. Children appear to be infected at a higher rate than would be expected in view of a presumed low rate of exposure. A Japanese study of 223 infants and children with pneumonia found that 2.2% were IgM-positive for *C psittaci* antibodies.

Infectivity is likely high among exposed humans: 44% of veterinary surgeons developed ornithosis after visiting a duck processing plant [83], and 49% of new employees in a duck-processing plant showed evidence of recent infection within 90 days of employment, although only 28% of them were clinically ill [84]. An Israeli study found that 81% of individuals exposed to diseased birds showed serologic evidence of acute infection. In a population with no recent outbreaks or avian illnesses, serology was positive in 43% of farm workers [85]. Screening of employees at an Australian duck processing plant in the wake of a *C psittaci* outbreak revealed that over 76% had serologic evidence of infection but only 12% had evidence of recent infection. Infection was usually acquired during the first year of employment [86].

Chlamydia pneumoniae

C pneumoniae exhibits a basic endemic rate and also shows periodic epidemicity. In contrast to *M pneumoniae*, it appears less likely to infect the young and more prone to infect the elderly [22]. In both adults and children, tropical regions have a higher prevalence of *C pneumoniae* than northern regions [22]. Seroprevalence studies show that more than 50% of U.S. residents have IgG to *C pneumoniae*, indicating past infection. Overall, it is responsible for approximately 10% of pneumonias, making it the third to fourth most common etiologic agent. In studies involving children, only 1% of children hospitalized with pneumonia (average age 3.7 years) had evidence of acute *C pneumoniae* infection, and in another study, only 5% of Japanese infants and children with pneumonia were IgM positive for *C pneumoniae* on microimmunofluorescence (MIF) testing [88]. After infancy, incidence rates rise rapidly. In one study, an annual attack rate of 6–9% was found in the 5- to 14-year-old age group

[90]. Many of these converters experienced minimal, if any, symptoms. Attack rates level off after the teenage years, and eventually 70% of older adults exhibit evidence of previous infection [89].

There is an unexplained gender difference, with males having positive serology at higher rates than females [90]. Experts feel that infection is likely universal, with the presence of negative antibodies indicating clearance after infection, and that reinfection is common [91]. Most likely due to its preferential infection of the elderly, 11.4% of all hospitalized patients with pneumonias are probably due to *C pneumoniae*. Other respiratory infections are also quite commonly due to the organism. Up to 20% of acute bronchitides are due to *C pneumoniae* [92], and the organism is also responsible for approximately 4% of exacerbations of chronic obstructive pulmonary disease (COPD) [93]. The relationship between chronic bronchitis and infection with *C pneumoniae* deserves attention, as 72% of COPD patients exhibit evidence of past infection [94]. Interestingly, infection with the pathogen causes ciliary stasis early on, which is believed to be responsible for frequent co-infections. These findings have led some to speculate that *C pneumoniae* has a pathogenetic role in chronic bronchitis [92,95].

Chlamydia trachomatis

Chlamydia trachomatis appears to be an exclusively human pathogen. It is the most common bacterial sexually transmitted disease (STD) in developed countries [96] and also has a high prevalence in developing nations. There is an incidence of approximately 4 million new cases in the United States each year [97]. High rates of prevalence are sustained by the fact that asymptomatic individuals may remain infectious for months, thereby infecting others without their knowledge [97].

Certain populations have extremely high rates of infection. For instance, 95% of commercial street-sex workers in Jamaica were MIF positive, indicating past or present infection, as opposed to 53% of blood donors, and active infection was found in 25% of these workers [98]. Sex workers in Istanbul had a much lower rate (12.9%) of seropositivity by DFA for unexplained reasons [99]. The high rates of infection that are sometimes seen in sex workers are felt to be due primarily to infection contracted while employed. High exposure rates in this population were illustrated by the finding that approximately 5% of seminal fluid samples recovered from a Copenhagen massage parlor demonstrated the presence of *C trachomatis* [100]. The overall prevalence of infection among sexually active asymptomatic men is approximately 10% [101]. Sexually active women have approximately a 15% prevalence rate [102]. Prevalence is highest among adolescent females and is also high among African-Americans, inner city residents, and the poor [97,206].

C trachomatis is also known to cause pneumonia. A Japanese study found 22% of children hospitalized with pneumonia to have IgM to *C trachomatis* [88]. This pathogen is also the cause of ocular trachoma and lymphogranuloma venereum (LGV). Ocular trachoma is a frequent cause of blindness, accounting for up to 9 million new cases per year and afflicting 500 million individuals worldwide [103]. LGV is caused by a distinct strain of *C trachomatis*, which exhibits high endemicity in South America, Africa, and Southeast Asia.

Coxiella burnetii

Coxiella burnetii is the agent of Q fever, existing in animal reservoirs such as sheep, goats, and cattle. The organism is prevalent throughout the world, with the exception of New Zealand [104]. The term *coxiellosis* has been applied to animal infection, which is usually asymptomatic. Abortion may result from infection with the organism in domestic animals. *C burnetii* is also found in fish, arthropods, birds, rodents, cats, and other livestock [105]. The organism can be found in the milk, urine, feces, and placentae of infected animals. The amniotic fluid and placenta can be the site of a tremendously high concentration of organisms [106], and not surprisingly, transmission appears to be highly correlated with parturition. It is believed that physiologic stress and the immunosuppression of pregnancy may encourage multiplication of the organism. Infected animals may continue to shed the organism for weeks [35]. Prevalence rates among livestock are often quite high. Sheep (24%) and goats (57%) were frequently seropositive in one California study [113], and commercial and noncommercial animals showed the same prevalence rates. Another study found that 82% of California dairy cows are antibody positive [107]. In cattle herds, serologic evidence of infection may be seen in 80% of animals [108].

Humans become infected via inhalation of infected aerosols, with the organism typically infecting monocytic cells. Males have a higher incidence than females, likely as a result of exposure differences [109]. In Nova Scotia, 12% of blood donors exhibited antibody to C burnetii [110], as did 49% of veterinarians and 35% of abattoir workers [111]. In Toronto, a more urban environment, only 0.6% of blood donors were positive, while 18% of staff at a Toronto animal research facility were infected, including 68% of the animal handlers. Of the 60 research lab workers in the Toronto study who had positive serology results, there were 12 cases of clinical illness, and two required hospital admission [112]. A study of the general population in California revealed positive serology results in 6% [113].

The incidence of the organism varies geographically; it is reported most frequently in regions where medical authorities are most vigilant. In countries without appropriate testing facilities, the reported incidence is quite low [114]. Due to the nonspecific nature of the illness and the fact that it is usually self-limited, many cases likely go undiagnosed. Highly endemic areas include parts of southern France, where the prevalence is felt to be 50 per 100,000 and 15% of cases of endocarditis are due to C burnetii. Spain, Switzerland, and Nova Scotia also have high prevalence rates. In other areas such as California and Great Britain, the rates have declined tremendously over the last 30–40 years [115]. A large survey of rural Welsh residents found only 21 individuals with positive serology, with a higher frequency in farmers [116]. In Carpathia, prevalence decreased from approximately 10% in the wake of a mid-1970s outbreak, to a 2–3% rate after 20 years [117]. Only 228 cases were reported in the United States between 1978 and 1986, half in California [118]. In regions where the main reservoir is sheep, such as the Basque region, a defined lambing period likely provides a seasonal variation to the incidence of acute Q fever, with the highest incidence in the spring and early summer [119]. The chronic forms of Q fever infection probably develop in only 1–10% of acute cases [120,121].

Rickettsia prowazekii

Rickettsia prowazekii, the agent of epidemic typhus, is unusual in that humans are the primary reservoir, with body lice (*Pediculus humanus corporis*) transmitting the organism from a rickettsemic individual to a new host. In the United States, the southern flying squirrel is also a reservoir [122]. Vertical transmission among animals has also been reported [123]. The infection is prominent in areas and settings that predispose humans to lice infestation, including the rural highlands of South and Central America, as well as Northeastern and Central Africa [124,125]. Periods of societal strife are also known to promote epidemics of infection. In wartime Bosnia and Herzegovina, for example, 4.3% of the general population were found to have antibodies to *R prowazekii* [126]. The potentially epidemic nature of the disease caused by this agent was illustrated by a recent outbreak of typhus in a jail in Burundi, followed by more extensive spread into refugee camps in Rwanda, Burundi, and Zaire [127]. The last U.S. typhus epidemic occurred in 1922 and since then, only rare, sporadic cases have been seen. Very few cases of epidemic typhus have been diagnosed in the United States, and by 1996 only 28 of these had been reported [36]. Among European immigrants after World War II, *R prowazekii* infection, almost always Brill-Zinsser disease, was seen with some frequency.

Rickettsia typhi

Rickettsia typhi has a worldwide distribution, especially in the warmer coastal areas, where its reservoir and vector abound [128]. Both sporadic cases and epidemics of murine typhus occur. During the 1940s, approximately 5,000 new U.S. cases were reported annually. By 1989, aggressive control measures had decreased this number to less than 100 [129]. U.S. prevalence is highest in California and Texas and varies seasonally, increasing during the warmer months [129]. In most of the world, infection is usually related to the indoor presence of rats and their infected fleas. Other factors that increase endemicity are those that promote increases in the rodent population. War, poor sanitation, and crowding appear to be problematic. In 1995, 61% of individuals in northeastern Bosnia and Herzegovina were found to have antibody to *R typhi* [126]. Other areas of high endemicity exist. For example, 28% of pregnant Tanzanian women were IFA-positive for *R typhi* [126]. In Malang, Indonesia, 36% of peridomestic rodents were seropositive for *R typhi*, and 35% of civilians also had antibodies [131]. Other areas of Africa (for example, Morocco) show much lower rates. A 1995 study found that only 1.7–4% of Moroccans were IFA positive for *R typhi* [132]. On the Greek island of Evia, 91% of *Rattus norvegicus* were antibody positive, as were 2.6% of the flea *Xenopsylla cheopis* [133]. Transmission in suburban areas may also be higher than generally expected. In suburban Bangkok, 8% of individuals showed evidence of recent *R typhi* infection [134]. In the southeastern United States, it is felt that a shift to a peridomestic cycle of transmission is occurring, with free-roaming dogs and cats, opossums, and their fleas now the predominant reservoirs and vectors [135].

Rickettsia rickettsii

R rickettsii (Rocky Mountain spotted fever) is transmitted via tick bite. RMSF is closely related to a number of other spotted fever illnesses, some of which occur in Asia, Australia, Brazil [136], and Europe [137]. RMSF is the second most common tick-borne disease in the United States. It is reported in every state except Vermont and Hawaii and can be contracted during any season [39]. The incidence of RMSF rose to a peak of 1,100 cases per year between 1977 and 1983. This increase was believed to be related to increased awareness of the disease as well as a population shift to more geographically remote areas [39]. The incidence declined thereafter, with only 590 annual cases reported in 1995 [138]. The true incidence of RMSF and murine typhus is probably underestimated by a factor of four or more [139]. The reported incidence within the United States varies regionally: 0.53 cases per 100,000 population in the West and South Central states, and 0.83 per 100,000 in the South Atlantic states [137]. For unknown reasons, more cases are now being seen in the Southeast: In 1994, 37% of all U.S. cases occurred in Georgia and the Carolinas. Most cases occur during the warmer months, likely reflecting levels of outdoor activity as well as seasonal variation in tick populations. Among the general population under the age of 65, infection rates appear to be similar in all age groups [138]. Men are more frequently infected, probably because of exposure differences. Infection rates during periods of intense exposure may be quite high. In a two-week training exercise in Arkansas, 38% of U.S. Army soldiers deployed in the field became infected [200].

Orientia tsutsugamushi

Scrub typhus is a disease of the Far East caused by the organism *Orientia tsutsugamushi*. It is prominent in Eastern Asia and the Western Pacific. One case report suggests that Africa may be a source as well [140]. The disease is transmitted by the bite of the larval stage of Trombiculidae mites, including *Leptotrombidium pallidum* and *Leptotrombidium scutellare*, which parasitize rodents. Humans are accidental hosts [141]. These vectors are prominent in scrub-like vegetation but can also be found in tall grass and other ecological niches [142]. It appears that the vector population itself is heavily infected. A Korean study of six different localities showed an overall chigger parasitization rate of 69%,with a wide geographic variation in prevalence and mite identity [141]. The incidence and prevalence of scrub typhus infection in humans can vary markedly according to geography, socioeconomic development, and age. Earlier studies showing sex differences likely reflect occupationally related exposure differences. In Thailand, as many as 59–77% of rural residents exhibit antibodies to *O tsutsugamushi*, indicating previous infection [143,144]. In metropolitan Bangkok, 21% of blood donors showed evidence of recent infection [145]. Evidence of antibody was found in approximately 20% of all civilian residents of the Pescadores Islands of Taiwan in the mid-1970s, with no sex difference. Infection before the age of 10 occurred in only 1%, but 41% had antibodies by age 50. Only 16% of urban dwellers had been infected, versus 38% of rural dwellers [46]. Among all Thai Army conscripts, the baseline seroprevalence rate varied between 6–18% but was higher in the Thai Rangers, who routinely perform patrol missions [146]. Febrile U.S. soldiers in Viet Nam were routinely screened for *O tsutsugamushi*, and 7% of a total of 1,650 were positive in one study [45]. The overall annual attack rate was calculated at 59 per 100,000, with 86% of cases occurring in certain heavily exposed combat units, which themselves accounted for less than 20% of the total military population. All documented exposures were noted to occur on the geographic "fringes" of the centers of population [45].

Bartonella

Bartonella quintana and *Bartonella henselae* are found worldwide. *B quintana* is probably transmitted by the body louse, *Pediculus humanus* [147], although scabies is a potential vector as well [148]. It is believed that the louse sheds the organism in its feces when it bites, which then inoculates the human host when the bite is scratched [149]. Interestingly, however, many of original victims do not have body lice, and efforts to isolate the organism from fleas have been unsuccessful [150]. *B henselae* is associated with cats, and possibly with cats' fleas [151,152]. *Bartonella* cases appear to be mostly sporadic; outbreaks are associated with conditions of poor sanitation and hygiene. Seropreva-lence is very dificult to determine, due to a lack of data; however, a serologic study performed in Seattle after a 1993 outbreak among the homeless found that 20% of homeless individuals had positive MIF titers for *B quintana*, versus 2% of random blood donors [153]. The importance of this high rate for other urban areas is not clear. Among veterinary professionals, seroprevalence for *Bartonella* infection is approximately 7% [202].

TRANSMISSION RISK FACTORS

Chlamydia psittaci

Transmission of *Chlamydia psittaci* between birds is heightened by stress, such as overcrowding, chilling, and malnutrition. Transmission to nestlings also occurs, along with potentially protective maternal antibodies [154]. The birds' clinical syndromes involve shedding of potentially infective material in copious ocular or nasal discharge, urate excretion, or diarrhea [16]. Direct contact by humans with these secretions or their aerosols results in infection in a high proportion of cases. These secretions and their aerosols are highly infectious and remain so for several months, as the organism is resistant to acid, alkali, and drying. Closer personal contact such as petting is risky [155], although relatively trivial exposure (e.g., aviary visits) is also a risk factor. The organism may also be transferred by bird bites and by handling the feathers of infected birds. Pre-existing skin injuries heighten susceptibility to transmission [54]. Among reported human cases, 70% of identified sources involved caged birds, and employment in situations where exposure was likely was also a risk [16]. In an outbreak among veterinary surgeons, handling of infected duck feathers was found to be a risk factor for transmission [115]. Handling the products of gestation of infected birds appear to be quite risky as well [246]. Interestingly, 25% of cases have no discernible avian exposure history [68,245], with infection likely due to an unnoticed transient exposure to infected droppings. Six serovars (A–F) have been isolated from birds [156], with differing degrees of virulence. Serovar D, for instance, was found to be highly pathogenic when inoculated into turkeys, and less so in other species [157]. The more virulent strains are believed to have larger and more numerous inclusions and to replicate more freely in the host cell's cytoplasm [157]. Certain orders of birds appear to be more susceptible to infection with a given serovar [158]. Psittacine and turkey strains are the most virulent for humans, resulting in more severe clinical symptomology [68]. Psittacosis can also be transmitted between humans, including nosocomially [159], and results in more clinically severe infection in these cases.

Chlamydia pneumoniae

Transmission of *Chlamydia pneumoniae* is believed to be exclusively human to human, with respiratory secretions the likely method of infection. Closed populations, including families, appear to be at risk for outbreaks. It appears that some asymptomatic individuals are capable of spreading the disease and some actively infected individuals are not [22]. Epidemic outbreaks occur in closed populations and may persist for six months at a time [22]. Patients with human immunodeficiency syndrome (HIV) appear to be more prone to infection with *C pneumoniae*, as evidenced by their higher seroprevalence rate, and the pathogen can be isolated from the bronchoalveolar lavage fluid (BALF) of 10% of HIV patients with pneumonia [160].

Chlamydia trachomatis

Chlamydia trachomatis is transmitted more easily from men to women [161]. Sex with a symptomatic partner poses a higher risk of transmission than with an asymptomatic one [162]. Pregnancy also appears to be a risk factor [163]. Concomitant infection with *Neisseria gonorrhoeae* increases the risk of transmission [164]. Higher frequency of sexual intercourse is correlated with increased rates of infection [165], and use of nonbarrier methods of contraception is a known risk factor [166]. Use of latex condoms decreases the risk of transmission and protects against viral pathogens such as HIV [100]. Condom breakage and slippage occur in a small percentage of encounters, resulting in potential pathogen exposure.

Vertical transmission is common, occurring in 60% of babies born to infected females. Infection in these cases causes inclusion conjunctivitis in 18% and pneumonia in 16% [167]. Pneumonia due to *C trachomatis* is seen most frequently in infants and is also prominent in immunocompromised patients [168].

Coxiella burnetii

Coxiella burnetii is transmitted to humans by inhalation of aerosols. *C burnetii* may remain in a spore-like state for months, resistant to drying and temperature extremes, and may remain viable in the soil for five months. Air samples may remain positive for two weeks after the local parturition of an infected animal [169]. Historically important sources of infection include domestic ungulates such as cattle, sheep, and goats. Cats, dogs, and deer are also potential sources [170]. In northern climates, parturient cats, particularly, have been noted to initiate outbreaks [171]. Infection typically occurs in proximity to a stationary source; however, more obscure sources have been seen. There have been reports of a high incidence in individuals living by roadsides over which infected animals and their products were transported [172,173]. These reports illustrate the high infectivity of the organism, which can, in fact, be transmitted by inoculation with a single organism [174]. Disease may also be transmitted via transfusion, gastrointestinal ingestion, drinking raw milk, skin trauma, sexual contact [175], vertically [176], and possibly ticks [114]. Person-to-person transmission occurs rarely [177]. There is one case of a physician who was infected after delivering the child of an infected patient [176]. Articles of clothing can become contaminated and thus infectious to those who do laundry or are otherwise exposed to clothing [178,179]. Only a handful of person-to-person instances of transmission have been reported [180,181]. High attack rates, short incubations, and more severe clinical syndromes are associated with exposure to the high inoculum involved in cleaning up the products of conception of infected parturient cats [182]. Patients who are immunocompromised due to HIV, neoplasia, or corticosteroid use are more susceptible to developing the chronic forms of the disease. Patients with pre-existing valvulopathy are more likely to develop Q fever endocarditis. Q fever can also be reactivated by the induction of immunosuppression [183].

Rickettsia

Rickettsia prowazekii is transmitted in conditions that favor lice infestation. Poor sanitation, crowding, infrequent washing, and infrequent changing of clothing are risk factors [37]. Periods of war, famine, and migration frequently foster these conditions. Epidemics of typhus were seen in Europe in the aftermath of World War I and in the concentration camps of World War II. *Rickettsia typhi* transmission is increased in regions and situations in which the rat population is high. As with *Rickettsia prowazekii*, war and periods of societal strife lead to conditions that favor outbreaks. One case of transmission due to a laboratory accident has been reported [184]. *Rickettsia rickettsii* transmission is higher in those with tick exposure [185] and is also possible in those who crush infected ticks between their fingers [137]. Pet ownership has not been found to be a risk factor, and person-to-person infection probably does not occur, except in cases of direct percutaneous inoculation [39].

Scrub typhus infection occurs in humans with environmental exposure to the chiggers (larval forms) of specific mites that infest rodents. Humans become infected as accidental hosts. Exposure occurs in proximity to the scrub-like vegetation that harbors populations of rodents, with both mice and rats potentially infected. Transmission occurs via the bite of a chigger. Infection rates rise during the early rainy season, due to a corresponding increase in arthropod population density. Soldiers who are deployed under simulated battlefield conditions are markedly susceptible to infection [146]. Outdoor activities such as hiking and mountain-climbing also put humans at risk for scrub typhus [186]. Sitting or lying on the ground in endemic areas places an individual at particular risk [289]. In addition to arthropod-to-human transmission, human-to-transmission may occur. Scrub typhus infection can be spread vertically [187] and via needlestick [188]. It appears that there are variations in strain virulence among *O tsutsugamushi* that likely affect the likelihood of disease transmission. These differences were actively exploited by the Japanese in the 1930s, who infected volunteers with the less virulent strains of the Pescadores, protecting them from the more virulent strains of Japan [189].

Bartonella

Bartonella quintana outbreaks also appear to be related to conditions that promote body louse infestation. The homeless, alcoholics, and HIV-infected seem most vulnerable. The risk for transmission of *Bartonella henselae* is believed to be increased by exposure to cats and their fleas. Ownership of kittens, cat bites, and cat scratches are risk factors [152].

OCCUPATIONAL RISK FACTORS

Psittacosis

Occupations associated with increased risk for acquiring psittacosis include veterinarians, veterinary technicians [190], poultry industry workers [191], farmers, zoo and aviary employees, laboratory workers [192], abattoir workers, and pet shop employees. Pigeon fanciers and other pet owners are particularly at risk, accounting for over 40% of all cases [16]. Although humans who have the most intimate contact with the animals or their products are at highest risk, microbial aerosols have been documented to infect employees who have had no direct animal contact [193]. Within a turkey processing plant, workers from the evisceration area or the "live hang" room were 5.6 and 3.4 times, respectively, as likely to become infected in the course of an outbreak than were individuals who worked in other areas of the plant, exhibiting 34% and 21% seropositivity rates, respectively. Mink room workers and deboning line workers also had high attack rates, and the clean-up crews in the deboning room had even higher rates of infection than the deboning line workers [205]. It was also noted that workers at a "further processing" plant became infected, proving that even a presumably trivial exposure to defeathered, eviscerated, chilled carcasses is potentially infectious [205].

Chlamydia pneumoniae Infection

Chlamydia pneumoniae presents a risk to closed populations such as military garrisons, schools, and families [92]. The attack rates among military garrisons during documented outbreaks ranges from 6% to 8% [23]. Physicians who care for these patients are presumably also at risk for infection as well as reinfection.

Chlamydia trachomatis Infection

Chlamydia trachomatis is an occupational hazard for commercial sex workers. Obviously, their clients are at risk as well. An interesting finding arose from a study of commercial sex workers in Copenhagen. It was found that due to a high rate of condom use by prostitutes when involved with paying customers, the rate of infection with *C trachomatis* was actually higher than that from encounters with nonpaying individuals, presumably spouses and lovers [100].

Q Fever

Coxiella burnetii presents potential risks for veterinarians, farmers, abattoir workers, wool processors [194], textile workers [192], laundry workers, and laboratory personnel. Outbreaks have occurred in meat-packing plants, dairies, and stockyards [108]. The outbreaks at research facilities are likely related to the use of goats and gravid sheep in experimental studies. Personnel who have direct contact with the animals or their products have the highest rates of infection. It is now known that any personnel with exposure to infected aerosols (including visitors) are also at relatively high risk for infection [195–197]. In the past, Q fever was studied by the U.S. military as a proposed agent for biologic warfare [198], and its potential to infect troops or even metropolitan areas with some impact has been explored [199].

Rickettsial Infections

Rickettsia prowazekii may be transmitted to individuals, such as prison guards, who work in close proximity to lice-infested individuals. *Rickettsia typhi* transmission to laboratory personnel is possible. The rate of *Rickettsia rickettsii* infection is believed to be higher in outdoor workers with heavy exposure to ticks. Soldiers may also contract the disease from exposure during field exercises [200]. Travelers to endemic areas are at risk for any of the rickettsioses [201].

Scrub Typhus

Those at risk for scrub typhus, *Orientia tsutsugamushi* infection, include individuals who have exposure to the mites *Leptotrombidium leptobromidium* and *Leptotrombidium scutellare* in endemic areas. Historically, this has included military personnel, outdoorsmen, unschooled children (who presumably spend a high proportion of time outdoors), and farmers [46].

Bartonella Infections

Individuals at risk for *Bartonella quintana* include soldiers, who may be exposed to prolonged conditions of poor sanitation and crowding. Cat owners and veterinarians are at risk for *Bartonella henselaea*. A random serologic survey of attendees at a veterinary conference revealed that 7% had antibodies to *B henselaea* or *B quintana*, suggesting a considerable incidence of occupational transmission [202].

Prevention and Control

ADMINISTRATIVE CONTROLS

Chlamydia psittaci

Importation of birds is overseen by the Veterinary Services of the Animal and Plant Health Inspection Service, U.S. Department of Agriculture (USDA). Previous to shipping, the importer requires an import permit from the USDA and a health certificate from a veterinarian of the exporting nation [204]. The USDA inspects all imports at the port of entry and enforces a 30-day quarantine to ensure freedom from infection. Ideally, birds are quarantined in the country of origin for 45 days prior to transport [203]. During U.S. quarantine, birds are fed a medicated feed containing 1% chlortetracycline to treat potential *Chlamydia psittaci* infection. An additional 15 days of this dietary therapy are strongly recommended to ensure adequate therapy. Birds with documented infection, or known exposure to *C psittaci*, should be placed in isolation. Treatment should be provided for all confirmed cases and possibly for all suspected ones. Isolation of the birds should be continued until all cases involving potential exposure are resolved, thus preventing the reinfection of a treated bird. Other procedures are described below:

- Overcrowding and malnutrition should be avoided, especially during transport.
- All parties involved in bird transactions should keep accurate records in order to allow retrospective identification of potential contacts and facilitate their treatment. This helps prevent propagation of an outbreak.
- Quarantine of all potentially infected birds from a site where infection has been known to occur should be implemented by the state's public health or animal authorities [204].
- At the discretion of public authorities, epidemiologic investigation may be undertaken to determine the source of infection and to alert all potentially exposed individuals. In cases involving newly acquired birds, elucidating the identity of the primary source of infection is vital. Important considerations in such inves-

tigations include the number and types of birds involved, human exposures and illnesses, condition of storage and transportation facilities, ventilation factors, and the treatments initiated, if any.

- Physicians should report cases of *C psittaci* infection to the appropriate health authorities. Suspected cases in birds should be referred to a veterinarian.
- Suspected outbreaks should be reported to the CDC's Childhood and Respiratory Diseases Branch, Division af Bacterial and Mycotic Diseases, National Center for Infectious Diseases: (404) 639-2215 [16].
- Industrial procesing of birds is generally overseen by state agencies and USDA meat inspectors. Ill-appearing birds should trigger serologic investigation for *C psittaci*, followed by treatment or sacrifice of the infected specimens [205]. Since infected birds may be asymptomatic and still remain infectious, routine screening of flocks prior to their processing, using a rapid and reliable test, is optimal.

Chlamydia trachomatis

Cases of *Chlamydia trachomatis* infection should be reported to the appropriate public health authorities. A high degree of coordination among health care professionals, educators, and outreach workers is required [97]. Health departments must ensure that all sexual partners of known cases are identified and notified and that adequate therapy and follow-up has been arranged. The CDC recommends that all states have laws that facilitate the collection of information regarding chlamydial cases. The CDC stresses primary and secondary prevention strategies:

- *Primary prevention* includes changes in behavior to include lower numbers of sexual partners, judicious partner selection, and the use of barrier methods of contraception.
- *Secondary prevention* includes (1) screening of women to identify and treat those at high risk for the sequelae of infection and (2) prompt and accurate recognition of chlamydial syndromes and timely, appropriate testing of those potentially infected.

Coxiella burnetii

Cases of *Coxiella burnetii* should be reported to the appropriate public health authorities so that an epidemiologic investigation may be initiated. Research facilities should be constructed with prevention of transmission in mind. Airtight segregation of potentially infectious laboratory specimens is imperative. Other procedures are:

- All laboratory animals should ideally be evaluated for *C burnetii* prior to transfer to research laboratories.
- In flocks of animals with significant prevalence (> 20%), culling and chemoprophylaxis should be strongly considered [113].
- Access to animal research facility should be limited, and visitation should be considered a risky practice.
- Accurate records of all animal transactions should be kept. Q fever is reportable in approximately 24 states [317].

Chlamydia trachomatis

Chlamydia trachomatis is reportable in many states. Notification of partners can be performed by the appropriate public health authorities if partner referral fails [206]. Counseling and education can be provided to infected individuals and their contacts at that time.

Rickettsia rickettsii

During the 1970s, a South Carolina program that attempted to test all submitted ticks for RMSF proved unsuccessful in decreasing the incidence of infection. However, the program was believed to have been beneficial insofar as it raised the public's and the medical profession's awareness of the importance of the disease [39].

Rickettsia typhi

Control of *Rickettsia typhi* may be achieved by eradication of rats and rat fleas. Insecticide-dusting campaigns are of some use in bringing epidemics under control [36]. Proper sanitation and waste disposal help prevent the conditions that encourage rat infestations [201].

SAFE WORK PRACTICES AND ENGINEERING CONTROLS

Chlamydia psittaci

Cages should be positioned so that material such as food and feathers cannot contaminate nearby cages. The sides of the cages should be solid, not mesh, and stacking of the cages is unwise. Cages and bowls should be cleaned daily (washed with soap and water), rinsed, disinfected, and rinsed again. The cage itself should be thoroughly disinfected between occupants, and exhaust ventilation should be adequate to prevent aerosol accumulation.

Newly acquired birds should be quarantined for 14–30 days before being added to a group. They should be treated prophylactically for *Chlamydia psittaci*, unless they have previously tested negative. Only birds who test negative for *C psittaci* should be accepted for boarding or consignment, and boarders should be maintained in an area with separate air-handling equipment.

In the case of an infected specimen, thorough cleaning of the cages that held the bird should be performed while the bird is held in isolation. The cage itself should be scrubbed with detergent, rinsed, disinfected, and rinsed again. Effective disinfectants include a 1:1,000 solution of quarternary ammonium compounds (alkyldimethylbenzylammonium chloride [Roccal, Zephiran]), 70% isopropyl alcohol, 1:100 dilution of household bleach (2.5 tbsp/gallon), chlorophenols, or 1% Lysol. The disinfectant should be allowed to have a minimum of 5 minutes' contact with the material being cleansed.

The cage itself should have a wire-mesh bottom, and litter that does not produce dust should be used. The litter should be moistened prior to removal and should be burned or double-bagged.

The room that housed the cage should also be cleaned and disinfected. Material not amenable to disinfection, such as litter and wooden perches, should be discarded. The floor should be mopped with disinfectant or an oil-impregnated sweeping compound.

The ventilation system also should be disinfected, since it may harbor the organism. During the cleaning of rooms and cages, ventilation and air currents should be minimized to prevent contamination of other areas. To prevent aerosolization of the organism, standard vacuum cleaners should not be used, and the floor itself should be disinfected or at least mopped with water.

The caretaker should observe the birds daily, weighing them every three to seven days.

Birds undergoing treatment should be segregated by sex.

Recommended antibiotic treatment protocol must be followed (see below).

Necropsy rooms in veterinary establishments should include a laminar flow hood to decrease the possibility of transmission [190].

Chlamydia trachomatis

Transmission of *Chlamydia trachomatis* during sexual intercourse can be reduced by the use of latex condoms. The male variety is preferred, athough the female condom may provide some protection (see page 285).

Coxiella burnetii

Coxiella burnetii presents a challenge to workplace prevention:

- Improved air handling to minimize exposure to infected aerosols must be achieved.
- Avoidance of infected animals is the key to prevention.
- Laboratories that culture *C burnetii* should do so under strictly controlled environmental control. This includes using sealed hoods, proper ventilation, and safe culturing techniques such as the shell-vial assay [357].
- Disinfection of the facility must be performed regularly.
- Excessive transport of specimens within the facility should be avoided [112].

Rickettsia prowazekii

Outbreaks of *Rickettsia prowazekii* in jail populations has been controlled by shaving and dusting all prisoners with 0.5% permethrin, changing mattresses and clothes, and cleaning the infected facility with cyfluthrin, for example [207]. Treating all personnel simultaneously with a single dose of doxycycline should minimize the potential for spread of the organism [207].

PERSONAL PROTECTIVE EQUIPMENT AND PREVENTIVE MEASURES

Chlamydia psittaci

Personnel who handle potentially infected birds should wear gloves, protective clothing, paper surgical hats, and a respirator with at least an N95 rating (a dust-mist mask may be substituted if the respirator is not available) [16].

Necropsies on potentially infected birds should be performed under a hood equipped with an exhaust fan. The carcass should be wetted with detergent and water to prevent aerosolization of infectious particles.

Coxiella burnetii

The use of protective equipment to reduce transmission is vitally important. Because clothing may also be contaminated when working with infected animals or their products, proper handling of potentially contaminated clothing is essential.

Vaccination of animals used in research would greatly diminish the possibility of zoonotic infection.

Careful laboratory technique can minimize the possibility of infection. Avoidance of mouth-pipetting and spills and prompt disposal of needles and syringes are important [208].

Rickettsial Infections

Outbreaks of *Rickettsia prowazekii* can be controlled by de-lousing programs. Infected individuals require de-lousing in order to effect cure. DDT, lindane powder, malathion, or carbaryl may be used [37] on the body, and permethrin may be used on articles of clothing. Prophylactic doxycycline may help prevent infection and interrupt the spread of an outbreak [36]. Correcting the conditions that promote lice infestation is quite important. Washing regularly, laundering, and use of insecticides are helpful. *Rickettsia typhi* infection rates can be decreased through aggressive rat and flea control. *Rickettsia rickettsii* infection can be prevented by the use of insect repellents and the wearing of protective clothing. DEET-containing products can be applied to the skin and clothing. Permethrin applied to clothing also helps prevent *Rickettsia rickettsii* infection. Avoidance of highly endemic areas is wise. Hair and skin survey after possible exposure is important, and pets should be inspected as well. Forceps removal of arthropods will help prevent transmission of tick-borne disease, as six hours of attachment are likely necessary for transmission. Proper technique requires anterior grasping of the ticks, with complete removal of all body parts, followed by washing the area with soap and water [39].

Orientia tsutsugamushi

Some measures for preventing scrub typhus include avoiding exposure to the tall grass and scrub vegetation that harbors the chiggers. Visitors to endemic areas should wear clothing that covers the arms and legs. Use of insect repellents, including application to the tops of boots and socks [209], should be encouraged. Using cots instead of placing sleeping bags on the ground also reduces exposure. Use of pesticides to control the population of mites may be considered if deployment and exposure are unavoidable [210]. Chemoprophylactic treatment with chloramphenicol (4 g orally each week, continued for four weeks after exposure) has been successful [211]. Weekly doses of doxycycline (200 mg orally) were found to be protective against experimental inoculation and are likely to be protective against susceptible strains for people visiting endemic areas [212]. Doxycycline has a favorable half-life and is likely to be better tolerated than chloramphenicol. Doxycycline prophyaxis should be continued for up to six weeks after exposure.

EMPLOYEE EDUCATION AND TRAINING

Chlamydia psittaci

Employees should be educated as to the highly infectious nature of *Chlamydia psittaci* and should be made aware of the routes of infection and the methods used to reduce risk. They should report any illnesses observed in birds to the appropriate veterinary authority immediately and should report any human illnesses promptly as well. Personnel involved in the sale of birds should be instructed never to sell an ill-appearing bird, or other animal. Physicians caring for infected patients should be alerted to the patient's exposure history and should use a low threshold to begin therapy. Patients with respiratory illnesses who have a known exposure to *C psittaci* should probably be started on empiric therapy while awaiting test results.

Chlamydia trachomatis

Commercial sex workers should be made aware of the benefit of using latex condoms. They should become well-skilled in the technical aspects of their usage so that breakage and slippage rates are decreased [213]. Proper use involves using a new condom before each act, using water-based lubricants only, and using correct methods for applying and removing condoms [206]. Female condoms can be used if male condom use is not possible [206]. The general population should be made aware of the intricacies of *C trachomatis* infection. Schools are a possible venue for the provision of information. The availability of confidential testing and treatment will enhance control efforts, especially among adolescents.

Coxiella burnetii

Individuals who handle animals or specimens potentially infected with *Coxiella burnetii* should become well-versed in the various manifestations of the disease and should understand the potential modes of transmission and methods used for prevention. In addition, they should be well acquainted with the proper procedures for ventilation, transport, and waste removal [112].

MEDICAL SURVEILLANCE

Chlamydia trachomatis

Screening for *Chlamydia trachomatis* in highly endemic areas may be of benefit, especially if the seroprevalence rate is greater than 5% [163]. The CDC recommends screening in a multitude of situations, listed in the next section.

Coxiella burnetii

Skin testing for *Coxiella burnetii* allows identification of individuals who are presumably not at risk for acute Q fever infection [113]. Identification of individuals with valvulopathy or immunosuppressive conditions allows potentially beneficial vaccination prior to exposure.

Bartonella quintana/Rickettsia prowazekii

Screening individuals for lice on a periodic basis, which may be performed in schools or as a public health measure during periods of societal strife, can be effective in detecting and eliminating lice infestation, thus eliminating the vectors of Bartonella quintana and Rickettsia prowazekii.

BIOLOGIC TESTING

Chlamydia psittaci

Testing of birds for AC should be performed prior to boarding or consignment, in cases of illness consistent with *Chlamydia psittaci*, and when possible exposure to AC has occurred.

Chlamydia trachomatis

The CDC recommends screening for *Chlamydia trachomatis* in [97]:

- Females less than 20 years old.
- Females, 20–24 years of age, who have had one or more new sex partners during the previous three months or do not consistently use barrier contraception.
- Women undergoing induced abortion.
- Women attending clinics for sexually transmitted diseases.
- Women in detention facilities.
- Women with mucopurulent cervicitis.
- Pregnant women (before third trimester).
- Sexually active adolescents [206].

IMMUNIZATION AND PROPHYLACTIC MEASURES

Pre- and Postexposure Measures

Chlamydia psittaci. Electron microscopy is being used to investigate potential targets of vaccine against *C psittaci,* with antigens on the elementary body of particular interest [214]. A lyophilized vaccine utilizing the temperature-sensitive 1B strain of *C psittaci* has been successfully used in ewes to prevent abortion [215]. Vaccines for cats are also under study [216]. No commercially available vaccine is available for birds. Previous *C psittaci* infection does not confer immunity.

Chlamydia trachomatis. Commercial sex workers in Turkey frequently use prophylactic antibiotics (Worm AM) effective against *C trachomatis.* One survey found that approximately 65% followed this practice. When infection is found in any individual, it is imperative that their sex partners be treated. Pregnant females who test positive can be treated with erythromycin, 250–500 mg orally four times daily for seven days, which reduces the chance of maternal-fetal transmission to 10% [163]. Perinatal application of erythromycin or tetracycline to prevent ocular trachoma is not effective [217], and the infected neonate should be treated with systemic erythromycin, as well as topical tetracycline if conjunctivitis is present [163].

Coxiella burnetii. Vaccine against *Coxiella burnetii* (Q-Vax) is commercially available in Australia and Eastern Europe. It is being given to Australian abattoir workers and Russian laboratory personnel [114]. Q-Vax proved to be 100% protective over a five-year period when given to 2,555 Australian abattoir workers [218]. U.S. efforts aimed at vaccine development continue [219]. A chloroform:methanol residue vaccine appears efficacious and should be less likely to result in sterile abscesses and granulomas [220]. Provision of vaccine to those likely to be exposed (see Table 4-5) may become more widespread. Individuals with known valvulopathy, diabetes mellitus, cancer, or other immunocompromised states may benefit most. A skin test to determine previous infection status will help avoid severe local reactions; ideally, it should be performed prior to vaccination [112].

Rickettsial Infections. Vaccine against *R prowazekii* is available. It is recommended for individuals who travel to endemic areas and live in close proximity to the indigenous populations (e.g., missionaries, anthropologists, and construction workers), medical personnel in endemic areas, and *R prowazekii* laboratory workers [221]. While no effective vaccine is available for *Rickettsia typhi,* infection results in long-lasting natural immunity. Vaccine against *Rickettsia rickettsii* is also not available, but research in this area continues [222].

Orientia tsutsugamushi. Effective vaccines against scrub typhus are not available, mostly because of the antigenic diversity among the various serotypes.

Metrics To Assess Adequacy of Preventive Measures

Coxiella burnetii. Air sampling to detect the Q fever pathogen is possible. Dust from air treatment ducts can also be tested for the presence of the organism.

Rickettsial Infections. Serologic surveys of domestic animals such as cats may provide useful information about the adequacy of measures designed to control *Rickettsia typhi* and *Rickettsia prowazekii* [223]. IFA and polymerase chain reaction (PCR) can be used to detect infection in fleas and rats [224], as well as ticks [225]. Ticks may also be tested for the presence of *Rickettsia rickettsii,* although the usefulness of such testing is in doubt [39].

SYMPTOMS AND SIGNS

Chlamydia psittaci

Chlamydia psittaci in birds (avian chlamydiosis) presents differently, depending on the virulence of the infecting strain as well as the species infected. Upper respiratory findings—mainly cough, dyspnea, sinusitis, poor flying performance, and nasal, conjunctival, and ocular discharge—are most frequent [226]. Ruffled feathers, lethargy, anorexia, yellow/green urate excretion, and diarrhea may also occur. Neurologic symptoms such as seizure and tremor are seen in many species [227]. Autopsy findings include rhinitis, airsacculitis, pneumonia, hepatosplenomegaly, and pericarditis [228].

Some species, such as chickens, are somewhat resistant to infection, and other species, such as pigeons and gulls [191], are often subclinically infected [15]. Ducks and geese may have unusual neurologic presentations such as disequilibrium [229]. Abortion is seen in sheep, cattle, goats, and horses. Conjunctivitis is noted in cats, cattle, sheep, hamsters, and guinea pigs, while enteritis has been reported in hares, cattle, and pigs. Arthritis may be a manifestation of infection in pigs, cattle, sheep, and horses [15].

The incubation period of *C psittaci* is six to 20 days in humans [83]. Rarely, the inoculum may directly infect the pulmonary parenchyma, resulting in an abbreviated one- to three-day incubation period [53]. Normally the bacteria infect the epithelial cells of the lower respiratory tract, then produce a two-stage bacteremia, which initially affect the reticuloendothelial cells of the liver and spleen and then involve the lungs [53]. Infection in humans may be asymptomatic or result in severe systemic infection with pneumonia [230]. The typical clinical scenario involves tracheobronchitis or atypical pneumonia manifested by the abrupt development of fever, chills, myalgia, headache, and dry cough. The headache may be severe. A "typical" pneumonia resembling that associated with community-acquired bacterial pathogens may occur [231]. Relative bradycardia and an unimpressive pulmonary examination (belying an impressive degree of pulmonary infiltrates) are often noted. Crackles may be heard in the lower lung fields [53]. Other presentations include a mononucleosis-like syndrome manifested by fever, pharyngitis, and lymphadenopathy [230,232], and a typhoid-like syndrome manifested by fever, malaise, and splenomegaly [12]. Rash, neurologic symptoms, and gastrointestinal symptoms have also been reported. Fever, pharyngitis, chest radiography shows pulmonary infiltrates in more than half the patients. Horder's spots, a pink maculopapular eruption, is seen in less than 50%. Unusual presentations are common, making for an extensive list of differential diagnoses. Unusual presentations include myopericarditis [233], endocarditis [234], hemorrhagic macular choroidopathy [235], psychiatric symptoms [236], hearing loss [237], intracranial hypertension [238], acute interstitial nephritis [239], acute glomerulonephritis [240], acute renal failure [241], transverse myelitis [242], cerebellar dysfunction [17], bilateral IVth nerve palsies [243], and elevated hepatic enzymes. These entities often occur in conjunction with the respiratory symptoms, confirming the systemic nature of the illness. In some cases, progression to severe hypoxemia, requiring mechanical ventilation, and ultimately death may occur [244]. In the pre-antibiotic area, mortality was likely 30–40% of patients with psittacosis [12]. Presently, overall mortality is estimated at 0.7% [245]. Gestational psittacosis appears to be particularly virulent. Transmitted from birds or sheep, it may present as a fulminant illness with pneumonia disseminated intravascular coagulation (DIC), elevated transaminases, and abnormal renal function [246]. In pregnant patients, placental insufficiency may result in miscarriage [247]. Chest radiography typically shows a unilobar infiltrate (90%), although migratory [248], multilobar, reticular [249], ground-glass [250], and miliary patterns have been reported. Hilar adenopathy is common [53].

Chlamydia pneumoniae

Chlamydia pneumoniae has a variety of presentations. In some cases, infection is asymptomatic, in others flu-like [92]. *C pneumoniae* most frequently causes bronchitis or pneumonia, which is usually symptomatic of reinfection. The severity of the clinical syndrome that emerges is heavily influenced by the presence of comorbid illlnesses and the patient's overall condition. In the elderly, pneumonitis occurs more commonly and is more likely to require hospitalization. In HIV-infected patients, a severe and ultimately fatal pneumonitis may ensue [353]. In some individuals, a prolonged syndrome characterized by bronchitic symptoms persisting for weeks may occur. Chronic infection that persists despite antibiotic therapy is seen in a small percentage of cases [251]. Pharyngitis, otitis, and sinusitis are frequent accompaniments to the respiratory tract symptoms [252]. Rarely, pharyngitis may be the sole manifestation of infection [30]. Reinfection is usually clinically milder, with less fever and a lower rate of hospitalization [29,253]. A typical clinical scenario for patients with *Chlamydia pneumoniae* infection is one of biphasic disease. First, pharyngitis and laryngitis occur, followed by cough after several days. Fever occurs early, especially in primary infection. The disease then enters a second phase involving lower respiratory tract symptoms, with rales and possibly wheezing [29]. Sinusitis, with sinus tenderness, may be seen. The onset of asthma may occur in the wake of a *C pneumoniae* infection, and there may be a pathogenetic role for the organism in this disease [254]. Other studies have shown that appropriate antibiotic treatment of asthmatics who are culture-positive for *C pneumoniae* results in improvement of their reactive airway disease [255] and that infected steroid-dependent asthmatics can be successfully weaned off oral steroids [256]. Rarely, neurologic syndromes, including Guillain-Barré, meningitis and cerebellar syndromes occur in patients with *C pneumoniae* infection [257]. Other associated findings may include erythema nodosum, fibromyalgia [258], arthritis [259], myocarditis, pericarditis, and endocarditis [22]. More recently, *C pneumoniae* has been serologically linked to atherosclerotic heart disease and myocardial infarction [260] and has been isolated from atheromatous plaques [261]. One study found 90% of patients with acute myocardial infarction to be MIF-IgG positive for *C pneumoniae* [262]. While some believe that the organism's presence itself promotes atherogenesis, the significance of these findings is currently being debated. *C pneumoniae* has also been detected by PCR in 49% of aortic valves which required replacement [263], and 45% of stroke/TIA patients were found to have antibody to *C pneumoniae*, versus 19.4% of controls [264]. Future investigations into the role of *C pneumoniae* in atherosclerotic and valvular heart disease offer the possibility that screening and treatment may eventually have an important role in the prevention of these diseases and their considerable morbidity and mortality.

Chlamydia trachomatis

Chlamydia trachomatis also has a variable presentation, depending on the strain involved, the age and sex of the infected individual, and the mode of transmission. The greatest danger posed by this pathogen is that it causes minimal, if any, symptoms in most of those it infects, whether men or women, and therefore may go undetected. Up to 70% of females who have endocervical infection exhibit minimal symptoms, typically experiencing various degrees of dysuria, vaginal discharge, or bleeding [265]. Examination at this point reveals cervical erythema and mucopurulent discharge [266]. Other manifestations in women include acute urethral syndrome and pelvic inflammatory disease (PID). Salpingitis develops in approximately 8% [267], which if untreated, can lead to female sterility [268]. In pregnant females, chorioamnionitis and premature delivery are possible [163]. In males, *C trachomatis* infection is usually asymptomatic. Some males develop urethritis, after a seven- to 14-day incubation. Dysuria and scant penile discharge may be noted. Males may also develop epididymitis and prostatitis [269], proctocolitis (in homosexuals) [270], arthritis [271], and conjunctivitis (presumably due to self-inoculation from genital infection) [272]. Other possible manifestations include neonatal inclusion conjunctivitis, pneumonia (seen in infants and immunocompromised patients) [273,274], and meningoencephalitis [275]. Lymphogranuloma venereum (LGV) is due to a strain of *C trachomatis* that rarely occurs in the United States. LGV typically causes a genital ulcer at the site of inoculation and later leads to inguinal and femoral adenopathy or perirectal disease [206].

Rickettsia Infections

Rickettsia prowazekii infection is heralded by one to three days of malaise, followed by severe headache, fever, chills, and prostration. A truncal rash typically appears in the region of the axillary folds and spreads centrifugally. Eventually only the palms, soles, and face are spared. The rash may be petechial or maculopapular [36]. Meningismus, delirium, and coma have been seen. Symptoms may last for two weeks or more, and convalescence may be prolonged [37]. Mortality occurs at variable frequency. Antibiotics shorten the febrile phase to 72 hours or less. Digital gangrene and cerebral thrombosis are potential adverse outcomes [36]. Thrombocytopenia and elevated transaminases may be seen.

Rickettsia typhi causes fever in almost all victims. Headache, rash, gastrointestinal symptoms, cough, and myalgia are seen in less than half of patients at presentation. The rash is truncal in 88%, when present. Anemia is seen in almost 65% of cases [129]. The elderly and those with comorbid conditions tend to have more severe symptoms, although murine typhus is generally milder than louse-born typhus.

Rickettsia rickettsii causes fever, headache, and rash in over 90% of those it infects. Rash typically begins on the wrists and ankles, and spreads centripetally. The organisms may infect and injure the microcirculation, leading to petechiae and gangrene. Meningismus and other neurologic abnormalities have been reported, and pulmonary manifestations such as pneumonia and pleural effusion are also seen [276]. Nausea and vomiting are frequently noted, and hepatosplenomegaly occurs in the more severe cases [39]. Conjunctivitis is seen in 30% or more, and periorbital edema may indicate severe infection in children [39].

Coxiella burnetii

Coxiellosis is the term used to describe *Coxiella burnetii* infection in animals. Infection in animals is usually asymptomatic, although abortion outbreaks have been noted. *C burnetii* produces symptoms in up to 50% of infected humans [108]. The presentation in humans appears to vary geographically for unknown reasons. For example, Q fever pneumonia is rare in Australia but is seen in up to 50% of cases in the United States and Great Britain [109]. In France, hepatitis is the most common presentation [277].

The typical incubation period after exposure is two to four weeks; the inoculum size affects the duration of incubation inversely [278]. Symptoms typically begin with a flu-like syndrome. Fever ranges up to 104°F, and the patient may experience chills, rigors, malaise, anorexia, myalgia, and headache. The fever may persist for three weeks. Relative bradycardia is often noted, and a severe retro-orbital headache [31] may be the most prominent symptom. A macular or purpuric exanthem is seen in 20% of patients with acute infection [277]. A vasculitic rash appearing later in the course of the disease, occurs in less than 10%.

Up to half of patients have pneumonia [279]. A dry cough is seen in up to 28% of the patients who have abnormal chest radiographs [280]. Dry crackles on lung auscultation are more typical than signs of consolidation [108]. Pleuritic chest pain occurs in up to 34% of infected individuals [174]. Pneumonia is usually mild but may progress to respiratory failure [35]. Radiographic films of the chest typically show patchy or rounded opacities in the lower lung fields. In one series, the lower lobes were involved in 100% of patients with pneumonia [281]. Multiple round lesions, effusions, air bronchograms, reticular infiltrates, hilar adenopathy, pseudotumor, and atelectasis have also been reported [35]. Clearing of the lungs may take more than 70 days [108]. Nausea, vomiting, and diarrhea are seen in a minority of patients. Hepatomegaly was seen in half of the patients in one series [109] and was absent in all patients in another study [284]. Splenomegaly also occurs in a small percentage of infected individuals [284].

Untreated, patients may develop a typhoidal state characterized by delirium and stupor. In the pre-antibiotic era, recovery took several weeks or even months.

Acute Q fever may also present as an isolated fever, pneumonia, meningitis, hepatitis, myocarditis, or pericarditis [114]. Other manifestations of acute Q fever include optic neuritis, choroidal neovascularization [282], rhabdomyolysis [283], thyroiditis, pancreatitis, syndrome of inappropriate antidiuretic hormone (SIADH), deep vein thrombosis, epididymitis, orchitis, abortion, and erythema nodosum [284]. The presentation of Q fever tends to vary geographically, perhaps reflecting differences in strain.

Chronic Q fever appears to develop more slowly and is more prominent in the elderly, the immunocompromised, and individuals with valvulopathy. Manifestations of chronic infection include endocarditis, osteomyelitis, abortion, and pseudotumor [114]. Endocarditis, which is usually indolent, is seen almost exclusively in those with pre-existing valvulopathy or prosthetic valves [285] and accounts for approximately 65% of chronic cases of Q fever [357]. Large vegetations and major embolic events have been noted, and fever with congestive heart failure is a frequent presentation [286]. Since routine blood cultures do not detect *C burnetii*, a high index of suspicion is required to make the diagnosis. Associated clues to the diagnosis include clubbing (seen in 37% of patients) [121], as well as indicators of an underlying inflammatory state, such as an elevated erythrocyte sedimentation rate, rashes, and splenomegaly [357].

Orientia tsutsugamushi

Orientia tsutsugamushi infection also has a variable clinical presentation. There appear to be considerable differences in virulence between different strains, with some causing a typically mild flu-like illness, and others leading to an overwhelming infection, resulting in death. Virulence factors are segregated geographically, so the result of infection varies dramatically with the area of endemicity. Host factors, specifically the issue of primary infection versus reinfection, are also important [287].

Infection with the agent of scrub typhus begins with inoculation of the host by the bite of the chigger. Within two days, a papule appears; it develops into a bulla and eventually ulcerates. Local multiplication of the organism often results in the formation of an eschar, a black crust surrounded by raised erythematous borders [45]. Asian patients appear less likely to have eschars, possibly due to a partial immunity derived from previous infection [288]. Lymphadenopathy begins regionally and becomes generalized in most patients. Only the nodes in close proximity to the inoculation site tend to be tender, however [45]. After an average of 16 days' incubation, symptoms begin in a characteristic flu-like manner. Fever of 104° F or more may be seen, along with myalgia, anorexia, and headache [289]. Dizziness is common [289].

In one study, fever and headache occurred in 100% of patients, chills in 80%, and cough in 45%. Adenopathy was noted in 85%, while an eschar was seen in only 46% [45]. When present, the eschar was on the leg or scrotum approximately 66% of the time [45]. In some patients, a generalized vasculitis ensues [291]. Other cutaneous manifestations include a macular or papular rash, which begins on the trunk, spreads to the extremities, and involves the palms and soles [289]. This rash may also reappear during clinical relapse, providing an important clue to therapeutic failure. The organism may also involve the central nervous system, causing mononuclear meningitis [290]. Many other clinical syndromes have been described: ocular problems such as conjunctival injection and subconjunctival hemorrhage [291], granulomatous hepatitis [292], "acute abdomen" [293], and interstitial pneumonitis [294]. Pleural and pericardial effusion [289], meningoencephalitis, and acute respiratory distress syndrome have also been reported [295]. Untreated, the illness lasts approximately two weeks, with a mortality that varies from 0% to 30%. Antimicrobial therapy shortens the clinical course of the infection, and decreases mortality to essentially zero [296]

Bartonella quintana and Bartonella henselaea

As with virtually all of the organisms discussed in this chapter, *Bartonella quintana* has an impressive variety of clinical presentations. *B quintana* causes trench fever, a bacteremic illness in which victims classically develop a single five-day fever. However, infected individuals may also remain afebrile, have recurrent episodes of five-day fever, or develop persistent fever [297]. Associated symptoms and signs, including myalgia, headache, bone pain, splenomegaly and evanescent maculopapular rash [298], are common. Shin pain may be a distinctive finding. *Bartonella henselaea* presentation also may involve recurrent fever, depending on the host's immune status. Disseminated infection by either species may cause bacillary angiomatosis, peliosis, or other inflammatory conditions [299]. *B henselaea* is also implicated as a cause of cat-scratch disease. Endocarditis has been reported with both species, as well as with *Bartonella elizabethae* [300]. Optic disc edema, retinal lesions, and optic nerve-head inflammatory masses have been seen with *B henselaea* [301,302]. While 50% of patients with *Bartonella* infections have self-limited disease, the remainder suffer relapses or develop more chronic forms of infection [149].

Differential Diagnosis

PSITTACOSIS

The differential diagnosis of psittacosis includes virtually any organism which can produce the clinical picture of atypical pneumonia. This would include *Coxiella burnetii, Mycoplasma pneumoniae, Chlamydia pneumoniae, Legionella, Francisella tularensis,* influenza, and other viruses. Epidemiologic clues may be obtained by thorough history-taking. Patients with psittacosis should always be questioned regarding exposure to animals, specifically birds. Q fever is suggested by a history of exposure to cats, goats, or other farm animals. Clinical clues are relatively nonspecific, being common to many of the illnesses listed above. With *C psittaci* infection, severe headache and dry cough are prominent. Photophobia, epistaxis, and Horder's spots, if present, are helpful diagnostically. Confirmation of *C psittaci* infection may not be available until serologic testing is complete; testing for complement fixation (CF) titers or indirect immunofluoresence (IFA) is particularly useful [303].

MYCOPLASMA PNEUMONIAE INFECTION

Like psittacosis, *Mycoplasma pneumoniae* infection also produces atypical pneumonia, with dry cough, malaise, and sore throat. Positive cold agglutinins are suggestive [304], and CF or immunoelectroprecipitation (IEP) of serum will detect antibody to *M pneumoniae* [303]. ELISA, which detects IgG or IgM to *M pneumoniae*, is also available and appears to be quite useful [306]. Legionnaires' disease may also present with atypical pneumonia, mental status changes, relative bradycardia, and high fever. Chills and rigors are less frequent symptoms in legionnaires' disease than in psittacosis, and pharyngitis is quite rare, in contrast to Q fever and *M pneumoniae* [35]. Specialized culture, direct fluorescent antibody (DFA) of sputum, or urine antigen detection can be used to diagnose *Legionella* [307,308].

Chlamydia pneumoniae tends to be less virulent than psittacosis [309]. Specialized serology is necessary to distinguish this infection from psittacosis, due to cross-reactivity among *Chlamydia* species. *Francisella tularensis* causes tularemia, which presents as pneumonia 7–20% of the time [310]. The diagnosis is suggested by a history of tick or deerfly bite, contact with wild rabbits, ulceroglandular lesions, or hilar adenopathy [311]. Diagnosis of tularemia may be accomplished serologically, using agglutination or ELISA assays [312]. Influenza and other viruses may also present with pneumonitis. Differentiation may be impossible on clinical grounds. Prominent upper respiratory symptoms and a typical seasonal attack pattern favor a diagnosis of viral infection, but ultimately culture and serology may be required [313]. Psittacosis may also present as culture-negative endocarditis, mimicking organisms of the HACEK (*Haemophilus parainfluenza*, *H aphrophilus*, *Actinobacillus*, *Cardiobacterium*, *Eikenella*, *Kingella*) group, or other fasitidious bacteria [53]. Gestational psittacosis may present with DIC, elevated transaminases, and abnormal renal function. These cases mimic some of the aspects of thrombotic thrombocytopenic purpura (TTP), hemolytic-uremic syndrome, and the HELLP (hemolysis, elevated liver function tests, low platelets) syndrome [246].

C pneumoniae typically presents as a mild respiratory illness. When pneumonia occurs, it may be confused with other causes of atypical pneumonia, as elucidated above. The age of the patient is a clue, as *Mycoplasma pneumoniae* is more likely in younger patients, as opposed to *C pneumoniae*, which is more prevalent in the elderly [90]. Prominent sore throat with laryngitis is, as noted, more common in patients with *C pneumoniae* infection than in those with *M pneumoniae* [24]. Viral causes of pharyngitis and bronchitis must also be considered. Respiratory viruses such as influenza, RSV, and adenovirus may present similarly.

Genital infection with *Chlamydia trachomatis*, when symptomatic, can be differentiated from *Neisseria gonorrhoeae* by a longer incubation, with less copious and purulent discharge [314]. Nongonococcal urethritis (NGU) can also be due to *Ureaplasma urealyticum* [315] or *Trichomonas vaginalis* [316]. PID can also be due to *Neisseria gonorrhoeae*, or anaerobic bacteria. *C trachomatis* should be included in the differential diagnosis of patients with suspected meningoencephalitis [243].

The differential diagnosis of Q fever depends on its presentation. When pneumonia is present, agents that cause atypical pneumonia should be considered, as detailed above. Differentiation between *Coxiella burnetii*, *Mycoplasma pneumoniae*, and *Legionella pneumophila* can be quite difficult. When flu-like symptoms predominate, influenza must be considered, especially during the brief winter flu season. Influenza typically exhibits a high attack rate in a given community for only a brief, two-week period each year. A history of exposure to domestic animals raises the possibility of brucellosis or leptospirosis [317]. When elevated transaminases are the presenting sign, confusion with viral hepatitis may occur. Chronic *C burnetii* infection may present as culture-negative endocarditis, raising the possibility of infection with fungus, *Chlamydia psittaci*, *Legionella*, or HACEK organisms. Other chronic vascular infections may be confused with chronic Q fever, and endocarditis with hepatomegaly may be confused with Q fever endocarditis.

The differential diagnosis of typhus includes exanthematous diseases. The rash of typhus typically begins in the axillary folds and progresses centrifugally, distinguishing it from the centripetal rash of RMSF, which classically begins on the wrists and ankles. Meningococcemia, measles, secondary syphylis, and rubella are other exanthematous diseases that should be considered in the differential of typhus [37]. Epidemiologic clues are often helpful, especially if the appearance of the rash is delayed.

Rickettsia typhi has a nonspecific clinical appearance, making it difficult to differentiate from other febrile illnesses even when rash is present. A central maculopapular rash develops in 70% of those infected with *R typhi* [201]. Epidemiologic evidence may be lacking, since the bite of the flea may not be recalled [137]. The differential diagnosis is similar to that for *Rickettsia prowazekii* and includes RMSF, secondary syphilis, ehrlichiosis, and Kawasaki's disease. Other rickettsioses, stroke, pneumonia, and gastroenteritis should also be considered [137]. The cutaneous signs of measles, rubella, or roseola may be mistaken for those of *R typhi* [201].

The differential diagnosis for *Rickettsia rickettsii* includes the other spotted fevers, typhoid fever, measles (especially if the rash is atypical), mononucleosis, and meningococcemia [137]. ITP and TTP enter the differential if thrombocytopenia develops. A presentation of fever and headache in the absence of rash poses great diagnostic difficulty, even during the expected seasonal period. The presence of pulmonary infiltrate may suggest other atypical pneumonia pathogens. The various spotted fevers may be distinguished from each other according to geographic clues.

The presentation of tsutsugamushi's disease may be clinically nonspecific. Infectious mononucleosis is a frequent misdiagnosis, as both illnesses may present with malaise, fever, and adenopathy. Diagnostic serologic tests, including the monospot test, are widely available and reliable [318]. The distinctive eschar is a useful diagnostic finding in patients with scrub typhus but is seen in fewer than half of patients [45]. Other diagnostic considerations include typhus, typhoid, brucellosis, leptospirosis, toxoplasmosis, and flavirus [37]. Typhus can be distinguished by the lack of an eschar, and a centrifugally spreading rash that emerges in the setting of lice infestation. Serologic testing, including ELISA and PCR, are helpful [319,320]. Typhoid fever is due to *Salmonella typhi* and may be clinically indistinguishable from typhus and scrub typhus. In patients with typhoid fever, cultures of blood, stool, and bone marrow as well as duodenal string culture should be performed. This will result in a diagnostic sensitivity of 90% [321], which is important, since serologic testing for typhoid is felt to be unreliable [322]. *Brucella* causes brucellosis, another zoonosis with nonspecific symptomology. A history of exposure to cows, camels, unpasteurized milk, or an occupational history of abattoir or veterinary work are helpful clues [323]. Diagnosis of brucellosis is usually achieved via isolation of the organism from blood or bone marrow [324]; serology may also be helpful [325]. Leptospirosis may also present in a flu-like fashion, with nonspecific findings. Conjunctival injection and hemorrhage, if present, are distinctive [326]. A history of exposure to dogs, rodents [327], or livestock, either recreationally or occupationally, is an important clue [328]. Isolation of *Leptospira* from blood, CSF, and urine is possible. Serologic tests for *Leptospira* are available and useful diagnostically [329,330]. Toxoplasmosis may present with lymphadenopathy and mimic mononucleosis. A history of exposure to cat feces or ingestion of undercooked meat may be present [331], and isolation of the organism in body fluids may be successful early in the course of the disease. A multitude of serologic tests are also available for toxoplasmosis, including PCR [332,333]. The flaviviruses may also present with fever, relative bradycardia, and myalgia [334]. CF, ELISA, and PCR testing are useful diagnostically.

Bartonella quintana and *Bartonella henselaea* must be differentiated from other causes of recurrent fever, including the diverse causes of endocarditis. Other arthropod-borne infections should be considered when infestation or bites are evident. In patients with HIV infection, the possibility of infection with fungal or mycobacterial organisms should be considered [52]. Infection after a cat scratch may be due to *Pasteurella multocida* or other organisms. When endocarditis is present, the wide differential of culture-negative endocarditis must be employed; this involves ruling out HACEK organisms, anaerobes, fungi, and fastidious organisms [335].

Diagnostic Evaluation

CHLAMYDIA PSITTACI

Avian Chlamydiosis

Avian chlamydiosis (AC) cases are classified by the CDC as suspected, probable, or confirmed [336].

- A *suspected* case involves:
  1. Clinical illness consistent with AC, with an epidemiologic link to another case of AC.
  2. Asymptomatic birds with equivocal serologic evidence of infection.
  3. Clinical illlness with a positive, nonstandardized laboratory test result.
  4. A clinical illness, consistent with AC, that responds well to antibiotic therapy.
- A *probable* case of AC involves an illness compatible with AC and either:
  1. A high serologic titer obtained after symptom onset.
  2. Fecal, cloacal, or respiratory/ocular exudate, which is ELISA- or fluorescent antibody (FA)–positive for *Chlamydia psittaci.*
- A *confirmed* case of AC requires either :
  1. Isolation of *Chlamydia psittaci* from a clinical specimen.
  2. ELISA- or FA-positive *Chlamydia psittaci* antigen in the bird's tissue.
  3. A serologic titer that increases more than fourfold in two specimens obtained at least two weeks apart.
  4. Giminez stain– or Machiavelo stain–positive AC organisms in the bird's tissues.

Methods of diagnosing AC include isolation of the organism from the bird's organs or secretions. While pharyngeal samples are the most likely to be positive, to increase sensitivity, sampling of multiple sites should be considered, especially if only a single animal is being investigated [337]. The sample is used to inoculate cell cultures, and staining subsequently reveals the organism's presence in the cellular inclusions. This can be accomplished by staining the tissue, using chromatic or immunologic stains. However, due to technical issues and safety concerns, few laboratories culture the organism. When sending specimens to these labs, pooling three to five days of specimens and transporting the specimens packed in ice is recommended. Culture of the organism is still considered the reference standard for antigen detection [15]. Antigen can be detected using ELISA [338], although the reliability of this test has been questioned. Other antigen-detection methods include cytologic staining [339], electron microscopy [340], PCR [341], elementary body-agglutination (EBA), immunoperoxidase [342], peroxidase anti-peroxidase [343], and microimmunofluorescence (MIF). In some studies, PCR assay was found to be more sensitive than culture and ELISA [344,345].

Serologic testing to detect antibodies to *Chlamydia psittaci* has several limitations. Chief among these is the fact that false-negative results are common early in the clinical course, due to low serum levels of antibody. Later, false-positive results are seen due to persistence of antibodies (CF detects both IgM and IgG) despite adequate therapy. Some authorities feel that serologic testing is most useful in epidemiologic studies and less useful in the clinical setting [15]. Serologic tests most commonly used to detect antibody to *Chlamydia psittaci* include complement-fixation (CF), which is sensitive but may remain elevated after treatment, and ELISA. Latex agglutination (LA) is also available; this test detects IgM to identify acute *Chlamydia psittaci* infection but fails to identify the more chronic forms of infection [62]. Elementary-body agglutination (EBA) is available but is performed in only one laboratory. Furthermore, EBA test results may remain positive despite therapy. In the absence of positive culture results, the most reliable diagnosis would be if a bird suspected to be a source of infection tests positive for both antibody and antigen. A fourfold increase in titer, or a positive titer with antigen detection, is generally considered significant.

Psittacosis

The CDC defines a *probable* case of psittacosis as:

1. Clinical findings consistent with psittacosis, with an epidemiologic link to a known case.
2. MIF or CF titer 1:32 after symptom onset.

A *confirmed* case of psittacosis requires:

1. Positive *Chlamydia psittaci* culture.
2. Clinical findings consistent with psittacosis: either a greater than fourfold increase in CF or MIF titer over two weeks or more, or MIF positive (> 1:32) for IgM.

Psittacosis is human infection with *C psittaci*. The disease presents the clinician with a diagnostic challenge. Rapid diagnosis is desirable, since delays may result in poor outcomes. One study found that because an average of eight days elapsed prior to diagnosis in five of eight patients with respiratory failure, they eventually died [244]. The diagnostician can be aided by epidemiologic clues, especially occupational or recreational exposures to birds. Such exposures are noted in 85% of patients with *C psittaci* infection and may prompt effective empiric antibiotic therapy [244].

Chest radiography is minimally useful due to its nonspecificity. While culture of the organism is possible, it is infrequently performed, mostly because of logistic and safety considerations. Specimens contaminated with C psittaci are quite infectious and therefore hazardous to laboratory personnel [53]. The usual diagnostic method for psittacosis involves finding a greater than fourfold rise in CF titer over more than a two-week period, although a single titer of 1:32 or greater is good presumptive evidence of infection, especially when the clinical findings are consistent with psittacosis. Microimmunofluoresence (MIF) assays are available and can distinguish between infection with the various chlamydial species. MIF also appears to be more sensitive than the standard CF titer (61% vs. 46%), but false-negative results may occur [346]. Direct fluorescent antibody (DFA), utilizing monoclonal antibodies against the antigens of C psittaci, is now available and allows much more rapid diagnosis [347]. DFA can be performed on sputum, for example, providing a means of rapid and accurate diagnosis. A false-positive result due to the presence of Chlamydia pneumonia or Chlamydia trachomatis infection is possible, and in such cases, the more species-specific MIF can be used. If results are equivocal because of a sluggish antibody response due to therapy, a third sample may be checked later in the clinical course of the infection. In cases of suspected endocarditis, culture of the organism may be performed, using the patient's serum; staining and immunofluorescence of the involved heart valve is another method for detecting the pathogen [348]. Bronchoalveolar lavage (BAL) fluid also yields the organism [349]. Lung biopsy tissue examined by direct immunofluorescence may also be positive [350].

Chlamydia trachomatis

Diagnosis of *Chlamydia trachomatis* requires a high index of suspicion, since most cases are subclinical. Specimens are best obtained from the endocervix in women and the urethra in men. Simultaneous urethral sampling in women increases sensitivity [351]. The most sensitive diagnostic method involves growing the organism in cell culture and staining with a species-specific fluorescein-labeled monoclonal antibody (FA) [97]. Lung tissue also can be cultured in cases of suspected *C trachomatis* pneumonia. While nonculture tests are felt to be acceptable in most circumstances, culture should be performed on rectal specimens, and on genital and nasopharyngeal specimens from infants [97]. Nonculture tests include the direct fluorescent antibody (DFA) test, ELISA, DNA probes, PCR, and MIF. DFA testing will detect chlamydial antigen in clinical specimens. ELISA, which utilizes an enzyme linked to a monoclonal antibody, is helpful, although use of chlamydial LPS as an antigen may render an ELISA assay non-species-specific. DNA probes involve the binding of luminescent DNA to chlamydial RNA. PCR is likely quite sensitive and specific; rapid (< 30 minutes) tests are available for office use. Nonspecificity is a problem, however. Specimens can also be obtained from the rectum, conjunctiva, urine, and serum [97]. Serologic testing for *C trachomatis* is available in some locations. An IgM MIF of ≥ 1:32 for *C trachomatis* is presumptive evidence of infection [206]. A presumptive diagnosis of *C trachomatis* should be made in patients with NGU, with PID, with epididymitis (if the patient is less than age 35), with sexual partners of known cases, and those with gonorrhea. In all cases, the treatment regimens should include antibiotics effective against *C trachomatis* infection. Despite a presumptive diagnosis, testing should still be performed for epidemiologic reasons as well as to determine appropriate care and follow-up [97].

Chlamydia pneumoniae

Chlamydia pneumoniae is usually a mild respiratory illness. Leukocytosis rarely occurs in patients with *C pneumoniae*, although an elevated ESR is common. A single subsegmental infiltrate on chest radiogram is seen most commonly [352], although a diffuse interstitial pattern has been noted in HIV-infected patients [353]. Pleural effusion secondary to *C pneumoniae* sometimes occurs, and the organism has been isolated from pleural fluid. However, the organism is best isolated using nasopharyngeal swabs to inoculate a cell culture. Fluorescent-antibody staining of the culture may be performed after several days of incubation; a positive result confirms the presence of *Chlamydia* species. Culture techniques are somewhat cumbersome, require several days of incubation, and are only 65% sensitive. These considerations have led to the development of several serologic diagnostic modalities. Complement fixation (CF) may be performed; the result is considered positive if there is a fourfold rise in titer or if a single titer is 1:64 or greater. Unfortunately, CF appears to be less sensitive than MIF and is genus-specific. Thus, a positive CF result does not distinguish between pneumonia due to *C pneumoniae*, *C psittaci*, or *C trachomatis* [22]. Using IgM- and IgG-specific MIF appears to be the most sensitive and specific method and can distinguish acute from previous infection [22]. Unfortunately, IgM is often absent in patients with reinfection and also in younger patients. IgA-specific MIF may help in cases of reinfection, however, as one study showed all individuals with reinfection to have MIF IgA titers of 1:64 or greater [29]. MIF may be considered positive if there is a fourfold rise in titer, if the IgM titer is 1:16 or greater, or if IgG is 1:512 or greater [22]. A new microimmunofluorescence test (MRL) appears to be somewhat more sensitive than the standard MIF test [354]. PCR appears to hold promise for rapid diagnosis and is believed to have acceptable sensitivity. PCR can be performed on throat swabs, bronchoalveolar lavage fluid (BALF), and other specimens [355,356].

Due to the mild, nonspecific nature of its presentation, Q fever can be difficult to diagnose. While a cluster of cases related to the same source may be seen, sporadic cases frequently occur. A history of occupational exposure and headache are important clues for the physician. The clinical presentation and laboratory findings are quite variable. *Coxiella burnetii* infection may present as pneumonitis, with interstitial or nodular infiltrates present in the lower lobes [192]. The white count is abnormal in approximately 30% of patients with this infection [35], thrombocytopenia is seen in 25% [108], and thrombocytosis due to platelet counts as high as 1,000,000 may be seen [284]. Elevated transaminases (2–3 times normal) are seen in approximately 50% of patients, while jaundice is rare [284]. Hemolytic anemia has been noted [109], and ESR may be elevated. Hypoxemia parallels the radiographic extent of disease. (In one study, 26% of patients had Pa_{O_2} less than 60 mmHg in one series [284].) CSF pleocytosis and elevated protein have also been seen in patients with *C burnetii* infection [109].

Infection can be confirmed by culture of the organism or, more commonly, by serologic methods. The organism can be grown in cell culture, chicken embryo, and in animals [357]. Due to a perceived hazard to laboratory personnel, culture is performed in very few laboratories, so diagnosis relies on serology. It is now possible to culture the organism more safely, using, for example, the shell-vial cell-culture technique. This method of culture may be performed on tissue biopsies and buffy coat samples; it requires only six days of incubation [357]. Culture techniques hold promise for cases in which early diagnosis is required, since, if *C burnetii* infection is present, the culture result is likely to be positive before serologic conversion occurs [358]. Serologic tests such as immunofluorescence (IFA) and complement fixation (CF) have classically been used to diagnose infection. A fourfold rise in titer was felt to indicate acute infection, while a single IFA of 1:256 or greater or CF of 1:64 or greater was also diagnostic [357]. Interestingly, testing for antibodies to phase II antigens is used to detect acute infection with CF, while testing for phase I antigens is useful in the detection of chronic infection [108]. It now appears that serologic diagnosis with microimmunofluorescence (MIF) is more helpful than CF or IFA. MIF can distinguish IgM, IgG, and IgA. MIF positive for IgM indicates acute infection, although positive titers of IgM may persist for one year [357]. Positive MIF for IgA and IgG ($\geq$ 1:800) to *C burnetii* phase I antigens indicates chronic infection with a high sensitivity and specificity [357]. A fourfold rise in ELISA may be used diagnostically but is believed by some to be less specific than MIF. One ELISA study, however, detailed an 89% positive predictive value and a 100% negative predictive value [114,359]. Another study that used ELISA specific for IgA and IgM antibodies to *C burnetii* found that diagnostic criteria requiring both to be positive resulted in a specificity of 100% without a decrease in sensitivity [360]. Antibody titers may wane over time, remaining positive for years in some patients [108]. Q fever endocarditis may be diagnosed by using the criteria of the Duke Endocarditis Service [361]. Analysis has shown that the sensitivity of this method is increased when a positive *C burnetii* blood culture or a high phase I titer of 1:800 or greater for IgG is considered the major diagnostic criterium [362]. PCR can be performed on valvular tissue or the supernatant of cell cultures but is currently less convenient than serology. *C burnetii* can also be detected directly, using immunologic staining methods in tissues such as heart valves. When Q fever hepatitis is present, autoantibodies to smooth muscle, a positive ANA, or a positive Coombs' test may be seen [357].

Prompt diagnosis of rickettsial diseases is important to decrease morbidity and mortality. Unfortunately, serologic diagnosis may not be timely, and serologic testing may be misleading in the early stages of infection. Epidemiologic clues, a high index of suspicion, and empiric therapy are important tools for the clinician. Skin biopsy may offer the best chance for early diagnosis of rickettsial infection, provided that rash is present. *Rickettsia prowazekii* may be diagnosed by culture, serologically, or by PCR [363]. ELISA testing for *R prowazekii* is available [319], as is MIF [127]. Immunohistochemical staining of tissues is possible and may be useful in acute cases [364].

Rickettsia typhi can be diagnosed serologically by IFA or LA. IFA remains the most widely used serologic test for the diagnosis of RMSF [320]. Indirect immunofluorescence (IFA) demonstrating titers of 1:128 or greater, or demonstration of a fourfold increase to 1:64 or greater, are considered positive [129], although results are not species-specific.

Immunohistologic identification of *R typhi* in tissue [365] and PCR [366] may become more widely available. Rapid diagnosis may also become more widely available through use of the Dip-S-Ticks, which has 88% sensitivity and 87% specificity for *R typhi* in testing IFA-positive sera [367]. *Rickettsia rickettsii* is potentially lethal, so early diagnosis is important. The pathology of the rash in RMSF is characteristic, revealing lymphohistiocytic capillaritis and venulitis, with extravasation of erythrocytes [368]. Timely diagnosis may be achieved by immunofluorescent staining of a punch biopsy of the rash. This technique has high specificity and 70% sensitivity [320]. Immunoperoxidase staining is less timely, since it is performed on a processed specimen, but exhibits the same sensitivity and specificity as immunofluorescent staining [369].

R rickettsii may cause nonspecific laboratory abnormalities such as anemia, thrombocytopenia, and hyponatremia [39]. The organism may be cultured from blood using the shell-vial assay, although some feel this poses a biohazard to lab personnel. Proper techniques make culture a much safer endeavor in the modern laboratory. Immunofluorescent staining of skin biopsies appears to be 70% sensitive and almost 100% specific [39]. Latex agglutination (LA) (≥ 1:64), IFA (≥ 1:64), CF, and indirect hemo-agglutination (≥ 1:128) are serologically diagnostic of RMSF [137]. The sensitivity of CF, LA, and IFA have been determined to be 63%, 71%, and 94%, respectively [370]. PCR also appears helpful, with greater sensitivity when skin biopsy specimens are used, as opposed to blood [139,371].

Historically, scrub typhus has been exquisitely responsive to appropriate antimicrobial therapy, so much so that a prompt response was felt to be diagnostic and a poor response to cast doubt on the diagnosis. The emergence of drug-resistant strains has made a serologic diagnosis more desirable [372]. Routine lab testing is of little help in diagnosing scrub typhus. Frequent findings include elevated ESR, serum lymphocytosis (> 50% lymphs in 70%), and increased transaminases [289]. Several serodiagnostic tests are available for diagnosing scrub typhus. In a study designed to compare the usefulness of currently available testing, the indirect immunoperoxidase (IIP) test (at a cutoff of 1:400) proved to be 90% sensitive and 100% specific; furthermore, it was more sensitive than the immunofluorescent antibody test (IFA) when acute sera was tested (80% vs. 68% sensitivity, respectively). A simpler ELISA test, known commercially as Dip-S-Ticks, proved to be 94% sensitive and 98% specific at a cutoff of one or more positive dots. The classic slide agglutination Weil-Felix reaction (cross-reactive antibodies to the *Proteus* X strain) was found to lack sensitivity [373]. PCR can also be used diagnostically [374] and may be positive when specific antibody tests are unrevealing [375].

Bartonella quintana and *Bartonella henselaea* are difficult to culture. Bone, skin, and blood specimens may yield the organism. When seeking *Bartonella* species, staining of the aerobic blood culture with acridine orange will allow identification of possible infection, and the appropriate subculture can then be performed [149]. A direct immunofluorescent antibody test was made available for *Bartonella* infection by the CDC in 1992 [335], with IFA titers of 1:64 or greater considered positive. Unfortunately the test does not differentiate between the two species. The sensitivity and specificity of IFA are felt to be 83% and 98%, respectively [376], although cross-reactivity with *Chlamydia pneumoniae* may occur [300]. PCR may become a useful tool for detection *Bartonella* organism but currently is not generally available [377,378]. The sensitivity and specificity of PCR have been measured at 61% and 100%, respectively [329].

Treatment and Rehabilitation

Treatment of avian chlamydiosis includes several established options. These include medicated feed impregnated with chlortetracycline (CTC), ideally maintaining a serum concentrations of 1 μg/mL [380]. Mash diets and pellets with greater than 1% CTC can be bought or mixed. White millet seed with CTC is available (e.g., Keet Life) and can be used to treat parakeets, canaries, finches, and budgerigars [62]. Larger psittacines and lovebirds require treatment with 1% CTC, either via medicated pellets (e.g., Psittacin, Psttavit) or a cooked mash [381] or nectar diet to which CTC powder (e.g., Cyanamid, Mix 66) has been added [62]. CTC can be added to hen feed to medicate pigeons [62]. Oral doxycycline, 25–50 mg/kg once a day, is another option for most psittacines. Doxycycline should probably be given at a dosage of 25–30 mg/kg each day for cockatoos and macaws, 25 mg/kg each day for African grey parrots, Goffin's cockatoos, and blue, gold, and green-winged macaws. A dose of 40–50 mg/kg each day is needed for cockatiels, Senegal parrots, and blue-fronted and orange-winged Amazon parrots. All these treatments should be continued for 45 days.

Adequate antibiotics cannot be provided via drinking water, since the psittacines have very low water requirements [62]. Turkeys require treatment with pelleted feed with CTC at a concentration of 400 g/ton, which should be continued for two weeks or more; the turkey should be held for at least two days prior to slaughter [62,229]. Intramuscular doxycycline is available in Europe and Canada. A dose of 75–100 mg/kg is injected into the pectoral muscle each day for four weeks and then every five days. Birds who are too ill to eat can be tried on injectable oxytetracycline; 75 mg/kg every three to four days has been successful in some species. Tissue necrosis is a problem with intramuscular CTC and oxytetracycline [380]. Quinolones and macrolides may be beneficial, but proof is lacking at present. Eno-floxacin is available for use and can be considered if other therapies have proved ineffective [382]. Supportive therapy with fluids, heat, and vitamins may also be helpful [383], and a diet low in calcium (< 0.7%) will allow for sufficient tetracycline absorption from the gastrointestinal tract.

Untreated psittacosis may result in a persistent fever for three to four weeks, often resulting in mortality [12]. Isolation of *Chlamydia psittaci* patients has not been traditional, due to a perceived low rate of infectivity, although transmission from patient to doctor or nurse has been described [12]. The CDC does not officially recommend patient isolation or prophylactic therapy of contacts [16]. Possible human-to-human transfer [159] suggests that respiratory isolation, or at least extreme care in handling the secretions and biological specimens of these patients, is prudent. Tetracyclines are the drugs of choice for the treatment psittacosis. Doxycycline, 100 mg orally twice daily, tetracycline, 500 mg orally twice daily, can be used. Treatment should be continued for at least 10–14 days after resolution of fever. Intravenous tetracycline at a dosage of 10–15 mg/kg/day can be used in the severely ill patient. Treatment with erythromycin may be effective; however, there are several reported cases in which the patient expired despite erythromycin therapy [244,384]. Erythromycin may be considered for pregnant females and children under age 9. Newer quinolones also may be useful [385], whereas sulfonamides are usually not. Appropriate therapy should result in clinical improvement within 48–72 hours. Although unusual, reinfection with *C psittaci* can occur [85].

Chlamydia pneumoniae is sensitive to tetracyclines, erythromycin, clarithromycin, and azithromycin [386]. It is not sensitive to sulfonamides and is less sensitive to quinolones [387]. Despite adequate therapy, relapse may occur, necessitating retreatment. Antibiotic resistance may develop in patients who are treated with azithromycin therapy [388] as well as those treated with doxycycline [389]. Some authorities have recommended 2 g per day of erythromycin or tetracycline, given in divided doses [22]. Animal studies suggest that short-term courses of antibiotics may become acceptable [390]. Patients with elevated IgA and IgG titers are considered to have chronic *C pneumoniae* infection and have been treated in one study with four months of doxycycline therapy without effect [391]. Optimum therapy for such cases remains to be determined.

Chlamydia trachomatis can be treated with doxycycline, 100 mg orally twice daily for seven days. The treatment of choice in uncomplicated cases is azithromycin, 1 g orally, which allows one-dose therapy. Alternatives to these two regimens for uncomplicated *C trachomatis* include ofloxacin (not for adolescent or pregnant patients), 300 mg orally twice daily for seven days, erythromycin base 500, mg orally four times daily for seven days (recommended in pregnant patients), erythromycin succinate, 800 mg orally four times daily for seven days [206], and sulfisoxazole, 500 mg orally four times daily for 0 days [97]. Pregnant patients who cannot tolerate erythromycin can be treated with amoxicillin, 500 mg orally twice daily for seven days [206]. Newer agents such as trovafloxacin [392] and dirithromycin [393] also appear effective. One study suggested that serovars, which tend to cause asymptomatic infection as opposed to cervicitis or PID, are more susceptible to doxycycline or azithromycin [394]. All strains of *C trachoma* exhibit susceptibility to sulfonamides. Rare cases of tetracycline resistance have been reported [395]. Therapy for PID should include the doxycycline regimen noted above, in order to cover infection and co-infection with *C trachomatis.* LGV requires doxycycline or erythromycin for 21 days. Bubo aspiration may be necessary [206]. Treatment of mucopurulent cervicitis should await test results, unless the patient is unlikely to return for follow-up [206]. The patient should be advised to observe sexual abstinence for seven days and until all partners have completed a full course of antibiotics. Testing for cure can be considered after three weeks. Ophthalmia neonatorum and infant pneumonia caused by *C trachomatis* can be treated with erythromycin, 50 mg/kg/day in four doses for 10–14 days. Mothers of newborns with *C trachomatis* pneumonia should also be screened and treated if necessary [206].

Although acute Q fever, including Q fever pneumonitis, is usually self-limited, treatment should be provided to reduce risk for chronic Q fever infection. Treatment of *Coxiella burnetii* is difficult due to the vacuolar location of the organism. Antibiotic sensitivities are somewhat heterogeneous; variable susceptibilities to quinolones, tetracyclines, rifampin, and erythromycin have been reported. Tetracycline antibiotics are the mainstay of therapy for acute Q fever, decreasing the duration of fever by 50% if started in the first 72 hours [396]. A dose of 25 mg/kg/day in four doses for a total of two to four weeks can be given to adults and children over the age of 8 with pneumonitis. Doxycycline, 100 mg orally twice weekly for two to three weeks, can be used in adults [108], while erythromycin, 500 mg orally four times daily for 10 days, also appears effective [397]. Other experts recommend combining doxycycline or erythromycin therapy with rifampin [35]. Using a macrolide with rifampin has the advantage of coverage for other atypical pathogens such as *Legionella* while awaiting serologic results [284]. Quinolones penetrate the CSF well and should be considered for patients with Q fever meningoencephalitis [357].

Chronic forms of Q fever such as endocarditis should theoretically be treated with a bactericidal agent. Traditionally, these entities have been treated with tetracyclines, sometimes in combination with other antibiotics. Rifampin with doxycycline or trimethoprim-sulfamethoxazole are options [357]. Another option is a combination of doxycycline and quinolone, with therapy extended to three years and more. Adding chloroquine, amantadine, or hydroxychloroquine to doxycycline increases the pH within the phagolysosome and may allow for regimens as short as 18 months [114,398]. Favorable outcomes have been reported [399]. Late relapses are frequent and result in a mortality of 60% [357]. Endocarditis therapy with combination regimens yields a mortality of 18% [285]. Some consider cure to have been achieved once phase I IgA and IgG are negative, with titers of 1:200 or less [357]. Monitoring serology seems the best approach to determining the length of therapy, with continuation of antibiotics if the patient remains positive [285]. Lifetime therapy may be necessary for some patients. Valve replacement has been used by some physicians in an attempt to cure Q fever endocarditis; however, the current consensus appears to be that it be considered only in cases of hemodynamic compromise or recurrent embolization [285,357]. In cases of prosthetic valve endocarditis, valve replacement after several weeks of antibiotic therapy is often required for cure [400].

Louse-borne typhus from *Rickettsia prowazekii* can be cured with a single dose of doxycycline, 100 mg orally [401]. Endogenously acquired *R prowazekii* (Brill-Zinsser disease) and *Rickettsia typhi* should be treated with doxycycline, 100 mg orally twice daily, chloramphenicol, 50 mg/kg/day in four divided doses, or tetracycline, 25 mg/kg/day in four divided doses [37]. *R typhi* also may be treated with quinolones. *Rickettsia rickettsii* can be treated with seven days of TCN, 25–50 mg/kg/day; chloramphenicol 50–75, mg/kg/day; or doxycycline, 100 mg orally twice daily [137]. Macrolides show some promise in vitro [402].

Mortality from scrub typhus in the pre-antibiotic era was approximately 50% but is now near zero when appropriate antibiotic therapy is instituted [372]. Treatment with tetracycline or chloramphenicol has been the mainstay of treatment for scrub typhus. Treatment with appropriate antimicrobials (TCN, 500 mg orally four times daily, or doxycycline, 100 mg orally twice daily for seven days) has historically been quite successful, leading to rapid defervescence, which is sufficiently characteristic to allow empiric diagnosis. In 60 U.S. servicemen who acquired scrub typhus in Viet Nam, the fever resolved within 28 hours [403]. No relapses were seen with 10 days of TCN therapy [45]. Virulent strains that are resistant to doxycycline and chloramphenicol have been found in Northern Thailand [372]. Drug-resistant strains may potentially be treated with ciprofloxacin [404], single or double-dose doxycycline [405], or short-course doxycycline (100 mg orally twice daily for three days). A Korean study found a 94% cure rate with three days of doxycycline, versus 100% with seven days of tetracycline ($p \geq 0.05$) [406]. Azithromycin proved successful even against a resistant strain in vitro, and may come to be important in the treatment of children and infected females [407]. Intravenous minocycline has been used in severe cases [295]. The occurrence of relapse was initially thought to be related to the initiation of therapy quite early in the course of the disease [211]. More recent studies do not support this concept, however; risk of relapse is now felt to be more likely due to the virulence of the infecting strain [406]. Some authorities recommend 14 days of antibiotic therapy to reduce this risk [44]. Reinfection with scrub typhus also may occur, necessitating retreatment [406].

Bartonella quintana and *Bartonella henselaea* seem highly susceptible to antibiotics in vitro; however, only the aminoglycosides have proved to be bactericidal for these organisms [402]. Erythromycin, 500 mg four times daily, is considered the current drug of choice; use of doxycycline or tetracycline is second-line therapy [50]. Erythromycin and azithromycin have been used with some success in cases of endocarditis [300,335]. Optimum therapy has not yet been established, however.

References

1. Moulder JW. Looking at *Chlamydiae* without looking at their hosts. *Am Soc Microbiol News* 1984; 50:353–62.
2. Moulder JW. Interaction of *Chlamydiae* and host cells in vitro. *Microbiol Rev* 1991;55:143–90.
3. Saah AJ. Rickettsiosis. In: Mandel GL, Bennett JE, Dolin R (eds). *Principles and Practice of Infectious Diseases*, 4th Ed. New York: Churchill Livingstone, 1995. Pp 1719–20.
4. Harris RL, Williams TL. Contribution to the question of pneumotyphus: a discussion of the original article by J. Ritter in 1880. *Rev Infect Dis* 1985;7:119–22.
5. Morange A. *De la psittacose, ou infection speciale determinee par les perruches.* PhD thesis, Academie de Paris, Paris, 1895.
6. Halberstaedter L, von Prowazek S. Zur aetiologie des trachoma. *Dtsch Med Wochensch* 1907;33:1285–7.
7. Coles AC. Micro-organisms in psittacosis. *Lancet* 1930;1:1011–2.
8. Macfarlane JT, Macrae AD. Psittacosis. *Med Bull* 1983;39:163–7.
9. Meyer KF, Eddie B. Characteristics of a psittacosis viral agent isolated from a turkey. *Proc Soc Exp Biol Med* 1932;83:99–101.
10. Haagen E, Mauer G. Dir psittacose in Deutschland. *Zentralb Bakteriol* 1938;143:81–2.
11. Pinkerton H, Swank RL. Recovery of virus morphologically identical with psittacosis from thiamin-deficient pigeons. *Proc Soc Exp Biol Med* 1940;45:704–6.
12. Wolins W. Ornithosis (psittacosis), a review with a report of eight cases resulting from contact with the domestic Pekin duck. *Am J Med Sci* 1948;216:551–64 .
13. Moulder JW. The relation of the psittacosis group (chlamydia) to bacteria and viruses. *Ann Rev Micro* 1966;20:107–30.
14. Schlossberg D. *Chlamydia psittaci* (psittacosis). In: Mandel GL, Bennett JE, Dolin R (eds), *Principles and Practice of Infectious Diseases*, 4th Ed. New York: Churchill Livingstone, 1995. Pp 1693–6.
15. Vanrompay D, Ducatelle R, Haesebrouck F. *Chlamydia psittaci* infections: a review with emphasis on avian chlamydiosis. *Vet Micro* 1995;45:93–119.
16. Compendium of psittacosis (chlamydiosis) control, 1997. *MMWR* 1997 (suppl);46(RR-13):1–13.
17. Korman TM, Turnidge JD, Grayson ML. *Clin Inf Dis* 1997;25(4):847–51.
18. Schacter J, Dawson CR. *Human Chlamydial Infections.* Littleton, MA: PSG Publishing, 1978. Pp 63–96.
19. Halberstaedter L, von Prowazek S. Ueber chlamydozoenbefunde bei blenorrhea neonatorum non gonorrhoica. *Klin Wochenschr* 1909;46:1839–40.
20. Heymann B. Ueber die fundorte der Prowazek'schen korperchen. *Berl Klin Wochenschr* 1910;47:663–6.
21. Lidner K. Zur atiologie der gonokokkenfrein urethritis. *Wien Klin Wochenschr* 1910;23:283–4.
22. Grayston JT. Infections caused by *Chlamydia pneumoniae* strain TWAR. *Clin Infect Dis* 1992; 15:757–63.
23. Saikku P, Wang SP, Kleemola M, et al. An epidemic of mild pneumonia due to an unusual strain of *Chlamydia psittaci. J Infect Dis* 1985;151:832–9.
24. Grayston JT, Kuo C-C, Wang S-P, et al. A new *Chlamydia psittaci* strain, TWAR, isolated in acute respiratory tract infections. *N Engl J Med* 1986;315:161–8.
25. Grayston JT, Kuo C-C, Campbell LA, Wang S-P. *Chlamydia pneumoniae* sp. nov. for *Chlamydia* sp. strain TWAR. *Int J Syst Bacteriol* 1989;39:88–90.
26. Mordhorst CH, Wang SP, Grayston JT. Epidemic 'ornithosis' and TWAR infection, Denmark 1976–85. In: Oriel D, Ridgway G, Schacter J, et al. (eds), *Chlamydial Infections.* Cambridge, Engl. Cambridge University Press, 1986. Pp 325–8.
27. Eng J, Flottorp A. Pra-ornithose; en epidemi av akutt luftveisinfeksjon med positiv Lygranum-KBR. *Tidsskr Nor Laegeforen* 1957;77:51–6.
28. Fraser PK, Hatch LA, Shell GN, et al. Minor respiratory illnesses caused by an agent of the psittacosis/lymphogranuloma-venereum group. *Lancet* 1964; 2:306–8.

29. Ekman M-R, Graystn JT, Visakorpi R, et al. An epidemic of infections due to *Chlamydia pneumoniae* in military conscripts. *Clin Infect Dis* 1993;17:420–5.

30. Grayston JT, Aldous MB, Easton A, et al. Evidence that *Chlamydia pneumoniae* causes pneumonia and bronchitis. *J Infect Dis* 1993;168:1231–5.

31. Derrick EH. "Q" fever, a new fever entity: clinical features, diagnosis and laboratory investigation. *Med J Aust* 1937;2:281–99.

32. Burnett FM, Freeman M. Experimental studies on the virus of "Q" fever. *Med J Aust* 1937;2:299–305.

33. Davis GE, Cox HR. A filter-passing infectious agent isolated from ticks: I. Isolation from *Dermacentor andersoni*, reactions in animals, and filtration experiments. *Public Health Rep* 1939;53:2259–67.

34. Leedom JM. Q fever; an update. In: Remington JS, Schwartz MN (eds), *Current Clinical Topics in Infectious Diseases.* New York: McGraw-Hill, 1980. Pp 304–31.

35. Marrie TJ. *Coxiella burnetii* (Q fever) pneumonia. *Clin Infect Dis* 1995;21(suppl 3):S253–64.

36. Baxter JD. The typhus group. *Clin Dermatol* 1996;14(3):271–8.

37. Saah, AJ. *Rickettsia prowazekii.* In: Mandel GL, Bennett JE, Dolin R (eds), *Principles and Practice of Infectious Diseases.* 4th Ed. New York: Churchill Livingstone, 1995. Pp 1735–7.

38. Azad AF. Epidemiology of murine typhus. *Ann Rev Entomol* 1990;35:553–69.

39. Silber JL. Rocky Mountain spotted fever. *Clin Derm* 1996;14:245–58.

40. Harden VA. Koch's postulates and the etiology of rickettsial diseases. *J Hist Med Allied Sci* 1987;42(3):277–95.

41. Tamura A, Ohashi N, Urakami H, et al. Classification of *Rickettsia tsutsugamushi* in a new genus, *Orientia* gen. nov., as *Orientia tsutsugamushi* comb. nov. *Int J Systematic Bacteriol* 1995;45(3):589–91.

42. Ohashi N, Kayama Y, Urakami N, et al. Demonstration of antigenic and genotypic variation in *Orientia tsutsugamushi* which were isolated in Japan, and their classification into type and subtype. *Microbiol Immunol* 1996;40(9):627–38.

43. Tamura A, Ohashi N, Koyama Y, et al. Characterization of *Orientia tsutsugamushi* isolated in Taiwan by immunofluorescence and restriction fragment length polymorphism analyses. *FEMS Microbiol Lett* 1997; 150(2):225–31.

44. Saah AJ. *Rickettsia tsutsugamushi* (scrub typhus). In: Mandel GL, Bennett JE, Dolin R (eds), *Principles and Practice of Infectious Diseases*, 4th Ed. New York: Churchill Livingstone, 1995. Pp 1740–1.

45. Berman SJ, Kundin WD. Scrub typhus in South Vietnam, a study of 87 cases. *Ann Intern Med* 1973;79:26–30.

46. Olson JG, Bourgeois AL. Changing risk of scrub typhus in relation to socio-economic development in the Pescadores Islands of Taiwan. *Am J Epidemiol* 1979;109:236–43.

47. Brown GW, Robinson DM, Huxsoll DL, et al. Scrub typhus: a common cause of illness in indigenous populations. *Trans R Soc Trop Med Hyg* 1976;70:444–8.

48. McNee JW, Renshaw A. "Trench fever": a relapsing fever occurring with the British troops in France. *Br Med J* 1916;1:225–34.

49. Tappero JW, Moele-Boetani J, Koehler J, et al. The epidemiology of bacterial angiomatosis and bacillary peliosis. *JAMA* 1993;269(6):770–5.

50. Daly JS. *Bartonella* species. In: Gorbach SL, Bartlett JG, Blacklow NR (eds), *Infectious Diseases.* Philadelphia: W.B. Saunders, 1998. Pp 1961–7.

51. Brenner DJ, O'Connor SP, Winkler HH, et al. Proposals to unify the genera *Bartonella* and *Rochalimea*, with descriptions of *Bartonella quintana* comb. nov., *Bartonella vinsonii* comb. nov., *Bartonella henselae* comb. nov., and *Bartonella elizabethae* comb. nov., and to remove the family Bartonellaceae from the order Rickettsiales. *Int J Syst Bacteriol* 1993;43:777–86.

52. Slater LN, Welch DF, Hensel D, et al. A newly recognized fastidious gram-negative pathogen as a cause of fever and bacteremia. *N Engl J Med* 1990;323:1587–89.

53. Gregory DW, Schaffner W. Psittacosis. *Sem Respir Med* 1997;12(1):7–11.

54. Anderson DC, Stoesz PA, Kaufmann AF. Psittacosis outbreak in employees of a turkey-processing plant. *Am J Epidemiol* 1978;107(2):140–8.

55. Wittenbrink MM, Mrozek M, Bisping W. Isolation of *Chlamydia psittaci* from a chicken egg: evidence of egg transmission. *Zentralblatt Fur Veterinarmedizin—Reihe B* 1993;40(6):451–2.

56. Williams AF, Beck NF, Williams SP. The production of EAE-free lambs from infected rams using multiple ovulation and embryo transfer. *Vet J* 1998;155(1):79–84.

57. Page LA. Experimental ornithosis in turkeys. *Avian Dis* 1959;3:51–66.

58. Papp JR, Shewen PE. Pregnancy failure following vaginal infection of sheep with *Chlamydia psittaci* prior to breeding. *Infect Immunol* 1996;64(4):1116–25.

59. Centers for Disease Control. *Psittacosis Surveillance, 1975–84.* Atlanta: CDC, June 1984.

60. Janeczek F, Gebermann H. Comparison of the cell culture method and ELISA for detection of *Chlamydia psittaci. Proc Symp Avian Dis, Munich* 1988:296–306.

61. Dorrestein GM, Wiegman LJJM. Inventaris onderzoek naar de uitscheiding van *Chlamydia psittaci* door parkieten in de omgeving van Utrecht door middel van ELISA. *Tijdschr Diergeneeskd* 1989;114:1227–32.

62. Vanrompay D, Butaye P, Van Nerom A, et al. The prevalence of *Chlamydia psittaci* infections in Belgian commercial turkey poults. *Vet Microbiol* 1997; 54(1):85–93.

63. Ryll M, Hinz KH, Neumann U, et al. Pilot study of the occurrence of *Chlamydia psittaci* infections in commercial Turkey flocks in Niedersachsen. *Deutsche Tierarztliche Wochenschrift* 1994;101(4):163–5.

64. Salibnas J, Caro MR, Cuello F. Antibody prevalence and isolation of *Chlamydia psittaci* from pigeons (*Columba livia*). *Avian Dis* 1993;37(2):523–7.

65. Gerbermann H, Korbel R. The occurrence of *Chlamydia psittaci* infections in raptors from wildlife preserves. *Tierartliche Praxis* 1993;21(3):217–24.

66. Psittacosis (editorial). *Br Med J* 1972;1:1–2.

67. Compendium of psittacosis (chlamydiosis) control. *MMWR* (suppl) 1997;46(RR-13):1–13.

68. Mair TS, Wills JM. *Chlamydia psittaci* infection in horses: results of a prevalence survey and experimental challenge. *Vet Record* 1992;130(19):417–9.

69. Miyamoto C, Takashima I, Karaiwa H, et al. Seroepidemiological survey of chlamydial infections in light horses from Japan. *J Vet Med Sci* 1993; 55(2):333–5.

70. Huchzermeyer FW, Gerdes GH, Foggin CM, et al. Hepatitis in farm hatchling Nile crocodiles (*Crocodylus niloticus*) due to chlamydial infection. *Tidjskr S Afr Vet Ver* 1994;65(1):20–2.

71. Papp JR, Shewen PE. Pregnancy failure following vaginal infection of sheep with *Chlamydia psittaci* prior to breeding. *Infect Immunol* 1996;64(4):1116–25.

72. Wittenbrink MM, Kirpal G, Thiele D, et al. Detection of *Chlamydia psittaci* in vaginal discharge of cows: a necessary enlargement of bacteriologic diagnosis for the etiologic clarification of fertility disorders in the female cow. *Zentralblatt Fur Veterinarmedizin—Reihe B* 1994;41(7–8):492–503.

73. Liao K, Chain CY, Lu YS, et al. Epizootic of *Chlamydia psittaci* infection in goats in Taiwan. *J Basic Microbiol* 1997;37(5): 327–33.

74. Thoma R, Guscetti F, Schiller I, et al. *Chlamydiae* in porcine abortion. *Vet Pathol* 1997;34(5):467–9.

75. Madic J, Huber D, Lugovic B. Serologic survey for selected viral and rickettsial agents of brown bears (*Ursus arctos*) in Croatia. *J Wildlife Dis* 1993; 29(4):572–6.

76. Gresham AC, Dixon CE, Bevan BJ. Domiciliary outbreak of psittacosis in dogs: potential for zoonotic infection. *Vet Record* 1996;138(25):622–3.

77. Kik MJ, van der Hage MH, Greydanus–van der Putten SW. Chlamydiosis in a fishing cat (*Felis viverrina*). *J Zoo Wildlife Med* 1997;28(2):212–4.

78. Martin JL, Cross GF. Comparison of the omp I gene of *Chlamydia psittaci* between isolates in Victorian koalas and other animal species. *Aust Vet J* 1997; 75(8):579–82.

79. Villemonteiz P, Agius G, Decroz B et al. Pregnancy complicated by severe *Chlamydia psittaci* infection acquired from a goat flock: A case report. *Eur J Obstet Gynecol Reprod Biol* 1990;37:91–4.

80. Barnes MG, Brainerd H. Pneumonitis with alveolar-capillary block in a cattle rancher exposed to epizootic bovine abortion. *N Engl J Med* 1964;271:981–5.

81. Lipman NS, Yan LL, Murphy JC. Probable transmission of *Chlamydia psittaci* from a macaw to a cat. *J Am Vet Med Assoc* 1994;204(9):1479–80.

82. Wreghitt T. Chlamydial infection of the respiratory tract. *Comm Dis Rep* 1993;3(9):R119–24.

83. Palmer SR. A common-source outbreak of ornithosis in veterinary surgeons. *Lancet* 1981;2:798–9.

84. Newman CP, Palmer SR, Kirby FD, et al. A prolonged outbreak of ornithosis in duck processors. *Epidemiol Infect* 1992;108(1):203–10.

85. Huminer D, Pitlik S, Kitayin D. Prevalence of *Chlamydia psittaci* infection among persons who work with birds. *Isr J Med Sci* 1992;28:739–41.

86. Hinton DG, Shipley A, Galvin JW, et al. Chlamydiosis in workers at a duck farm and processing plant. *Aust Vet J* 1993;70(5):174–6.

87. Jantos CA, Wienpahl B, Schiefer HG, et al. Infection with *Chlamydia pneumoniae* in infants and children with acute lower respiratory tract disease. *Pediatr Infect Dis J* 1995;14:117–22.

88. Numazaki K, Chiba S, Umetsu M. Detection of IgM antibodies to *Chlamydia trachomatis*, *Chlamydia pneumoniae*, and *Chlamydia psittaci* from Japanese infants and children with pneumonia. *In Vivo* 1992;6(6):601–4.

89. Thom DH, Wang SP, Grayston JT, et al. *Chlamydia pneumoniae* strain TWAR and angiographically demonstrated coronary artery disease. *Arterio Throm* 1991;11:547–51.

90. Aldous MB, Grayston JT, Wang S-P, et al. Seroepidemiology of *Chlamydia pneumoniae* in Seattle families, 1966–79. *J Infect Dis* 1992;166:646–9.

91. Thom DH, Grayston JT, Campbell LA, et al. Respiratory infection with *Chlamydia pneumoniae* in middle-aged and adult outpatients. *Eur J Clin Microbiol Infect Dis* 1994;13(10):785–92.

92. Cosentini R, Blasi F. New pathogens for respiratory infections. *Curr Opin Pulmon Med* 1996;2(3):174–80.

93. Blasi F, Legnani D, Lombardo VM, et al. *Chlamydia pneumoniae* infections in acute exacerbations of COPD. *Eur Respir J* 1993;6:19–22.

94. Verkooyen NA, van Lent NA, Mousavi Joulandan SA, et al. Diagnosis of *Chlamydia pneumoniae* infection in patients with chronic obstructive pulmonary disease by micro-immunofluorescence and ELISA. *J Med Microbiol* 1997;46:959–64.

95. Maaertens G, Lewis SJ, de Goveia C, et al. Atypical bacteria are common cause of community-acquired pneumonia in hospitalized adults. *S Afr Med J* 1994;84:678–82.

96. Ronsmans C, Bulut A, Yolsal N, et al. Clinical algorithms for the screening of *Chlamydia trachomatis* in Turkish women. *Genitourin Med* 1996;72:182–6.

97. Recommendations for the prevention and management of *Chlamydia trachomatis* infections, 1993. *MMWR* 1993;42:1–39.

98. Dowe G, King SD, Brathwaite AR, et al. Genital *Chlamydia trachomatis* (serotypes D-K) infection in Jamaican commercial street sex workers. *Genitourin Med* 1997;73:362–4.

99. Agacfidan A, Chow JM, Pashazade H, et al. Screening of sex workers in Turkey for *Chlamydia trachomatis*. *Sex Trans Dis* 1997;10:573–5.

100. Worm AM, Lauritzen E, Jensen IP, et al. Markers of sexually transmitted disease in seminal fluid of male clients of female sex workers. *Genitourin Med* 1997;73:284–7.

101. Karam GH, Martin DH, Flotte R, et al. Asymptomatic *Chlamydia trachomatis* infections among sexually active men. *J Infect Dis* 1986;154:900–3.

102. Cates W, Wasserheit JN. Genital chlamydial infections: epidemiology and reproductive sequellae. *Am J Obstet Gynecol* 1991;164:1771–81.

103. Thylefors B. Development of trachoma control programs and the involvement of national resources. *Rev Infect Dis* 1985;7:774–6.

104. Hilbink F, Penrose M, Kovacova E, et al. Q fever is absent from New Zealand. *Int J Epidemiol* 1993; 22:945–9.

105. Baca OG, Paretsky D. Q fever and *Coxiella burnetti:* a model for host-parasite interaction. *Microbiol Rev* 1983;47:127–49.

106. Babudieri B. Q fever: a zoonosis. *Adv Vet Sci Comp Med* 1959;5:82–182.

107. Biberstein EL, Behymer DE, Bushnell R, et al. A survey of Q fever (*Coxiella burnetti*) in California dairy cows. *Am J Vet Res*1974;35:1577–82.

108. Antony SJ, Schaffner W. Q fever pneumonia. *Sem Respir Infect* 1997;12(1):2–6.

109. Spelman DW. Q fever: a study of 111 consecutive cases. *Med J Aust* 1982;1:547–53.

110. Marrie TJ, Van Buren J, Faulkner RS, et al. Seroepidemiology of Q fever in Nova Scotia and Prince Edward Island. *Can J Microbiol* 1984;30:129–34.

111. Marrie TJ, Fraser J. Prevalence of antibodies to *Coxiella burnetti* among veterinarians and slaughterhouse workers in Nova Scotia. *Can Vet J Res* 1985;26: 181–4.

112. Simor AE, Brunton JL, Salit IE, et al. Q fever: hazard form sheep used in research. *Can Med Assoc J* 1984;130:1013–6.

113. Ruppanner R, Brooks D, Morrish D, et al. Q fever hazards from sheep and goats used in research. *Arch Environ Health* 1982;37(2):103–10.

114. Raoult D. Q fever: still a query after all these years (edit). *J Med Microbiol* 1996;44(2):77–8.

115. Palmer SR, Young SE. Q-fever endocarditis in England and Wales. *Lancet* 1982;2:1448–9.

116. Davies TR, Edwards Y, Margan A, et al. Prevalence of Q fever in a rural practice. *J Public Health Med* 1997;19(3):324–7.

117. Klymchuk MD, Kushnir ZH, Kiriiak OP, et al. The characteristics of the spread of *Coxiella burnetii* in the Carpathian region. *Mikrobiolohichnyi Zhurnal* 1997;59(5):46–52.

118. Sawyer LA, Fishbein DB, McDade JE. Q fever: current concepts. *Rev Infect Dis* 1987;9:935–46.

119. Pascual F, Carrascosa M. The epidemiology of Q fever (letter). *Eur Heart J* 1997;18:1190.

120. Brouqui PB, Dupont HT, Drancourt M, et al. Chronic Q fever. *Arch Intern Med* 1993;153(5):642–8.

121. Stein A, Raoult D. Q fever endocarditis. *Eur Heart J* 1995;16(suppl B):19–23.

122. Bozeman FM, Masiello SA, Williams MS, et al. Epidemic typhus rickettsiae isolated from flying squirrels. *Nature* 1975;255:545–7.

123. Kurganova II, Klimchuk ND. Transplacental transmission of the causative agent in experimental rickettsial infection. *Mikrobiolohichnyi Zhurnal* 1996;58(4): 80–5.

124. Perine RL, Chandler BP, Krause DK, et al. A clinico-epidemiological study of epidemic typhus in Africa. *Clin Infect Dis* 1992;14(5):1149–58.

125. Saah AJ. *Rickettsia prowazekii* (Epidemic or louse-born typhus). In: Mandel GL, Bennett JE, Dolin R (eds), *Principles and Practice of Infectious Diseases*, 4th Ed. New York: Churchill Livingstone, 1995. Pp 1735–7.

126. Punda-Polic V, Leko-Brbic J, Radulovic S. Prevalence of antibodies to rickettsiae in the north-western part of Bosnia and Herzegovina. *Eur J Epidemiol* 1995; 11(6):697–9.

127. Raoult D, Roux V, Ndihokubwayo JB, et al. Jail fever (epidemic typhus) outbreak in Burundi. *Emerging Infect Dis* 1997;3(3):357–60.

128. Dumler JS, Walker DH. Murine typhus. In: Mandel GL, Bennett JE, Dolin R (eds), *Principles and Practice of Infectious Diseases*, 4th Ed. New York: Churchill Livingstone, 1995. Pp 1737–9.

129. Dumler JS, Taylor JP, Walker DH. Clinical and laboratory features of murine typhus in South Texas, 1980 through 1987. *JAMA* 1991;266:1365–70.

130. Anstey NM, Tissot Dupont H, Hahn CG, et al. Seroepidemiology of *Rickettsia typhi*, spotted fever group Rickettsiae, and *Coxiella burnetii* infection in pregnant women from urban Tanzania. *Am J Trop Med Hyg* 1997;57(2):187–9.

131. Richards AL, Soeatmadji DW, Widodo MA, et al. Seroepidemiologic evidence for murine and scrub typhus in Malang, Indonesia. *Am J Trop Med Hyg* 1997;57(1):91–5.

132. Meskini M, Beati L, Benslimane A, et al. Seroepidemiology of rickettsial infections in Morocco. *Eur J Epidemiol* 1995;11(6):655–60.

133. Chaniotis B, Psarulaki A, Chaliotis G, et al. Transmission cycle of murine typhus in Greece. *Ann Trop Med Parasitol* 1994;88(6):645–7.

134. Strickman D, Tanksul P, Eamsila C, et al. Prevalence of antibodies to Rickettsiae in the human population of suburban Bangkok. *Am J Trop Med Hyg* 1994; 51(2):149–53.

135. Azad AF, Radulovic S, Higgins JA, et al. Flea-borne rickettsioses: ecologic considerations. *Emerging Infect Dis* 1997;3(3):319–27.

136. deLemos ER, Machado RD, Coura JR. Rocky Mountain spotted fever in an endemic area in Minas Gerais, Brazil. *Memorias do Instituto Oswaldo Cruz* 1994; 89(4):497–501.

137. Walker DH, Raoult D. *Rickettsia rickettsii* and other spotted fever group Rickettsiae (Rocky Mountain spotted fever and other spotted fevers). In: Mandel GL, Bennett JE, Dolin R (eds), *Principles and Practice of Infectious Diseases*, 4th Ed. New York: Churchill Livingstone, 1995. Pp 1721–7.

138. Summary of notifiable diseases, United States, 1995. *MMWR* 1996;44:1

139. Walker DH, Dumler JS. Emerging and reemerging rickettsial diseases (editorial). *N Engl J Med* 1994; 331(24):1651–2.

140. Ghorbani RP, Ghorbani AJ, Jain MK, et al. A case of scrub typhus probably acquired in Africa. *Clin Infect Dis* 1997;25(6):1473–4.

141. Song HJ, Kim KH, Kim SC, et al. Population density of chigger mites, the vector of tsutsugamushi disease in Chollanam-do, Korea. *Korean J Parasitol* 1996; 34(1):27–33.

142. Traub R, Wisseman CL Jr. The ecology of chigger-borne rickettsiosis (scrub typhus). *J Med Entomol* 1974;11:237.

143. Takada N, Khamboonruang C, Yamaguchi T, et al. Scrub typhus and chiggers in northern Thailand. *Southeast Asian J Trop Med Public Health* 1984; 15:402–6.

144. Johnson DE, Crumm JW, Hanchalay S, et al. Seroepidemiological survey of *Rickettsia tsutsugamushi* infection in a rural Thai village. *Trans R Soc Trop Med Hyg* 1982;76:1–3.

145. Strickman D, Tanskul P, Eamsila C, et al. Prevalence of antibodies to rickettsiae in the human population of suburban Bangkok. *Am J Trop Med Hyg* 1994; 1(2):149–53.

146. Eamsila C, Singsawat P, Duangvaraporn A, et al. Antibodies to *Orientia tsutsugamushi* in Thai soldiers. *Am J Trop Med Hyg* 1996;55(5):556–9.

147. Vinson JW, Fuller HS. Studies on trench fever. I. Propagation of rickettsia-like organisms from a patient's blood. *Pathol Microbiol* 1961;24 (suppl): 152–5.

148. Spach DO, Candor AS, Dougherty MJ, et al. *Bartonella (Rochalimaea) quintana* bacteremia in inner-city patients with chronic alcoholism. *N Engl J Med* 1995;332:424–8.

149. Gluckman SJ. Q fever and trench fever. *Clin Dermatol* 1996;14(3):283–7.

150. Maurin M, Raoult D. *Bartonella (Rochalimea) quintana* infections. *Clin Microbiol Rev* 1996; 9(3):273–92.

151. Koehler JE, Glaser CA, Tappero JW. *Rochalimea henselaea* infection: a new zoonosis with the domestic cat as a reservoir. *JAMA* 1994;16:553–4.

152. Zangwill KM, Hamilton DH, Perkins BA, et al. Cat-scratch disease in Connecticut. *N Engl J Med* 1993;329:8–13.

153. Jackson LA, Spach DH, Kippen DA, et al. Seroprevalence to *Bartonella quintana* among patients at a community clinic in downtown Seattle. *J Infect Dis* 1996;173(4):1023–6.

154. Kocianova E, Rehacek J, Lisak V. Transmission of antibodies to *Chlamydia psittaci* and *Coxiella burnetti* through eggs and "crop milk" in pigeons. *Eur J Epidemiol* 1993;9(2):209–12.

155. Bano Aracil M, Gonzalez Moran F, Bertomeu Blanch F, et al. Familial outbreak of pneumonia by psittacosis. *Medicina Clinica* 1992;99(7):258–60.

156. Andersen AA. The serotyping of *Chlamydia psittaci* isolates using serovar-specific monoclonal antibodies with the micro-immunofluoroscence test. *J Clin Microbiol* 1991;29:707–11.

157. Vanrompay D. Avian *Chlamydia psittaci* phyla and their pathogenic significance for turkeys. *Verhandelingen—Koninklijke Academie voor Geneeskunde van Belgie* 1996;58(6):701–9.

158. Vanrompay D, Andersenn AA, Ducatelle R, et al. Serotyping of European isolates of *Chlamydia psittaci* from poultry and other birds. *J Clin Microbiol* 1993;31(1):134–7.

159. Hughes C, Maharg P, Rosario P, et al. Possible nosocomial transmission of psittacosis. *Infect Cont Hosp Epidemiol* 1997;18(3):165–8.

160. Augenbraun MH, Robin MR, Chirwing K, et al. Isolation of *Chlamydia pneumoniae* from lungs of patients infected with the human immunodeficiency virus. *J Clin Microbiol* 1991;29:401–2.

161. Katz BP, Caine VA, Jones RB. Estimation of transmission probabilities for chlamydial infection. In: Bowie WR, Calswell HD, Jones RP, et al. (eds), *Chlamydial Infections*. Cambridge, Engl: Cambridge University Press, 1990. Pp 567–70.

162. Ramstedt K, Forssman L, Giesecke J, et al. Epidemiologic characteristics of two different populations of women with *Chlamydia trachomatis* infection and their male partners. *Sex Transm Dis* 1991;18:205–10.

163. Smith JR, Taylor-Robinson D. Infections due to *Chlamydia trachomatis* in pregnancy and the newborn. *Baillieres Clin Obstet Gynecol* 1993;7(1):237–55.

164. Batteiger BE, Fraiz J, Newhall WJ, et al. Association of recurrent chlamydial infection with gonorrhea. *J Infect Dis* 1989;159:661–9.

165. Blythe MJ, Katz BP, Orr DP, et al. Historical and clinical factors associated with *Chlamydia trachomatis* genitourinary infection in female adolescents. *J Pediatr* 1988;112:1000–4.

166. Mardh PA, Paavonen J, Puolakkainen M. *Chlamydia*. New York: Plenum Press, 1989.

167. Schachter J, Grossman M, Sweet RL, et al. Prospective study of perinatal transmission of *Chlamydia trachomatis*. *JAMA* 1986;255:3374–7.

168. Meyers JD, Hackman RC, Stamm WE. *Chlamydia trachomatis* infection as a cause of pneumonia after human bone marrow transplantation. *Transplantation* 1983;36(2):130–4.

169. Lennette EH, Welsh HH. Q fever in California. Recovery of *Coxiella burnetti* from the air of premises harboring infected goats. *Am J Hyg* 1951;54:44–9.

170. Marrie TJ. Epidemiology of Q fever. In: Marrie TJ (ed), *Q fever: The Disease*. Vol 1. Boca Raton, FL: CRC Press, 1990. Pp 49–70.

171. Marrie TJ, Haldane EV, Faulkner RS, et al. The importance of *C burnetii* as a cause of pneumonia in Nova Scotia. *Can J Public Health* 1985;76:233–6.

172. Q fever outbreak—Switzerland. *MMWR* 1984; 33:355–61.

173. Salmon MM, Howells B, Glencross EJF, et al. Q fever in an urban area. *Lancet* 1982;1:1002–4.

174. Sawyer LA, Fishbein DB, McDade JE. Q fever: current concepts. *Rev Infect Dis* 1987;9:935–46.

175. Kruszewska D, Tylewska-Wierzbanowska SK. *Coxiella burnetii* penetration into the reproductive system of male mice, promoting sexual transmission of infection. *Infect Immunol* 1993;61:1448–95.

176. Raoult D, Stein A. Q fever during pregnancy—a risk for women, fetuses and obstetricians (letter). *N Engl J Med* 1994;330:371.

177. Deutsch DL, Petersen ET. Q fever: transmission form one human being to another. *JAMA* 1950;1943:348–50.

178. Laughlin T, Waag D, Williams J, et al. Q fever: from deer to dog to man (letter). *Lancet* 1991;337:676–7.

179. Marrie TJ, Langille D, Papukna V, et al. Truckin' pneumonia—an outbreak of Q fever in a truck repair plant probably due to aerosols from clothing contaminated by contact with newborn kittens. *Epidemiol Infect* 1989;102:119–27.

180. Mann JS, Douglas JG, Inglis JM, et al. Q fever: person-to-person transmission within a family. *Thorax* 1986;41:974–5.

181. Deutsch DL, Peterson ET. Q fever: transmission from one human being to others. *JAMA* 1950;143:348–50.

182. Marrie TJ, Durant H, Williams JC, et al. Exposure to parturient cats: a risk factor for acquisition of Q fever in maritime Canada. *J Infect Dis* 1988;158:101–8.

183. Sidwell RW, Thorpe BD, Gebhardt LP. Studies of latent Q fever infections. II. Effects of multiple cortisone infections. *Am J Hyg* 1964;79:320–7.

184. Norazah A, Mazlah A, Cheong YM, et al. Laboratory-acquired murine typhus—a case report. *Med J Malaysia* 1995;50(2):177–9.

185. Wilfert CM, McCormack JN, Kleeman K, et al. Epidemiology of Rocky Mountain spotted fever as determined by active surveillance. *J Infect Dis* 1984; 150:469–79.

186. Kitahama S, Suzuki J, Kawakami Y. A case of tsutsugamushi disease infected by mountain climbing in the Republic of Korea. *Kansenshogaku Zasshi (J Jap Assoc Infect Dis)* 1996;70(5):516–9.

187. Suntharassaj T, Janjindamai W, Krisanapan S. Pregnancy with scrub typhus and verical transmission: a case report. *J Obstet Gynecol Res* 1997;23(1):75–8.

188. Jee HG, Chung MH, Lee SG, et al. Transmission of scrub typhus by needlestick from a patient receiving perfloxacin. *Scand J Infect Dis* 1996;28(4):411–2.

189. Kawamura R, Kasahara S, Toyama T, et al. On the prevention of tsutsugamushi disease (2nd report). Results of preventive inoculations for people in the endemic regions and laboratory tests with the Pescadores strain. *Tokyo Iji Shinshi* 1938;3115: 3323–6.

190. Filstein MR, Ley AB, Vernon MS. Epidemic of psittacosis in a college of veterinary medicine. *J Am Vet Med Assoc* 1981;179(6):569–72.

191. Durfee PT, Pullen MM, Currier RW, et al. Human psittacosis associated with commercial processing of turkeys. *J Am Vet Assoc* 1975;167(9):804–8.

192. Esposito AL. Pulmonary infections acquired in the workplace. *Clin Chest Med* 1992;13(2):355–65.

193. Buchanan TM, Hendricks SL, Patton CM, et al. Brucellosis in the United States, 1960–72: an abattoir-associated disease. *Medicine* 1974;53(6):427–39.

194. Sigel MM, McNair Scott TF, Henle W. Q fever in a wool and hair processing plant. *Am J Public Health* 1950;40:524–32.

195. Hall CJ, Richmond SJ, Caul EO, et al. Laboratory outbreak of Q fever acquired from sheep. *Lancet* 1982;1:1004–6.

196. Meiklejohn G, Reimer LG, Graves PS, et al. Cryptic epidemic of Q fever in a medical school. *J Infect Dis* 1981;144(2);107–13.

197. Dupuis G, Petite J, Peter O, et al. An important outbreak of human Q fever in a Swiss Alpine valley. *Int J Epidemiol* 1987;16:282–7.

198. Vol. II, Feb 24, 1977. Unclassified document; *U.S. Army Activity on the U.S. Biological Warfare Programs.* L–3,4,5,6.

199. Franz DR, Jahrling PB, Friedlander AM, et al. Clinical recognition and management of patients exposed to biological warfare agents. *JAMA* 1997;278(5):399–411.

200. Sanchez JL, Candler WH, Fishbein DB, et al. A cluster of tick-borne infections: association with military training and asymptomatic infections due to *Rickettsia rickettsii*. *Trans R Soc Trop Med Hyg* 1992;86: 321–5.

201. McDonald JC, MacLean JD, McDade JE. Imported rickettsial disease: clinical and epidemiologic features. *Am J Med* 1988;85:799–805.

202. Noah DL, Kramer CM, Verbsky MP, et al. Survey of veterinary professionals and other veterinary conference attendees for antibodies to *Bartonella henselaea* and *B quintana*. *J Am Vet Assoc* 1997;210(3):342–4.

203. Compendium of chlamydiosis (psittacosis) control. *J Am Vet Med Assoc* 1994;203:1673–80.

204. U.S. Dept of Agiculture, Animal and Plant Health Inspection Service. *Importation of Certain Animals, Birds, and Poultry and Certain Animal, Bird and Poultry Products: Requirements for Means of Conveyance and Shipping Containers.* CFR Title 9, Part 92. 101–7, Jan 1, 1997.

205. Hedberg K. An outbreak of psittacosis in Minnesota turkey industry workers: implications for modes of transmission and control. *Am J Epidemiol* 1989; 130:569–77.

206. 1998 guidelines for treatment of sexually transmitted diseases. *MMWR* 1998;47(RR-1):1–116.

207. Bise G, Coninx R. Epidemic typhus in a prison in Burundi. *Trans R Soc Trop Med Hyg* 1997;91(2): 133–4.

208. Pike RM. Past and present hazards of working with infectious agents. *Arch Path Lab Med* 1978;102: 333–6.

209. Mehr ZA, Rutledge LC, Echano NM, et al. U.S. Army soldiers' perceptions of arthropod pests and their effects on military missions. *Milit Med* 1997;162(12): 804–7.

210. Ho TM, Fauziah MK, Saleh I. Laboratory evaluation of five pesticides for control of *Leptobromidium fletcheri* (Acari: Trombiculidae). *Southeast J Trop Med Public Health* 1992;23(1):125–7.

211. Smadel JE, Traub R, Frick L, et al. Chloramphenicol (chloromycetin) in the chemoprophylaxis of scrub typhus (tsutsugamushi disease). III. Suppression of overt disease by prophylactic regimens of four-week duration. *Am J Hyg* 1950;51:216–28.

212. Twartz JC, Shirai A, Selvaraju G, et al. Doxycycline prophylaxis for human scrub typhus. *J Infect Dis* 1982;146:811–8.

213. deGraaf R, Vanwesenbeeck I, van Zessen G, et al. The effectiveness of condom use in heterosexual prostitution in the Netherlands. *AIDS* 1993;7:265–9.

214. Buendia AJ, Salinas J, Sanchez J, et al. Localization by electron microscopy of antigens of *Chlamydia psittaci* suitable for diagnosis or vaccine development. *FEMS Microbiol Lett* 1997;150(1):113–9.

215. Chalmers WS, Simpson J, Lee SJ, et al. Use of a live chlamydial vaccine to prevent ovine enzootic abortion. *Vet Record* 1997;141(3):63–7.

216. Sturgess CP, Gruffydd-Jones TJ, Harbour DA, et al. Studies on the safety of *Chlamydia psittaci* vaccination in cats. *Vet Record* 1995;137(26):668–9.

217. Hammerschlag MR, Cummings C, Roblin PM, et al. Efficacy of neonatal ocular prophylaxis for the prevention of chlamydial and gonococcal conjunctivitis. *N Engl J Med* 1989;320:769–72.

218. Acklund JR, Worswick DA, Marmion BP. Vaccine prophylaxis of Q fever. *Med J Aust* 1994;160:704–8.

219. Marmion BP, Ormsbee RA, Krykor M. Vaccine prophylaxis of abattoir-associated Q fever. *Epidemiol Infect* 1990;104:275–87.

220. Waag DM, England MJ, Pitt ML. Comparative efficacy of a *Coxiella burnetii* chloroform: methanol residue (CMR) vaccine and a licensed cellular vaccine (Q-Vax) in rodents challenged by aerosol. *Vaccine* 1997;15(16):1779–83.

221. Typhus vaccine. *MMWR* 1978;27:189.

222. Dumler JS, Wisseman CL Jr, Fiset P, et al. Cell-mediated immune responses of adults to vaccination, challenge with *Rickettsia rickettsii*, or both. *Am J Trop Med Hyg* 1992;46(2):105–15.

223. Matthewman L, Kelly P, Hayter D, et al. Domestic cats as indicators of the presence of spotted fever and typhus group Rickettsiae. *Eur J Epidemiol* 1997;13(1): 109–11.

224. Tselentis Y, Psaroulaki A, Maniatis J, et al. Genotypic identification of murine typhus *Rickettsia* in rats and their fleas in an endemic area of Greece by the polymerase chain reaction and restriction fragment length polymorphism. *Am J Trop Med Hyg* 1996;54(4): 413–7.

225. Gage KL, Gilmore RD, Karstens RH, et al. Detection of *Rickettsia rickettsii* in saliva, hemolymph and triturated tissues of infected *Dermacentor andersoni* ticks by polymerase chain reaction. *Mol Cell Probes* 1992;6(4):333–41.

226. Harrison GJ. A practitioner's view of the problem of avian chlamydiosis. *J Am Vet Assoc* 1989;195:1525–8.

227. Wages DP. Diseases of pigeons. *Vet Clin North Am* 1987;37:1089–107.

228. Vanrompay D, Ducatelle R, Haesebrouck F, et al. Primary pathogenicity of a European isolate of *Chlamydia psittaci* from turkey poults. *Vet Microbiol* 1993;38(1–2):103–13.

229. Grimes JE, Wyrick PB. Chlamydiosis (ornithosis). In: Calnek BW (ed), *Diseases of Poulty.* 9th Ed. Iowa State University Press, 1991. Pp 311–25.

230. Schaffner W, Drutz DJ, Duncan GW, et al. The clinical spectrum of endemic psittacosis. *Arch Intern Med* 1967;119:433–43.

231. Monsieur I, Maysman M, Vincken W, et al. Severe community-acquired pneumonia caused by atypical organisms. *Acta Clinica Belgia* 1997;52(2):112–5.

232. Byrom NP, Walls J, Mair HJ. Fulminant psittacosis. *Lancet* 1979;1:353–6.
233. Diaz F, Collazos J. Myopericarditis due to *Chlamydia psittaci*: the role of autoimmunity. *Scand J Infect Dis* 1997;29(1):93–4.
234. Lamaury J, Sotto A, Le Quellec A, et al. *Chlamydia psittaci* as a cause of lethal bacterial endocarditis. *Clin Infect Dis* 1993;17(4):821–2.
235. Duprat F, Akoum N, Le Hoang P. Hemorrhagic macular choroidopathy in young adults. *J Francais d' Opthal* 1995;18(3):226–9.
236. Hain C, Demisch S, Langer B. Organically-induced delusional syndrome in psittacosis. *Psychiatrische Praxis* 1997;24(4):198–9.
237. Brewis C, McFerran DJ. "Farmer's ear": sudden sensorineural hearing loss due to *Chlamydia psittaci* infection. *J Laryngol Otol* 1997;111(9):855–7.
238. Prevett M, Harding AE. Intracranial hypertension following psittacosis (letter). *J Neurol Neurosurg Psychol* 1993;56(4):425–6.
239. Branley P, Speed B. Acute interstitial nephritis due to *Chlamydia psittaci* (letter). *Aust NZ J Med* 1995;25 (4):365.
240. Jeffrey RF, More IA, Carington D, et al. Acute glomerulonephritis following infection with *Chlamydia psittaci*. *Am J Kidney Dis* 1992;20(1):94–6.
241. Mason AB, Jenkins P. Acute renal failure in fulminant psittacosis. *Respir Med* 1994;88(3):239–40.
242. Crook T, Bannister B. Acute transverse myelitis associated with *Chlamydia psittaci* infection. *J Infection* 1996;32(2):151–2.
243. Newton P, Lalvani A, Conlon CP. Psittacosis associated with bilateral 4th cranial nerve palsies. *J Infection* 1996;32(1):63–5.
244. Verweij P, Meis JF, Eijk R, et al. Severe human psittacosis requiring artificial ventilation: case report and review. *Clin Infect Dis* 1995;20(2):440–2.
245. Centers for Disease Control. *Psittacosis surveillance. Annual summary 1975–84.* Atlanta: CDC, June 1987.
246. Hyde SR, Benirschke K. Gestational psittacosis: case report and literature review. *Modern Pathology* 1997;10(6):602–7.
247. Jorgensen DM. Gestational psittacosis in a Montana sheep rancher. *Emerging Infect Dis* 1997;3(2):191–4.
248. Yamato H, Segawa K, Tsuda T, et al. A case of psittacosis with migratory infiltrates. *Japan J Thorac Dis* 1992;30(1):100–5.
249. Taniguchi H, Mukae N, Ihibashi H, et al. A case of fulminant psittacosis necessitating mechanical ventilation diagnosed by chlamydial isolation from BALF. *J Japan Assoc Infect Dis* 1995;69(12):1396–401.
250. Miyashita Y, Nakamori Y. A family outbreak of *Chlamydia psittaci* infection. *J Japan Assoc Infect Dis* 1996;70(4):377–81.
251. Hammerschlag MR, Chirgwin K, Roblin PM. Persistent infection with *Chlamydia pneumoniae* following acute respiratory illness. *Clin Infect Dis* 1992; 14(1):178–82.
252. Ekman MR, Grayston JT, Visakorpi R. An epidemic of infections due to *Chlamydia pneumoniae* in military conscripts. *Clin Infect Dis* 1993;17:420–5.
253. Thom D, Grayston JT, Campbell LA, et al. Respiratory infection with *Chlamydia pneumoniae* in middle-aged and older adult patients. *Eur J Clin Microbiol Infect Dis* 1994;13:785–92.
254. Hahn DL, Dodge RW, Galugjatnikov R. Association of *Chlamydia pneumoniae* (strain TWAR) infection with wheezing, asthmatic bronchitis, and adult-onset asthma. *JAMA* 1991;266:225–30.
255. Emre U, Roblin PM, Gelling M, et al. The association of *Chlamydia pneumoniae* infection and reactive airways disease in children. *Arch Pediatr Adoles Med* 1994;148(7):341–2.
256. Hahn DL, Bukstein D, Luskin A, et al. Evidence for *Chlamydia pneumoniae* infection in steroid-dependent asthma. *Ann Allergy Asthma Immunol* 1998;80(1): 45–9.
257. Korman TM, Turnidge JD, Grayson ML. Neurological complications of chlamydial infections: case report and review. *Clin Infect Dis* 1997;25:847–51.
258. Machtey I. *Chlamydia pneumoniae* antibodies in myalgia of unknown cause (including fibromyalgia) (letter). *Br J Rheumatol* 1996;36(10):1189–90.
259. Moling O, Pegoretti S, Rielli M, et al. *Chlamydia pneumoniae*-reactive arthritis and persistent infection. *Br J Rheumatol* 1996;35(11):1189–90.
260. Naidu BR, Ngeow YF, Kannan P, et al. Evidence of *Chlamydia pneumoniae* infection obtained by the polymerase chain reaction in patients with acute myocardial infarction and coronary heart disease. *J Infect* 1997;35:199–203.
261. Shor A, Kuo C-C, Patton DL. Detection of *Chlamydia pneumoniae* in coronary artery fatty streaks and atheromatous plaques. *S Afr Med J* 1992;82:158–61.
262. Mazzoli S, Tofani N, Fantini A. *Chlamydia pneumoniae* antibody response in patients with acute myocardial infarction and their follow-up. *Am Heart J* 1998;135:15–20.
263. Nystrom-Rosander C, Thelin S, Hjelm E, et al. High incidence of *Chlamydia pneumoniae* in sclerotic heart valves of patients undergoing aortic valve replacement. *Scand J Infect Dis* 1997;29(4):361–5.
264. Cook PJ, Honeybourne D, Lip GY, et al. *Chlamydia pneumoniae* antibody titers are significantly associated with acute stroke and transient cerebral ischemia: the West Birmingham Stroke Project. *Stroke* 1998; 29(2):404–10.
265. Cates W, Wasserheit JN. Genital chlamydial infections: epidemiology and reproductive sequellae. *Am J Obstet Gynecol* 1991;164:1771–81.
266. Brunham RC, Paavonen J, Stevens CE, et al. Mucopurulent cervicitis: the ignored counterpart in women of urethritis in men. *N Eng J Med* 1984;311:1–6.

267. Westrom L, Svensson L, Wolner-Hanssen P, et al. Chlamydial and gonococcal infections in a defined population of women. *Scand J Infect Dis* 1982; 32(suppl):157–62.

268. Paavonen J. Genital *Chlamydia trachomatis* infections in the female. *J Infect Dis* 1992;25(suppl 1):39–45.

269. Berger RE, Alexander ER, Harnisch JP, et al. Etiology, manifestations and therapy of acute epididymitis: prospective study of 50 cases. *J Urol* 1979;121: 750–4.

270. Quinn TC, Goodell SE, Mkrtichian E, et al. *Chlamydia trachomatis* proctitis. *N Engl J Med* 1981; 305:195–200.

271. Keat A. Extra-genital *Chlamydia trachomatis* infection as sexually-acquired reactive arthritis. *J Infect* 1992;25(suppl 1):47–9.

272. Stenberg K, Mardh P-A. Genital infection with *Chlamydia trachomatis* in patients with chlamydial conjunctivitis: unexplained results. *Sex Transm Dis* 1991;18:1–4.

273. Schacter J, Grossman M, Sweet RL, et al. Prospective study of perinatal transmission of *Chlamydia trachomatis. JAMA* 1986;255:3374–7.

274. Ito JI, Comess KA, Alexander ER, et al. Pneumonia due to *Chlamydia trachomatis* in an immunocompromised adult. *N Engl J Med* 1982;307:95–8.

275. Goldman JM, McIntosh CS, Calver GP, et al. Meningoencephalitis associated with *Chlamydia trachomatis* infection. *Br Med J* 1983;286:517–8.

276. Helmick CG, Bernard KW, D'Angelo LJ. Rocky Mountain spotted fever: clinical, laboratory, and epidemiologic features of 262 cases. *J Infect Dis* 1984;150:480–6.

277. Tissot Dupont H, Raoult D, Brouqui P, et al. Epidemiologic features and clinical presentations of acute Q fever in hospitalized patients. *Am J Med* 1992; 93:427–34.

278. Tiggert WD, Benenson AS. Studies of Q fever in man. *Trans Assoc Am Physicians* 1956;69:98–104.

279. Dupont HT, Raoult D, Broqui P. Epidemiological features and clinical presentations of acute Q fever in hospitalized patients: 323 French patients. *Am J Med* 1992;93:427–34.

280. Feinstein M, Yesner R, Marks JL. Epidemic of Q fever among troops returning from Italy in the spring of 1945: clinical aspects of the epidemic at Fort Patrick Henry, Virginia. *Am J Hyg* 1946;44:72–87.

281. Sobradillo V, Ansola P, Baranda F, Corral C. Q fever pneumonia: a review of 164 community-acquired cases in the Basque country. *Eur Respir J* 1989;2:263–6.

282. Ruiz-Moreno JM. Choroidal neovascularization in the course of Q fever. *Retina, J Ret Vitr Dis* 1997;17(6): 553–5.

283. Carrascosa M, Pascual F, Borobia MV, et al. Rhabdomyolysis associated with acute Q fever. *Clin Infect Dis* 1997;25:1243–4.

284. Marrie TJ. Q fever pneumonia. *Semin Respir Infect* 1989;4(1):47–55.

285. Siegman-Igra Y, Kaufman O, Keysary A, et al. Q fever endocarditis in Israel and a worldwide review. *Scand J Infect Dis* 1997;29:41–9.

286. Tunkel AR, Kaye D. Endocarditis with negative blood cultures (letter). *N Engl J Med* 1992.326(18): 1215–6.

287. Shiga K, Ogawa M, Ono T, et al. Analysis of clinical severity of tsutsugamushi disease according to the serotype of pathogenic rickettsia. *Kansenshogaku Zasshi—J Japan Assoc Infect Dis* 1997;71(4):299–306.

288. Smadel JE, Traub R, Ley HL, et al. Chloramphenicol (chloromycetin) in the chemoprophylaxis of scrub typhus (tsutsugamushi disease). II. Results with volunteers exposed in hyperendemic areas of scrub typhus. *Am J Hyg* 1949;50:75–91.

289. Marschang A, Nothdurft HD, Kumlien S, von Sonnenburg F. Imported rickettsioses in German travellers. *Infection* 1995;23(2):94–7.

290. Pai H, Sohn S, Seong Y, et al. Central nervous system involvement in patients with scrub typhus. *Clin Infect Dis* 1997;24(3):436–40.

291. Kato T, Watanabe K, Katori M, et al. Conjunctival injection, episcleral vessel dilation, and subconjunctival hemorrhage in patients with new tsutsugamushi disease. *Japan J Opthal* 1997;41(3):196–9.

292. Chien RN, Liu NJ, Lin PY, et al. Granulomatous hepatitis associated with scrub typhus. *J Gastro Hepat* 1995;10(4):484–7.

293. Yang CH, Young TG, Peng MY, et al. Unusual presentation of acute abdomen in scrub typhus: a report of two cases. *Chin Med J* 1995;55(5):401–4.

294. Chan CH, Lai F, Daly B, et al. Scrub typhus pneumonitis with delayed resolution. *J Trop Med Hyg* 1995;98(2):114–6.

295. Fang CT, Ferng WF, Hwang JJ, et al. Life-threatening scrub typhus with meningoencephalitis and acute respiratory distress syndrome. *J Formosan Med Assoc* 1997;96(5):390.

296. Saah AJ. *Rickettsia tsutsugamushi* (scrub typhus). In: Mandel GL, Bennett JE, Dolin R (eds), *Principles and Practice of Infectious Diseases*, 4th Ed. New York: Churchill Livingstone, 1995. Pp 1740–1.

297. Liu WT. Trench fever: a resume of literature and a note on some obscure phases of the disease. *Chin Med J* 1984;97:179–90.

298. Relman DA. Has trench fever returned? *N Engl J Med* 1995;332(7):463–4.

299. Slater LN, Welch DF. *Rochalimaea* species (recently renamed *Bartonella*). In: Mandel GL, Bennett JE, Dolin R (eds), *Principles and Practice of Infectious Diseases*, 4th Ed. New York: Churchill Livingstone, 1995. Pp 1741–7.

300. Drancourt M, Mainardi JL, Brouqui P, et al. *Bartonella (Rochalimaea) quintana* endocarditis in three homeless men. *N Engl J Med* 1995;332:419–23.

301. Bafna S, Lee AG. Bilateral optic disc edema and multifocal retinal lesions without loss of vision in cat-scratch disease (letter). *Arch Ophthal* 1996;114(8): 1016–7.

302. Cunningham ET Jr, McDonald HR, Schatz H, et al. Inflammatory mass of the optic nerve head associated with systemic *Bartonella henselaea* infection. *Arch Ophthal* 1997;115(12):1596–7.

303. Peter O, Dupuis G, Burgdorfer W, et al. Evaluation of the complement fixation and indirect immunofluorescence tests in the early diagnosis of primary Q fever. *Eur J Clin Microbiol* 1985;4:394–6.

304. Leo A, Enders G, Roelcke D. Increase of post-infection cold agglutinins after infection with *Mycoplasma pneumoniae*, varicella-zoster and rubella virus. *Beitrage Zur Infusionstherapie und Transfusionsmedizin* 1994;32:197–9.

305. Rastawicki W, Jagielski M. Enzyme-linked immunosorbent assay, complement fixation test and immuno-electroprecipitation test in the diagnosis of *Mycoplasma pneumoniae* infections—comparative analysis. *Zentralblattt fur Bakteriologie* 1996; 283(4):477–84.

306. Uldum SJ, Jensen JS, Sondergard-Andersen J, et al. Enzyme immunoassay for detection of immunoglobulin M (IgM) and IgG antibodies to *Mycoplasma pneumoniae*. *J Clin Microbiol* 1992;30:1198.

307. Kashuba AD, Ballow CH. Legionella urinary antigen testing: potential impact on diagnosis and antibiotic therapy. *Diag Microbiol Infect Dis* 1996;24(3):129–39.

308. Kazandjian D, Chiew R, Gilbert GL. Rapid diagnosis of *Legionella pneumophila* serogroup 1 infection with the Binax enzyme immunoassay urinary antigen test. *J Clin Microbiol* 1997;35(4):954–6.

309. Chirgwin K, Roblin PM, Gelling M, et al. Infection with *Chlamydia pneumonia* in Brooklyn. *J Infect Dis* 1991;163:757–61.

310. Cox SK, Everett ED. Tularemia. An analysis of 25 cases. *Missouri Med* 1981;78:70–4.

311. Gill V, Cunha BA. Tularemia pneumonia. *Semin Respir Infect* 1997;12(1):61–7.

312. Snyder MJ. Immune responses to *Francisella tularensis*. In: Rose NR, Friedman H, Fahey JL (eds), *Manual of Clinical Laboratory Immunology*. Washington, DC: American Society of Microbiology, 1986. Pp 377–8.

313. George RB, Ziskind MM, Rasch JR, et al. Mycoplasma and adenovirus pneumonias: comparison with other atypical pneumonias in a military population. *Ann Intern Med* 1966;65:931–42.

314. Stamm WE, Koutsky LA, Benedetti JK, et al. *Chlamydia trachomatis* urethral infections in men. Prevalence, risk factors, and clinical manifestations. *Ann Intern Med* 1984;100:47–51.

315. Bowie WR, Wang SP, Alexander ER, et al. Etiology of nongonococcal urethritis. Evidence for *Chlamydia trachomatis* and *Ureaplasma urealyticum*. *J Clin Invest* 1977;59:735–42.

316. Krieger JN, Verdon M, Siegel N, et al. Risk assessment and laboratory diagnosis of trichomoniasis in men. *J Infect Dis* 1992;166:1362–6.

317. Q fever among slaughterhouse workers—California. *MMWR* 1986;35(14):223–4.

318. Sevic S. Serologic diagnosis of acute infectious mononucleosis. *Medicin Pregled* 1997;50(9–10):403–8.

319. Bise G, Coninx R. Epidemic typhus in a prison in Burundi. *Trans R Soc Trop Med Hyg* 1997; 1(2):133–4.

320. Kostman JR. Laboratory diagnosis of rickettsial diseases. *Clin Dermatol* 1996;14(3):301–6.

321. Gilman RH, Terminel M, Levine MM, et al. Relative efficacy of blood, urine, rectal swab, bone-marrow and rose-spot cultures for recovery of *Salmonella typhi* in typhoid fever. *Lancet* 1975;1:1211–3.

322. Wicks ACB, Cruickshank JG, Musewe N. Observations of the diagnosis of typhoid fever in an endemic area. *S Afr Med J* 1974;48:1368–70.

323. Applebaum GD, Mathisen G. Spinal brucellosis in a southern California resident. *West J Med* 1997; 166(1):61–5.

324. Gotuzzo E, Carrillo C, Guerra J, et al. An evaluation of diagnostic methods for brucellosis: the value of bone marrow cultures. *J Infect Dis* 1986;153:122–5.

325. Young EJ. Serologic diagnosis of human brucellosis: analysis of 214 cases by agglutination tests and review of the literature. *Rev Infect Dis* 1991;13:359–72.

326. Saltoglu N, Aksu HZ, Tasova Y, et al. Leptospirosis: twelve Turkish patients with the Weil syndrome. *Acta Medica Okayama* 1997;51(6):339–42.

327. Vinetz JM, Glass GE, Flexner CE, et al. Sporadic urban leptospirosis. *Ann Intern Med* 1996;125(10): 794–8.

328. Katz AR, Sasaki DM, Mumm AH, et al. Leptospirosis on Oahu: an outbreak among military personnel associated with recreational exposure. *Milit Med* 1997; 162(2):101–4.

329. Petchclai B, Hiranras S, Potha U. Gold immunoblot analysis of IgM-specific antibody in the diagnosis of human leptospirosis. *Am J Trop Med Hyg* 1991; 45:672–5.

330. Gussenhoven GC, van der Hoorn MA, Goris MG, et al. LEPTO dipstick, a dipstick assay for detection of *Leptospira*-specific immunoglobulin M antibodies in human sera. *J Clin Microbiol* 1997;35(1):92–7.

331. Wallace GD. The role of the cat in the natural history of *Toxoplasma gondii*. *Am J Trop Med Hyg* 1973; 22:313–22.

332. Szenasi Z, Nagy E, Ozsvar Z, et al. Serodiagnosis of toxoplasmosis. *Orvosi Hetilap* 1997;138(51):3241–7.

333. Bretagne S, Costa JM, Kuentz M, et al. Late toxoplasmosis evidenced by PCR in a marrow transplant recipient. *Bone Marrow Trans* 1995;15(5):809–11.

334. Zaki AM. Isolation of a flavivirus related to the tick-borne encephalitis complex from human cases in Saudi Arabia. *Trans R Soc Trop Med Hyg* 1997;91(2):179–81.

335. Case records of the Massachusetts General Hospital. Weekly clinicopathological exercises. Case 2-1997. A 38-year-old man with digital clubbing, low-grade fever, and a murmur. *N Engl J Med* 1997;336(3):205–10.

336. Case definitions for infectious conditions under public health surveillance. *MMWR* 1997;46(No. RR-10):27.

337. Andersen AA. Comparison of pharyngeal, fecal, and cloacal samples for the isolation of *Chlamydia psittaci* from experimentally infected cockatiels and turkeys. *J Vet Diag Invest* 1996;8(4):448–50.

338. Fudge AM, Connely F. Diagnosis of avian chlamydiosis infections using enzyme immunoassay methods. *Proc Assoc Avian Vet* 1990;263–9.

339. Stamp JT, McEwen AG, Watt JAA, et al. Enzootic abortion in ewes. *Vet Rec* 1950;62:251–4.

340. Grimes JE, Daft BE, Grumbles LC, et al. *A Manual of Methods for Laboratory Diagnosis of Avian Chlamydiosis.* Kennet Square, PA: American Association of Avian Pathology, 1987.

341. Hewinson RG, Griffiths PC, Bevan BJ, et al. Detection of *Chlamydia psittaci* from avian field samples using the PCR. *Vet Rec* 1991;199:129–30.

342. Tappe JP, Andersen AA, Cheville NF. Respiratory and pericardial lesions in turkeys infected with avian or mammalian strains of *Chlamydia psittaci. Vet Pathol* 1989;26:386–95.

343. Moore FM, McMillan MC, Margaret L, et al. Comparison of culture, peroxidase-antiperoxidase reaction and serum latex agglutination methods for the diagnosis of chlamydiosis in pet birds. *J Am Vet Med Assoc* 1991;199:71–73.

344. Messmer TO, Skelton SK, Moroney JF, et al. Application of a nested, multiplex PCR to psittacosis outbreaks. *J Clin Microbiol* 1997;35(8):2043–6.

345. Hewinson RG, Griffiths PC, Bevan BJ, et al. Detection of *Chlamydia psittaci* DNA in avian clinical samples by polymerase chain reaction. *Vet Microbiol* 1997;54(2):155–66.

346. Wong KH, Skelton SK, Daugharty H. Utility of complement fixation and microimmunofluorescence assays for detecting serologic responses in patients with clinically diagnosed psittacosis. *J Clin Microbiol* 1994;32(10):2417–21.

347. Oldach DW, Gaydos CA, Mundy LM, et al. Rapid diagnosis of *Chlamydia psittaci* pneumonia. *Clin Infect Dis* 1993;17(3):338–43.

348. Shapiro DS, Kenney SC, Johnson M, et al. Brief report: *Chlamydia psittaci* endocarditis diagnosed by blood culture. *N Engl J Med* 1992;326(18):1192–5.

349. Taniguchi H, Mukae H, Ihiboshi H, et al. A case of fulminant psittacosis necessitating mechanical ventilation diagnosed by chlamydial isolation from BALF. *J Japan Assoc Infect Dis* 1995;69(12):1396–401.

350. Essig A, Zucs P, Susa M, et al. Diagnosis of ornithosis by cell culture and polymerase chain reaction in a patient with chronic pneumonia. *Clin Infect Dis* 1995;21(6):1495–7.

351. Jones RB, Katz BP, Van Der Pol B, et al. Effect of blind passage and multiple sampling on recovery of *Chlamydia trachomatis* from urogenital specimens. *J Clin Microbiol* 1986;24:1029–33.

352. Cook PJ, Honeybourne D. *Chlamydia pneumoniae. J Antimicrob Chemother* 1994;34:859–73.

353. Comandini UV, Maggi P, Santopadre P, et al. *Chlamydia pneumoniae* respiratory infections among patients infected with the human immunodeficiency virus. *Eur J Clin Microbiol Infect Dis* 1997;16(10):720–6.

354. Freidank HM, Vogele H, Eckert K. Evaluation of a new commercial microimmunofluorescence test for detection of antibodies to *Chlamydia pneumoniae, Chlamydia trachomatis,* and *Chlamydia psittaci. Eur J Clin Microbiol Infect Dis* 1997;16(9):685–8.

355. Tong CYW, Sillis M. Detection of *Chlamydia pneumoniae* and *Chlamydia psittaci* in sputum samples by PCR. *J Clin Pathol* 1993;46:313–7.

356. Maass M, Dalhoff K. Comparison of sample preparation methods for detection of *Chlamydia pneumoniae* in bronchoalveolar lavage fluid by PCR. *J Clin Microbiol* 1994;32:2616–9.

357. Raoult D, Marrie T. Q fever. *Clin Infect Dis* 1995;20:489–96.

358. Kostman JR. Laboratory diagnosis of rickettsial diseases. *Clin Dermatol* 1996;14(3):301–6.

359. Uhaa IJ, Fishbein DB, Olson JG, et al. Evaluation of specificity of indirect enzyme-linked immunosorbent assay for the diagnosis of human Q fever. *J Clin Microbiol* 1994;32:1560–5.

360. Devine P, Doyle C, Lampkin G. Combined determination of *Coxiella burnetii*–specific immunoglobulin M (IgM) and IgA improves specificity in the diagnosis of Q fever. *Clin Diag Lab Immunol* 1997;4(3):384–6.

361. Durack DT, Lukes AS, Bright DK. New criteria for diagnosis of infective endocarditis: utilization of specific echocardiographic findings. *Am J Med* 1994;96:200–9.

362. Fournier PE, Casalta JP, Habib G, et al. Modification of the diagnostic criteria proposed by the Duke Endocarditis Service to permit improved diagnosis of Q fever endocarditis. *Am J Med* 1996;100:629–33.

363. Aniskovich LP, Motin VL, Lichoded LJ, et al. Identification of *Rickettsia prowazekii* using the polymerase chain reaction. *Eur J Epidemiol* 1993;9(6):645–9.

364. Walker DH, Feng HM, Ladner S, et al. Immunohistochemical diagnosis of typhus rickettsioses using an anti-lipopolysaccharide monoclonal antibody. *Modern Path* 1997;10(10):1038–42.

365. Walker DH, Parks FM, Betz TB, et al. Histopathology and immunohistologic demonstration of the distribution of *Rickettsia typhi* in fatal murine typhus. *Am J Clin Pathol* 1989;91:720–4.

366. Carl M, Tibbs CW, Dobson ME, et al. Diagnosis of acute typhus infection using the polymerase chain reaction. *J Infect Dis* 1990;161:791–3.

367. Kelly DJ, Chan CT, Paxton H, et al. Comparative evaluation of a commercial enzyme immunossay for the detection of human antibody to *Rickettsia typhi. Clin Diag Lab Immunol* 1995;2(3):356–60.

368. Kao GF, Evancho CD, Ioffe O, et al. Cutaneous histopathology of Rocky Mountain spotted fever. *J Cutan Pathol* 1997;24(10):604–10.

369. Procop GW, Burchette JL Jr, Howell DN, Sexton DJ. Immunoperoxidase and immunofluorescent staining of *Rickettsia rickettsii* in skin biopsies. A comparative study. *Arch Pathol Lab Med* 1997;121(8):894–9.

370. Kaplan JE, Schonberger LB. The sensitivity of various serologic tests in the diagnosis of Rocky Mountain spotted fever. *Am J Trop Med Hyg* 1986;35:840–4.

371. Sexton DJ, Kanj SS, Wilson K, et al. The use of a polymerase chain reaction as a diagnostic test for Rocky Mountain spotted fever. *Am J Trop Med Hyg* 1994;50(1):59–63.

372. Watt G, Chouriyagune C, Ruangweerayud R, et al. Scrub typhus poorly responsive to antibiotics in northern Thailand. *Lancet* 1996;348(9020):86–9.

373. Pradutkanchana J, Silpapojakul K, Paxton H, et al. Comparative evaluation of four serodiagnostic tests for scrub typhus in Thailand. *Trans R Soc Trop Med Hyg* 1997;91(4):425–8.

374. Shieh GJ, Chen HL, Chen HY, et al. Detection of *Rickettsia tsutsugamushi*–specific DNA from the lymphocyte of patients by polymerase chain reaction. *Proc Natl Sci Counc Repub China B, Life Sciences* 1995; 19(1):43–6.

375. Furuya Y, Katayama T, Hara M, et al. The patients without specific antibodies were diagnosed by PCR as tsutsugamushi disease. *J Japan Assoc Infect Dis* 1997;71(5):474–6.

376. Szelc-Kelly CM, Goral S, Perez-Perez GI, et al. Serologic responses to *Bartonella* and *Afipia* antigens in patients with cat scratch disease. *J Pediatr* 1995; 127:23–6.

377. Rodriguez-Barradas MC, Hamill RJ, Houston ED, et al. Genomic fingerprinting of *Bartonella* species by repetitive element PCR for distinguishing species and isolates. *J Clin Microbiol* 1995;33:1089–93.

378. Breathnach AS, Hoare JM, Eykyn SJ. Culture-negative endocarditis: contribution of *Bartonella* infections. *Heart* 1997;77(5):474–6.

379. Goldenberger D, Zbinden R, Perschii I, et al. Detection of *Bartonella (Rochalimaea)henselae/B quintana* by polymerase chain reaction. *Schweizerische Medizinische Wochenschrift. Journal Suisse de Medecine* 1996;126(6):207–13.

380. Flammer K. Treatment of avian chlamydiosis in exotic birds in the United States. *J Am Vet Med Asoc* 1989;195:569–72.

381. McDonald SE, Bayer EV. Psittacosis in pet birds. *Calif Vet* 1981;4:6–17.

382. Lindensruth H. Feldversuch zur Wirksamkeits-und Vertraglichkeitsprufung von Baytril bei importierten Psittaciden im Rahmen der Staatlichen Psittakoseprophylaxe und therapie. *Vet Med Diss, Giessen*, 1992.

383. Harrison GJ. A practitioner's view of the problem of avian chlamydiosis. *J Am Vet Med Assoc* 1989; 195:1525–8.

384. van Berkel M, Dik H, van der Meer JW, et al. Acute respiratory insufficiency from psittacosis. *Br Med J* 1985;290:1503–4.

385. Miyashita N, Niki Y, Kishimoto T, et al. In vitro and in vivo antichlamydial activities of HSR-903, a new fluoroquinolone antibiotic. *Antimicrob Agents Chemother* 1997;41(4):857–9.

386. Roblin PM, Montalban G, Hammerschlag MR. Susceptibilities to clarithromycin and erythromycin of isolates of *Chlamydia pneumoniae* from children with pneumonia. *Antimicrob Agents Chemother* 1994; 38(7): 1588–9.

387. Roblin PM, Kutlin A, Hammerschlag MR. In vitro activity of trovafloxacin against *Chlamydia pneumoniae. Antimicrob Agents Chemother* 1997;41(9): 2033–4.

388. Roblin PM, Hammerschlag MR. Microbiologic efficacy of azithromycin and susceptibilities to azithromycin of isolates of *Chlamydia pneumoniae* from adults and children with community-acquired pneumonia. *Antimicrob Agents Chemother* 1998;42(1):194–6.

389. Nystrom-Rosander C, Hulten K, Gustavsson I, et al. Susceptibility of *Chlamydia pneumoniae* to azithromycin and doxycycline: methodological aspects in the determination of minimal inhibitory and minimal bactericidal concentrations. *Scand J Infect Dis* 1997; 29(5):513–6.

390. Malinveerni R, Kuo C-C, Campbell LA, et al. Effects of two antibiotic regimens on course and persistence of experimental *Chlamydia pneumoniae* TWAR pneumonitis. *Antimicrob Agents Chemother* 1995;39(1): 45–9.

391. Sinisalo J, Mattila K, Nieminen MS, et al. The effect of prolonged doxycycline therapy on *Chlamydia pneumoniae* serological markers, coronary heart disease risk factors and forearm basal nitric oxide production. *J Antimicrob Chemother* 1998;41(1):85–92.

392. Jones RB, Van der Pol B, Johnson RB. Susceptibility of *Chlamydia trachomatis* to trovafloxacin. *J Antimicrob Chemother* 1997;39(suppl B):63–5.

393. Roblin PM, Kutlin A, Sokolovskaya N, et al. In-vitro activity of dirithromycin against *Chlamydia trachomatis. J Antimicrob Chemother* 1997;39(5):647–9.

394. Rice RJ, Bhullar V, Mitchell SH, et al. Susceptibilities of *Chlamydia trachomatis* isolates causing uncomplicated female genital tract infections and pelvic inflammatory disease. *Antimicrob Agents Chemother* 1995; 39(3):760–2.

395. Lefevre JC, Lepargneur JP, Guion D, et al. Tetracycline-resistant *Chlamydia trachomatis* in Toulouse, France. *Pathol Biol* 1997;45(5):376–8.

396. Powell OW, Kennedy KP, McIver M, et al. Tetracycline in the treatment of Q fever. *Aust Ann Med* 1962;11:184–8.

397. Sobradillo V, Zalacain R, Capelastegui A, et al. Antibiotic treatment in pneumonia due to fever. *Thorax* 1992;47:276–8.

398. Maurin M, Benoliel AM, Bongrand P, et al. Phagolysosomal alkalinization and the bactericidal effects of antibiotics: the *Coxiella burnetii* paradigm. *J Infect Dis* 1992;66:1097–102.

399. Lupoglazoff JM, Brouqui P, Magnier S, et al. Q fever tricuspid valve endocarditis. *Arch Dis Child* 1997; 77(5):448–9.

400. Berbari EF, Cockerill FR, Steckelberg JM. Infective endocarditis due to unusual or fastidious organisms. *Mayo Clin Proc* 1997;72:532–42.

401. Perine PL, Krause DW, Awoke A, et al. Single-dose doxycycline treatment of louse-born relapsing fever and epidemic typhus. *Lancet* 1974;2:742–4.

402. Maurin M, Raoult D. In vitro susceptibilities of spotted fever group *Rickettsiae* and *Coxiella burnetii* to clarithromycin. *Antimicrob Agents Chemother* 1993; 37(12):2633–7.

403. Sheehy TW, Hazlett D, Turk RE. Scrub typhus: a comparison of chloramphenicol and doxycycline in its treatment. *Arch Intern Med* 1973;132:77–80.

404. McClain JB, Joshi B, Rice R. Chloramphenicol, gentamicin, and ciprofloxacin against murine scrub typhus. *Antimicrob Agents Chemother* 1998;32:285–6.

405. Brown GW, Saunders JP, Singh S, et al. Single dose doxycycline therapy for scrub typhus. *Trans R Soc Trop Med Hyg* 1978;72:412–6.

406. Song JH, Lee C, Chang WH, et al. Short-course doxycycline treatment versus conventional tetracycline therapy for scrub typhus: a multicenter randomized trial. *Clin Infect Dis* 1995;21(3):506–10.

407. Strickman D, Sheer T, Salata K, et al. In vitro effectiveness of azithromycin against doxycycline-resistant and susceptible strains of *Rickettsia tsutsugamushi*, etiologic agent of scrub typhus. *Antimicrob Agents Chemother* 1995;39(11):2406–10.

13 / Occupational Fungal Respiratory Infections

David R. Trawick

Although human exposure to fungal species is universal, the development and expression of pulmonary disease is contingent on a number of variables. First is the level of exposure. If the spore count is increased, such as during hospital renovations or with contamination of hospital duct systems, nosocomial outbreaks of fungal pneumonias have occurred. In occupational settings involving exposure to moldy hay or during the malt-brewing process, intense exposure of healthy individuals may result in various allergic phenomenon. The second factor is the presence of underlying lung disease or damage to the lung parenchyma that predisposes to colonization with fungus, e.g., *Aspergillus*. Third, the level of immunocompetence in the host influences its response to fungal exposure. Prolonged neutropenia places individuals at risk for opportunistic fungal disease, whereas immune deficiencies involving T cells predispose to progressive infection with endemic fungi. Fourth, the use of antibiotics may alter bacterial ecology, allowing overgrowth of saprophytic fungi and potentiating an invasive state [1]. Finally, a history of atopy can increase vulnerability to allergic phenomenon such as asthma or allergic bronchopulmonary aspergillosis [2].

The spectrum of pulmonary manifestations of fungal lung disease is exemplified by the diseases caused by *Aspergillus*. Common practice has resulted in a division of *Aspergillus* lung disease into saprophytic, hypersensitivity, and invasive categories, but overlap among the categories is recognized. For example, a patient may show evidence of both hypersensitivity and invasive disease.

Occupational fungal lung disease may occur along a similar spectrum of manifestations. In general, one can arbitrarily divide these manifestation between infectious and noninfectious phenomena. Concerning the former, the most important example is fungal pneumonia. Among the latter, allergic bronchopulmonary aspergillosis, hypersensitivity pneumonitis, and asthma account for significant fungus-related pulmonary morbidity. This chapter specifically examines fungal pneumonias and their relation to occupation.

Fungal Pneumonia

Fungal pneumonias are relatively uncommon despite the ubiquitous presence of spores in the environment. Davies has divided fungal pneumonias into two categories, with seven organisms accounting for the majority of infections [3]. The *pathogenic infections* are caused by the endemic mycoses: histoplasmosis, blastomycosis, coccidioidomycosis, and paracoccidioidomycosis. Cryptococcus is also included in this group. The infectious particles of these organisms are not killed by neutrophils. Therefore, any nonimmune host is susceptible to infection unless ultimately controlled by T cells (which is usually the case). Normal hosts usually recover from infection unless overwhelmed by a large number of infectious particles. In the face of T-cell deficiency, however, progressive disease occurs.

The *opportunistic infections* are caused by aspergillosis, mucormycosis, and candidiasis [3]. The spores of the first two are regularly inhaled by humans. All three possess spores that are killed by neutrophils. Therefore, a potent nonimmune barrier prevents infection. Even in the presence of immune deficiency such as acquired immunodeficiency syndrome (AIDS), the risk of invasive disease is small. When phagocyte number is compromised, however, such as in prolonged neutropenia following chemotherapy, or when phagocyte function is impaired, as in chronic granulomatous disease, invasive infections occur quite frequently.

Although candidiasis is included among the opportunistic fungal infections, it differs from the others in that it is not a soil organism but rather part of the endogenous flora that colonize the skin, mucous membranes, and gastrointestinal tract. Transmigration across the bowel and invasion from the skin, rather than inhalation, are the usual means of candidal infection.

This chapter examines the three most common endemic *pathogenic* fungal pneumonias.

HISTOPLASMOSIS

Epidemiology

Histoplasma capsulatum is a dimorphic soil fungus that grows as hyphae in nature. The infective particles are spores of which there are two types: micronidia, which are 2–6 µm in diameter, and the larger, macronidia, which are 6–14 µm [4]. The smaller spores are more numerous and more likely to be deposited in the lungs. The fungus grows throughout the world, but the major river valleys of the central United States exhibit the highest prevalence of histoplasmosis [4]. Soil enriched by bird and bat excrement fosters growth of the organism. Bats may also harbor the fungus in their intestinal tract and spread the disease from their habitat in trees, caves, and attics [5,6].

Pathogenesis

Infection occurs through inhalation of the spores. At human body temperatures, the spores germinate and release yeast forms, which are phagocytized but not killed by the macrophages. The organism multiplies within the macrophages and spreads to draining lymph nodes and throughout the body [3,4]. Generally, within two weeks, specific lymphocyte-mediated cellular immunity develops, enabling the macrophages to kill off or encapsulate the fungus. Positive skin results are seen at this time. Granulomas and necrosis may occur in both the lung and at distant sites. Calcified lesions may be found in the liver and spleen, even after mild infections [3,4].

Clinical Presentation

In the majority of individuals, acute pulmonary histoplasmosis is an asymptomatic, self-limited illness. On the other hand, 0.5% of individuals who have experienced intense exposure may present with flu-like symptoms, including fever, chills, headache, and a nonproductive cough. Usually, these symptoms last from a few days to as long as three weeks and then resolve. In some cases, such as in infants or the elderly, there is inadequate cellular immunity and progressive disseminated disease develops [4].

Diagnosis

The majority of cases of histoplasmosis go undiagnosed. In the appropriate clinical scenario, testing for serum complement fixation titers against the histoplasma yeast antigen may be the best single most effective tool for the diagnosis of acute infections. However, this method has only 70% sensitivity and diagnostically sufficient increases in titers may take up to one month [7]. Ultrasensitive assays for specific histoplasma polysaccharide antigen in the urine are useful for diagnosing progressive disseminated disease, especially in AIDS patients. Patients with chronic cavitary disease usually have positive sputum cultures [3].

Treatment

Treatment is generally required only for acute, life-threatening conditions, prolonged infections, or patients with progressive disseminated disease. Amphotericin B is the drug of choice in acute, life-threatening situations and for progressive disseminated disease. Itraconazole is often effective for chronic cavitary disease [3].

Occupational Hazards

Immunocompetent individuals who have symptomatic infections often experience intense point-source exposure, such as after cleaning a chicken house or an attic. A classic example, which has been studied through the years, involves the case of a farmer and his two sons, ages 5 and 21, all of whom became acutely ill three weeks after cleaning a silo. All manifested bilateral non-segmental areas of consolidation on chest radiographs, the resolution of which took months, and all demonstrated diffuse calcifications on repeat radiographs done years later. The father was the most ill; *H capsulatum* was cultured from both his sputum and bone marrow [8].

BLASTOMYCOSIS

Epidemiology

Blastomyces dermatitidis, such as *H capsulatum*, is a dimorphic soil fungus that exists as a mycelial form in nature but converts to a yeast form in tissue. It, too, is endemic within the great river valleys, but its range, unlike histoplasmosis, extends to the east along the coastal areas of the Carolinas and further to the northwest toward northern Wisconsin, Minnesota, and Canada [3]. Since no accurate skin test exists, however, the endemic area has generally been mapped by case reports. Clinical illness is estimated to occur only one tenth as often as histoplasmosis [3]. *B dermatitidis* is also very difficult to isolate and culture from soil, which has hindered investigations of areas that epidemiologic evidence suggests may be a common source for exposure [9]. In epidemics, isolation of the fungus has been associated with bodies of water, but it is not known whether the water is a primary factor or an explanation for greater exposure from recreational activities [10].

Pathogenesis

Infection begins with inhaling the spores, followed by clearing of the organism by bronchopulmonary phagocytes. After undergoing transition to the yeast phase, the fungus may spread to other organs through the bloodstream. Unlike histoplasmosis, blastomycosis infections may spread to skin and bone at any stage of the infection and with any type of pulmonary involvement [3,9]. As immunity evolves, there is development of granulomas that are distinctive of blastomycosis and generally do not caseate [9]. Although spontaneous resolution of pneumonia may occur, it is possible that the infection reactivates both in pulmonary and extrapulmonary sites, with or without previous therapy [11].

Clinical Presentation

Blastomycosis occurs four to five times more frequently in males than in females. The typical patient is male, age 25–50, who works outdoors or has numerous outdoor activities or recreations. In an epidemic, however, women and children are as likely to be infected. Otherwise, diagnoses in children are rare. Symptoms of infection are relatively nonspecific, including malaise, weight loss, and fever. The acute pneumonia of blastomycosis presents in a fashion similar to bacterial pneumonia: fever, chills, and a productive cough [9]. The natural history of pulmonary blastomycosis ranges from an asymptomatic infiltrate, to acute pneumonia, chronic fibrocavitary pneumonia resembling tuberculosis (TB), or, occasionally, indolent mass-like entities resembling bronchogenic carcinoma [3].

Diagnosis

In contrast to histoplasmosis, blastomycosis produces gross purulent sputum that usually contains the characteristic yeast forms. The organisms can be viewed in 10% potassium-hydroxide-treated preparations of sputum as well as cytology specimens prepared with Papanicolaou's stain [12]. Cultures of sputum and infected tissue also have a high yield, but culture results may not be available for several weeks [3]. Skin testing is neither sensitive nor specific and is generally not readily available clinically [9]. Immuno-diffusion tests, complement fixation methods, and enzyme immunoassays have all undergone evaluation, but none has yet proved to have the diagnostic utility of the antigen testing described by Wheat for *H capsulatum* [13].

Treatment

The first decision the clinician must make is whether to treat the patient immediately with an antifungal agent or observe the individual for a time. Certainly, there have been reports of blastomycosis epidemics in which most patients exhibited self-limited disease [14]. Davies argues for treating the majority of patients presenting with blastomycosis, while Bradsher favors observation and treatment for clinical deterioration and/or progression [3,9]. In either case, if treatment does occur, itraconazole, 400 mg/day for six months, is very effective for mild to moderate cases [15]. Severely ill patients require amphotericin.

Occupational Hazards

In 1998, two cases of pulmonary blastomycosis were reported in immunocompetent males who had worked together on a prairie-dog relocation project in Colorado [16]. One man was age 25, the other 35. Work practices included using a gasoline-powered auger and hand trowels to excavate abandoned prairie dog burrows that were used by many animal species. The workers did not use protective clothing or masks. The ill workers had spent six to seven hours each day digging, creating large amounts of dust, with their faces close to the dirt. Rain was frequent during the project. Only the two ill workers had abnormalities on chest radiographs.

These were the first reported case of blastomycosis acquired in Colorado. Two factors may have contributed to the development of fungal pneumonia in these workers [16]. *B dermatitidis* is more common in soils with high nitrogen and organic content, which may have been fostered by the stored food and fecal matter of animals living in the burrows [17]. Second, the rainfall that occurred during the excavation may have contributed to the reproduction of the fungus [18].

COCCIDIOIDOMYCOSIS

Epidemiology

Coccidioides immitis is a fungus endemic in the lower Sonoran Desert of the southwestern United States. It also inhabits adjacent areas of northern Mexico and desert areas of Central America and South America. The areas of highest concentration are the southern San Joaquin Valley of California and southern Arizona. In young adults moving to these areas for the first time, asymptomatic skin conversion rates are reported to be 2.5–3.5% per year [19]. *C immitis* grows in the mycelial form in the desert soil in a semiarid climate in which the summers are hot and dry, the winters mild, and the rainfall moderate [3]. Spore formation occurs along the hyphae that break from the mycelium and are carried by the wind. Infection occurs by inhalation of the spores (anthroconidia). Outbreaks of coccidioidomycosis have occurred during archeologic digs, construction, and oil exploration in areas where anthroconidia density in the soil is high [20].

Pathogenesis

The inhalation of anthroconidia into the alveoli initiates a predominately neutrophilic inflammatory response. The neutrophils, however, are incapable of killing the spores, which grow into spherules of 30–80 μm in diameter [3]. Each spherule reproduces by progressive cleavage of the cytoplasm, forming endospores (endosporulation). Eventually, the spherule ruptures, releasing endospores into the tissue, with each endospore possessing the potential to become another spherule.

Specific cell-mediated immunity is the main mechanism by which the body resists infection, which generally occurs within two weeks [20]. Therefore, individuals with reduced function or numbers of T cells are at risk for progressive disease [20].

Clinical Presentation

Coccidioidomycosis may present as primary pulmonary infection, progressive pulmonary disease, or disseminated disease [20]. Sixty percent of individuals with the primary pulmonary disease have no symptoms [21]; the remaining 40% have influenza-like symptoms lasting one to three weeks. Approximately 25% of the symptomatic individuals exhibit more severe manifestations, including pleuritic chest pain [20]. Erythema nodosum and erythema multiforme may occur in primary disease but do not portend a better outcome, as previously thought. A symmetric arthritis, predominantly in the ankles but potentially involving several joints, may evolve during the primary infection as an immune complex phenomenon. This *desert rheumatism,* as it is known because of the geographic regions where coccidioidomycosis is most prevalent, is generally self-limited [20].

Chest radiography usually exhibits an alveolar infiltrate or nodular density. The infiltrate often is subpleural and may abut the fissure. Approximately, 5% of patients develop chronic changes such as nodules or thin-walled cavities.

Chronic progressive coccidioidal pneumonia, which resembles tuberculosis, is rare. Although it may evolve from the primary infection, it often occurs subsequent to apparent healing of the primary infection, progressing in an indolent fashion.

Disseminated disease occurs in less than 1% of coccidioidal infections and may involve every organ except the gastrointestinal tract. It may represent progression of a primary infection or reactivation of a quiescent focus [22]. The skin is the most common site of dissemination in which granulomas are observed. The joints and bones are the second most common sites. Meningitis accounts for the majority of deaths from disseminated disease [20].

Diagnosis

A positive skin test will develop in most individuals within two weeks of infection. Unfortunately, this may simply reflect prior infection, especially if the individual lives in an endemic area. Direct examination of sputum smears after 10% KOH treatment or Papanicolaou staining may be diagnostic but is not very sensitive. Histologic examination of infected tissues may demonstrate organisms when special stains are employed. Culture results are more sensitive than direct histopathologic examination, with culture growth usually occurring within the first week. The mycelial growth form is highly infective, and laboratory personnel working with specimens should be forewarned to take appropriate safety measures. Fortunately, serologic diagnostic methods for coccidioidomycosis are more advanced than those for other pathogenic mycoses [23]. A finding of positive IgM titers is consistent with acute infection. Complement-fixing (IgG) antibodies occur later in the course of the disease in most patients [3]. Although testing for antibodies is highly specific when the results are positive, false-negative results may occur early in the course of the disease [23].

Treatment

Treatment is generally not required for mild to moderate primary pulmonary coccidioidomycosis. It should be considered, however, for patients who are at risk for disseminated disease, including immunosuppressed patients, diabetics, and pregnant women [3]. In addition, some ethnic groups (African-Americans and Filipinos) are more predisposed to disseminated disease.

Treatment should always be undertaken in patients with severe primary infections or persistent, progressive disease. In addition, disseminated disease always requires urgent therapy. Fluconazole, 400 mg/day for six to 12 months, should be used in high-risk patients. Shorter courses of fluconazole have been used in low-risk patients, as has itraconazole. Amphotericin may be used in severe primary and disseminated disease [3].

Occupational Hazards

A coccidioidomycosis outbreak from a common-point source, confirmed by soil cultures, occurred during the summer of 1970 among archeology students excavating Indian ruins near Chico, California [24]. The outbreak involved at least 61 of the 103 students and faculty members participating in a five-week summer archeology course sponsored by Queens College of the City University of New York and Chico State College. Most had never been in areas known to be endemic for coccidioidomycosis. The work involved shoveling dry dirt through screens to sift out artifacts. Dust clouds often obscured vision or provoked coughing spells. No precautions were taken, and no masks were used. The conditions were hot and dry, with temperatures often reaching 43°C. The first confirmed illness occurred 13 days after the first exposure to soil. One particularly ill woman presented with fever, shaking chills, headache, malaise, and a generalized maculopapular, pruritic rash. Chest radiography revealed extensive bilateral pneumonia with hilar adenopathy.

This report emphasized dust control to reduce the degree of exposure of archeologic workers. It also served as a basis for providing workers with informed consent regarding the hazards of the work and encouraged skin testing of all workers without previous positive reactions and close observation of individuals more predisposed to serious infections.

Prevention and Control

Since the risk for developing symptomatic fungal pneumonia remains small, few public health measures have been developed. However, measures for protecting workers against histoplasmosis have been reported by the Centers for Disease Control and Prevention (CDC) and are considered applicable to the prevention of blastomycosis and coccidioidomycosis [16,25]. These measures include:

1. Use of a CDC-approved N-95 disposable half-facepiece filtering respirator (or equivalent) and protective clothing and shoe covers by all persons engaged in soil-disturbing activities.
2. Employer-provided instruction of all workers who may possibly be engaged in soil-disturbing activities as to the proper fitting and wearing of recommended face masks.
3. Implementation of respiratory protection programs for employees.
4. Education of workers about clinical signs and symptoms of disease and treatment options.

References

1. Addis E. Pulmonary mycotic disease. In: Haselton P, (ed), *Spencer's Pathology of the Lung*. 5th Ed. New York: McGraw-Hill, 1996. Pp 257–304.
2. Trawick D, White D. When to suspect and treat *Aspergillus* lung disease. *Contemp Intern Med* 1996;8:66–77.
3. Davies S, Sarosi G. Pulmonary mycoses. In: Bone R (ed), *Textbook of Pulmonary and Critical Care Medicine*, 1996.
4. Gurney J, Conces D Jr. Pulmonary histoplasmosis. *Radiology* 1996;199:297–306.
5. Greer D, McMurray D. Pathogenesis of experimental histoplasmosis in the bat, artibeus lituratus. *Am J Trop Med Hyg* 1981;30:653–9.
6. Hasenclever H, Shackette M, Young R, et al. The natural occurrence of *Histoplama capsulatum* in a cave. I. Epidemiologic aspects. *Am J Epidemiol* 1967;86:238–45.
7. Davies S. Serodiagnosis of histoplasmosis. *Semin Respir Infect* 1986;1:9–15.
8. Procknow J. Pulmonary histoplasmosis in a farm family: fifteen years later. *Am Rev Respir Dis* 1967;95:171–88.
9. Bradsher R. Blastomycosis. *Clin Infect Dis* 1992;14:S82–S90.
10. Bradsher R. Water and blastomycosis: don't blame the beaver. *Am Rev Respir Dis* 1987;136:1324–6.
11. Recht L, Philips J, Eckman M, et al. Self-limited blastomycosis: a report of 13 cases. *Am Rev Respir Dis* 1979;120:1109–12.
12. Sutliff W, Cruthirds T. *Blastomyces dermatitidis* in cytological preparations. *Am Rev Respir Dis* 1973;108:149–51.
13. Wheat L, Kohler R, Tewari R. Diagnosis of disseminated histoplasmosis by detection of *Histoplasma capsulatum* antigen in serum and urine specimens. *N Engl J Med* 1986;314:136–42.
14. Klein B, Vergeront J, Davis J. Epidemiologic aspects of blastomycosis, the enigmatic systemic mycoses. *Semin Respir Infect* 1986;1:29–39.
15. Dismukes W, Bradsher R Jr, Cloud G, et al. Itraconazole therapy for blastomycosis and histoplamosis: NAID Mycoses Study Group. *Am J Med* 1992;93:489–97.
16. Blastomycosis acquired occupationally during prairie dog relocation—Colorado, 1998. *MMWR* 1999;48:98–100.
17. Klein B, Vergeront J, Weeks R, et al. Isolation of *Blastomyces dermatitidis* in soil associated with a large outbreak of blastomycosis in Wisconsin. *N Engl J Med* 1986;314:529–34.
18. Davies S, Sarosi G. Epidemiological and clinical features of pulmonary blastomycosis. *Seminars in Respiratory Infections* 1997;12:206–18.
19. Kerrick S, Lundergan L, Galgiani J. Coccidioidomycosis at a university health service. *Am Rev Respir Dis* 1985;131:100–2.
20. Einstein H, Johnson R. Coccidioidomycosis: new aspects of epidemiology and therapy. *Clin Infect Dis* 1993;16:349–56.
21. Drutz D, Catanzaro A. Coccidioidomycosis. Part I. *Am Rev Respir Dis* 1978;117:559–85.
22. Bayer A, Yoshikawa T, Guze L. Chronic progressive coccidioidal pneumonitis. Report of 6 cases with clinical, roentgenographic, serologic, and therapeutic features. *Arch Int Med* 1979;139:536–40.
23. Gagliani J. Coccidioidomycosis: a regional disease of national importance. *Ann Intern Med* 1999;130:293–300.
24. Werner S, Pappagianis D, Heindl I, et al. An epidemic of coccidioidomycosis among archeology students in northern California. *N Engl J Med* 1972;286:507–12.
25. Lenhart S, Schafer M, Mitchell S, et al. *Histoplasmosis: Protecting Workers at Risk.* DHHS (NIOSH) publication no. 97-146. Atlanta: Centers for Disease Control, 1997. Pp 1–23.

14 / Occupational Upper Respiratory Tract Infections

Paul C. Levy

Infections of the upper respiratory tract include a broad variety of illnesses caused by a large number of different viruses and bacteria. Often referred to as the *common cold* by health care professionals as well as by members of society at large, symptoms include varying degrees of nasal stuffiness, rhinorrhea, sore or scratchy throat, cough, and chest congestion. Despite having similar clinical symptoms and signs, a large number of specific agents have been identified as causing this illness (Table 14-1). The majority of these infections are caused by viruses from the rhinovirus, coronavirus, parainfluenza, and respiratory syncytial virus groups [1,2]. Importantly, bacterial respiratory infections, such as those caused by group A beta-hemolytic streptococci, can be indistinguishable on clinical grounds from viral causes of colds. In about one third of patients, no identifiable infectious agent can be identified. Fortunately, the majority of upper respiratory tract infections (URIs) are self-limited and rarely lead to significant morbidity or mortality. Nevertheless, URIs are one of the most common causes for absenteeism and reduced worker productivity. Estimates of the economic costs of the common cold run in the billions of dollars, largely the result of restricted work activity, additional visits to health care providers, and treatment costs.

This chapter reviews the most common causes of URIs and their associated clinical syndromes. It discusses their role in occupation-related illness as well as measures targeted at their prevention, control, and treatment. The spectrum and occupational issues related to influenza virus infection are discussed in Chapter 11.

Epidemiology

Infections of the upper respiratory tract occur in all age groups. In general, children average six to eight colds per year, while the rate for adults is roughly half that observed in children. There is a clear seasonal variation in attack rates throughout the world, with the majority of infections occurring during the months of September through April [2], the colder months in the United States. However, attack rates are similar in warmer regions. It is a common misunderstanding that exposure to cold predisposes to infection. Studies have failed to demonstrate increased rates of infections in otherwise healthy individuals after controlled exposure to cold temperatures. Occupationally acquired URIs have not been well studied. Reports of outbreaks caused by specific agents are largely confined to military recruits and health care facilities [3].

ORGANISMS ASSOCIATED WITH UPPER RESPIRATORY TRACT INFECTIONS

Rhinoviruses

Rhinoviruses are the most common cause of the common cold, accounting for upwards of 40–50% of infections in adults [1,2]. These viruses are composed of single-strand RNA and are members of the Picornaviridae family. There are approximately 100 antigenic serotypes, all of which are capable of causing disease in humans. The prevalence of rhinovirus-neutralizing antibody first appears in childhood and tends to peak in young adults. In older adults, the prevalence

Table 14-1
Infectious Agents Associated with Upper Respiratory Tract Infections

Viruses	Nonviral Pathogens
Rhinovirus	*Mycoplasma pneumoniae*
Coronavirus	Group A beta-hemolytic streptococci
Parainfluenza virus	*Branhamella catarrhalis*
Respiratory syncytial virus	
Influenza virus	
Adenovirus	

declines somewhat, probably as a result of reduced exposure. Although rhinoviruses cause infections of the upper respiratory tract throughout the year, there are usually peaks in the fall and spring in the United States. In the tropics infection tends to occur during the rainy season. The reasons for seasonal and geographic variation in the prevalence of rhinovirus infections are not entirely clear, although changes in living conditions (e.g., indoor crowding) and conditions of higher humidity may play a role [2].

It appears close contact is required for rhinovirus to spread. Infected nasal secretions are typically spread by direct contact (e.g., from hand to hand) followed by self-inoculation of mucosal surfaces such as the nose and conjunctiva. Inhalation of infected aerosols will also result in transmission of infection, but this mechanism is felt to be a less important means of spread than direct contact. The slightly lower temperature of the nasal passages (33–34°C) provides a more favorable temperature to support growth than that found in the lower respiratory tract. In fact, core body temperatures of 37°C or higher may actually inhibit viral replication. Recent data have shown that rhinoviruses infect mucosal cells by first attaching to a specific surface protein, intercellular adhesion molecule 1 (ICAM-1). Methods to inhibit cellular attachment of the virus are currently under study and may provide a novel way to prevent infection in the future.

A typical rhinovirus infection lasts seven days, although 25% of individuals may have symptoms for up to two weeks. In general, symptoms of rhinorrhea, sore or scratchy throat, and nasal stuffiness are most common. Complications include bacterial sinusitis and otitis media. Individuals with underlying asthma and chronic obstructive pulmonary disease are at an increased risk of an acute exacerbation of lower respiratory symptoms during rhinovirus infection.

Parainfluenza Virus

Human parainfluenza virus infections are found worldwide [4]. In addition to causing URIs, parainfluenza virus infections are a primary cause of lower respiratory tract diseases in the very young, the elderly, and individuals with compromised immune systems. Parainfluenza virus infections are responsible for approximately one third of lower respiratory tract infections in children under five years of age.

Parainfluenza virus is an enveloped, single-stranded RNA virus. The viral envelope is embedded with two different proteins. These envelope proteins possess neuraminidase and hemagglutinin activity similar to that of influenza virus and have been used in serotyping. The distinct serotypes have antigens in common with several other members of the Paramyxoviridae family and have been linked with specific patterns of respiratory tract disease [4]. Type 1 is most commonly associated with croup (laryngeal tracheobronchitis) but has also been associated with bronchiolitis and pneumonia in young children. Parainfluenza virus type 2 is associated with similar symptoms as type 1, with a peak incidence in young children approximately 2 years of age. Type 3 parainfluenza virus produces a spectrum of symptoms similar to respiratory syncytial virus (RSV) and is the second leading cause of bronchiolitis and pneumonia in young infants. Type 4 parainfluenza virus infections have been less well studied, but seroprevalence surveys suggest that approximately 50% of young children ages 3–5 have been infected.

The clinical symptoms of parainfluenza virus infections include those often associated with the common cold, such as rhinitis, pharyngitis, and conjunctivitis. In addition, symptoms associated with infection of the lower respiratory tract such as cough, wheeze, and sputum production may also appear. The clinical spectrum of parainfluenza virus infections tends to bear a closer similarity to infections caused by RSV than do those usually associated with rhinoviruses.

Adenovirus

Adenoviruses are best known clinically for their ability to cause infection in both the upper respiratory tract and the conjunctiva [5]. In contrast to most viruses associated with URIs, adenoviruses are composed of double-stranded DNA. The outer protein coat is made up of 252 capsomere subunits. These viruses belong to the genus *Mastadenovirus*, and at least 47 distinct serotypes have been identified. Human adenoviruses have been further classified into six subgenera (A through F). Adenoviruses interact with human cells in three distinct ways. When human epithelial cells are infected, the virus goes through a replicative cycle producing a large number of viral progeny. In addition, a latent or chronic infection that produces very few infectious particles has been described in lymphoid cells. Last, adenovirus has been shown to integrate itself into certain host-cell DNA. This integration is termed oncogenic transformation, in which viral DNA is replicated with host cell division but no infectious particles are produced [5].

Adenoviruses are found worldwide. Infection usually occurs from fall to spring, but sporadic cases may occur throughout the year. Over half of adenovirus infections do not lead to clinical symptoms. Approximately 2% of acute respiratory tract infections in adults and 5% in children are caused by adenoviruses. The high prevalence of serum antibodies to multiple serotypes in adults suggests frequent exposure throughout an individual's life span. The different serotypes are associated with age-specific infections [5]. For example, types 1, 2, 5, and 6 are often found in young children, whereas types 3, 4, and 7 are more often observed in young adults. Certain serotypes have been linked with outbreaks in military recruits.

Adenoviruses cause a wide spectrum of illnesses. The symptoms of clinically apparent respiratory tract infections are very similar to those observed with influenza and RSV—rhinorrhea, fever, sore throat, and cough. Typically, these symptoms subside within seven days. Lower respiratory tract involvement is more likely to occur in infants and children, but this is much less common than with RSV. A whooping cough-like syndrome has been described in patients with adenovirus infection, although a direct causal link has not been firmly established.

A broad variety of additional clinical infections are caused by adenoviruses [5,6]. Pharyngoconjunctival fever occurs in small outbreaks and is associated with conjunctivitis and adenopathy in addition to the URI symptoms described above. Environmental sources such as contaminated swimming pools and ponds have been associated with outbreaks of adenovirus infection. Epidemic keratoconjunctivitis is caused by adenovirus and is associated with types 8, 19, and 37. Symptoms of bilateral conjunctivitis and periauricular lymphadenopathy can last from one to four weeks. Hemorrhagic cystitis, diarrhea, and intussusception syndromes in children and infections of the central nervous system (encephalitis and meningoencephalitis) have been caused by adenoviruses.

Coronaviruses

Coronaviruses account for approximately 10–15% of upper respiratory tract infections. Similar to rhinoviruses, coronaviruses are also single-stranded RNA viruses but are much more difficult to culture. Only four antigenic types have been characterized. The seasonal prevalence of coronavirus is different from that of rhinoviruses; it is most commonly observed in late fall, winter, and early spring.

Respiratory Syncytial Virus

Respiratory syncytial virus (RSV) is an enveloped, single-negative-stranded RNA virus from the Paramyxoviridae family, which derives its name from the characteristic syncytia observed in pathologic specimens [7]. Replication of the virus within host cells results in fusion of neighboring cells into large multinucleate syncytia. A lipid envelope bearing two important glycoproteins surrounds the viral genome. These proteins, G and F, facilitate attachment and fusion, respectively, of the virus to the host cell. The clinical significance of the two distinct antigenic groups and different subtypes is not yet known.

RSV is a major cause of respiratory tract disease in infants and young children, with the highest infection rates observed in babies during the first six months of life. Annual epidemics can last more than five months and occur worldwide. In the United States, infections may develop as early as November or December but not uncommonly may be delayed until spring. When outbreaks occur in day care centers, attack rates are very high, with nearly 100% of susceptible infants being infected. Lower respiratory tract disease develops in more than 40% of infants infected with RSV, leading to clinical pneumonia, bronchiolitis, or tracheobronchitis. Repeated infections are common throughout all age groups, with attack rates over 50% reported in studies of second exposure.

Adults are also at risk for infection with RSV. The illness is usually milder than that observed in children with symptoms similar to those associated with the common cold. Severe lower respiratory tract disease may develop in adults, especially individuals with significant co-morbid health problems and transplant patients receiving immunosuppressive therapy. Complications of severe bronchitis, prolonged cough, and pneumonia are not uncommon.

Branhamella catarrhalis *(Moraxella catarrhalis)*

Branhamella catarrhalis is a gram-negative diplococcal organism that has been recognized only in recent decades as an important cause of upper and lower respiratory tract disease in humans [8]. Originally classified as a species of the genus *Neisseria*, it has been reclassified several times, based on studies of its fatty acids and DNA content. Some authorities have classified this organism as a subgenus of *Moraxella*, although this remains controversial because organisms in this category tend not to cause disease in humans and are rod shaped.

Approximately 5% or more of healthy adults are colonized by *B catarrhalis* in the upper respiratory tract. Colonization is more common, however, in children, the elderly, and individuals with underlying medical conditions. Similar to other upper respiratory tract infections, *Branhamella* infections are observed more commonly in the winter months. Recent studies have demonstrated that colonization is a dynamic process, with frequent elimination and recolonization cycles occurring spontaneously among carriers.

In general, *Branhamella* has been implicated in causing disease in both the upper and lower respiratory tract. Upper tract disease is more common in children, among whom *Branhamella* has been frequently linked with sinusitis and otitis media. Conditions of the lower respiratory tract that are observed most commonly are exacerbations of chronic obstructive pulmonary disease (COPD), pneumonia in the elderly, and nosocomial pneumonia [8].

The generally accepted criteria for implicating *B catarrhalis* as causing an exacerbation of COPD rely on securing sputum smears showing a predominance of intracellular gram-negative diplococci and/or sputum cultures. Even when these criteria are fulfilled, however, it is often unclear whether the organism is a colonizer or a true pathogen. The frequency with which *Branha-mella* infections are associated with bronchitis and worsening COPD has been estimated to run as high as 30% of patients. *Branhamella* may also be responsible for upward of 10% of cases of pneumonia in the elderly. Generally, these patients have associated medical conditions such as COPD, heart failure, or diabetes. On clinical grounds alone, it is not possible to differentiate pneumonia caused by *Branhamella* from other causes of pneumonia. Diagnosis requires culture of the organism from sputum, blood, or pleural fluid (if present).

Mycoplasma pneumonia

Mycoplasma pneumoniae is one of 14 different mycoplasmal species found in humans [9]. Additional species infect plants and animals. Species of *Mycoplasma* are the smallest known free-living organisms. The small size of the *Mycoplasma* genome, which limits biosynthetic capabilities, explains these organisms' complex nutritional requirements. They must first attach themselves to host cells in order for colonization or disease to occur. While the majority of mycoplasmas remain attached to the cell surface, intracellular translocation has been described and may protect the organism from the host's immune response.

Children and young adults are especially prone to disease caused by *M pneumoniae*. Approximately 10–20% of pneumonias that originate in the community setting are attributable to *Mycoplasma* infections. The incubation period is long (two to four weeks) prior to the development of fever, chills, headache, and sore throat. Cough is usually moderate to severe, especially worse at night and generally nonproductive. Cough symptoms can often dominate the clinical picture and may persist for three to four weeks. While most patients develop only tracheobronchitis, about 3% of individuals have findings of pneumonia on chest radiographs. A number of extrapulmonary complications have been reported, including aseptic meningitis, meningoencephalitis, hemolytic anemia, arthritis, myopericarditis and heart failure, among others. Mucocutaneous lesions can be observed in 25% or more of infected individuals.

A diagnosis of infection with *Mycoplasma* is usually made on clinical grounds, since serologic markers may not develop until the second or third week of the illness. Cold agglutinin titers of 1:64 or greater are supportive of a diagnosis but are observed in fewer than 50% of cases and thus are nonspecific. Paired specimens, obtained two to four weeks apart, that demonstrate significant titers of IgM and/or IgG antibody are diagnostic. Unfortunately, the clinical utility of serologic testing for early detection is limited. Therapy is usually empiric, since there are no readily available and reliable diagnostic tests that will detect infection with *Mycoplasma* early in the illness [9,10]. Treatment guidelines are discussed below.

Streptococcus pyogenes *(Group A Streptococci)*

Although *Streptococcus pyogenes* is the only species in the Lancefield group A streptococci, this organism is responsible for a wide variety of diseases in humans [11]. The more common clinical infections are streptococcal pharyngitis, impetigo, pneumonia, and empyema. Recently, it has been recognized that exotoxin-producing strains of group A streptococci can trigger a toxic, shock-like syndrome with clinical characteristics very similar to the better known staphylococcal toxic shock syndrome. In addition, the postinfectious syndromes of acute rheumatic fever and poststreptococcal glomerular nephritis can follow infection by *S pyogenes*. With respect to URIs, this chapter focuses on pharyngitis caused by *S pyogenes*. The reader is referred elsewhere for a more thorough discussion of the entire spectrum of disease caused by group A streptococci [11,12].

Group A streptococcal pharyngitis, which is spread by contact with an infected individual, is one of the most common bacterial infections in childhood. Although infection can also develop after contact with an asymptomatic carrier, this is thought to occur much less commonly. Outbreaks described in military barracks have been well characterized, showing that likelihood of developing an infection is directly linked with the distance between one's bunk and the nearest carrier. Surveillance cultures have shown that about 15% of the population are asymptomatic carriers of group A streptococci. The incubation period is brief, with only one to four days between significant exposure and development of symptoms. The posterior pharynx usually appears reddened and swollen, and the tonsils often display a mottled grayish-white exudate. Tender lymph nodes are frequently found at the angle of the jaw and along the anterior cervical chain.

A number of investigators have tried to develop clinical criteria, such as exudative pharyngitis, tender adenopathy and fever, to predict whether or not a patient's symptoms are due to infection by group A streptococci. Unfortunately, the sensitivity and specificity of these criteria have ranged between 50% and 75%. The recently available rapid diagnostic testing kits tend to be highly specific (about 90–95%) but less sensitive (50–90%). Thus, it is reasonable to initiate treatment on the basis of a positive rapid test, but a negative test should be confirmed by a properly obtained throat culture.

Prevention and Infection Control

Prevention of transmission of the broad group of infections discussed above is a major challenge. Although many of these agents have predictable seasonal attack rates, they all are ubiquitous in the environment. Simple measures in areas providing clinical care to patients are effective at reducing risk of transmission. Unfortunately, these strategies require a large amount of time and effort, making them impractical in schools, day care centers, or other areas outside of patient care settings. In addition, there are few well-designed studies on the prevention and control of URIs outside of health care settings. The recommendations detailed in Table 14-2 and discussed below have been best studied in hospital settings and have been developed by the Hospital Infection Control Practices Advisory Committee (HICPAC) and the Centers for Disease Control and Prevention [13,14].

The backbone of infection control in hospitals is education and periodic monitoring of employee compliance with precautions, for employee knowledge and adherence to infection-control recommendations are essential. HICPAC recently recommended a two-tiered approach to infection control. The first tier, termed *Standard Precautions*, details precautions that should be implemented in all clinical areas. Standard Precautions include hand washing, before and after patient contact, and wearing gloves when touching blood, body fluids, secretions, and contaminated items. Employees should wash their hands, regardless of the patient's diagnosis or presumed infectious status and regardless of whether gloves are worn [13,14].

While hand washing has been shown to reduce transmission from direct contact and autoinoculation, individuals with URIs can also spread infection through the generation of infectious aerosols (i.e., usually particle sizes of more than 5 μm in diameter) when coughing, sneezing, or talking. Transmission to health care workers or patient visitors can occur when infectious droplets come in contact with mucous membranes. Thus, the second tier of infection control is *Transmission-based Precautions*, which are used in the care of patients with known or suspected specific pathogens [13]. Transmission-based Precautions include three categories: Airborne, Contact, and Droplet Precautions. These more intensive preventive measures are important in minimizing the risk of acquiring infection from an ill patient as well as reducing the possible spread of infection from a clinical provider. Since most of the agents that cause URI are spread by contact and/or droplet formation, Droplet Precautions are recommended in addition to Standard Precautions for the care of patients with URIs.

Droplet Precautions for hospitalized patients with URI include placement in a private room (when available) or a room with another patient who has active infection with the same organism. Masks should also be worn by health care workers when working within three feet of these patients. From a logistical standpoint, however, these should be in place upon entering a patient's room. Masks and eye protection (goggles or face shields) as well as clean, nonsterile gowns should be used during encounters or procedures that may expose providers to splashes or sprays of body

Table 14-2
Isolation Precautions To Reduce Transmission of Infections to Employees

Organism	Isolation Precautions	Duration of Precautions
Rhinovirus	Standard	None specified
Adenovirus[a]	Standard + Droplet	Duration of illness
Parainfluenza	Standard + Contact	Duration of illness
Respiratory syncytial virus[b]	Standard + Contact	Duration of illness
Mycoplasma pneumoniae	Standard + Droplet	Duration of illness
Branhamella catarrhalis	Standard	None specified
Streptococcus pyogenes[c]	Standard + Droplet	24 hours after effective therapy initiated

[a] It is also important to eliminate potential environmental reservoirs such as solutions and/or equipment in eye clinics.
[b] Eye/nose goggles should be used for all contact with potentially infected patients. Use of masks alone may not protect conjunctivae. Gowns should be used if soiling is likely.
[c] In the event that a nosocomial case of group A streptococcal disease is identified, culture specimens of pharyngeal, rectal, vaginal, and/or skin lesions should be obtained, as appropriate, from employees who are potential sources.

fluids or secretions. Currently recommended precautions for the individual infectious agents discussed in this chapter are outlined in Table 14-2.

PREVENTION OF SPECIFIC INFECTIONS IN THE WORKPLACE

Respiratory Syncytial Virus

During seasonal community-wide RSV infections, health care workers are at increased risk of acquiring the infection themselves. Several studies have shown that a large number of clinical staff become infected in community outbreaks of RSV [6]. In general, implementation of infection control procedures such as hand washing, eye/nose goggles, patient isolation, and use of gowns and gloves reduces nosocomial spread. In one small prospective study, when use of eye/nose goggles in combination with Standard Precautions were compared with use of Standard Precautions alone, the infection rate of clinical staff was markedly reduced in the former [15]. Only 8% of staff became infected with RSV, as determined by viral isolation and/or serology, compared to 34% of staff when eye/nose goggles were not routinely used. Additional outbreaks have been reported in long-term care facilities, bone marrow transplant centers, and intensive care units.

The incubation period for RSV ranges from two to eight days, and viral shedding can last as long as three to four weeks. Compliance with Contact Precautions markedly reduces nosocomial spread. Most hospitals have found it impractical to restrict the work activity of health care employees with symptomatic viral upper respiratory tract infections. HICPAC suggests, however, that in the setting of a community outbreak of RSV or influenza, providers with symptoms of URI should be assigned to duties other than the care of high-risk patients until acute symptoms resolve [14].

Adenovirus

Infections caused by adenovirus may be especially difficult to control. Adenoviral keratoconjunctivitis is highly contagious, with outbreaks reported in ophthalmology clinics [6] as well as in hospitals and long-term care facilities [14]. In ophthalmology clinic outbreaks, attack rates were highest in persons evaluated for eye problems (21% of those at risk) and was especially high for those who underwent procedures that resulted in manipulation of the eyelids, tonometry (74%), or minor surgery (38%). Respiratory symptoms of URI are common but do not always accompany eye symptoms. The incubation period ranges from five to 12 days, and shedding of infectious virus may continue for two weeks after the onset of symptoms. Although HICPAC recommends that an infected health care worker be relieved of their job responsibilities for as long as the worker remains symptomatic, the long period of viral shedding suggests that it may be reasonable to minimize high-risk patient contact for a more extended period. To minimize risk to care providers, Standard Precautions as well as Contact Precautions should be observed in the care of patients with adenovirus [13,14].

Group A Streptococcus

Patients with group A streptococcal infections can transmit infection to care providers by contact and/or through aerosols, although the latter mechanism is thought to be less common. Care providers who become infected may develop a wide variety of manifestations of group A streptococcal disease, including pharyngitis, cellulitis, and the group A toxic-shock-like syndrome. Rarely have asymptomatic carriers been linked to nosocomial outbreaks of infection [16], although asymptomatic hospital personnel have been found to carry the organism in the pharynx, skin, rectum, and female genital tract.

The incubation period for group A streptococcus pharyngitis is two to five days. Other illnesses caused by group A streptococcus have different incubation periods. Culture surveys of hospital personnel are not recommended unless an outbreak triggers the need for epidemiologic investigation. If an employee is identified as a carrier through culture surveys, the individual's activities should be restricted until 24 hours after starting appropriate therapy. Workers who are discovered to be carriers in the absence of a hospital outbreak are generally not treated, nor is there any need to restrict their patient care activities [14,16].

TREATMENT

Employees with uncomplicated URI caused by the respiratory viruses discussed above generally need only supportive care [2,17,18]. Antihistamines are usually effective in reducing rhinorrhea and sneezing. Topical as well as systemic decongestants may provide symptomatic relief of nasal obstruction but should be used with caution in patients with hypertension. If topical decongestants are used consistently for more than three or four days, symptoms may rebound when they are discontinued (rhinitis medicamentosa). More recently, topical use of anticholinergic medications (e.g., ipratropium bromide) has been shown to reduce symptoms of rhinitis and nasal congestion due to URIs.

These recommendations include a few important exceptions that pertain to individuals with impaired immune function. Workers who have received bone marrow transplantation and those who are immunosuppressed because of solid organ transplantation are at a particularly high risk for developing lower respiratory tract disease. The associated risks for severe disease in workers infected with human immunodeficiency virus 1 (HIV1) appear to be less than that of organ transplant patients. Although there are no specific guidelines regarding these populations of workers, common sense dictates that individuals with these associated health problems should make strong efforts to avoid situations in which they would need to provide care for patients potentially infected with RSV. There are currently no definitive recommendations as to whether prophylactic use of ribavirin should be given to high-risk individuals in the event of significant exposure [7].

A number of additional treatments for the common cold have been studied, but their potential benefits are controversial. Unproven therapies include inhalation of steam, large doses of vitamin C (e.g., greater than 1 g/day), zinc supplements, and nonsteroidal anti-inflammatory medications. Data on these treatments are mixed. Some studies suggest a therapeutic benefit, while others do not [17,18].

Antibiotics are not indicated in the treatment of an uncomplicated cold. Despite this well-known fact, overuse of antibiotics runs rampant in many primary care office settings. It has been estimated that over 20% of antibiotic prescriptions in the United States are for "treatment" of upper respiratory tract infections. Ideally, antibiotic use should be reserved for treatment of specific complications such as bacterial sinusitis and pneumonia. More liberal use of antibiotics has been recommended in patients with underlying obstructive airways disease, especially if patients experience increased dyspnea and a change in sputum color or volume [19].

Antibiotic regimens recommended for individuals with *Mycoplasma pneumoniae* include the use of doxycycline or macrolide antibiotics (i.e., erythromycin, clarithromycin, or azithromycin). An extended course of two to three weeks has been recommended to minimize the risk of relapse. A fluoroquinolone medication can be used as an alternative [9,10].

Branhamella catarrhalis susceptibility to antibiotics has evolved over the past 25 years. Beta-lactam antibiotics were highly effective until the development of resistance. Recently, upward of 90% of isolates from both the United States and Europe produce beta-lactamase. Antibiotics currently recommended for treatment of *B catarrhalis* include second- or third-generation cephalosporins, trimethoprim-sulfamethoxazole, and ampicillin-clavulanate. Alternative agents are macrolide antibiotics or fluoroquinolones [8,10].

Treatment of group A streptococcal pharyngitis consists of a single dose of penicillin given intramuscularly (penicillin G benzathine, 1.2 million units IM) or a 10-day course of oral penicillin V, 250 mg [11]. Erythromycin is recommended for individuals who are allergic to penicillin. It is worth emphasizing that treatment with penicillin reduces the incidence of rheumatic fever and suppurative complications of group A streptococcus, such as peritonsillar abscess, lymphadenitis and sinusitis, but does not significantly affect the duration of symptoms. There are no definitive guidelines for the management of individuals who have persistent carriage of group A streptococcus despite treatment with penicillin. Most authorities do not recommend retreatment of asymptomatic carriers unless the carrier is thought to be a potential source of infection to others. Penicillin in combination with rifampin has been used to eradicate pharyngeal carriage, but data in this area are not extensive [11,16].

References

1. Makela MJ, Puhakka T, Ruuskanen O. Viruses and bacteria in the etiology of the common cold. *J Clin Microbiol* 1998;36:539–42.
2. Gwaltney JM Jr. The common cold. In: Mandell GL, Bennett JE, Dolin R (eds), *Principles and Practice of Infectious Diseases*, 4th Ed. New York: Churchill Livingstone, 1995. Chap 39.
3. Wald TG, Shult P, Krause P, et al. A rhinovirus outbreak among residents of a long-term care facility. *Ann Intern Med* 1995;123:588–93.
4. Henrickson K, Ray R, Belshe R. Parainfluenza viruses. In: Mandell GL, Bennett JE, Dolin R (eds), *Principles and Practice of Infectious Diseases*, 4th Ed. New York: Churchill Livingstone, 1995. Chap 134.
5. Baum SG. Adenoviridae. In: Mandell GL, Bennett JE, Dolin R (eds), *Principles and Practice of Infectious Diseases*, 4th Ed. New York: Churchill Livingstone, 1995. Chap 121, pp 1282–387.
6. Dawson C, Darrell R. Infections due to adenovirus type 8 in the United States. I. An outbreak of epidemic keratoconjunctivitis originating in a physician's office. *N Engl J Med* 1963;268(19):1031–7.
7. Hall CB, McCarthy CA. In: Mandell GL, Bennett JE, Dolin R (eds), *Principles and Practice of Infectious Diseases*, 4th Ed. New York: Churchill Livingstone, 1995. Chap 136, pp 1501–19.
8. Murphy TF. Lung infections—2: *Branhamella catarrhalis:* epidemiological and clinical aspects of a human respiratory tract pathogen. *Thorax* 1998;53(2):124–8.
9. Baum SG. Mycoplasma pneumoniae and atypical pneumonia. In: Mandell GL, Bennett JE, Dolin R (eds), *Principles and Practice of Infectious Diseases*, 4th Ed. New York: Churchill Livingstone, 1995. Chap 161, pp 1704–13.
10. Bartlett JG, Breiman RF, Mandell LA, et al. Guidelines from the Infectious Diseases Society of America. Community-acquired pneumonia in adults: guidelines for management. *Clin Infect Dis* 1998;26:811–38.
11. Wessels MR. Streptococcal and enterococcal infections. In: Fauci AS, Braunwald E, Isselbacher KJ, et al. (eds.), *Principles of Internal Medicine*, 14th Ed. New York: McGraw-Hill, 1998. Pp 885–92.
12. Bisno AL. Streptococcus pyogenes. In: Mandell GL, Bennett JE, Dolin R (eds), *Principles and Practice of Infectious Diseases*, 4th Ed. New York: Churchill Livingstone, 1995. Chap 76, pp 1786–99.
13. Centers for Disease Control and Prevention, Hospital Infection Control Practices Advisory Committee, Hierholzer WJ Jr. (Chairperson), et al. Guideline for isolation precautions in hospitals. Part I and II. Recommendations for isolation precautions in hospitals. *Am J Infect Control* 1996;24:24–52.
14. Centers for Disease Control and Prevention, Hospital Infection Control Practices Advisory Committee, Hierholzer WJ Jr. (Chairperson), et al. Guideline for infection control in healthcare personnel. *Infect Control Hosp Epidemiol* 1998;19(6):407–63.
15. Gala CL, Hall CB, Schnabel KC, et al. The use of eye-nose goggles to control nosocomial respiratory syncytial virus infection. *JAMA* 1986;256(19):2706–8.
16. Nosocomial Group A streptococcal infections associated with asymptomatic health-care workers—Maryland and California, 1997. *MMWR* 1999;48(08):163–6.
17. Spector SL. The common cold: current therapy and natural history. *J Allergy Clin Immunol* 1995;95: 1133–8.
18. Mossad SB. Clinical review: fortnightly review—treatment of the common cold. *Br Med J* 1998;317:33–6.
19. British Thoracic Society Guidelines for the Management of Chronic Obstructive Pulmonary Disease. The COPD Guidelines Group of the Standards of Care Committee of the BTS. *Thorax* 19;52(5):S1–28.

15 / Occupational Plague

Andrew W. Artenstein and Daniel R. Lucey

Historically known as "The Plague" or "the Black Death," plague continues to evoke fear and panic that appear out of proportion to the relatively low number of annually reported cases. This may be due to the tendency of the disease to flare up periodically in epidemic foci throughout the world. Four distinct pandemics have been recorded to date: 542 to 600 AD involving the entire Roman empire; the "Black Death" of fourteenth-century Europe, which is estimated to have killed one fourth of the population there; the European pandemic of the fifteenth, sixteenth, and seventeenth centuries, and the present one [1]. The current pandemic is believed to have begun in the late nineteenth century near the China-Tibet border and reached the ports of Hong Kong in 1894 [1]. From there, it spread via commercial ships to countries all over the world, including the United States, where a major epidemic occurred in the San Francisco area during the first part of the twentieth century [1]. During the U.S. involvement in the Vietnam War, more than 10,000 cases of plague were reported from that country [2].

Pathogenesis

Plague is caused by the organism *Yersinia pestis*, named for Alexandre Yersin, who is credited with its discovery in Hong Kong in 1894 [2]. The organism is a gram-negative bipolar staining bacillus that belongs to the family Enterobacteriaceae. The bipolar staining pattern may sometimes result in the characteristic "safety pin" appearance in stained smears of clinical specimens. *Y pestis* grows aerobically on most culture media, does not ferment lactose, and can be distinguished from other species of *Yersiniae* by its profile of biochemical reactions [3]. The organism harbors a number of virulence factors, including an antiphagocytic capsule-type structure, a coagulase enzyme, and a lipopolysaccharide endotoxin [3].

Epidemiology

INCIDENCE AND PREVALENCE

Human plague occurs worldwide, with more than 18,000 cases and greater than 1,800 plague-related deaths reported during the 15-year period 1980–1994 [4]. Urban plague continues in parts of Africa and Asia. At least six countries annually report cases of human plague: Vietnam, Myanmar, Madagascar, Tanzania, Brazil, and the United States [5]. The number of cases reported worldwide in the first half of this decade is greater than that reported during the entire 1980s, with recent outbreaks occurring in Madagascar, Peru, and India [6]. During the outbreak in southern India between late August and October 1994, there were 5,150 suspected cases and 53 deaths reported, although the reason for the unexpectedly low case-fatality ratio is not clear [7].

Unlike other parts of the world, it is felt that nearly all of the diagnosed cases of human plague in the United States are reported to public health authorities. The occurrence of plague in the United States is sporadic, with the highest incidence of cases during the spring and summer months, when people spend more time outdoors and are more likely to come into contact with the vector. During the 50-year period 1947–1996, 390 cases of human plague were reported in the United States, with 60 (15%) deaths [8]. All of these cases occurred in 10 states (in descending order): New Mexico, California, Arizona, Colorado, Utah, Oregon, Idaho, Nevada, Wyoming, and Texas [2]. Over the 26-year period 1970–1995 an average of 13 cases per year were reported to the Centers for Disease Control (CDC); nearly 90% of these occurred in New Mexico, Arizona, Colorado, and California [4].

TRANSMISSION

Plague is primarily a zoonotic disease; humans are an incidental host. Rodents serve as the primary host for plague and are the major source of human exposure. Natural animal reservoirs include dozens of wild and domestic mammal species, most notably wild urban and sylvatic rodents and larger predators/carnivores [9]. Throughout the world, rats are the most important urban reservoir of plague, although other important sylvatic reservoirs include ground squirrels [10], rock squirrels [2], prairie dogs [11,12], mice, bobcats, rabbits, voles, and chipmunks [2]. Domestic cats have become an increasingly recognized source of human infection [13–15].

Plague is transmitted among its animal reservoirs by the bite of infected fleas or, less commonly, by ingestion of contaminated animal tissues by the host. Fleas are the only arthropod vectors known to transmit *Y pestis* in nature, and more than 30 species of fleas can perform this task, although the Oriental rat flea, *Xenopsylla cheopsis*, may be the most important [16]. Transmission usually occurs once the bacteria have multiplied in the proventriculus of the flea to such an extent during repetitive blood meals that the flea gut becomes obstructed by the bacilli and infected blood is regurgitated into the wound of the host [2]. The coagulase enzyme of *Y pestis* contributes to this "blocking" of the flea gut by causing ingested blood to clot [2]. The flea continues to feed, and the cycle of regurgitation continues, increasing the vector's efficiency of transmission. Other potential mechanisms of flea-borne transmission include penetration of infected flea feces into abraded skin, either directly or through inoculation by scratching, or mechanical transmission via contaminated flea mouth parts [2].

Human infection with plague occurs when infected fleas leave their small mammal hosts and infest man. The greatest risk, historically, exists when epizootics cause high mortality in rodent populations ("ratfall"), as fleas will leave a dead rat upon cooling of its body temperature and tend to seek alternative hosts in close proximity. This explains the increased incidence of human urban plague during times of war, social upheaval, and natural disaster, all settings that lead to crowding and unsanitary conditions. In the United States, most human cases are acquired in or around the patient's residence through the bite of an infected flea either from a sylvatic source [2] or a domestic cat or dog [2,13,14]. Because domestic cats may develop clinical plague and die of overwhelming infection, they may represent an additional human risk factor during epizootics; in fact, primary plague pneumonia has been reported to be transmitted directly from cats to humans [15].

Human cases of plague in the southwestern United States are therefore most closely associated with activities that result in contact with infected fleas or their hosts, such as camping, hunting, or working in enzootic areas. Additional risk factors associated with acquiring plague in endemic areas include the presence of harborage and food sources for wild rodents in close proximity to the home and, possibly, failure to control fleas on pet cats and dogs [2]. Native American peoples, especially the Navajo, account for a disproportionate share of the reported cases, probably because of socioeconomic and cultural factors that place them in close contact with infected animals [2,17]. Human plague may also occur as a result of direct inoculation with body fluids or tissues of infected animals, which may take place during the skinning or consuming of dead squirrels or rabbits [2,17]. Entry appears to be through breaks in the skin or mucosa of the susceptible host. Finally, human-to-human transmission of plague pneumonia is theoretically possible but has not been reported from the United States since the Los Angeles outbreak of 1924 [18], although the recent epidemic in India heightens concern about this mode of transmission and spread [7].

OCCUPATIONAL RISK FACTORS

Aside from the obvious occupational risks for hunters, taxidermists, archeologists, veterinarians, and other animal handlers, there have been rare reports of laboratory-acquired infection in humans. The first report, in 1901, was of a medical student working to prepare plague antiserum with samples from the San Francisco outbreak [1]. Burmeister and colleagues reviewed the extant literature in 1962 and presented four additional cases of laboratory-acquired pneumonic plague and one secondary case in one of the contacts [19]. The likely portal of entry was inhalation, and the resulting illness was similar to the naturally occurring disease.

Prevention and Control

PREVENTIVE MEASURES (NONBIOLOGIC)

The CDC recommends various nonbiologic preventive measures against plague, depending on an individual's risk status [4]. Residents of enzootic areas or places where recent plague cases have occurred in animals or humans should eliminate sources of food and shelter (e.g., brush piles and junk heaps) for rodents near their homes; modify homes to prevent rodent access; avoid contact with sick or dead animals; treat domestic cats and dogs weekly with appropriate insecticides; restrict pets from wandering; and handle sick cats with extreme caution to avoid exposure to potentially infectious secretions [15]. Hunters, hikers, campers, and others who participate in outdoor recreational activities in endemic areas should follow the same precautions. Veterinary workers and others who may come into contact with infected animals should be educated on ways to minimize exposure to infection and should wear gloves and eye protection when handling animals [4]. Respiratory Precautions, including masks, should be taken when treating severely ill domestic cats [4].

Laboratory work involving cultures of *Y. pestis* should be carried out using biosafety level 2 practices, including the use of biologic safety cabinets and other containment equipment during manipulation of plague cultures, handling infectious materials, or conducting necropsies on infected animals [4]. Immunization with inactivated plague vaccine (see below) is recommended in this setting.

Patients diagnosed with bubonic plague without pulmonary involvement warrant Universal Precautions only. Individuals suspected of having plague pneumonia should be placed in strict respiratory isolation for at least 48 hours after the institution of appropriate antimicrobial therapy. Those with confirmed plague pneumonia should be kept in respiratory isolation until their sputum cultures are negative. Although there are scant scientifically generated data concerning the efficacy of face masks in the prevention of pneumonic spread of plague, recommendations have been proposed, based on studies of operating-room masks in the prevention of surgical wound infections [20]. Masks, covering the nostrils and mouth, should be worn continuously during potential exposures; masks should be changed at least every 30–40 minutes, as they may become a nidus for aerosolized organisms; and multilayer masks or high efficiency filters may be needed to limit entry of small particles.

Prophylactic antimicrobial therapy is recommended for medical personnel and others who have had close exposure to a case of suspected or proven pneumonic plague [4]. *Close exposure* is generally defined as within 2 meters (approximately 6.5 feet) of the patient, and these prophylaxis recommendations usually apply to family contacts as well [2,4]. The current recommendations for adult chemoprophylaxis are doxycycline, 100–200 mg/day orally in two equal doses every 12 hours for seven days, or tetracycline, 2 g/day in two or four equal doses at 12- or six-hour intervals, respectively, for seven days [4]. Trimethoprim-sulfamethoxazole, 1.6–3.2 g/day of the sulfa component in two equal doses at 12-hour intervals, is a reasonable alternative for adults and may be the preferred therapy for children (at pediatric doses).

MEDICAL SURVEILLANCE

Because of the high case-fatality rate and the potential for epidemic disease, plague has been designated a class I notifiable disease and is therefore subject to regulations that require mandatory reporting of suspected cases to state health departments [4]. These authorities are required to investigate cases and subsequently report to the CDC, under whose authority further investigation is carried out. Laboratory-confirmed cases are subsequently reported to the World

Health Organisation (WHO) in Geneva, Switzerland.

Once sporadic cases in humans have been confirmed, epidemiologic surveillance must be undertaken to identify potential geographic areas of risk and to assess the potential for additional cases. Such surveillance measures may include detailed risk and exposure histories from cases and contacts; assessment of the environment where a case has occurred; evaluation of the geographic vicinity for evidence of epizootic disease, such as obtaining information about rodent die-offs, performing autopsies of dead rodents and other potential hosts, and trapping live animals for serologic testing as well as flea assessments [2]. Environmental control measures should be carried out in concert with surveillance. Education of those at risk, maintenance of strict hygienic standards, vector control by insecticide use, rodent control by rodenticides and trapping, rat-proofing of houses, and vaccination of high-risk individuals are all strategies believed to be effective in the control of plague [2]. The CDC and WHO have also continued to reassess and enhance international surveillance systems for the detection and control of epidemic plague [2,21], most recently, in response to the Indian epidemic of 1994 [7].

IMMUNIZATION

Plague vaccine (available from Greer Laboratories, Lenoir, NC; telephone 800-438-0088 or 704-754-5327), a formalin-inactivated (killed) product is the only licensed vaccine against plague. It is recommended for persons at high risk for plague exposure, such as laboratory personnel who work with live *Y pestis* organisms and individuals (e.g., animal handlers and environmental field workers) who have regular contact with wild rodents or their fleas in enzootic areas [4]. Routine vaccination is not recommended for health care workers, travelers, or persons residing in enzootic areas unless they are at high risk for exposure by virtue of other activities. The vaccine is given as a primary series of three intramuscular (deltoid) immunizations over a six-month interval, with booster doses depending on the level of ongoing risk [4]. Although local reactions to the vaccine are relatively common, severe reactions are unusual. Immunization does not obviate the need for antimicrobial prophylaxis when indicated (see above), since there are limited efficacy data concerning the vaccine in humans.

Symptoms and Signs

Clinically, plague can present, at least initially, in a variety of ways. Bubonic plague is the most common form of the disease, accounting for more than 80% of cases in the United States [4], although in a recent review of 27 cases of plague that occurred over a 25-year period at the Gallup Indian Medical Center in New Mexico, only 37% presented with classic bubonic symptoms and signs [22]. During an incubation period that averages two to eight days following the bite of an infected flea, bacteria proliferate in regional lymph nodes. The patient subsequently develops an abrupt onset of fevers, rigors, malaise, prostration, and headache, sometimes with prominent gastrointestinal symptoms, followed within 24 hours by a bubo, a one- to 10-centimeter exquisitely tender, firm mass of lymph nodes in the area draining the site of infection [23]. Buboes most commonly occur in the groin (femoral nodes are more frequently affected than inguinal nodes); axillary or cervical lymph nodes are less commonly involved [17]. Involvement of intra-abdominal nodes may mimic a surgical abdomen. Skin lesions are not common in bubonic plague, and the typical absence of a lesion at the site of the flea bites, as well as the absence of an ascending lymphangitis, may distinguish this form of plague from other bacterial infections [3]. Occasionally, vasculitic lesions of the distal extremities occur as a result of the sepsis syndrome that patients typically display. The bubonic presentation of plague can result in a fulminant clinical course progressing rapidly to death in 50–60% of untreated patients [4], but because of its distinctive clinical presentation in endemic areas, the majority of patients are treated appropriately and early, and more than 85% survive [3].

Septicemia in plague infection can occur during the course of bubonic disease or, less frequently, can develop without detectable lymphadenopathy. Primary septicemic plague presents as a nonspecific febrile illness and tends to progress to septic shock and death in approximately 50% of cases, largely the result of delays in diagnosis and treatment [22].

Primary pneumonic plague, acquired via the inhalation route from a patient or domestic animal (such as a cat) with pneumonic plague or exposure to aerosols of plague cultures in a laboratory, is rare and is associated with an exceedingly high mortality. Secondary pneumonic plague accounted for more than 90% of the 36 reported cases of pneumonic plague in the United States between 1950 and 1983 [24]. The infection results from hematogenous dissemination of bacteria from the bubo and presents in the setting of fever and lymphadenopathy with cough and/or hemoptysis; pleuritic chest pain; patchy bronchopneumonia, cavities, or confluent consolidation radiographically; and purulent sputum containing plague bacilli [3]. Pneumonic plague is highly contagious by the airborne route.

Plague meningitis is a rare complication of inadequately treated bubonic plague and presents with symptoms and signs similar to other forms of bacterial meningitis. It is associated with a high mortality rate. Plague can also present as a pharyngitis or tonsillitis and is thought to rarely occur in this form following inhalation or ingestion of bacilli [2]. Nearly 20% of the cases in a recent series presented in this fashion and mortality was high, owing to diagnostic delays [22].

Differential Diagnosis

The finding of a bubo, especially of the groin, in concert with constitutional symptoms and a potential exposure history in an endemic area, is highly suggestive of plague and certainly warrants empiric treatment for this diagnosis. Other potential causes of inguinal lymphadenitis include secondary syphilis, lymphogranuloma venereum, granuloma inguinale, chancroid, primary genital herpes, cat scratch disease, loiasis, onchocerciasis, and tularemia [25]. The latter infection shares many characteristics of plague, including exposure history and systemic signs, but it usually presents as an ulceroglandular syndrome with an ulcer or pustule at the site of vector inoculation and affects the axillary or epitrochlear chains more commonly than the groin [2].

The differential diagnosis of bubonic plague involving the axillary or cervical lymph nodes includes acute pyogenic infections caused by streptococci and staphylococci; scrofula, either due to tuberculosis or nontuberculous mycobacteria [26]; cat scratch disease; tularemia; deep mycotic infections; toxoplasmosis; and typical and atypical forms of viral mononucleosis [25]. Plague pharyngitis typically presents as a bacterial pharyngitis, tonsillitis, or sinusitis and therefore the symptoms are frequently attributed to streptococcal disease. In the series of Crook and colleagues, all of the patients who presented with pharyngitis were initially treated with penicillin, thus resulting in a therapeutic delay and, subsequently, a higher mortality [22]. The clinical presentation of patients with pneumonic plague is similar to that of other severe, typical and atypical forms of community-acquired pneumonia as well as to pneumonia due to tularemia, psittacosis, Q fever, and influenza. When pneumonia occurs following dissemination from a bubo, the diagnosis is generally apparent.

Patients with primary septicemic plague, i.e., the absence of buboes, present similarly to those with sepsis from other causes. A history of potential exposure in an endemic area should raise the possibility of both plague and septicemic tularemia. In patients who present with a predominance of gastrointestinal symptoms and signs, an intra-abdominal source of sepsis, such as appendicitis, cholecystitis, or bowel obstruction, must be considered.

Diagnostic Evaluation

The diagnosis of plague should be considered in patients experiencing febrile illness who have a history of potential exposure to rodents or other small mammals in known endemic regions. This includes febrile patients who seek medical attention in the eastern two thirds of the United States but who have recently traveled to western states. Routine laboratory data are generally consistent with those of a systemic infection but are otherwise nondiagnostic [22]. Blood cultures were noted to be positive for *Y. pestis* in 96% of cases in a recent series of mixed clinical presentations using standard bacteriologic media [22], but in the early stages of bubonic plague, 27% of blood cultures were found to be positive in previous reports [2].

A bacteriologic diagnosis may be accomplished in more than 75% of cases through smear and culture of a bubo aspirate or sputum (in cases of pneumonic disease) [2,22]. Because buboes are not typically fluctuant, aspirates may require an initial injection of a small amount of saline. Aspirated sanguineous material should undergo Gram's staining to identify gram-negative coccobacilli or bacilli, Giemsa or Wright's staining to look for the characteristic "safety-pin" appearance, and culture for definitive identification. Microbiologic confirmation can be obtained through the Centers for Disease Control and Prevention, Plague Branch, P.O. Box 2087, Fort Collins, Colorado 80522 (telephone 303-221-6450). A fluorescent antibody test can be applied to bubo aspirates and sputum for rapid diagnosis, and a passive hemagglutination test using fraction I of *Y pestis* can be performed on acute- and convalescent-phase serum at the CDC laboratory [3]. Serologic testing may be used to diagnose plague in those with negative cultures; a fourfold or greater increase in titer or a single titer of 1:16 or greater is presumptive evidence of infection.

Treatment

In order to avoid excessive mortality, early administration of antimicrobial therapy effective against *Y pestis* is essential [22]. Streptomycin has been the drug of choice for plague for more than 50 years and is usually administered in two divided doses of 15 mg/kg, each given intramuscularly for 10 days [3,22]. Other aminoglycosides demonstrate variable activity against *Y pestis* but are not as effective as streptomycin [2]. While most patients show rapid improvement with therapy and become afebrile within three days, a 10-day course should be completed, because buboes may continue to harbor viable bacteria after clinical improvement [2]. An alternative to streptomycin for allergic individuals or those for whom an oral agent is desired, is tetracycline given orally as 2–4 g per day in four divided doses for 10 days. Chloramphenicol given intravenously at a loading dose of 25 mg per kilogram of body weight, followed by 60 mg/kg per day in four divided doses is another alternative and is the drug of choice for plague meningitis [2,3]. Penicillins and cephalosporins have not proved effective in the treatment of plague [22]. Recently, multidrug resistance has been reported in a strain of *Y pestis* isolated from a patient with bubonic plague in Madagascar [27,28]. Because this resistance was mediated by a plasmid transferable among strains, the report raises concerns about clinical and public health issues.

Occupational Considerations

As discussed above, plague is an uncommon occupational disease of hunters, taxidermists, veterinarians, animal handlers, and others whose livelihood or avocations place them in potential contact with the bacterial hosts or their vectors in endemic areas. There are also rare reports of plague as a laboratory-acquired infection [19]. The major risk factors in the laboratory setting include direct contact with cultures or infectious materials from humans or small mammal hosts; infectious aerosols generated during manipulation of cultures or infected animal tissues; and percutaneous injuries from contaminated laboratory equipment [29]. The appropriate prevention and control measures are discussed above. Plague may also be viewed as an occupational disease risk of health care providers, most notably in regard to pneumonic disease; however, as discussed above, person-to-person transmission is rare in sporadic disease.

References

1. Link VB. *A History of Plague in the United States.* Washington, DC: U.S. Department of Health, Education, and Welfare, Public Health Service, 1955.
2. Butler T. *Plague and Other Yersinia Infections.* New York: Plenum Publishing Corporation, 1983.
3. Butler T. Yersinia species (including plague). In: Mandell GL, Bennett JE, Dolin R (eds), *Principles and Practice of Infectious Diseases,* 4th Ed. New York: Churchill Livingstone, 1995. Pp 2070–6.

4. Centers for Disease Control and Prevention. Prevention of plague: recommendations of the Advisory Committee on Immunization Practices (ACIP). *MMWR* 1996;45(RR-14):1–15.

5. Walker DH, Barbour AG, Oliver JH, et al. Emerging bacterial zoonotic and vector-borne diseases: ecological and epidemiological factors. *JAMA* 1996;275: 463–9.

6. Dennis DT, Hughes JM. Multidrug resistance in plague. *N Engl J Med* 1997;337:702–4.

7. Centers for Disease Control and Prevention. Human plague—India, 1994. *MMWR* 1994;43:689–91.

8. Centers for Disease Control and Prevention. Fatal human plague—Arizona and Colorado, 1996. *MMWR* 1997;46:617–20.

9. Madon MB, Hitchcock JC, Davis RM, et al. An overview of plague in the United States and a report of investigations of two human cases in Kern County, California, 1995. *J Vector Ecology* 1997;22:77–82.

10. Craven RB, Maupin GO, Beard ML, et al. Reported cases of human plague infections in the United States, 1970–1991. *J Med Entomol* 1993;30:758–61.

11. Anderson SH, Williams ES. Plague in a complex of white-tailed prairie dogs and associated small mammals in Wyoming. *J Wildlife Dis* 1997;33:720–32.

12. Cully JF Jr, Barnes AM, Quan TJ, et al. Dynamics of plague in a Gunnison's prairie dog colony complex from New Mexico. *J Wildlife Dis* 1997;33:706–19.

13. Kaufmann AF, Mann JM, Gardiner TM, et al. Public health implications of plague in domestic cats. *J Am Vet Med Assoc* 1981;179:875–8.

14. Eidson M, Tierney LA, Rollag OJ, et al. Feline plague in New Mexico: risk factors and transmission to humans. *Am J Public Health* 1988;78:1333–5.

15. Werner SB, Weidmer CE, Nelson BC, et al. Primary plague pneumonia contracted from a domestic cat at South lake Tahoe, Calif. *JAMA* 1984;251:929–31.

16. Wilson ME. The power of plague. *Epidemiology* 1995;6:458–60.

17. Cleri DJ, Vernaleo JR, Lombardi LJ, et al. Plague pneumonia disease caused by *Yersinia pestis. Semin Respir Infect* 1997;12:12–23.

18. Centers for Disease Control and Prevention. Human plague—United States, 1981. *MMWR* 1982;31:74–6.

19. Burmeister RW, Tigertt WD, Overholt EL. Laboratory-acquired pneumonic plague: report of a case and review of previous cases. *Ann Intern Med* 1962;56:789–800.

20. Mohan A, Misra A. Use of face masks during a plague epidemic. *Postgrad Med J* 1996;72:127.

21. Fritz CL, Dennis DT, Tipple MA, et al. Surveillance for pneumonic plague in the United States during an international emergency: a model for control of imported emerging diseases. *Emerging Infect Dis* 1996;2:30–6.

22. Crook LD, Tempest B. Plague: a clinical review of 27 cases. *Arch Intern Med* 1992;152:1253–6.

23. Butler T. Yersinia infections: centennial of the discovery of the plague bacillus. *Clin Infect Dis* 1994;19:655–63.

24. Barnes AM, Poland JD. Plague in the United States. 1983. *MMWR* 1984;33:15SS–21SS.

25. Swartz MN. Lymphadenitis and lymphangitis. In: Mandell GL, Bennett JE, Dolin R (eds), *Principles and Practice of Infectious Diseases*, 4th Ed. New York: Churchill Livingstone, 1995. Pp 936–44.

26. Artenstein AW, Kim JH, Williams WJ, et al. Isolated peripheral tuberculous lymphadenitis in adults: current clinical and diagnostic issues. *Clin Infect Dis* 1995; 20:876–82.

27. Galimand M, Guiyoule A, Gerbaud G, et al. Multidrug resistance in *Yersinia pestis* mediated by a transferable plasmid. *N Engl J Med* 1997;337:677–80.

28. Dennis DT, Hughes JM. Multidrug resistance in plague. *N Engl J Med* 1997;337:702–4.

29. Richmond JY, McKinney RW. *Biosafety in Microbiological and Biomedical Laboratories*, 3rd Ed. Washington, DC: U.S. Department of Health and Human Services Public Health Service, 1993.

16 / Occupational Hantavirus Pulmonary Syndrome

Randall L. Updegrove

Viruses classified into the hantavirus genus [1] of the family Bunyaviridae were first isolated in Korea in 1978. However, sporadic epidemics have been attributed to these viruses since the 1930s and, possibly, earlier. The hantaviruses are trisegmented, single-stranded RNA viruses that are lipid enveloped. During the Korean conflict in the 1950s, some 3,000 members of the United Nations forces developed an illness characterized by fever, hemorrhage, and acute renal failure. This illness complex became known by several names, including *Songo fever*, *hemorrhagic nephrosonephritis*, *Korean hemorrhagic fever*, *Manchurian fever*, and *epidemic hemorrhagic fever*. Since then, the illness has been classified as hemorrhagic fever with renal syndrome (HFRS). In 1993, intense multi-agency collaborative efforts led to the identification and characterization of a second illness, first seen in the southwestern United States, caused by a different hantaviral type, known as hantavirus with pulmonary symptoms, or HPS. Information as to the nature of these illnesses, as well as the causative viruses, continues to be refined and expanded, and ongoing research is identifying new viral hosts and viral serotypes of this genus.

Hantavirus pulmonary syndrome (HPS) was first identified in May 1993, after an outbreak of a fatal respiratory illness in the southwestern United States. The first cases were reported in New Mexico, when two Native American residents of the same house died within five days of each other. Over the next months, several other states throughout the southwest, including Arizona, Colorado and Utah, reported similar cases. Using nucleotide sequence analysis and polymerase chain reaction on extracted RNA from autopsy specimens, as well as the identification of antibodies cross-reactive to rodent-borne hantaviruses responsible for HFRS in Eurasia [1], suspicion grew that there was a probable association of this disease with HFRS. The patterns of cross-reactivity in the human convalescent and rodent serum specimens, clinical syndrome dissimilar to that of HFRS, and the pattern of immunohistochemical reactivity associated with this disease, led to the identification of a previously unrecognized hantavirus. Shortly thereafter, the clinical and pathologic features of this syndrome were clarified, risk factors for infection identified, and the primary rodent host found [2–5]. The virus was named the *Four Corners virus* and later, the *Sin Nombre virus*, or *Muerto Canyon virus*. Molecular diagnostic assays as well as serologic testing were quickly developed.

Epidemiology

Although HPS was first identified in 1993, retrospective serologic testing showed evidence of a case as early as 1959 [6], with another case retroactively identified from 1978. Up until 1996, the Centers for Disease Control and Prevention had confirmed 131 cases of HPS in the United States, with an overall case-fatality rate of 49.6%. Of confirmed cases, the mean age is 35 years, with a range of 11 to 69 years. Gender analysis shows no predilection for either sex, with approximately 50% of cases male and 50% female. Cases have occurred in Caucasians as well as African Americans. Any racial or age variations in infection rates are most likely attributable to differences in activities that facilitate exposure to the rodent reservoir for the hantavirus, which is usually in rural settings.

Although the initial cases occurred in the Southwest among Native Americans, 24 additional states have reported cases since 1993. Although most of these cases are west of the Mississippi River, cases have been reported in Rhode Island, New York, Florida, and Louisiana. Outside of the United States, HPS has been identified in Argentina, Canada, Brazil, and Paraguay [7].

TRANSMISSION RISK FACTORS

HPS appears to be caused by multiple agents that together form a distinctive evolutionary class [8]. Three hantavirus serotypes have been identified that cause HPS: Sin Nombre virus (SNV), Black Creek Canal virus (BCCV), and Bayou virus (BV). The Sin Nombre virus has been associated with a case fatality rate 10 times that of the other hantaviruses. SNV is the prototypical HPS and was the first virus isolated from HPS patients, in the spring and summer of 1993 [9]. BCCV has been associated with HPS in Florida [10]. Antigens and viral sequencing of patients with HPS in Texas and Louisiana have identified the presence of BV in that area. In 1993, nucleotide sequence analysis of amplified DNA products from three polymerase chain reaction (PCR) positive humans, and six PCR-positive rodents of the deer mouse species (*Peromycus maniculatus*) showed a closely related, direct genetic link between the hantavirus sequences in the rodents and the human cases. The deer mouse is found throughout the United States, except in the Southeast. It is the principal reservoir for the hantavirus responsible for HPS, carrying SNV.

Rodent infection parallels that found with the hantaviruses associated with HFRS, with the virus shed in saliva, urine, and feces. Human infection occurs in ways similar to that of the HFRS viruses, primarily through transmission by aerosolized virus inhaled from rodent excreta that have inoculated arid materials. In addition, transmission can occur when dried materials contaminated with rodent saliva are disturbed and introduced into disrupted skin, the conjunctivae, or contaminated water or food. Human-to-human transmission has not been seen. The deer mouse is the primary reservoir for the virus in the southwestern United States and Canada [4]. The white-footed mouse (*Peromyscus leucopus*) acts as the main host for a SNV-like virus in the eastern United States [11]. In southern Florida, the cotton rat (*Sigmodon hispidus*) is the reservoir for BCCV, and the rice rat (*Oryzomys palustris*) is the reservoir for the Bayou virus [12]. In addition, hantavirus antibodies have been found in the pinon mouse (*Peromyscus truei*), chipmunk (*Eutamias dorsalis*), the brush mouse (*Peromyscus boylii*), and the western chipmunk (*Tamias* species).

Similar to HFRS virus, outbreaks of HPS appear to be geographically and seasonally influenced, and parallel rodent migrations and eradication efforts. Although little is known about activities that lead to a high risk of infection, studies indicate that entering buildings or areas that are infrequently opened or disturbed contributes to increasing risk [2]. The number of rodents in a house or building obviously contributes to this risk, with rodent-infested structures found to be associated with several cases [13]. Geographic distribution of HPS cases in the United States is strongly tied to more frequent close proximity of humans and the habitats of certain rodent species. For example, the deer mouse and white-footed deer mouse often live near residents and domestic settings. Therefore, the density of their populations can be high in areas frequently visited by humans. Additionally, the rodents tend to migrate indoors, particularly during colder months, and to farms during the fall and spring. Seeking cooler areas, rodents may move to forested areas in the warmer summer months.

OCCUPATIONS AT RISK

Occupations found to be at risk for HPS viral infection, therefore, are those that place workers in the proximity of higher rodent populations during higher risk seasons. Clustering of cases is common. Fortunately, cases of occupationally related HPS virus infection are infrequent [14,15]. Occupations at risk include grain farmers, farm workers, laborers, repairmen, construction workers, animal-pest-control workers, livestock specialists, field biologists, forestry workers, park rangers, mill workers, utility workers, feedlot workers, various technicians, hikers, and service industry workers, as well as others (Table 16-1). In 1994, a study showed the presence of antibody to SNV in six of 528 mammologists and rodent workers in the United States with varying degrees of rodent exposures [15]. Although person-to-person transmission, particularly among hospital employees and patients, has not occurred, infection has occurred in laboratory workers handling rodents. Some of these cases may have involved transmission of the virus via rodent bite.

Prevention and Control

ADMINISTRATIVE CONTROLS

Recommendations to decrease the risk for hantavirus exposure include precautions for individuals or groups working in occupations associated with rodent, rodent excreta, or contaminated dust exposure [16]. In addition, state health departments and the Centers for Disease Control and Prevention (CDC) have formed the *HPS Registry*, through which the effectiveness and usefulness of recommended risk-reduction efforts are assessed. Reporting of new cases by health care providers to these agencies remains paramount for the identification of additional pathogenic hantaviruses, rodent hosts, and risk factors for infection.

Table 16-1
Occupations at Risk for Hantavirus Pulmonary Syndrome

Laboratory workers	Farm workers
Service repairmen	Technicians
Ranch workers	Service industry
Shepherds	Longshoremen
Pest control workers	Immunologists
Maintenance workers	Plumbers
Animal handlers	Granary workers
Construction workers	Mammologists
Field biologists	Park rangers
Mill workers	Utility employees
Laborers	

Prevention and effective treatment of HPS, as well as HFRS, is based on three strategies: minimization of rodent population clusters in the workplace, avoidance of exposure to contaminated materials or aerosolized excreta, and awareness of the early signs of disease, to allow for rapid treatment and medical support. Prevention begins with public awareness, particularly among occupational groups at risk for exposure, who routinely engage in higher risk activities. Some of these activities include living in previously vacant buildings; field crop harvesting or planting; barn cleaning; disturbing rodent-infested areas while in woods or fields; or residing or working in areas with an increasing or relatively high rodent population (including laboratories). Eradication of the rodent reservoirs, however, is infeasible. Risk can be reduced, however, through proper environmental hygiene that deters rodents from colonizing the work area. The CDC has issued recommendations for eliminating rodent infestations by rodent-proofing urban and suburban buildings, and reducing the rodent populations via modification of the rodent habitat and sanitation [17,18] (Table 16-2).

The CDC has also issued general precautions for residents of affected areas, including ways to reduce the rodent population of a residence or workplace. These are primary prevention strategies to reduce risk for hantavirus (Table 16-3). The cleanup of rodent-contaminated areas also involves adherence to recommended procedural steps (Table 16-4).

For individuals working with vacant dwellings that contain large numbers of rodents, or in areas previously occupied by an individual with a confirmed hantavirus infection, the CDC recommends the following precautions (Table 16-5).

MEDICAL SURVEILLANCE

Individuals who work in areas where rodents are likely to congregate, work with rodents directly (particularly those identified as frequent harbingers of the hantavirus), or are involved in cleanup operations or in any other capacity, are associated with a high risk of hantavirus exposure (see above), should undergo medical surveillance for early signs of infection. Medical surveillance is

Table 16-2
CDC Recommendations for Elimination of Rodent Infestations

- Before rodent elimination work begins, ventilate closed buildings or areas inside buildings by opening doors and windows for at least 30 minutes. Use an exhaust fan or cross-ventilation if possible. Leave the area until the airing-out period is finished. This airing may help remove any aerosolized virus inside the closed-in structure.
- Seal, screen, or otherwise cover all openings into the home that have a diameter of <¼ inch. Then, set rodent traps inside the building, using peanut butter as bait. Use only spring-loaded traps that kill rodents.
- Treat the interior of the structure with an insecticide labeled for flea control; follow label instructions. Insecticide sprays or powders can be used in place of aerosols if they are appropriately labeled for flea control. Rodenticides may also be used while the interior is being treated, as outlined below.
- Remove captured rodents from the traps. Wear rubber or plastic gloves while handling rodents. Place the carcasses in a plastic bag containing a sufficient amount of a general-purpose household disinfectant to thoroughly wet the carcasses. Seal the bag, then dispose of it by burying in a 2- to 3-foot-deep hole or by burning. If burying or burning are not feasible, contact the local or state health department about other appropriate disposal methods. Rebait and reset all sprung traps.
- Before removing the gloves, wash gloved hands in a general household disinfectant, then in soap and water. A hypochlorite solution (prepared by mixing three tablespoons of household bleach in 1 gallon of water) may be used in lieu of a commercial disinfectant. When using the chlorine solution, avoid spilling the mixture on clothing or other items that may be damaged. Thoroughly wash hands with soap and water after removing the gloves.
- Leave several baited spring-loaded traps inside the house at all times as a further precaution against rodent reinfestation. Examine the traps regularly. Disinfect traps no longer in use by washing in a general household disinfectant or the hypochlorite solution. Disinfect and wash gloves as described above, and wash hands thoroughly with soap and water before beginning other activities.

From U.S. Dept. of Health and Human Services, Public Health Service. Hantavirus infection—southwestern United States: interim recommendations for risk reduction. MMWR 1993;42(RR-11):1–13.

based on a combination of worker education and early detection (Table 16-6).

Laboratory workers handling rodents should take additional precautions. Certain high-risk techniques, such as intubation of laboratory animals or other activities that tend to generate aerosols, should be completed in biologic safety cabinets with proper exhaust ventilation and filter systems [19]. Laboratory work that may result in propagation of hantaviruses should be conducted in a biosafety level 3 facility [20], with BSL-2 practices recommended for handling clinical specimens, and BSL-3 practices recommended for handling infected tissue and viral cell cultures [21]. In general, however, laboratory workers practicing Universal Precautions while processing routine clinical specimens (blood, urine, or respiratory secretions) are not considered to be at increased risk for hantavirus infection.

BIOLOGIC TESTING

For all workers whose occupations place them in a high-risk group for hantavirus exposure, a baseline serum sample should be obtained and stored at –20°C. In the event of infection, this sample can be tested (along with acute sera) for presence of the hantavirus antigen and antibodies. In addition, convalescent serum is obtained from infected individuals. Analysis using enzyme-linked immunosorbent assay (ELISA) can be used to detect the presence of immunoglobulin M (IgM) and/or rising titers of immunoglobulin G (IgG) antibodies, which are indicative of acute infection. In laboratories, frequent serologic testing of laboratory rats and replacement of infected rodents with seronegative animals are recommended [19]. Serologic surveillance of laboratory personnel is also useful to identify early hantavirus infection. It should be noted that studies have demonstrated evidence of hantavirus antibodies (to SNV and Hantaan virus) in asymptomatic laboratory workers and mammologists with varying degrees of rodent exposure.

IMMUNIZATION

At present, there is no immunization available to the different serotypes of hantavirus.

Table 16-3
CDC Recommendations for Reducing Rodent Populations

- Keep all food and water covered and stored in rodent-proof containers with tight-fitting lids.
- Store all garbage inside the building or in outbuildings in rodent-proof metal or thick plastic containers with tight-fitting lids.
- Wash dishes and cooking utensils immediately after use, and remove all spilled food.
- Dispose of trash and clutter.
- Use spring-loaded rodent traps continuously.
- For an adjunct to traps, use rodenticide with bait under a plywood or plastic shelter (covered bait station) on an ongoing basis inside the house.
- Keep rodents from entering the building:
  - Use steel wool or cement to seal, screen, or otherwise cover all openings into the home that have a diameter of > ¼ inch.
  - Place metal roof flashing as a rodent barrier around the base of wooden, earthen, or adobe dwelling up to a height of 12 inches and buried in the soil to a depth of 6 inches.
  - Place 3 inches of gravel under the base of homes or under mobile homes to discourage rodent burrowing.
- Within 100 feet of the building, reduce food and shelter sources for rodents:
  - Used raised cement foundations in new construction of sheds, barns, outbuildings, or woodpiles.
  - When possible, place woodpiles 100 feet or more from the house, and elevate wood at least 12 inches from the ground.
  - Store grains and animal feed in rodent-proof containers.
  - Near buildings, remove food sources that might attract rodents, or store food and water in rodent-proof containers.
  - Store hay on pallets, and use traps or rodenticide continuously to keep hay free of rodents.
  - Do not leave pet food in feeding dishes.
  - Dispose of garbage and trash in rodent-proof containers that are elevated at least 12 inches off the ground.
  - Haul away trash, abandoned vehicles, discarded tires, and other items that may serve as rodent nesting sites.
  - Cut grass, brush, and dense shrubbery within 100 feet of the home.
  - Place spring-loaded rodent traps at likely spots for rodent shelter within 100 feet around the building, and use continuously.
  - Use an EPA-registered rodenticide approved for outside use in covered bait stations at places likely to shelter rodents within 100 feet of the building.

From U.S. Dept. of Health and Human Services, Public Health Service. Hantavirus infection—southwestern United States: interim recommendations for risk reduction. *MMWR* 1993;42(RR-11):1–13.

Table 16-4
CDC Recommendations for Cleanup of Contaminated Areas

- Persons involved in the cleanup should wear rubber or plastic gloves.
- Spray dead rodents, nests, droppings, foods, or other items that have been tainted by rodents with a general-purpose household disinfectant. Soak the material thoroughly, and place in a plastic bag. When cleanup is complete, or when the bag is full, seal the bag. Then, place the sealed bag into a second plastic bag and seal it. Dispose of the bagged material by burying in a two- to three-foot-deep hole, or by burning. If these alternatives are not feasible, contact the local or state health department concerning other appropriate disposal methods.
- After the above items have been removed, mop floors with a solution of water, detergent, and disinfectant. Spray dirt floors with a disinfectant solution. A second mopping or spraying of floors with a general-purpose household disinfectant is optional. Carpets can be effectively disinfected with household disinfectants or by commercial-grade steam cleaning or shampooing. To avoid generating potentially infectious aerosols, do not vacuum or sweep dry surfaces before mopping.
- Disinfect countertops, cabinets, drawers, and other durable surfaces by washing them with a solution of detergent, water, and disinfectant, followed by an optional wiping-down with a general-purpose household disinfectant.
- Rugs and upholstered furniture should be steam cleaned or shampooed. If rodents have nested inside furniture and the nests are not accessible for decontamination, the furniture should be removed and burned.
- Launder potentially contaminated bedding and clothing with hot water and detergent, handling the dirty laundry with rubber or plastic gloves, then washing or disinfecting the gloves. Machine-dry laundry at a high setting or hang out to air dry in the sun.

From U.S. Dept. of Health and Human Services, Public Health Service. Hantavirus infection—southwestern United States: interim recommendations for risk reduction. *MMWR* 1993;42(RR-11):1–13.

Table 16-5
CDC Recommendations for Work in Contaminated Areas

- A baseline serum sample, preferably drawn at the time these activities are initiated, should be available for all persons conducting the cleanup of homes or building with heavy rodent infestation. The serum sample should be stored at –20°C.
- Persons involved in the cleanup should wear coveralls (disposable if possible), rubber boots or disposable shoe covers, rubber or plastic gloves, protective goggles, and an appropriate respiratory protection device (half-mask air-purifying (or negative-pressure) respirator with a high-efficiency particulate air (HEPA) filter, or a powered air-purifying respirator (PAPR) with HEPA filters). Respirators (even positive-pressure types) are not considered protective if facial hair interferes with the facial seal, since proper fit cannot be assured. Respirator practices should follow a comprehensive user program and be supervised by a knowledgeable person [21, art 9].
- Personal protective equipment (PPE) should be decontaminated upon removal at the end of the day. If the coveralls are not disposable, they should be laundered on site. If no laundry facilities are available, the coveralls should be immersed in liquid disinfectant until they can be washed.
- All potentially infective waste material (including respirator filters) from clean-up operations that cannot be burned or deep buried on site should be double bagged in appropriate plastic bags. The bagged material should then be labeled as infectious (if it is to be transported) and disposed of in accordance with local requirements for infectious waste.
- Workers who develop a febrile or respiratory illness within 45 days of the last potential exposure should immediately seek medical attention and inform the attending physician of the potential occupational risk of hantavirus infection. The physician should contact local health authorities promptly if hantavirus-associated illness is suspected. A blood sample should be obtained and forwarded with the baseline serum through the state health department to CDC for hantavirus antibody testing [art 9].

From U.S. Dept. of Health and Human Services, Public Health Service. Hantavirus infection—southwestern United States: interim recommendations for risk reduction. *MMWR* 1993;42(RR-11):1–13.

Case Study: Hantavirus Pulmonary Syndrome

Two days prior to hospital admission, a 30-year-old plumber sought care at an emergency room complaining of a two-day history of fever, chills, headache, myalgia, nausea with vomiting, and a dry, nonproductive cough. Shortly prior to the onset of symptoms, he recalled working in an old basement, where he noticed several piles of rodent droppings adjacent to pipes. His oral temperature on admission was 103°F (39°C), and his pulse rate 118 bpm. Complete blood count indicated a white blood cell count of 6,600/mm^3 (normal: 4,500–11,000/mm^3) and a decreased platelet count of 117,000/mm^3 (normal: 130,000–400,000/mm^3). A chest radiograph was normal. The man was diagnosed with an acute febrile illness, treated symptomatically, and released to outpatient follow-up.

Two days later, the patient again presented to the emergency room, this time with a persistent fever of 101°F to 104°F, tachycardia (heart rate of 140 bpm), and hypotension (blood pressure of 70/50 mm Hg). On repeat laboratory testing, his white blood cell count had risen mildly to 12,000/mm^3, with a cell differential of 18% neutrophils, 55% bands, 18% lymphocytes, and 2% immature granulocytes. His platelet count had dropped to 35,000/mm^3. Additional laboratory testing showed BUN 38 mg/dL (consistent with mild azotemia), creatinine 2.0 mg/dL (mild elevation), and elevated serum liver enzyme levels (LDH 2487 U/L [normal: 297–628 U/L], AST 226 U/L [normal: 14–50 U/L], and ALT 152 [normal: 7–56 U/L]). Hypoal-buminnemia was present (serum albumin level of 2.0 g/dL). Serum lipase and amylase levels were elevated, at 771 U/L and 226 U/L, respectively, although the patient did not complain of abdominal pain and had a normal abdominal physical examination. Chest radiography performed upon hospital admission showed perihilar interstitial infiltrates. He was hypoxic, with oxygen saturation (room air) of 80%. Over the next three days, he became progressively hypoxemic and developed pulmonary edema and oliguria. With supportive care, including careful fluid monitoring, his symptoms resolved and he was released.

Symptoms and Signs

The spectrum of disease, including severity as well as clinical presentation, is distinctly different in

Table 16-6
CDC Recommendations for Medical Surveillance of Workers in High-Risk Areas

- Obtain a baseline serum sample (at time of hire) and store at –20°C.
- Educational program(s) should be organized and provided to all workers to be involved in potentially high-risk jobs. This program should include, as a minimum, details regarding the types of work associated with the virus, the CDC recommendations for disease prevention as well as cleanup of high-risk sites, and signs and symptoms associated with the disease (both HFRS and HPS).
- High-risk workers who develop a febrile or respiratory illness within 45 days of the last potential exposure should be instructed to seek immediate medical attention and inform the treating health care provider of the possible risk of hantavirus infection. If the provider then suspects hantavirus infection, he/she should alert local health authorities. A serum sample should be obtained and sent to the state health department for forwarding to the CDC for antibody testing for hantavirus.
- Employers should mandate the wearing of half-face air-purifying respirator or PAPR equipped with HEPA filters when removing rodents from traps or handling rodents in the affected area(s). The use of respirators should be in conjunction with a full respirator protection program at the workplace. Therefore, any hantavirus surveillance program should also include a concurrent medical clearance evaluation of respirators, based on the anticipated environmental conditions of use, and the respirator types to be worn.

From U.S. Dept. of Health and Human Services, Public Health Service. Hantavirus infection—southwestern United States: interim recommendations for risk reduction. *MMWR* 1993;42(RR-11):1–13.

patients with HPS compared to those with HFRS. At the time of presentation, no defined set of signs and symptoms dependably distinguishes HPS from other types of noncardiogenic pulmonary edema or adult respiratory distress syndrome (ARDS). HPS patients commonly present with a prodromal illness consisting of *myalgia*, *fever*, *cough*, and *headache* (similar to that of HFRS). Although gastrointestinal symptoms (abdominal pain, nausea, and vomiting) may occur, they are atypical. The initial symptoms usually persist for up to five days prior to hospitalization. Evidence of *respiratory distress*, including tachypnea and tachycardia, develop quite abruptly, with laboratory findings of leukocytosis, vascular volume contraction with hemoconcentration (76% of cases), hypoalbuminemia, and thrombocytopenia (71% of cases). In addition, a moderate increase in serum creatinine (> 2.5 mg/dL) may be seen but is present in only 10% of all fatal cases. Rhabdomyolysis and lactic acidosis may also occur. Although hemorrhagic signs may be evident in patients with HPS, they are not usually as significant as they are in those with HFRS. Chest radiographic findings may initially be lacking (during the prodromal phase), but later they typically provide a picture of evolving pulmonary edema, with extensive bibasilar or perhilar airspace disease found in 70% of cases, and pleural effusions in 60% [22].

The two major life-threatening pathophysiologic changes in HPS are (1) increased permeability pulmonary edema and (2) an atypical form of septic shock, caused by myocardial depression and hypovolemia [23]. Hypoxia is progressive and can be rapid (as can the development of pulmonary edema), not infrequently occurring within the first 24 hours of admission. Survival is threatened with the development of hypotension or hypoxia, with death more likely if both develop. Hypotension is not necessarily a direct consequence of hypoxia, for patients may be able to maintain adequate oxygenation while developing progressive hypoxia [24,25]. Patients develop severe pulmonary capillary leak syndrome with abnormal gas exchange. Although this can sometimes be reversed by mechanical ventilation, patients frequently die as a result of cardiovascular collapse [26]. Myocardial involvement secondary to infection is suggested by the onset of death, often secondary to diminished cardiac output and terminal electromechanical dissociation, with dysrhythmias preterminally [27]. The mortality rate of HPS is approximately 50%. In those who survive, recovery is usually complete.

Pulmonary histology of patients with HPS shows alveoli engorged with proteinaceous fluid, with few inflammatory cells. Heart and kidney tissue, however, show no evidence of necrosis or inflammation [28].

In addition to clinical diagnosis, serologic tests (detection of Four Corners virus-specific antibodies in serum by Western blot assays), in combination with reverse transcriptase-polymerase chain reaction (RT-PCR) (to identify Four Corners virus RNA in peripheral blood mononuclear cells) and detection of hantavirus antigen by immunohistochemistry (IHC), should be used to confirm the clinical diagnosis of acute infection. Detection of hantavirus IgM antibodies in serum, or a fourfold or greater rise in serum IgG antibodies to hantavirus, confirms the diagnosis.

The CDC, in an attempt to alert clinicians to the usual presentation of this initially nondescript illness, has identified clinical features that help to identify cases (Table 16-7).

Treatment

There is no definitive treatment for HPS at present, but the foundations of treatment include early recognition and rapid provision of full supportive measures. Rapid recognition of likely hantavirus infection and immediate institution of full supportive measures in an intensive care unit setting have been associated with better patient outcome. Prolonged periods of hypoxia or hypotension prior to stabilization portend a higher risk of death [24]. Mechanical ventilation or supplemental oxygen is frequently necessary. To maintain adequate cardiac output, inotropic and pressor agents, with judicious fluid administration, are often used; central pressure and cardiac monitoring is important when using these agents. Ribavirin, an antiviral agent, has been used with mixed results in vivo but has been found to be active against hantavirus in vitro. To date, however, ribavirin has not been shown to improve mortality from HPS, although it may have some use in treatment in the future. Adverse effects of ribavirin have necessitated blood transfusions in several patients [26,29].

Differential Diagnosis

Particularly in the early stages of disease, hantavirus is very easily misdiagnosed, owing to

Table 16-7
CDC Screening Criteria for Hantavirus Pulmonary Syndrome in Persons with Unexplained Respiratory Illness

Potential case-patients must have one of the following:

- A febrile illness (>101° F (38.3°C) occurring in a previously healthy person characterized by unexplained adult respiratory distress syndrome, *or* bilateral interstitial pulmonary infiltrates developing within one week of hospitalization with respiratory compromise requiring supplemental oxygen

  or

- An unexplained respiratory illness resulting in death in conjunction with an autopsy examination demonstrating noncardiogenic pulmonary edema without an identifiable specific cause of death

Potential case-patients are to be ***excluded*** if they have any of the following:

- A predisposing underlying medical condition (e.g., severe underlying pulmonary disease, solid tumors or hematological malignancies, congenital or acquired immunodeficiency disorders, or medical conditions [e.g., rheumatoid arthritis or organ transplant recipients] requiring immunosuppressive drug therapy [e.g., steroids or cytotoxic chemotherapy])
- An acute illness that provides a likely explanation for the respiratory illness (e.g., recent major trauma, burn, or surgery; recent seizures or history of aspiration; bacterial sepsis; another respiratory disorder such as respiratory syncytial virus in young children; influenza; or legionella pneumonia)

Confirmed case-patients must have the following:

- At least one specimen (e.g., serum and/or tissue) available for laboratory testing for evidence of hantavirus infection

  and

- In a patient with a compatible clinical illness, either serology (presence of hantavirus-specific immunoglobulin M or rising titers of immunoglobulin G), polymerase chain reaction for hantavirus ribonucleic acid, or immunohistochemistry for hantavirus antigen is positive its nonspecific symptoms. The hantavirus prodrome very closely resembles the symptoms of influenza, namely fever, myalgias, headache, and chills. Influenza cases, however, are more likely to present sore throat and cough [30]. Patients with severe abdominal pain are sometimes misdiagnosed with acute abdomen, and occasionally these hantavirus patients are admitted to surgical wards. Aseptic meningitis can present similarly; however, the absence of sore throat, coryza, and meningismus are distinguishing factors. Patients with pneumococcal pneumonia can usually be distinguished from those with HPS because lobar infiltrates on CXR are more likely in pneumococcal pneumonia than in HPS [30]. In one study, multivariate discriminate analysis revealed that three clinical characteristics at admission (nausea and/or vomiting, lack of cough, and dizziness), along with three initial laboratory abnormalities (decreased platelet count, serum bicarbonate level, and increased hematocrit level), were key to identifying all patients with HPS and in excluding HPS in at least 80% of patients with unexplained ARDS [30]. The classic hantavirus pulmonary virus infection is marked by a nonspecific prodrome, followed by *abrupt* deterioration of pulmonary function and development of ARDS and hypotension. This pattern of infection, along with characteristic laboratory findings (noted above) and confirmation of hantavirus antibodies, along with strong clinical suspicion and a recent history consistent with probable rodent excreta exposure, allows astute clinicians to distinguish HPS from several other infectious agents (Table 16-8).

Table 16-8
Differential Diagnosis of Hantavirus Pulmonary Syndrome

Influenza	Aseptic meningitis
Unexplained ARDS	Pneumonic plague
Pneumococcal bacteremia	Psittacosis
Histoplasmosis	Severe mycoplasma pneumonia
Tularemia (pulmonary)	Legionellosis
Meningococcemia	Leptospirosis
Disseminated fungal infection	Rickettsial infection

Hemorrhagic Fever with Renal Syndrome

EPIDEMIOLOGY

The hantaviruses associated with HFRS generally cause an acute interstitial nephropathy with fever, hemorrhage of variable severity, and renal insufficiency, which frequently lead to hypotension and shock [31–34]. Historically, hantaviruses have fallen into four types: Hantaan (the protypical hantavirus), Seoul, Puumala, and Prospect Hill. Five additional serotypes (Dobrava/Belgrade, Leakey, Thailand, Thotta-payalam) have been identified as additional serotypes [4,34–38]. A fairly unique feature of the hantaviruses (among the other members of the Bunyaviridae family) is their high specificity for rodent species. The hantaviruses are rarely transmitted by arthropod vectors [39]. The viruses are, then, endemic to regions with rodent populations that are associated with specific hantavirus types. The first hantavirus was discovered in 1976, although hantavirus-induced disease has been identified since the 1930s [39,40].

Study of the epizootology of the hantavirus types responsible for HFRS unveils a large distribution throughout the world. Hantaan virus (HV) is most often found in rodents in Asia. Puumula virus (PV), on the other hand, is found in Scandinavia and eastern Europe, including eastern Russia, again in rodent hosts [41]. Prospect Hill virus (PHV) was first isolated in Maryland [41,42]. Seoul virus is found in the common rat, which is why it has the largest geographic distribution of all of the hantaviruses, thanks largely to worldwide shipping [39]. Phylogenetically, HV and SV are most closely related, and PV and PHV are the most closely linked [43].

The primary reservoir for the hantaviruses are rodents [39]. Exposure to nesting materials heavily contaminated with infectious secretions and excretions, grooming behavior, and intraspecies wounding by biting are significant factors in the continuation of the enzootic cycle [33,44]. Rats weighing in excess of 300 g—that is, reproductively mature—and displaying aggressive behavior appear to have a higher seroprevalence of infection [45–48].

The individual viral serotypes are rodent-specific, and the rodents are carriers but have no apparent disease [49]. The virus appears to persist in the reservoir animals and is shed very slowly. Once rodent infection occurs, viremia ensues for a short period of time, with the production of host antibodies to the virus and with viral dissemination to the lungs, salivary glands, and kidneys. Although the antibodies probably remain for the rest of the host's life and protect the host from acquiring disease, viral shedding persists.

Human infection usually occurs after disruption of reservoir rodent populations, primarily via inhalation of aerosolized infected rodent excreta, although rodent saliva also contains virus, making bites another route of transmission to humans. In addition, direct contamination of food or household items with infected rodent excreta can lead to transmission to humans.

The severity of infection varies significantly, depending on the causative virus involved. For example, although antibodies for the Prospect Hill virus (PH) have been frequently identified in individuals' sera, no manifestations of illness have been associated with the virus to date. Prior to the identification of HPS, PH was the only indigenous North American hantavirus. Of the four major serotypes, Hantaan, Puumala, and Seoul are known human pathogens. The Puumala virus is associated with a mild form of disease (without shock and hemorrhage), known as nephropathia epidemica [4, art 3]. Although usually associated with mild disease, infection by the Seoul virus occasionally leads to severe illness and death in humans. HFRS due to Hantaan virus infection usually begins with an abrupt onset and progresses through five stages before resolution. The Dobrava virus has been identified mostly in the Balkans, where it can also be associated with severe HFRS.

Person-to-person transmission of any of the hantaviruses has not been reported. Health care workers, therefore, do not appear to be vulnerable to infection via treatment of infected patients [1]. However, laboratory workers handling infected laboratory rodents have been found to be at risk [45,50–52].

Although no confirmed cases of HFRS have been identified in North America, the illness is well known in various other regions of the world. In China, cases of HFRS have been retrospectively identified from 1931 to 1942, among Japanese soldiers. It was known as *atypical scarlet fever*, *acute nephritis*, *hemorrhagic typhus*, and others [53]. From 1950 to 1990, 904,995 people residing in China became infected with the disease; the average morbidity was 2.69/100,000, with 38,965 deaths (case fatality rate of 4.31%) [53]. Currently, outbreaks of HFRS continue to occur in approximately 30 Chinese areas.

In addition to being region-specific in its distribution, hantavirus infection is also seasonal. A periodicity of infection and epidemics exists, related to host ecology, human control efforts, and human and (host) animal natural immunity [54]. Generally, epidemic peaks occur in winter (rural regions), summer (forest regions), and spring (urban regions). The reason for this lies in the host ecology. In the spring and fall (less harsh months), rodents prefer to live in fields. In the summer, the forests provide a cool respite from the hot sun's rays. In the winter months, however, many rodents seek warmer, more pleasant shelter indoors. This migration of the host provides the foundation for the relatively increased incidence of human infection in the spring and fall months in farm workers, in park rangers and hikers in the summer, and in indoor workers in the winter months. Eradication efforts aimed at minimizing the rodent population have been successful at lowering the incidence of disease, while large rodent populations in areas with no or poor population reduction efforts have led to increased incidence of infection.

Hantavirus-induced HFRS is found in eastern Russia, Korea, and China. The distribution parallels the range of the striped field mouse [39,41]. HV-infected mice in Korea display a seasonal movement pattern that mirrors the HV disease rates in that country. The mice are reproductively active in the fall and spring, producing large numbers of gravid mice, which excrete more urine than nongravid mice, leading to higher amounts of aerosolized virus in the air during these seasons. Fall and spring also happen to be the planting and harvesting times [28]. The combination of increased aerosolized virus in the fields and increased time in the fields by agricultural workers (during planting and harvesting) leads to greater potential viral exposure and infection risk. In Sweden, PV is found in the bank vole, and disease incidence has been correlated with the size of the vole population for a given year [41]. In HFRS-endemic areas in eastern Europe, Asia and Scandinavia, well-demarcated "microfoci" of disease are found, making this a "place disease" [55].

In 1976, Lee and Lee first isolated Hantaan virus in the lung tissue of striped field mice from a region of Korea endemic for HFRS. Following this discovery, serologic diagnosis of HV infection identified several genera of rodents in varied geographic areas that harbor the virus [32] (Table 16-9). The principal reservoirs of hantaviruses are rodents of the superfamily Muroidea and the family Muridae (genera: *Apodemus*, *Mus*, and *Rattus*) and the family Arvicolidae (genera: *Microtus* and *Clethrionomys*). *Rattus Norvegicus* (Norway rats), as well

Table 16-9
Hantavirus Infection in the United States: Rodent and Mammal Hosts

Region	Species
Northeast	
New York City	*R norvegicus*
Philadelphia	*R norvegicus*
Pennsylvania	*M pennsylvanicus*
Mid-Atlantic	
Baltimore	*R norvegicus*
	M pennsylvanicus
	P leucopus
	M musculus
	Tamias striatus
	B brevicauda
	Sciurus carolinensis
Fairfax, Virginia	
Frederick, Maryland	*M pennsylvanicus*
	M leucopus
	Tamiasciurus hudsonicus
	B brevicauda
	Pitymys pinetorum
West Virginia	*M pennsylvanicus*
	P maniculatus
	Microtus chrotorrhinus
	P leucopus
	C gapperi
Pocahontus, West Virginia	*C gapperi*
Southeast	
New Orleans	*R norvegicus*
Miami	*R norvegicus*
Houston	R norvegicus
Galveston, Texas	*R norvegicus*
Arkansas	*R norvegicus*
Del Rio and Leakey, Texas	*Perognathus flavus*
	P hispidus
	M musculus
	S hispidus
Southwest	
Los Angeles	*R norvegicus*
New Mexico	*P maniculatus*
	M californicus
	P truei
	Peromyscus boylii
	Peromyscus crinitus
	N cinerea
	P difficilis
	N mexicana
West	
San Francisco	*R norvegicus*
Denver	*R norvegicus*
Seattle	*R norvegicus*
Tacoma, Washington	*R norvegicus*
Portland, Oregon	*R norvegicus*
Sacramento, California	*R norvegicus*
Oakland, California	*R norvegicus*
Monterey, California	*M californicus*
San Mateo, California	*M californicus*
California (General), Colorado (General), and New Mexico (General)	*P maniculatus*
	N mexicana
	N cinerea
	P californicus
	P truei
	P difficilis
	M californicus
	Peromyscus crinitus
	Peromyscus boylii
Snow Canyon, Utah	*P boylii*
	Peromyscus eremicus
	P crinitus
	Onychomys torridus
	Dipodomys merriami
	Neotoma lepida
Far West	
Alaska	*C rutilus*
	M pennsylvanicus
Hawaii (Hilo, Oahu, Maui)	*R norvegicus*

as some species of *Clethrionomys* and *Microtus*, are found in Scandinavia and the Americas. The prototypical rodent Hantaan virus reservoir, *Apodemus* (mouse) genus, is not found in the Americas. However, serologic evidence of a relative of the Hantaan virus, the Prospect Hill virus, has been isolated from the meadow vole (*Microtus pennsylvanicus*), particularly those weighing more than 50 g [56,57]. Also, the Seoul virus has been isolated from Norway rats found in the United States, in Philadelphia, Houston, New Orleans, and Baltimore [58–61]. Although no verified cases of HFRS have occurred in the United States to date, hantaviruses found in members of the *Rattus* genus were identical to hantaviruses in Japan and Korea responsible for causing disease [1,51,52]. Hantavirus-infected rats have also been identified in other areas of the United States, including Columbus, Ohio, New York City, Honolulu, and San Francisco. Leakey, Texas is the home of the Leakey virus, identified in a mouse frequently found in homes, *Mus musculus*, and antigenically dissimilar from the previously recognized hantavirus serotypes [35]. Prospect-Hill-like hantavirus antibodies have also been found in other species, including *Clethrionomys rutilus*, *Peromyscus difficilis*, *Peromyscus truei*, *Neotoma mexicana*, *Neotoma cinerea*, *Peromyscus maniculatus*, *Peromyscus californicus*, and *Clethrionomys gapperi*, *Microtus californicus*, and *Peromyscus leucopus* in Virginia, West Virginia, California, Minnesota, Colorado, Alaska, Maryland, and New Mexico [46–48,56–58,62].

In addition to rodents, other animals have been associated with hantavirus and HFRS. In Maryland, for example, cats (*Felis catus*) have shown antibodies to hantavirus, while in China, musk shrews (*Suncus murinus*) have been implicated in the spread of disease [63]. Other small mammals (the short-tailed shrew *Blarina brevicauda* and the long-tailed weasel *Mustela frenata*) [47,48,57], as well as bats [64] may harbor hantavirus-related viruses (Table 16-9).

Case Study: HFRS

Two weeks prior to presentation, the patient, a 25-year-old college student, had participated in the restoration of an old barn at his parents' vacation home in Sweden. He felt well until three days before presentation, when he developed a headache, fever, abdominal and lower back pain, and a reddened face. Just prior to being seen by a physician, he also developed cutaneous hemorrhage. When first evaluated, his temperature was 38° C; his blood pressure was 120/78. He was initially treated empirically with antibiotics but returned the next day feeling worse and with persistent fever. Admission laboratory tests indicated hemoconcentration, thrombocytopenia, and leukocytosis and elevated serum creatinine, with proteinuria and hematuria. Shortly after admission to the hospital, he abruptly developed renal failure and hypovolemic shock (over 24 hours). A Swan-Ganz catheter was placed, with findings of low cardiac output and increased systemic vascular resistance. He was treated with judicious use of intravenous fluid therapy as well as inotropic agents. His renal function improved over the next few days, although diuresis requiring potassium replacement was noted. He continued to improve over the next few weeks and dieresis ceased. He was released three weeks after admission; no sequelae were noted at a follow-up visit.

Clinical Manifestations

Each of the hantavirus types infects a single rodent species, with lifelong asymptomatic infection. The virus is transmitted horizontally among rodents, and infected rodents shed virus in saliva, urine, and feces for several weeks after infection. The incubation period for human infections ranges from four days to six weeks (average 12–16 days), and the duration of disease, from 11 to 42 days.

HANTAAN VIRUS

The most severe form of HFRS occurs with infection by the Hantaan virus; fatality rates are 5–15%. This virus occurs in Asia and is the prototypical model of HFRS. HFRS caused by HV is usually abrupt in onset. Five distinct clinical phases have been described, as infection progresses in an infected individual: *febrile*, *hy-*

potensive, *oliguric*, *diuretic*, and *convalescent*. The delineation of these phases may be less evident in milder infections. Severe infection usually occurs with the Dobrava virus.

The first, or febrile, phase usually spans three to five days and is marked by the onset of headache, widespread petechiae, facial flushing, and lumbar and abdominal pain. This is followed by the hypotensive phase, marked by the onset of shock, with low cardiac output and increased systemic vascular resistance. The cause of shock is unknown; however, involvement of several mediators, including kinin activation, have been studied [22]. During this phase, thrombocytopenia, hemoconcentration, and leukocytosis are seen. The oliguric phase follows, with associated hypertension. If careful fluid monitoring is not conducted, pulmonary edema and respiratory distress can occur, as a result of volume overload. Hemorrhagic complications and DIC can occur during this phase, as during the preceding two stages. If the patient survives the first three stages, the diuretic phase ensues, marked by possible electrolyte abnormalities. Hyposthenuria marks the beginning of the final, convalescent phase, often persisting for weeks. Full recovery is common.

SEOUL AND PUUMULA VIRUSES

Infection with the Seoul or Puumula virus usually leads to a milder form of HFRS than that with the Hantaan virus, with fatality rates of less than 1%. The Seoul virus is distributed worldwide, although no reported cases of infection have been reported in the United States. The Puumula virus, identified in Scandinavia and several European countries, is associated with a form of HFRS known as nephropathia epidemica [64–66]. This infection is characterized by fever, abdominal pain, back pain, and renal impairment. Nephropathia epidemica usually carries a favorable prognosis, but permanent renal effects may occur. The Prospect Hill virus, indigenous to North America, is currently not associated with disease, but serologic evidence of infection has been identified in individuals. Mild cases of HFRS may have occurred in the United States but had been overlooked or attributed to other causes. Additionally, several other strains of hantavirus, such as the Girard Point virus (isolated from *Rattus norvegicus* in Philadelphia and Houston [60]) and the Baltimore isolate [59], have been identified, although their contribution to disease is unclear.

As noted above, in HFRS, as in HPS, the reservoirs for the viruses are rodents. In addition, the mode of transmission from rodent to human is identical. Therefore, recommended methods of disease control, safe work practices, preventive and medical treatment measures, as well as the occupational groups at risk are similar for both diseases. Additionally, treatment measures are the same, based on early recognition and intensive supportive measures. The reader is therefore referred to the above discussion regarding these topics (see Hantavirus pulmonary syndrome) for further review.

References

1. Schmaljohn CS, Hasty SE, Dalrymple JM, et al. Antigenic and genetic properties of viruses linked to hemorrhagic fever with renal syndrome. *Science* 1985; 227:1041–4.
2. Zeitz PS, Butler JC, Cheek JE, et al. A case-control study of hantavirus pulmonary syndrome during an outbreak in the southwestern United States. *J Infect Dis* 1995;171:864–70.
3. Duchin JS, Koster FT, Peters CJ, et al. Hantavirus pulmonary syndrome: a clinical description of 17 patients with a newly recognized disease. *N Engl J Med* 1994;14:949–1005.
4. Childs JE, Ksiazek TG, Spiropoulou CF, et al. Serologic and genetic identification of *Peromyscus maniculatus* as the primary rodent reservoir for a new hantavirus in the southwestern United States. *J Infect Dis* 1994;169:1271–80.
5. Zaki SR, Greer PW, Coffield LM, et al. Hantavirus pulmonary syndrome: pathogenesis of an emerging infectious disease. *Am J Pathol* 1995;146:552–79.
6. Frampton JW, Lanser S, Nichols CR, et al. Sin Nombre virus infection in 1959. *Lancet* 1995;346:781–2.
7. Laboratory Centre for Disease Control. First reported cases of hantavirus pulmonary syndrome in Canada. *Canada Communicable Dis Rep* 1994;20:121–8.
8. Hjelle B, Krolikowske J, Torrez-Martinez N, et al. Phylogenetically distinct hantavirus implicated in a case of hantavirus pulmonary syndrome in the northeastern United States. *J Med Virol* 1995;46(1):21–7.
9. Elliott LH, Ksiazek TG, Rollin PE, et al. Isolation of the causative agent of hantavirus pulmonary syndrome. *Am J Trop Med Hyg* 1994;51:102–8.

10. Khan AS, Spiropoulou CF, Morzunov S, et al. Fatal illness associated with a new hantavirus in Louisiana. *J Med Virol* 1995;46:281–6.
11. Song JW, Lack LJ, Gajdusek DC, et al. Isolation of pathogenic hantavirus from white-footed mouse (*Peromyscus leucopus*). *Lancet* 1994;344:1637.
12. Torrez-Martinez N, Hjelle B. Enzootic of Bayou hantavirus in rice rats (*Oryzomys palustris*) in 1983. *Lancet* 1994;344:1637.
13. Armstrong LR, Zaki SR, Goldoft MW, et al. Hantavirus pulmonary syndrome associated with entering or cleaning rarely used, rodent-infested structures. *J Infect Dis* 1995;172:1166.
14. Zeitz PS, Graber JM, Voorhees RA, et al. Assessment of occupational risk for hantavirus infection in mammalogists and rodent workers (Abstract no. H57). Abstracts of the 35th Interscience Conference on Antimicrobial Agents and Chemotherapy. Washington, DC: American Society for Microbiology 1995. P 190.
15. Armstrong LR, Khabbaz RF, Childs JE, et al. Occupational exposure to hantavirus in mammalogists and rodent workers (Abstract). *Am J Trop Med Hyg* 1994; 51(suppl):94.
16. Centers for Disease Control. Hantavirus infection—southwestern United States: interim recommendations for risk reduction. *MMWR* 1993;42(no. RR-11).
17. Pratt HD, Brown RZ. *Biological factors in domestic rodent control.* Washington, DC: U.S. Government Printing Office, DHEW Publication No. (CDC) 79-8144, 1979.
18. Scott HG, Borom MR. *Rodent-borne disease control through rodent stoppage.* Washington, DC: U.S. Government Printing Office, DHEW Publication No. (CDC) 77-8343, 1977.
19. Wong TW, Chan YC, Yap EH, et al. Serological evidence of hantavirus infection in laboratory rats and personnel. *Int J Epidemiol* 1988;17:887–90.
20. Centers for Disease Control/National Institutes of Health. *Biosafety in microbiological and biomedical laboratories*, 2nd Ed. DHHS publication no. (CDC) 88-8395. Atlanta: CDC, 1988.
21. Sewell DL. Laboratory-associated infections and biosafety. *Clin Microbiol Rev* 1995;8:389–405.
22. Butler JC, Peters CJ. Hantaviruses and hantavirus pulmonary syndrome. *Clin Infect Dis* 1994;19:387–95.
23. Hallin GW, Simpson SQ, Crowell RE, et al. Cardiopulmonary manifestations of hantavirus pulmonary syndrome. *Crit Care Med* 1996;24(2):252–8.
24. Centers for Disease Control. Update: hantavirus pulmonary syndrome—United States, 1993. *MMWR* 1993;42:816–20.
25. Duchin JS, Koster FT, Peters CJ, et al. Hantavirus pulmonary syndrome: a clinical description of 17 patients with a newly recognized disease. *N Engl J Med* 1994;330:949–55.
26. Levy H. Clinical Course: Management and Pathology of Hantavirus Pulmonary Syndrome (Abstract from Session 67). Presented at the American Society for Microbiology's 34th Interscience Conference on Antimicrobial Agents and Chemotherapy, Orlando, FL, October 4–7, 1994.
27. Jenison S, Hjelle B, Simpson S, et al. Hantavirus pulmonary syndrome: clinical, diagnostic, and virologic aspects. *Semin Respir Infect* 1995;10(4):259–69.
28. Morrison YY, Rathbun RC. Hantavirus pulmonary syndrome: the four corners disease. *Ann Pharmacol* 1995;29:57–63.
29. Chapman LE, Mertz G, Khan AS, et al. Open Label Intravenous Ribavirin for Hantavirus Pulmonary Syndrome (Abstract H111). Presented at the American Society for Microbiology's 34th Interscience Conference on Antimicrobial Agents and Chemotherapy, Orlando, FL, October 4–7, 1994.
30. Moolenaar RL, Dalton C, Lipman HB, et al. Clinical features that differentiate hantavirus pulmonary syndrome from three other acute respiratory illnesses. *Clin Infect Dis* 1995;21(3):643–9.
31. Lahdevirta J. Nephropathia epidemica in Finland: a clinical, histological and epidemiological study. *Ann Clin Res* 1971;3(suppl 8):1–154.
32. Yanagihara R, Gajdusek DC. Hemorrhagic fever with renal syndrome: a historical perspective and review of recent advances. In: Gear JHS (ed), *CRC Handbook of Viral and Rickettsial Hemorrhagic Fevers.* Boca Raton, FL: CRC Press, 1988. Pp 151–88.
33. Lee HW, Lee PW. Korean hemorrhagic fever. II. Isolation of etiologic agent. *Korean J Virol* 1977;7:19–29.
34. Xiao SY, LeDuc JW, Chu YK, et al. Phylogenetic analyses of virus isolates in the genus *Hantavirus*, family Bunyaviridae. *Virology* 1994;198:205-17.
35. Baek LJ, Yanagihara R, Gibbs CJ Jr, et al. Leakey virus: a new hantavirus isolated from *Mus musculus* in the United States. *J Gen Virol* 1988;69:3129–32.
36. Avsic-Zupanc T, Xiao SY, Stojanovic R, et al. Characterization of Dobrava virus: a hantavirus from Slovenia, Yugoslavia. *J Infect Dis* 1992;38:132–7.
37. Gligic A, Dimkovic N, Xiao SY, et al. Belgrade virus: a new hantavirus causing severe hemorrhagic fever with renal syndrome in Yugoslavia. *J Infect Dis* 1992; 166:113–20.
38. Chu YK, Rossi C, LeDuc JW, et al. Serological relationships among viruses in the *Hantavirus* genus, family Bunyaviridae. *Virology* 1994;198:196–204.
39. LeDuc JW, Childs JE, Glass GE. The hantaviruses, etiologic agents of hemorrhagic fever with renal syndrome: a possible cause of hypertension and chronic renal disease in the United States. *Ann Rev Public Health* 1992;13:79–98.
40. Lee HW, Lee PW, Johnson KM. Isolation of the etiologic agent of Korean hemorrhagic fever. *J Infect Dis* 1978;137:298–308.
41. LeDuc JW. Epidemiology of Hantaan and related viruses. *Lab Anim Sci* 1987;37:413–8.

42. Lee PW, Amyx HL, Gajdusek DC, et al. New hemorrhagic fever with renal syndrome-related virus in indigenous wild rodents in United States (letter). *Lancet* 1982;2:1405.
43. Nichol ST, Spiropoulou CF, Morzunov S, et al. Genetic identification of a hantavirus associated with an outbreak of acute respiratory illness. *Science* 1993;262: 914–7.
44. Glass GE, Childs JE, Korch GW, et al. Association of intraspecific wounding with hantaviral infection in wild rats (*Rattus norvegicus*). *Epidemiol Infect* 1988;101: 459–72.
45. Childs JE, Korch GW, Smith GA, et al. Geographical distribution and age-related prevalence of Hantaan-like virus in rat populations of Baltimore, Maryland, U.S.A. *Am J Trop Med Hyg* 1985;34:385–7.
46. Korch GW, Childs JE, Glass GE, et al. Serological evidence of hantaviral infections within small mammal communities of Baltimore, Maryland: spatial and temporal patterns and host range. *Am J Trop Med Hyg* 1989;41:230–40.
47. Childs JE, Glass GE, Korch GW, et al. Prospective seroepidemiology of hantaviruses and population dynamics of small mammal communities of Baltimore, Maryland. *Am J Trop Med Hyg* 1987;37:648–52.
48. Childs JE, Glass GE, Korch GW, et al. The ecology and epizootiology of hantaviral infections in small mammal communities of Baltimore, Maryland: a review and synthesis. *Bull Soc Vector Ecol* 1988;13:113–22.
49. Lee HW, Baek LJ, Johnson KM. Isolation of Hantaan virus, the etiologic agent of Korean hemorrhagic fever, from wild urban rats. *J Infect Dis* 1982;146:638–44.
50. Lee PW, Gibbs CJ Jr, Gajdusek DC, et al. Serotypic classification of hantaviruses by indirect immunofluorescent antibody and plaque reduction neutralization tests. *J Clin Microbiol* 1985;22:940–4.
51. Dantas JR Jr, Okuno Y, Tanishita O, et al. Viruses of hemorrhagic fever with renal syndrome (HFRS) grouped by immunoprecipitation and hemagglutination inhibition. *Intervirology* 1987;27:161–5.
52. Sugiyama K, Matsuura Y, Morita C, et al. Determination of immune adherence HA of the antigenic relationship between *Rattus*- and *Apodemus*-borne viruses causing hemorrhagic fever with renal syndrome. *J Infect Dis* 1984;149:472.
53. Chen HX, Qiu FX. Epidemiological survey: epidemiologic surveillance on the hemorrhagic fever with renal syndrome in China. *Chinese Med J* 1993;106(11):857–63.
54. Chen HX, Qiu FX, Dong BJ, et al. Epidemiological studies on hemorrhagic fever with renal syndrome in China. *J Infect Dis* 1986;154:394.
55. Smadel JE. Epidemic hemorrhagic fever. *Am J Public Health* 1953;43:1327–30.
56. Lee PW, Amyx HL, Gajdusek DC, et al. New hemorrhagic fever with renal syndrome-related virus in indigenous wild rodents in United States. *Lancet* 1982; 2:1405.
57. Lee PW, Amyx HL, Yanagihara R, et al. Partial characterization of Prospect Hill virus isolated from meadow voles in the United States. *J Infect Dis* 1985;152: 826–9.
58. Tsai TF, Bauer SP, Sasso DR, et al. Epizootiologic and epidemiologic investigations of Hantaan virus-related infections in the United States. In: Bender TR, Diwan AR, Raymond JS (eds), Hemorrhagic fever with renal syndrome. Honolulu: School of Public Health, University of Hawaii, 1985:18–22.
59. Childs JE, Korch GW, Glass GE, et al. Epizootiology of hantavirus infections in Baltimore: isolation of a virus from Norway rats and characteristics of infected rat populations. *Am J Epidemiol* 1987;126:55–68.
60. LeDuc JW, Smith GA, Johnson KM. Hantaan-like viruses from domestic rats captured in the United States. *Am J Trop Med Hyg* 1984;33:992–8.
61. LeDuc JW, Smith GA, Johnson KM, et al. Urban rats as hosts of Hantaan-like viruses in the Americas. In: Bender TR, Diwan AR, Raymond JS (eds), *Hemorrhagic fever with renal syndrome*. Honolulu: School of Public Health, University of Hawaii, 1985;15–7.
62. Lee PW, Yanagihara R, Franko MC, et al. Preliminary evidence that Hantaan or a closely related virus is enzootic in domestic rodents. *N Engl J Med* 1982; 307:624–5.
63. Tang YW, Xu ZY, Zhu ZY, et al. Isolation of a haemorrhagic fever with renal (HFRS) virus from Suncus Murinus, an insectivore. *Lancet* 1985;1:513–4.
64. Kim GR, Lee YT, Park CH. A new natural reservoir of hantavirus: isolation of hantaviruses from lung tissues of bats. *Arch Virol* 1994;134(1–2):85–95.
65. Gajdusek DC. Virus hemorrhagic fevers–special reference to hemorrhagic fever with renal syndrome (epidemic hemorrhagic fever). *J Pediatr* 1962;60:841–57.
66. Settergren B. Nephropathia epidemica (hemorrhagic fever with renal syndrome) in Scandinavia. *Rev Infect Dis* 1991;13:736–44.

17 / Occupational Hepatitis

Daniel A. Nackley

Hepatitis is a general term that indicates hepatic inflammation. *Viral hepatitis* is reserved for diseases characterized by inflammation of the liver due to several infectious viruses [1].

Hepatitis may be inapparent, with a subclinical presentation, or may cause a period of self-limited incapacitation. Depending on the etiology, the disease may become chronic. In rare instances, it progresses to fulminant hepatic inflammation [2].

Infectious hepatitis is not unique to any one population or group, but it was the emergence of the AIDS epidemic in the early 1980s that drew renewed attention to the significant risks of hepatitis and other infectious diseases in health care workers. Increasing attention was focused on the use of Universal Precautions (which have now been replaced with Standard Precautions), as well as immunizing health care workers against hepatitis B. Several landmark pieces of legislation and recommendations were promulgated by the National Institutes of Occupational Health and Safety (NIOSH) and by Congress. These included the Guidelines for Protecting the Safety and Health of Health Care Workers (NIOSH); Public Law 100-607; the Health Omnibus Programs Extension Act of 1988, Title II, Programs with Respect to Acquired Immune Deficiency Syndrome; and Guidelines for Prevention of Transmission of Human Immunodeficiency Virus and Hepatitis B Virus to Health-Care and Public Safety Workers: A Response to P.L. 100-607, the Health Omnibus Programs Extension Act of 1988.

These pieces of legislation and agency recommendations culminated in the OSHA Bloodborne Pathogens Standard. Today, countless numbers of workers benefit from this landmark legislation. However, there is a constant influx of new information that emanates from the isolation of new bacteria and viruses as well as from improved understanding of the pathogen, host, and transmission/vector relationships. There exist new means of preventing and treating diseases, with new vaccines, immunobiologics, and medications. In addition, populations and groups other than health care workers—day care workers, law enforcement officers, and penal corrections employees—are affected. Thus, occupational medicine physicians are challenged by the increasing array of work settings and types of jobs that put workers at risk for contracting hepatitis. This challenge expands the scope of traditional occupational medicine practice to the arena of infectious disease, infection control, and public health.

In addition to the clinical and laboratory features of occupationally acquired infectious hepatitis, this chapter reviews the historical aspects, epidemiology, prevention, and treatment of viral hepatitis as well as other infectious viral and nonviral sources of hepatic inflammation. There is also an in-depth discussion of special populations with unique risks for contracting hepatitis (with which the author has had extensive experience). These are the populations that have the greatest risk of contracting work-related viral hepatitis. The chapter also briefly discusses work accommodations for employees who have hepatitis and current recommendations for the work management of infected individuals who perform invasive procedures. The chapter closes with a review of the prevention of occupational infectious hepatitis.

General Principles

Viral hepatitis is caused by a pathogenic virus that invades hepatocytes. Viruses responsible for viral hepatitis are hepatitis A, B, C, D, and E. Other viruses that may cause hepatic inflammation, one characteristic of the disease process, are Epstein-Barr virus, cytomegalovirus, herpes simplex virus, yellow fever virus, and rubella virus.

Pathologically and histologically, the typical lesion consists of necrosis of the hepatocyte, with a mononuclear lymphocytic inflammatory response. However, these features are not specific for any one particular infective agent, or cause, of hepatic inflammation [2].

Clinical and Laboratory Manifestations

Symptoms of acute viral hepatitis are nonspecific and predominantly constitutional and gastrointestinal. Prodromal symptoms include malaise, fatigue, anorexia, nausea, vomiting, and arthralgias. Following the prodromal symptoms, there is an icteric phase characterized by hepatic inflammation, abdominal pain, and jaundice. Symptoms often lessen during the icteral phase, particularly in children.

Physical manifestations may include mild fever, hepatomegaly, splenomegaly, jaundice, and pruritus. Spider nevi and telangiectasia may be present in chronic cases as a result of hepatic insufficiency that results in an estrogenic effect.

The hallmark of laboratory studies is significant elevation of the serum aminotransferases. The alanine aminotransferase (ALT) elevation often exceeds that of the aspartate aminotransferase (AST). Other laboratory manifestations include elevations of serum bilirubin, alkaline phosphatase, and prothrombin time. There may be a decrease in the serum albumin, resulting in hyperglobulinemia. Hemolysis may occur, and urinalysis often reveals the presence of bilirubin.

Among the possible complications of viral hepatitis are massive hepatic necrosis, cholestatic hepatitis, aplastic anemia, vasculitis, and pancreatitis. In cases of hepatitis B, C, and D, the process may evolve to chronic hepatitis [2].

Historical Aspects

Awareness of hepatitis dates back many centuries. References to disorders characterized by jaundice appear in the literature of the ancient Greeks, Babylonians, and Chinese [3].

It was not until 1963 that the Australian antigen of hepatitis B was characterized by Blumberg [4]. Since then, testing methodologies have expanded to include specific serologic tests of the host antibody response, the characterization of seven different viral hepatitides, and the development of polymerase chain-reaction technology in characterizing various strains of a given virus.

Hepatitis A

BACKGROUND AND EPIDEMIOLOGY

Hepatitis A (HAV) is a 27-nm RNA *Hepatovirus*, a member of the family Picornaviridae. While HAV occurs worldwide, it tends to occur in sporadic and epidemic proportions in developed portions of the world. It is historically a disease associated with poor public sanitation or poor hygiene. In developing countries, adults are typically immune, and the disease occurs as part of the endemic illnesses. Humans and nonhuman primates are the reservoirs for the virus. The typical modes of transmission are person to person (via the fecal-oral route), common source (through food or water), sexual, and blood/intravenous [5–7].

In developed parts of the world, where there are good sanitation and public health practices, most adults do not contract HAV infection. As a result, when an outbreak does occur, it tends to be proportionally more epidemic. Transmission rates are high in day care centers, long-term residential facilities, and other settings where there is high risk of fecal-oral transmission [5]. In the United States, epidemic cycles appeared to have ended by the 1980s. Since 1983, however, HAV rates have increased, with one of the most recent epidemics occurring in 1997 due to contaminated strawberries from Mexico [5,6]. In the United States, other outbreaks have been attributed to common-source vectors, that is, food or water contamination.

The incubation period averages 28 to 30 days, but may range from 15 to 50 days. The period of communicability begins in the latter half of the incubation period and continues into the first few days of the onset of jaundice [5].

WORK ISSUES

If hepatitis A infection is detected during the incubation period, the infected individual should be placed on enteric precautions during the first two weeks of illness but for no more than one week after the onset of jaundice. Quarantine is not required. After the period of communicability, accommodation may be required: Individuals with resolving infection may need to be placed on light duty, with frequent rest breaks or an abbreviated work day or work week. Typically, recovery is complete after HAV infection [5].

ACTIVE AND PASSIVE IMMUNIZATION

There are two variants of hepatitis A vaccine licensed for use in the United States: Havrix and Vaqta. Each is highly effective in individuals over 18 years of age when administered according to the manufacturer's direction. The high immunogenicity of the two vaccines makes postvaccination serologic testing unnecessary. In addition, standard commercially available assays may not detect neutralizing antibodies to HAV in actively immunized individuals, since the HAV vaccine induces an antibody response much weaker than that due to natural infection [7].

The vaccines' long-term effectiveness has not been fully characterized, but it appears that protective levels of anti-HAV are sustained for 20 years or more. Typically, the majority of HAV vaccine recipients are immune within two weeks after the first immunization; 100% of recipients are immune within four weeks after the first vaccination. Current recommendations are for vaccination four weeks prior to anticipated exposure (travel to an endemic area). The full vaccination series consists of two vaccines over six months.

Before hepatitis A vaccine was available, passive immunization with serum immune globulin (IG) was the method of protecting individuals, both pre-exposure and postexposure. If an individual plans to travel to an endemic area within four weeks after active immunization with HAV vaccine, current recommendations are that he/she receive 0.02 mL/kg of IG, which will provide up to three months of protection. HAV vaccine may be administered concurrently with IG, but different injection sites should be used. While concurrent administration may reduce the immunogenicity of HAV vaccine, the effect is not considered to be clinically significant.

POSTEXPOSURE PROPHYLAXIS

When exposure to hepatitis A is likely or anticipated, such as when traveling to an endemic area, active immunization with hepatitis A vaccine is preferable. When nonimmune individuals are exposed to hepatitis A, a single dose of intramuscular IG is recommended because of its high level of efficacy in preventing disease. The standard dose of IG is 0.02 mL/kg. Current guidelines recommend the use of IG for postexposure prophylaxis as soon as possible. It may be administered up to two weeks after HAV exposure. Efficacy after two weeks' postexposure is not known [7].

IG is prepared by the pooling of human plasma that has been screened for hepatitis B surface antigen, HIV, and anti-HCV. There has been no documented transmission of any bloodborne infectious disease with immune globulin for intramuscular injection (IGIM). In 1994, however, the CDC reported outbreaks of hepatitis C infection among individuals who had received certain lots of intravenous immune globulin (IGIV) for primary immunodeficiency disorder. After this outbreak, the contaminated lots of IGIV were removed from the medical marketplace [8]. Since that time there has been a market shortage of IGIM. IGIM, however, has an excellent track record, with no documented cases of transmission of bloodborne infection. There are currently two providers of IGIM in the United States: Michigan Biologics Institutes (1-800-843-7477) and the Massachusetts Public Health Biologic Laboratories via the American Red Cross, New England Region (1-617-461-2000). Currently, IGIM should be reserved for cases of postexposure prophylaxis. Now that there is a safe and effective vaccine against hepatitis A, pre-exposure prophylaxis with the vaccine is preferable to using IGIM. Using hepatitis A vaccine in cases of potential exposure ensures that the current supplies of IGIM will be adequate when it is needed for postexposure prophylaxis. Table 17-1 details the recommended doses of IG for

Table 17-1
Recommended Doses of Immune Globulin (IG)

Setting	Duration of Coverage	IG Dose[a]
Pre-exposure	Short-term (1–2 months)	0.02 mL/kg
	Long-term (3–5 months)	0.06 mL/kg[b]
Postexposure	—	0.02 mL/kg

[a] IG should be administered by intramuscular injection into either the deltoid or gluteal muscle. For children <24 months of age, IG can be administered in the anterolateral thigh muscle.
[b] Repeat every 5 months if continued exposure to HAV occurs.
From Prevention of hepatitis A through active or passive immunization: recommendations of the Immunization Practices Advisory Committee. *MMWR* 1996;45(No. RR-15).

hepatitis A pre-exposure and postexposure prophylaxis [9].

Hepatitis B

BACKGROUND AND EPIDEMIOLOGY

It is now known that there are at least two viruses responsible for bloodborne hepatitis: hepatitis B virus and hepatitis C virus. Hepatitis B virus (HBV) was formerly referred to as *serum hepatitis*. It is a 27-nm DNA virus in the family Hepadnaviridae. HBV may be transmitted via the bloodborne (percutaneous, intravenous) perinatal, or sexual route [5]. Humans are the natural reservoir for the virus. Worldwide, HBV is a major cause of acute and chronic hepatitis, cirrhosis, and primary hepatocellular carcinoma. Five percent of the adult U.S. population is anti-HBcore positive and 0.5% is HBsAg positive (infectious).

Infectious hepatitis B virions have been found in nearly all human bodily fluids; however, only blood, blood products, semen, saliva, and vaginal fluids are considered to be infectious. The incubation of HBV ranges from 45 to 180 days, with an average of 60–90 days [5]. Infectious individuals can infect others for many weeks before the onset of symptoms and throughout the clinical phase. Unlike hepatitis A, which has a fairly typical disease course followed by complete resolution, HBV infection has a variety of clinical outcomes. Approximately 95% of healthy adults with acute HBV infection recover completely, but 5–10% remain HBsAg positive after resolution of symptoms and are at risk for developing chronic hepatitis.

All seronegative individuals are susceptible to HBV infection. The risk of contracting infection after a bloodborne exposure ranges from 2% to 40%, depending on the absence or presence of hepatitis E antigen in the infectious source. Overall, the attack rate is 30% [5,10].

Individuals with serologic resolution of previous infection have lifelong immunity. Immunity is characterized serologically by the following findings on blood studies: anti-HBs positive, HBsAg negative, and anti-HBcore positive. Typically, the anti-HBs and anti-HBcore serologic findings are lifelong.

PREVENTION

Individuals who have received the complete series of one of the three commercially available vaccines and who demonstrate serologic evidence of immunity are protected (i.e., anti-HBs positive). The three vaccines for hepatitis B that have been used in the United States are: Heptavax (made from pooled sera of HBV carriers, no longer available in the United States); Engerix HB; and Recombivax. It is not certain how long protection lasts, but it is anticipated to be indefinite in individuals who are known responders.

Hepatitis B vaccine-induced antibodies to HBV are known to wane gradually, and many individuals (60% or more) of the initial responders lose detectable antibodies within 12 years. However, among adults who responded to the initial series, even with declining or undetectable levels of antibody, booster doses are considered to be unnecessary and are not recommended by some clinicians. However, previously published recommendations by the CDC have recommended that anti-HBs be tested unless an adequate level has been demonstrated within the past 24 months. If the anti-HBs is considered to be inadequate, a booster dose of hepatitis B vaccine should be administered [11–13].

Some individuals who have been documented responders to hepatitis B immunization have nonetheless developed asymptomatic HBV infection, demonstrated by the presence of anti-HBcore, with no subsequent development of HBsAg. These individuals with mild, asymptomatic infection have not demonstrated any of the sequelae associated with either acute or chronic HBV infections [12–14].

Hepatitis B vaccine is typically administered to adults in three doses. After the initial dose, subsequent doses are administered at one and six months. Postvaccination testing is not mandatory; however, in populations in which there is a high rate of HBV carriage or where the risk of exposure is significant (e.g., health care workers), postvaccination testing should be considered.

TREATMENT OF NONRESPONDERS TO THE PRIMARY VACCINE SERIES

Serologic response rates are highest in individuals who receive the vaccination in the first and second decades of life. More than 90% of healthy adults and 95% of infants, children, and adolescents develop protective antibody responses from the primary series [11]. However, with each successive decade of life, the response rate lessens. Only 80–85% of the vaccine recipients who receive the primary series at the age of 40 to 45 years develop protective antibodies. Smoking and obesity also lessen the immunologic response to the primary series.

Fifteen percent to 20% of individuals who are nonresponders to the primary vaccine series develop adequate antibody response after one additional dose of hepatitis B vaccine (one booster, lifetime total of four hepatitis B vaccines), and 30–50% after three additional doses (three boosters, lifetime total of six hepatitis B vaccines) [13]. If an individual sustains an exposure and is a known nonresponder, serologic testing for HBsAg should be performed to determine if the individual is a chronic carrier.

In addition, because of the possible waning of immunity with time in those who have previously been vaccinated with hepatitis B vaccine, some clinicians perform periodic serologic testing of previously vaccinated responders to ensure that they are immune when a significant exposure occurs. Current CDC recommendations, however, do not recommend such an approach in previously vaccinated known responders, since follow-up studies have revealed no clinical hepatitis B illness in this population. With a continuing focus on cost-effective medicine, follow-up testing in previously known responders (even with exposure to a HBsAg source) appears to be unnecessary.

The Centers for Disease Control and Prevention (CDC) has published guidelines for post-exposure prophylaxis for percutaneous or mucosal exposure to hepatitis B virus(Table 17-2) [12].

PASSIVE IMMUNIZATION WITH HBIG

Hepatitis B immune globulin (HBIG) should be utilized in individuals who have not been vaccinated or who are nonresponders to the hepatitis B vaccine. HBIG provides an instant method of protection, which lasts approximately three months. Current recommendations for the use of HBIG as postexposure prophylaxis are that it be administered at a dose of 0.06 mL/kg intramuscularly as soon as possible after exposure. It is recommended that the total HBIG dose be split into two equally divided doses and then injected in each gluteal muscle. Hepatitis B vaccine series should be initiated concurrently. If hepatitis B vaccine is not initiated, then HBIG should be repeated in one month [12].

HBIG should be administered no later than seven days after exposure, for there are no data as to its efficacy after seven days [12]. In addition, there are uncertainties as to the maximum recommended doses of HBIG. Previous recommendations have cited a maximum dose of 5 mL in adults [14]. However, at a dose of 0.06 mL/kg, individuals over 80 kg (176 lb) would require larger doses. Thus, for large or obese adults, some physicians may exceed the 5-mL maximum dose.

As part of counseling after an exposure, the treating physician should thoroughly inform the

Table 17-2
Recommended Postexposure Prophylaxis for Percutaneous or Permucosal Exposure to Hepatitis B Virus, United States

Vaccination and Antibody Response Status of Exposed Person	Treatment When Source Is: HBsAG[a] Positive	HBsAg Negative	Source Not Tested or Status Unknown
Unvaccinated	HBIG[b] × 1; initiate HB vaccine series[c]	Initiate HB vaccine series	Initiate HB vaccine series
Previously vaccinated:			
Known responder[d]	No treatment	No treatment	No treatment
Known nonresponder	HBIG × 2 or HBIG × 1 and initiate revaccination	No treatment	If known high-risk source, treat as if source were HBsAg positive
Antibody response unknown	Test exposed person for anti-HBs[e] 1. If adequate,[d] no treatment 2. If inadequate,[d] HBIG × 1 and vaccine booster	No treatment	Test exposed person for anti-HBs 1. If adequate,[d] no treatment 2. If inadequate,[d] initiate revaccination

[a] Hepatitis B surface antigen.
[b] Hepatitis B immune globulin; dose 0.06 mL/kg intramuscularly.
[c] Hepatitis B vaccine.
[d] Responder is defined as a person with adequate levels of serum antibody to hepatitis B surface antigen (i.e., anti-HBs ≥ 10 mIU/mL); inadequate response to vaccination defined as serum anti-HBs < 10 mIU/mL.
[e] Antibody to hepatitis B surface antigen.
From Immunization of health-care workers: recommendations of the Advisory Committee on Immunization Practices (ACIP) and the Hospital Infection Control Practices Advisory Committee (HICPAC). *MMWR* 1997;46(No. RR-18):3–8.

exposed worker about the risks of contracting disease or infection, a follow-up plan, and precautions. The precautions relevant to hepatitis B, C, and D and HIV include avoiding childbearing for up to one year after exposure and refraining from donations of blood, from breast feeding, and from sharing of razor blades or toothbrushes. In addition, the physician should counsel exposed individuals to use a latex condom (in a monogamous relationship) or refrain from sexual intercourse and high-risk sexual practices (if not in a monogamous relationship).

Often, the spouse or sexual partner may have questions that need to be answered by the physician.

Hepatitis C

BACKGROUND AND EPIDEMIOLOGY

Hepatitis C (HCV) has historically been called *non-A, non-B hepatitis (NANB)*. Prior to 1989, the etiologic agent was unknown and there were no serologic markers. The infectious agent, HCV, was later identified using serum of chimpanzees who carried NANB hepatitis [1,2] and has been characterized as an RNA virus, with a genome similar to that of *Flavivirus* and *Pestivirus*, each a genus in the Flaviridae family [2].

HCV has six genotypes, with subtypes within each genotype. As a result, there are several perplexing issues regarding the diagnosis, presentation, and treatment of HCV [1].

1. The difficulty in identifying infection by serologic tests—even with the resultant development of second- and third-generation tests, which attempt to increase the sensitivity and specificity.
2. Naturally acquired infection with HCV apparently does not lead to immunity against reinfection secondary to the genomic varia-bility.
3. As a result of the genome variability of HCV, it has been difficult to develop a vaccine to prevent infection.

ROUTES OF TRANSMISSION

HCV can be found in serum, saliva, semen, urine, stool, and vaginal secretions. Typically, transmission is via large volume inoculation, such as that which occurs with blood transfusion. However, HCV can be spread via perinatal or sexual contact.

Hepatitis C (HCV) is commonly transmitted by way of intravenous drug abuse, renal dialysis, and administration of untreated clotting factor concentrates. Approximately 0.5% of blood donors in the United States are positive for HCV antibodies. It has been found that about 40% of acute sporadic cases of HCV are not associated with any risk factors. Thus, while interpersonal spread may occur, the mechanism has not been determined.

The incubation period for HCV may range from two weeks to six months but commonly is 6–9 weeks. The attack rate is considered to be 3%, with a range of 1.2 to 10.05 per percutaneous exposure [10]. Infected individuals may be contagious prior to the development of ALT elevation, and infectiousness may persist indefinitely. HCV titers appear to be low, and ALT activity correlates with peaks in virus concentration [2,5].

Occupational exposure to HCV is of equal concern as with HBV. At least 85% of persons with HCV infection develop chronic infection, and of these, approximately 70% develop chronic liver disease and enzyme elevation [15].

Individuals with chronic HCV infection are at increased risk for cirrhosis of the liver. In addition, chronic HCV infection appears to be associated with hepatocellular carcinoma [16].

Currently, there is no pre-exposure or postexposure prophylaxis and no effective therapy for those with chronic HCV infection. The means of transmission are not well defined in sexual or household contacts; thus, it is somewhat difficult to recommend specific guidelines to prevent secondary transmission (other than avoidance of sharing toothbrushes or razor blades).

Prevention of exposure in susceptible individuals is the current preventive approach. Health care workers and workers in long-term residential facilities or correctional systems should adhere to Standard Precautions. Current postexposure guidelines are as follows [10,15]:

1. Source testing for antibody to anti-HCV and ALT should be performed.
2. Individuals exposed to anti-HCV positive source should have baseline testing for anti-HCV, ALT.
3. Confirmation of anti-HCV positive results should be obtained by supplemental assay.
4. Immune globulin has not been shown to be efficacious in postexposure prophylaxis against HCV.
5. Some authorities advocate the use of alpha-interferon in early cases of HCV infection. It has been proposed that using polymerase chain reaction (PCR) testing for HCV RNA will detect infections earlier, thus leading to early treatment with interferon. However, PCR is currently not a licensed assay, and there is a high degree of variability in the results. There are no data to demonstrate the efficacy of alpha-interferon early in the course of infection rather than the use of standard therapy for chronic HCV.
6. Follow-up surveillance testing should be performed for six to nine months following exposure.

Hepatitis D

BACKGROUND AND EPIDEMIOLOGY

Hepatitis D virus (HDV) is also known as the *delta hepatitis agent* [1]. It is a defective RNA virus that utilizes HBsAg for its structural protein sheath. HDV requires coinfection in an individual who is HBsAg positive, either acute or chronically [16]. HDV can occur as one of two entities: (1) acute coinfection of HDV simultaneous with acute HBV; or (2) acute HDV superinfection concomitant with chronic HBV.

Acute Simultaneous HDV Coinfection

Patients with acute simultaneous coinfection of HDV with acute HBV typically have a better prognosis. Less than 5% of cases of acute HDV infection result in chronic delta hepatitis. Coinfection is typically characterized by a low-level titer of anti-HDV and is short lived. Thus, anti-HDV tests typically may not detect HBV/HDV coinfection secondary to low titers.

Acute HDV Superinfection Concomitant with Chronic HBV

This entity runs a more virulent course than simultaneous HDV coinfection: 70% of all HDV superinfections result in chronic hepatitis. HDV superinfection with chronic HBV is more easily detected than acute simultaneous HDV confection because there are higher levels of anti-HDV.

HDV infection (where coinfection or superinfection) runs a more severe course than isolated HBV or HCV infection. Acute infection with HDV has a mortality of 2–20%. In chronic HDV hepatitis, 60–70% of patients develop cirrhosis within 15 to 20 years.

EPIDEMIOLOGY

Hepatitis D infection occurs worldwide. Humans are the natural reservoir. Experimentally, HDV can be transmitted in chimpanzees infected with HBV. HDV can also be modeled experimentally in the woodchuck infected with woodchuck hepatitis virus. Although there is evidence of intrafamilial spread and sexual infection, HDV is more commonly and easily spread by parenteral exposure. The incubation period is two to eight weeks.

The primary means of preventing HDV infection is the prevention of HBV through HBV vaccination. In individuals who already have HBV infection, whether acute or chronic, avoidance of risks for HDV exposures is the only effective means of preventing the disease [5].

Hepatitis E

BACKGROUND AND EPIDEMIOLOGY

Hepatitis E virus (HEV) is a 32-nm RNA virus that is structurally similar to calicivirus [16] and similar epidemiologically to HAV. HEV has been referred to as *enterically transmitted non-A, non-B hepatitis (ETNANB)*. The infection was first documented in New Delhi, India, during a 1955 epidemic. It is transmitted by the fecal-oral route; contaminated drinking water is the typical vehicle for outbreaks [16,17].

Usually, the incubation period is two to nine weeks, with a mean of 45 days. During epidemics, however, the incubation period is 15–64 days, with a mean of 26–42 days. The actual period of communicability is not well defined, but HEV has been detected in stool samples for up to 14 days after the onset of jaundice. The reservoir is unknown, but it is known that HEV is transmissible to chimpanzees, cynomolgus macaques, tamarins, and pigs [5].

The attack rate is highest in the 15- to 40-year-old population. There is a 15–20% case fatality rate among pregnant women; the greatest risk is during the third trimester [1,5,17].

Prevention of HEV is best achieved via strict adherence to hygienic and dietary principles one follows to avoid infectious diarrhea—avoidance of local water in endemic areas (unless boiled or carbonated), avoidance of uncooked foods, and avoidance of fruits that one does not peel. In the United States, the use of immunoglobulin is unlikely to prevent HEV secondary to the country's low endemic rate [17].

Hepatitis F

Hepatitis F is a recently characterized enteric agent isolated from human stool. The agent has experimentally been transmitted to primates. Prevention is similar to that for hepatitis A [18].

Hepatitis G

Hepatitis G is a bloodborne virus that appears to have transmission characteristics in common with hepatitis C. The virus and its epidemiology have not been well defined. It has a serologic occurrence rate of 15 per 1,000 blood donors (1.5%). Clearly, much remains to be discovered with hepatitis G [1].

Other Sources of Infectious Hepatic Inflammation

Various viral and nonviral infectious diseases can cause hepatic inflammation. These diseases should be included, along with noninfectious etiologies (e.g., drug, chemical, autoimmune), in the differential diagnosis of workers with elevated liver enzymes [1]. For purposes of discussion of infectious hepatitis, the classification can be considered as (1) acute hepatitis due to other viruses and (2) hepatitis due to nonviral infectious agents [16].

ACUTE HEPATITIS DUE TO OTHER VIRUSES

The liver may be affected by several viral agents. One of the most common causes of hepatic inflammation is Epstein-Barr virus (EBV), the etiologic agent associated with heterophile-positive infectious mononucleosis. Other viruses that can cause hepatic inflammation are cytomegalovirus (heterophile-negative mononucleosis syndrome), rubella, rubeola, mumps, and Coxsackie B virus.

Typically, in these cases of viral infection, the hepatic inflammation is mild, with liver enzymes ranging from two to five times normal and with little if any jaundice. With EBV-associated hepatitis, an acute icteric syndrome can occur, although this is relatively uncommon. In the immunocompromised host with a systemic viral infection, however, hepatic inflammation can be severe, resulting in hepatic necrosis and possibly death from hepatic failure. This scenario has been associated with herpes simplex virus, cytomegalovirus, and varicella-zoster virus [16]. Yellow fever, a zoonosis transmitted by several variants of mosquito [5], also can cause severe hepatitis, resulting in significant elevations in the liver enzymes and mortality approaching 20–50%. While yellow fever is not endemic in the United States, it is endemic in Central America, South America, and Central Africa.

HEPATITIS DUE TO NONVIRAL INFECTIOUS AGENTS

Liver inflammation and dysfunction can result from bacteria, mycobacteria, rickettsia, fungi, brucellosis, tularemia, plague, bacterial sepsis, and legionnaires' disease. There are three nonviral infectious agents that can produce an acute hepatitis syndrome: syphilis, leptospirosis, and Q fever [16].

Syphilis

Primary and early secondary syphilis can cause ALT and AST elevations of four to eight times normal. The diagnosis of syphilis-related hepatitis is made on the basis of the history, physical examination, and serologic tests for syphilis.

Leptospirosis

Leptospirosis is a febrile illness caused by the spirochete *Leptospira*, which occurs worldwide. *Leptospira* infection has protean manifestations, including sudden and severe onset of fever, headache, chills, severe myalgias, rash and severe myalgia, and may affect the hepatic and pulmonary systems. Leptospirosis has a relatively low case-fatality rate, but in affected individuals with hepatic and renal involvement, the rate is over 20%. Leptospirosis is contracted by exposure to water contaminated with the urine of infected animals, typically infected rats. It is an occupational hazard for sewage workers, farmers, veterinarians, and those with potential exposure to infected waters. It is an unusual cause of jaundice in the United States [5].

Q Fever

Q fever is a rickettsial disease caused by *Coxiella burnetii*. The natural reservoirs are infected farm animals, some wild animals, and ticks. The infection is transmitted by the airborne route, with contaminated airborne dust or other particles containing the rickettsia. It can also be transmitted by ingestion of contaminated raw milk. Direct transmission by blood or bone marrow transfusion has been reported [6]. The hepatic manifestations of Q fever range from subclinical hepatic involvement and inflammation (the typical course) to overt jaundice. It is transmitted by infected farm animals.

Special Populations with Unique Risk for Exposure

SEWAGE WORKERS

The health of sewage workers has been of concern for centuries. Bernardino Ramazzini, the Father of Occupational Medicine, described the plight of sewage workers in *Diseases of Workers*

(De Morbis Artficium). In particular, he described the maladies of those who clean privies and cesspits [19]. There have been several illnesses described in sewage workers. These descriptions range from "sewage worker's syndrome" [20] to various bacterial, parasitic, and enteric infections contracted through exposure to sewage [21,22].

Several authorities have suggested an epidemiologic link between hepatitis A seroprevalence exposure to sewage at work. Skinhoj and colleagues described an increased prevalence of anti-HAV in sewage workers, compared to gardeners and municipal clerks [23], and several investigators have recommended immunization of sewage workers with hepatitis A vaccine [24–27]. Formal recommendations by the CDC or Advisory Committee on Immunization Practices (ACIP) have not been publicly promulgated, however. It is reasonable to consider vaccination of sewage workers with hepatitis A vaccine, considering the low endemic rate in the U.S. population and relatively low cost of the vaccine compared with the health care costs associated with hepatitis A illness. This view is not universally accepted, however, and several authors do not support vaccination of sewage workers against hepatitis A [28–30]. Another hepatic risk for sewage workers is leptospirosis, but the hepatic inflammation associated with it is often subclinical and is usually not the focal aspect of the disease.

HEALTH CARE WORKERS

Hepatitis B is a major threat to health care workers (along with HIV and hepatitis C). In 1993, there were an estimated 1,450 cases of occupationally acquired HBV infection in health care workers (HCWs). This represents a 90% decrease from the estimated number of HBV infections in HCWs in 1985 [12]. The decrease in incidence is attributable to wide-scale voluntary immunization of HCWs with the hepatitis B vaccine.

In 1991, the OSHA Bloodborne Pathogens Standard became law, and health care institutions were required to provide active hepatitis B immunization to susceptible employees with potential exposure to blood or other potentially infectious bodily fluids. This mandatory provision for the protection of HCWs has greatly contributed to the significant decline in occupationally acquired HBV infection in HCWs.

LAW ENFORCEMENT AND CORRECTIONAL DEPARTMENT PERSONNEL

Hepatitis B is highly prevalent in the criminal population, especially in individuals with a history of intravenous drug use (IDU). By virtue of the antisocial and violent tendencies of the criminal population, law enforcement and correctional department personnel are often subjected to injuries to the skin and are exposed to bodily fluids such as blood and saliva. Many police departments and correctional institutions have instituted HBV vaccination programs since the inception of the OSHA Bloodborne Pathogens Standard, but these programs are not mandatory because these employees are not technically considered health care workers.

When law enforcement and correctional personnel are exposed to a source of bodily fluids in the line of work, it is often difficult (if not impossible) to test the source of the exposure in a timely manner. Often, the arrestee, suspect, or inmate (source) refuses voluntary testing for HBV, HCV, and HIV, and some states do not have statutory authority for the testing of bloodborne pathogens in the criminal population. When such authority exists, it is argued that the source's confidentiality is breached when the source is tested and the results revealed to law enforcement and correctional personnel. Because of the real threat of litigation against municipal and state law enforcement departments and correctional departments by the source for attempted testing, many departments have chosen not to aggressively pursue source testing. Often, the exposed law enforcement or correctional workers have to pursue legal action to test the source, either at their own expense or with the assistance of the labor union.

In these instances, the treating physician and the exposed law or correctional worker need to discuss the pros and cons of using HBIG. The theoretical risks and expense of HBIG passive immunization to that of contracting HBV (as well as postexposure prophylaxis for HIV) should also be discussed.

WORKERS IN LONG-TERM RESIDENTIAL FACILITIES

Historically, long-term residential facilities have been associated with diseases transmitted by the fecal/oral route, the respiratory route, fomites, and several other routes and vectors of transmission. Individuals residing in, and those working in, these facilities are at significant risk for contracting one of several communicable diseases. Contributing factors include poor hygiene, close living conditions, and individuals with overall poor health and/or physical conditioning.

Hepatitis A is common in day care centers with children in diapers. In addition, among adults in crowded living conditions, where spread is a greater risk, transmission can be rapid if an infectious source/index case becomes available. This is often the situation in long-term residential facilities for the developmentally disabled.

Hepatitis B also has been linked to institutional clients and staff. Hepatitis B is most commonly transmitted via perinatal, sexual, and bloodborne routes. However, it also appears to be transmitted by household contacts. Thus, hepatitis B is also of concern in long-term residential facilities [5].

OTHER POPULATIONS AT RISK FOR ABRASIONS TO THE SKIN WHERE HBV IS PRESENT

Any situation in which an employee can sustain a cut or abrasion of the skin, with subsequent exposure to blood or infectious bodily fluids at the portal of entry (cut, abrasion, or exposed mucous membrane), puts the individual at risk for HBV. Mevorach, Eliakim, and Brezis reported a case of horizontal transmission of HBV in Israeli meat cutters who shared knives in the butcher shop where they worked. These authors make the case that hepatitis B vaccination should be universal and not reserved just for what have historically been considered high-risk groups [31].

Work Issues with Enteric Hepatitis (Hepatitis A, E, and F)

Food handlers can transmit either hepatitis A or E. Food handlers infected with hepatitis A should not be allowed to prepare or serve food until they are no longer infectious. This is typically seven days after the onset of jaundice [12]. Current CDC recommendations include IGIM treatment for other food handlers at the same location as the index case; IGIM administration to patrons should also be considered if the index-case food handler was involved in the preparation of foods to be eaten uncooked, or was involved in the preparation or serving of foods after cooking and had diarrhea or poor hygiene practices. This assumes that the potentially exposed patrons can be identified within two weeks after exposure [7].

Because of the low prevalence of HEV infection in the United States, this disease is of less concern in this country. Individuals with HEV may be infectious for 14 days after the onset of jaundice (the period of infectivity has not been completely characterized). One should consider handling the worker infected with hepatitis E, using well-established precautions for hepatitis A.

Hepatitis F has not been well characterized. Until more is understood about this disorder, similar precautions should be followed as those for hepatitis A.

Health care workers with hepatitis A should be restricted from patient contact until seven days after the onset of jaundice [12].

Work Issues with Bloodborne Hepatitis (Hepatitis B, C, D, and G)

In a work environment, individuals with hepatitis B, C, D, or G may be of concern both to management and to co-workers. Those with acute infection are typically too ill to work. Special accommodations may be necessary for those who are able to work or who may be in the recovery or convalescent phase. Accommodation may be in the form of minimal exertion or an abbreviated workday.

Workers with acute and/or chronic infection who do not perform exposure-prone invasive procedures require no specific restrictions, provided that there is no epidemiologic link for transmission of infection to contacts [12]. Standard Precautions should be utilized (see Prevention below) [32].

Workers with acute and/or chronic infection who perform exposure-prone invasive procedures require more careful work placement. These workers should not perform exposure-prone invasive procedures until counsel has been sought from an expert review panel who evaluate the particular disorder and skill level of the worker, relevant to the specific procedure of concern [12]. Long-term accommodation may be necessary in these instances. These are often difficult decisions and reflect a balance between the rights of the infected employee and the duty to protect the public.

Prevention

As previously stated, pre-exposure vaccination against hepatitis A and B is very effective in preventing these infections. There is currently no vaccine available for hepatitis C, D, E, F, or G.

Because of the increasing recognition of the threat of bloodborne diseases, it is generally accepted that precautions should be utilized in health care settings, especially to prevent the transmission of currently known diseases for which there is no effective pre-exposure therapy.

Prior to the recognition of HIV-related illnesses, patients who were suspected of having communicable disease, such as hepatitis A or B, were placed on isolation. Those with suspected hepatitis A were placed on enteric precautions, and those with serum hepatitis (hepatitis B) were placed on blood precautions.

When etiologic factors associated with HIV infection were recognized, Universal Precautions were initiated for all HCWs who potentially could be exposed to patients' blood or bodily fluids. Universal Precautions were applied only to those fluids known to transmit bloodborne diseases and to bodily fluids with visible blood. Universal Precautions have since been replaced by Standard Precautions [32].

Standard Precautions are now taken by HCWs when they are exposed to patients' blood, bodily fluids, secretions, and excretions (except for sweat) and when contacting patients' mucous membranes and nonintact skin.

Personal protective equipment that helps prevent exposure to pathogens includes gloves, facial protection, and gowns. Hand washing is used after doffing gloves, between patients, and for any contact with blood, bodily fluids, secretions, or excretions.

Although Standard Precautions (a form of administrative controls) and personal protective equipment provide some protection to the worker, engineering controls are clearly the most desirable means of preventing exposure. On that front, significant technologic advances have been made in the design of needleless drug-delivery systems. Similarly, vascular access systems that minimize the risk of accidental needlesticks (self-sheathing systems) are also available. These should be utilized in an organized, methodical approach to preventing exposures.

Future Challenges

In the past three decades, tremendous progress has clearly been made in the characterization and understanding of viral and nonviral hepatitides. Our knowledge base has expanded from an understanding of the epidemiologic determinants of disease to characterization of the etiologic agents, the risks for infection, and the prevention of infection through immunobiologics. In addition, improved therapies are becoming available as a better understanding of the molecular biology of these diseases is gained. Furthermore, tremendous strides have been made in legislative protections for workers who are in the highest risk groups. With the emergence and discovery of new agents of hepatic inflammation, challenges remain, however. This, coupled with continual development of improved treatments of infectious hepatitis, will continue to challenge occupational medicine physicians into the next millennium.

References

1. Dienstag JL, Isselbacher KJH. Acute viral hepatitis. In: Fauci AS, Braunwald E, Isselbacher KJ, et al. (eds), *Harrison's Principles of Internal Medicine*, 14th Ed. New York: McGraw Hill, 1998. Pp 1677–92.
2. Ockner RK. Acute viral hepatitis. In: Bennett JC, Plum F (eds), *Cecil Textbook of Medicine*, 20th Ed, Vol 1. Philadelphia: WB Saunders, 1996. Pp 762–72.
3. Hollinger FB. Serologic evaluation of viral hepatitis. *Hosp Pract* 1987;Feb 15:101–14.
4. Carey WD, Patel G. Viral hepatitis in the 1990s, part I: current principles of management. *Cleve Clin J Med* 1992;59(3):317–25.
5. Benenson AS (ed). *Control of Communicable Diseases Manual*, 16th Ed. Washington, DC: APHA, 1995. Pp 217–33.
6. Hepatitis A associated with consumption of frozen strawberries—Michigan, March 1997. *MMWR* 1997; 46:288–95.
7. Prevention of hepatitis A through active or passive immunization: recommendations of the Immunization Practices Advisory Committee (ACIP). *MMWR* 1996;45(No. RR-15).
8. Outbreak of hepatitis C associated with intravenous immunoglobulin administration—United States, October 1993–June 1994. *MMWR* 1994;43:505–9.
9. Fleming DW. Immune Globulin Shortage—health care provider information. (Letter, Sept 6, 1996.) Document #221060. Atlanta: Centers for Disease Control and Prevention, Oct 9, 1996.
10. Swinker M. Occupational infections in health care workers: prevention and intervention. *Am Fam Physician* 1997;56:2291–9.
11. Wood RC, MacDonald KL, White KE, et al. Risk factors for lack of detectable antibody following hepatitis B vaccination of Minnesota health care workers. *JAMA* 1993;270:2935–9.
12. Immunization of health-care workers: recommendations of the Advisory Committee on Immunization Practices (ACIP) and the Hospital Infection Control Practices Advisory Committee (HICPAC). *MMWR* 1997;46(No. RR-18):3–8.
13. Hepatitis B virus: a comprehensive strategy for eliminating transmission in the United States through universal childhood vaccination: recommendations of the Advisory Committee on Immunization Practices (ACIP). *MMWR* 1991;40(RR-13).
14. Update on adult immunization: recommendations of the Immunization Practices Advisory Committee (ACIP). *MMWR* 1991;40(No. RR-12):9–10, 31, 47.
15. Recommendations for follow-up of health-care workers after occupational exposure to hepatitis C virus. *MMWR* 1997;46:603–7.
16. Hsu HH, Feinstone SM, Hoofnagle JH. Acute viral hepatitis. In: Mandell GL, Bennett JE, Dolin R (eds), *Principles and Practice of Infectious Diseases*, 4th Ed. New York: Churchill Livingstone, 1994. Pp 1136–53.
17. CDC. Hepatitis E among U.S. travelers, 1980–1992. *MMWR* 1993;42:1–4.
18. Bowden DS, Moaven LD, Locarnini SA. New hepatitis virus: are there enough letters in the alphabet? *Med J Aust* 1996;164:87–9.
19. Ramazzini, B. *Diseases of Workers*. Thunder Bay, Canada: OH&S Press, 1993. Pp 86–91. (Translated from the Latin text *De Morbis Artificium* of 1713 by Wilmer Cave Wright.)
20. Rylander R, Andersson K, Belin L, et al. Sewage worker's syndrome. *Lancet* 1976;28:478–9.
21. Sumathipala RW, Morrison GW. Campylobacter enteritis after falling into sewage. *Br Med J* 1983;286:1356.
22. Sehgal R, Mahajan RC. Occupational risks in sewage work. *Lancet* 1991;33:1404.
23. Skinhoj O, Hollinger FB, Hovind-Hougen K, et al. Infectious liver diseases in three groups of Copenhagen workers: correlation of hepatitis A infection to sewage exposure. *Arch Environ Health* 1981;36:139–43.
24. DeSerres G, Levesque B, Higgins R, et al. Need for vaccination of sewer workers against leptospirosis and hepatitis A. *Occup Environ Med* 1995;52:505–7.
25. Poole CJM, Shakespeare AT. Should sewage workers and carers for people with learning disabilities be vaccinated for hepatitis A? *Br Med J* 1993;306:1102.
26. Donoghue AM, Hancox B. Hepatitis A vaccination for sewage workers. *N Z Med J* 1995;108(100):235–6.
27. Longsen PJ. Hepatitis A vaccine. *Br Med J* 1992; 305:888.
28. Warken AA, Hoff GL. Hepatitis A in waste water treatment plant workers: is vaccination necessary?. *J Occup Environ Med* 1998;40:515–7.
29. Maguire H. Hepatitis A virus infection: risk to sewage workers unproved. *Br Med J* 1993;307:561.
30. California Department of Health. Illness in sewage workers/recommendations for prevention. *California Morbidity* 1992;#35/#36.
31. Mevorach D, Eliakim R, Brezis M. Hepatitis B—an occupational risk for butchers? (Letters.) *N Engl J Med* 1992;116(5):428.
32. Garner JS. Guideline for isolation precautions in hospitals. *Infect Control Hosp Epidemiol* 1996;17:53–80.

18 / Occupational Gastroenteritis

Alain J. Couturier and Wendell Perry

Infectious gastroenteritis is difficult to define without knowledge of the causative organism. In general, the term suggests only infectious inflammation of the mid- or lower intestine resulting in diffuse epigastric pain, fever, nausea, and vomiting in the early stages of infection. As the inflammation progresses, cramping and secretory diarrhea, accompanied by hyperactive bowel sounds, develop.

The constellation of pathogens that can cause infectious gastroenteritis accounts for millions of dollars in lost work time and medical costs. Occupational health professionals are concerned principally with *Salmonella*, *Shigella*, enteroinvasive *Escherichia coli*, *Campylobacter jejuni*, *Yersinia*, *Vibrio*, *Clostridium difficile*, *Giardia lamblia*, *Cryptosporidiosis*, *Helicobacter pylori*, hepatitis A, rotavirus, and Norwalk virus. Workers especially likely to be affected by these organisms are hospital employees, nursing home workers, day care employees, wastewater workers, military personnel confined to closed spaces, food handlers, and animal handlers. Those who are charged with treating individuals with work-related gastroenteritis should have a good understanding of how these bacterial and viral pathogens are transmitted and of risk factors for infection. These and other organisms implicated in occupational gastroenteritis and their modes of transmission are summarized in Table 18-1 [1].

Epidemiology

RISK FACTORS FOR TRANSMISSION

The organisms most often involved in occupational gastrointestinal infections find their way to the host through a variety of routes. Most commonly, transmission is achieved through food or water, of which the oral-fecal and person-to-person routes are important subsets. A summary of this data is given in Table 18-1.

INCIDENCE AND PREVALENCE

Each of the organisms profiled in Table 18-1 falls somewhere along a continuum that ranks its influence in creating debilitating gastrointestinal symptoms among discrete sectors of the work force. The impact of these organisms and their victims can now be addressed individually [2]:

- Hepatitis A virus. Fully 35–54% of nursing home staff, ICU personnel, orphanage personnel, day care workers, and other health care workers will test positive for past exposure to this virus. Janitorial staff are particularly vulnerable.
- Norwalk virus. Nurses and nursing assistants who work in nursing homes have the highest incidence of occupational infection from this virus. During acute outbreaks, 30–50% of nursing home staff may be affected. One interesting study describes an outbreak of Norwalk-like virus (small round-structured virus, SRSV) aboard a U.S. aircraft carrier where overcrowding was blamed for ease of transmission [13].
- *Salmonella*. Employees who staff hospitals, nursing homes, institutions for children, and restaurants are at higher risk for developing *Salmonella* infection.
- *Shigella*. Crowding and poor personal hygiene are believed to be responsible for facilitating transmission of *Shigella*.

Table 18-1
Modes of Transmission of Organisms that Cause Occupational Gastroenteritis

Organism	How Transmitted
Giardia lamblia	Fecal-oral; by contaminated food or water or person-to person
Listeria monocytogenes	Food-borne; by contaminated hospital equipment
Shigella	Fecal-oral; by contaminated food or person to person
Salmonella	Food-borne; fecal-oral, person to person; contaminated hospital equipment
E coli 0157:H7 (EHEC strains)	Food-borne, waterborne; person to person
E coli (ETEC strains)	Food-borne, waterborne
E coli (EIEC strains)	Food-borne
E coli (EPEC strains)	Food-borne; person to person
Cryptosporidium parvum	Food-borne, waterborne; fecal-oral, animal to person, and person to person
Vibrio cholerae	Waterborne, food-borne
Campylobacter jejuni	Food-borne, waterborne; animal to person
Helicobacter pylori	Oral-oral, fecal-oral; contaminated medical equipment
Clostridium difficile	Person to person
Yersinia frederiksenii	Food-borne; waterborne
Rotavirus	Fecal-oral; questionable waterborne; respiratory droplets
Hepatitis A virus	Fecal-oral; person to person; needle sharing
Norwalk virus	Fecal-oral; person to person

- *Helicobacter pylori.* Internists and endoscopists are at increased risk for contracting this infection, mainly as a result of contact with contaminated medical equipment.
- *Giardia lamblia.* Infection with this organism appears principally among day care workers in the 25- to 39-year-old age group. Infection rates are highest from July through October. The incidence of infection can range from 1% to 50%, depending on the population being sampled.
- *Cryptosporidium parvum.* In the general population, prevalence is less than 1–4.5% in a survey of stool samples. The rate is higher, however, for animal handlers, health care workers, and day care employees.
- *Campylobacter jejuni.* Prevalence is probably highest among workers with the greatest risk of contact with uncooked or undercooked chicken, unpasteurized milk, and nonchlorinated water. Such workers include food factory processors and poultry handlers.
- *Clostridium difficile.* Although infection with this organism is most frequently associated with patients receiving antibiotic therapy, hospital workers can be infected through contaminated materials and person-to-person contact.
- *Listeria monocytogenes.* Prevalence of this infection in the general population is roughly 4.5 per million. Nosocomial infections are substantially higher in adults over 40 years of age.
- *Eschericia coli* 0157:H7 (EHEC strains). In unusual settings, such as logging camps, where there is the possibility of consuming inadequately cooked meat and drinking unpasteurized milk, workers are at increased risk for *E coli* infection from this strain of the bacteria.
- *Yersinia.* This infection appears among hospital workers who have consumed contaminated water, meat, or dairy products.
- Rotavirus. Day care and nursing home employees are particularly susceptible to rotavirus infections.

Occupational Risk Factors

Clearly, some vocations require that workers place themselves at increased risk for job-related gastorenteritis. These are discussed below.

HEALTH CARE WORKERS

The wide spectrum of health care occupations and professions includes physicians, nurses, nursing assistants, technicians, laboratory personnel, and housekeeping staff. As a broad category of workers, they are the most likely to contract infectious diseases, and gastrointestinal infections are no exception. Some reported incidents are outlined below; they provide a good overview of the organisms transmitted and the circumstances that contribute to their transmission.

Ironically, health care workers are one of the most uncooperative populations when it comes to appreciating the hazards to which they are exposed and taking appropriate precautions. One author cites the prevailing belief among hospital workers that their specialized knowledge and training is, in some way, armor against infectious diseases. In other cases, the zeal for research and medical advancement can blind some hospital workers to the personal dangers inherent in their profession. Gestal observes, "Despite the many serious dangers present in hospitals and medical research centres, health and safety regulations are frequently ignored" [3].

One article describes a hospital epidemic, principally among nursing staff, of a diarrheal illness due to *Cryptosporidium* originating with a single immunocompromised patient. This case history looks retrospectively at the likely modes of transmission and possible breakdown of infection-control standards. The authors conclude that although meticulous infection-control procedures and equipment were in place at the facility, lapses in such matters as hand washing techniques, use of protective clothing, and reporting of symptoms had occurred. Staff had not maintained rigid adherence to procedures. Conspicuous among the procedural violations were relaxed attitudes toward consuming food and drink at nursing stations. Since *Cryptosporidium* is transmitted by the fecal-oral route, there was a clear cause-and-effect consequence of these actions [4].

Another study looks at an outbreak of gastroenteritis caused by SRSV among hospital nursing staff. According to Caceres and Kim [5], these viruses "have been implicated frequently in closed communities, such as nursing homes, hospitals, cruise ships, and dormitories." This investigation demonstrated that SRSV infection can be transmitted person to person (the precise route was not established, but the respiratory route was a strong likelihood) as well as via food-borne or waterborne means. This study also showed that strictly observed infection-control measures (including use of gowns and gloves, use of face masks, frequent hand washing, and isolation of sick staff members) are effective in protecting patients. Even so, close person-to-person contact among infected staff members who relaxed their vigilance with each other resulted in an employee epidemic of gastroenteritis. The practical implications of this study led Caceres and Kim to two conclusions: (1) "casual contact between staff may spread SRSVs and cause gastroenteritis outbreaks in institutional settings" and (2) "staff should not work while ill with gastroenteritis and, optimally, should not return to work until completely free of symptoms" [5].

NURSING HOME PERSONNEL

The need to exclude ill employees from health care facilities is especially important in the case of nursing homes. Many nursing home residents are debilitated and suffer compromise of their immune system. This makes them particularly vulnerable to nosocomial infection, including gastroenteritis. In fact, each year more deaths due to diarrhea occur among the elderly than among children. By the same token, the tendency of infectious diseases to be more widespread in nursing facilities makes employees proportionally susceptible to acquiring infections—and to transmitting them.

Epidemics of gastroenteritis in nursing homes can be swift and severe, affecting up to 50% of staff and residents. In one reported case, an outbreak of viral gastroenteritis in a nursing home accounted for three hospitalizations and two deaths among 121 residents. In this instance, two staff members continued to work while symptomatic. Some of the recommendations stemming from this study include "stopping new admissions and readmissions during the outbreak period, excluding symptomatic employees from patient care and food handling until 48 hours after resolution of diarrhea and vomiting, handling fecally contaminated laundry as little as possible and transporting such laundry in an enclosed and sanitary manner, wearing masks when cleaning vomitus or stool, and informing visitors of the outbreak." As always, this study reemphasizes the recurrent theme of strict adherence to good and frequent hand washing techniques [6].

Gellert's study chronicles an unusually long (two-week) outbreak of acute gastroenteritis among staff and residents of a Los Angeles nursing home. The etiologic agent was identified as an SRSV related to Norwalk-like agents. The study was revealing in two ways. First, it raised the possibility that forms of acute gastroenteritis may be transmitted by airborne aerosolized vomitus as well as by the more commonly recognized person-to-person transmission. Second, the study gave rise to the novel recommendation that investigations of respiratory precautions be undertaken in such circumstances. It also underscored the time-honored infection control measure often echoed in these cases: To minimize personnel crossover from infected and uninfected wards, strict enforcement of employee sick leave during illness and careful hand washing are critical [7,8].

In his study of a Norwalk virus outbreak in a nursing home, Stevenson emphasizes the importance of primary prevention, that is, eliminating the common source of the outbreak rather than simply implementing infection-control measures once the epidemic has gained a foothold. In this instance, contamination of cold foods by kitchen staff was the etiologic event. Therefore, preventive measures such as exclusion of affected staff, good cleaning in the food preparation area, reinforcement of good hygiene practices, and elimination of higher risk cold foods were stressed over isolation techniques and respiratory precautions. The author argued that once the outbreak became established, little could be done to prevent it from running its course. This line of thinking gained increasing popularity with Chadwick and other authorities who came to believe that advocates of certain fastidious infection-control methods had overstated their case [9–11].

WASTEWATER TREATMENT WORKERS

Studies that compare prevalence of infectious disease symptoms among various professions have shown that there is a statistically significant imbalance favoring gastrointestinal symptoms in wastewater workers. Clearly, workers who are exposed to the spectrum of wastewater products, from raw sewage to highly treated wastewater, encounter an impressive array of pathogens. Although specific bacterial, parasitic, fungal, and viral agents are not always recoverable from stool samples, manifestation of gastrointestinal symptoms—and possibly their subclinical disease counterparts—predominate in wastewater workers. Most studies have been disappointing in the yield of specific pathogens gathered from ill workers. There is, however, a strong relationship between level of exposure to wastewater and severity and frequency of symptoms such as abdominal bloating, cramping, and diarrhea [12].

MILITARY PERSONNEL

Military recruits in basic training have long been cited as examples of how infectious disease can spread rapidly among those confined to close spaces and subjected to overcrowding. Sharp and Hyams [13] provide an illustration of this phenomenon in a study examining an epidemic of gastroenteritis that swept through the enlisted spaces aboard a U.S. aircraft carrier. Significant findings from this study revealed that the outbreak of gastroenteritis—defined by nausea, vomiting, or watery stool—was more prevalent among those who had eaten in dining areas served by infected food handlers and two to three times greater among those who occupied berthing compartments accommodating more than 50 crew members. This data led the authors to allow for the possibility of both food-borne and waterborne transmission of disease as well as spread through person-to-person contact. Not unimportant was the statistic that one to two work days were lost by ill crew members [13].

FOOD HANDLERS

As discussed previously, kitchen workers and food handlers in hospitals and nursing homes have been strongly implicated in the transmission of various gastrointestinal illnesses to fellow workers and residents. In the case of SRSV, a single ill worker can become a common infection source capable of contaminating food and water sources available to employees and institutional residents. Person-to-person transmission can then accelerate the epidemic. One interesting study [14] raised the possibility that a presymptomatic food handler shed SRSV in the kitchen of a hospital and contaminated cold lunch items that were subsequently consumed by both employees and residents who later became ill. Alternatively, the authors were also willing to consider the possibility that the virus was transmitted mechanically from the clothing of the worker who had handled a sick child at home. In any case, the heretofore overlooked possibility that presymptomatic kitchen workers were able to contaminate their work environment, gave rise to infection-control precautions never before implemented. For example, an educational program was created that emphasized awareness that employees could contaminate food *before* becoming symptomatic, merely by coming into contact with a sick relative at home. That emphasis was designed to provide a rationale for taking particular care to follow good kitchen-hygiene practices such as meticulous hand washing, changing into clean overclothing prior to beginning a shift, enforced sick leave for symptomatic workers, and destruction of food that symptomatic workers have handled [14].

In another notable case, a food-producing company instituted elaborate infection-control and surveillance measures following a devastating outbreak of *Campylobacter* infection among workers at its plant [15]. Their new policy mandated that employees with gastrointestinal disturbances or anyone who had possible exposure to patients with such illnesses must have stool testing and must have follow-up and be cleared before returning to work. Anyone with positive stool specimens was barred from work, with full pay. Moreover, when an employee has an episode of gastroenteritis symptoms, the worker is seen by a company physician who takes a thorough history, aided by a detailed questionnaire [15].

ANIMAL HANDLERS

Gastrointestinal zoonoses (diseases that infect both humans and animals) are found in workers who come in contact with potentially infected animals, such as slaughterhouse (abattoir) workers and veterinarians. One illustration of how these infections can occur appears in a Swedish case in which abattoir workers contracted *Campylobacter* gastroenteritis during a particularly large holiday slaughter of poultry. Extenuating circumstances such as the youth and inexperience of the workers exacerbated what would probably otherwise have been only a minor outbreak [16].

A similar case in another Scandinavian country involved veterinary students who, in this instance, engaged in experimental work with calves intentionally injected with *Cryptosporidium*. In spite of what they believed to be adequate protection through protective clothing and hand washing, all five students became infected and symptomatic with *Cryptosporidium* gastroenteritis, most probably through the fecal-oral route. The researchers conclude that cryptosporidiosis is a highly contagious cattle-borne zoonosis that "can certainly be considered an occupational risk for farmers, animal handlers, veterinary students and surgeons, laboratory personnel, and research workers . . . capable of crossing the interface between man and animals" [17]. As a footnote, other reports cite *Streptococcus suis* as a zoonotic pathogen occasionally seen in farmers who come into close contact with pigs. In humans, this disease is manifested as copious diarrhea that can occasionally result in acute dehydration.

WORKERS IN REMOTE LOGGING AND INDUSTRIAL CAMPS

Workers who are forced to operate in primitive, remote areas often enjoy less-than-hygienic work and living conditions. Most of these cases are "typical," and many of the circumstances are striking in their similarities. One case involved workers at a gas drilling rig in a remote wilderness area of British Columbia. There, 21 persons suffered a sudden attack of vomiting, abdominal cramps, and diarrhea. Investigators determined that the water supply was situated 18 meters from a crude, unlined sewage pit. It was surmised that contaminated drinking water was the culprit in this epidemic of gastroenteritis. Once water was transported from a municipal system and bacteriologic testing was implemented, there were no recurrences [18,19].

Prevention and Control

ADMINISTRATIVE CONTROLS AND EMPLOYEE EDUCATION AND TRAINING

Written plans or administrative controls that define policies to defeat the spread of infectious gastroenteritis in the workplace will have varying levels of effectiveness, depending on the causative organism, mode of transmission, and the occupation affected. At a minimum, these programs should address contingency behaviors in the event of an institutional outbreak of gastroenteritis, and ideally they should cover preventive measures such as symptom reporting, isolation of infected and uninfected, personal protective equipment, removal and cleanup practices, proper laundry and food handling, employee surveillance, and, where practical, immunization. Ideally, such employee training should take place at the time of hiring and at regular intervals thereafter.

SAFE WORK PRACTICES AND ENGINEERING CONTROLS

The purpose of any rational engineering control strategy is to effectively separate the worker from any infectious agents (particularly those described above) that have become part of the work environment. Specific methodologies in this arena may include purely mechanical ones, such as protective clothing, hand washing, isolation techniques, food and laundry handling procedures, and cleanup and disinfection techniques; or they may involve more elaborate plans such as reporting sick contacts, preemptive notification of potential contacts, and elaborate employee surveillance methods.

It is difficult to be specific about some of these strategies because the many organisms incriminated in the etiology of infectious gastroenteritis possess unique properties. However, the following discussion addresses some of the unique features regarding prophylactic measures and immunization to prevent infectious gastroenteritis.

PERSONAL PROTECTIVE EQUIPMENT

Personal protective equipment has a role to play when a gastrointestinal pathogen has been documented—whether in an institutional setting or in a less controlled environment such as a logging camp. The need for personal protective equipment is often a tacit concession that engineering control methods and other preventive measures have already broken down. That is not to say that personal protective equipment is not a very useful protective tool standing between a vulnerable employee population and almost certain infection.

When examining our armamentarium of protective equipment, we must consider the entry points that an organism may exploit. Near total coverage must include, as a minimum, gowns, caps, facemask, footcovers, goggles, and gloves. Clearly, this whole array of protection is not practical in all situations—remote camps and military maneuvers come to mind. It does make sense, however, when the microbial "cat is out of the bag" in a given environment and risks to employees are high, for instance, in a research situation where a spill has occurred.

MEDICAL SURVEILLANCE AND BIOLOGIC TESTING

In most cases of occupational gastroenteritis, a retrospective look at epidemiologic and etiologic factors would not lead us to conclude that comprehensive medical monitoring or surveillance of employees would have been a practical or cost-effective preventive measure. Ongoing or frequently scheduled employee physical examinations and laboratory work in, for example, nursing homes, in the absence of suspicious symptoms or at least incriminating risk factors, would never pass the test of frugality in this cost-conscious medical culture. In any event, the efficacy of these strategies is, as yet, unproved for the prevention of rapidly spreading diseases such as the infectious forms of gastroenteritis.

A possible exception to this general statement may be the special circumstances of animal handlers who are constantly and chronically exposed to zoonoses that may be more readily detectable by methods such as fecal leukocytes, complete blood count, and fecal ova and parasites.

Similarly, well-intentioned biologic testing of potentially contaminated sources such as food and water supplies will probably not be sufficient to prevent such easily contagious and rapidly transmissible diseases as most forms of infectious gastroenteritis.

IMMUNIZATION AND PROPHYLACTIC MEASURES

Hepatitis A is probably the only pathogen discussed so far that is susceptible to both preexposure and postexposure chemoprophylaxis. Hepatitis A immune globulin (IG) has proved to be an effective agent of prevention when administered within two weeks of suspected exposure to the virus. Also, the recently developed vaccine against hepatitis A would be a logical prophylactic choice for the wastewater worker who risks exposure to this virus on a daily basis.

The newly implemented rotavirus vaccine may have applications for day care workers as well as for the children for whom they care. Unfortunately, technical and economic stumbling blocks have left few other preventive agents in the battle against occupational gastroenteritis. In short, the chemoprophylactic arsenal against this class of microbe is relatively meager. Our efforts should be focused on some of the preventive measures discussed earlier rather than on chemoprophylaxis.

Symptoms and Signs

Anyone who has suffered or witnessed a bout of gastroenteritis will have no difficulty identifying its symptoms and signs. As stated previously, some key elements of the syndrome include nausea, vomiting, abdominal cramping, flatulence, and explosive and/or watery or bloody diarrhea. Other constitutional symptoms such as fever, chills, headache, malaise, and myalgias may accompany the more prominent gastrointestinal symptoms. Table 18-2 reviews some of the major gastrointestinal pathogens and the symptoms associated with infection.

Differential Diagnosis

When reviewing the differential diagnosis of acute gastroenteritis, the common occupationally acquired organisms discussed above must obviously be considered, but to be thorough in the assessment of ill workers, other nonoccupational causes of gastrointestinal symptoms must be considered as well, including:

- Laxative-induced diarrhea.
- Antibiotic-induced diarrhea.
- Other medication-induced diarrhea, such as that cause by iron- or manganese-containing compounds; high-dose salicylate, quinidine, NSAIDs, beta blockers, methyldopa, digitalis, or phenothiazine.
- Toxin-mediated diarrhea.
- Inflammatory bowel disease.
- Irritable bowel syndrome.
- Lactase deficiency.
- Diabetes.
- Hyperthyroidism.
- Malabsorptive states.

Diagnostic Evaluation

All diagnostic work-ups involve a detailed medical history, physical examination, and laboratory evaluation.

In some settings, it has been useful to provide the ill employee with a detailed questionnaire chronicling sick contacts, work environments, adherence to preventive procedures, record of ingestions of food and fluids, prior illnesses, chronic illnesses, medications, etc. Obviously, this should never be used as a substitute for a thorough history taken by a medical professional.

Typical presentations of gastroenteritis include nausea, vomiting, diarrhea, bloating, cramping, flatulence, and a host of associated constitutional symptoms such as fever, chills, headache, malaise, and myalgias.

In these cases, the physical exam should focus on vital signs, which may show elevated temperature, extremes of blood pressure, respiratory dis-

Table 18-2
Signs and Symptoms Associated with Gastrointestinal Pathogens

Organism	Signs and Symptoms
Giardia lamblia	Nausea; epigastric distress; flatulence; nonbloody diarrhea
Listeria monocytogenes	Acute, mild febrile illness with influenza-like symptoms
Shigella	Early watery and then bloody diarrhea; tenesmus
Salmonella	Watery or bloody diarrhea with or without systemic symptoms
E coli	Diarrhea with watery explosive onset; nausea, chills, cramps
Cryptosporidium parvum	Crampy, profuse, watery diarrhea, sometimes with anorexia and vomiting
Vibrio cholerae	Abrupt, explosive rice-water stool; severe electrolyte and fluid depletion; no abdominal pain or fever
Campylobacter jejuni	Prodrome of headaches, malaise, myalgias, fever, bloody diarrhea
Helicobacter pylori	Dyspepsia associated with epigastric or substernal "burning," early satiety; abdominal fullness
Clostridium difficile	Profuse watery diarrhea; fever; abdominal pain; leukocytosis
Yersinia frederiksenii	Simulates Crohn's disease and appendicitis; joint complaints
Rotavirus	Vomiting; watery diarrhea; fever; occasionally dehydration
Hepatitis A virus	Minor flu-like illness: anorexia, malaise, nausea, vomiting, and fever
Norwalk virus	Diarrheal illness often severe enough to cause dehydration

tress, and tachycardia or arrhythmias. General appearance, alertness level, or listlessness may herald more serious complications, namely electrolyte imbalance and dehydration. Evaluation of skin turgor, mucosal hydration, heart rate, peripheral capillary refill findings, and mental status may give clues to dehydration.

In the laboratory work-up, a complete blood count can be quite revealing in the areas of elevated polymorphonuclear leukocytes or depressed lymphocytes. These findings can sometime distinguish a viral disease from a bacterial one. A basic electrolyte panel will reveal serious electrolyte imbalances caused by severe diarrhea and vomiting. Stool studies are occasionally useful in determining the precise etiology of infective gastroenteritis. In general, however, they have been quite disappointing in identifying specific agents.

Treatment

Most bouts of acute gastroenteritis are short-lived and self-limited. These diseases often respond well to fluid resuscitation and gastrointestinal "rest." Bland diets and bismuth products are useful in providing symptomatic relief, but occasionally a prolonged illness will require intervention with antibiotics and electrolyte supplements. Table 18-3 outlines proposed first-line antibiotics recommended for specific infectious organisms.

Occupational Considerations

Although infectious gastroenteritis is not an obvious topic for most discussions of occupational diseases, little imagination is required to identify several occupations where there is clear cause and effect between job responsibilities and employee infection. Prominent among these occupations are the health professions and their supporting staff. Fortunately, most health institutions have well-developed prevention and contingency plans to meet the challenges of occupational disease. This efficiency may be motivated as much by economic incentives as by humanitarian impulses. Long regarded as merely an annoying illness that offers no serious, long-lasting health risk to the host, gastroenteritis is taken seriously in the occupational setting, principally as a drain on employer resources.

The price of employee sick leave attributable to illness is a major expense for most health care facilities, and the problems of infectious gastroenteritis pose a particularly vexing set of problems. The frustrations in dealing with this disease entity are its unpredictiblity, rapid spread,

Table 18-3
Antibiotics Recommended for Specific Organisms

Organism	Antibiotic
Giardia lamblia	Metronidazole
Listeria monocytogenes	IV ampicillin
Shigella	Cipro
Salmonella	Cipro
E coli	Antibiotics contraindicated
Vibrio cholerae	Cipro or Norflox
Campylobacter jejuni	Cipro or Norflox
Helicobacter pylori	Antibiotic combinations, which can include ampicillin, amoxicillin, biaxin in concert with other GI agents
Clostridium difficile	Metronidazole
Yersinia frederiksenii	Cipro or Norflox

and acutely debilitating symptoms. As noted earlier, chemoprophylaxis is not an important weapon against most of the causative organisms. In many cases, we have been forced to *react* to epidemics and hope that our efforts will stem a serious outbreak. This does not mean that prevention has no place in dealing with infectious gastroenteritis—quite the contrary. Prevention, of course, does not imply complete eradication of gastrointestinal illness in an institution for all time. Rather, it suggests somewhat smaller victories, such as limiting the spread of disease to residents, outside contacts, and employees. Also, implementation of routine preventive practices such as hand washing and hygienic food and water handling may obviate such heavy reliance on containment policies.

The health care industry, in particular, has gained valuable experience and subsequently provided leadership in controlling gastroenteritis outbreaks in their institutions. As outlined previously, most hospitals and nursing homes have developed some, all, or combinations of the following preventive techniques: (1) limitations on admissions to and discharge from wards where outbreaks are occurring; (2) involvement of the infection-control department; (3) restrictions on visitors; (4) strict enforcement of staff sick leave; (5) thorough use of personal protective equipment; (6) frequent and thorough hand washing; (7) restriction of patient movements during an outbreak; (8) no cross staffing between infected and uninfected wards; (9) liberal use of sodium hyperchloride disinfectant by dedicated cleaning staff; and (10) care in handling of soiled linen and other contaminated items [20].

It is hoped that other professions may learn to develop their own approach to preventing and halting outbreaks of occupational gastroenteritis. As a starting point, there is much useful data to borrow from the health care professions if only because they have been on the forefront of groundbreaking experiences in this arena.

References

1. Fleming LE. Unusual occupational gastrointestinal and hepatic disorders. *Occ Med: State of the Art Reviews* 1992;7(3):43.
2. Sepkowitz KA. Occupationally acquired infections in health care workers (part II). *Ann Intern Med* 1996;125(11):917–28.
3. Gestal JJ. Occupational hazards in hospitals: risk of infection. *Br J Ind Med* 1987;44:435–42.
4. Gardner G. An outbreak of hospital-acquired cryptosporidiosis. *Br J Nurs* 1994;3(4):152–8.
5. Caceres VM, Kim DK. A viral gastroenteritis outbreak associated with person-to- person spread among hospital staff. *Infect Contr Hosp Epidemiol* 1998;19(3):162–7.
6. Rodriguez EM, Parrott C. An outbreak of viral gastroenteritis in a nursing home: importance of excluding ill employees. *Infect Contr Hosp Epidemiol* 1996;17(9): 587–92.
7. Standaert SM, Hutcheson RH. Nosocomial transmission of Salmonella gastroenteritis to laundry workers in a nursing home. *Infect Control Hosp Epidemiol* 1994;15(1):22–6.

8. Gellert GA, Waterman SH. An outbreak of acute gastroenteritis caused by a small round structured virus in a geriatric convalescent facility. *Infect Control Hosp Epidemiol* 1990;11(9):459–64.
9. Stevenson P, McCann R. A hospital outbreak due to Norwalk virus. *J Hosp Infect* 1994;26:261–72.
10. Chadwick PR, McCann R. Transmission of a small round-structured virus by vomiting during a hospital outbreak of gastroenteritis. *J Hosp Med* 1994;26: 251–9.
11. Augustin AK, Simor AE. Outbreaks of gastroenteritis due to Norwalk-like virus in two long-term care facilities for the elderly. *Can J Infect Control* 1995; 10(4):111–3.
12. Khuder SA, Arthur T. Prevalence of infectious diseases and associated symptoms in wastewater treatment workers. *Am J Ind Med* 1998;33:571–7.
13. Sharp TW, Hyams KC. Epidemiology of Norwalk virus during an outbreak of acute gastroenteritis aboard a US aircraft carrier. *J Med Virol* 1995;45:61–7.
14. Lo SV, Connolly AM. The role of pre-symptomatic food handler in a common source outbreak of food-borne SRSV gastroenteritis in a group of hospitals. *Epidemiol Infect* 1994;113:513–21.
15. Jones A. Campylobacter enteritis in a food factory. *Lancet* 1979;Mar 17:611.
16. Christenson B, Ringner A. An outbreak of Campylobacter enteritis among the staff of a poultry abattoir in Sweden. *Scand J Infect Dis* 1983;15:167–72.
17. Pohjola S, Okasanen H. Outbreak of Cryptosporidiosis among veterinary students. *Scand J Infect Dis* 1986; 18:173–8.
18. Glover D. Gastroenteritis outbreak at an industrial camp—British Columbia. *BC Dis Surveillance* 1991; 89(3):66–8.
19. Werner SB. Gastroenteritis following ingestion of sewage-polluted water: an outbreak at a logging camp on the Olympic Peninsula. *Am J Epidemiol* 1968; 89(3): 277–85.
20. Russo PL, Spelman DW. Hospital outbreak of a Norwalk-like virus. *Infect Control Hosp Epidemiol* 1997;18(8):576.

19 / Occupational Tetanus

Philip E. Fisher and Alain J. Couturier

Given our present understanding of tetanus, the management of occupational tetanus infection is primarily an issue of prevention. If proper immunization practices are in place and prompt and proper wound care is administered, occupational tetanus could truly become a disease of the past. Although the bacterial culprit is ubiquitous, the unique mechanism of tetanus infection and disease permits several means of easy and effective intervention, both prior to and following exposure to this potentially deadly pathogen.

Epidemiology

INCIDENCE

Tetanus infection remains the leading cause of neonatal death in developing countries [1]. In early 1998, the disease was estimated to be killing well over half a million children each year in the developing world, most commonly through neonatal tetanus, which had a reported incidence of about 6 per 1,000 live births [2]. These neonatal infections are believed to result from the dressing of umbilical stumps with dung and to neonatal circumcision performed in primitive conditions. The infant mortality rate from tetanus in developing countries is reported to be 90% [3].

In Europe and North America, the disease is extremely rare as a result of better hygiene, improved wound care management, and higher immunization rates. It is increasingly becoming a disease of the elderly and is thought to be secondary to their impaired local responses to infection and to poorly maintained immunity [4]. The average annual incidence of tetanus in the United States during 1989–1990 was 0.02 per 100,000 people. This is considerably less than the rate of 0.39 per 100,000 reported in 1947. Similarly, the overall case fatality rate for this same time period declined from 91% in 1947 to 24% in 1989–1990 [5].

Another source [6] reports an incidence in the United States of 90 new cases per year and states that most of these cases involved individuals age 55 years or older and that virtually all affected individuals were either unimmunized or inadequately immunized. Given the considerable mortality rate that still exists today, this is clearly a disease that can and should be prevented, rather than permitted to occur and claim the lives of such a large number of its victims.

RISK FACTORS FOR TRANSMISSION

Tetanus infection is not a contagious disease. Rather, the spores of the *Clostridium tetani* organism reside in the soil and in the feces of domestic animals and humans. The organism is found most commonly in warmer climates and in highly cultivated rural areas. Infection takes place when the spores are deposited into an anaerobic environment and then germinate into toxin-producing organisms. Although typically introduced by deep puncture wounds, in many cases no apparent wound is found, making it likely that very minor, unnoticed (and hence unreported) trauma can also be the portal of entry [7]. The disease manifests when these organisms release their toxin. The toxin is a protein that diffuses away from the infected wound, enters the circulation, and then travels along nerves to the spinal cord. There it binds to inhibitory neurons, resulting in violent, spasmodic contraction of opposing muscle groups. Jaw muscles are commonly involved, giving rise to "lockjaw"—the common name for tetanus disease.

Adding to the virulence of this bacteria is the fact that its spores may remain dormant in the infected tissue, only to germinate later and begin producing and releasing their toxin after the initial wound has healed. Furthermore, the growth of other bacteria or the presence of foreign material such as dirt can enhance the anaerobic conditions that permit germination of the spores [8]. Both considerations are important in the proper management of tetanus and its prevention following penetrating trauma.

OCCUPATIONAL RISKS FACTORS

The single most important occupational risk factor for tetanus is absent or inadequate immunization status. It is therefore imperative that every effort be made to maintain tetanus immunity among all at-risk employees.

Tetanus is a potential problem in any outdoor occupation, especially those in which minor skin trauma is frequent. Agricultural workers account for the largest percentage of exposed individuals in the United States [7].

Prevention and Control

ADMINISTRATIVE CONTROLS

All employers must develop a method for assessing the immune status of their at-risk employees at the time of hiring and should arrange for the immediate correction of any deficiencies before the worker begins employment. Further, it is the employer's responsibility to track its employees and to notify them when the need arises (every 10 years) to boost their immunization with another dose of tetanus toxoid [9].

EMPLOYEE EDUCATION AND TRAINING

Employee training in tetanus prevention should focus on the need for adequate immunization and the importance of immediately reporting any work-related traumatic injury, particularly penetrating trauma or trauma associated with a high-risk or "dirty" wound. High-risk (tetanus-prone) wounds are:

- Wounds for which more than six hours have elapsed between injury and treatment.
- Wounds in which there is retention of devitalized tissue or foreign bodies.
- Any deep puncture wound.
- Missile wounds.
- Burns.
- Frostbite.
- Crush injuries.
- Avulsion injuries.

IMMUNIZATION AND PROPHYLACTIC MEASURES

Proper immunization involves both pre- and postexposure measures. Pre-exposure, all individuals should ideally have completed their initial immunization series, followed by a booster dose given every 10 years for life. The initial series is ideally begun in infancy with three doses of adsorbed tetanus toxoid given no less than one month apart, then a booster given 12 months following dose number three, and a fifth dose upon entering school [4].

Following injury, preventive measures include surgery to remove dead tissue and any foreign bodies. In cases in which the wound is considered "tetanus prone" (Table 19-1), prevention also includes the administration of human tetanus immune globulin. Immunoglobulin should also be given to patients with incomplete or unknown vaccine history and to patients with humoral immunosuppression, including HIV infection.

Symptoms and Signs

Patients with tetanus initially present with restlessness, irritability, stiffness of the neck, contraction of the muscles of the jaw, and sometimes convulsions. As additional muscle groups become involved, cramp-like pain develops and grows

Table 19-1
Treatment of Tetanus (Summary)

(1) Passive immunization (antitoxin): human tetanus immunoglobulin (HTIG) 500 IU injected into the deltoid muscle STAT.

(2) Active immunization: booster dose of tetanus toxoid (or initial of series if no previous), 0.5 mL of Td injected into the deltoid muscle of the arm opposite that into which HTIG injected.

(3) Antimicrobials: metronidazole, 500 mg intravenously or orally every eight hours.

(4) Symptomatic measures:
   (a) Dysphagia/airway management: intubate with a cuffed endotracheal tube upon first suspicion of dysphagia; often, elective tracheostomy under general anesthesia is necessary.
   (b) Muscle rigidity: diazepam, 10 mg given intravenously every three to four hours.
   (c) Paralyzed when intubated: pancuronium is the agent of choice for critically ill patients requiring artificial ventilation [10].
   (d) Anxiety (may be conscious although paretic): benzodiazepines offer sedation, amnesia, and muscle relaxation in addition to their anxiolytic effects.

(5) Wound debridement and/or excision: Do AFTER giving antitoxin.

(6) Nutrition:
   (a) If mild, feed orally.
   (b) If dysphagic, pass a nasogastric tube while under general anesthesia for tracheostomy, then NG feed (2,500 cal/day).
   (c) If paralytic ileus, hyperalimentation.

(7) Hydration: Complicated by heavy insensible fluid losses from sweating and unswallowed saliva:
   (a) Weigh daily.
   (b) Give enough fluid (orally and/or intravenously) to maintain a urine output of 1.5–2.0 L/day and a urine specific gravity ≤ 1.015.

(8) DVT/PE risk (due to dehydration and prolonged immobilization once paralyzed): anticoagulation therapy starting 24 hours after tracheostomy.

(9) Autonomic and cardiovascular instability:
   (a) Arterial and central venous pressure monitoring in an intensive care setting.
   (b) No standardized approach proposed (due to the lack of comparative trials and the limitations of case reports).
   (c) Consider magnesium sulfate, 4 g intravenous bolus, then 2–3 g/hour [11].
   (d) Consider adrenergic blocker—propranolol, 10 mg every three to six hours via nasogastric tube until heart rate averages < 100.
   (e) If hypertension persists, consider labetalol, 50–100 mg every six hours via nasogastric tube or by continuous intravenous infusion (0.25–1.0 mg/min).

more severe, and breathing becomes labored. Untreated, the pain is almost unbearable, and the patient often dies of aspiration pneumonia.

Once the tetanus toxin has bound to the spinal neurons, any minor stimulus can trigger the simultaneous contraction of opposing muscle groups, giving rise to trismus (or "lockjaw") or risus sardonicus (a "sardonic smile") if the facial muscles are involved, or opisthotonos (backward arching) with back muscle involvement. With loss of sympathetic inhibition, the heart rate and blood pressure are both affected, giving rise to dangerous cardiovascular instability. As the toxin is unable to cross the blood-brain barrier, the unmedicated patient's alertness and mentation remain tragically intact throughout the course of the illness. The clinical presentation of tetanus has been divided into three categories:

- Mild tetanus, in which there is muscle rigidity that may be generalized or may affect only one limb (so-called local tetanus). There is often trismus and/or a change in facial expression.
- Moderate tetanus, in which there is more severe rigidity, giving rise to risus sardonicus and opisthotonos. The diagnostic characteristic of a moderate case, however, is dysphagia secondary to pharyngeal muscle involvement.
- Severe tetanus, in which there are intense reflex spasms. Untreated, these can result in vertebral fracture. The back spasms are accompanied by spasms of the laryngeal muscles, the diaphragm, and the intercostal muscles—spasms that impede or prevent adequate ventilation. Severe tetanus also frequently presents with varying degrees of autonomic dysfunction. Cardiovascular responses to such stimuli as aspiration of secretions become exaggerated and systolic blood pressures in excess of 300 mm Hg are not uncommon. There is profuse sweating and extreme peripheral vasoconstriction. Catecholamine levels rise, and the sympathetic nervous system becomes grossly overactive and incoordinate, giving rise to such cardiovascular complications as supraventricular tachycardia, multifocal ventricular ectopy, unresponsive hypotension, sudden bradycardia, and cardiac arrest [4].

Differential Diagnosis

Fortunately few conditions present similarly to the disease of tetanus. Strychnine poisoning is about the only true mimic. Overdose or sensitivity to phenothiazines can be confused, but with these one typically sees both grimacing and facial movements where the jaw is widely opened [4].

Diagnostic Evaluation

Tetanus is a presumptive diagnosis made exclusively on history and physical examination. If the diagnosis is even suspected, attention should turn to immediate treatment. Once the tetanus toxin has bound to a neuron, the antitoxin will not neutralize its action. It is therefore imperative to administer the antitoxin as soon as possible, so that it can bind with and neutralize the toxin before the toxin has a chance to bind with the nerve cells.

Treatment and Rehabilitation

The management of tetanus infection depends on the severity of the illness. In all cases, the physician must remain alert for progression of symptoms, and hospitalization in an intensive care setting is therefore always indicated [7].

Table 19-1 outlines the management strategy for tetanus. Ideally, one would typically endeavor to enlist the consultation services of one or more intensivists to assist in the management of the paralysis, mechanical ventilation, tracheostomy, cardiac instability, and the infectious process. Time is of the essence, however, with regard to the administration of the antitoxin, and one should err on the side of giving it without delay in marginal situations. Human (not equine) tetanus immunoglobulin is much preferred, for severe and sometimes fatal anaphylactic reactions have been relatively common with the equine but are extremely rare with the human immunoglobulin [4].

References

1. Davies-Adetugbo AA, Torimiro SE, Ako-Nai KA. Prognostic factors in neonatal tetanus. *Trop Med Internat Health* 1998;3(1):9–13.
2. Thayaparan B, Nicoll A. Prevention and control of tetanus in childhood [review]. *Curr Opin Pediatr* 1998;10(1):4–8.
3. Ernst ME, Klepser ME, Fouts M, et al. Tetanus: pathophysiology and management [review]. *Ann Pharmacother* 1997;31(12):1507–13.
4. Wyngaarden JB, Smith LH (eds). *Cecil Textbook of Medicine*, 17th Ed. Philadelphia: Saunders Company, 1985. Pp 1579–82.
5. Prevots R, Suter RW, Strebel PM, et al. Tetanus surveillance—United States, 1989–90. *MMWR* 1992;41(SS-8):1–9.
6. Branch WT (ed). *Office Practice of Medicine*, 2nd Ed. Philadelphia: Saunders, 1987. Pp 1256, 1259.
7. Wald PH, Stave GM (eds). *Physical and Biological Hazards of the Workplace*. New York: Van Nostrand Reinhold, 1994. Pp 334–6.
8. Nester EW, Roberts CE, Lidstrom ME, et al (eds). *Microbiology*, 3rd Ed. Philadelphia: CBS College Publishing, 1983. Pp 583–85, 835.
9. Lewy R, Brown T, Christenson WN, et al. American College of Occupational and Environmental Medicine Guidelines—employee health services in health care institutions. *J Occup Med* 1986;28(7).
10. Shapiro BA, Warren J, Egol AB, et al. Practice parameters for sustained neuromuscular blockade in the adult critically ill patient: an executive summary. *Crit Care Med* 1995;23:1601–5.
11. Lipman J, James MF, Erskine J, et al. Autonomic dysfunction in severe tetanus: magnesium sulfate as an adjunct to deep sedation. *Crit Care Med* 1987;15:987–8.

20 / Occupational Rabies

Carl N. Zenz, Jr.

Although only a few cases of human rabies occur annually in the United States, the increase in international travel and foreign assignments, along with recent improvements in vaccines, has greatly enhanced pre- and post-exposure strategies for this deadly virus. Rabies has plagued mankind for centuries. In the fourth century BC, Aristotle wrote "that dogs suffer from the madness. This causes them to become very irritable and all animals they bite become diseased" [1]. Hippocrates supposedly refers to rabies when he says that "persons in a frenzy drink very little, are disturbed and frightened, tremble at the least noise, or are seized with convulsions."

Aulus Comaelius Celsus, in 100 AD, contradicted Aristotle's assertion that humans were exempt from rabies and was the first to suggest treatment by excision and cautery of the bite inflicted by a rabid animal [2]. Girolamo Fracastoro, a sixteenth-century Italian physician wrote a description of the aspects of human disease. It was in 1804 that Zinke first demonstrated that rabies could be transmitted by saliva. Numerous researchers in the 1800s, such as Krugelstein and Ekstrom, studied the pathogenesis and treatment of rabies [3].

Pasteur discovered that the true infectious agent of rabies could be obtained and transmitted from the brains of animals dying of the disease. He published his first report in 1881. He reported induction of rabies by the central nervous system material and spinal fluid, thus demonstrating that the source of the virus was not limited to saliva. Pasteur noted that the virus was found not only in the lower centers of the brain, but also in the spinal cord. He also differentiated "dumb rabies," characterized by paralysis, and "furious rabies" in which the animal attacked everything.

In 1884, Pasteur reported that the clinical signs produced were somewhat dependent upon the dose of infective material and that infections of small amounts of virus did not produce immunity. He also reviewed the hypothesis of the passage of the virus from the periphery to the central nervous system via the nerves versus that of the distribution of the virus by the bloodstream. Additionally, he discussed the theoretic basis of immunizing injections [4].

Pasteur gave his first detailed report in 1885 to the Academy of Science on his method of rabies prophylaxis. The immunization was carried out by injecting a dog subcutaneously with a syringe of broth to which was added a small portion of rabid rabbit cord, beginning with one that was dried long enough to be avirulent and successively using more virulent material until a virulent cord was finally reached. The dog was then refractory to rabies.

During that summer, a 9-year-old boy was referred to him. The boy, who had been bitten 14 times by a rabid dog, was examined by Doctors Grancher and Valpian, who believed he had received a fatal inoculation of rabies virus. Pasteur went on to say, "The death of this child seemed inevitable, and I decided not without lively and cruel doubts, as one can believe, to try in Joseph Meister, the method which had been successful in dogs. Consequently, on July 6 at 8:00 in the evening, 60 hours after the bites, in the presence of Doctors Valpian and Grancher, we inoculated under a skin fold in the right hypochrondrium of the little Meister a half syringe of the cord of a rabid rabbit preserved in a flask of dry air for 15 days." Thirteen successive inoculations were made with the cords of increasing virulence. The patient survived [5]. These findings laid the foundation for a better understanding of the pathogenesis of the disease and development of improved vaccines.

The rabies virus belongs to the family Rhabdoviridae, genus *Lyssavirus.* The *Lyssavirus* genus is now considered to contain seven viruses, of which rabies is an enveloped, single, nonsegmented, negative-stranded ribonucleic acid virus [6,7].

The extremely poor prognosis for rabies encephalitis has hastened the development of vaccines to safely prevent the development of the disease as well as provide effective postexposure therapy. The importance of preventive measures remains the cornerstone for controlling rabies.

Epidemiology

INCIDENCE AND PREVALENCE

It is difficult to evaluate the true mortality rate due to rabies worldwide. Most recent estimates by the World Health Organization are over 50,000 deaths annually, with probable significant underreporting [8]. An estimated 600,000 to 2 million dog bites occur yearly in the United States, and 30,000 people annually receive treatment for rabies prevention following potential exposures [9,10]. Four cases of human rabies were documented in the United States during 1997 [11]. The only documented cases of rabies due to human-to-human transmission occurred in patients who received corneal transplants from persons who died of undiagnosed rabies [12]. It has been estimated that 99% of all human deaths from rabies occur in the tropical zone [13].

TRANSMISSION RISK FACTORS

The transmission of the rabies virus to a human is usually through the bite of an infected animal. Other means include the inhalation of infected bat secretions, infected-animal licks on mucous membranes, and receiving corneal grafts from infected donors. The primary reservoirs of the virus are cats, dogs, foxes, coyotes, skunks, raccoons, jackals, wolves, and bats. In countries where domestic animal rabies has not been adequately controlled, dogs account for 90% or more of the reported cases in which there has been animal-to-human transmission. Within areas of good domestic-animal rabies programs (such as the United States, Canada, and European countries), dogs account for less than 5% of cases.

OCCUPATIONAL RISK FACTORS

Occupations that expose the workers to potential infectious sources of this virus may be categorized into four groups, based on risk. These categories are continuous, frequent, infrequent (but greater than the population at large), and rare (no greater than the population at large). Workers that fall into the continuous risk category include rabies research laboratory workers and rabies biologics production workers. Other potentially exposed workers include veterinarians and staff, animal-control and wildlife workers in rabies-enzootic areas, rabies diagnostic laboratory workers, and mail delivery workers. Travelers, such as field engineers working in areas where rabies is enzootic and immediate access to adequate medical care (with biologics) is limited, are also at risk and should be immunized (Table 20-1) [14].

PREVENTION AND CONTROL

Education of potentially exposed workers with primary or pre-exposure vaccination is the key to preventing this disease. Workers need to be aware of the transmission modes of the rabies virus, the need for immunization, depending upon their job functions, and the necessity for immediate therapeutic intervention following an exposure incident.

Pre-exposure prophylaxis does not eliminate the need for additional therapy after exposure; however, it eliminates the use of rabies immune globulin (RIG) and decreases the number of doses needed. Additionally, if postexposure therapy is delayed, the primary series might protect those individuals.

IMMUNIZATION AND PROPHYLATIC MEASURES

Primary vaccination may be done via intramuscular or intradermal injections. Three 1.0-mL

Table 20-1
Rabies Pre-exposure Prophylaxis Guide—United States, 1999

Risk Category	Nature of Risk	Typical Populations	Pre-exposure Recommendations
Continuous	Virus present continuously, often in high concentrations. Specific exposures likely vaccination if antibody to go unrecognized. Bite, nonbite, or aerosol exposure.	Rabies research laboratory workers;[b] rabies biologics production workers.	Primary course. Serologic testing every 6 months: booster vaccination if antibody titer below acceptable level.
Frequent	Exposure usually episodic, with source recognized. Bite, nonbite, or aerosol.	Rabies diagnostic lab workers,[a] spelunkers, Veterinarians and staff, and wildlife workers in rabies-enzootic areas.	Primary course. Serologic testing every 2 years: booster vaccination if antibody titer is below acceptable level[b] exposure.
Infrequent (greater than population at large)	Exposure nearly always episodic with source recognized. Bite or nonbite exposure.	Veterinarians and animal-control and wildlife workers in areas with low rabies rates. Veterinary students. Travelers visiting areas where rabies is enzootic and immediate access to appropriate medical care, including biologics, is limited.	Primary course. No serologic testing or booster vaccination.
Rare (population at large)	Exposure always episodic with source recognized. Bite or nonbite exposure.	U.S. population at large, including persons in rabies-epizootic areas.	No vaccination necessary.

[a] Judgment of relative risk and extra monitoring of vaccination status of laboratory workers is the responsibility of the laboratory supervisor.
[b] Minimum acceptable antibody level is complete virus neutralization at a 1:5 serum dilution by the rapid fluorescent focus inhibition test. A booster dose should be administered if the titer falls below this level.
Adapted from Centers for Disease Control and Prevention. Human rabies prevention—United States, 1999: recommendations of the Advisory Committee on Immunization Practices (ACIP). *MMWR* 1999;48(No. RR-1):1–21.

injections into the deltoid muscle of human diploid cell vaccine (HDCV), rabies vaccine adsorbed (RVA), or purified chick embryo cell vaccine (PCEC) on days 0, 7, and 21 or 28 may be used (Table 20-2).

The intradermal regimen of three 0.1-mL ID doses of HDCV on days 0, 7, and 21 or 28 is also used for pre-exposure vaccination. HDCV should not be administered intradermally to individuals receiving antimalarial chemoprophylaxis, since this may inhibit antibody production.

Individuals who work in research laboratories or vaccine-production facilities are at high risk for inapparent exposures. These individuals should have rabies antibody tests every six months.

SYMPTOMS AND SIGNS

Human rabies evolves through five clinical phases: (1) incubation period, (2) prodrome, (3) acute neurologic phase, (4) coma, and (5) death or recovery [15]. Recovery is rare, and infected individuals usually succumb in the later stages of the disease. The development of rabies depends on the type of exposure, the animal involved, and pre- and postexposure treatment received. The rabies virus usually enters the body through skin broken by a bite or scratch; however, it can also enter through intact mucous membrane and may be inhaled as an aerosol or be transplanted through infected corneal grafts.

Table 20-2
Rabies Biologics—United States, 1999

Human Rabies Vaccine	Product Name	Manufacturer
Human diploid cell vaccine (HDCV)		Pasteur-Meneux Serum et Vaccins, Connaught Laboratories, Inc., phone: (800) VACCINE (822-2463)
Intramuscular	ImovaxG Rabies	
Intradermal	Imovax Rabies I.D.	
Rabies vaccine adsorbed (RVA), intramuscular	Rabies vaccine adsorbed (RVA)	BioPort Corporation, phone: (517) 335-Ri 20
Purified chick embryo cell vaccine (PCEC), intramuscular	RaoAvert	Chiron Corporation, phone: (800) CHIRONE (244-7668)
Rabies immune globulin (RIG)	Imogam Rabies-HI	Pasteur-Meneux Serum et Vaccins, Connaught Laboratories, Inc., phone: (800) VACCINE (822-2463)
	BayRab	Bayer Corporation Pharmaceutical Div., phone: (800) 288-8370

Adapted from Centers for Disease Control and Prevention. Human rabies prevention—United States, 1999: recommendations of the Advisory Committee on Immunization Practices (ACIP). *MMWR* 1999;48(No. RR-1):1–21.

The incubation time in human rabies is variable. It may be as short as nine days to as long as a year or more. The mean incubation period is 30 to 78 days. Approximately 14% of cases have longer incubations. Short incubation is seen in patients with more severe exposure and with bite exposures to the face and head [16]. The patient is asymptomatic during incubation.

PRODROMAL SYMPTOMS

The earliest symptoms of rabies are generally nonspecific and may suggest another illness. Symptoms include malaise, headache, gastrointestinal symptoms, dyspnea, fatigue, and anorexia. Most patients are febrile: More than 50% in one series had a temperature greater than 101° F (38.3°C). Chills may accompany the fever. The most common early gastrointestinal symptoms include nausea, vomiting, abdominal cramping, and diarrhea. Other presenting symptoms may include sore throat, photophobia, headache, and dizziness. Pain or paresthesia at the site of the bite is the only relatively specific prodromal symptom. Itching may occur at the site of a healed bite wound or involve the whole bitten limb and may be so intense as to result in excoriation of the skin by scratching. The explanation for local paresthesia may be the multiplication of the virus in the dorsal root ganglion of the sensory nerve supplying the area of the bite. Three of four patients who had acquired rabies via corneal transplant noted pain referable to the eye receiving the infected cornea [17].

THE ACUTE NEUROLOGIC PHASE

This phase includes a wide variety of systemic disorders. The symptoms are varied and may include aerophobia and hydrophobia. The onset is two to 10 days after the prodromal symptoms; the individual develops signs of nervous system involvement, including hyperactivity, hallucinations, disorientation, seizures, nuchal stiffness, bizarre behavior, and paralysis. A period of marked hyperactivity may last from hours to days, with periods of agitation, thrashing, and biting; this is known as *"furious" rabies.* This hyperactivity may occur spontaneously or be precipitated by tactile, auditory, visual, or olfactory stimuli. Between episodes, the patient is usually lucid and cooperative but often is anxious.

Hydrophobia, the most characteristic symptom, occurs in up to 50% of patients. An intense psychic response, even terror, induced by attempts to drink or even the sight of water, is typical. Severe, painful spasms of the pharynx and larynx produce choking, gagging, and fear. Inspiratory spasms lasting 5 to 15 seconds are part of the hydrophobic response, and these may lead to respiratory arrest or generalized fatal convulsions. Warrel and colleagues have suggested that the respiratory signs may be related to respiratory myoclonus and be caused by brain stem lesions rather than occurring as a conditioned reflex arising from throat pain [18].

Abnormalities that may appear during this period of hyperactivity include muscle fasciculations (especially near the site of exposure), hyperventilation, hypersalivation, and focal or generalized convulsions. The majority of patients manifest signs of delirium. Other neurologic signs may include meningismus, cranial nerve pareses leading to diplopia, ptosis, dysphagia, and dysarthria. Limb paresis (at times with clear signs of pyramidal tract lesions) and reflex alterations also may be present.

Autonomic changes such as hyperpyrexia, hypotension, excessive sweating, piloerection, pupil dilation, hypersalivation, and tachycardia frequently develop. In about 20% of patients, a second clinical form of rabies infection presents as paralysis. The entire clinical course is similar neurologically to the Landry-Guillain-Barré syndrome. This course of rabies has been described as *"dumb" rabies* (or *rage tranquil*). The paralysis may be diffuse and symmetric or an ascending paralysis. The acute neurologic period usually lasts for one week.

COMA

During this phase of rabies, the previous signs of hydrophobia are replaced by irregular respiration and prolonged periods of apnea. Respiratory arrest resulting in death may occur during this time. The duration of coma may range from hours to months, depending on the intensity of care the patient receives. Supplemental trials of corticosteroids, interferon, and other antivirals have not positively affected the outcomes.

RECOVERY

Very few patients have recovered from a documented rabies virus infection, even with aggressive treatment.

Differential Diagnosis

Patients with encephalopathy of unknown origin should have rabies infection considered in the differential diagnosis, even without known exposure to the virus through an animal bite. In a review of all 32 rabies cases reported in the United States between 1980 and 1996, Noah and colleagues found that a lack of clinical suspicion of rabies delayed the diagnosis. Since no postexposure prophylaxis was received, all 32 individuals succumbed [19]. There is little to distinguish rabies from other viral encephalitides. A history of exposure is the most helpful diagnostic clue. Other possible conditions include poliomyelitis, Landry-Guillain-Barré syndrome, and hysterical reactions to animal bites (pseudohydrophobia). Neuroparalytic reactions from postexposure courses of rabies prophylaxis consisting of CNS-tissue vaccines may still occur in parts of the world where this type of vaccine is utilized.

DIAGNOSTIC EVALUATION

Because laboratory diagnosis is usually not possible during the first week of illness, the appearance of symptoms plus a history of exposure to a rabid animal strongly support the diagnosis of rabies. Individuals without a history of vaccination develop serum antibodies that are first detectable on the tenth day of illness (with a rapid rise thereafter to high levels). Detectable antibodies appear in the cerebrospinal fluid (CSF) later in the clinical course (approximately the third week). Since vaccination does not induce CSF antibodies, high CSF titers support the diagnosis.

Fluorescent antibody staining techniques enable the detection of rabies antigen in nuchal skin biopsies. Saliva and skin samples may be analyzed by reverse-transcriptase polymerase chain reaction (RT-PCR) assay. Rabies virus neutralizing antibody titers from serum and CSF samples can be obtained by the rapid fluorescent focus inhibition test (RFFIT). Virus isolation can be done to confirm other positive test results by tissue culture or intracerebral inoculation of mice [20].

Treatment

Postexposure prophylaxis following a possible exposure may be categorized into two groups: those with previous vaccinations and those without.

Previously vaccinated persons are those who have received one of the recommend courses of HDCV, RVA, or PCEC. These individuals should receive two intramuscular doses (1.0 mL each) of vaccine, one immediately and one three days later.

Physicians need to evaluate each possible exposure to rabies and the need for rabies prophylaxis (Table 20-3).

Immediate washing of all bite wounds with soap and water and a virucidal agent (e.g., povidone-iodine solution) is important. Postexposure rabies vaccination should include both passive antibody and vaccine in previously unimmunized individuals. The recommended dose of human RIG is 20 IU/kg body weight, and if feasible, the full dose should be infiltrated in the area around and into the wound. (Any remaining volume should be injected intramuscularly at a site distant from vaccine administration.) The first dose of a five-dose course (1 mL of HDCV, RVA, or PCEC) should be given intramuscularly as soon as possible after exposure. The remaining doses should be given on days 3, 7, 14, and 28 after the first vaccination (Table 20-4).

Advances in the understanding of the immunology of the rabies virus has promoted the development of even more efficacious vaccines, along with an improved dosage schedule for both primary and postexposure immunizations. Routine pre-exposure vaccination should be contemplated for a variety of occupations, depending on multiple issues, such as risk of exposure (as in laboratory workers) and location of the individual's work activities (as in the tropics). The availability of vaccines and rabies immune globulin for follow-up treatment in certain parts of the world where rabies is endemic is another key consideration. For high-risk activities, serum antibody levels may be drawn to monitor the worker's protective levels. Due to the extreme mortality rate associated with this virus, a high degree of employee awareness about the need for follow-up in postexposure situations is mandatory, as well as routine preventive administration of these vaccines for high-risk overseas workers.

References

1. Fleming G. *Rabies and Hydrophobia*. London: Chapman and Hall, 1872. P 7.
2. Smithcors JF. The history of some current problems in animal disease. VII Rabies (Part 1). *Vet Med* 1958; 53:149.

Table 20-3
Rabies Postexposure Prophylaxis Guide—United States, 1999

Animal Type	Evaluation and Disposition of Animal	Postexposure Prophylax Recommendations
Dogs, cats, and ferrets	Healthy and available for 10 days' observation	Persons should not begin prophylaxis unless animal develops clinical signs of rabies.[a]
	Rabid or suspected rabid, unknown (e.g., escaped)	Vaccinate immediately. Consult public health officials.
Skunks, raccoons, foxes, and most other carnivores; bats	Regarded as rabid unless animal proven negative by laboratory tests[b]	Consider immediate vaccination.
Livestock, small rodents, lagomorphs (rabbits and hares), large rodents (woodchucks and beavers), and other mammals	Consider individually	Consult public health officials. Bites of squirrels, hamsters, guinea pigs, gerbils, chipmunks, rats, mice, other small rodents, rabbits, and hares almost never require antirabies postexposure prophylaxis.

[a] During the 10-day observation period, begin postexposure prophylaxis at the first sign of rabies in a dog, cat, or ferret that has bitten someone. If the animal exhibits clinical signs of rabies, it should be euthanized immediately and tested.

[b] The animal should be euthanized and tested as soon as possible. Holding it for observation is not recommended. Discontinue vaccine if results of immunofluorescence testing of the animal are negative.

Adapted from Centers for Disease Control and Prevention. Human rabies prevention—United States, 1999: recommendations of the Advisory Committee on Immunization Practices (ACIP). *MMWR* 1999;48(No. RR-1):1–21.

Table 20-4
Rabies Postexposure Prophylaxis Schedule—United States, 1999

Vaccination Status	Treatment	Regimen[a]
Not previously vaccinated	Wound cleansing	All postexposure treatment should begin with immediate thorough cleansing of all wounds with soap and water. If available, a virucidal agent such as a povidone-iodine solution should be used to irrigate the wounds.
	RIG	Administer 20 IU/kg body weight. If anatomically feasible, the full dose should be infiltrated around the wound(s) and any remaining volume should be administered IM at an anatomic site, distant from vaccine administration. Also, RIG should not be administered in the same syringe as vaccine. Because RIG might partially suppress active production of antibody, no more than the recommended dose should be given.
	Vaccine	HDCV, RVA, or PCEC 1.0 mL, IM (deltoid area[b]), one dose each on days 0[c], 3, 7, 14, and 28.
Previously vaccinated[d]	Wound cleansing	All postexposure treatment should begin with immediate thorough cleansing of all wounds with soap and water. If available, a virucidal agent such as a povidone-iodine solution should be used to irrigate the wounds.
	RIG	RIG should not be administered.
	Vaccine	HDCV, RVA, or PCEC 1.0 mL, IM (deltoid area[b]), one dose each on days 0[c] and 3.

HDCV = human diploid cell vaccine; *PCEC* = purified chick embryo cell vaccine; *RIG* = rabies immune globulin; *RVA* = rabies vaccine adsorbed; *IM* = intramuscular.

[a] These regimens are applicable for all age groups, including children.

[b] The deltoid area is the only acceptable site of vaccination for adults and older children. For younger children, the outer aspect of the thigh may be used. Vaccine should never be administered in the gluteal area.

[c] Day 0 is the day the first dose of vaccine is administered.

[d] Any person with history of pre-exposure vaccination with HDCV, RVA, or PCEC; prior postexposure prophylaxis with HDCV, RVA, or PCEC; or previous vaccination with any other type of rabies vaccine and a documented history of antibody response to the prior vaccination.

Adapted from Centers for Disease Control and Prevention. Human rabies prevention—United States, 1999: recommendations of the Advisory Committee on Immunization Practices (ACIP). *MMWR* 1999;48(No. RR-1):1–21.

3. Fernandez PJ. History of rabies and global aspects. In: Baer GM (ed), *The Natural History of Rabies,* 2nd Ed. Boca Raton, FL: CRC Press, 1991. Pp 1–24.
4. Pasteur L, Chamferland CE, Roux M. Nouvelle communication sur la rage. *CR Acad Sci* 1884;98;457.
5. Pasteur L. Sur la rage. *CR Acad Sci* 1881;92:1259.
6. Plotkin SA, Rupprecht CE, Koprowski H. Rabies vaccine. *Vaccines*, 3rd Ed. New York: Saunders, 1999. Pp 744–5.
7. Bourky H, Kissi B, Tordo N. Molecular diversity of the lyssavirus genus. *Virology* 1993;194:70–81.
8. Wilde H, Mitmoonpitak C. Canine rabies in Thailand. *World Health Magazine* 1998(4):10–11.
9. Hildreth EA. Prevention of rabies on the decline of Sirius. *Ann Intern Med* 1963;88:883–96.
10. Parish HM, Clark FB, Brobst D, et al. Epidemiology of dog bites. *Public Health Rep* 1967;82:1009–18.
11. Human rabies—Texas and New Jersey, 1997. *MMWR* 1998;47(1):1–5.
12. Warrell DA, Warrell MJ. *Human Rabies and Its Prevention: An Overview, Reviews of Infectious Diseases,* Vol 10, Suppl. 4. Chicago: University of Chicago, 1998.

13. Acha PN, Arambulo PV II. Rabies in the tropics—history and current status. In: Kuwert E, Merieux C, Loprowski H, et al. (eds), *Rabies in the Tropics.* Berlin: Springer-Verlag, 1985. Pp 343–59.
14. Centers for Disease Control and Prevention. Human rabies prevention—United States, 1999: recommendations of the Advisory Committee on Immunization Practices (ACIP). *MMWR* 1999:48(No RR-1):1–21.
15. Robinson PA. Rabies virus. In: Belshe RB (ed), *Textbook of Human Virology*, 2nd Ed. New York: Mosby Year Book, 1991. Chap 19.
16. Warrell DA. The clinical picture of rabies in man. *Trans R Soc Trop Med Hyg* 1976;70:188–95.
17. Centers for Disease Control. Human-to-human transmission of rabies via corneal transplant—Thailand. *MMWR* 1981;30:472–4.
18. Miller A, Nathanson N. Rabies: recent advances in pathogenesis and control. *Ann Neurol* 1977;2:511–9.
19. Noah D, et al. Review of rabies cases reported in the U.S. between 1980 and 1996. *Ann Intern Med* 1998;128(11):922–30.
20. Human rabies—Virginia, 1998. *MMWR* 1999;48:95–7. *JAMA* 1999;281(10):891–2.

21 / Occupational Infectious Diseases with Dermatologic Features

Boris D. Lushniak

Occupational dermatology is the facet of dermatology that deals with skin diseases whose etiology or aggravation is related to some exposure in the workplace. By its nature, occupational dermatology is also related to occupational and preventive medicine. The ideal role of a medical practitioner involved in occupational dermatology is not only to diagnose and treat patients, but also to determine the etiology of the occupational skin disease and to make recommendations for its prevention. Occupational dermatology covers a wide variety of skin diseases, including allergic contact dermatitis, irritant contact dermatitis, pigmentary disorders, skin cancer, as well as infectious diseases. Many general references on occupational skin disorders are available [1–3].

In general, the causes of occupational skin disorders can be grouped into the following categories:

1. Physical insults (friction, pressure, trauma, vibration, heat, cold, variations in humidity, ultraviolet/visible/infrared radiation, ionizing radiation, and electric current).
2. Chemical insults (water, soaps/detergents, inorganic acids, alkalis, salts of heavy metals, aliphatic acids, aldehydes, alcohols, esters, hydrocarbons, solvents, metallo-organic compounds, lipids, aromatic and polycyclic compounds, resin monomers, and proteins).
3. Biologic causes (plants, arthropods, bacteria, Rickettsiae, viruses, fungi, and parasites).

Diseases in the biologic category include occupational dermatologic infectious diseases. These are diseases that have a major manifestation on the cutaneous surface and result from exposure to an infectious agent found in a workplace setting. This exposure can occur through direct skin contact (epicutaneous), inoculation (percutaneous), or through the respiratory system (inhalational).

Epidemiology

Epidemiologic data specifically related to occupational dermatologic infectious diseases are very limited. Other than limited descriptions in case presentations, case studies, and epidemic investigation reports, little is known about the epidemiology of most of these diseases in the United States. For the infectious diseases that are nationally reportable, it is impossible to determine what proportion are due to occupational exposures. In many cases, it is difficult to definitively prove that the disease process is occupationally related. The accuracy of the diagnosis is related to the skill level, experience, and knowledge of the medical professional who makes the diagnosis and then confirms the relationship with a workplace exposure. The questions to be answered by the clinician include the following: (1) Is the patient's condition a dermatologic infectious disease? (2) Is the organism found in the patient's workplace environment? (3) Was there an opportunity for the worker to become infected in the workplace? (4) What other nonoccupational exposures (e.g., recreational activities) must be considered [4]?

The public health importance of a disease can be measured in several ways, using statistical, clinical, and economic measures [5]. These measures include the absolute number of cases, the incidence rate, the prevalence rate, the prognosis and preventability of the disease, and the economic impact of the disease (e.g., medical costs and days away from work). There are many gaps in this information for occupational dermatologic infectious diseases.

As of 1997, 52 infectious diseases were designated as notifiable at the national level in the United States [6]. Of the diseases discussed in this chapter, the following number of cases were reported for 1996 and 1997: anthrax—0/0 cases; brucellosis—112/98; Lyme disease—16,455/12,801; measles—508/138; Rocky Mountain spotted fever—831/409; rubella—238/181; rubella congenital syndrome—4/5; varicella—83,511/98,727 [6,7]. Although tularemia was dropped as a notifiable condition in 1995, 36 states maintain it as a notifiable condition. These states reported 105 cases in 1997 [6].

National occupational injury and illness data are available from the U.S. Bureau of Labor Statistics (BLS). The BLS conducts annual surveys of approximately 250,000 employers, selected to represent all private industries in the United States [8]. The survey results are then projected to estimate the numbers and incidence rates of injuries and illnesses in the American working population. BLS data are limited in that they exclude self-employed individuals, small farms, and government agencies; depend on misinterpretable definitions of reportable occupational injuries and illnesses; rely to a large extent on employees' reporting conditions to the employer; do not provide information on the etiology of the skin disease; and are considered underestimates of the true number of cases [9–12].

There is limited information on occupational dermatologic infectious diseases in the BLS data. In 1993, there were an estimated 60,200 cases of occupational skin diseases or disorders, or 7.6 per 10,000 workers [8]. Of these, 12,613 cases, 1.6 per 10,000 workers, resulted in one or more days away from work [13]. The majority of these (70%) were due to the most common occupational skin disease—dermatitis. Infections of the skin and subcutaneous tissue accounted for 20% of the 12,613 cases or 2,458 cases (0.31 per 10,000 workers). Most of these were listed as cellulitis and abscess (1,305 cases); the others included unspecified (596), not elsewhere classified (416) and pilonidal cyst (98) [8]. The median days away from work for workers with these skin infections were five days. In 1993, under a separate category of infectious and parasitic diseases, the BLS recorded 3,346 cases, which resulted in at least one day away from work [8]. Few diagnoses were listed, but diagnoses with potential skin manifestations included viral diseases accompanied by exanthem (1,206 cases), chickenpox (1,018), scabies/chiggers/mites (367), herpes zoster (111), dermatophytosis (including athlete's foot and tinea) (71), and coccidioidomycosis (53).

Finland has a more advanced surveillance system for occupational diseases. In 1996, of 1,097 cases of occupational skin diseases, 68% were due to dermatitis, while 8% (92 cases) were due to skin infections [14]. The etiologies of these infections included mites (64 cases), dermatophytosis (10), poxvirus (9), not specified bacteria (3), other known bacteria (2), molds (1), eubacteria (1), herpesvirus (1), and unknown (1).

Overview

Many of the occupational dermatologic infectious diseases result in not only cutaneous signs and symptoms but also in systemic effects as well. The cutaneous manifestations will be stressed in this chapter. Infections such as impetigo, erysipelas, cellulitis, folliculitis, furuncles, carbuncles, and abscesses caused by common organisms such as group A streptococci or *Staphylococcus aureus* will not be discussed. Traumatic wounds or infestations secondarily infected with these common pathogens will not be emphasized in this chapter. Finally, sexually transmitted diseases, many of which have cutaneous manifestations and can be considered to be occupational diseases in the sex trades, will not be included here.

The occupational dermatologic infectious diseases covered in this chapter range from very common diseases in the United States, both in occupational and nonoccupational settings (e.g., candidiasis and dermatophytosis), to very rare diseases in the United States (e.g., anthrax and tularemia), to diseases never seen in the United States. Some of these occur only outside of the United States and are seen here only as rare cases of imported occupational diseases in workers exposed overseas.

In general, risk of infection can be associated with individual worker susceptibility (e.g., immune status, trauma to the protective barrier of the skin), the existence of the pathogen in the environment (e.g., endemic geographic locations), and occupational exposure to the pathogen, its reservoir, or fomites or to work conditions in which the pathogens thrive. Reservoirs and fomites of the pathogens include people (coworkers, clients, patients, or children), animals or animal products, soil or plant materials, ticks/insects, water, and marine life. Conditions in which pathogens can thrive and increase worker susceptibility include wet work and hot and humid environments. The occupational dermatologic infectious diseases associated with these sources and conditions are listed in Tables 21-1 through 21-6. In addition, laboratory workers are at risk of infection with the pathogens with which they are working.

The specific diseases will be described by pathogen category. Occupational dermatologic infectious diseases can be grouped by etiologic agent into the following disease categories: (1) bacterial, (2) rickettsial, (3) viral, (4) superficial fungal, (5) subcutaneous fungal, (6) systemic fungal, and (7) parasitic.

Table 21-1
Occupational Dermatologic Infectious Diseases Associated with Exposures to Patients or Children

Cutaneous tuberculosis
Herpetic whitlow
Warts
Measles
Rubella
Chickenpox
Herpes zoster (shingles)
Hand-foot-mouth disease
Erythema infectiosum (fifth disease)
Dermatophytes (anthropophilic)
Scabies

Table 21-2
Occupational Dermatologic Infectious Diseases Associated with Exposures to Animal and Animal Products

Anthrax
Brucellosis
Cat scratch disease
Erysipeloid
Cutaneous tuberculosis
Tularemia
Orf
Milker's nodules
Cowpox
Warts
Dermatophytes (zoophilic)

BACTERIAL DISEASES

Anthrax

Anthrax is caused by *Bacillus anthracis*, a large, aerobic, spore-forming gram-positive rod. The disease is infrequently seen in most industrialized countries, but worldwide there are an estimated 20,000 to 100,000 cases of human anthrax annually [15]. Humans are infected as a result of direct inoculation, usually through abrasions, during contact with infected domestic and wild animals (cattle, sheep, goats, pigs, horses, and others) or animal products (e.g., hide, wool, hair, and bone). Infected animals shed the bacteria in hemorrhages or spilt blood. The spores can remain viable for years in soil, dried animal skin and hides, and animal products. High-risk occupations include abattoir (slaughterhouse) workers, farmers, hunters, laboratory workers, veterinarians, wildlife workers, wool workers, and

Table 21-3
Occupational Dermatologic Infectious Diseases Associated with Exposures to Soil and Plants

Anthrax
Dermatophytes (geophilic)
Chromomycosis
Mycetoma
Sporotrichosis
Blastomycosis
Paracoccidioidomycosis
Cutaneous larva migrans

Table 21-4
Occupational Dermatologic Infectious Diseases Associated with Exposures to Ticks and Insects

Lyme disease
Tularemia
Spotted fevers
Typhus
Ehrlichiosis
Rocky Mountain spotted fever
Leishmaniases

any workers exposed to animal hair (especially goat hair), hides, or animal products, especially from the Middle East, Asia, Africa, South and Central America, and southern and eastern Europe [16,17]. These workers include longshoremen, freight handlers, and tannery workers. Inhalation or ingestion of spores can cause severe respiratory disease (woolsorter's disease) or intestinal disease.

The cutaneous form of the disease is usually seen on the head, forearms, and hands. Two to three days after inoculation a red patch appears, which later becomes a painless, purplish-red, raised, boggy, vesicular or pustular nodule ("malignant pustule"). After a few days, this lesion becomes necrotic with an evident black eschar and surrounding edema. Satellite lesions can form around the primary lesion. Systemic signs include high fever, malaise, and weakness. Regional lymph nodes may become enlarged and septicemia is possible. Untreated cutaneous anthrax has a case-fatality rate of 5% to 20% [17]. The diagnosis is made by clinical signs, known exposures, serology, and Gram's stain and culture of the blood, lesion, or discharges. Treatment options include penicillin, erythromycin, chloramphenicol, and tetracycline. Preventive measures include immunizing high-risk workers, immunizing the animals, sterilizing or disinfecting the fomites, educating high-risk workers, controlling dusts and ventilating high-risk work areas, using protective clothing, and emphasizing workplace hygiene [17–21].

Table 21-5
Occupational Dermatologic Infectious Diseases Associated with Water, Marine Fish, and Shellfish Exposures

Erysipeloid
Mycobacterium marinum granuloma
Tularemia
Vibrio vulnificus infection
Aeromonas hydrophila infection
Vibrio parahaemolyticus infection
Pseudomonas aeruginosa infection
Warts
Cercarial dermatitis

Table 21-6
Occupational Dermatologic Infectious Diseases Associated with Exposures to Wet Work and Hot and Moist Environments

Candidiasis
Dermatophytoses
Tinea versicolor

Brucellosis

Brucellosis is caused by gram-negative coccobacillary rods, *Brucella abortus* (in cattle), *Brucella suis* (in pigs), *Brucella canis* (in dogs), or *Brucella melitensis* (in goats and sheep), found on animals or animal blood, urine, and discharges. The organisms are found worldwide, especially in the Mediterranean countries of Europe and Africa, the Middle East, India, central Asia, Mexico, and Central and South America [17]. Humans are infected as a result of direct inoculation, usually through abrasions, during contact with infected domestic animals, their secretions, or animal products. Humans can also be infected by ingestion of unpasteurized milk or cheese. High-risk occupations include those handling infected animals, such as abattoir workers, meat packers, livestock handlers, and veterinarians [17,22].

The incubation period is one to 10 weeks, after which there is an onset of an acute febrile illness. Systemic signs of infection can be severe and include chills, fever, headache, and weakness. Characteristic findings include lymphadenopathy, hepatosplenomegaly, and arthritis. The dermatologic manifestations are nonspecific and appear in less than 10% of those infected [15]. They include papulopustular, maculopapular, urticarial, or vesicular eruptions, at times petechial, at times ulcerated. The diagnosis is confirmed by serology or culture. Treatment is with tetracycline, doxycycline, rifampin, or streptomycin. Relapses can occur in 3% to 10% of treated patients. Preventive measures include eliminating infected animals, immunizing animals, educating high-risk workers, using protective clothing, and emphasizing workplace hygiene [17].

Cat Scratch Disease

Cat scratch disease is caused by *Bartonella* (formerly *Rochalimaea*) *henselae* and can occur in animal handlers and veterinarians [17,23,24]. It is a benign, usually self-limited, disease, which can appear worldwide. It usually occurs after a bite or scratch from a kitten or cat, but has been reported after contact with dogs, monkeys, and chickens [25]. A papule, nodule, pustule, or ulceration develops after three to 14 days at the scratch or bite site, and this is followed by enlargement of the regional lymph nodes, which is the hallmark of the disease. One-third of patients have no skin lesions and develop only lymphadenopathy [25]. Myalgias, fevers, chills, and headaches can occur; encephalopathy occurs rarely. The diagnosis is made by history and clinical findings, culture, and serology. The therapeutic effectiveness of antibiotics is unclear. Preventive measures include educating high-risk workers, using protective clothing, and thorough cleaning of cat bites and scratches [17].

Erysipeloid

Erysipeloid ("fish poisoning," "crab poisoning," "shrimp picker's disease") is caused by *Erysipelothrix rhusiopathiae*, a gram-positive bacillus found in fish, crabs, and other shellfish in fresh and salt water environments, cattle, pigs, sheep, poultry, and rabbits [15]. High-risk occupations include fishermen, butchers, cooks, and poultry and farm workers. One to seven days after inoculation (usually on the hand), burning, itching, and pain develop, along with tender, erythematous, violet, or purplish plaques. Oftentimes, there is slow peripheral spread and central clearing with rare lymphangitis. Constitutional signs and symptoms are usually mild, with low-grade fever and malaise. Arthritis, septicemia, and endocarditis are rare findings. The diagnosis is made on clinical findings, and isolation of the pathogen may be difficult, often requiring full-thickness biopsies. The treatments include systemic penicillin, cephalosporins, and erythromycin. Preventive measures include the elimination of decaying nitrogenous material, which is the main source of infection, worker education, and use of protective clothing [16].

Lyme Disease

Lyme disease is caused by the spirochete *Borrelia burgdorferi* which is transmitted by the bite of the tick *Ixodes scapularis* (the black-legged or deer tick found in the eastern United States) and *Ixodes pacifici* (the western black-legged tick found in the western United States) [26,27]. High-risk occupations include outdoor workers in endemic areas whose activities include farming, hunting, trapping, surveying, landscaping, brush clearing, forestry, and wildlife and parks management [28–31]. Endemic areas in the United States include the northeastern, mid-Atlantic, and the upper north-central regions, as well as scattered areas in northwestern California [32]. The disease can also be found in Canada, Europe, China, and Japan [17].

An initial manifestation, seen in up to two-thirds of cases and developing days to weeks after the tick bite, is a distinct lesion of erythema migrans. This lesion begins as an erythematous macule or papule at the site of the tick bite, slowly enlarges to beyond 5 cm in size, and then develops central clearing. The untreated skin lesion can last up to several weeks. The other manifestations of Lyme disease are varied and include fever, headache, myalgia, arthralgia, lymphadenopathy, and neurologic and cardiac abnormalities. The diagnosis can be difficult and is usually made on clinical criteria and known exposures in combination with serology. Antibiotics such as doxycycline, tetracycline, and amoxicillin are used for therapy. Prevention strategies include worker education, avoidance of tick-infested habitats—usually wooded, brushy, or overgrown grassy areas, especially in spring and summer—use of repellants or insecticides (DEET or permethrin), use of protective clothing (long-sleeve shirts, boots, and high socks with pants tucked into socks), and prompt inspection for ticks and correct tick removal (grasp as close to the skin as possible with forceps and apply gentle traction) [33]. With the recent introduction of a vaccine, immunization of high-risk workers in endemic areas is now recommended [34].

Mycobacterium marinum *Granuloma*

Mycobacterium marinum, an acid-fast photochromogen rod (Runyon Group I), is the causative organism in a condition referred to as "swimming pool granuloma" or "fish tank granuloma" [35]. High-risk occupations include fishermen, butchers, and fish tank workers, and those exposed to contaminated water [36,37]. A papule develops four to six weeks after trauma and exposure to the organism in water. This evolves into a warty, ulcerating nodule or plaque, usually on the hand, knee, or elbow, with some spread along the lymphatics (a sporotrichoid pattern). Definitive diagnosis is by tissue culture; the organism grows best at 30° to 32°C. Treatment regimens include surgical excision, heat therapy, minocycline, tetracycline, doxycycline, trimethoprim-sulfamethoxazole, and rifampin plus ethambutol [38]. Preventive measures include worker education and use of protective clothing.

Cutaneous Tuberculosis

Mycobacterium tuberculosis can rarely cause both primary inoculation tuberculosis (tuberculous chancre) and a verrucous condition in previously sensitized individuals called "prosector's wart," "anatomic tubercle," or "necrogenic wart" (tuberculosis verrucosa cutis). In both conditions, the pathogen can be introduced at the sites of minor abrasions or wounds. Tuberculous chancre can be found in health care workers, and tuberculosis verrucosa cutis had been historically seen in pathologists, morgue attendants, and surgeons [39]. Similar lesions caused by *Mycobacterium bovis* from cattle can affect veterinarians, butchers, and farmers.

Tuberculous chancre presents as a papule or scab that does not heal and develops into a large, painless ulcer with ragged edges. Regional lymphadenopathy can follow the skin manifestations. Tuberculosis verrucosa cutis begins as a indurated nodule with a warty surface, which then extends in a serpiginous manner, resulting in a red-brown, warty plaque, with central clearing. The diagnosis can be difficult; diagnostic options include acid-fast staining, culture of lesions or skin biopsies, and polymerase chain reaction of specimens [40]. The treatment of cutaneous tuberculosis is similar to that of pulmonary tuberculosis. Prevention includes worker education, workplace hygiene, and the use of protective clothing.

Tularemia

The causative organism in tularemia is a gram-negative coccobacillus *Francisella tularensis*, found in rabbits, deer, beavers, squirrels, skunks, and muskrats. It is transmitted through abrasions by contaminated water, blood, or tissue, or inoculation from the wood tick (*Dermacentor andersoni*), dog tick (*Dermacentor variabilis*), lone star tick (*Amblyomma americanum*), or rarely the deerfly (*Chrysops discalis*), and the mosquito (*Aedes cinereus* in Russia and Sweden) [15,17]. It can also be transmitted by ingestion and inhalation. The disease is seen in North America, Europe, the former Soviet Union, China, Japan, and Mexico [17]. High-risk workers include abattoir workers, butchers, farmers, foresters, hunters (especially those skinning rabbit hides), and veterinarians.

The clinical manifestations fall into six categories—glandular, ulceroglandular, oculoglandular, typhoidal, pulmonary, and oropharyngeal [15]. The most common manifestation is ulceroglandular tularemia, in which a tender papule develops three to five days after inoculation and progresses into an ulcer with black eschar. Infection is associated with fever, enlarged lymph nodes, and splenomegaly. The diagnosis is made by serology or culture, and treatment is with streptomycin, tetracycline, chloramphenicol, or gentamicin [15,16]. Preventive measures include worker education, avoidance of tick-infested habitats, use of repellants and insecticides, use of protective clothing. An investigational live attenuated vaccine is available for high-risk groups [17].

Other Waterborne Infections

Vibrio vulnificus is an important waterborne pathogen that can cause severe wound infections with direct contact and a primary septicemia if ingested (usually in raw shellfish). The case-fatality rate can be up to 50% in disseminated disease [15]. The organism is commonly found in sediments in salt water and estuaries, in fish, and in shellfish. Fishermen, crabbers, shrimp workers, and those exposed to contaminated water are at risk. Wound infections due to *V vulnificus* usually follow cuts on the hand while cleaning crabs or shrimp, or from entry of the pathogen through an open wound exposed to sea water. Infections are endemic along the coast of the Gulf of Mexico and in warmer waters of the Pacific and Atlantic coasts [41,42]. The wound infections can appear as pustules with cellulitis and lymphangitis; they may be rapidly progressive with extensive skin necrosis and gangrene [15]. The diagnosis is made by culturing the organism from blood or the wound. Treatment of the wound infections include tetracycline or chloramphenicol, and an aminoglycoside. Prevention strategies include worker education and protective clothing.

Similar wound infections sustained in fresh water, with manifestations of a bullous cellulitis, fasciitis, and myonecrosis, may be caused by *Aeromonas hydrophila*. In addition, *V parahaemolyticus* can also induce wound infections after lacerations are exposed to shellfish or sea water [41]. *Pseudomonas aeruginosa* skin infections (folliculitis, ecthyma gangrenosum, cellulitis) have been associated with the use of hot tubs, whirlpools, saunas, and swimming pools. In addition, cases have been described in ocean divers [43,44].

Rickettsial Diseases

Rickettsiae are coccobacillary obligate intracellular parasites and are transmitted to humans by arthropods, such as ticks, mites, fleas, and lice. Transmission occurs by inoculation at the time of the bite (ticks and mites) or by insect defecation near the bite (lice and fleas) [45]. The infections caused by rickettsiae include a variety of spotted fevers (usually with generalized rashes including lesions on palms and soles), Q fever (no cutaneous signs), typhus (truncal rash), and ehrlichiosis (maculopapular or petechial rash on trunk and proximal extremities). Workers at high risk for these diseases include outdoor workers such as farmers, foresters, rangers, trappers, hunters, construction workers, and surveyors [16].

Rocky Mountain Spotted Fever

The most common rickettsial infection in the United States is Rocky Mountain spotted fever, which is caused by *Rickettsia rickettsii*. The infection is seen in the southeastern and south-central United States, Canada, and Central and South America [17]. The illness ranges from asymptomatic disease to a fulminant disease with significant mortality, ranging from 20% to 80% in untreated patients [45]. The organism is transmitted by a tick bite from the Rocky Mountain wood tick (*Dermacentor andersoni*) in the western United States, the American dog tick *(Dermacentor variabilis)* in the eastern and southern United States, and the Lone Star tick (*Amblyomma americanum*) in the southwestern United States [17].

One to 14 days after a tick bite, severe headaches, fevers, chills, and arthralgias develop. On the fourth to sixth day, blanching macules followed by petechiae and ecchymoses (an infectious vasculitis) appear on the wrists and ankles, spread to the palms and soles, and later generalize and become purpuric [45]. The diagnosis is confirmed by serology and immunofluorescent staining of biopsy specimens. The treatment is with tetracycline or chloramphenicol. Prevention strategies include worker education, avoidance of tick-infested habitats especially in spring and summer, use of repellants and insecticides, use of protective clothing, and prompt inspection for ticks and correct tick removal [17].

VIRAL DISEASES

Herpetic Whitlow

Medical and dental professionals and staff are at risk for developing herpetic whitlow, caused by herpes simplex virus type I or type II [46,47]. This condition presents two to 12 days after direct skin contact with a patient's lesion or with a carrier of herpes. The lesion usually occurs on a finger as a recurrent, painful vesicle(s) on an erythematous base. The diagnosis can be made clinically and confirmed by microscopically examining unroofed vesicle scrapings for multinucleated giant cells (Tzanck test), by viral culture, and by serology. If left untreated, the lesions usually heal within one to two weeks but are often reactivated. Antiviral oral medications such as acyclovir, famciclovir, or valacyclovir can shorten the course and induce long-term suppression. Prevention is achieved by worker education, workplace hygiene, and protective clothing, especially gloves [17].

Orf, Milker's Nodules, Cowpox

Viral infections contracted from direct exposure to infected livestock can occur in abattoir workers, shearers, milkers, veterinarians, and farm workers. Orf (ecthyma contagiosum) appears worldwide and is caused by a virus belonging to the genus *Parapoxvirus.* It is transmitted by direct contact with the lesions of infected sheep and goats or from contaminated objects such as fences, barn doors, feeding troughs, and shears [48,49]. Milker's nodules are also caused by a *Parapoxvirus* and occur after contact with infected dairy cattle. Lesions of orf and milker's nodules are similar. After an incubation period of three to seven days, infection results in a solitary, painless, flat, or dome-shaped papule, vesicle, or bulla with a central umbilicated crust, usually on the hands, fingers, and forearms. These lesions usually evolve over one to two months through a variety of stages, each lasting a week (maculopapular, targetoid, weeping, regenerative, papillomatous, and regressive stages) [16,48]. Multiple lesions can occur as well. These two infections differ from cowpox, which is a rare but potentially severe disease caused by an *Orthopoxvirus.* Painful, hemorrhagic pustules or black eschars can be found on the hand or face [50]. In all three infections, there can be regional lymphadenopathy, fever, and malaise.

The diagnosis of orf and milker's nodules is based on clinical presentation, exposure history, and serology. Confirmation is made by viral culture or electron microscopic confirmation of the viruses. Lesions usually resolve within two months, and treatment is ordinarily not necessary. Persistent lesions may be electrodesiccated and curettaged or excised. Prevention strategies include worker education, maintaining cleanliness of animal housing areas, good personal hygiene, washing exposed areas with soap and water, and use of protective clothing [17].

Warts

Warts accounted for over 3 million visits to nonfederal office-based physicians in the United States in 1995 [51]. The proportion of these caused by occupational exposures is unknown. Warts are caused by any of a variety of the over 70 human papillomaviruses (HPV), which are found worldwide. High-risk workers include meat handlers, fish handlers, and poultry processing workers, who can develop verrucous papules usually on the hands [52–55]. These are usually caused by HPV type 7, but other types may be involved as well [56]. There is a suggestion that HPV type 7 is widely distributed in the environment, but an unknown factor in meat enhances viral replication [57]. The diagnosis is usually made by clinical appearance, which can vary from dome-shaped papules to filiform papules to flat-topped papules or macules. There is no reliable cure for warts; most treatments rely on destruction (electrodesiccation and curettage, liquid nitrogen, keratolytics, and laser). Prevention strategies include worker education and use of protective clothing. During destruction of warts using laser or electrosurgery, medical personnel may put themselves at risk because of exposure to aerosolized HPV, which can induce laryngeal warts [58,59]. Facemasks and control of smoke through ventilation and work practices are recommended [60].

Other Viral Infections

Other viruses with important skin manifestations are usually seen in the pediatric population but may be important to susceptible health care, school, and childcare workers [61–67]. These include measles, rubella, chickenpox (varicella-zoster), hand-foot-mouth disease, and erythema infectiosum. Transmission of these diseases is person to person through direct contact with secretions, droplet, or airborne routes. These diseases tend to be more severe in adults. Vaccinations are available for the first three diseases.

Measles (rubeola) is caused by infection with a paramyxovirus. Typical measles has a prodrome of two to four days of fever, respiratory congestion, conjunctivitis, and cough. This is followed by tiny white or blue-gray Koplik spots on the buccal mucosa and then by nonpruritic, erythematous papules that begin behind the ear, spread to the whole body, become confluent, and last from four to seven days. Rubella is caused by a togavirus, which can cause a mild illness with a variable rash, usually a faint pink macular eruption that spreads from the face to the trunk and proximal extremities. Its most feared complication is congenital rubella syndrome. Varicella (chickenpox) is characterized by the abrupt onset of faint erythematous macules that progress to vesicles over one to two days. Old lesions crust over with new lesions forming in the course of seven to 10 days. Perinatal disease can be serious. Reactivation in adults can lead to herpes zoster (shingles), with painful vesicles occurring in dermatomal patterns. Hand-foot-mouth disease, caused by several coxsackievirus group A enteroviruses, is characterized by the abrupt onset of papules that progress to vesicles in an acral distribution. Erythema infectiosum (fifth disease) is caused by the human parvovirus B19. The typical presentation is the initial "slapped cheek" erythematous patches or plaques on the face, followed in one to four days by lacy, reticulated macules and papules on the extremities. The skin lesions may wax and wane for days to weeks. The clinical presentation of the adult infection may vary and may be confused with rubella or an allergic reaction. Fever, malaise, and headache may occur. The infection can cause arthritis in adults and can induce fetal death (hydrops fetalis) [67].

The diagnosis of these viral diseases is usually based on clinical manifestations and serology. There is no specific treatment for measles, rubella, hand-foot-mouth disease, and erythema infectiosum. Antiviral medications and immune globulins have been used in varicella-zoster infections. Prevention strategies include worker education, vaccination, reducing person-to-person contact (isolation), proper ventilation, and promotion of hygienic measures [17,68].

SUPERFICIAL FUNGAL DISEASES

Fungal infections accounted for nearly 2 million visits to nonfederal office-based physicians in the United States in 1995 [51]. The proportion of these infections caused by occupational exposures is unknown.

Candidiasis

Paronychial and interdigital candidal infection caused by *Candida albicans* is the most common fungal disease of occupational origin and can be seen in those engaged in wet work, such as food service personnel, dishwashers, housekeepers, and bartenders [16]. The presentation includes swollen, erythematous, tender skin in the nail folds or interdigital spaces, often with a serous or purulent discharge. In paronychial infections, malformation of the proximal nail plate can occur. Candidal infection can also occur in skin fold areas (intertrigo) in workers working in hot and humid environments. The diagnosis of candidal infections can be made by microscopic examination of scale immersed in potassium hydroxide (KOH) or culture. Oftentimes, multiple organisms can be involved in paronychial infection, including *Pseudomonas aeruginosa* and *Staphylococcus aureus.* Treatment regimens include topical and oral antifungal agents. Patient education is very important to eliminate the predisposing factors (trauma, wet work, hot and humid environments) and to introduce healing and prevention strategies. Keeping the hands dry through the use of appropriate gloves is key.

Dermatophytosis

Dermatophytosis, also known as tinea or ringworm infections, can be caused by a variety of species of *Epidermophyton*, *Microsporum*, and *Trichophyton*. These species can reside on humans (anthropophilic), animals (zoophilic), or in the soil (geophilic). Medical and dental workers, school and childcare workers, veterinarians, animal handlers, and agricultural and construction workers are at risk. Anthropophilic dermatophytes (e.g., *Trichophyton rubrum*, *Trichophyton mentagrophytes*) can cause fungal infection on the body or the feet. These can occur in medical or childcare environments or in workplaces in association with sweaty foot environments (e.g., use of protective boots) or where there are common shower areas [16,69]. *Trichophyton verrucosum* (cattle) and *Microsporum canis* (small animals), both zoophilic dermatophytes, can infect farmers, cattle handlers, veterinarians, and animal handlers [16,70]. *Microsporum gypseum*, found in clay or sandy soil, can infect agricultural and construction workers. The general clinical appearance of dermatophyte infections is that of annular, scaling erythematous plaques, but presentations can vary by body site and can be highly inflammatory at times. Locations of involvement include the scalp (tinea capitis), the bearded areas (tinea barbae), general glabrous skin (tinea corporis), the groin (tinea cruris), the feet (tinea pedis), the hands (tinea manuum), and the nails (tinea unguium/onychomycosis). The diagnosis can be made by microscopic examination of scale immersed in KOH or culture. Treatment regimens include topical and oral antifungal agents (e.g., griseofulvin, imidazoles, and the triazoles). Preventive measures include worker education, using fungicidal agents to clean showers and dressing rooms, maintaining personal hygiene including the use of fungicidal powders on feet and in shoes and socks, and using protective clothing [17,69].

Tinea Versicolor

Tinea versicolor (pityriasis versicolor), a common skin disorder caused by *Malassezia furfur (Pityrosporum orbiculare)*, can be seen in workers who work in hot and humid environments [71]. Heat, humidity, occlusion, and sweat contribute to this condition. Clinically it presents as asymptomatic, hypopigmented or hyperpigmented (red-brown) macules or patches with fine, dustlike scales. The usual areas of involvement include the chest, neck, back, abdomen, and proximal extremities. The diagnosis can be made by microscopic examination of scale immersed in KOH, which gives the typical "spaghetti and meatballs" appearance of the hyphae and spores. Treatment regimens include topical and oral antifungal agents and selenium sulfide washes, but relapses are common. Prevention strategies are limited and include improving the ambient work conditions as well as selenium sulfide body washes.

SUBCUTANEOUS FUNGAL DISEASES

Chromomycosis

Chromomycosis (chromoblastomycosis) is a chronic skin disease that results from traumatic implantation of the pathogenic agent from soil, plant debris, wood fragments, or other environmental debris into the skin [72]. The disease, which can be caused by a variety of demataceous (pigmented) fungi (including *Fonsecaea pedrosoi*, *Cladosporium carrionii*, *Fonsecaea compactum*, *Rhinocladiella aquaspersa*, and *Phialophora verrucosa*), can be found worldwide, but is usually seen in tropical and subtropical areas. The disease usually affects the rural poor who are exposed to the soil in outdoor occupations. The skin manifestations usually are seen on the lower legs and feet, and begin as pink, scaly papules, which evolve into verrucous nodules and plaques with classic "black dots" (transepithelial elimination) on their surfaces. The diagnosis is confirmed through culturing the organism and skin biopsies (special fungal stains to look for sclerotic or Medlar bodies) [72]. Treatment can include wide excision and oral antifungal agents such as ketoconazole, itraconazole, 5-fluorocytosine, and amphotericin B. Relapses and partial cures are common. Prevention strategies include worker education, personal hygiene, and protective clothing (especially shoes) [17].

Mycetoma

Mycetoma (Madura foot) is caused by either multiple species of aerobic actinomycetes (actinomycetoma) or true fungi (eumycetoma) found in soil [16]. After traumatic inoculation, usually into the foot, hand, or back (from carrying contaminated materials), slowly enlarging, painless, subcutaneous nodules form. Ultimately, these evolve into slowly progressive, chronic, indurated plaques with sinus tracts. Agricultural workers in tropical and subtropical areas are at risk. The diagnosis is made by direct microscopic study of biopsy specimens and culture. Actinomycetoma has been treated with streptomycin sulfate, trimethoprim-sulfamethoxazole, and dapsone, although relapse is not unusual. Eumycetoma is more difficult to treat, and surgical excision and oral antifungals are used. Prevention strategies include worker education, personal hygiene, and protective clothing (especially shoes) [17].

Sporotrichosis

Sporotrichosis usually occurs in the skin and the lymph nodes, and can be recurring if not treated. The organism causing the disease, *Sporothrix schenkii*, a dimorphic fungus, is found in soil, timber, sphagnum moss, and other plant material, and appears in most temperate and tropical climates of the world [73]. Agricultural and forestry workers, gardeners, florists, greenhouse workers, and miners are at risk. An epidemic among gold miners in South Africa affected over 3,000 workers; the source was fungus growing on mine timbers [17]. An outbreak in 1988 in the United States affected 84 people in 14 states; many of those infected were forestry or nursery workers handling sphagnum moss [74]. The disease usually occurs three weeks after traumatic implantation of the fungus through thorns, splinters, or straw. It most often presents as an ulcerating papule with nodules forming along the paths of the draining lymphatics (lymphocutaneous form with sporotrichoid spread). There is also a fixed form of the disease with no sporotrichoid spread. The diagnosis can be confirmed through culturing the organism and serology; diagnosis from microscopic examination of skin biopsies is more difficult. Treatments include oral potassium iodide, ketoconazole, itraconazole, or amphotericin B. Prevention strategies include worker education, decontamination of fomites with fungicides, and use of protective clothing [17,75].

SYSTEMIC FUNGAL INFECTIONS

A variety of systemic mycoses have rare cutaneous manifestations (usually in disseminated disease) including coccidioidomycosis, histoplasmosis, paracoccidioidomycosis, and blastomycosis. The most distinctive lesions can be seen in paracoccidioidomycosis and blastomycosis.

Blastomycosis

Blastomycosis (North American blastomycosis) is an uncommon disease caused by the thermal dimorphic fungus, *Blastomyces dermatitidis.* The fungus is found in the soil or near the soil (decaying wood or animal manure), and most cases occur in the central and southeastern United States, Africa, India, and the Middle East [17]. Farming, forestry, construction, and other outdoor workers may be at risk [16,76]. The infection is usually acquired as a primary pulmonary infection, though cutaneous disease is its most common nonpulmonary manifestation. The earliest lesions are papulopustules or nodules, which progress to arciform, serpiginous plaques with a raised edge. These can ulcerate and form microabscesses. The diagnosis can be confirmed through culturing the organism (which is very difficult), serology, and skin biopsies (using routine or special fungal stains). Treatments include ketoconazole, itraconazole, and amphotericin B. There are no known successful prevention strategies for this disease.

Paracoccidioidomycosis

Paracoccidioidomycosis (South American blastomycosis) is caused by *Paracoccidioides brasiliensis* found in the soil in tropical and subtropical areas of Mexico, and Central and South America [17]. Workers in contact with the soil, such as farmers, laborers, and construction workers, are at risk. The fungus is introduced into the lungs and disseminates to other organs such as the skin. The skin manifestations include painful ulcers in the mouth or around the mouth and nose. The diagnosis can be made by culture or microscopic examination of sputum or pus. Treatments include ketoconazole, itraconazole, and amphotericin B. There are no known successful prevention strategies for this disease.

PARASITIC DISEASES

Cercarial Dermatitis

"Swimmer's itch," "swamp itch," or "clamdigger's itch" (cercarial dermatitis) is caused by avian schistosomes, which penetrate the skin causing a pruritic papular eruption [16]. This condition can occur worldwide, including the Great Lakes region and the California coast, and can be seen in divers, lifeguards, and dock workers exposed to sea-level fresh water or brackish seawater. Infection results in urticarial papules on exposed skin surfaces, which subside usually within weeks. The diagnosis is based on clinical appearance and exposure history. Treatment is symptomatic. Prevention strategies include worker education and protective clothing. Sea bather's eruption is often confused with swimmer's itch. This condition occurs only in salt water and is a very pruritic, macular, maculopapular, or vesicular eruption limited to areas covered by swimwear. It is not considered an infectious disease and is caused by larval forms of marine cnidarians [77].

Cutaneous Larva Migrans

The dog and cat intestinal hookworms, *Ancylostoma ceylonicum and Ancylostoma caninum,* can produce mobile, serpiginous linear, pruritic plaques, usually on the feet (creeping eruption). The organisms can migrate several centimeters in a day. Those at risk include workers exposed to contaminated sand or dirt on subtropical and tropical beaches, farmers, sewer workers, lifeguards, and construction workers. The diagnosis is usually made by clinical appearance of the lesion and a history of exposure. Treatment includes cryotherapy and topical and oral thiabendazole [78]. Prevention strategies include worker education and protective clothing.

Other nematodes that rarely cause occupational skin diseases include trichinosis, dracunculiasis, filariasis, loiasis, onchocerciasis, enterobiasis, strongyloidiasis, and toxocariasis [16].

Leishmaniases

The leishmaniases are a variety of diseases caused by species of the protozoa Leishmania, transmitted from zoonotic reservoir hosts to humans by several species of sandflies (Phlebotomus, Lutzomyia). The infection is found in Asia, the Middle East, in the Mediterranean region, sub-Saharan Africa, south-central Texas, and Central and South America [17,79]. Farmers and other outdoor workers working in forested areas are at risk [17]. Its forms include visceral, mucocutaneous, and cutaneous (old world and new world) leishmaniases. The skin lesions can vary and include pruritic papules, nodules, and ulcerated craters. The diagnosis is confirmed by identifying organisms in smears or biopsy specimens or by culture. Lesions may be treated with local excision, cryotherapy, and with pentavalent antimonials. Prevention strategies include covering exposed skin and applying repellents and insecticides to minimize sandfly bites in endemic areas.

Mite Infestations

Human scabies is a contagious disease caused by the mite *Sarcoptes scabiei* and is spread by direct skin-to-skin contact and through fomites such as clothing and linen. High-risk groups include medical personnel, nursing home workers, and childcare workers [80]. This condition is marked by intensely pruritic vesicles and burrows, usually found on interdigital webs, elbows, feet, genitalia, buttocks, and axillae. Other clinical forms include nodular and crusted (Norwegian) scabies. The diagnosis of scabies is made by demonstrating mites, eggs, or feces (scybala) on scrapings from affected skin. Treatment includes topical scabeticides and oral ivermectin. Prevention strategies include worker education, good workplace hygiene, and protective clothing.

Mites that bite humans, but do not generally infest the body, include grain mites, straw mites, rat mites, fowl or avian mites, and dog/cat/rabbit mites [81]. These can produce pruritic papules or papular urticaria. Animal caretakers and agricultural workers are at risk.

Public Health Perspective

The clinician should view each patient with a potential occupational dermatologic infectious disease from a broader public health perspective. The worker with an occupational dermatologic infectious disease should be viewed as a "sentinel health event" [82–84]. This recognition and resulting action by the clinician, in consultation with public health authorities, can lead to potential disease prevention in other workers. This can only occur with proper diagnosis of the worker, a high level of suspicion on the part of the clinician in suspecting workplace exposures, ultimate confirmation of the association to the workplace exposures that caused the disease, and, finally, steps taken to modify those exposures [84]. If successful, this approach would lead to the prevention of relapses and of new cases of occupational dermatologic infectious diseases.

ACKNOWLEDGMENT

Funding support: This chapter was written as part of the author's official duties as a government officer and thus cannot be copyrighted.

References

1. Adams RM (ed). *Occupational Skin Disease*, 2nd Ed. Philadelphia: Saunders, 1990.
2. Hogan DJ (ed). *Occupational Skin Disorders*. New York: Igaku-Shoin, 1994.
3. Marks JG, DeLeo VA. *Contact and Occupational Dermatology*. St. Louis: Mosby Year Book, 1992.
4. Di Salvo AF (ed). *Occupational Mycoses*. Philadelphia: Lea & Febiger, 1983.
5. Lushniak BD. The epidemiology of occupational contact dermatitis. *Dermatol Clin* 1995;13:671–80.
6. Centers for Disease Control and Prevention. Summary of notifiable diseases, United States, 1997. *MMWR* 1997;46(54):3.
7. Centers for Disease Control and Prevention. Summary of notifiable diseases, United States, 1996. *MMWR* 1996;45(53):3.
8. Bureau of Labor Statistics (BLS). *Occupational injuries and illnesses in the United States*. Washington, DC: US Department of Labor, Bulletin 2478, 1996.
9. Mathias CGT, Morrison JH. Occupational skin disease, United States. *Arch Dermatol* 1988;124:1519–24.
10. Mathias CGT, Sinks TH, Seligman PJ, et al. Surveillance of occupational skin disease—a method utilizing workers' compensation claims. *Am J Ind Med* 1990;17: 363–70.
11. National Institute for Occupational Safety and Health (NIOSH). *National Occupational Survey—Pilot study for development of an occupational disease surveillance method*. Rockville, MD: U.S. Department of Health, Education, and Welfare, HEW Publication (NIOSH) 75-162, 1975.
12. Taylor JS. Occupational disease statistics—in perspective. *Arch Dermatol* 1988;124:1557–8.
13. Burnett CA, Lushniak BD, McCarthy W, et al. Occupational dermatitis causing days away from work in U.S. private industry. *Am J Ind Med* 1998;34:568–73.
14. Karjolainin A, Aalto L, Jolanki L, et al. *Occupational diseases in Finland, 1996*. Helsinki: Finnish Institute of Occupational Health, 1998.
15. Swartz MN, Weinberg AN. Miscellaneous bacterial infections with cutaneous manifestations. In: Fitzpatrick TB, Arthur AZ, Wolff K, et al (eds), *Dermatology in General Medicine*, 4th Ed. New York: McGraw-Hill, 1993. Pp 2354–70.
16. Ancona AA. Biologic causes. In: Adams RM (ed), *Occupational Skin Disease*, 2nd Ed. Philadelphia: Saunders, 1990. Pp 89–112.
17. Benenson AS (ed). *Control of Communicable Diseases Manual*, 16th Ed. Washington: American Public Health Association, 1995.
18. Briggs PM, Delta BG, Keener SR, et al. Human cutaneous anthrax—North Carolina, 1987. *MMWR* 1988;37:413–4.
19. LaForce FM. Anthrax. *Clin Infect Dis* 1994;19:1009–13.
20. Anonymous. Anthrax: memorandum from a WHO meeting. *Bull WHO* 1996;74:465–70.
21. Hanna P. Anthrax pathogenesis and host response. *Curr Top Microbiol Immunol* 1998;225:13–35.
22. Trout D, Gomez TM, Bernard BP, et al. Outbreak of brucellosis at a United States pork packing plant. *J Occup Environ Med* 1995;37:697–703.
23. Zangwill KM, Hamilton DH, Perkins BA, et al. Cat scratch disease in Connecticut—epidemiology, risk factors, and evaluation of new diagnostic test. *N Engl J Med* 1993;329:8–13.
24. Noah DL, Kramer CM, Verbsky MP, et al. Survey of veterinary professionals and other veterinary conference attendees for antibodies to *Bartonella henselae* and *B quintana*. *J Am Vet Med Assoc* 1997;210:342–4.
25. Freedberg IM. Cat-scratch disease. In: Fitzpatrick TB, Arthur AZ, Wolff K, et al. (eds), *Dermatology in General Medicine*, 4th Ed. New York: McGraw-Hill, 1993. Pp 2351–3.
26. Dennis DT. Lyme disease. *Dermatol Clin* 1995;13:537–51.
27. Sarpa C, Trevisan G, Stinco G. Lyme borreliosis. *Dermatol Clin* 1994;12:669–85.
28. Goldstein MD, Schwartz BS, Friedman C. Lyme disease in New Jersey outdoor workers: a statewide survey of seroprevalence and tick exposure. *Am J Public Health* 1990;80:1225–9.
29. Schwartz BS, Goldstein MD, Childs JE. Antibodies to *Borrelia burgdorferi* and tick salivary gland proteins in New Jersey outdoor workers. *Am J Public Health* 1993;83:1746–8.
30. Schwartz BS, Goldstein MD, Childs JE. Longitudinal study of *Borrelia burgdorferi* infection in New Jersey outdoor workers, 1988–1991. *Am J Epidemiol* 1994;139:504–12.
31. Bowen SG, Schultze TL, Hayne C, et al. A focus of Lyme disease in Monmouth County, New Jersey. *Am J Epidemiol* 1984;120:387–94.
32. Anonymous. Appendix methods used for creating a national Lyme disease risk map. *MMWR* 1999;48 (RR07):21–4.
33. Abele DC, Anders KH. The many faces and phases of borreliosis I. Lyme disease. *J Am Acad Dermatol* 1990;23:167–86.
34. Anonymous. Recommendations for the use of Lyme disease vaccine—Recommendations of the Advisory Committee on Immunization Practices. *MMWR* 1999;48(RR07):1–17.
35. Hautmann G, Lotti T. Atypical mycobacterial infections of the skin. *Dermatol Clin* 1994;12:657–68.
36. Miller WC, Toon R. *Mycobacterium marinum* in Gulf fishermen. *Arch Environ Health* 1973;27:8–10.
37. Cole G. Mycobacterium marinum infection in a mechanic. *Contact Dermatitis* 1987;16:283.

38. Edelstein H. *Mycobacterium marinum* skin infections: report of 31 cases and review of the literature. *Arch Intern Med* 1994;154:1359–64.
39. Sehgal V. Cutaneous tuberculosis. *Dermatol Clin* 1994;12:645–53.
40. Penneys NS, Leonardi CL, Cook S, et al. Identification of *Mycobacterium tuberculosis* DNA in five different types of cutaneous lesions by polymerase chain reaction. *Arch Dermatol* 1993;129:1594–8.
41. Bonner JR. Spectrum of *Vibrio* infections in a Gulf Coast community. *Ann Intern Med* 1983;99:464.
42. Hlady WG, Klontz KC. The epidemiology of *Vibrio* infections in Florida, 1981–1993. *J Infect Dis* 1996;173:1176–83.
43. Lacour JP, El Baze P, Castanet J, et al. Diving suit dermatitis caused by *Pseudomonas aeruginosa*: two cases. *J Am Acad Dermatol* 1994;31:1055–6.
44. Ahlen C, Mandal LH, Iverson OJ. Identification of infectious *Pseudomonas aeruginosa* strains in an occupational saturation diving environment. *Occup Environ Med* 1998;55:480–4.
45. Schaffner W. Rickettsial diseases. In: Fitzpatrick TB, Arthur AZ, Wolff K, et al. (eds), *Dermatology in General Medicine*, 4th Ed. New York: McGraw-Hill, 1993. Pp 2499–506.
46. Jones JG. Herpetic whitlow: an infectious occupational hazard. *J Occup Med* 1985;10:725–8.
47. Rowe N, Heine C, Kowalsky C. Herpetic whitlow: an occupational disease of practicing dentists. *JAMA* 1981;105:471–3.
48. Bodnar MG, Miller OF, Tyler WB. Facial orf. *J Am Acad Dermatol* 1999;40:815–7.
49. Ruxin TA, Taylor JS. Other occupational dermatoses: acne, pigmentary disorders, skin cancer, infection, reactions to temperature and humidity, scleroderma, and nail changes. In: Hogan DJ (ed), *Occupational Skin Disorders.* New York: Igaku-Shoin, 1994. Pp 96–9.
50. Baxby D, Bennett M, Getty B. Human cowpox 1969–93: a review based on 54 cases. *Br J Dermatol* 1994;131:598–607.
51. Weinstock MA, Boyle MM. Statistics of interest to dermatologists. In: Thiers BH, Lang PG (eds), *Yearbook of Dermatology and Dermatologic Surgery 1998.* St. Louis: Mosby, 1998. P 21.
52. Vittorio CC, Schiffman MH, Weinstock MA. Epidemiology of human papillomaviruses. *Dermatol Clin* 1995;13:561–74.
53. Rudlinger R, Bunney MH, Grob R, et al. Warts in fish handlers. *Br J Dermatol* 1989;120:375–81.
54. Jablonska S, Obalek S, Golebiowska A. Epidemiology of butcher's warts. *Arch Dermatol Res* 1988;280 (suppl):S24–S28.
55. Stehr-Green PA, Hewer P, Meekin GE, et al. The aetiology and risk factors for warts among poultry processing workers. *Int J Epidemiol* 1993;22:294–8.
56. Keefe M, al-Ghambi A, Coggon D, et al. Cutaneous warts in butchers. *Br J Dermatol* 1994;130:9–14.
57. Keefe M, al-Ghambi A, Coggon D, et al. Butchers' warts: no evidence for person-to-person transmission of HPV7. *Br J Dermatol* 1994;130:15–7.
58. Bergbrandt IM, Samuelsson L, Olofsson S, et al. Polymerase chain reaction for monitoring human papillomavirus contamination of medical personnel during treatment of genital warts with CO_2 laser and electrocoagulation. *Acta Derm Venereol (Stockh)* 1994;74: 393–5.
59. Gloster HM, Roenigk RK. Risk of acquiring human papillomavirus from the plume produced by the carbon dioxide laser in the treatment of warts. *J Am Acad Dermatol* 1995;32:436–41.
60. National Institute for Occupational Safety and Health (NIOSH). *Hazard Controls—Control of smoke from laser/electric surgical procedures.* Cincinnati: U.S. Department of Health and Human Services, DHHS (NIOSH) Publication 96-128, 1996.
61. Sepkowitz KA. Occupationally acquired infections in health care workers. *Ann Intern Med* 1996;125:826–34.
62. Memar O, Tyring SK. Cutaneous viral infections. *J Am Acad Dermatol* 1995;33:279–87.
63. Johnston JM, Burke JP. Nosocomial outbreak of hand-foot-mouth disease among operating suite personnel. *Infect Control* 1986;7:172–6.
64. Harrison J, Jones CE. Human parvovirus B19 infection in healthcare workers. *Occup Med* 1995;45:93–6.
65. Gillespie SM, Cartter ML, Asch S, et al. Occupational risk of human parvovirus B19 infection for school and day-care personnel during an outbreak of erythema infectiosum. *JAMA* 1990;263:2061–5.
66. Atkinson WL, Markowitz LE, Adams NC, et al. Transmission of measles in medical settings. *Am J Med* 1991;91:320S–324S.
67. Valeur-Jensen AK, Pedersen CB, Westergaard T, et al. Risk factors for parvovirus B19 infection in pregnancy. *JAMA* 1999;281:1099–105.
68. Weber DJ, Rutala WA, Hamilton H. Prevention and control of varicella-zoster infections in healthcare facilities. *Infect Control Hosp Epidemiol* 1996;17:694–705.
69. Arnow PM, Houchins SG, Pugliese G. An outbreak of tinea corporis in hospital personnel caused by a patient with *Trichophyton tonsurans* infection. *Pediatr Infect Dis J* 1991;10:355–9.
70. Philpot CM. The role of animals in the spread of fungal skin infections in humans. In: Marks R, Plewig G (eds), *The Environmental Threat to the Skin*. London: Martin Dunitz, 1992. Pp 377–80.
71. Tucker SB, Watsky KL. Other dermatoses. In: Rosenstock L, Cullen MR (eds), *Textbook of Clinical Occupational and Environmental Medicine*. Philadelphia: Saunders, 1994. Pp 530–42.

72. Al-Doory Y. Chromomycosis. In: Di Salvo AF (ed), *Occupational Mycoses*. Philadelphia: Lea & Febiger, 1983. Pp 95–122.

73. Goodman NL. Sporotrichosis. In: Di Salvo AF (ed), *Occupational Mycoses*. Philadelphia: Lea & Febiger, 1983. Pp 65–78.

74. England T, Kasten MJ, Martin R, et al. Multistate outbreak of sporotrichosis in seedling handlers, 1988. *MMWR* 1988;37:652–3.

75. Hajjeh R, McDonnell S, Reef S, et al. Outbreak of sporotrichosis among tree nursery workers. *J Infect Dis* 1997;176:499–504.

76. Lenaway DD, Bailey AM, Smith H, et al. Blastomycosis acquired occupationally during prairie dog relocation—Colorado, 1998. *MMWR* 1999;48:98–100.

77. Tomchik RS, Russell MT, Szmant AM, et al. Clinical perspectives on seabather's eruption, also known as sea lice. *JAMA* 1993;269:1669–72.

78. Davies HD, Sakuls P, Keystone JS. Creeping eruption: A review of a clinical presentation and management of 60 cases presenting to a tropical disease unit. *Arch Dermatol* 1993;129:588–91.

79. Magill AJ. Epidemiology of the leishmaniases. *Dermatol Clinics* 1995;13:505–23.

80. Jimenez-Lucho VE, Fallon F, Caputo C, et al. Role of prolonged surveillance in the eradication of nosocomial scabies in an extended care Veterans Affairs medical center. *Am J Infect Control* 1995;23:44–9.

81. Krinski WL. Dermatoses associated with the bites of mites and ticks. *Int J Dermatol* 1983;22:75–91.

82. Newman LS. Occupational illness. *N Engl J Med* 1995;333:1128–34.

83. Landrigan PJ, Baker DB. The recognition and control of occupational disease. *JAMA* 1991;266:676–80.

84. Rutstein DD, Mullan RJ, Frazier TM, et al. Sentinel health events (occupational): a basis for physician recognition and public health surveillance. *Am J Public Health* 1983;73:1054–62.

22 / Occupational Slow Virus Infection

Jonathan S. Rutchik

Slow infection is a term used to describe a group of illnesses in animals and humans that result from a transmissible prion protein, PrP. Known as *transmissible spongiform encephalopathies (TSE)* [1], this group includes scrapies in sheep, bovine spongiform encephalopathy (BSE) in cattle, and Creutzfeldt-Jakob disease (CJD), Gerstmann-Straussler-Shenker syndrome (GSS), fatal familial insomnia (FFI), and atypical prion disease in humans. Prusiner and colleagues have demonstrated that PrP is a slowly infectious proteinaceous particle that is devoid of nucleic acid, resists the action of enzymes that destroy RNA and DNA, and has a structure that is unlike a virus [2]. The term *spongiform* refers to the classic neuropathology changes found in the cerebral and cerebellar cortices at autopsy.

CJD is the most important of the TSEs in humans; GSS, FFI, and atypical prion disease are inheritable and extremely rare. CJD is a fatal dementing neurodegenerative illness that presents most commonly in late middle age. Neurologic and psychological symptoms are common, but clinical findings vary substantially. Progressive dementia and myoclonus are the most constant clinical signs. When symptoms develop, however, death ensues within one year. CJD is predominantly sporadic, but prion disease has both infective and genetic properties. By injecting brain tissue from patients with this disorder, researchers have demonstrated that the agent responsible is transmissible from humans to primates [3]. CJD does not appear to be spontaneously contagious, but iatrogenic transmission has been reported in many instances [2]. Incubation periods for these cases have varied from months to decades [4]. Corneal transplantation, implantation of cerebral depth encephalography electrodes, implantation of dura mater grafts, and human growth hormone therapy [5] have been suggested as modes of transmission.

Occupations in which contact with human or animal neural tissues is common pose risk for exposure. These include histopathologists, laboratory technicians, veterinarian neuroscientists, pathologists, anatomists, neurosurgeons, and other surgeons as well as morticians and others in health-related professions. Since CJD has been reported in animal handlers who may have been exposed to neural tissues, butchers and farmers may also have increased risk for exposure [6,7]. Proper preparations, precautions, and handling techniques are discussed below.

Recently a new variant of CJD (nvCJD) has been discovered in younger patients, predominantly in the United Kingdom. This nvCJD has been characterized by a specific pathologic profile as well as the pathognomic spongiform changes found on histologic examination of the brain in patients with CJD [8]. Ten years prior to this, the UK experienced an epizootic BSE [9] thought to be secondary to exposure of calves to contaminated rendered cattle carcasses in the form of meat and bone-meal nutritional supplements. This has raised concerns over whether transmission from animal to man may occur by means other than contact with neural tissues [10]. A UK government expert panel announced that the agent responsible for BSE might have spread to humans, based on the recognition of 10 persons with nvCJD [11]. The United States has begun active surveillance; the CDC reported no nvCJD in the United States in 1996 [9]. Although there is no clear evidence that supports transmission by blood, bodily fluid or tissues from outside the central nervous system transmission, UK epidemiologists in one study have reported an increased incidence of CJD in dairy farmers in the UK and other countries. These authors underscore that mouse-transmission studies presently under way will help reveal whether the causative agent for BSE has infected humans [11].

Incidence and Prevalence

The annual incidence of CJD has been reported to be one to two cases per million of the population [2]. The incidence is higher in Israelis of Libyan descent, North African immigrants to France, and Slovakians. A small proportion (5–15%) of cases are familial, suggesting that some genetic susceptibility exists [12]. The high frequency in Libyan Jews is now known to be due to a codon 200 mutation in the PrP gene in affected families [13]. The CDC reported annual death rates during 1979–1994 to be stable at approximately 1 case per million population. The number of deaths attributed to CJD among those under 45 years old ranged from 0 in 1984 to 8 in 1981 and 1993. In most years, none were reported in those under age 30. One of these died and had been previously identified as a recipient of a pituitary-derived human growth hormone; the other had negative neuropathology. Between 1991 and 1995, the annual number of deaths remained stable; the average annual death rate was 1.2 per million. Nine were under age 55, one of these was under 45, and none were under 30. None of these had neuropathology characteristics of nvCJD [9].

A statistically significant excess of cases among dairy farmers and their spouses, and among people at increased risk of contact with live cattle infected with BSE, was noted between 1970 and 1996 in a study performed in the United Kingdom [11]. This high incidence, however, was comparable to that observed in dairy farmers in countries where BSE is rare or nonexistent. The authors speculated that individuals in this occupation in countries where they collected data may be at increased risk of CJD for reasons other than exposure to the causative agent of the bovine disease. They also remarked, however, that the absolute risk was noted to be extremely low—well below 10 cases per million.

Transmission and Occupational Risk Factors

A European collaborative study group assessed occupational and historical risk factors retrospectively for 405 patients with definite or probable CJD between 1993 and 1995 in Belgium, France, Germany, Italy, the Netherlands, and the United Kingdom. They reported no increased risk in relation to a history of surgery or blood transfusion or an association between CJD and specific animal-source food consumption (not with beef, veal, lamb, cheese, or milk). No association was noted between CJD and occupational exposure to animals or leather. Positive findings were as follows: ingestion of raw meat (RR 1.63, CI 1.18–2.23); ingestion of brain (RR 1.68, CI 1.18–2.39); frequent exposure to leather products (RR 1.94, CI 1.13–3.33); and exposure to fertilizer consisting of hoofs and horns (RR 2.32, CI 1.38–2.91). Also, the study found evidence of familial aggregation of CJD, with dementia, due to causes other than CJD [10].

CJD has been reported in six physicians and 24 health care workers, many of them with documented exposure to animal or human brain tissue [4]. A 61-year-old dairy farmer presented with atypical dementia and died three months after hospital admission. Postmortem neuropathology examination identified spongiform changes typical of CJD. This patient had a documented case of BSE in his herd of cattle (the animal had been potentially exposed to contaminated feed before July 1988) but had no contact with the cow's internal organs or tissues. He had, however, drunk pooled milk from the herd. The authors suggested continued surveillance of specific occupational groups because of the risk of direct inoculation from bovine tissue, but they remarked that this was likely a chance finding and that a causal link was conjectural [6]. A 59-year-old cattle farmer was diagnosed with CJD. He also had a single case of BSE in the cattle on his farm in 1991. Sheep were also on the farm, but none were known to have scrapie. The farmer had been involved in calving and had assisted the veterinarian with cesarean sectioning. It was not known if he assisted with the BSE-infected cow, but he had otherwise not been involved in any other procedure with the animal. He had not had contact with meat or bone meal and denied ever tasting animal feed. He also denied drinking unpasteurized milk since before 1972. In this case, the clinical presentation and pathologic confirmation was consistent with the sporadic form of CJD, not with the new variant [7]. Other authors reiterated that two large epidemiology surveys—one a French 15-year investigation [14] and the other a British case control study conducted between 1980 and 1984 [15]—failed to find a link between occupation and CJD [16].

A 62-year-old woman had been employed in a neuropathology laboratory for 22 years. Her duties included rinsing formalin-fixed brains and processing, cutting, and staining sections of brain without participating in actual brain cutting. She became ill and died one year later. Autopsy confirmed a neuropathologic diagnosis of CJD [17]. Review of department log books revealed that she had worked on brain specimens of two persons who had been diagnosed with CJD. These cases were seen 16 and 11 years prior to the onset of her symptoms. The neuropathologist who worked on those brains remains healthy and active. The author of this case study acknowledged the occupational risks of the neuropathology profession but suspected a chance occurrence. A 75-year-old histologist developed CJD [18]. This was pathologically demonstrated and confirmed. Questioning of the patient's family revealed that he had worked with animal and human brains before 1969: In 1963 and 1964, he had performed sheep dissections. This author considered the occupational exposure a possible causative factor in the patient's illness.

The first pathologist diagnosed with CJD was reported in 1992. Records were not available to elucidate whether he had performed or assisted with any autopsies for which CJD was the diagnosis. The authors of this case study emphasized care and precautions in handling potential contaminated material at autopsy, especially for cadavers of patients with dementia of unknown or cytogenic origin [19].

A review article included a case report of an internist who had received 12 months of training in pathology in 1959 and died of CJD [20]. The patient's father had had Alzheimer's disease. The author of the article mentioned that it is unlikely that clinical illness invariably follows exposure to the infectious agent, since there is a potentially high rate of exposure and only a small number of health care workers who have been reported to have had CJD. A genetic susceptibility may be required, however.

Prevention and Controls

The pathogen responsible for CJD withstands many customary sterilization methods, including heat, formaldehyde and ultraviolet radiation, which typically eradicate viral and bacterial pathogens [21]. Since many neurologic and psychological symptoms may herald CJD's clinical onset, pathologists and laboratory staff must exercise extreme caution when handling cadavers with unclear neurologic or psychiatric diagnoses.

It is possible to transmit CJD to nonhuman primates and small laboratory animals by intercerebral, subcutaneous, intraperitoneal, intramuscular, and intravenous inoculation and by ocular transplantation. Subcutaneous and intramuscular routes of inoculation are said to be less efficient methods of inoculation than the intracerebral route in producing disease. Also, other tissues with a lower titer of infectivity are still transmissible, including liver, lung, lymph node, kidney, and leukocytes. Blood has been infectious in both human [22] and experimental CJD; urine has also been found to be infectious in humans. Saliva, external secretions, and stool have not been found to contain the pathogen. Conjugal cases, which have been reported, indicate a common source of infection rather than cross-contamination.

Many methods of disinfection have been tested [22]. *Ineffective* procedures include boiling, ultraviolet irradiation, ethylene oxide sterilization, ethanol, formalin, beta propiolactone, detergents, quaternary ammonium compounds, lysol, alcoholic iodine, acetone, and potassium permanganate. Formaldehyde, diluted to 10%, has also been shown to be ineffective. A 1.0 Eq/L solution of sodium hydroxide bathed for 60 minutes, then steamed at 121°C for 30 minutes, has proved effective in at least two studies [24,25]. Steam autoclaving for one hour at 132° C is the other fully effective, recommended procedure. A more recent study instructs that instruments should be disposable or decontaminated by soaking in 1N sodium hydroxide (40 g/L) or in undiluted sodium hypochlorite for one hour and then submitted to autoclaving at 134°C for one hour [26]. The study further describes that tissues should be blocked thinly for histologic analysis and soaked in concentrated formic acid for one hour, then in 4% formaldehyde solution for at least 48 hours. It is noteworthy that formalin-fixed tissues embedded in paraffin stored at room temperature may be infectious for years and thus should always be handled with caution.

The above-described disinfection procedures must be used for venipuncture needles, forceps, scissors, lumbar puncture needles, and for any other instruments used on a patient with probable CJD. Discarded clothing worn during these procedures also should be collected and autoclaved. Specimens submitted to laboratories should be clearly marked as coming from patients with definite or suspected CJD. Disposable gloves should be worn, and skin contact with any possible infectious material should be followed by washing the skin with 1N sodium hydroxide for several minutes. Universal Precautions, including use of gown, glasses, masks and gloves, should be used by those performing autopsy or necropsy on tissues possibly contaminated with PrP. The autopsy and brain-cutting work areas should be restricted to only those necessary to perform the work. Also, a manual saw should be used for cutting of the skull, taking care not to cut into the brain or spinal cord tissue. If an electric saw is used, a towel should cover it to reduce aerosolization. The autopsy drain should be closed and the water collected and decontaminated. The cadaver should be washed with 1N of sodium hydroxide, the wash water sterilized, and appropriate precautions communicated to the mortician. Organs and trimmed tissues need to be meticulously collected and completely incinerated [23,27].

If accidental puncture occurs, the wound should be cleaned with iodine (Betadine), phenolic antiseptic (hexachlorophene or 5% Lysol), or 0.5% sodium hypochlorite (Dakin's fluid or household bleach) or should be swabbed with a 1:3,000 solution of potassium permanganate [27].

Clearly, patients with CJD must not be blood or organ transplant donors or sources of human tissue for preparation of biologic products to be used in humans, such as dura mater, pituitary hormones, and human interferon.

Symptoms and Signs

Eighty percent of sporadic cases of TSE are diagnosed in persons between 50 and 70 years of age. TSE may be sporadic, infectious, or familial and has recently been reported in young adults. Both genders are equally affected. One third of a large series of patients had prodromal symptoms of fatigue, depression, weight loss, and disorders of sleep and appetite that lasted several weeks. Another third initially had neurologic symptoms such as memory loss, confusion, or uncharacteristic behavior, and one third initially had focal signs such as ataxia, aphasia, visual loss, hemiparesis, or amyotrophy. Early aspects of the disease vary greatly, but changes in behavior, emotional response and intellectual function, together with abnormalities of cerebellar and visual function, are most common. Early symptoms may confuse the diagnostician. Progression, however, is rapid, and myoclonic contractions appear in all cases; this is associated with a striking startle response. Ataxia and dysarthria also become prominent. Stupor and coma usually follow, and myoclonus often continues until death. Akinetic-mutism is also common in the late stage of the disease [1,28].

The electroencephalographic picture is often characterized by diffuse and nonspecific slowing, accompanied occasionally by stereotypical high-voltage slow (1–2 Hz) and sharp-wave complexes on an increasingly slow and low-voltage background. The high-voltage sharp waves are synchronous with the myoclonus but may persist in its absence. EEG reveals this characteristic pattern in 60–90% of patients, depending on the disease phase and the number of EEGs performed [29].

Blood and CSF are often normal. Specific diagnostic protein markers of the CSF, such as neuron-specific enolase, have been shown to be good diagnostic tools. CSF levels above 35 ng/mL were noted to be 80% sensitive and 92% specific for CJD [30]. Blood measurement of PrP, in conjunction with a clinical diagnosis, confirms the diagnosis of CJD due to heritable causes.

The classic constellation of neuropathologic changes in CJD consists of spongiform degeneration, neuronal loss, and astrocytic gliosis. Only spongiform degeneration is specific for CJD, however. The disease usually affects the cerebral and cerebellar cortices diffusely. In some cases, occipitoparietal regions are almost exclusively involved; in others, the cerebellum is most seriously affected. Light microscopy of pathologic specimens typically leads to a definitive diagnosis. Immunohistochemistry using antibodies against the prion protein is preferable in all suspected cases of CJD and is mandatory whenever a routine histologic work-up does not yield definitive results [29].

A description of features of nvCJD was derived from a series of 10 patients in Great Britain. The mean age of onset was 29, and the median duration of illness was 14 months. All patients presented with early psychiatric symptoms, most often depression. Eight developed early sensory symptoms, which were persistent and painful. All patients developed ataxia and involuntary movements, and by the end, most had akinetic mutism. EEGs were abnormal in most, but none had characteristic features. Findings of cerebral imaging were normal [31]. Recently, PrP was found to be present in the biopsied tonsillary tissue of 20 patients with this clinical and pathologic variant of CJD; patients with the sporadic form of CJD were negative for tonsillary PrP. In late stages of nvCJD, this biopsy technique may prove sensitive and specific [32].

Differential Diagnosis

Lithium intoxication, metabolic encephalopathies, carcinomatous meningitis, viral encephalitides, and diffuse central demyelinating disease, a type of multiple sclerosis called *Schilder's disease*, may mimic the presentation of TSE in the early aspects of the illness. Diffuse Lewy body disease and atypical Alzheimer's disease may also present with early mental changes and may also progress to myoclonus. Subacute sclerosing panencephalitis may resemble TSE but is mainly seen in children or young adults. Limbic encephalitis and AIDS dementia are also on the differential diagnostic list. Myoclonus and dementia may be present in cerebral lipidoses in children and young adults but is chronic and includes retinal changes, which do not occur in TSE [1]. Because of the recent case reports of TSE in patients under the age of 45, a high index of suspicion is warranted for progressive atypical dementia in younger age groups.

Diagnostic Evaluation, Treatment, and Rehabilitation

Diagnostic evaluation for TSE includes a complete neurologic examination. Special attention should be given to assessment of mental status and visual and cerebellar function. Electroencephalography is suggested. MRI may not be helpful. Neuron-specific enolase may be useful if obtained from the cerebrospinal fluid. Brain biopsy is diagnostic; the specimen should be taken from an area of the brain whose function reflects the prominent clinical features of the patient.

Because of the disease's rapidly progressive nature, no treatment or rehabilitation is possible. Antiviral agents have been ineffective [1].

References

1. Viral Infections of the Nervous System. In: Adams RD, Victor M, Ropper AH (eds), *Principals of Neurology*, 6th Ed. New York: McGraw Hill. 1997. Chap 33.
2. Prusiner SB. Genetic and infectious prion disease. *Arch Neurol* 1993;50:1129.
3. Gibbs CJ, Gadjusek DC, Asher OM. CJD (spongiform encephalopathy): transmission to the chimpanzee. *Science* 1968;161:388–9.
4. Brown P. Iatrogenic CJD. *Aust NZ J Med* 1990;20: 633–4.

5. Billette de Villemeur T, Deslys JP, Pradel A, et al. CJD from contaminated growth hormone extracts in France. *Neurology* 1996;47:690–5.
6. Sawcer SJ, Yuill GM, Esmonde TF. CJD in an individual occupational exposed to BSE. *Lancet* 1993; 341:642.
7. Young GR, Fletcher NA, Zeidler M, et al. CJD in a beef farmer. *Lancet* 1996;348:610–11.
8. Will RG, Ironside JW, Zeidler M. A new variant of CJD in the UK. *Lancet* 1996;347:921–5.
9. Surveillance for CJD—United States. *MMWR* 1996; 45:665–8.
10. Van Duijn, Delasnerie-Laupretre N, Masulla C, et al. Case control study of risk factors of CJD in Europe during 1993–1995. *Lancet* 1998;351:1081–5.
11. Cousens SN, Zeidler M, Esmende TF, et al. Sporadic CJD in the United Kingdom: analysis of epidemiological surveillance data for 1970–1996. *Br Med J* 1997;315:389–96.
12. Masters CL, Harris JO, Gadjusek DC, et al. CJD: patterns of worldwide occurrence and the significance of familial and sporadic clustering. *Ann Neurol* 1979; 5:177.
13. Hsiao K, Meiner Z, Kahana E. Mutation of the prion protein in Libyan Jews with CJD. *N Engl J Med* 1991;324:1091–7.
14. Brown P, Cathala F, Raubertas RF, et al. The epidemiology of CJD: conclusions of a 15-year investigation in France and a review of the world literature. *Neurology* 1987;37:895–904.
15. Harries-Jones R, Knight R, Will RG. CJD in England and Wales, 1980–1984; a case control study of potential risk factors. *J Neurol Neurosurg Psychiatry* 1988;51:1113–9.
16. Ridley RM, Baker RF. Occupational risk of CJD. *Lancet* 1993;341:641.
17. Miller DC. CJD in histopathology technicians. *N Engl J Med* 1988;318:853–4.
18. Sitwell L, Lach B, Atack E, et al. CJD disease in histopathology technician. *Neurology* 1988;318(13):854.
19. Gorman DG, Benson F, Vogel DG, et al. CJD in a pathologist. *Neurology* 1992;42:463.
20. Berger JR, David NJ. CJD in a physician: a review of the disorder in health care workers. *Neurology* 1993;43:205–6.
21. Steelman VM. Creutzfeldt-Jakob disease: recommendation for infection control. *Am J Infect Control* 1994;22:312–8.
22. Patry D, Curry B, Easton D, et al. CJD after blood product transfusion from a donor with CJD. *Neurology* 1998;50:1872–3.
23. Brown P, Gibbs CJ, Amyx HL, et al. Chemical disinfection of Creutzfeldt-Jakob disease virus. *N Engl J Med* 1982;306:21:1279–82.
24. Taguchi F, Tamai T, Uchida K. Proposal for a procedure for complete inactivation of the CJD agent. *Arch Virol* 1991;119:297–301.
25. Committee on Health Care Issues, American Neurological Association. Precautions in handling tissues, fluids and other contaminated materials from patients with documented or suspected CJD. *Neurology* 1986; 19(1):75–7.
26. Budka H, Aguzzi A, Brown P, et al. Tissue handling in suspected CJD and other human spongiform encephalopathies (prion disease). *Brain Pathol* 1995;5(3):319–22.
27. Gadjusek DC, Gibbs CJ, Asher DM, et al. Precautions of medical care of and in handling materials from patients with transmissible virus dementia (CJD). *N Engl J Med* 1977;297:1253–8.
28. Johnson RT, Gibbs CJ. Medical progress: CJD and related transmissible spongiform encephalopathies. *N Engl J Med* 1998;339(27):1994–2004.
29. Kreztschmar HA, Ironside JW, DeArmond SJ, et al. Diagnostic criteria for sporadic CJD. *Arch Neurol* 1996;53:913–20.
30. Zerr I, Bodemer M, Recker S. Cerebrospinal fluid concentration of neuron specific enolase in diagnosis of CJD. *Lancet* 1995;345:1609.
31. Zeidler M, Stewart GE, Barraclagh CR, et al. New variant CJD: neurological features and diagnostic tests. *Lancet* 1997;350:903–7.
32. Hill AF, Butterworth RJ, Joiner S, et al. Investigation of variant Creutzfeldt-Jakob disease and other human prion diseases with tonsil biopsy sample. *Lancet* 1999;353(9148):183–9.

23 / Occupational Meningitis

Robert C. Godefroi

The gram-negative diplococci *Neisseria meningitidis* and the gram-negative bacillus *Haemophilus influenzae* type b (Hib) can result in either asymptomatic upper respiratory tract colonization or potentially fatal invasive disease. Meningitis is the most common presentation of *N meningitidis* and is a rare complication of *Haemophilus influenzae* infection in adults. Since the introduction of the Hib vaccine in 1991, Hib meningitis in children has become exceedingly rare. Despite the availability of the meningococcal quadrivalent polysaccharide vaccine, however, the incidence of invasive meningococcal disease has remained stable in recent years [1]. The mortality of meningococcal disease is higher than that of Hib disease but is similar to that of meningitis. In contrast to Hib infections, which occur only sporadically, meningococcal disease occurs both sporadically and in outbreaks. *N meningitidis* serogroup A, rare in the United States, causes widespread epidemics in Africa and Asia. Recently, in the United States, *N meningitidis* serogroup C outbreaks have occurred, for unknown reasons, with increased frequency. Meningococcal cases and outbreaks generate considerable fear among family members, health care providers, and community members alike. Cases must be diagnosed early, and the management of outbreaks remains a great challenge requiring significant public health resources.

Epidemiology

Meningococcal disease occurs in a worldwide distribution as endemic disease or in epidemics. Three serogroups—A, B, and C—account for more than 90% of cases of meningococcal disease [2]. Serogroups B and C each account for approximately 45% of cases in the United States, where most are due to endemic disease [3]. In the 15 U.S. outbreaks of serogroup C meningococcal disease (SCMD) reported between 1989 and 1993, school-age children and young adults were most commonly affected [2]. Although virtually nonexistent in the United States, group A strains are responsible for large epidemics worldwide. In the sub-Saharan region of Africa known as the *Meningitis Belt*, epidemic attack rates have approached 1%. In the United States, major epidemics are rare, the last one occurring in 1945 [4]. When group A epidemics occur in industrialized nations, they are generally small and mainly involve lower socioeconomic groups [5].

The majority of the estimated 2,600 annual cases of meningococcal disease occur sporadically. In the United States, outbreaks of serogroup C meningococcal disease have occurred frequently in the 1980s and early 1990s. An increase has been reported as well in Canada, Denmark, the United Kingdom, and Spain [2]. The rate of endemic SCMD in the United States has remained unchanged, however, as approximately 25 cases per 100,000 population occur. Secondary cases of SCMD occur occasionally among people in close contact with victims of the primary disease, but these cases are rare, primarily because those in close contact now receive appropriate chemoprophylactic antibiotics [6]. SCMD outbreaks have different epidemiologic characteristics from those of endemic SCMD. These outbreaks are characterized by the increased transmission of disease among persons who share a common organizational affiliation or live in the same community and yet do not have close personal contact [6]. Organization-based outbreaks have recently occurred in schools, universities, and correctional facilities [2].

Serogroup B primarily causes sporadic disease, but it can cause outbreaks, although these have been infrequently reported in the United States [7]. Since the 1970s, a group of closely related strains of serogroup B, designated the ET5 complex, has caused substantially elevated rates of disease in Europe, Cuba, and several South American countries [8].

In developed countries, endemic or sporadic meningococcal disease incident rates are 1 to 3 per 100,000 persons, whereas endemic rates in many developing countries range from 10 to 25 per 100,000 persons [4]. In the United States between 1989 and 1991, the average annual incidence of meningococcal disease was 1.1 per 100,000, with 46% of cases occurring in children less than two years of age [9]. In the United States, a significantly higher incidence of infection has been observed in blacks: 1.5 compared to 1.1 (in nonblacks) in 100,000 [9]. In temperate climates, meningococcal infection due to both serogroup B and serogroup C strains has a seasonal peak, with most cases occurring during the first quarter of the year.

N meningitidis is a normal commensal of the human respiratory tract. Colonization of the nasopharynx follows inhalation of infected aerosolized droplets from a previously colonized individual. Meningococcal colonization is a benign condition; 25–40% of young adults in temperate climates have meningococcal colonies in their throats without disease [10]. In Europe, the overall carriage rate is about 10% [11]. Some *Neisseria* meningitis strains, however, do possess pathogenic potential, which is expressed in certain individuals. It is the noncarrier who is at greatest risk.

The majority of persons who are exposed to pathogenic meningococci become carriers and do not develop invasive disease. For example, although the prevalence of carriers can be as high as 95% in military recruits during group A epidemics, less than 1% actually develop systemic disease [12]. It is the asymptomatic carrier that is the major source of transmission of pathogenic strains [11], for most cases of meningococcal disease have not had direct contact with another such patient.

Known risk factors for meningococcal carriage include living in a household with a person with meningococcal disease or a carrier [13,14] and household or institutional crowding [15,16]. Other semiclosed populations such as people living in college dormitories or chronic care hospitals and persons in nursery schools are at increased risk of infection [17]. Campus bar workers have also been found to have increased prevalence of meningococcal carriage [18]. Increased carriage has also been noted among public transportation workers [11]. In all of these work environments, close person-to-person contact takes place. Despite being exposed to patients with meningococcal infection, health care workers do not have a greater risk of acquiring this infection than the general public [17].

Smokers of 20 or more cigarettes per day have an odds ratio for meningococcal carriage of 5.3 relative to nonsmokers [19]. Exposure to passive smoking in the home has also been independently associated with increased risk of meningococcal carriage [11,15].

Individual host factors that increase an individual's susceptibility to invasive meningococcal disease are well known: The most common are deficiencies in the complement system [4]. Meningococcal infections in persons with properdin deficiency is associated with a case fatality rate of 75% [20]. Certain infectious agents may increase the risk of bacterial disease by suppression of the immune system. Investigators have also found a link between bacterial meningitis and mycoplasma infection [21,22] as well as a number of viral infections, including influenza, adenovirus, parainfluenza, and respiratory syncytial virus [4].

The risk of developing meningococcal disease increases 500- to 1,200-fold in household contacts during the 30–60 days following a case, as compared with the general population [23,24]. Without intervention, the overall risk is 4–5% [14]. The risk of household transmission is greatest in the first week following contact [14,23].

The predilection of meningococcal disease for military personnel has been noted historically. In World War I and World War II, meningitis selectively attacked new draftees in recruit camps. Since the end of World War II and the introduction of the polysaccharide vaccination program for U.S. military recruits, meningococcal disease has been less of a problem for the armed services.

In the Korean War, there were only seven cases of meningitis among U.S. troops [25]. During the Vietnam War, however, meningococcal disease in U.S. Army recruits once again became a problem.

Nosocomial transmission of *N meningitidis* occurs rarely and is probably associated more frequently with cases of meningococcal pneumonia than meningitis or meningococcal disease [26,27]. Between 1975 and 1997, only five cases occurred in health care workers [23]. Four cases involved mouth-to-mouth resuscitation, and one case involved intubation of a patient with meningococcal infections [28,29]. One case of a laboratory researcher who contracted meningococcal disease while working with significant quantities of serogroup B *N meningitidis* has been reported [30].

Health care providers who have been exposed to children during meningococcal outbreaks are often anxious about bringing *N meningitidis* home to their own children. The children of health care providers, however, are probably not at an increased risk of colonization with *N meningitidis* during an outbreak [31].

Signs and Symptoms of Meningococcal Disease

The most common clinical presentations of meningococcal disease are meningitis and meningococcal septicemia, otherwise called *meningococcemia*. Occasionally, the disease presents as occult bacteremia, primary pneumonia, oral pharyngitis, or conjunctivitis. Acute meningococcemia is frequently preceded by an acute infection of the upper respiratory tract. Common initial symptoms are fever, chills, malaise, myalgias, arthralgias, and headache. Acute meningococcal disease is usually an illness of rapid onset, and patients frequently deteriorate quickly. Patients who present with meningococcal meningitis but without meningococcal septicemia may have a less dramatic clinical presentation. The classic clinical presentation of meningococcal meningitis, like other types of bacterial meningitis, includes headache, fever, and meningismus, often with signs of cerebral dysfunction. Photophobia, abdominal pain, and diarrhea also may occur. Skin rashes often develop and may be the initial signs of meningococcemia. Petechiae are present in approximately 50% of patients and are the most common skin finding, but macular and macular papular rashes may also occur [32]. Petechiae often appear on the ankles, wrists, and axilla and may progress to involve any part of the body, but the palms and soles are usually spared [33]. The number of petechial lesions may increase dramatically and continue to increase for up to 24 hours after microbial therapy has begun [33]. Purpuric lesions can occur in fulminant infections and are more specific for meningococcal septicemia than petechiae [32]. Therefore, when a patient presents with fever and petechiae, and/or purpuric lesions, meningococcal disease must be strongly considered in the differential diagnosis. The differential diagnosis of patients presenting with fever and petechiae or purpuric lesions also includes endocarditis, disseminated gonococcal disease, murine and epidemic typhus, parvovirus, B19 infection, Epstein-Barr virus, cytomegalovirus, viral hemorrhagic fevers, and rickettsial infections such as Rocky Mountain spotted fever [34]. Fulminant progressive meningococcemia is often referred to as *Waterhouse-Friderichsen syndrome*. Delirium may develop quickly, and congestive heart failure also may ensue.

Features of septic shock often predominate in the presentation of patients with Waterhouse-Friderichsen syndrome. Acute renal failure, hypotension, cyanosis, and disseminated intravascular coagulation (DIC) may occur. Meningococcal arthritis complicates bacteremia in 2–10% of cases involving adults [32]. In patients that survive meningococcemia, a variety of neurologic complications may occur.

Signs of meningitis include positive Kernig's and Brudzinski's signs. Kernig's sign is elicited by extension of the knee while the hip is flexed and the patient is supine. It is considered a positive sign if knee extension causes pain in the upper back or neck. Brudzinski's sign is a reflex flexion of the hips and knees on neck flexion with the patient sitting with legs straight. Meningitis may occur without specific signs in the elderly or in immunocompromised individuals.

The differential diagnosis of the neck stiffness seen in meningitis includes cervical spondylitis, cervical osteomyelitis, and soft-tissue inflammation, of which painful cervical lymphadenopathy is by far the most common during the illness. Conjunctivitis may be one of the presenting features in up to 2% of patients of meningococcal septicemia or meningitis [35].

N meningitidis also causes lower and upper respiratory tract infections. Primary meningococcal pneumonia is a well-recognized entity. In an outbreak in a military camp, 10 of 16 patients with meningococcemia or meningitis had concurrent pneumonia [36]. In one study of 162 individuals with community-acquired pneumonia, *N meningitidis* was the etiologic agent in only 6% of the cases [37].

Diagnostic Evaluation

The diagnosis of meningococcal septicemia is confirmed by isolation of *N meningitidis* from a blood culture specimen. If possible, blood culture results should be obtained before antibiotics are given, but delay in administering antibiotics is associated with increased mortality [38]. *N meningitidis* may also be isolated from the cerebral spinal fluid (CSF). Gram-stain smears from petechial skin lesions may reveal *N meningitidis* in up to 70% of cases [33]. Because asymptomatic carriage is common, the diagnosis of meningococcal disease cannot be made by culturing *N meningitidis* from the oral pharynx. Rapid serologic tests are available to detect *N meningitidis* capsular polysaccharide antigen in the cerebrospinal fluid (CSF) and urine.

The cerebrospinal fluid in meningococcal meningitis is usually under increased pressure and thus appears cloudy, and CSF pleocytosis is present. CSF glucose is usually reduced to below 1.5 mmol/L, or less than 40% of the value of the plasma glucose obtained concomitantly [39]. The CSF protein concentration is elevated in virtually all cases. A CSF glucose of less than 40% of the plasma value and an elevated protein concentration are not features of viral meningitis but are found in more than 80% of cases of bacterial meningitis [40].

Direct microscopy often demonstrates the presence of gram-negative diplococci. In cases in which a gram stain of CSF fluid does not demonstrate organisms, the CSF leukocyte differential count is helpful in diagnosing bacterial meningitis. The presence of polymorphonuclear cells suggests bacterial etiology, but these cells may rarely be found in early viral meningitis as well. A lymphocyte pleocytosis is unusual in meningococcal meningitis, although it has been reported [41]. Overall, in cases of bacterial meningitis, only 10% of patients initially present with a predominance of lymphocytes in the CSF [42].

The role of CT scanning in the diagnosis of meningitis is controversial. Patients with meningitis rarely have major abnormalities on CT scanning in the absence of focal neurologic findings [43]. In patients with suspected meningitis and signs of increased intercranial pressure or focal findings on neurologic examination, a CT scan is indicated before the performance of lumbar puncture. Antibiotic therapy should be initiated before any patient with suspected meningitis is sent for a CT scan.

Mortality in Acute Meningococcal Disease

Disseminated meningococcal disease carries with it a significant risk of death. The mortality rate in developed countries is about 7–8% in adults [41]. There are several clinical features associated with a poor prognosis: the presence of shock, the appearance of a rash, and an altered level of consciousness. In addition, death from acute me-ningococcal disease is associated with hypotension upon presentation. Patients with a purpuric rash are significantly more likely to be hypotensive, have DIC, and to succumb to the illness [44]. Additional clinical findings associated with poor prognosis include the presence of coma, seizures, or metabolic acidosis [45] and age greater than 60 [46].

Treatment

Early recognition and prompt treatment with appropriate antibiotics are crucial in treating meningococcal septicemia or meningitis. Ideally, blood cultures should be obtained before beginning antibiotic therapy, unless this significantly delays the administration of antibiotics. Penicillin is the antibiotic of choice for invasive meningococcal disease; the adult dose is 12–24 million units per day in divided doses every four hours. Relative resistance to penicillin has been reported from a significant number of countries, including the United States and Canada [4,47,48]. Although treatment with penicillin is still effective against these relatively resistant strains [49,50], it has been recommended that higher doses of penicillin be used [50]. Complete resistance has also been reported in a small number of cases [47]. Broad-spectrum cephalosporins are used frequently in the treatment of meningitis and are active against moderately susceptible strains of meningococci [47].

Beta-lactamase production in patients with meningococci is extremely rare but has been reported [47]. Chloramphenicol achieves high concentrations in the CSF [4] and remains an alternative to penicillin for the treatment of meningococcal meningitis. Resistance to sulfonamides is now widespread, and they should not be used for treatment of meningococcal infection or carriage [4]. Data on the use of adjuvant corticosteroid therapy for the treatment of meningococcal meningitis are limited. In one study, there was no difference in the frequency of neurologic sequelae observed in the group receiving corticosteroids versus the placebo group [51].

Even with the introduction of newer antimicrobial agents, the mortality among adults with gram-positive bacillary meningitis remains high. With the advent of broad-spectrum cephalosporins, gram-negative bacillary meningitis mortality may be decreasing. In one hospital study conducted in the 1980s, almost one fourth of adults with meningitis died [46].

Prevention and Control

Effective control of meningococcal disease outbreaks is important because of the high morbidity and mortality connected with the disease. An outbreak is defined as two or more cases occurring simultaneously in the same place. The incubation period is between two and 10 days, and epidemics occur quickly. Outbreaks usually cause considerable public anxiety, and the management of both cases and contacts as well as public relations is extremely important. In this section, the main emphasis is on the prevention and control of cases and on organizational outbreaks of serogroup B and C meningococcal disease in technologically developed countries, not serogroup A epidemics that occur in Africa.

MENINGOCOCCAL VACCINE

The quadrivalent A,C,Y,W-135 vaccine (Menomune A,C,Y,W-135, manufactured by Connaught Laboratories) is the only formulation now available in the United States. The recommended dose of this vaccine is a single 0.5-mL subcutaneous injection. The immunogenicity and clinical effectiveness of serogroup A and C meningococcal vaccines are well known. The serogroup C vaccine is poorly immunogenic in children under 18–24 months of age [52,53]. The serogroup A and C vaccines have demonstrated excellent clinical effectiveness in older children and adults and are useful in controlling epidemics [54,55]. Serogroup Y and W-135 polysaccharide vaccines are safe and effective in adults and children greater than 2 years of age [53,56]. Antibody levels against group A and C polysaccharides decrease dramatically after three years following a single dose of vaccine [6]. In the United States, the routine vaccination of civilians with the quadrivalent meningococcal polysaccharide vaccine is not recommended because of its relative ineffectiveness in children less than 2 years of age, who carry the highest risk of endemic disease, and because of its short duration of protection. However, the polysaccharide meningococcal vaccine is recommended to control serogroup C meningococcal outbreaks. The Advisory Committee on Immunization Practice (ACIP) recommends routine vaccination with the meningococcal quadrivalent vaccine for certain high-risk groups including (1) persons who have a terminal complement component deficiency, (2) persons with asplenia, and (3) research and clinical laboratory personnel who are exposed to *N meningitidis* in the laboratory setting [6].

FOREIGN TRAVEL

Quadrivalent vaccine should also be offered to people traveling to countries where *N menin-*

gitidis is either highly endemic or epidemic, such as the sub-Saharan African region and Nepal.

Individuals at particularly increased risk include health care providers, refugee camp aides, individuals making contact with people with traditional lifestyles where the disease is endemic, and individuals who travel extensively and unpredictably, such as field service engineers and military and intelligence personnel [57]. Vaccination is not recommended for short-term business trips or vacations to areas of endemic meningococcal activity if travelers are not expected to have exposure to resident populations and crowded conditions.

Revaccination may be indicated for persons who continue to be at high risk for infection. In older children and adults, revaccination may be considered after three to five years [6]. Adverse reactions are generally mild and consist of local reactions at the injection site. Serogroup B vaccines are moderately effective in older children and adults [58,59], but no serogroup B meningococcal vaccines are currently licensed for use in the United States.

SPORADIC CASE MANAGEMENT

In the United States, the main method of prevention and control of meningococcal disease is antimicrobial chemoprophylaxis for close contacts of sporadic cases of disease. Close contacts include household members, day-care-center contacts, and anybody directly exposed to a patient's oral secretions. *Close contacts* may be defined as people sleeping in the same household as the index case, anyone who has mild kissing contact with the patient, and health care personnel performing endotracheal intubation or endotracheal tube management of index cases. The attack rate for household contacts has been estimated to be 4 per 1,000 persons exposed [60]. The rate of secondary disease in close contacts is highest during the first few days after the onset of symptoms in the index case. Oral pharyngeal swabs are not helpful in determining the need for chemoprophylaxis and may unnecessarily delay the beginning of antibiotic treatment.

Currently, rifampin is the drug of choice for chemoprophylaxis (Table 23-1). Resistance to rifampin, however, has occurred in 10–27% of treated patients [61]. There is concern that widespread use of rifampin for prophylaxis in outbreaks may lead to further problems with microbial resistance [62]. Other antimicrobial agents are effective in reducing nasopharyngeal carriage of *N meningitidis*. These include ciprofloxin and ceftriaxone. Minicycline also successfully eradicates nasochondrial carriage; because of its high incidence of vestibular side effects, however, it is not a first-line drug of choice [34]. Close contact of cases caused by serogroup A or C strains should receive a single dose of the quadrivalent polysaccharide vaccine. The decision to vaccinate close contacts of cases for which the serogroup is not known, should be based on local epidemiology of the disease and be made by appropriate public health officials.

Swabbing

If the effectiveness of chemoprophylaxis antibiotics is to be monitored, culturing of nasopharyngeal swabs of close contacts should take place four to seven days after the course of antibiotics is completed [63]. Swabbing to check for the elimination of carriage, however, is of limited value, as a single negative swab does not guarantee freedom from nasopharyngeal carriage. However, if a repeat swab is positive, additional chemoprophylaxis antibiotics are indicated. Swabbing of close contacts in order to determine who should receive chemoprophylaxis is inappropriate and is not recommended. However, swabs taken from close family contacts may be used for diagnostic purposes in suspected cases of meningococcal disease if penicillin has been given to the patient prior to hospital admission. Swabbing of family contacts may also afford an isolate for serogroup and serotype determination.

Subtyping of *N meningitidis* isolates may be useful in determining whether a group of cases actually represents an outbreak. SCMD outbreaks are usually caused by closely related strains. If strains from a group of patients have different subtypes, then the group of cases probably represents a cluster of cases and not an outbreak. Subtyping is time consuming and can be done only in specialized reference laboratories. Outbreak control efforts should not be delayed pending results of subtyping.

Table 23-1
Schedule for Administering Chemoprophylaxis Against Meningococcal Disease

Drug	Age Group	Dosage	Duration and Route of Administration[a]
Rifampin	Adults	600 mg every 12 hr	2 days
Ciprofloxacin	Adults	500 mg	Single dose
Ceftriaxone	Adults	250 mg	Single intramuscular dose

[a] Oral administration unless indicated otherwise.
Adapted from Centers for Disease Control and Prevention. Control and prevention of meningococcal disease and control and prevention of serogroup C meningococcal disease: evaluation and management of suspected outbreaks. Recommendations of the Advisory Committee on Immunization Practices (ACIP). *MMWR* 1997;46(RR-5):1–21.

OUTBREAK MANAGEMENT

In the United States, the routine use of meningococcal vaccine during outbreaks is not recommended because 50% of meningococcal disease is caused by serogroup B, for which an effective vaccine is not licensed in the United States. Serogroup B outbreaks and sporadic cases are controlled by administration of chemoprophylaxis antibiotics to close contacts. The polysaccharide meningococcal vaccine, however, is useful for controlling serogroup C meningococcal outbreaks. Because meningococcal vaccine takes seven to 10 days to precipitate protective antibody response, close contacts should also receive immediate chemoprophylaxis. Family contacts of index cases have the greatest risk and should receive priority for vaccination during epidemics. Moreover, after a few weeks, family contacts may be at risk for disease despite adequate chemoprophylaxis [64].

Currently, ACIP does not recommend mass chemoprophylaxis for institutional or organizational outbreaks, citing a lack of effectiveness in most settings in which an outbreak has occurred. In small organizational outbreaks of SCMD, however, ACIP suggests that mass chemoprophylaxis be considered. The latter recommendation is based in part on a recent study of school-based outbreaks of meningococcal disease in the United States, suggesting that the initiation of mass chemoprophylaxis may prevent some subsequent cases from occurring [65]. Disadvantages of the broad usage of antimicrobial drugs for chemoprophylaxis include the cost of the drug and its administration, the inherent difficulty of administering chemoprophylaxis antimicrobial drugs to large populations, the potential side effects of the medication, and the possible development of resistant microbes. There are no recommendations at this time to control SCMD outbreaks by closing schools and colleges or by canceling community events like athletic contests.

MANAGEMENT OF SUSPECTED CASES

Patients with suspected meningococcal disease should be given parental penicillin before hospital admission [66]. Upon admission, HICPAC isolation procedures require respiratory isolation for at least 24 hours after antibiotic treatment [67]. CSF cultures, blood cultures, and nasopharyngeal swab cultures for meningococci should be obtained [63]. Blood and CSF cultures should be taken as soon as possible if parental penicillin was given prior to hospital admission. All meningococcal isolates should be sent to a reference laboratory for serogrouping, serotyping, and antibiotic sensitivity testing. Public health officials should be immediately notified about suspected cases of meningitis. The stimulus for notification should always be clinical suspicion and not the laboratory diagnosis of disease.

MANAGEMENT OF HEALTH CARE WORKERS SUSPECTED TO BE EXPOSED TO MENINGOCOCCAL DISEASE

Individuals are considered exposed to *N meningitidis* if they have had prolonged contact with a patient with meningococcal disease while unmasked or if they have had contact with an infected patient's respiratory secretions. Exposed individuals need chemoprophylaxis and antibiotics within 24 hours of exposure [68]. After a patient is diagnosed with meningococcal disease, infection control specialists should determine which health care providers require chemoprophylaxis and refer them to employee health services immediately for implementation of therapy.

Lymphocytic Choriomeningitis

Human disease due to infection with lymphocytic choriomeningitis (LCM) virus has occurred in sporadic outbreaks in Europe, Asia, and the Americas. Vectors are various rodents. Outbreaks have occurred among personnel in medical research institutions where hamsters reside. Disease caused by LCM is almost never fatal. The clinical syndrome varies from an acute febrile illness to aseptic meningitis and mild encephalitis. At present, there is no specific treatment and no vaccine available for LCM infection. The testing of hamster colonies in research laboratories is recommended to avoid human contact with this pathogen [69].

Epidemiology of *Haemophilus influenzae*

The species *H influenzae* encompasses a group of pleomorphic gram-negative human pathogens. *H influenzae* is a commensal of the upper respiratory tract. There are six capsular serotypes of *H influenzae*, although *H influenzae* serotype B (Hib) is the capsular serotype most frequently associated with human disease. Unencapsulated *H influenzae* strains are termed *nontypeable H influenzae*. Before the introduction of the Hib vaccine in the United States in 1991, approximately 10,000 cases of meningitis occurred annually in children. The widespread usage of conjugate type-B vaccine in the routine immunization schedule of children has resulted in the near elimination of invasive type-B disease in young children in the United States [70]. *H influenzae* infections also cause morbidity and mortality in the adult population. In one recent study, invasive *H influenzae* infections in adults had an annual incidence of 5.6 cases per 100,000 individuals [71]. However, *H influenzae* is a relatively uncommon cause of meningitis in adults, and approximately 50% of the isolates are nontypeable [72]. Epidemics of Hib infection occur in day care centers and among persons in close populations such as in geriatric units [73,74]. In one large study of 1,147 cases of *H influenzae* meningitis, eight associated cases of meningitis occurred in family members, a 500-fold increase when compared to the general public. No secondary cases occurred in contacts over age 6 [75], however.

Prior infection with influenza and other viruses probably facilitates invasive *H influenzae* infection [76]. In a large study conducted by the Centers for Disease Control, the majority of invasive adult infections occurred in patients with significant pre-existing conditions, which included chronic lung disease, malignancy, alcoholism, pregnancy, advanced age, immunosupressive drug treatment, splenectomy, and HIV infection [71]. Two outbreaks of *H influenzae* infection caused by nonencapsulated strains have occurred since 1990 in the United Kingdom. Both outbreaks involved nosocomial transmission in pulmonary units [77,78]. In one large series, *H influenzae* was responsible for 4% of community-acquired and 4% of nosocomial cases in adults [46] with nontypeable strains predominating [79].

PREVENTION AND CONTROL

HICPAC respiratory isolation procedures should be followed when a person suspected to have invasive *H influenzae* infection is admitted to the hospital. Nasopharyngeal culturing is of little value, as mentioned above, for *H influenzae* is a normal inhabitant of the upper respiratory tract. Meningitis may result from hematogenous spread but has also been associated with cranial trauma [80].

SYMPTOMS AND SIGNS

The clinical presentation of meningitis due to Hib and nontypeable *H influenzae* is similar to that of other bacterial pathogens, including *N meningitidis*. An additional suppurative focus of infection, such as otitis media, sinusitis or pneumonia, appears in approximately 30% of cases of *H influenzae* meningitis [42].

DIAGNOSTIC EVALUATION

As stated above, the nasopharyngeal culturing of *H influenzae* is not recommended because of the high carriage rate among healthy individuals. The diagnosis is made by cultures of blood or CSF. Cultures should be performed even if antibiotic therapy has been already initiated. In some cases, tympanocentesis or needle aspiration of the maxillary sinus cavity or margins of an area of cellulitis or involved lung may help to obtain specimens for bacterial isolation studies. In about 70% of cases of meningitis, CSF smears reveal the *H influenzae* organism. Detection of capsular antigen in serum or CSF by using immunoelectrophoresis, latex agglutination, or enzyme-linked immunosorbent assay (ELISA) is diagnostic in up to 90% of culture-proven cases of meningitis [42].

TREATMENT

Like other cases of bacterial meningitis, Hib meningitis can be rapidly fatal if not aggressively treated. Historically, ampicillin has been the drug of choice, but in recent times, resistant strains have become common. Resistance is almost always mediated by beta-lactamase production [81]. In the United States, chloramphenicol has historically produced excellent results in severe infections due to *H influenzae* and is still a first-line therapy. Chloramphenicol, 75 to 100 mg/kg/day divided into four doses, is given. Because drug resistance has recently occurred in the United States and Europe, however, routine susceptibility testing is recommended [82]. Chloramphenicol has as its major side effect, dose-related reversible toxicity to the bone marrow. Other treatment options include a third-generation cephalosporin and trimethoprim/sulfamethoxazole [82].

CONTROL AND PREVENTION

Chemoprophylaxis is effective in preventing secondary cases [83–85] and is recommended for household residents and other individuals who have close contact with an index case. These include adult members of a household, especially if another susceptible child is a resident. Rifampin is the drug usually recommended for prophylaxis of Hib meningitis. The currently recommended dose for adults is 600 mg twice daily for four days.

Future Outlook for the Prevention and Treatment of Meningitis

N meningitidis is the leading cause of bacterial meningitis in young adults in the United States. Hib meningitis, common in children before the advent of the Hib vaccine, is a rare cause of meningitis in adults. The quadrivalent meningococcal vaccine is used for control of serogroup A and C outbreaks in certain high-risk individuals and for travelers to foreign areas with increased meningococcal activity. No vaccine effective for serogroup B is currently licensed in the United States. In the United States, chemoprophylaxis for close contacts of sporadic cases of meningococcal disease is the primary measure to prevent meningococcal infection. In spite of the advent of broad-spectrum antibiotics, the case fatality rate for bacterial meningitis remains high at approximately 25%. In the future, effective prevention of meningococcemia in technologically developed countries will probably result from the development of an improved conjugate vaccine similar to the Hib vaccine that is administered as part of a routine infant immunization program. For now, it is imperative that physicians have a high index of suspicion in diagnosing meningococcal meningitis and report all suspected cases promptly to appropriate public health officials.

References

1. Moore KA. Meningococcal disease and public health practice, a complicated roadmap. *JAMA* 1998;279:472–3.
2. Jackson LA, Schuchat A, Reeves MW, et al. Serogroup C meningococcal outbreaks in the United States: an emerging threat. *JAMA* 1995;273:383.
3. Centers for Disease Control and Prevention. Laboratory-based surveillance for meningococcal disease in

selected areas—United States, 1989–1991. *MMWR* 1993;42:21.

4. Riedo FX, Plikaytis BD, Broome CV. Epidemiology and prevention of meningococcal disease. *Pediatr Infect Dis J* 1995;14(8):643–56.
5. Boslego JW, Tramont EC. Neisseria meningitidis. In: Gorbach SL, Bartlett JG, Blacklow NR (eds), *Infectious Diseases.* Philadelphia: Saunders, 1992. P 1452.
6. Centers for Disease Control and Prevention. Control and prevention of meningococcal disease and control and prevention of serogroup C meningococcal disease: evaluation and management of suspected outbreaks. Recommendations of the advisory committee on immunization practices (ACIP). *MMWR* 1997;46(RR-5):1–21.
7. Jackson LA, Alexander ER, Debolt CA, et al. Evaluation of the use of mass chemoprophylaxis during a school outbreak of enzyme type 5 serogroup B meningococcal disease. *Pediatr Infect Dis J* 1996:15(11): 992–8.
8. Pinner RW. Addressing the challenges of emerging infectious diseases. *Am J Med Sci* 1996;311(1):3–8.
9. Jackson LA, Wenger JD. Laboratory-based surveillance for meningococcal disease in selected areas: United States, 1989–1991. *MMWR* 1993;42:21–30.
10. Griffiss JM. Mechanisms of host immunity. In: Cartwright K (ed), *Meningococcal Disease.* West Sussex, Engl: John Wiley & Sons, 1995.
11. Caugant DA, Hoiby EA, Magnus P, et al. Asymptomatic carriage of *Neisseria* meningitis in a randomly sampled population. *J Clin Microbiol* 1994;32:323–30.
12. Goldschneider I, Gotschlich EC, Artenstein MS. Human immunity to the meningococcus. *J Exp Med* 1969;129:1307.
13. Broome CD. The carrier state: *Neisseria* meningitis. *J Antimicrob Chemother* 1996;18(Suppl A):25–34.
14. Munford RS, Taunay AE, de Mornais JS, et al. Spread of meningococcal infection within households. *Lancet* 1974;1:1275–8.
15. Thomas JC, Bendana MS, Waterman SH, et al. Risk factors for carriage of meningococcus in the Los Angeles men's jail system. *Am J Epidemiol* 1991;133:286–95.
16. Le Saux N, Ashton F, Rahman M, et al. Carriage of *Neisseria* species in communities with different rates of meningococcal disease. *Can J Infect Dis* 1992;3:60–4.
17. Apicella MA. Neisseria meningitides. In: Mandell Gl, Douglas RG, Bennett JE (eds), *Principles and Practice of Infectious Diseases,* 3rd Ed. New York, NY: Churchill Livingstone, 1990. Pp 1896–1909.
18. Imrey PB, Jackson LA, Ludwanski PH, et al. Meningococcal carriage, alcohol consumption, and campus bar patronage in a serogroup C meningococcal disease outbreak. *J Clin Microbiol* 1995;33(12):3133–7.
19. Stuart JM, Cartwright KAV, Robinson PM, et al. The effect of smoking on meningococcal carriage. *Lancet* 1989(ii):723–5.
20. Densen P, Weiler JM, Griffiss JM, et al. Familial properdin deficiency and fatal meningococcemia. *N Engl J Med* 1997;316:922–6.
21. Krasinski K, Nelson JD, Butler S, et al. Possible association of mycoplasma and viral respiratory infections with bacterial meningitis. *Am J Epidemiol* 1987;125:499–508.
22. Moore PS, Hierholzer J, Dewitt W, et al. Respiratory viruses and mycoplasma as cofactors for epidemic group A meningococcal meningitis. *JAMA* 1990;264:1271–5.
23. De Wals P, Hetoghe L, Borlee-Grimee I, et al. Meningococcal disease in Belgium, secondary attack rate among household daycare nursery, and pre-elementary school contacts. *J Infect* 1981;3(Suppl 1):53.
24. Meningococcal Disease Surveillance Group. Analysis of endemic meningococcal disease serogroup and evaluation of chemoprophylaxis. *J Infect Dis* 1976;134:201.
25. Cowdrey AE. *The Medics' War.* Washington, DC: Center of Military History, United States Army, 1987. P 147.
26. Rose HD, Lenz IE, Sheth NK. Meningococcal pneumonia: a source of nosocomial infection. *Arch Intern Med* 1981;141:575–7.
27. Cohen MS, Steere AC, Baltimore R, et al. Possible nosocomial transmission of group Y *Neisseria meningitidis* among oncology patients. *Ann Intern Med* 1979;91:7–12.
28. Nosocomial meningococcemia—Wisconsin. CDC. *MMWR* 1978;27:358–63.
29. Feldman HA. Some recollections of the meningococcal diseases. (The First Harry F. Dowling Lecture.) *JAMA* 1972;220:1107–12.
30. Stephens DS, Hajjeh RA, Baughman WS, et al. Sporadic meningococcal disease in adults: results of a five-year population-based study. *Ann Intern Med* 1995; 123:937–40.
31. King WJ, MacDonald NE, Wells G, et al. Relationship between parental occupation and children's oral pharyngeal colonization with *Neisseria meningitidis. J Pediatr* 1995;126(6):937–9.
32. Glode MP, Smith AL. Meningococcal disease. In: Feigin RD, Cherry JD (eds), *Textbook of Pediatric Infectious Diseases,* 3rd Ed.. Philadelphia: Saunders, 1992. P 1185.
33. Boslego JW, Tramont EC. *Neisseria meningitidis.* In: Gorbach SL, Bartlett JG, Blacklow NR (eds), *Infectious Diseases.* Philadelphia: Saunders, 1992. P 1452.
34. Salzman MB, Rubin LG. Meningococcemia. *Infect Dis Clin North Am* 1996;10(4):709–25.
35. Odegaard A. Primary meningococcal conjunctivitis followed by meningitis and septicemia. *NIPH Ann* 1983;6:55–7.
36. Hoppes GM, Ellenbogen C, Gebhart RJ. Group Y meningococcal disease in United States Air Force recruits. *Am J Med* 1977;62:661–6.
37. Kertulla Y, Leinonen M, Koskela M, et al. The aetiolgy of pneumonia: application of bacterial serology and basic laboratory methods. *J Infect* 1987;14:21–30.

38. Strang JR, Pugh EJ. Meningococcal infections: reducing the case fatality rate by giving penicillin before admission to hospital. *Br Med J* 1992;305:141.
39. Olcen P, Barr J, Kjellander J. Meningitis and bacteremia due to *Neisseria meningitidis*: clinical and laboratory findings in 69 cases from Orebro County, 1965–1977. *Scand J Infect Dis* 1979;11:111–9.
40. Nye FJ. The value of initial laboratory investigations in the management of meningitis. *J Infect* 1993;7:31–8.
41. Steven N, Wood M. The clinical spectrum of meningococcal disease. In: Cartwright K (ed), *Meningococcal Disease*. West Sussex, Engl: John Wiley & Sons, 1995.
42. Scheld WM. Bacterial meningitis and brain abscess. In: Harrison TR (ed), *Harrison's Principles of Internal Medicine*, 13th Ed. New York: McGraw-Hill, 1994.
43. Cabral DA, Flodmark O, Farrell K, et al. Prospective study of computed tomography in acute bacterial meningitis. *Pediatrics* 1997;111:201–5.
44. Toews WH, Bass JW. Skin manifestations of meningococcal infection: an immediate indicator of prognosis. *Am J Dis Child* 1974;127:173–6.
45. Yabek SM. Meningococcal meningitis presenting as acute cerebellar ataxia. *Pediatrics* 1973;52:718–20.
46. Durand ML, Calderwood SB, Weber DJ, et al. Acute bacterial meningitis in adults. *N Engl J Med* 1993;328 (1):21–8.
47. Oppenheim BA. Antibiotic resistance in *Neisseria meningitidis*. *Clin Infect Dis* 1997;24(suppl 1):S98–101.
48. Van Esso D, Fontanals D, Uriz S, et al. *Neisseria meningitidis* strains with decreased susceptibility to penicillin. *Pediatr Infect Dis J* 1997;6:438–9.
49. Saez-Nieto JA, Fontanals D, Garcia de Jalon J, et al. Isolation of *Neisseria meningitidis* strains with increased penicillin minimal inhibitory concentrations. *Epidemiol Infect* 1987;99:463–9.
50. Jones DM, Sutcliff EM. Meningococci with reduced susceptibility to penicillin (letter). *Lancet* 1990;335: 863–4.
51. Girgis NI, Farid Z, Mikhail IA, et al. Dexamethasone treatment for bacterial meningitis in children and adults. *Pediatr Infec Dis J* 1989;8:848–51.
52. Peltola H, Kayhty H, Kuronen T, et al. Meningococcus group A vaccine in children three months to five years of age: adverse reactions and immunogenicity related to endotoxin content and molecular weight of the polysaccharide. *J Pediatr* 1978;92:818–22.
53. Gold R, Lepow ML, Goldschneider I, et al. Kinetics of antibody production to group A and group C meningococcal polysaccharide vaccines administered during the first six years of life: prospects for routine immunization of infants and children. *J Infect Dis* 1979;140: 690–7.
54. Pinner RW, Onyango F, Perkins BA, et al. Epidemic meningococcal disease in Nairobi, Kenya, 1989. *J Infect Dis* 1992;166:359–64.
55. Cochi SL, Markowitz LE, Joshi DD, et al. Control of epidemic group A meningococcal meningitis in Nepal. *Int J Epidemiol* 1997;16:91–7.
56. Zangwill KM, Stout RW, Carlone GM, et al. Duration of antibody response after meningococcal polysaccharide vaccination in U.S. airforce personnel. *J Infect Dis* 1994;169:847–52.
57. Statement on meningococcal vaccination for travelers. *Can Communic Dis Rep* 1995;21:25–9.
58. Sierra GVG, Campa HC, Varcacel NM, et al. Vaccine against group B *Neisseria meningitidis*: protection trial and mass vaccination result in Cuba. *NIPH Ann* 1991;14:195–207.
59. Bjune G, Hoiby EA, Gronnesby JK, et al. Effect of outer membrane vesicle vaccine against group B meningococcal disease in Norway. *Lancet* 1991;338:1093–6.
60. Meningococcal Disease Surveillance Group. Analysis of endemic meningococcal disease by serogroup in evaluation of chemoprophylaxis. *J Infect Dis* 1976;134: 201–4.
61. Weidner CE, Dunkel TB, Pettyjohn FS, et al. Effectiveness of rifampin in eradicating a meningococcal carrier state in a relatively closed population: emergence of resistant strains. *J Infect Dis* 1971;124:172.
62. Guttler RB, Counts GW, Avent CK, et al. Effect of rifampin and minicyclin on meningococcal carrier states. *J Infect Dis* 1971;124:199.
63. PHLS Meningococcal Infections Working Party. The epidemiology and control of meningococcal disease. *Communic Dis Rep* 1989;(8):3–6. (Internal publication of the public health laboratory service, London.)
64. Stuart JM, Cartwright K, Robinson PM, et al. Does eradication of meningococcal carriage in household contact prevent secondary cases of meningococcal disease? *Br Med J* 1989;298:569–70.
65. Zangwill KM, Schuchat A, Riedo FX, et al. School-based clusters of meningococcal disease in the United States. *JAMA* 1997;277:389–95.
66. Cartwright K, Reilly S, Whit D, et al. Management of early meningococcal disease. *Lancet* 1993;342:985–6.
67. Guideline for isolation precautions in hospitals part one: evolution of isolation practices. *Am J Infect Control* 1996;24:24–52.
68. Committee on Infectious Diseases, American Academy of Pediatrics. 1994. *Redbook: Report of the Committee on Infectious Diseases*, 23rd Ed. Elk Grove Village, IL: American Academy of Pediatrics, 1994.
69. Last JM. *Public Health and Preventive Medicine*, 12th Ed. Norwalk, CT: Appleton-Century-Crofts, 1986. P 343.
70. Adams G, Deaver KA, Cochi SL, et al. Decline of childhood hemophilus influenza type B (Hib) disease in the Hib vaccine era. *JAMA* 1993;269:221–6.
71. Farley MM, Stephens DS, Brachman PS Jr, et al. Invasive hemophilus influenza disease in adults: a prospective, population-based surveillance. *Ann Intern Med* 1992;116(10):806–12.

72. Apicella MA. Infections due to hemophilus influenza, hacek group, capnocytophaga, and *H ducreyi*. In: Harrison TR (ed), *Harrison's Principles of Internal Medicine*, 13th Ed. New York: McGraw-Hill, 1994.

73. Johnston RB, Anderson P, Newman S. Opsonization and phagocytosis of hemophilus influenza type B. In: Sell SH, Karzon DT (eds), *Hemophilus Influenza*. Nashville: Vanderbilt University Press, 1973. Pp 99–112.

74. Peltola H, Kayhty H, Virtanen M, et al. Prevention of hemophilus influenza type B bacteremic infections with the capsular polysaccharide vaccine. *N Engl J Med* 1984;310:1561–6.

75. Eskola J, Peltola H, Takala AK, et al. Efficacy of hemophilus influenza type B polysaccharide-diphtheria toxoid conjugate vaccine in infancy. *N Engl J Med* 1987;317:717–22.

76. Michaels RH, Myerowitz RL, Klaw R. Potentiation of experimental meningitis due to hemophilus influenza by influenza a virus. *J Infect Dis* 1977;135:641–5.

77. Sturm AW, Mostert R, Rouing PJ, et al. Outbreak of multiresistant non-encapsulated hemophilus influenza infections in a pulmonary rehabilitation center. *Lancet* 1990;335(8683):214–6.

78. Gough J, Kraak WA, Anderson EC, et al. Cross infection by non-encapsulated hemophilus influenza. *Lancet* 1990;336(8708):159–60.

79. Spagnuolo PJ, Ellner JJ, Lerner PI, et al. Hemophilus influenza meningitis: the spectrum of disease in adults. *Medicine* 1982,61:74–85.

80. Strausbaugh LJ. Hemophilus influenza infections in adults. *Postgrad Med* 1997;101(2):191–200.

81. Doern GV. Trends in antimicrobial susceptibility of bacterial pathogens of the respiratory tract. *Am J Med* 1995;99(Suppl 6b):3–7S.

82. Moxon ER. Hemophilus influenza. In: Harrison TR (ed), *Harrison's Principles of Internal Medicine*, 13th Ed. New York: McGraw-Hill, 1994.

83. Band JD, Frazier DW, Ajello G. Prevention of hemophilus influenza type b disease. *JAMA* 1984;251: 2381.

84. Fleming DW, Leibenhaut MH, Albanes D, et al. Secondary hemophilus influenza type B in daycare facilities: risk factors and prevention. *JAMA* 1985;254:509.

85. Shapiro ED, Wald ER. Efficacy of rifampin in eliminating pharyngeal carriage of *Haemophilus* influenza type B. *Pediatrics* 1980;66:5.

24 / Occupational HIV Infection

Lynn G. Stansbury and Alain J. Couturier

Occupational transmission of the human immunodeficiency virus (HIV) has been documented so far only in health care workers and prostitutes. Worldwide, commercial sex workers and those who patronize them run the greatest risk of occupational HIV infection and its end stage, acquired immunodeficiency syndrome (AIDS). This is particularly true in Africa and Asia, where prevalence rates have been documented as high as 35% in long-distance truckers and 80–90% in travel-route-associated prostitutes [1–6]. The incidence of occupational HIV infection in health care workers (HCW) is a fraction of that in commercial sex workers (CSW) but is a major source of concern for that group. Health care workers are also the only occupational group among whom postexposure prophylaxis has been evaluated [7,8].

Epidemiology

Occupational risk of exposure to HIV is proportional to the prevalence of HIV infection in the community, biophysiologic transmission factors of both pathogen and host, and the exposure potential inherent in the work being done.

Incidence and Prevalence

The HIV pandemic shows remarkable local differences in epidemiologic rates and patterns. Some of this appears due to biologic factors [9,10], but the spread of HIV requires intimate contact and thus is tightly bound to personal, social, and economic decision-making.

In the industrialized world, there has been an early shift to an endemic pattern: Incidence and prevalence, although still disproportionately affecting the poor and marginalized, are relatively low by world standards and defined more by prevalence than incidence. In the United States, in particular, the prevalence of "people living with AIDS" increased by 12% from 1992 through 1997 [11]. This occurred over a period when incidence actually fell, from highs of about 80,000 new cases (with roughly equivalent new HIV seroconversions identified) per year in the early to mid-1990s to about 20,000 new AIDS cases currently diagnosed per year (again, with roughly the same number of new HIV seroconversions), or a crude AIDS incidence rate of 22.1 per 100,000 per year. Some of this increased prevalence is attributed to expanded case definitions for AIDS, primarily to ensure inclusion of the increasing numbers of women with later-stage HIV infection. However, the major factor is believed to be decreasing mortality due to improvements in medical treatment, particularly direct antiviral treatment—multidrug "cocktails" and the protease inhibitors—which slow the progression of immunodeficiency [12,13].

In contrast to the situation in the wealthier nations, most of the rest of the world is still experiencing an expanding epidemic defined by an incidence that is high and still rising. Prevalence rates are also high but describe a churning reservoir of individuals who become infected, stay in the prevalence pool for 5–7 years, and then die with little more than palliative care. This figure is a rough average of the typical eight- to 10-year natural history of HIV infection in adults and the much shorter, two- to five-year course of congenital infection [14,15]. The most brutal recent illustration of these national differences comes from the Southern Hemisphere. In 1998, Australia and New Zealand, credited with good

HIV/AIDS prevention programs but also benefitting from the overall better health of industrial societies, together reported 600 new cases of HIV/AIDS, a crude incidence rate of between 2 and 3 per 100,000 population. In South Africa, in the same period, 700,000 new infections were recorded, for a crude incidence of 1,970 per 100,000, more than 750 times the rate in Australia/New Zealand [16–18]. Although the prohibitive expense of AIDS treatment for poorer nations has received lay media attention recently [19], other factors are involved in these extraordinary differences and will have to be addressed nationally and internationally [20].

Transmission Risk Factors

BIOMOLECULAR ISSUES IN TRANSMISSION

HIV is a retrovirus of the subfamily Lentivirus, a group of viruses that cause chronic cytopathic infections of the immune system of various vertebrate species. HIV is closely related to the immunodeficiency viruses of nonhuman primates. With the extraordinary growth in the human population in the last half of the twentieth century, human penetration into remote forest habitats, and rapid transit, this virus appears to have made a successful species jump in the relatively recent past and has been rapidly propagated and amplified by human behavior and susceptibility [21–23].

Humans are the only known reservoir of HIV. Transmission requires intimate contact between susceptible host target cells and free virus or virus contained in inflammatory cells, either suspended in human blood or present in other body fluids or tissues. Transmission does not occur via vectors or fomites, intact skin to intact skin, the airborne/respiratory route, or fecal/oral contact. Particularly in transmission by sexual contact, initial infection is most likely through direct cell-to-cell passage, with syncitium formation or other forms of cellular trafficking [24]. However, the dominant and characteristic form of ongoing viral infection and pathogenesis occurs with binding of the virus-specific envelope protein complex, gp120/gp41, to the CD4 molecule expressed on the surface of helper T-lymphocytes as part of T-cell responsiveness to foreign antigens [25]. Binding then initiates the stages of the viral life cycle: penetration, conversion of the RNA genome to DNA by the unique viral enzyme reverse transcriptase, integration of viral with host cell DNA, expression of viral messenger RNA and proteins, then virion assembly and budding from the cell membrane [26].

To date, of the various biomolecular steps in transmission and propagation of infection, the only portions that have proved vulnerable to interference are the viral envelope itself and two of the enzyme-mediated steps. The plasma-membrane-derived lipid bi-layer viral envelope is easily disrupted by solvents and the usual range of antiseptic agents and processes, including drying, heating, and freezing. The nucleoside analogues, of which the best known is azidothymidine (AZT), interfere with reverse transcriptase conversion of genomic RNA to the proviral DNA. The protease inhibitors interfere with the final steps that produce infective viral units.

Polymerase chain reaction (PCR) and related techniques for measuring HIV RNA circulating in plasma demonstrate that a newly infected individual can transmit infection within days, as viral titers skyrocket before the immune response activates sufficiently—usually at four to six weeks following infection—to moderate the replication of virus and produce measurable antibody [27–31]. Infection through sexual contact carries the double risk of successful local transmission, owing to the concentration of virus in contiguous lymphatic tissue, as well as bloodborne transmission owing to escalating viremia. Percutaneous transmission appears to result in primary infection of regional nodes, which then become propagation sites for eventual generalized disease [14,32].

CLINICAL ISSUES IN TRANSMISSION

Clinically, the likelihood of transmission centers around three issues: the viral titer of the source and the volume and mode of contact of the infectious material. Virus can be recovered eventually from most body fluids and tissues [33], but only blood products, sexual fluids, breast milk, and visibly bloody fluids have been associated with transmission [8,32–36]. Viral titers are determined by the natural stage of infection, treatment, treatment failure, and individual factors, but in general they are highest about four weeks after infection and in late-stage infection or when a particular antiviral regimen is failing [37]. Not surprisingly, clinical and epidemiologic observations document that transmission more often occurs from contact with infected individuals just prior to seroconversion, in late-stage disease, or with persistent high viral titers despite treatment [38,39].

Transfusion-associated infection is the most obvious example of the importance of volume in assessing the risk of an exposure. Transfusion with infected blood conveys the highest risk of transmission of HIV, essentially 100% [40, 41]. Perinatal exposure conveys the next most extreme risk, one neonatal infection in two to six births to infected mothers [34,42]. The exact mode by which transmission to the fetus and/or neonate occurs is still not clear but is most likely a combination of intrauterine blood-to-blood or blood-to-tissue contacts over time and birth-canal exposure to blood and inflammatory cells. Elective caesarean section, before rupture of membranes or onset of labor, reduces the rate of transmission by more than half [42,43].

Percutaneous exposure—in the conventional sense of puncture with a sharp object rather than transfusion—is consistently reported to result in seroconversion in about 1 in 300 contacts. However, the risk of actual contacts clearly varies with exposure factors and can be as high as 1 in 20 with penetration of highly infective material into highly vascular tissue [44–46]. See Table 24-1.

Table 24-1
Factors Predicting Transmission of HIV to Health Care Providers after Percutaneous Exposure

Factor	Adjusted Odds Ratio[a] (95% CI)[b]
Deep (intramuscular) injury	16.1 (6.1 to 44.6)
Visible blood on sharp device	5.2 (1.8 to 17.7)
Needle used to enter blood vessel	5.1 (1.8 to 14.8)
Source patient with terminal AIDS	6.4 (2.2 to 18.9)
Zidovudine prophylaxis used	0.2 (0.1 to 0.6)

[a] All were significant at $p < 0.01$.
[b] Confidence interval.
Adapted from Centers for Disease Control. Case-control study of HIV seroconversion in health care workers after percutaneous exposure to HIV-infected blood—France, United Kingdom, and United States, January 1988–August 1994 *MMWR* 1995; (44)50:931.

Mucosal contact—genital and oral—is of course the route of sexual transmission. Early published estimates of the risk of mucosal exposure focused on anogenital contact studies in stable, HIV-antibody discordant couples. These estimates varied but suggested that mucosal contact was a less efficient route of transmission than deep percutaneous injection and vastly less risky than transfusion, between 1 per 1,000 contacts with an infected individual with preclinical disease (and presumably, in the light of recent understanding, low viral titer) to 1 in 50 with someone with late stage disease [2,38]. More recent estimates take into account the synergistic effects of concurrent inflammation—such as co-existing STDs, helminthic infections, or periodontal disease—in a promiscuous heterosexual context and suggest that mucosal transmission—both anogenital and oral—is much more efficient in some circumstances than previously understood [33,47].

In the health care setting, blood splashes to oral mucosa and nonintact skin have been associated—albeit very rarely—with transmission [48-50]. See Table 24-2. The normal concentration of inflammatory cells in the human mouth could be expected to support receptive transmission, but saliva itself is inhibitory to virus, and the very rare reports of transmissions—only one health-care-related—due to bites emphasize both the extent of inflammatory disease and the presence of blood in the mouth of the biter [51,52]. Transmission has not been associated with ocular mucosal contact alone.

Likewise, transmission has not been associated with contact of infectious material with intact skin. Langerhans' cells, however, the bone-marrow-derived, immunologically competent cell population that make up 2–4% of the epidermis, express CD4, can be infected with HIV in vitro, and are probably one of the vehicles, along with dermal capillary injection, for shallow percutaneous infection or infection via abraded or otherwise nonintact skin [53]. Transmission in this

Table 24-2
Risk Assessment for Health Care Workers' Occupational Exposure to HIV

Risk of Transmission by Percutaneous Injury	Mucosal Contact or Contact with Nonintact Skin	Bite Wounds
0.2–0.5%	Not quantified. (Transmission by this route has been documented pooled risk estimate, 0.1% [46])	Not quantified. (Possible route of transmission in three nonoccupational exposures) [52,53]
Risk of Transmission by Potentially Infected Material		
Documented	**Possible**[a]	**Unlikely**
Blood, blood products, blood fluids	Semen, vaginal fluid, cerebrospinal fluid, breast milk, exudates, serosa fluids, amniotic fluid, saliva (during dental procedures)	Saliva, urine, feces

[a] These fluids have not yet been implicated in health care transmission but are likely to contain virus and have been implicated in other modes of transmission.
Adapted from Gerberding JL. Occupational exposure to blood-borne viruses. *N Engl J Med* 1995;332(7):444–51; used by permission, Copyright Clearance Center, Inc.

way is not as frequent as via deep muscular injection but has occurred [8,48].

Occupational Risk Factors

Despite widespread early concern, documented occupational transmission of HIV has remained confined to two work groups, prostitutes and health care workers. See Table 24-3. Public safety work, professional sports, and the military also have significant potential for adverse and uncontrolled exposure to infected blood or tissues, but occupational infection has not been reported in these groups [54]. In contrast, long-distance truck driving does not intrinsically impose such risks. However, long-distance trucking is clearly associated with the risk for and the spread of HIV/AIDS through much of Africa and Asia, as a result of extrafamilial sexual contact and the social conditions surrounding nontraditional intimate and economic relationships. HIV infection must therefore be considered a significant occupationally-related risk in this group and educational and preventive efforts must be directed toward them [55–57].

Among prostitutes, except in Islamic countries where tight community control over the lives of both men and women may be a factor in relatively low HIV prevalence, the prevalence of HIV in any given community appears to be in reverse proportion to the social and legal status of commercial sex workers (CSW) in general and of women in particular. As examples, in the United States, where the status of women is advanced, individual communities in the state of Nevada have legalized brothels and state law mandates condom use in commercial sex [58]. Coupled with active community concern and support—albeit primarily for local economic reasons—Nevada has never recorded a case of occupationally acquired HIV in a registered CSW [59]. In contrast, prostitution is illegal in Thailand, despite that country's international reputation for commercial sex, the status of women remains poor, the overall burden of disease remains great, and the prevalence of HIV in CSWs in some areas has reached 65% [17]. Additional risk factors for HIV infection in CSWs include patronage by long-distance truckers, street versus brothel work, low income, increased number of partners, the likelihood that the CSW and/or preferred personal partner are intravenous drug users, inconsistent or no use of condoms, and the likelihood of violence or refusal to pay if condom use is requested [60–66].

Among health care workers, occupational risk of HIV is almost entirely associated with the use of bedside, laboratory, or other clinical instrumentation that may cause percutaneous injury with contamination by infected blood. In general, the more such procedures are associated with a particular health care subgroup, the greater the risk [8,45]. See Table 24-3.

Prevention and Control

PRIMARY PREVENTION

Administrative Controls

In classic occupational health practice, administrative—typically, staffing—controls are the first level of risk-reduction. This is not broadly relevant to occupational risk of HIV, but some examples are possible. In its unusually pro-active approach to HIV risk in prostitutes, along with the provisions outlined above, the state of Nevada has also legislated that HIV-positive individuals may not be licensed as CSWs. While this somewhat draconian approach does not solve many of the issues surrounding CSWs and HIV infection, it does make clear the community position on the issue of HIV transmission in the course of their work [58]. Army regulations address HIV-positive soldiers mainly in terms of fitness-for-duty (see below). However, in an attempt to reduce duty-related risk of HIV transmission to fellow soldiers, HIV-positive soldiers cannot be deployed overseas. This avoids the potential both for blood exchange in the course of battle and contamination of the "walking blood bank" on which forward units depend for donors [67].

Engineering Controls, Safe Work Practices, and Personal Protective Equipment

Safe work practices have proved far more important in reducing occupational HIV exposure than engineering controls. For health care workers, manufacturers have enthusiastically promoted needleless and other risk-reducing systems. However, the only two strategies shown to significantly reduce percutaneous injury among health care workers have been (1) placing impervious disposal containers within arm's reach of any areas—including the bedside—where percutaneous procedures are done and (2) stopping the common practice of recapping used needles [68–70].

Table 24-3
Number of U.S. Health Care Workers with Documented and Possible Occupationally Acquired HIV Infection, Reported through June 1996

Occupation	Documented Occupational Transmission	Possible Occupational Transmission
Dental worker, including dentist	0	7
Embalmer/morgue technician	0	3
Emergency medical technician/ paramedic	0	10
Health aide/attendant	1	12
Housekeeper/maintenance worker	1	7
Laboratory technician, clinical	16	16
Laboratory technician, nonclinical	3	0
Nurse	20	27
Physician, nonsurgical	6	11
Physician, surgical	0	4
Respiratory therapist	1	2
Technician, dialysis	1	2
Technician, surgical	2	1
Technician/therapist, other than those listed above	0	5
Other health care occupations	0	1
Total	51	108

Adapted from Centers for Disease Control. *HIV/AIDS Surveillance Report* 1996;8(1):15.

Standard (Universal) Precautions are the basic safe work practices addressing risk for bloodborne pathogen transmission. (See also discussion in Chapter 34) Based on the presumption that all human blood and body fluids are infectious, Standard Precautions mandate frequent handwashing and the use of appropriate barriers to avoid contact with blood, high-risk body fluids, mucosa, or nonintact skin. Any barrier between infectious material and a portal of entry decreases the risk of transmission of HIV to some extent, but impermeable barriers are the most dependable and efficient. Gloving, usually with latex, is the best-accepted barrier protection, along with frequent glove changes and double gloving when the likelihood of percutaneous injury is great. However, consistent use of face-shields or masks/goggles to avoid splashes to eyes or mouth are also important. Unfortunately, as the use of natural rubber latex as a barrier protection across a wide range of occupations has increased, both in terms of numbers of users and frequency of use, reactivity to latex has emerged as a secondary occupational problem. Irritant contact dermatitis, delayed hypersensitivity, and immediate hypersensitivity—true allergy—have all been described, including fatal anaphylactic reactions [71].

Employee Education, Training, and Compliance

The most effective methods for reducing the risk of occupational HIV transmission are simple, cheap, familiar, and readily available. However, even with extensive efforts at education, compliance among those at greatest occupational risk for HIV—commercial sex workers in the Third World—will continue to be minimal without significant changes in the behavioral, economic, and legal conditions that surround their lives [72]. For other workers at risk for blood and body fluid exposure, ensuring compliance with safe work practices, once these were defined, has been less of a problem than providing adequate information to foster appropriate personal and professional responses to HIV issues.

As noted above, in at least three theoretically high-risk work groups—contact professional sports, public safety, and the military—occupational transmission of HIV has not occurred. Whatever the actual risk of transmission in these groups, early efforts were undertaken to educate and, where necessary, to change behaviors to avoid transmission. Professional boxing mandated the use of impermeable gloves for ringside attendants for fighters within a few years of the onset of the epidemic. Early in 1992, a consortium of professional sports associations, including the NBA, the NFL, the NHL, and baseball and high school and college groups, informally adopted the WHO Consensus Statement on AIDS and Sports. This guideline, which agrees with the American Academy of Pediatrics Commission on Sports Medicine and Fitness, does not restrict HIV-positive athletes from playing but does mandate common sense on-field blood/body fluid management and education of HIV-positive athletes about the potential for transmission in contact sports [73–75].

The concern and the learning curve of public safety workers about the HIV epidemic closely followed that of the general public. At the same time in the mid-1980s when school children with HIV were being excluded from academic classes, police officers were requesting hazardous materials outfitting when confronting AIDS activists [76]. An unprecedented Public Health Service education project in 1988, including material mailed to all U.S. households, resulted in demonstrable improvement in public knowledge about HIV infection and a general calming of public behavior and discourse [77,78]. For public safety workers, this period of increasing community enlightenment was coupled with increasingly reassuring evidence that a sub-epidemic of infection in their group was not occurring. In 1989, the CDC published recommendations for occupational risk reduction in public safety work [79]. Along with the by-now-familiar Standard Precautions, these included awareness of special risks, such as the potential for exposures to sharps in the searching of vehicles and extraction of victims from wrecked vehicles.

Attitudes of health care workers mirrored and to some extent amplified those of the general public and of public safety workers. However, the anticipated hepatitis B–like epidemic did not emerge in this group either, and simple primary preventive measures—nonrecapping of needles, immediate disposal of "sharps," and appropriate barrier methods—have been incorporated readily and effectively into bedside and laboratory practice.

IMMUNIZATION

As of this writing, fully successful immunization against HIV infection cannot be demonstrated, naturally or artificially. The virus's ability to rapidly express variability while retaining pathogenicity, the targeting of the immune system by infection, and the role of the immune system itself in amplifying the infection once it is established, all complicate the search for effective immunizing agents. In addition, the complexity of the pathogenic process and its proximity to simian infections has made the elucidation and analysis of animal models especially difficult. However, after some notable failures in the mid-1990s, vaccine research appears to be gaining some momentum again [80–82].

SECONDARY PREVENTION

Wound Care

When a percutaneous injury or mucosal splash occurs with potentially HIV-infected blood or body fluids, the first step is copious irrigation. If blood can be expressed from a puncture wound, that is useful both to assess the depth of the wound and to potentially express transmitted virus as well, but this procedure should not be prolonged at the expense of scrubbing. Wounds should be scrubbed for 15 minute with some form of antibacterial solution such as povidone iodine or chlorhexidine gluconate and a surgical scrub brush/sponge. Povidone iodine at 1/4 the concentration found in common clinical solutions will effectively kill HIV [83]. Pouring isopropyl alcohol into open wounds or otherwise damaging tissue is not advised. Mucosal exposures such as mouth or eyes should be irrigated for 15 minutes with sterile normal saline.

Postexposure Prophylaxis

Recent advances in understanding the early natural history of HIV infection and the availability of effective treatments to temper viral replication have catapulted postexposure prophylaxis (PEP) from wishful thinking to the community standard of care [84–87]. Once infection is established, although viral replication in many individuals can be greatly reduced as long as a given treatment regimen remains effective, infection has never been eliminated. However, prenatal treatment of infected mothers and even relatively brief treatment begun within the first 48 hours after birth of infants born to untreated infected mothers, are both associated with dramatic reductions in perinatal infection [88–90]. This suggests that at some point in the initial stages of transmission, perhaps before viral replication has greatly accelerated, the recipient immune system can, in some situations and in some individuals, clear the infection. Clinical data on PEP in both neonates and health care workers show that, as a very broad generalization, it prevents between two out of three to four out of five expected infections [10,85]. Results in neonates and animal models suggest that timing is critical: Efficacy clearly decreases the longer after exposure PEP is initiated [89–91].

At the present time, PEP is recommended only for those with conventional—typically, health care associated—occupational exposure. See Table 24-4. Offering PEP after high-risk sexual exposure has been discussed [92], although clearly in the context of personal, rather than occupational, behavior and health care. However, the fundamental issues and recommendations remain the same (Table 24-5). Once the high-risk status of the source and exposure are understood as likely and the offer of PEP appropriate, every effort must be made, while remaining sensitive to the emotional impact of the circumstances and recommendations, to begin the medication promptly. Concern about source confidentiality is appropriate, but the need for the injured worker to know the HIV status of the source is paramount. In addition, every effort must be made to protect the confidentiality of the exposed worker. Even if, on second thought or with additional information or with the onset of unacceptable side effects, follow-up doses are never taken, the optimal timing associated with the first minutes to hours after exposure will never be recovered. In general, in current practice, prophylaxis is generally not offered more than 72 hours after exposure, although there is no absolutely established cutoff [87,92].

The data on which postexposure prophylaxis is based reflect experience with AZT alone and include treatment failures despite appropriate timing and dosage [93]. Acknowledging widespread drug-resistant HIV, the current recommendation is to combine agents. This multidrug

Table 24-4
Advice on Prophylaxis after Occupational Exposure to HIV at San Francisco General Hospital and the Warren G. Magnuson Clinical Center of the National Institutes of Health

	Attributes of the Source Patient		
Attributes of the Exposure	**Asymptomatic, Known Low Titer**	**AIDS, Symptomatic Infection**	**AIDS, Preterminal, Acute Infection, Known High Titer**
Percutaneous injuries			
Superficial injury	Offer	Recommend	Strongly encourage
Visibly bloody device used in artery or vein	Recommend	Recommend	Strongly encourage
Deep intramuscular injury or actual injection	Recommend	Strongly encourage	Strongly encourage
Mucosal contacts			
Small volume and brief contact	Offer	Offer	Offer
Large volume or prolonged contact	Offer	Recommend	Recommend
Large volume and prolonged contact	Recommend	Recommend	Strongly encourage
Cutaneous contacts			
Small volume and brief contact	Offer if obvious portal of entry	Offer if obvious portal of entry	Offer if obvious portal of entry
Large volume or prolonged contact	Offer (recommend if obvious portal of entry)	Offer (recommend if obvious portal of entry)	Offer (recommend if obvious portal of entry)
Large volume and prolonged contact	Offer (recommend if obvious portal of entry)	Offer (recommend if obvious portal of entry)	Offer (recommend if obvious portal of entry)

Adapted from Gerberding JL. Prophylaxis for occupational exposure to HIV. *Ann Intern Med* 1996;125(6):497–501; used by permission.

approach includes the use of AZT and 3TC (lamivudine) as baseline agents, with the addition of protease inhibitors if the nature of the exposure or source warrant. The 1998 CDC recommendations on PEP in HCW [87] and the paper by Katz and Gerberding on PEP after high-risk sexual exposure, cited above [92], also include important discussions on the counseling and emotional support that must be provided to any individual for whom PEP is recommended or provided, as well as more detailed recommendations on clinical and laboratory follow-up.

SURVEILLANCE

Medical Surveillance and Biologic Testing

Serologic testing for HIV was standardized by the U.S. military by the late 1980s [94]. The combination of an enzyme-linked immunosorbent assay (ELISA) for screening and the Western blot electrophoretic assay for confirmation provided overall sensitivity and specificity of greater than 99% [95] and—in the absence of an immunization that could provide a more proactive approach to the community risks imposed by the HIV epidemic—was incorporated into mandatory surveillance for military personnel. At the National Institutes of Health, the Occupational Medical Service offers a voluntary program for at-risk employees to monitor the potential for seroconversion to the primary retroviruses—most importantly, HIV—under study in laboratory and clinical research programs in the various institutes. The mainstay of such a program is periodic testing—yearly for clinical and semi-annually for laboratory personnel working directly with the viruses. Any institution wishing to establish such a program must be prepared to organize data and record keeping with the most stringent confidentiality and attention to detail. Among other things, this involves clear understanding and plan-

Table 24-5
Treatment Protocol for Postexposure Prophylaxis

Treatment regimen (4 weeks):	AZT (zidovudine):	200 mg orally three times per day
	3TC (lamivudine):	150 mg orally twice a day

If source has a high viral load (> 50,000 copies/mL), has advanced HIV disease, or has been previously treated with one or both of the nucleoside analogues, consider adding:

	indinavir	800 mg orally every eight hours on an empty stomach
	or nelfinavir	750 mg orally every eight hours, with a meal

Initiate therapy as soon as possible after known or possible exposure, ideally, within the first two hours after exposure.

Toxicity monitoring:
- Symptoms
- Focused physical examination (mouth, cervical/axillary/inguinal nodes, liver/spleen)
- Laboratory testing: CBC, liver function tests, amylase, BUN/creatinine, urinalysis

Monitoring frequency:
Every two weeks while receiving treatment; at six weeks, three months, six months, 12 months

HIV monitoring:
- HIV antibody test at baseline, six months, and 12 months (required)
- HIV antibody test at six weeks and three months (optional)
- HIV antigen test, HIV polymerase chain reaction (PCR), and culture if symptoms of acute retrovirus illness occur in a seronegative health care worker.

In addition, if the source is known to be hepatitis B or C antigen positive, the exposed worker should be tested for the appropriate antibodies, offered hepatitis B immune globulin if appropriate and monitored for seroconversion.

Pregnancy testing should be offered if appropriate and counseling provided regarding the avoidance of pregnancy during the follow-up period. However, pregnancy is not a contraindication to the offer of PEP, although, at this time, only AZT/3TC can be recommended.

Adapted from Gerberding JL. Prophylaxis for occupational exposure to HIV. *Ann Intern Med* 1996;125:497–501; Katz, Gerberding. The care of persons with recent sexual exposure to HIV. *Ann Intern Med* 1998;128:306–12.

ning for follow-up of both positive and "indeterminate" Western blot results, including communication, counseling, and, when necessary, referral of involved employees.

Metrics

Postexposure prophylaxis protocols and surveillance programs both generate data on repeat, periodic serologic testing. Large institutions like the U.S. military or the NIH are able to depend on dedicated computer data bases. Steps to ensure the preservation and confidentiality of these data bases are integral to these programs. They also permit statistical review and analysis. However, outside of these major institutions, which are at once powerful and committed by their nature to a longer view than many other public and private enterprises, it may be much more difficult to collect or to make appropriate use of data regarding occupational HIV infection. For-profit health care institutions may be particularly shy about overtly generating data that might be reviewed to their legal or financial disadvantage. And whereas AIDS is a reportable disease consistently throughout the United States, only 29 states and the Virgin Islands collect so-called confidential name-based data on HIV seroconversion in adults and adolescents. Within those limits, however, any occupational medical service or practitioner planning PEP and/or HIV exposure surveillance can and should explore community, state, and CDC public health data collection processes for support.

Clinical Considerations

Workers confirmed as HIV-antibody-positive, whether or not as a result of occupational exposure, must be referred promptly for appropriate evaluation and follow-up. About 80% of newly antibody positive individuals recall a brief, mononucleosis-like illness, the so-called *acute retroviral syndrome*, which can occur shortly after transmission and 10 to 21 days before seroconversion [27,28,96]. The clinical manifestations of HIV infection associated with chronic and progressive immunocompromise—AIDS—are not expected for at least many months, more commonly years, and occasionally a decade or more. However, the emotional support, the physical and hematologic work-up, and, more recently, the treatment appropriate for preclinical HIV infection are beyond the capabilities of most occupational medical services. Further, the nature of these services, at least in the United States at the present time, is such that attempting to provide even preclinical care for HIV infection in a work-based setting risks an unacceptable violation of privacy.

Occupational Considerations

FITNESS FOR DUTY

The acknowledged risks and the social control inherent in military life have permitted the U.S. Army to define fitness-for-duty issues more clearly for HIV-positive soldiers than has been possible for any other occupational group. Except when deployed for action, a soldier's life tends to be administrative and sedentary but with the need to maintain and be able to regularly demonstrate physical fitness to clear standards. The Army approach to these issues, then, may be of use across many employment settings as a considered assessment of what employers may reasonably expect and plan for with HIV-positive employees.

Army regulations stipulate that HIV positive soldiers are fully capable of assigned duties with the following exceptions. Although they may reenlist if they meet standard qualifications, they may not sign up for training that incurs additional service. As noted above, HIV-positive soldiers may not be deployed overseas (other than to their home of record, such as Guam or Puerto Rico). In part, this is to reduce uninfected soldiers' risk of battle- or transfusion-associated exposure. However, experience with vaccinia suggests that HIV-positive individuals cannot be safely immunized with live-virus vaccines [97] and so cannot be immunized appropriately for overseas duty. In addition, the availability of appropriate medical care at forward centers cannot be guaranteed. As clinical disease requiring more frequent medical follow-up evolves, HIV-positive soldiers may not be assigned to posts distant from a military medical center (for example, as a recruiter). Only with the onset of progressive clinical illness or profound immunodeficiency are medical discharge procedures begun [67].

Private-sector data collected over three years, 1990–1992, showed that workers with both clinical (AIDS) and preclinical HIV infection lost excess time from work. Those with AIDS lost about a month more than comparable uninfected individuals, and those with preclinical HIV infection, a little less than two weeks more than comparable workers [98]. How recent advances in treatment will change this picture remains to be seen. Although decreased morbidity from opportunistic infection and other consequences of late-stage infection might be expected to decrease time loss among workers with AIDS, the treatments themselves require close follow-up and are not without significant side effects. Similarly, current recommendations to begin antiretroviral treatment in the earliest stages of recognized infection [27,28] can be expected to result in increased time required for clinical office and laboratory visits and illness attributable to side effects of medication.

The Infected Health Care Worker: How Much Risk?

Over the almost two decades of the HIV epidemic, transmission from infected health care workers to their patients remains exquisitely rare but has been documented. The first instance involved six patients in the practice of an American dentist, but the precise means of transmission was never identified [99]. A French orthopedic surgeon was diagnosed with AIDS encephalopathy in 1994. He had probably been infected with HIV in 1983 by a needlestick injury during surgery on a patient who had had multiple transfusions. A retrospective review of the surgeon's practice identified a single instance of transmission in more than 1,900 patients, an elderly woman on whom the surgeon had done a hip replacement in 1992, at which point the surgeon's subsequent history suggests that his viral titer was likely to have been high. Although the records of the surgery noted no particular incident, it was lengthier than ususal. The surgeon recalled finding blood inside his gloves after surgeries at least weekly, despite his latterly practice of double gloving, and described routine handling—rather than using instruments to manipulate— sharp metal materials and objects [100]. In a third instance, infection appears to have been propagated from one HIV-positive patient to four others who had outpatient surgical procedures done in a single day in a clinical practice in Australia, but the means of transmission was never identified [101].

Summary and Conclusions

The physical devastation and inevitable mortality associated with HIV infection make it the most feared of potentially occupationally acquired infections and one of enormous economic significance worldwide. However, HIV is not highly contagious, when compared to other bloodborne pathogens, and is not transmitted by casual workplace contact. Simple, cheap, effective, and familiar primary preventive methods are readily available and easily incorporated into all work situations where transmission has been shown to occur. At least for health care workers in the industrialized world, effective postexposure treatment is also available. Extension of the social and economic commitment that has been dedicated to the welfare of these workers to primary and secondary prevention for commercial sex workers would be an important step toward controlling the global HIV/AIDS pandemic.

Acknowledgment

The author is indebted to John R. Hess, M.D., Walter Reed Army Institute of Research, and to James M. Schmitt, M.D., and the staff of the National Institutes of Health Occupational Medical Service for their advice and support during the preparation of this chapter.

References

1. Kreiss JK, Koech D, Plummer FA, et al. AIDS virus infection in Nairobi prostitutes: spread of the epidemic to East Africa. *N Engl J Med* 1986;314:414–8.
2. Piot P, Kreiss JK, Ndinya-Achola JO, et al. Heterosexual transmission of AIDS. *AIDS* 1987;1:199–206.
3. Carswell JW, Lloyd G, Howells J. Prevalence of HIV-1 in East African lorry drivers. *AIDS* 1989;3:759–61.
4. George S, Jacob M, John TJ. A case-control analysis of risk factors in HIV transmission in South India. *J Acquir Immune Defic Syndr Hum Retrovirol* 1997;14 (3):290–3.
5. Bwayo J, Plummer F, Omari M, et al. Human immunodeficiency virus infection in long-distance truck drivers in east Africa. *Arch Intern Med* 1994;154:1391–6.
6. Mbugua GG, Muthami LN, Mutura CS, et al. Epidemiology of HIV infection among long distance truck drivers in Kenya. *East Afr Med J* 1995;72(8):515–8.
7. Centers for Disease Control. Case-control study of HIV seroconversion in health-care-workers after percutaneous exposure to HIV-infected blood—France, United Kingdom, and United States, January 1988–August 1994. *MMWR* 1995;44:929–33.
8. Bell DM. Occupational risk of human immunodeficiency virus infection in healthcare workers: an overview. *Am J Med* 1997;102(5B):9–15.
9. Riu R, Paxton WA, Choe S, et al. Homozygous defect in HIV-1 coreceptor accounts for resistance of some multiply-exposed individuals to HIV-1 infection. *Cell* 1996;86:367–77.
10. Bentwich Z, Kalinkovich A, Weisman Z. Immune activation is a dominant factor in the pathogenesis of African AIDS. *Immunol Today* 1995;16:187–91.
11. Centers for Disease Control and Prevention. *HIV/AIDS surveillance report, year-end edition.* 1998;(December)10:1–43.
12. Centers for Disease Control. *HIV/AIDS surveillance report. National AIDS Clearinghouse* 1996;8:5.
13. Palella FJ Jr, Delaney KM, Moorman AC, et al. Declining morbidity and mortality among patients with advanced human immunodeficiency virus infection. *N Engl J Med* 1998;338:853–60.
14. Panteleo G, Graziosi C, Fauci AS. The immuno-pathogenesis of human immunodeficiency virus infection. *N Engl J Med* 1993;328:327–35.
15. Galli L, de Martino M, Tovo P-A, et al. Onset of clinical signs in children with HIV-1 perinatal infection. *AIDS* 1995;9:455–61.
16. Central Intelligence Agency. *The World Fact Book*, 1998.

17. Balter M. AIDS now world's fourth biggest killer. *Science* 1999;284(5417):1101.
18. Balter M. On world AIDS day, a shadow looms over southern Africa. *Science* 1998;282(5395):1790–1.
19. Rosenberg D, Barry J. No money, no meds. *Newsweek* 1999 July 12:32–3.
20. Lurie P, Hintzen P, Lowe RA. Socioeconomic obstacles to HIV prevention and treatment in developing countries: the roles of the International Monetary Fund and the World Bank. *AIDS* 1995;9:539–46.
21. Sharp PM, Li WH. Understanding the origins of AIDS viruses. *Nature* 1988;336:315.
22. Myers G, MacInnes K, Korber B. The emergence of simian/human immunodeficiency viruses. *AIDS Res Hum Retroviruses* 1992;8:373–86.
23. McCutchin FE. Global diversification of HIV. In: Crandall KA (ed), *The Evolution of HIV.* Baltimore: Johns Hopkins University Press, 1999. Pp 41–101.
24. Phillips MD. The role of cell-to-cell transmission in HIV infection. *AIDS* 1994;8:719–31.
25. Barker E, Barnett SW, Stamatatos L, et al. The human immunodeficiency viruses. In: Levy JA (ed), *The Retroviridae*, Vol 4. New York: Plenum Press, 1995. Pp 1–67.
26. Folks TM, Hart CE. The life cycle of human immunodeficiency virus type 1. In: De Vita VT, Hellman S, Rosenberg S (eds), *AIDS: Etiology, Diagnosis, Treatment and Prevention*, 4th Ed. Philadelphia: Lippincott-Raven, 1997. Pp 29–43.
27. Kahn JO, Walker BD. Acute human immunodeficiency virus type 1 infection. *N Engl J Med* 1998;339:33–9.
28. Quinn TC. Acute primary HIV infection. *JAMA* 1997;278:58–62.
29. Mellors JW, Rinaldo CR Jr, Gupta P, et al. Prognosis in HIV-1 infection predicted by the quantity of virus in plasma. *Science* 1997;275:14.
30. Mellors JW, Munoz A, Giorgi JV, et al. Plasma viral load and CD4 lymphocytes as prognostic markers of HIV-1 infection. *Ann Intern Med* 1997;126:946–54.
31. O'Brien WA, Hartigan PM, Martin D, et al. Changes in plasma HIV-1 RNA and CD4+ lymphocyte counts and the risk of progression to AIDS. *N Engl J Med* 1996;334:426–31.
32. Royce RA, Sena A, Cates W Jr, Cohen MS. Sexual transmission of HIV. *N Engl J Med* 1997;336:1072–8.
33. Levy JA. The transmission of HIV and factors influencing progression to AIDS. *Am J Med* 1993;95:86–100.
34. Van den Perre P, Simonon A, Msellati P, et al. Postnatal transmission of human immunodeficiency virus type-1 from mother to infant. A prospective cohort study in Kigali Rwanda. *N Engl J Med* 1991;325:593–8.
35. Fischl M, Dickenson GM, Scott GB, et al. Evaluation of heterosexual partners, children and household contacts of adults with AIDS. *JAMA* 1987;257:640.
36. Gershon R, Vlahov D, Nelson K. The risk of transmission of HIV-1 through non-percutaneous, non-sexual modes—a review. *AIDS* 1990;4:645–50.
37. Saag MS, Holodniy M, Kuritzkes DR, et al. HIV viral load markers in clinical practice. *Nat Med* 1996; 2(6):625–9.
38. de Vicenzi I. A longitudinal study of human immunodeficiency virus transmission by heterosexual partners. European Study Group on Heterosexual Transmission of HIV. *N Engl J Med* 1994;331:341–6.
39. Dickover RE, Garratty EM, Herman SA, et al. Identification of levels of maternal HIV-1 RNA associated with risk of perinatal transmission. Effect of maternal zidovudine treatment on viral load. *JAMA* 1996; 275:599–605.
40. Ward JW, Deppe DA, Samson S. Risk of human immunodeficiency virus infection from blood donors who later developed the acquired immunodeficiency virus syndrome. *Ann Intern Med* 1987;106:61–2.
41. Donegan E, Stuart M, Niland JC, et al. Infection with human immuno-deficiency virus type 1 (HIV-1) among recipients of antibody-positive blood donations. *Ann Intern Med* 1990;113:733–9.
42. Tovo P-A, de Martino M, Gabiano C, et al. Mode of delivery and gestational age influence perinatal HIV-1 transmission. *J Acquir Immune Defic Syndr Hum Retrovirol* 1996;11:88–94.
43. The International Perinatal HIV Group. The mode of delivery and the risk of vertical transmission of human immunodeficiency virus type-1. *N Engl J Med* 1999;340:977–87.
44. McEvoy M, Porter K, Mortimer P, et al. Prospective study of clinical, laboratory, and ancillary staff with accidental exposures to blood or body fluids from patients infected with HIV. *Br Med J* 1987;292:1595–7.
45. Henderson DK, Fahey B, Wiley M, et al. Risk for occupational transmission of human immunodeficiency virus type 1(HIV-1) associated with clinical exposures: a prospective study. *Ann Intern Med* 1990;113:740–6.
46. Tokars JI, Marcus R, Culver DH, et al. Surveillance of HIV infection and zidovudine use among health care workers after occupational exposure to HIV-infected blood. *Ann Intern Med* 1993;118:913–9.
47. Mastro TD, Kitayaporn D. Transmission probabilities: estimates from epidemiologic studies. *AIDS Res Hum Retroviruses* 1998;14(Suppl 3):S223–7.
48. Centers for Disease Control. Update: human immunodeficiency virus infections in health-care workers exposed to blood of infected patients. *MMWR* 1987;36:285–9.
49. Gioannini P, Sinicco A, Cariti G, et al. HIV infection acquired by a nurse. *Eur J Epidemiol* 1988;4:119–20.
50. Gerberding JL. Occupational exposure to blood-borne viruses. *N Engl J Med* 1995;332(7):444–51.
51. Anonymous. Transmission of HIV by human bite. *Lancet* 1987;2:522.

52. Vidmar L, Poljak M, Tomazic J. Transmission of HIV-1 by human bite. *Lancet* 1996;347:1762–3.

53. Blauvelt A. The role of skin dendritic cells in the initiation of human innumodeficiency virus infection. *Am J Med* 1997;102(5B):16–20.

54. Stansbury L, Schmitt JM, Markowitz M. HIV in the workplace. In: Rom WM (ed), *Environmental and Occupational Medicine*, 3rd Ed. Philadelphia: Lippincott-Raven, 1998. Pp 775–95.

55. Rakwar J, Lavreys L, Thompson ML, et al. Cofactors for the acquisition of HIV-1 among heterosexual men: prospective cohort study of trucking company workers in Kenya. *AIDS* 1999;13:607–14.

56. Martin HL Jr, Jackson DJ, Mandaliya K, et al. Preparation for AIDS vaccine evaluation in Mombasa, Kenya: establishment of seronegative cohorts of commercial sex workers and trucking company employees. *AIDS Res Hum Retroviruses* 1994;10(Suppl 2):S235–7.

57. Bansal RK, Nia AB. Truck crew and risk of contraction of STSs, including HIV: encouraging the use of condoms by the method of applying theories. *Indian J Med Sci* 1998;52(6):253–64.

58. Albert AE, Warner DL, Hatcher RA, et al. Condom use among female commercial sex workers in Nevada's legal brothels. *Am J Public Health* 1995;85:1514–20.

59. Stein ZA. More on women and the prevention of HIV infection. *Am J Public Health* 1995;85:1485–7.

60. Padian N. Prostitute women and AIDS: epidemiology. *AIDS* 1988;2:413–9.

61. Karim Q, Karim SSA, Soldan K, et al. Reducing the risk of HIV infection among South African sex workers: socioeconomic and gender barriers. *Am J Public Health* 1995;85:1521–5.

62. Singh YN, Mlaviya AN. Experience of HIV prevention interventions among female sex workers in Delhi, India. *Int J STD AIDS* 1994;5:56–7.

63. Morris M, Pramvalratana A, Podhisita C. Determinants of condom use with commercial sex partners in Thailand. *AIDS* 1994;8:504–15.

64. Kilmarx PH, Limpakarnjanarat K, Maestro NTD, et al. HIV-1 Seroconversion in a prospective study of female sex workers in northern Thailand: continued high incidence among brothel-based women. *AIDS* 1998;12(14):1889–98.

65. Van den Hoek J, Coutinho RA, van Haastrecht HJA, et al. Prevalence and risk factors of HIV infections among drug users and drug-using prostitutes in Amsterdam. *AIDS* 1988;2:55–60.

66. Aim G, DeVincenzi I, Ancelle-Park R, et al. HIV infection among French prostitutes. *AIDS* 1989;3: 767–8.

67. Department of the Army. Identification, surveillance, and administration of personnel infected with human immunodeficiency virus (HIV), revised, 1994. *Army Regulations* 1988:600–11.

68. Whitby M, Stead P, Saiman J. Needlestick injury: impact of a recapping device and an associated education program. *Infect Control Hosp Epidemiol* 1991; 12:220–5.

69. Beekman SE, Vlahov D, Koziol DC, et al. Temporal association between implementation of universal precautions and a sustained, progressive decrease in percutaneous exposures to blood. *Clin Infect Dis* 1994;18:562–9.

70. Haiduven D, DeMaio T, Stevens D. A five year study of needlestick injuries; significant reduction associated with communication, education, and convenient placement of sharps containers. *Infect Control Hosp Epidemiol* 1992;13:265–71.

71. Sussman GL, Beezhold DH. Allergy to latex rubber. *Ann Intern Med* 1995;122:43–6.

72. Alexander P. Sex work and health: a question of safety in the workplace. *J Am Med Women's Assoc* 1998; 53:77–82.

73. Gunby P. Boxing: AIDS? *JAMA* 1988;259:1613.

74. Goldsmith MF. When sports and HIV share the bill, smart money goes on common sense. *JAMA* 1992; 67:1311–4.

75. American Academy of Pediatrics Committee on Sports Medicine and Fitness. Human immunodeficiency virus [acquired immunodeficiency syndrome (AIDS) virus] in the athletic setting. *Pediatrics* 1991;88:640–1.

76. Shilts R. *And the Band Played On*. New York: Penguin Books, 1988. P 600.

77. Centers for Disease Control. Understanding AIDS: an information brochure being mailed to all U.S. households. *MMWR* 1988;37:261–9.

78. Centers for Disease Control. HIV epidemic and AIDS: trends in knowledge—United States. *MMWR* 1989;38:353–8, 363.

79. Centers for Disease Control. Guidelines for prevention of transmission of human immunodeficiency virus and hepatitis B virus to health care and public safety workers. *MMWR* 1989;38:S6.

80. Vasil S, Thakallapally R, Pillai S, et al. Reagents for HIV/SIV vaccine studies. In: *Human Retroviruses and AIDS 1998*. Los Alamos: Los Alamos National Laboratory. Vol III, Pp 91–101.

81. Barnett SW, Klinger JM, Doe B, et al. Prime-boost immunization strategies against HIV. *AIDS Res Hum Retroviruses* 1998;14(Suppl 3):299–309.

82. Cohen J. Glimmerings of hope from the bottom of the well. *Science* 1999;285:656–7.

83. Kaplan JC, Crawford DC, Durno AG, et al. Inactivation of human immunodeficiency virus by Betadine. *Infect Control* 1987;8:412–4.

84. Centers for Disease Control. Public Health Service statement on management of occupational exposure to human immunodeficiency virus, including considerations regarding zidovudine postexposure use. *MMWR* 1990;39(RR-1):1–14.

85. Gerberding J. Prophylaxis for occupational exposure to HIV. *Ann Intern Med* 1996;125:497–501.

86. Centers for Disease Control. Update: provisional Public Health Service recommendations for chemoprophylaxis after occupational exposure to HIV. *MMWR* 1996;45(22):468–72.

87. Centers for Disease Control. Public Health Service guidelines for the management of health care worker exposures to HIV and recommendations for postexposure prophylaxis. *MMWR* 1998;47:(RR-7).

88. Connor EM, Sperling RS, Geiber R, et al. Reduction of maternal-infant transmission of human immunodeficiency virus type 1 with zidovudine treatment. *N Engl J Med* 1994;331:1173–80.

89. Wade NA, Birkhead GS, Warren BL, et al. Abbreviated regimens of zidovudine prophylaxis and perinatal transmission of the human immunodeficiency virus. *N Engl J Med* 1998;339:1409–14.

90. Fiscus SA, Schoenbach VJ, Wilfert C. Short courses of zidovudine and perinatal transmissions of HIV. *N Engl J Med* 1999;340:1040–1.

91. Tavares L, Roneker C, Johnston K, et al. 3′-azido-3′ deoxythymidine in feline leukemia-infected cats: a model of therapy and prophylaxis of AIDS. *Cancer Res* 1987;47:3190–4.

92. Katz MH, Gerberding JL. The care of persons with recent sexual exposure to HIV. *Ann Intern Med* 1998;128:306–12.

93. Jochimsen EM. Failures of zidovudine post-exposure prophylaxis. *Am J Med* 1997;102(5B):52–5.

94. Brown AA, Brundage JF, Tomlinson JP, et al. The US Army HIV testing program: the first decade. *Milit Med* 1996;161:117–22.

95. Damato JJ, O'Bryen BN, Fuller SA, et al. Resolution of indeterminate HIV-1 test data using the Department of Defense HIV-1 testing program. *Lab Med* 1991;22:107–13.

96. Schacker T, Colier AC, Hughes J, et al. Clinical and epidemiologic features of primary HIV infection. *Ann Intern Med* 1996;125:257–64.

97. Redfield RR, Wright DC, James WD, et al. Disseminated vaccinia in a military recruit with HTLV-III disease. *N Engl J Med* 1987;316:673–6.

98. Leigh JP, Lubeck DP, Farnham P, et al. Potential and actual workdays lost among patients with HIV. *J Acquir Immune Defic Syndr Hum Retrovirol* 1995;8(4):392–8.

99. Ciesielski C, Marianos D, Ou CY, et al. Transmission of human immunodeficiency virus in a dental practice. *Ann Intern Med* 1992;116:798–805.

100. Lot F, Seguier JC, Fegueux S, et al. Probable transmission of HIV from an orthopedic surgeon to a patient in France. *Ann Intern Med* 1999;130:1–6.

101. Chant K, Lowe D, Rubin G, et al. Patient-to-patient transmission of HIV in private surgical consulting rooms. *Lancet* 1993;342:1548–9.

25 / Occupational Malaria

Bruce A. Barron and Mark J. Utell

Malaria is a tropical parasitic infection that has successfully evaded scientific advances in prevention, control, and treatment. Although the incidence of vector-borne malaria in the United States is exceptionally low, international travelers account for more than 1,000 imported cases annually [1–3]. Occupational malaria, for the most part, is an acquired illness resulting from travel to malaria-endemic regions of the world (Figure 25-1). Employees (both military and civilian) traveling to regions having high transmission rates, drug-resistant parasites, and/or insecticide-resistant mosquitoes are at the greatest risk of contracting this disease [4].

Malaria was first described by Hippocrates during the fourth century BC, and despite its long history, the etiology and natural course of the disease were not completely delineated until the early twentieth century. Clear delineation of the malaria parasite life cycle has also been crucial to our understanding of transmission risk factors (Table 25-1), which are both complex and multifactorial. Ultimately, transmission risks depend on a delicate balance between the plasmodium agent, mosquito vector, susceptible human host, and environmental conditions, as shown in Figure 25-2. Each facet of this balance is reviewed in this chapter.

Plasmodium Organisms

The *Plasmodium* life cycle follows a pattern of asexual reproduction in the human host and sexual reproduction in the mosquito vector. There are four species of the *Plasmodium* agent that naturally infect humans: *Plasmodium falciparum*, *Plasmodium vivax*, *Plasmodium ovale*, and *Plasmodium malariae*.

P falciparum is the most virulent of the species. It accounts for nearly half of the world's malaria infections and more than 95% of deaths due to malaria [5]. *P falciparum* is most abundant in sub-Saharan Africa, New Guinea, and Haiti [5,6]. *P vivax* predominates in the Indian subcontinent, Middle East, and Central America [5,6]. The prevalence of these two species is similar in Southeast Asia, Oceana, and South America. *P malariae* and *P ovale* infections are relatively unusual outside of Africa [5,6]. *P malariae* is remarkable because this species has the ability to persist in the circulatory system for years without causing symptoms. These infectious agents have gained renewed public health interest as a result of the recent emergence of drug-resistant strains, which have precipitated in an increased incidence and geographic distribution of the disease [7].

There are no free-living forms of this parasite. Human hosts represent the only significant reservoir for the organism [8]. Although other primate malarias can infect humans, natural transmission is extremely rare [9]. Transmission of malaria from infected mosquitoes to humans is strongly dependent on the sporozoite rate (i.e., the ratio of infective to noninfective female anopheline mosquitoes), while the sporozoite rate is dependent on the mosquito vector's susceptibility to parasitic infection, in vivo parasite replication, vector longevity, and vector population densities [10].

As a host, humans serve an important role in the life cycle of the malaria parasite. Even though malaria can be transmitted congenitally [11], through blood transfusions [12], or through exposure to bloodborne pathogens [13,14], the preponderance of the disease is transmitted through the bite of an infective female *Anopheles*

Figure 25-1
Approximate Geographic Distribution of Malaria

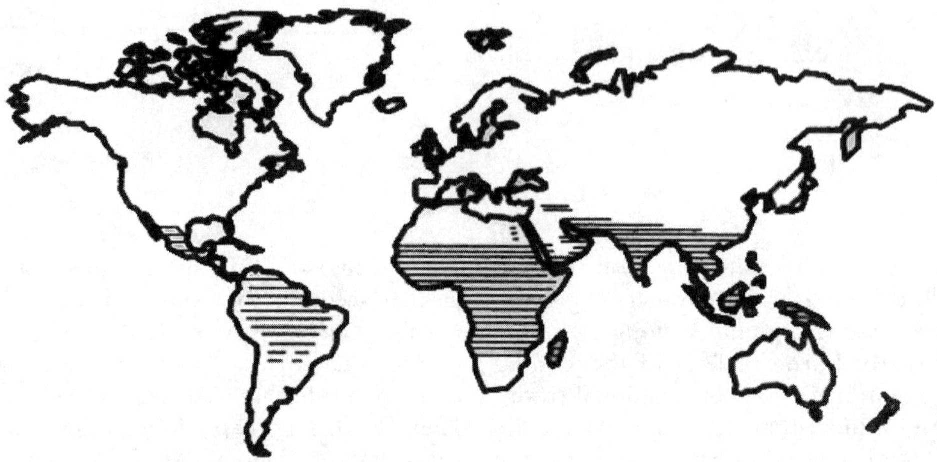

= (approximate) malaria endemic regions of the world.

species mosquito. This mosquito is the only known vector for malaria [8,15]. Although these mosquitoes feed from dusk until dawn, their feeding activity may vary considerably throughout the night, depending on the species [6,15,16]. Conversely, it is important for occupational physicians to realize that mosquitoes that bite during the day do not transmit malaria [15,16]. *Anopheles gambiae* mosquitoes are effective vectors because this species is ubiquitous, long-lived (5–25% daily mortality rate), and anthropophilic (have a preference for human hosts) [8,17]. These factors make them especially effective vectors [18,19].

There are other highly anthropophilic and long-lived anophelines, such as the *Anopheles dirus* found in Southeast Asia. Fortunately the *A dirus* mosquitoes breed in small forest pools and usually are not a problem in domestic environments. This is unlike the *A gambiae*, which are well adapted to human habitats. Studies suggest that rural villagers living in high-transmission areas may be bitten 50–100 times per night by *A gambiae* mosquitoes (having a 5% sporozoite rate). Since these mosquitoes rest after blood meals on house walls (i.e., endophilic), they are susceptible to malaria vector control measures (e.g., spraying the house with a residual insecticide) [20]. *Anopheles* mosquitoes also have a broad geographic distribution. This species can still be found in the United States and has recently been implicated in three outbreaks of vector-borne malaria from infected migrant workers in Texas, New Jersey, and California [1,3,21,22].

Malaria transmission depends on a number of environmental factors, including geographic location, season, climate, deforestation, irrigation, and pest-control measures. Unfortunately, many anopheline mosquitoes have developed resistance to chlorinated insecticides, organophosphates, and carbamates [23]. Ambient temperature and ground elevation are also important determinants of transmission risk because sporogeny cannot take place in temperatures below 16° C or above 33° C, or in extremely arid climates, heavy rains, or altitudes above 2,000 meters [8,13,14]. Transmission rates are higher during the rainy seasons, since the moisture fosters mosquito breeding sites [14,24].

Plasmodium Life Cycle

The *Plasmodium* life cycle begins when a female *Anopheles* mosquito ingests infected human blood containing the sexual stages of the parasite (gametocytes) as depicted in Figure 25-3. Male and female gametocytes unite to form the ookinete inside the mosquito's stomach. The ookinete

Table 25-1
Malaria Transmission Risk Factors in Traveling Employees

Environmental	
Geographic region (high to low risk)	
West Africa	
East Africa	
Indian subcontinent	
Far East	
South America	
Central America	
Rainy seasons	
Regions with poor pest control	
Ambient temperatures between 16°C and 33°C	
Elevations less than 2,000 meters	
Mosquito vector	
Anopheles gambiae, *arabiensis*, and *funestus*	
Mosquito vector population densities (high)	
Mosquito vector longevity (prolonged)	
Mosquito insecticide resistance	
Plasmodium agent	
Plasmodium falciparum (greater than nonfalciparum forms)	
Plasmodium drug resistance	
Sporozoite rates (high)	
Human host	
Repeated or prolonged trips to malaria-endemic areas	
Repeated or prolonged nighttime exposure in malaria-endemic areas	
Inadequate antimosquito measures and chemoprophylaxis	
Poor compliance with antimosquito measures and chemoprophylaxis	
Poor health status/pre-existing systemic illness	
Sensitivities/allergies to chemoprophylactic and therapeutic agents	
Nonimmune status	
Pregnancy	

subsequently penetrates the stomach wall and forms a cyst containing thousands of sporozoites on its outer surface. This process requires eight to 35 days depending on the species of parasite and the vector's ambient temperature. Sporozoites migrate to the salivary glands and other organs in the infected mosquito, rendering them infective for life. Infective mosquitoes inject between 5 and one hundred motile sporozoites into the human host during a blood meal. The sporozoites rapidly invade hepatocytes and develop into exoerythrocytic schizonts. After the sporozoites mature, the hepatocytes rupture and release between 10^5 and 10^6 asexual parasites (merozoites) into the hepatic sinusoids and vascular system.

In *P vivax* and *P ovale* infections, a small number of organisms lie dormant in the liver for several months to years before multiplying. These sleeping forms of the parasite (known as hypnozoites) can cause either delayed primary attacks or relapses in the future [25]. It is for this reason that *P vivax* and *P ovale* infections have been labeled "relapsing malarias." Conversely, *P falciparum* and *P malariae* do not form hypnozoites, and as a result, relapses do not occur.

The merozoites (released by hepatocyte rupture) quickly invade susceptible circulating red cells, where they grow and multiply cyclically [26]. Most of the merozoites develop into asexual forms. Merozoites differentiate from early trophozoites (ring forms) to mature blood schizonts that rupture the red cell, releasing eight to 30 free merozoites, which invade other red cells. This process takes 48 hours for *P falciparum*, *P vivax*, and *P ovale* infections (tertian fevers) and 72 hours for *P malariae* infections (quartan fever). Clinical symptoms parallel the rupture of red cell schizonts.

After three to 15 days, red-cell merozoites that did not differentiate into asexual forms may develop into male (microgametocyte) or female (macrogametocyte) sexual forms. Gametocytes do not cause symptoms. These sexual forms may circulate for months to years in the bloodstream until they are ingested by an anopheline mosquito during a blood meal. Within the mosquito's midgut, thousands of new infective sporozoites are formed, and the life cycle begins again [8,13].

In summary, the mosquito must feed twice on humans in order to transmit malaria. They must first ingest human blood infected with the sexual stages of the parasite, survive eight to 35 days for the gametocytes to mature to sporozoites, and then bite another susceptible human host in order to transmit the disease [18,19].

Epidemiology

Its global impact on morbidity and mortality makes malaria one of the most important tropical diseases. This parasitic disease is endemic in

Figure 25-2
Major Factors Affecting Malaria Transmission in Travelers. (Transmission risk depends on the interactions and relative balance of each factor. See text for details.)

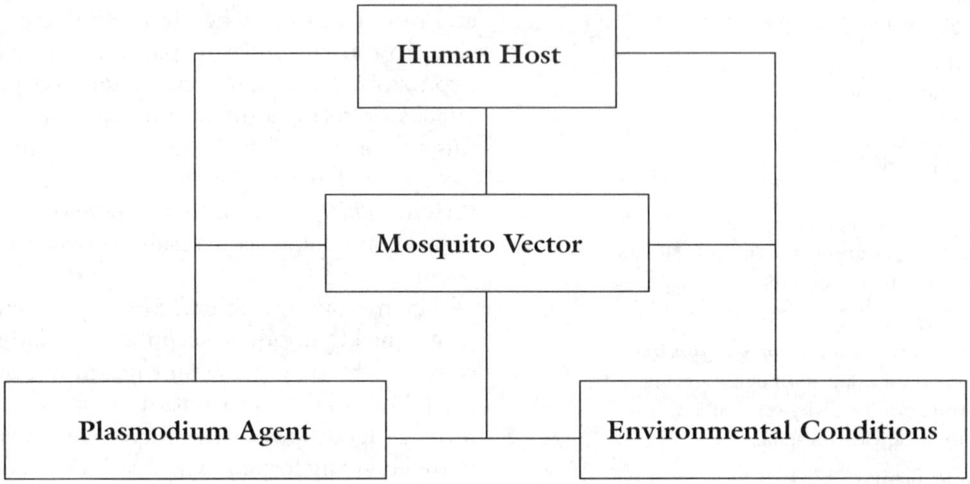

more than 100 countries, and nearly 40% of the world's population live in endemic tropical regions [9]. Malaria has an estimated prevalence of 300–500 million persons and accounts for more than 1 million deaths annually [5,6]. Although malaria has been eradicated from North America, Europe, and Russia, the emergence of drug-resistant parasites and pesticide-resistant mosquitoes has resulted in a resurgence of the disease in the tropics [27–29]. Despite significant advances in malaria prevention and control, the burden of disease has increased dramatically over the past several decades [30–32].

Each year, about 8 million U.S. civilians travel to malaria-endemic countries, and nearly 30,000 contract malaria [33–35]. Longitudinal studies of North American and European travelers in Africa reveal an incidence of 15 cases per 1,000 travelers per month and a 2–4% mortality rate [4,36–39]. Malaria in the United States is, for the most part, limited to imported cases in travelers, military personnel, and immigrants from malaria endemic countries [40]. Non-imported infections in the United States have rarely been acquired through the bite of an infected *Anopheles* mosquito entering the country in aircraft returning from malaria-endemic regions (airport malaria) [41–44], congenitally from an infected mother, iatrogenically through blood transfusion (induced malaria), and by local transmission (autochthonous malaria) from persons with imported disease who serve as the reservoir for local vector mosquitoes [1,3,21,22]. From an occupational perspective, individuals at highest risk include military personnel, traveling federal employees, foreign service diplomats, corporate travelers, expatriated business executives, commercial airline crews, airport employees, and maritime employees.

Prevention and Control

It is important to remember that occupational malaria is a preventable disease. The risk of contracting this disease within a given geographic region depends on the presence of malaria parasites, vector mosquitoes, susceptible human hosts, and favorable environmental conditions. Interventions designed to eliminate or control one or more of these risk factors significantly decrease the incidence of disease in the occupational setting.

Although both genetic resistance and immunity decrease the morbidity of malaria, these traits are unlikely to be significant factors in the prevention of occupational malaria. Resistance to infection occurs in employees who have sickle cell trait, hereditary ovalocytosis, or absent Duffy

Figure 25-3
The Plasmodium Life Cycle. (The left side of the figure summarizes the sexual [mosquito] phase and the right side of the figure summarizes the asexual [human] phase of the life cycle.)

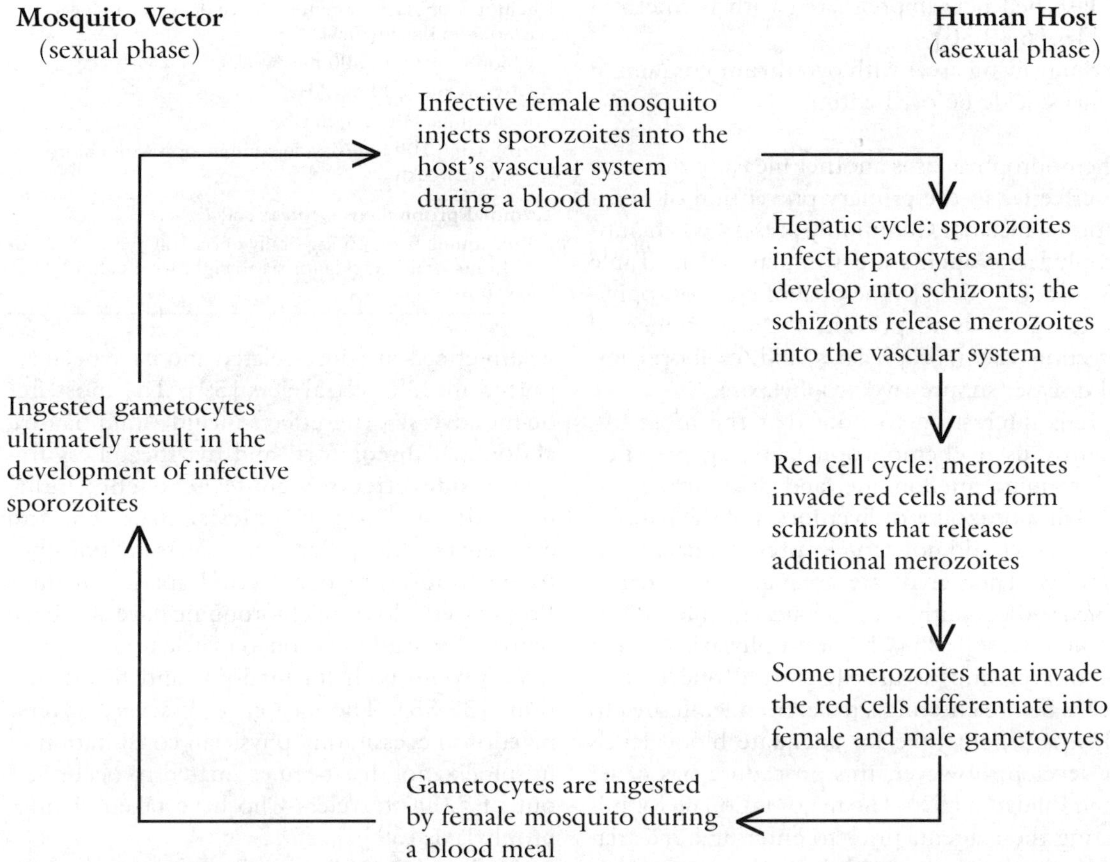

blood group antigen on their red cells, but this population represents a small proportion of the traveling work force at any given point in time [45,46]. Natural immunity in U.S. travelers is also unlikely, since this requires prolonged residence in hyperendemic regions and repeated infections. Natural immunity is species-specific, strain-specific, and stage-specific (asexual forms of the parasite), and it is acquired gradually [47]. Natural immunity confers only partial immunity (semi-immunity) and subsequent attacks can still occur, albeit at decreased frequency and severity. Most tropical residents have asymptomatic infections by 10 years of age through the development of antitoxic immunity or premunition (a state in which an active low-grade infection establishes resistance to reinfection). Since the nonimmune traveler usually lacks genetic resistance, partial homologous immunity (immunity derived from members of a single species) and premunition, occupationally acquired infections are more likely to be fulminant and lethal.

Education, training, and appropriate application of antimosquito measures are important factors in preventing occupational malaria. Since anopheline mosquitoes are endophilic and bite from dusk to dawn, traveling employees should be encouraged to observe the following antimosquito measures [48]:

- Remain in air-conditioned and/or well-screened facilities after sunset.
- Avoid the use of perfumes that would attract mosquitoes.
- Wear protective long-sleeved clothes (sprayed with permethrin insecticide when feasible).

- Apply a topical insecticide such as 30% to 35% diethyltoluamide (DEET) to exposed skin areas [6,15].
- Use bed nets impregnated with permethrin [15,16,49,50].
- Spray living areas with pyrethrum-containing insecticide before bedtime.

Chemoprophylaxis is another measure that may be effective in the primary prevention of occupational malaria. Commonly prescribed chemoprophylactic agents are summarized in Table 25-2 [6,13–16,34]. The goal of chemoprophylactic agents is to prevent the occurrence of infection (causal prophylaxis) and/or abort clinical disease (suppressive prophylaxis).

It is interesting to note that the most frequently used chemoprophylactic agents (i.e., chloroquine, mefloquine, and doxycycline) do not kill sporozoites or liver forms of the parasite and, as such, do not actually prevent malaria infections. They eradicate asexual blood forms, which subsequently aborts clinical manifestations of the disease [51]. Chemoprophylaxis (except for doxycycline) is usually started one to two weeks before entering a malaria-endemic area to allow sufficient time for adequate blood levels to develop; however, this procedure has never been validated [52]. The major rationale for initiating these agents prior to entering a malaria-endemic area is to establish the habit of taking the medication and to identify adverse drug effects prior to departure. Chemoprophylactic agents should be continued during the exposure and for a four-week period after departure from the malaria-endemic area. This allows sufficient time for the incubating liver forms to mature and be released into the bloodstream, where suppressive drugs are biologically active [9,15–17,34].

Chloroquine is the prophylactic agent of choice for travel to countries not exhibiting chloroquine-resistant parasites [9,15,17,34,53]. It has a serum half-life of seven to ten days, and the usual dose is 500 mg of chloroquine phosphate (300 mg base) once weekly. Chloroquine's exact mechanism of action has not been fully elucidated; however, this drug appears to exert its antimalarial activity on the hemoglobin-containing digestive vesicles of the parasite. Although chloroquine is usually well tolerated, adverse health effects are dose-related and have been reported in 23% of travelers [39]. The most frequent adverse drug effects include mild nausea, abdominal discomfort, and diarrhea. Less frequent side effects include headache, lightheadedness, fatigue, emesis, pruritus, and erythema [39,54]. Rare side effects include photosensitization, myopathy, and aplastic anemia. Prophylactic doses of chloroquine have also been reported to cause neuropsychiatric toxicity (e.g., toxic psychosis, hallucinations, and disorientation) [39,55]. The incidence of severe adverse reactions necessitating physician consultation or hospitalization has been estimated to occur in 1 out of 7,000 travelers who have taken chemoprophylaxis [39].

Table 25-2
Medications Commonly Used in the Prevention of Malaria

Chemoprophylactic agents (choice depends on local plasmodium sensitivities)
Chloroquine salt, 500 mg/week
Doxycycline, 100 mg/day
Mefloquine salt, 250 mg/week
Proguanil, 200 mg/day, in combination with chloroquine weekly
Terminal prophylaxis (*P vivax* and *P ovale*)
Primaquine base, 15 mg orally once daily for 14 days, or 45 mg orally weekly for six to eight weeks after exposure

Mefloquine, 250-mg salt once weekly, is the chemoprophylactic agent of choice for employees traveling to geographic regions harboring chloroquine-resistant *P falciparum* and *P vivax.* It should be started one to two weeks prior to travel and taken weekly during the exposure and for four weeks after departure from the malarious area. Although mefloquine had initially been reported to be 90–95% effective in preventing malaria [6,14,53,56], a recent meta-analysis reported significantly lower efficacy rates [57]. The rate of adverse drug effects (e.g., depression, dreams, fatigue, headache, insomnia, anorexia, abdominal discomfort, nausea, vomiting, fever, and pruritus) and drug discontinuance were high in most of the studies analyzed. The authors concluded this outcome was likely to impair mefloquine's effectiveness and precluded its routine use for chemoprophylaxis in travelers [57]. It is important to note that chemoprophylactic doses of mefloquine may cause the same severe neuropsychiatric effects found in therapeutic doses, but much less frequently (1:10,000 travelers) [39,55].

Doxycycline, 100 mg daily, is reportedly 88% to 100% effective in preventing malaria and is the preferred chemoprophylactic agent for individuals unable to take mefloquine (e.g., pilots, mefloquine-intolerant employees) traveling to geographic regions with chloroquine-resistant malaria. It is also the drug of choice for travelers to Thailand where *P falciparum* is mefloquine-resistant. Doxycycline should be taken two to three days before travel, daily during the exposure, and for four weeks after exposure. The most commonly reported side effects are nausea, epigastric distress, and vaginal candidiasis. Doxycycline may cause severe photosensitivity reactions; therefore, it should be prescribed in conjunction with a sunscreen. Pregnant women and other travelers who are unable to take doxycycline or mefloquine should be advised not to travel to geographic regions of chloroquine or mefloquine resistance because there are no safe and effective chemoprophylactic alternatives [6,15–17,34].

Since chloroquine, mefloquine, and doxycycline are not active against hypnozoites, travelers to areas of the world where *P vivax* and *P ovale* are indigenous species must follow these agents with a two-week course of primaquine (terminal prophylaxis) in order to prevent relapse [6,14–16,53]. Relapses can occur weeks or months after discontinuing schizonticidal drugs; thus, terminal prophylaxis should at least partially overlap the terminal weeks of chloroquine, mefloquine, or doxycycline prophylaxis. Although primaquine is usually well tolerated, the most common adverse drug effects include abdominal discomfort, nausea, headache, and pruritus. Since primaquine is a potent oxidant, it can cause severe hemolytic anemia in persons with glucose-6-phosphate dehydrogenase (G6PD) deficiency. This is primaquine's most common serious adverse effect; therefore, the G6PD status of an employee must be established prior to its administration. This drug must be taken daily (26.3-mg primaquine phosphate tablets are equivalent to 15-mg primaquine base tablets) for 14 days, or three primaquine phosphate tablets must be taken once weekly for eight weeks.

According to Behrens and Curtis, the efficacy of chemoprophylactic agents measured in terms of percent risk reduction compared with unmedicated controls was 66% for chloroquine and 61% for doxycycline, assuming 100% compliance [58]. One should note that these efficacy calculations assumed 100% compliance and that compliance itself was a major confounder of the data. Studies assessing drug compliance have yielded high *noncompliance* rates, ranging from 23% in travelers visiting West Africa [59], 72% in hospitalized patients with confirmed malaria [58], and 75% in airline flight attendants [60]. Compliance in U.S. travelers has also been reportedly low [61]. Some 51% of American travelers who developed malaria did not take chemoprophylaxis, while another 30% did not take the appropriate prophylactic regimen suggested by the Centers for Disease Control and Prevention (CDC). Furthermore, only two thirds of travelers continued chemoprophylaxis for a full four weeks after their departure from malaria-endemic regions [39].

The emergence of drug-resistant parasites and insecticide-resistant vectors has made vaccine development more compelling. Although a considerable amount of research and funding has been directed toward vaccine development during the past two decades, an effective antimalarial vaccine has not been formulated [62]. Many vaccines in current use have been developed against diseases for which natural infection confers lifelong immunity; however, malaria infections do not routinely confer such prolonged immunity. The partial immunity conferred by infection is not only temporary, but also species-, strain-, and stage-specific [17,63]. Ultimately, a vaccine that proves effective most likely stimulates both humoral and cell-mediated immunity and contains antigens from all three malarial stages: sporozoite, merozoite, and gametocyte.

Symptoms and Signs

The early recognition and diagnosis of malaria can be quite challenging because the initial symptoms are nonspecific and similar to those of many other infections (e.g., fever, chills, general malaise, fatigue, headache, myalgias, and mild abdominal discomfort). The acute symptoms of malaria typically occur after an incubation period of eight to 16 days. The average time interval between infective bites and onset of symptoms is approximately seven to 14 days for *P falciparum*, seven to 30 days for *P malariae*, and eight to 14 days for *P vivax* and *P ovale*. Infected employees may complain of fatigue, headache, myalgias, arthralgias, vague abdominal discomfort, and dysphoria [64–66]. To those unfamiliar with the disease (e.g., nonimmune patients and nontropical physicians) these nonspecific symptoms are frequently attributed to flulike illnesses, while semi-immune persons often recognize them as an early prodrome of the disease.

The classic malarial paroxysm has three stages: (1) The chill stage begins with a sudden shaking chill that lasts 15 to 90 minutes; (2) the hot stage is associated with temperature spikes up to 42° C; and (3) the sweating stage begins as the temperature falls below 39° C and the victim sweats profusely. The paroxysm usually subsides four to eight hours later and is followed by fatigue and sleep. Table 25-3 summarizes the most common signs and symptoms of imported malaria observed in military and civilian tropical travelers [9]. Nearly all travelers complained of fever, chills, rigors, diaphoresis and headache, but only one third presented with classic paroxysms.

Complicated malaria is almost always caused by *P falciparum*. The risk of complicated malaria increases as parasitemias rise above 2% in nonimmune or pregnant employees and above 5% in semi-immune hosts. The most frequent complications include coma, seizures, renal failure, hemoglobinuria (blackwater fever), noncardiogenic pulmonary edema, profound hypoglycemia, bleeding, coagulopathy, and jaundice [9]. The mortality rate for patients with complicated malaria exceeds 30% even when treated in intensive care units [17]. Table 25-4 summarizes clinical and laboratory findings associated with high mortality rates [67,68].

Special emphasis should be placed on the early recognition and treatment of cerebral malaria because this complication can be fatal within six to 24 hours after the onset of fever. The mortality rate in those who develop this complication is almost 100% in untreated and 20% in treated individuals [68]. Approximately 3% of survivors experience permanent sequelae (e.g., mental retardation, cortical blindness, deafness, cerebellar ataxia, hemiparesis, and spasticity) such that their quality of life and employability are severely impaired [69]. Clinically, this complication resembles a toxic encephalopathy, and as such, meningismus and nuchal rigidity do not occur. Focal and lateralizing neurologic signs are uncommon. Delirium, stupor, hypertonicity, extensor plantar responses, brainstem dysfunction, frontal lobe release signs, and retinal hemorrhages may be present, but papilledema is notably ab-

Table 25-3
Common Clinical Manifestations of Imported Malaria

Symptoms (decreasing order of frequency)
Fever
Chills and sweats
Headache
General malaise, fatigue, and anorexia
Arthralgias and myalgias
Nausea, vomiting, diarrhea, and abdominal pain
Dyspnea
Chest pain
Altered mental status
Rash
Signs (decreasing order of frequency)
Elevated temperature
Splenomegaly
Hepatomegaly
Orthostatic hypotension
Jaundice
Abdominal tenderness

Table 25-4
Clinical and Laboratory Prognostic Indicators of Death

Clinical prognostic indicators
Hemodynamic shock
Coma
Recurrent seizures
Concomitant bacterial superinfections
Laboratory prognostic indicators
Parasitemias greater than 500,000/μL
Lactic acidosis
Hypoglycemia
Azotemia
Severe anemia
Coagulopathy

sent [68]. Lumbar puncture, which should be performed to exclude bacterial meningitis, is usually unremarkable except for increased lactate and protein levels. Similarly CT and MR imaging may show mild cerebral edema, but cerebral hemorrhages and infarctions are quite rare [17].

DIFFERENTIAL DIAGNOSIS

Malaria mimics many infectious diseases, and therefore the differential diagnosis is quite extensive (Table 25-5) [70–72]. Although malaria is a relatively common disease among tropical travelers, the diagnosis is frequently missed by nontropical physicians [9,36,64,66]. Studies have shown that fever in returning travelers rarely represents an unusual tropical disease; therefore, a positive travel history should be enough to prompt nontropical clinicians to include malaria in the differential diagnosis [70–72]. This point was substantiated by investigators at the McGill Centre for Tropical Diseases, who reported the following diagnoses in 587 febrile travelers: malaria (32%), hepatitis (6%), viral upper respiratory infection (6%), pyelonephritis (4%), pneumonia (3%), dengue (2%), enteric fever (2%), shigellosis (2%), nontyphoidal salmonellosis (2%), infectious mononucleosis (2%), and acute bronchitis (2%) [72].

DIAGNOSTIC EVALUATION

Timely and accurate diagnosis starts with a comprehensive health history and physical examination. A negative travel history (recent and remote), transfusion history, illicit drug history, and residence more than two miles from an international airport or migrant housing renders the di-

Table 25-5
Differential Diagnosis of Fever in Tropical Travelers (Partial List)

Common causes
- Viral syndrome
- Upper respiratory infections
- Gastroenteritis
- Food-related illnesses and toxins
- Infectious mononucleosis
- Hepatitis A
- Drug fever

Cyclic fever
- African trypanosomiasis
- Brucellosis
- Dengue
- Endocarditis
- Malaria
- Relapsing fever
- Sepsis
- Visceral leishmaniasis

Fever and splenomegaly
- Babesiosis
- Brucellosis
- Endocarditis
- Enteric fever
- Epidemic typhus
- Infectious mononucleosis
- Leptospirosis
- Malaria
- Relapsing fever
- Schistosomiasis (acute)
- Toxoplasmosis
- Visceral leishmaniasis

Fever and hepatomegaly
- Amebic liver abscess
- Cytomegalovirus infection
- Hepatitis A, B, C, D, E
- Lassa fever
- Leptospirosis
- Malaria
- Q fever
- Relapsing fever
- Yellow fever
- Visceral leishmaniasis

Fever and anemia/thrombocytopenia
- Cytomegalovirus infection
- Dengue
- Drug fever
- Endocarditis
- Enteric fever
- Hemorrhagic fever
- Human immunodeficiency virus syndrome (acute)
- Infectious mononucleosis
- Malaria
- Meningococcemia
- Q fever
- Sepsis
- Visceral leishmaniasis

agnosis of malaria highly unlikely [3,21,41–44]. Conversely, a positive travel history should prompt the occupational physician to order thick and thin blood smears in tropical travelers presenting with fever or flu-like syndromes.

Thick and thin blood smears are minimally invasive, simple, and cost effective. Their sensitivity and specificity exceed 90% in most instances [13,17,19]. It is essential for these smears to be interpreted by experienced personnel who are able to differentiate species through the visualization of distinct morphologic features. Clinically, the most important aspect of species identification is the differentiation of *P falciparum* from *P vivax*, *P ovale*, and *P malariae*. The thin smear is also useful in quantifying the percentage of parasitized red cells, since this finding has important prognostic implications. A single set of negative thick and thin blood smears does not exclude malaria. Thick and thin blood smears should be repeated every six to 12 hours for 48 hours [13,34]. The probability of malaria becomes quite low when repeated thick and thin blood smears remain negative [17].

In addition to thick and thin blood smears, molecular probes have recently been developed for rapid diagnosis. These probes were designed to detect parasitic DNA and protein antigens. One rapid direct reading dipstick test was recently field tested. The investigators reported an 80–100% range for test sensitivity and specificity as compared to blood smears [73]. Despite these promising results, blood smears remain the test of choice for diagnosis, species differentiation, and parasite counts.

Serologic testing for malaria is useful from an epidemiologic but not a diagnostic perspective because it cannot differentiate acute from chronic infection and protective from nonprotective antibody [47]. Although *P falciparum* parasites can be cultured in vitro to test for drug sensitivities, cultures are not used for diagnostic purposes.

Treatment

Occupational health professionals must consider the diagnosis of malaria in all traveling employees who develop flu-like symptoms or fever on return to the United States, since a delay in diagnosis and treatment could be fatal in 12 to 24 hours [36,37]. Studies have shown that with the advent of rapid transmeridian flight approximately 90% of transient tropical travelers become symptomatic on return to the United States [37,70, 74–76]. The potential for suboptimal clinical outcomes is further compounded by the fact that nontropical physicians have been shown to misdiagnose malaria almost 40% of the time in fatal cases [36]. Until an accurate diagnosis has been established, a presumptive diagnosis of malaria should be considered in all tropical travelers who present with fever, flu-like symptoms, or systemic illness.

The treatment of malaria can be quite complex, since it depends on the type of infection, severity of infection, level of parasitemia, presence of malarial complications, probability of parasite drug resistance, and host health status (e.g., age, allergies, medications, and confounding medical conditions) [53]. Some basic treatment strategies include (1) treating as a *P falciparum* infection until proved otherwise, (2) assuming chloroquine resistance until drug sensitivities are known, and (3) assuming chloroquine and mefloquine resistance in travelers to Southeast Asia until drug sensitivities are known.

All nonimmune and pregnant employees with *P falciparum* malaria should be admitted to the hospital. Nonimmune employees with falciparum parasitemias greater than 2%, semi-immune employees with falciparum parasitemias greater than 5%, and any employee with complicated malaria should be admitted to an intensive care unit. Reliable semi-immune adults with mild *P vivax*, *P ovale*, or *P malariae* infections may be treated on an outpatient basis, provided daily parasite counts can be obtained until the infection has been adequately controlled [8,13,17,34,77].

There are a substantial number of therapeutic agents in the antimalarial drug armamentarium. They can be categorized by medication class and mechanism of action, as depicted in Table 25-6 [8,13,14,77]. Treatment strategies for stand-by treatment (SBT), uncomplicated malaria, uncomplicated drug-resistant malaria, and complicated malaria are summarized in Table 25-7 and Table 25-8 [13,34,53,77]. The therapeutic agents most commonly used in the United States are briefly discussed in the following paragraphs.

Table 25-6
Categorization of Antimalarial Drugs

Drug classification schema
Quinoline-related compounds
- Chloroquine
- Halofantrine
- Mefloquine
- Primaquine
- Quinidine
- Quinine

Antifolates
- Proguanil
- Pyrimethamine

Qinghaosu/artemisinin derivatives
- Arteether
- Artemether
- Artesunate

Antimicrobial agents
- Azithromycin
- Clindamycin
- Dapsone
- Sulfonamides
- Tetracycline

Mechanism of action schema
Blood schizonticides (eradicate parasites in red cells)
- Fast-acting/potent
  - Artemisinin
  - Chloroquine
  - Halofantrine
  - Mefloquine
  - Quinidine
  - Quinine
- Slower-acting (added for synergism)
  - Clindamycin
  - Doxycycline
  - Sulfonamides
  - Tetracycline
- Hepatic schizonticides (eradicate intrahepatic parasites)
  - Primaquine
  - Proguanil
  - Pyrimethamine
- Gametocides (eradicate blood sexual form of parasite)
  - Primaquine
  - Pyrimethamine

STAND-BY TREATMENT

Stand-by treatment as defined by the World Health Organization (WHO) is the self-administration of antimalarial medication for treatment of fever or flu-like symptoms when prompt medical attention is unavailable [78]. The risks of adverse drug effects are ostensibly mitigated because self-treatment is considered a life-saving intervention in complicated falciparum infections. Therefore, employees must be well educated regarding prodromal symptoms and indications for self-treatment. SBT should not be considered during the first week of exposure, since the incubation period for malaria is at least seven days. Employees should also be advised that symptoms may first develop after leaving malaria-endemic zones and on return to the United States. As soon as possible after initiating SBT, definitive medical attention must be sought for further evaluation and treatment, as indicated. SBT may be used separately or in conjunction with chemoprophylaxis. Recommended SBT indications and therapeutic agents are summarized in Table 25-7 [79].

Table 25-7
Stand-by Treatment for Nonimmune Travelers

Indications for stand-by treatment (SBT)
1. SBT without chemoprophylaxis
   - Low-risk areas having limited medical availability
   - Short-term travelers in which the efficacy of chemoprophylaxis is not clearly defined
   - Brief repeated exposures in which the risks of long-term chemoprophylaxis are not acceptable
2. SBT with chemoprophylaxis
   - High-risk areas

Stand-by treatment (regimen depends on parasite type, parasite drug resistance, transmission risks, drug toxicities, and employee health status)
1. Chloroquine-sensitive malaria endemic areas
   - Chloroquine, 1,000 mg orally initially, followed by 500 mg orally 6 hours later, then 500 mg orally once daily for two days
2. Chloroquine-resistant malaria endemic areas
   - Mefloquine, 500 mg orally followed by 500 mg orally 12 hours later, or fansidar 3 tablets orally as a single dose, or halofantrine, 500 mg orally every six hours for three doses
3. Multidrug-resistant malaria endemic areas
   - Quinine, 650 mg orally every eight hours for seven days, or doxycycline, 100 mg orally once daily for seven days

UNCOMPLICATED MALARIA

Chloroquine is the drug of choice for all uncomplicated chloroquine-sensitive infections. The usual dosage is 25 mg base per kilogram administered over a 72-hour period, as summarized in Table 25-8. Cure rates exceed 95% when this regimen is employed [53]. Chloroquine must be followed by a two-week course of primaquine in order to eradicate *P vivax* and *P ovale* hypno-

Table 25-8
Medications Commonly Used in the Treatment of Malaria

Therapeutic agents (choice depends on sensitivities and drug availability)
Uncomplicated malaria infections
Chloroquine base, 10 mg/kg orally (600 mg, max) followed by 5 mg/kg orally (300 mg max) at six hours, 24 hours, and 48 hours
Quinine sulfate 10 mg/kg (usually 650 mg) orally three times daily for seven days *plus*
Tetracycline, 250 mg orally four times daily for seven days, *or*
Clindamycin, 10 mg/kg orally (900 mg max) every eight hours for three to five days, *or*
Pyrimethamine, 25 mg/sulfadoxine 500 mg (per tablet), three tablets orally as a single dose
Mefloquine base, 15 mg/kg orally (usually 750 mg) followed by 10 mg/kg orally (usually 500 mg) six to eight hours after the initial dose (maximum recommended total dose is 1,250 mg)
Halofantrine base, 8 mg/kg orally every six hours for three doses (500 mg maximum/dose); repeat after seven days for nonimmune employees
Artesunate, 4 mg/kg orally once daily for three days plus mefloquine or tetracycline
Complicated malaria infections (plus other adjunctive agents and modalities as indicated)
Chloroquine base 10 mg/kg iv over 8 hours (600 mg max), then 15 mg/kg iv over 24 hours (900 mg max)
Quinidine gluconate base 10 mg/kg iv load over 1–2 hours, followed by 0.02 mg/kg/min iv until parasitemia is less than 1% and employee can tolerate oral medications
Artemether 3.2 mg/kg im followed by 1.6 mg/kg im q 24 hours until employee can tolerate oral medications
Artesunate 2.4 mg/kg iv load followed by 1.2 mg/kg iv at 12 hours and 24 hours, then 1.2 mg/kg iv q 24 hours until employee can tolerate oral medications
Exchange transfusion for parasitemias greater than 10% in conjunction with altered mental status

zoites and prevent relapse (radical cure) [53,77]. As previously noted, primaquine may cause severe oxidant hemolysis in employees with glucose-6-phosphate dehydrogenase (G-6-PD) deficiency. Although primaquine is contraindicated in severe G-6-PD deficiency, it may be administered once weekly to employees with mild deficiency under close observation for a period of six to eight weeks [77].

UNCOMPLICATED DRUG-RESISTANT MALARIA

Uncomplicated chloroquine resistant *P falciparum* malaria is best treated with one of three regimens: quinine sulfate plus tetracycline (clindamycin should be substituted for pregnant women); quinine sulfate plus pyrimethamine/sulfadoxine; or pyrimethamine/sulfadoxine monotherapy [53,80]. In geographic regions where pyrimethamine/sulfadoxine resistance is uncontrolled, chloroquine-resistant *P falciparum* infections should be treated with quinine sulfate plus tetracycline, mefloquine, or halofantrine [53,81]. Nonimmune travelers to Thailand, other parts of Southeast Asia, or the Amazon should receive a full seven-day course of treatment, because *P falciparum* parasites are less sensitive to quinine in these geographic regions [81–83].

Clinicians should be aware that despite reportedly high cure rates, the effectiveness of these therapeutic agents is often limited by adverse drug effects. Some of the more notable adverse effects include (1) quinine—bitter taste, cinchonism, and hyperinsulinemic hypoglycemia [8,51,53]; (2) pyrimethamine/sulfadoxine—severe exfoliative dermatitis, erythema multiforme, and Stevens-Johnson syndrome [17,51]; (3) mefloquine—emesis, dysrhythmia, and toxic encephalopathy [51,53,83,84]; and (4) halofantrine—dose-dependent atrioventricular conduction delay, QTc prolongation, and sudden death [84,85].

Chloroquine-resistant *P vivax* can be effectively treated with mefloquine or quinine sulfate plus tetracycline. Pyrimethamine/sulfadoxine has proved to be less effective [17,53,77], and higher doses of pyrimethamine (22.5 to 30 mg base/day for 14 days) are required to eradicate hypnozoites and prevent relapses [53,86].

UNCOMPLICATED MULTIDRUG-RESISTANT MALARIA

Quinine sulfate plus tetracycline (clindamycin in pregnant employees) is recommended for the treatment of uncomplicated mefloquine-resistant *P falciparum* infections [51,53,83]. Although the artemisinin compounds are fast acting and effective, they have not been licensed for use in the

United States. These compounds have been highly effective in the treatment of multidrug-resistant falciparum infections and have become the drugs of choice for quinine-resistant *P falciparum* elsewhere in the world [51,87–89].

COMPLICATED MALARIA

The treatment of choice for complicated malaria is strongly dependent on parasite sensitivities. Parenteral chloroquine is the drug of choice for severe chloroquine-sensitive malaria infections [34,53]. Quinidine gluconate is recommended for treatment of severe chloroquine-resistant and mefloquine-resistant *P falciparum* infections, since parenteral quinine dihydrochloride is no longer available in the United States [53,90]. Although a number of regimens have proven effective, the one most commonly employed in the United States is quinidine gluconate 10 mg/kg intravenously over one to two hours followed by a continuous infusion of 0.02 mg/kg/minute. The rate of infusion must be titrated according to clinical response, and the rate should be decreased by 30–50% after 48 hours in hyperparasitemic patients [53]. Major toxicities include hypotension, dysrhythmias, and hyperinsulinemic hypoglycemia [53].

In many countries, parenteral artemisinin and tetracycline or mefloquine are recommended for treatment of quinine-resistant *P falciparum*; however, in the United States, parenteral quinidine plus tetracycline remains the treatment of choice, since artemisinin agents are not available [53,88].

Whether complicated or uncomplicated, malaria treatment interventions must be closely monitored. Most employees with uncomplicated or drug-sensitive malaria show marked clinical improvement within 48 hours and defervesce within 96 hours [13,17,34]. Examination of thick and thin blood smears every 12 hours is recommended until the parasitemia proportion is less than 1% [17]. Drug resistance is indicated by parasitemia levels that fail to decline by 75% after 48 hours or persist beyond eight days of treatment [17,77]. The presence of circulating gametocytes during the treatment phase does not indicate drug resistance or treatment failure [77].

Since the risk of death from malaria is directly proportional to the degree of parasitemia [67,91], exchange transfusion (ET) should be considered in all critically ill patients who have not responded adequately to other therapeutic interventions [91,92]. Although ET has not been shown to improve survival rates in randomized clinical trials, it is currently recommended as an adjunct in patients with *P falciparum* parasitemias exceeding 10%, coma, respiratory failure, coagulopathy, or renal failure [93]. Once initiated, exchange transfusions should be continued until parasitemia levels have fallen to less than 5%.

Severe malaria should be managed in an intensive care unit to monitor and maintain fluid and electrolyte balance [68]. In addition to ET, other therapeutic interventions previously shown to be clinically effective in the treatment of complicated malaria include acetaminophen for fever [17], prophylactic phenobarbital to prevent seizures [94], benzodiazepines to treat seizures [77], early hemodialysis or peritoneal dialysis for oligouric renal failure [95], positive pressure ventilation for noncardiogenic pulmonary edema [96], and glucose supplementation for hypoglycemia [17].

Occupational Considerations

In summary, occupational malaria is primarily a concern in employees and military personnel traveling to malaria-endemic geographic regions. Pretravel health assessments are recommended at least one month prior to departure in order to identify pre-existing medical conditions that may adversely impact the employee's health and safety while in a travel status. It is paramount for the occupational health professional to be adequately informed regarding travel itineraries because methods of prevention must be tailored on an individual basis. The occupational health professional must also closely monitor CDC and WHO preventive and treatment recommendations because of frequent changes in the distribution of malaria and parasite drug resistance. Additionally, it is important to realize that evolving environmental changes such as global warming may significantly alter the geographic distribution of malaria and vectorial densities in the future [97]. As previously noted, allergic, pregnant, and other employees who are unable to take or comply with chemoprophylactic regimens recommended by the CDC, WHO, or U.S. Public Health Service should not be medically cleared for travel to high-risk areas unless there are mitigating circumstances.

It is also strongly recommended that pretravel health assessments include employee education and training regarding the risks of malarial disease, antimosquito measures, malaria chemoprophylaxis (including terminal prophylaxis), signs and symptoms of disease, stand-by treatment, postexposure procedures and prophylaxis, and the necessity to comply with preventive recommendations as delineated in Table 25-9. Additionally, employees should be encouraged to minimize exposure risks whenever feasible, since it is possible to acquire malaria despite the appropriate application of antimosquito measures and use of chemoprophylactic agents. As a final measure, employees who become ill after returning to the United States should be instructed to inform their physicians that they have been traveling and potentially exposed to malaria parasites.

Since occupational malaria usually results from employee travel to malaria-endemic zones on business, most cases will be compensable, and appropriate claims will need to be filed. Compensability may be more difficult to ascertain in rare situations such as runway malaria and airport malaria; however, these and other possibilities (e.g., autochthonous malaria) should be considered when a causal link is not obvious during the disability case review [41–44,98–101].

Finally, there is very little in the scientific literature regarding malaria-associated disability in traveling employees; however, uncomplicated imported malaria infections typically defervesce after two to three days of hospitalization [102]. Most employees return to work in approximately one week, depending on workplace demands and premorbid health status, without permanent impairment or disability [101]. Conversely, complicated infections (usually *P falciparum*) may result in prolonged hospitalizations, extended disability, permanent impairment, and death. Therefore, early recognition and treatment are critical in preserving employee health, performance, and productivity.

Table 25-9
Employee Personal Protective Measures

Antimosquito measures
Wear long-sleeved shirts and trousers
Apply DEET to exposed areas at dusk
Spray "knock-down" insecticide in living and sleeping areas at dusk
Use electrically operated insecticide generators containing pyrethroids or mosquito coils
Stay in air-conditioned/screened rooms after sunset
Use permethrin impregnated bed nets
Employee behavior patterns
Limit activities in malaria-endemic areas when feasible
Avoid unprotected nighttime exposures when feasible
Comply with recommended chemoprophylaxis and stand-by treatment
Pregnant females and employees who are unable to comply with recommended preventive measures due to medication allergies or poor health should not travel to malaria endemic areas unless absolutely necessary
Employees should be well educated regarding the signs and symptoms of malaria
Employees should be aware that malaria symptoms may start during or after exposure

References

1. Centers for Disease Control. Mosquito-transmitted malaria—California and Florida, 1990. *MMWR* 1991;40:106–8.
2. Centers for Disease Control. Summary of notifiable diseases, United States, 1990. *MMWR* 1991;39:55–61.
3. Centers for Disease Control and Prevention. Local transmission of *Plasmodium vivax* malaria—Houston, Texas, 1994. *MMWR* 1994;44:295.
4. Steffen R, Fuchs E, Schildknecht J, et al. Mefloquine compared with other malaria chemoprophylaxis regimens in tourists visiting East Africa. *Lancet* 1993; 341:1299–1303.
5. World Health Organization. World malaria situation in 1993. *Wkly Epidemiol Rec* 1996;71:17–24.
6. Centers for Disease Control and Prevention. *Health information for international travel—1995.* Atlanta: CDC, 1995.
7. Barat LM, Bloland PB. Drug resistance among malaria and other parasites. *Infect Dis Clin North Am* 1997;11:969–87.

8. Miller LH. Malaria. In: Warren KS, Mahmoud AAF (eds), *Tropical and Geographical Medicine*. New York: McGraw-Hill, 1994. Pp 223–39.
9. Stanley J. Malaria. *Em Med Clin North Am* 1997; 15:113–55.
10. Beier JC, Copeland RS, Mtalib R, et al. Ookinete rates in Afrotropical mosquitoes as a measure of human malaria infectionousness. *Am J Trop Med Hyg* 1992;47:41–6.
11. Quinn TC, Jacobs RF, Mertz GJ, et al. Congenital malaria: a report of four cases and a review. *Clin Lab Obstet* 1982;10:229.
12. Bruce-Chwatt LJ. Transfusion malaria revisited. *Trop Dis Bull* 1982;79:827–40.
13. Zucker JR, Campbell CC. Malaria: principles of prevention and treatment. *Infect Dis Clin North Am* 1993;7:547–67.
14. Schwartz IK. Prevention of malaria. *Infect Dis Clin North Am* 1992;6:313–31.
15. Centers for Disease Control. Recommendations for the prevention of malaria among travelers. *MMWR* 1990;39:1–10.
16. Advice for travelers. *Med Lett* 1995;37:99–108.
17. White NJ. Malaria. In: Cook GC (ed), *Manson's Tropical Diseases*, 2nd Ed. Philadelphia: Saunders, 1996. Pp 1087–164.
18. MacDonald G. *The Epidemiology and Control of Malaria*. London: Oxford University Press, 1957. Pp 5–35.
19. Jones C, Grab B. The assessment of insecticidal impact on the malaria mosquito's vectorial capacity from data on the proportion of parous females. *Bull WHO* 1965;31:71–86.
20. Curtis CF. Introduction I: an overview of mosquito biology, behaviour and importance. In: Bock GR and Cardew G (eds), *Olfaction in Mosquito-Host Interactions*. New York: John Wiley & Sons, 1996. Pp 3–7.
21. Brook JH, Genese CA, Blotand PB, et al. Brief report: malaria probably locally acquired in New Jersey. *N Engl J Med* 1994;331:22–3.
22. Brillman J. Plasmodium vivax malaria in Mexico—a problem in the United States. *West J Med* 1994; 147:469–73.
23. Wyler DJ. Malaria—resurgence, resistance, and research. *N Engl J Med* 1983;308:875–8.
24. Harries AD. Malaria: keeping the mosquitoes at bay. *Lancet* 1993;342:506–7.
25. Krotoski WA. Discovery of the hypnozoite and a new theory of malaria relapse. *Trans R Soc Trop Med Hyg* 1985;79:1–11.
26. White NJ, Ho M. The pathophysiology of malaria. *Adv Parasitol* 1992,31:34–173.
27. Wernsdorfer WH. Epidemiology of drug resistance in malaria. *Acta Trop* 1994;56:143–56.
28. World Health Organization. Insecticide resistance and vector control. Seventeenth report of the WHO Expert Committee on Insecticides. WHO Technical Report Series no. 443. Geneva, Switzerland: WHO, 1970.
29. Krogstad DJ. Malaria as a reemerging disease. *Epidemiol Rev* 1996;18:77–89.
30. Centers for Disease Control and Prevention. Epidemic malaria—Tadjikistan. *MMWR* 1996;45:513–6.
31. Quinn TC, Plorde JJ. The resurgence of malaria. *Arch Int Med* 1981;141:1123–4.
32. Brillman J. Plasmodium vivax malaria from Mexico—a problem in the United States. *West J Med* 1994;147: 469–73.
33. Freedman DO. Imported malaria—here to stay. *Am J Med* 1992;93:239–42.
34. Hoffman SL. Diagnosis, treatment, and prevention of malaria. *Med Clin North Am* 1992;76:1327–55.
35. Zucker JR, Barber AM, Paxton LA, et al. Malaria surveillance—United States, 1992. *MMWR* 1995;44:1–17.
36. Greenberg AE, Lobel HO. Mortality from *Plasmodium falciparum* malaria in travelers from the United States, 1959–1987. *Ann Intern Med* 1990;113:326–7.
37. Lobel HO, Campbell CC, Schwartz, et al. Recent trends in the importation of malaria caused by *Plasmodium falciparum* into the United States from Africa. *J Infect Dis* 1986;152:613–7.
38. Lobel HO, Phillips-Howard PA, Brandling-Bennett AD, et al. Malaria incidence and prevention among European and North American travellers to Kenya. *Bull WHO* 1990;68:209–15.
39. Steffen R, Heusser R, Machlon R, et al. Malaria chemoprophylaxis among European tourists in tropical Africa: use, adverse reactions, and efficacy. *Bull WHO* 1990;68:313.
40. Olliaro P, Cattani J, Wirth D. Malaria, the submerged disease. *JAMA* 1996;275(3):230–3.
41. Holvoet G, Michielsen P, Vandepitte J. Airport malaria in Belgium. *Lancet* 1982;ii:881–2.
42. Smeaton MJ, Slater PJ, Robson P. Malaria from a "commuter" mosquito. *Lancet* 1984;i:845–6.
43. Whitefield D, Curtis CF, White GB, et al. Two cases of falciparum malaria acquired in Britain. *Br Med J* 1984;289:1607–9.
44. Isaacson M. Airport malaria: a review. *Bull WHO* 1989;67:737–43.
45. Miller LH, Mason SJ, Clyde DF, et al. The resistance factor to *Plasmodium vivax* in blacks. *N Engl J Med* 1976;295:302–4.
46. Nagel RL, Roth EF. Malaria and red cell genetic defects. *Blood* 1989;74:1213–21.
47. Deans JA, Cohen S. Immunology of malaria. *Ann Rev Microbiol* 1983;37:25–49.
48. Wolfe MS. Protection of travelers. *Clin Infect Dis* 1997;25:177–86.
49. Beach RF, Ruebush TR, Sexton JD. Effectiveness of permethrin-impregnated bed nets and curtains for

malaria control in a holoendemic area of Western Kenya. *Am J Trop Med Hyg* 1993;49:290–300.

50. D'Alessandro U, Olaleye BO, McGuire W, et al. Mortality and morbidity from malaria in Gambian children after introduction of an impregnated bed-net programme. *Lancet* 1995;345:479–83.
51. Kain KC. Chemotherapy and prevention of drug-resistant malaria. *Wilderness Env Med* 1995;6:307–24.
52. Navy Medical Department. *Guide to Malaria Prevention and Control.* Norfolk, VA: Navy Environmental Health Center, 1995. Pp 62–9.
53. Drugs for parasitic infections. *Med Lett* 1995;37:99–108.
54. Harries AD, Chugh KS. Chloroquine-induced pruritus in Nigerian medical and nursing students. *Ann Trop Med Parasitol* 1986;80:479–80.
55. Phillips-Howard PA, terKuile FO. CNS adverse events associated with antimalarial agents—fact or fiction? *Drug Safety* 1995;12:370–83.
56. Magill AJ, Smoak BL. Failure of mefloquine chemoprophylaxis for malaria in Somalia. *N Engl J Med* 1993;329:1206.
57. Croft A, Garner P. Mefloquine to prevent malaria: a systematic review of trials. *Br Med J* 1997;315:1412–6.
58. Behrens RH, Curtis CF. Malaria in travelers: epidemiology and prevention. *Br Med Bull* 1993;49:363–81.
59. Phillips-Howard PA, Radalowicz A, Mitchell J, et al. Risk of malaria in British residents returning from malarious areas. *Br Med J* 1990;300:499–503.
60. Steffen R, Holdener F, Wyss R, et al. Malaria prophylaxis and self-therapy in airline crews. *Aviat Space Environ Med* 1990;61:942–5.
61. Centers for Disease Control and Prevention. Malaria surveillance—United States, 1992. *MMWR* 1995; 44(Suppl SS-5).
62. Amador R, Patarroyo ME. Malaria vaccines. *J Clin Immunol* 1996;16(4):183–9.
63. Wyler DJ. Malaria—resurgence, resistance, and research. *N Engl J Med* 1983;308:875–8.
64. Froude JRL, Weiss LM, Tanowitz HB, et al. Imported malaria in the Bronx: review of 51 cases recorded from 1986–1991. *Clin Infect Dis* 1992;15:774–80.
65. Gordon S, Brennessel DJ, Goldstein JA, et al. Malaria: a city hospital experience. *Arch Intern Med* 1988;148:1569–71.
66. Wiest PM, Opal S, Romulo RL, et al. Malaria in travelers in Rhode Island: a review of 26 cases. *Am J Med* 1990;91:30–6.
67. Field JW. Blood examination and prognosis in acute falciparum malaria. *Trans R Soc Trop Med Hyg* 1949;43:33–68.
68. Warrell DA, Molyneaux ME, Beales PF. Severe and complicated malaria. *Trans R Soc Trop Med Hyg* 1990;84(Suppl):1–65.
69. Brewster DR, Kwiatowski D, White NJ. Neurological sequelae of cerebral malaria in children. *Lancet* 1990;336:1039–43.
70. Svenson JE, Gyozrkos TW, MacLean JD. Diagnosis of malaria in the febrile traveler. *Am J Trop Med Hyg* 1995;53:518–21.
71. Gasser RA, Magill AJ, Oster CN, et al. The threat of infectious disease in Americans returning from Operation Desert Storm. *N Engl J Med* 1991;324:857–64.
72. Strickland GT. Fever in the returned traveler. In: Wolfe MS (ed), Travel Medicine. *Med Clin North Am* 1992;76:1375–92.
73. Beadle C, Long GW, Weiss WR, et al. Diagnosis of malaria by detection of *Plasmodium falciparum* HRP-2 antigen with a rapid dipstick antigen-capture assay. *Lancet* 1994;334:564–8.
74. Maegraith B. Unde venis. *Lancet* 1963;1:401–4.
75. Baker PB, Dronen SC. Vivax malaria. *Am J Emerg Med* 1986;4:52–8.
76. Stair T, Ricci R, Pedicano J, et al. Malaria in the emergency department. *Ann Emerg Med* 1983;12:422–5.
77. White NJ. The treatment of malaria. *N Engl J Med* 1996;335:800–6.
78. World Health Organization. Health risks and their avoidance. In: International Travel and Health. Geneva: *WHO,* 1993.
79. World Health Organization. Development of recommendations for the protection of short-term travellers to malaria endemic areas: memorandum from two WHO meetings. *Bull WHO* 1988;66:177–9.
80. Dobertslyn EB, Phintuyothim P, Noeypatimondh S, et al. Single-dose therapy of falciparum malaria with mefloquine or pyrimethamine-sulfadoxine. *Bull WHO* 1979;57:275–9.
81. Watt G, Loesuttiribool L, Shanks GD, et al. Quinine with tetracycline for the treatment of drug resistant falciparum malaria in Thailand. *Am J Trop Med Hyg* 1992;47:108–11.
82. Looareesuwan S, Charoenpan P, Ho M. Fatal *Plasmodium falciparum* malaria after an inadequate response to quinine treatment. *J Infect Dis* 1990;161:577.
83. Patchen LC, Campbell CC, Williams SB. Neurologic reactions after a therapeutic dose of mefloquine. *N Engl J Med* 1989;321:1415–6.
84. terKuile FO, Dolan G, Nosten F, et al. Halofantrine versus mefloquine in treatment of multidrug resistant falciparum malaria. *Lancet* 1993;341:1044–9.
85. Nosten F, terKuile FO, Luxemburger C, et al. Cardiac effects of antimalarial treatment with halofantrine. *Lancet* 1991;341:1054–6.
86. Krotoski WA. Frequency of relapse and primaquine resistance in Southeast Asian vivax malaria. *N Engl J Med* 1980;303:587–92.
87. Hien TT, White NJ. Qinghaosu. *Lancet* 1993; 341:603–8.

88. White NJ. Artemisinin: current status. *Trans R Soc Trop Med Hyg* 1994;88(Suppl):3–4.

89. Looareesuwan S, Wiravan C, Vanijanonta S, et al. Randomized trial of artesunate and mefloquine alone and in sequence for acute uncomplicated falciparum malaria. *Lancet* 1992;339:821–4.

90. Miller KD, Greenberg AE, Campbell CC. Treatment of severe malaria in the United States with a continuous infusion of quinidine gluconate and exchange transfusion. *N Engl J Med* 1989;321:65–70.

91. Marik PE. Severe falciparum malaria: survival without exchange transfusion. *Am J Trop Med Hyg* 1989; 1:627–9.

92. Phillips P, Nantel S, Benny WB. Exchange transfusion as an adjunct to the treatment of severe falciparum malaria: case report and review. *Rev Infect Dis* 1990;12:1100.

93. Miller KD, Greenberg AE, Campbell CC. Treatment of severe malaria in the United States with a continuous infusion of quinidine gluconate and exchange transfusion. *N Engl J Med* 1989;321:65–70.

94. White NJ, Looareesuwan S, Phillips RE, et al. Single-dose phenobarbitone prevents convulsions in cerebral malaria. *Lancet* 1988;2:64–6.

95. Tran TMT, Nguyen HP, Ha V, et al. Acute renal failure in patients with severe falciparum malaria. *Clin Infect Dis* 1992;15:874–80.

96. Brooks MH, Kiel FW, Sheehy TW, et al. Acute pulmonary edema in falciparum malaria: a clinicopathological correlation. *N Engl J Med* 1968;279:732–7.

97. Intergovernmental Panel on Climate Change, Working Group II. Summary for Policymakers: Scientific-Technical Analyses of Impacts, Adaptations, and Mitigation of Climate Change. Cambridge: Cambridge University Press, 1995.

98. Conlon CP, Berendt AR, Dawson K, et al. Runway malaria. *Lancet* 1990;335:472.

99. Bada JL, Cabezos J, Fernandez-Roure JL. Runway malaria. *Lancet* 1990;335:881.

100. Connor MP, Green AD. Runway malaria in a British serviceman. *J Royal Soc Med* 1995;88:415P–416P.

101. Oswald G, Lawrence EP. Runway malaria. *Lancet* 1990;335:1537.

102. Official Disability Guidelines, 1998. Corpus Christi, Texas: Work-Loss Data Institute, 1997. Pp 125–6.

26 / Occupational Lyme Disease

Michael D. Goldstein and Brian S. Schwartz

Lyme disease is a tick-borne infection caused by the spirochete *Borrelia burgdorferi*. It was first recognized as a clinical entity in 1975 after an outbreak of cases of juvenile rheumatoid arthritis in Old Lyme, Connecticut [1]. In retrospect, persons with acute illnesses and skin rashes compatible with erythema migrans (EM), the hallmark rash of early Lyme disease, have been reported in Europe since the early twentieth century [2]. Since 1975, reported cases of Lyme disease in the United States have increased dramatically, reaching approximately 16,000 cases in 1996, the last year for which national data are available, and the illness has become an important public health problem in many parts of the world.

The spirochetal agent of the disease was first isolated in 1982 from *Ixodes scapularis* ticks, collected on Shelter Island, New York [3]. This spirochete was subsequently linked serologically to patients with clinical Lyme disease. The organism was cultured from the blood and cerebrospinal fluid of patients, and specific IgG and IgM antibody responses were demonstrated [4,5].

Lyme disease has been associated with a constellation of clinical manifestations including skin rash, erythema migrans, fever, arthralgias, myalgias, arthritis, carditis, and nervous system abnormalities. Various antibiotic regimens have been used to treat the infection successfully.

A number of epidemiologic studies have addressed the incidence and prevalence of the infection in persons at risk of tick exposure by virtue of their employment and have found significantly elevated odds ratios for outdoor workers, compared to workers who are not involved in outdoor work. Several preventive strategies have been used successfully to decrease the risk of tick bites, such as protective clothing and insect repellents, and the application of acaricides to certain brush and tall-grass areas, but the effectiveness of these measures has not been rigorously demonstrated. In late 1998, a vaccine based on recombinant OspA (outer surface protein A) was approved by the Food and Drug Administration for use in adults at risk for the disease. While several questions remain unanswered concerning the use of the vaccines, these hold promise as being a significant addition to the public health arsenal in the prevention of the disease.

Vector and Transmission

The primary vectors of Lyme disease are very small ticks (much smaller than the common dog and cattle ticks) of the *Ixodes ricinus* complex. In particular, the disease is transmitted by *I scapularis* in the northeastern and midwestern United States, *Ixodes pacificus* in the western United States, *I ricinus* in Europe and western portions of the former Soviet Union, and *Ixodes persulcatus* in China, Japan, and eastern Russia [6].

Ticks seek host animals from the tips of tall grasses and shrubs and transfer to animals or persons who brush against this vegetation. Ticks can attach to any part of the body but often crawl to the more hidden or hairy areas, such as the groin, armpits, and scalp. Ticks feed on blood by inserting their mouth parts into the host's skin. As they feed on the blood (a complete meal can take up to several days), infected ticks may transmit the spirochete to the host. Knowledge of the life cycle of the tick can be helpful in efforts to minimize exposure risk. Ticks, like other arthropods, pass through three life stages—larva, nymph, and adult. Tick larvae rarely carry the infection at the time of feeding. The most important vector of the disease is the nymph, which appears during the spring, when people are beginning to increase their outdoor activities and are wearing fewer layers of clothing. The nymph is difficult to detect because of its small size (less than 2 mm). Transmission of the spirochete to the host occurs after 24 to 48 hours of feeding [7].

The life cycle of these hard-body ticks comprises a two-year span. Adult ticks feed and mate on large animals, especially deer, in the fall and early spring. Female ticks then drop off these animals to lay eggs on the ground. During the summer, eggs hatch into larvae. Larvae feed on mice, other small mammals, and birds in the summer and fall. They are then inactive until the next spring, when they molt into nymphs. Nymphs feed on small rodents, other mammals, and birds in the late spring and summer and then molt into adults in the fall, completing the two-year life cycle. Ticks acquire *B burgdorferi* when they feed on infected small animals, most importantly the white-footed mouse, the key reservoir of the disease in nature. Because "year two" nymphs appear before "year one" larvae in any given year, they are able to transmit the spirochetes that were acquired during their larval feeding the prior year to newly born mice the next spring. This allows larvae to acquire the spirochete each year. Infected nymphs and adults can transmit the spirochete to other host animals, including humans, during the course of their normal feeding behavior. Humans are incidental hosts.

Epidemiology

Lyme disease transmission cycles occur in many of the northern temperate regions of the world including Europe, Russia, China, and Japan. In the United States, the highest incidence of cases has been reported in the Northeast, the Midwest (particularly Wisconsin and Minnesota), and the West (particularly northern California). In the United States, the Centers for Disease Control and Prevention has documented an increasing number of cases over the past two decades, with over 16,000 reported cases in 1996 [8].

Numerous studies of outdoor employees from around the world, commonly forestry and park workers, have documented the increased risk for infection by *B burgdorferi* [9–21]. Outdoor workers have been reported to have a two- to sixfold elevation of risk for *B burgdorferi* infection in comparison to populations not involved in outdoor work. Many of these studies have evaluated the prevalence of anti-*B burgdorferi* antibody or the annual incidence of seroconver-sion, using enzyme-linked immunosorbent assay (ELISA), without confirmation, as currently recommended, and Western blot analysis. Seroprevalence rates have ranged from 5% to 28% in various populations, and annual incidence of seroconversion has ranged from 5% to 7% [18,22]. These data suggest that a large number of seropositive workers do not have a history of clinical Lyme disease, suggesting that seroconversion can occur asymptomatically (in 72–100% of cases). Alternatively, it is possible that the reliance on ELISA without Western blot could lead to a large number of false-positive serologic test results. The body of literature, however, clearly indicates that outdoor work increases the risk of infection with *B burgdorferi*. This point has both clinical and legal implications.

Clinical Course

Lyme disease may progress through a series of clinical stages. The earliest form of the disease starts at the site of spirochete inoculation into the skin. This phase, termed *early localized* disease, is characterized by skin rash at the site of the bite. Shortly thereafter an *early disseminated* form of the illness involving flu-like symptoms may occur. Within weeks to months, a *later disseminated* phase of the illness can occur, often involving infection of the nervous system or heart. Without treatment, the *late chronic* form of the disease ensues, with arthritis and late neurologic manifestations. It is important to note that not all infected individuals pass through each of these stages. Some individuals may develop late disease without ever exhibiting, or perhaps not noticing, the signs and symptoms of early disease.

EARLY LOCALIZED INFECTION

Erythema migrans (EM) is a red circular rash that appears on the skin at the site of the tick bite. This lesion begins as a small papule at the bite site. The papule forms into a slowly enlarging ring, while the central erythema usually fades gradually to a normal skin color but may become slightly blue. The ring remains flat, blanches with pressure, and does not generally desquamate, vesiculate, or have scale at the periphery, as ringworm does. The lesion tends to be nonpruritic and is not painful [23]. Any rash that starts as a papule and expands over several days to weeks, eventually reaching over 5 cm in diameter, should be considered as possible erythema migrans. Although classically described as a "target," only a minority of patients have such a rash; the majority of EM rashes are solid without central clearing. Within days of the onset of EM, half the patients develop secondary annular lesions, signaling early dissemination of the spirochete [6]. Infecting organisms can sometimes be isolated on culture of the secondary lesions. Both EM and the secondary lesions disappear spontaneously over a period of several weeks, even without treatment.

EARLY DISSEMINATED INFECTION

Early disseminated infection often presents as flulike symptoms, which may accompany or appear independently of EM. Symptoms may include fatigue, headache, fever, chills, myalgias, arthralgias, and lymphadenopathy. The generalized arthralgic joint pains common in this phase of the illness are often migratory, may involve several joints, and rarely include swelling. This should be differentiated from frank arthritis, which does not typically present until the late infection phase noted below.

LATE DISSEMINATED INFECTION

Late disseminated infection typically occurs several weeks to months after the initial tick bite. The cardinal manifestations are neurologic and cardiac. Involvement of the nervous system (e.g., facial palsy and other cranial neuropathies, aseptic meningitis, motor or sensory radiculoneuritis, myelitis, encephalitis) occurs in approximately 15% of cases [24], and cardiac abnormalities (e.g., atrioventricular block, myopericarditis) in approximately 8% of cases [25].

LATE (CHRONIC) INFECTION

Late infection is typically defined as having a duration of greater than one year. There are three primary manifestations of late disease: arthritis, neurologic disease, and an unusual skin manifestation. Lyme arthritis may appear from several weeks to two years after the onset of illness and occurs in approximately 60% of untreated patients who have had EM [26]. The arthritis, most commonly monoarticular, has a predilection for the large joints, with the knees often affected. Individual attacks of arthritis may persist for a week to several months, alternating with a symptom-free period of time of similar duration. Late neurologic manifestations are rare but may include neuropsychiatric symptoms affecting mood and concentration as well as focal central nervous system lesions, such as focal encephalitis, transverse myelitis, a multiple sclerosis–like syndrome, and vestibular or optic neuritis [27]. Late disease may also be accompanied by incapacitating fatigue. Acrodermatitis chronica atrophicans, the late skin manifestation, is well documented in Europe but is still rare in the United States. This lesion appears to result from chronic persistence of infection in the skin. The lesions begin as violaceous plaques or nodules on the extensor surfaces of the extremities, which eventually progress to epidermal and dermal atrophy.

Diagnosis

The diagnosis of Lyme disease can be difficult to make because its signs and symptoms mimic those of many other illnesses. The diagnosis of Lyme disease should take the following into account:

- *History of possible exposure to ticks*: A careful history is very helpful. Have there been recent visits or residential exposures to grassy, wooded settings in endemic regions? Does the individual recall finding a tick on the body, and was it embedded in the skin? If so, for approximately how long? How was it removed?

- *Signs and symptoms of disease*: Does the patient report flu-like symptoms occurring in the spring or summer? Is there a history of a rash compatible with EM? Has the patient had other characteristic signs or symptoms of Lyme disease (as previously described)?
- *Appropriate use of laboratory testing*, as described below.

DIFFERENTIAL DIAGNOSIS

Several illnesses—fibromyalgia, erhlichiosis, babesiosis, Rocky Mountain spotted fever—deserve special consideration when establishing a differential diagnosis in a suspected case of Lyme disease.

Fibromyalgia

Fibromyalgia and Lyme disease share several clinical manifestations and are often confused with one another. Although fibromyalgia occasionally occurs as a sequel of Lyme disease, it is not an indication of persistent infection. Lyme disease is only one of many triggers for the development of fibromyalgia. Improper diagnosis of fibromyalgia as Lyme disease can lead to significant overdiagnosis of the latter condition [6,28–31].

Ehrlichiosis

Ehrlichiosis is a systemic illness caused by rickettsial organisms of the genus *Ehrlichia*. In the United States, the two illnesses of particular concern are human granulocytic ehrlichiosis (HGE) and human monocytic ehrlichiosis (HME). These infections are transmitted by a tick bite (often *Amblyomma americanum* for HME and *I scapularis* for HGE) and occur primarily during the summer months. HGE is typically caused by the rickettsiae, *Ehrlichia equi* and *Ehrlichia phagocytophila*, while HME is often caused by the rickettsia *Ehrlichia chaffeensis*. HGE shares many epidemiologic features with HME, including history of tick exposure, rural residence, and spring-summer seasonality. Geographically, HGE cases tend to occur in the upper-midwestern and northeastern United States, while cases of HME have been reported primarily from the southern states. There are no clinical features that consistently distinguish HGE from HME, and for case management, it is not necessary to differentiate between them. In 50% of patients, systemic symptoms, including fever, chills, headache, myalgia, nausea and vomiting, may be accompanied by a rash (commonly involving the trunk). Leukopenia, thrombocytopenia, and elevated liver function tests are common. Diagnostic confirmation is based on analysis of acute and convalescent serologies [32,33].

Cases of co-infection with both the agent of HGE and *B burgdorferi* have been reported. Some authors have recently advocated that empiric therapy for both Lyme disease and ehrlichiosis should be considered in any patient suspected of having a tick-borne illness and presenting with signs and symptoms compatible with both infections [11]. It should be noted that doxycycline is the initial treatment of choice for ehrlichiosis.

Babesiosis

Babesiosis is another illness transmitted by *I scapularis* and is caused by the intraerythrocytic protozoan *Babesia microti*. Gradual onset of malaise, anorexia, and fatigue are followed by intermittent fevers (as high as 104°F) as well as chills, myalgias, arthralgias, and nausea and/or vomiting. The illness can last for a few weeks to several months. Babesiosis is diagnosed by microscopic identification of the organism on Giemsa- or Wright-stained blood smears. Serologic tests for detection of anti-*Babesia* antibodies are available through the CDC and several research laboratories [34].

Rocky Mountain Spotted Fever

Rocky Mountain spotted fever is a serious, potentially fatal vasculitis due to infection with *Rickettsia rickettsii*. Most cases are reported in the southeastern and south central states. The dog, wood, and Lone Star ticks (*Dermacentor variabilis*, *Dermacentor andersoni*, and *Amblyomma americanum*, respectively) are the primary vectors. Most reported cases occur during the summer months. A diffuse maculopapular rash (which begins on wrists and ankles and spreads centrally) with development of petechiae is seen in 90% of patients after three to four days of fever, headaches, and myalgias. Thrombocytopenia and elevated liver function tests are common. Diagnostic confirmation requires immunofluorescent staining of skin biopsy specimens or analysis of acute and convalescent serologies [32].

LABORATORY TESTING

Lyme disease has been associated with a variety of nonspecific laboratory abnormalities early in the disease [35,36]. These include elevated erythrocyte sedimentation rate (ESR), elevated serum total IgM level, elevated alanine aminotransferase (ALT), and aspartate aminotranferase (AST) levels, and mild anemia. In terms of disease-specific testing, no one method is the gold standard, but several useful tools are available.

Cultures

While *B burgdorferi* is uncommonly cultured from blood or cerebrospinal fluid [37], it can sometimes be recovered from skin biopsies of EM or secondary annular lesions [38].

Serologic Testing

Serologic testing can be helpful in the diagnosis of Lyme disease when used by a practitioner with a clear understanding of the benefits and shortcomings of such testing. There is currently no standardization of serologic tests, and many have been shown to have low sensitivity and specificity [39–41]. Indiscriminant use of these tests in patients with a low pretest probability of disease will result in a very low predictive value and many false-positive test results. The U.S. Centers for Disease Control and Prevention (CDC) is currently spearheading an effort to standardize testing for Lyme disease.

Currently, there are three widely available types of antibody testing: indirect fluorescent antibody (IFA), ELISA, and Western blot. ELISA tends to be more accurate than IFA and is typically the initial test of choice when performing serologic testing. It should be noted that IgM antibody does not peak until three to six weeks after the onset of disease and IgG antibodies are generally highest only months or years later [27]. The Western blot (a more expensive but more specific test than ELISA or IFA) is useful as a confirmatory test following a positive, borderline, or suspected false-positive ELISA test result. It should be noted that individuals with syphilis (VDRL positive) may have positive Lyme disease serologic studies by ELISA or IFA, although this is less of a problem with currently available tests. The CDC recommend follow-up of any positive first-stage antibody test with a Western blot test. Specific IgM bands can be evaluated during the first few weeks of the disease, with IgG bands evaluated thereafter. Specific CDC criteria for determining serologic positivity have been formulated [42]. In our experience, the IgM Western blot is a problematic test, with a higher rate of false-positive test results because of its less stringent criterion for positivity (two of three bands rather than five of 10 for IgG). A common scenario is that of a patient being evaluated for possible late disease who has a positive ELISA, an IgG Western blot with zero or one band, and an IgM Western blot with two or three bands. This is likely a false-positive IgM Western blot test result.

A recent research advance in the diagnosis of Lyme disease involves the use of the polymerase chain reaction (PCR) to detect *B burgdorferi* DNA at sites of active infection (e.g., joint fluid) [43,44]. This test is not currently widely available. PCR testing of the urine has recently been the focus of intensive scientific evaluation. Studies reveal that while this testing may have some utility in monitoring the efficacy of treatment, it has not yet been appropriately validated and is not suitable for use as a stand-alone test in the diagnosis of Lyme disease [45–48].

TREATMENT

Determination of the appropriate treatment modality for an individual patient depends on a variety of factors, including the certainty of diagnosis and stage of illness. It is important to reassure patients that all stages of the disease are curable with antibiotics. The issue of chronic infection is controversial and is discussed below. It is recommended that the occupational medicine physician consult with specialists trained in infectious diseases if therapeutic modalities beyond initial treatment with oral antibiotics are required (e.g., patients refractory to oral antibiotics and/or late stage cases).

Early Infection

Early disease is typically treated with doxycycline, 100 mg twice daily for three to four weeks. Amoxicillin is preferred for pregnant or lactating women and young children.

Later Stages of the Disease

Later stages may, in some cases, be treated initially with oral doxycycline or amoxicillin. More serious or refractory illness may require treatment with a course of intravenous antibiotics such as penicillin or ceftriaxone.

Prevention

TICK CONTROL

Various methods have been utilized to minimize the density and distribution of vector ticks in the environment. The first and simplest method entails removing leaves, brush, and tall grasses around residences and gardens. This limits the possibility of human exposure to ticks. More active tick control methods have recently been investigated by the U.S. Department of Agriculture [49]. Investigators compared area-wide application of an acaricide (e.g., a "tick-toxic" substance such as permethrin) with acaricide self-application to mice (e.g., using permethrin-impregnated cotton that is used for nesting materials) and deer (e.g., via deer feeders that paint the deer with permethrin, as they stick their heads between two rollers to feed), vegetation reduction, and reducing the density of white-tailed deer populations. Their results indicate that area-wide acaricide application or vegetation reduction is most effective for short-term management of small recreational or residential sites. Acaricide self-application to deer appears to be the most cost-effective technology for the long-term management of large geographic areas.

PERSONAL PROTECTION

The CDC recommend [8] that individuals observe the following precautions prior to, during, and immediately after leaving a potentially tick-infested area:

- Avoid tick-infested areas, to the extent feasible, especially during the summer months.
- Wear light colored clothing so that ticks can be spotted more easily.
- Tuck pant legs into socks or boots and shirts into pants.
- Tape the area where pants and socks meet so that ticks cannot crawl under clothing.
- Spray insect repellent containing DEET on clothes and on exposed skin other than the face, or treat clothes (especially pants, socks, and shoes) with permethrin, which kills ticks on contact.
- Wear a hat and a long-sleeve shirt.
- Walk in the center of trails to avoid overhanging grass and brush.
- After being outdoors, remove clothing and wash and dry it at a high temperature.
- Inspect body carefully and remove attached ticks with tweezers, grasping the tick as close to the skin surface as possible and pulling straight back with a slow steady force to avoid crushing the tick's body.

It is unclear whether these measures actually decrease the risk of Lyme disease, but at least two studies not specifically designed to address the issue [19,21] concluded that preventive behaviors (e.g., protective clothing, insect repellents) appear to decrease the risk for infection by the spirochete.

VACCINATION

Considerable effort has recently been focused on the development of a Lyme disease vaccine. Two recent studies [50,51] investigated the efficacy of two similar vaccines utilizing injections of recombinant outer surface protein A (OspA) of the spirochete. In the investigation by Steere and colleagues, 10,936 individuals were randomly assigned to receive either the vaccine or an inactive placebo. The results revealed that three injections of the vaccine over a twelve-month period prevented most cases of Lyme disease or asymptomatic *B burgdorferi* infection, and had an acceptable rate of local or systemic side effects (e.g., self-limited soreness at injection site, mild flu-like symptoms). In a second randomized, placebo-controlled study of 10,305 subjects by Sigal and colleagues, the OspA vaccine also proved to be safe and effective in the prevention of Lyme disease.

Vaccine efficacy was noted to be between 49% (Steere et al.) and 62% (Sigal et al.) following administration of the first two injections, and increased to between 76% (Steere et al.) and 92% (Sigal et al.) following the third injection, at the end of 12 months. The vaccine evaluated in the study by Steere et al. developed by SmithKline Beecham, received approval by the Food and Drug Administration in December 1998. The second vaccine application is likely to be submitted by Pasteur Merieux Connaught in early 1999.

An accompanying editorial and subsequent published correspondence [52,53] emphasized that the vaccination of persons with frequent or prolonged exposure to tick habitats in areas where the disease is endemic is likely to be an important preventive strategy. The vaccine should not, however, be put into widespread use. The efficacy of the vaccines in children is yet to be established, as are the need for booster vaccinations and the duration of protection. Furthermore, whether vaccination is more cost effective than early diagnosis and treatment of Lyme disease has not been established. In addition, concerns have been raised that vaccination may cause individuals in high-risk areas to neglect personal protection efforts against tick bites. This could result in increased risk for infection by other tick-borne diseases (e.g., RMSF, HGE, babesiosis). Continuing analysis of the vaccine's benefit in populations at risk is recommended.

Controversies

PROPHYLACTIC ANTIBIOTICS FOR TICK BITE

There is often great pressure on the treating physician to provide antibiotics to a patient following a tick bite. While there is still controversy regarding the need for antibiotics in this situation [27,54,55], several factors should be taken into account when making this decision:

- Was the tick a vector tick (e.g., *Ixodes scapularis*) or a different species?
- Was the tick mobile when found, or was it attached to the skin (embedded)?
- How long was the tick likely to be embedded? Was the tick fully engorged? This is important because transmission of the spirochete typically occurs only after 24 to 48 hours of feeding.
- Was the tick acquired from an endemic area?

A reasonable approach may be to offer empiric antibiotics after a tick bite to patients who remove a highly engorged tick from an endemic area and who are very concerned about the development of Lyme disease, are not deemed reliable to follow-up if symptoms develop, or are at considerable risk of the disease does develop (e.g., pregnant women). If antibiotics are not prescribed, the physician should alert patients to the symptoms of early Lyme disease and advise them to return for re-evaluation if symptoms occur.

PATIENTS WITH FIBROMYALGIA, CHRONIC FATIGUE SYNDROME, AND OTHER ILLNESS ENTITIES CHARACTERIZED BY NONSPECIFIC SYMPTOMS

Fibromyalgia, chronic fatigue syndrome (CFS), and Lyme disease can share several overlapping clinical manifestations (e.g., fatigue, arthralgias, myalgias, sleep disturbances, and a perception of diminished mental function) and are often confused with one another [56].

Although fibromyalgia occurs occasionally as a sequel to Lyme disease, it is not an indication of persistent infection. Lyme disease is only one of many triggers for the development of fibromyalgia. In regard to CFS there is no convincing evidence that it can be "triggered" by pre-existing Lyme disease. Neither fibromyalgia nor CFS have clear etiologies. Medication regimens are therefore symptom-focused and include nonsteroidal anti-inflammatories as well as antidepressants. Antibiotics have not proved to be effective for the treatment of either of these two illnesses.

It is important to note that Lyme disease has received a good deal of attention in the lay press. There are a number of Lyme disease patient advocacy groups that perform a number of very beneficial services in public education and patient support. Unfortunately, some of these groups occasionally disseminate information without the proper context. Individuals with vague or nonspecific symptoms may depend on some of this information to diagnose themselves with Lyme disease. They may, for example, go on the Internet, get lists of symptoms associated with Lyme disease, identify one or two (e.g., fatigue, arthralgias), which they may have had at some point, and become convinced that they have Lyme disease.

The physician needs to keep in mind that improper diagnosis of patients with fibromyalgia, CFS, and other illness entities with nonspecific symptoms, can lead to a significant overdiagnosis of Lyme disease. Serologic testing and subsequent antibiotic treatment of patients should therefore be reserved for instances in which there is a strong suspicion of *B burgdorferi* infection, based upon exposure history, clinical signs, and symptoms [6,28–31,42].

"CHRONIC" LYME DISEASE

The late stages of Lyme disease were once referred to as *chronic Lyme disease*. This was a bit of a misnomer. All stages of Lyme disease are potentially curable. It should be emphasized that there is no convincing data to suggest that very long-duration antibiotic regimens are beneficial.

In some cases, individuals have been misclassified as having chronic Lyme disease because of persistently elevated antibody levels (which typically remain positive for years after the active infection has been cured), and have been treated with antibiotics for years on end. The treating physician needs to remember that the diagnosis and treatment of Lyme disease should be based primarily on clinical signs and symptoms. Laboratory test results should serve solely as an adjunct to the clinical determination.

ATYPICAL ANTIBIOTIC TREATMENT REGIMENS

Certain individual physicians and patient groups have advocated the use of alternative therapies for the treatment of Lyme disease. These include long-term (months or years) oral or intravenous antibiotics, pulse therapy (e.g., parenteral antibiotics once weekly), and iatrogenic induction of malaria. While standard antibiotic regimens are usually, although not universally, effective in curing disease and preventing progression [40], these alternative regimens have not been shown to be safe and efficacious. No clinical trials have determined the need for, or effectiveness of, courses longer than four weeks for any stage of Lyme disease [6].

PERSISTENT SYMPTOMS AFTER APPROPRIATE TREATMENT

Persistent symptoms after appropriate treatment are not uncommon. At all stages, symptom resolution may be slow and lag behind antibiotic therapy [6]. Self-limited nonspecific symptoms may persist for six months or more following treatment [42]. Persistent symptoms beyond this point may be due to permanent damage (e.g., following arthritis), incorrect initial diagnosis, and/or other concurrent illness (e.g., fibromyalgia, depression). Some have raised concerns about the possibility of resistant strains of *B burgdorferi* or the persistence of organisms in isolated foci [42].

Physicians caring for many Lyme disease patients have noted in a small group of patients (with indisputable Lyme disease) that a month of treatment is not curative. This failure may be due to poor compliance with an oral antibiotic regimen. Alternatively, in some patients with unrelieved joint pain and swelling following intravenous therapy, the finding of *B burgdorferi* DNA in joint fluids by PCR indicates that further antibiotic therapy may be beneficial. Those who do not have a positive PCR finding do not benefit from further treatment [56].

It should be re-emphasized however that in general, there is no convincing evidence that treatment regimens administered longer than one month are clinically prudent or beneficial.

Role of Occupational Health Professions and Future Advances in Prevention

During the last 20 years, Lyme disease has increased in incidence and has now become a social phenomenon as well. It is now the most common vector-borne disease in the United States. Much attention has been focused on Lyme disease by the media and various Lyme disease support groups. Therefore, it is more important than ever that physicians be familiar with the details of the epidemiology, clinical management, and controversial issues surrounding the disease. When evaluating patients with suspected *B burgdorferi* infection, testing and treatment decisions must balance sound medical science with the needs of the patient.

By virtue of outdoor work in endemic areas, many occupations are at an increased risk for tick exposure. Studies of occupational groups in outdoor settings indicate that *B burgdorferi* infection is clearly a hazard of outdoor work; the relative risk may be as high as sixfold. Simple preventive practices involving tick-control measures or personal precautions such as careful daily skin searching for ticks and possibly application of permethrin or DEET to clothing or skin, respectively, may decrease the risk of Lyme disease in high-risk workers. The very recent development of a vaccine provides promise of being an important new public health approach for the prevention of Lyme disease.

References

1. Steere AC, Malawista SE, Snydman DR, et al. Lyme arthritis: an epidemic of oligoarticular arthritis in children and adults in three Connecticut communities. *Arthritis Rheum* 1977;20(1):7–17.
2. Steere AC, Grodzicki RL, Kornblatt AN, et al. The spirochetal etiology of Lyme disease. *N Engl J Med* 1983;308(13):733–40.
3. Burgdorfer W, Barbour AG, Hayes SF, et al. Lyme disease—a tick-borne spirochetosis? *Science* 1982; 216(4552):1317–9.
4. Steere AC, Grodzicki RL, Kornblatt AN, et al. The spirochetal etiology of Lyme disease. *N Engl J Med* 1983;308(13):733–40.
5. Benach JL, Bosler EM, Hanrahan JP, et al. Spirochetes isolated from the blood of two patients with Lyme disease. *N Engl J Med* 1983;308(13):740–2.
6. Rahn DW, Malawista SE. Lyme disease. In: Koopman (ed), *Arthritis and Allied Conditions*, 13th Ed. Baltimore: Williams & Wilkins, 1997. Pp 2321–39.
7. Piesman J, Mather TN, Sinsky RJ, et al. Duration of tick attachment and *Borrelia burgdorferi* transmission. *J Clin Microbiol* 1987;25(3):557–8.
8. Centers for Disease Control and Prevention, Public Information Guide for Lyme Disease, available on Internet at *www.cdc.gov/ncidod/disease/lyme/lyme.htm*.
9. Zhioua E, Rodhain F, Binet P, et al. Prevalence of antibodies to *Borrelia burgdorferi* in forestry workers of Ile de France, France. *Eur J Epidemiol* 1997;13(8):959–62.
10. Rath PM, Ibershoff B, Mohnhaupt A, et al. Seroprevalence of Lyme borreliosis in forestry workers from Brandenburg, Germany. *Eur J Clin Microbiol Infect Dis* 1996;15(5):372–7.
11. Ahkee S, Ramirez J. A case of concurrent Lyme meningitis with ehrlichiosis. *Scand J Infect Dis* 1996; 28(5):527–8.
12. Ikushima M, Kawahashi S, Okuyama Y, et al. The survey of prevalence of Lyme borreliosis in forestry workers in Saitama prefecture. *Kansenshogaku Zasshi* 1995;69(2):139–44.
13. Nakama H, Muramatsu K, Uchikama K, et al. Possibility of Lyme disease as an occupational disease—seroepidemiological study of regional residents and forestry workers. *Asia Pac J Public Health* 1994;7(4):214–7.
14. Moll van Charante AW, Groen J, Osterhaus AD. Risk of infections transmitted by arthropods and rodents in forestry workers. *Eur J Epidemiol* 1994;10(3):349–51.
15. Rees DH, Axford JS. Evidence for Lyme disease in urban park workers: a potential new health hazard for city inhabitants. *Br J Rheumatol* 1994;33(2):123–8.
16. Schwartz BS, Goldstein MD, Childs JE. Longitudinal study of *Borrelia burgdorferi* infection in New Jersey outdoor workers, 1988–1991. *Am J Epidemiol* 1994; 139(5):504–12.
17. Nuti M, Amaddeo D, Crovatto M, et al. Infections in an Alpine environment: antibodies to hantaviruses, leptospira, rickettsiae, and *Borrelia burgdorferi* in defined Italian populations. *Am J Trop Med Hyg* 1993;48(1): 20–5.
18. Kuiper H, van Dam AP, Moll van Charante AW, et al. One year follow-up study to assess the prevalence and incidence of Lyme borreliosis among Dutch forestry workers. *Eur J Clin Microbiol Infect Dis* 1993;2(6): 413–8.
19. Parrott C, Johnson K, Strauss S, et al. Lyme disease in outdoor workers on Assateague Island: high tick-exposure but low disease risk. *MD Med J* 1993;42(2):165–8.
20. Kuiper H, de Jongh BM, Nauta AP, et al. Lyme borreliosis in Dutch forestry workers. *J Infect* 1991;23(3):279–86.
21. Schwartz BS, Goldstein MD. Lyme disease in outdoor workers: risk factors, preventive measures, and tick removal methods [see comments]. *Am J Epidemiol* 1990;131(5):877–85.
22. Rath PM, Ibershoff B, Mohnhaupt A, et al. Seroprevalence of Lyme borreliosis in forestry workers from Brandenburg, Germany. *Eur J Clin Microbiol Infect Dis* 1996;15(5):372–7.

23. Habif TP. *Clinical Dermatology*, 3rd Ed. St. Louis Mosby Year Book, 1996. Pp 464–72.
24. Reik L, Steere AC, Bartenhagen NH, et al. Neurologic abnormalities of Lyme disease. *Medicine (Baltimore)* 1979;58(4):281–94.
25. Luft BJ, Dattwyler RJ. Lyme borreliosis. *Curr Clin Top Infect Dis* 1989;10:56–81.
26. Duffy J. Lyme disease. *Infect Dis Clin North Am* 1987;1(3):511–27.
27. Weil HFC, et al. Lyme disease. In: Reese RE, Betts RF (eds), *Practical Approach to Infectious Diseases*, 4th Ed. Baltimore: Lippincott-Raven, 1996. Pp 878–902.
28. Sigal LH. Summary of the first 100 patients seen at a Lyme disease referral center. *Am J Med* 1990;88 (6):577–81.
29. Dinerman H, Steere AC. Fibromyalgia following Lyme disease: association with neurologic involvement and lack of response to antibiotic therapy [abstract]. *Arthritis Rheum* 1990;33(Suppl):S136.
30. Steere AC, Taylor E, McHugh GL, et al. The overdiagnosis of Lyme disease *JAMA* 1993;269 (14):1812–6.
31. Hsu VM, Patella SJ, Sigal LH. "Chronic Lyme disease" as the incorrect diagnosis in patients with fibromyalgia [see comments]. *Arthritis Rheum* 1993;36(11):1493–500.
32. Carey CS, Lee HH, Woeltje KS (eds). *Washington University Manual of Medical Therapeutics*, 29th Ed. Philadelphia: Lippincott-Raven, 1998.
33. Fritz CL, Glaser CA. Ehrlichiosis. *Infect Dis Clin North Am* 1998;12(1):122–36.
34. American Academy of Pediatrics. *AAP 1997 Red Book: Report of the Committee on Infectious Diseases*, 24th Ed. 1997. Pp 146–7.
35. Steere AC, Malawista SE, Bartenhagen NH, et al. The clinical spectrum and treatment of Lyme disease. *Yale J Biol Med* 1984;57(4):453–64.
36. Steere AC, Bartenhagen NH, Craft JE, et al. The early clinical manifestations of Lyme disease. *Ann Intern Med* 1983;99(1):76–82.
37. Steere AC. Lyme disease [see comments]. *N Engl J Med* 1989;321(9):586–96.
38. Nadelman RB, Nowakowski J, Forseter G, et al. Failure to isolate *Borrelia burgdorferi* after antimicrobial therapy in culture-documented Lyme borreliosis associated with erythema migrans: report of a prospective study. *Am J Med* 1993;94(6):583–8.
39. Schwartz BS, Goldstein MD, Ribeiro JM, et al. Antibody testing in Lyme disease. A comparison of results in four laboratories [see comments]. *JAMA* 1989;262 (24):3431–4.
40. Luger SW, Krauss E. Serologic tests for Lyme disease. Interlaboratory variability [see comments]. *Arch Intern Med* 1990;150(4):761–3.
41. Magnarelli LA, Miller JN, Anderson JF, et al. Cross-reactivity of nonspecific treponemal antibody in serologic tests for Lyme disease. *J Clin Microbiol* 1990;28 (6):1276–9.
42. Sigal LH. Pitfalls in the diagnosis and management of Lyme disease. *Rheumatology* 1998;41(2):195–204.
43. Nocton JJ, Dressler F, Rutledge BJ, et al. Detection of *Borrelia burgdorferi* DNA by polymerase chain reaction in synovial fluid from patients with Lyme arthritis [see comments]. *N Engl J Med* 1994;330(4):229–34.
44. Keller TL, Halperin JJ, Whitman M. PCR detection of *Borrelia burgdorferi* DNA in cerebrospinal fluid of Lyme neuroborreliosis patients [see comments]. *Neurology* 1992;42(1):32–42.
45. Brettschneider S, Bruckbauer H, Klugbauer N, et al. Diagnostic value of PCR for detection of *Borrelia burgdorferi* in skin biopsy and urine samples from patients with skin borreliosis. *J Clin Microbiol* 1998;36 (9):2658–65.
46. Mercier G, Burckel A, Lucotte G. Detection of *Borrelia burgdorferi* DNA by polymerase chain reaction in urine specimens of patients with erythema migrans lesions. *Cell Probes* 1997;11(2):89–94.
47. Bayer ME, Zhang L, Bayer MH. *Borrelia burgdorferi* DNA in the urine of treated patients with chronic Lyme disease symptoms: a PCR study of 97 cases. *Infection* 1996;24(5):347–53.
48. Schmidt B, Muellegger RR, Stockenhuber C, et al. Detection of *Borrelia burgdorferi*-specific DNA in urine specimens from patients with erythema migrans before and after antibiotic therapy. *J Clin Microbiol* 1996;34 (6):1359–63.
49. Mount GA, Haile DG, Daniels E. Simulation of management strategies for the blacklegged tick (Acari: Ixodidae) and the Lyme disease spirochete, *Borrelia burgdorferi*. *J Med Entomol* 1997;34(6):672–83.
50. Steere AC, Sikand VK, Meurice F, et al. Vaccination against Lyme disease with recombinant *Borrelia burgdorferi* outer-surface lipoprotein A with adjuvant. Lyme Disease Vaccine Study Group [see comments]. *N Engl J Med* 1998;339(4):209–15.
51. Sigal LH, Zahradnik JM, Lavin P, et al. A vaccine consisting of recombinant *Borrelia burgdorferi* outer-surface protein A to prevent Lyme disease. Recombinant Outer-Surface Protein A Lyme Disease Vaccine Study Consortium [see comments] [published erratum appears in *N Engl J Med* 1998;339(8):571]. *N Engl J Med* 1998;339 (4):216–22.
52. Steigbigel RT, Benach JL. Immunization against Lyme disease—an important first step [editorial; comment]. *N Engl J Med* 1998;339(4):263–4.
53. Correspondence. Immunization against Lyme disease [letters]. *N Engl J Med* 1998;339(22):1637–9.
54. Magid D, Schwartz B, Craft J, et al. Prevention of Lyme disease after tick bites. A cost-effectiveness analysis [see comments]. *N Engl J Med* 1992;327(8):534–41.
55. Medical Letter. Treatment of Lyme disease. *Med Lett Drugs Ther* 1992;34:95–7.
56. Barbour AG. *Lyme Disease: The Cause, the Cure, the Controversy*. Baltimore: Johns Hopkins University Press, 1996. Pp. 172–3.

27 / Viral Travel-Related Infections

Eric P. Wohlrab

Travel is booming, and there is no sign of a slowdown. It is estimated that well over one billion people travel by air yearly. International travel is also increasingly common and now a way of life for thousands of workers. The speed and penetration of various forms of travel are fueling the geometric increases in the total volume of worldwide travelers. While the global economy is expanding, the geographic world seems to be shrinking. Even exotic travel locations are within easy reach. Diminishing economic and political barriers are bringing civilizations closer and opening new frontiers for corporate development and profit.

The exploration of every new horizon presents additional challenges and associated risks. Among the medical challenges in this new global village are the emergence and re-emergence of infectious diseases and the need to protect travelers and workers from infectious agents and environmental risks [1]. Complicating this medical challenge is the recent failure of the worldwide public health infrastructure to check the spread of some common and exotic infectious diseases [2,3]. In the United States alone, the temporary resurgence of tuberculosis (TB) in the early 90s is now attributed not only to an increasing number of immunocompromised hosts, but also to loss of public health funding and professional complacency in several state-run TB programs. As we enter the twenty-first century, we still see infectious diseases accounting for 33% of the mortality throughout the world [4]. Nature does not stand still. Since the eradication of smallpox, over 30 new infectious diseases have arisen globally to plague man and beast. For humans, these new illnesses include Ebola, *Hantavirus,* and AIDS/HIV to name only a few [4,5].

Infected travelers and resistant microorganisms can now span the continents in just hours. Travel-related infection could potentially include the whole range of known and, as of yet, undiscovered human pathogens. Travelers can return home from distant parts of the world within the incubation period of every known infectious disease.

The risk of acquiring travel-related infections depends as much on the behavior of the traveler as on the itinerary of the trip. To ascertain the true health risks to travelers and to interrupt the possible adverse health sequelae, the clinician must know many things about individual travelers and their trips and understand the classic public health approach of reviewing the triad of agent, host, and environment [6,7].

This chapter addresses the health concerns of people who travel for business and those whom the traveler contacts. It focuses on the occupational aspects of viral-related diseases and on relevant strategies for prevention.

Epidemiology

Proper consideration of travel-related risks of infection includes:

- Knowledge of the traveler's personal health history.
- Purpose of travel.
- Duration of travel.
- Final destination and in-route stops.
- Mode of travel.
- Local endemic conditions.

In addition, the analysis of travel-related disease risk requires a careful review of the classic epidemiologic triad of agent, host, and environment.

Occupational infections are human diseases (host factors) that are caused by work (environmental factors) associated with exposure to various biologically active agents (agent factors). Occupational infection can result from person-to-person contact by infectious individuals, as in health care workers; with infected animal or human tissue or bodily fluids as in laboratory workers; with unknown or asymptomatic contagious individuals or other agents as in travel; or with infected animals as in agriculture [8].

INCIDENCE AND PREVALENCE

Infectious disease has no respect for international boundaries. The continuing worldwide outbreaks of infectious disease have clearly supported the 1992 Institute of Medicine Report on the increasing frequency of emerging infection [4]. Compound these outbreaks with the threats of biologic weapons by rogue nations or terrorist groups, and the risk of infectious disease for the international traveler is more than theoretical. Although exact statistics on the number of new or existing viral illnesses are seldom available for calculation of true incidence and prevalence rates, several countries do measure and track trends in the number of new or outbreak cases reported. It has been estimated that 55 million patients suffer some travel-related illness every time they travel [9,10]. Several international efforts are under way to intensify efforts systematically in the surveillance and control of emerging infectious diseases worldwide. The World Health Organization, based on a mandate by its 190 member states, is developing a strategy, in collaboration with the CDC, to strengthen and coordinate its response to global emerging disease [6].

Despite a less than robust global surveillance system, there is usually enough health information available to determine if certain infectious agents are present at endemic versus epidemic levels in most regions of the world. The CDC Yellow Book, *Travel for the International Traveler*, which is available in paperback and on the Internet, contains pertinent information on the major health risks for travelers around the globe. This text is a core resource for any occupational medicine practice that provides travel medicine services.

Over 400 distinct viruses infect humans [11]. They produce diseases ranging from subclinical and mild self-limiting infections to common systemic infections and overwhelming, highly lethal infections such as meningoencephalitis or hemorrhagic fever with shock. An in-depth review of all viral associated diseases is beyond the scope of this chapter. However, the more prevalent and problematic viral travel-associated diseases warrant special discussion. These select viral diseases (Table 27-1) are presented on the basis of their three primary modes of transmission: person to person, arthropod vector to person, and animal to person (zoonoses).

TRANSMISSION RISK FACTORS

The etiology, pathogenesis, clinical picture, diagnosis, and treatment of occupational and nonoccupational illness are, for all practical purposes, the same, but the epidemiology, control, and prevention of occupational illnesses are frequently more complex. Water purification, waste sanitation, food preparation, vector control, recreational activities, and personal hygiene of the traveler strongly influence exposure and health risk. The risks associated with international travel vary with the locations visited, the duration of the trip, and the traveler's age, health, and activities while abroad. In general, travelers going to Australia, Canada, Western Europe, Japan, New Zealand, and the United States require no special prophylactic measures. In contrast, visitors to developing areas may be exposed to serious and sometimes life-threatening infections.

Viruses produce cell injury by a number of different mechanisms [11,12]. They can directly lyse cells by viral replication, by induced antiviral antibody and complement, or by cell-mediated immune mechanisms that recognize infected host cells. As virus infection spreads and sufficient numbers of cells are injured, disease results. Additionally, products of inflammation, released from sites of cell injury, and circulating interferon and other lymphokines may contribute to the signs and symptoms of viral infections. A second mode of injury occurs when a viral infection transforms the cell, causing it to proliferate continuously and form tumors, sometimes as a result of the presence of viral oncogenes in the virus.

Table 27-1
Modes of Transmission of Viral Diseases

Person to Person	Arthropod to Person (Arboviral)	Animal to Person (Zoonotic)
Ebola-Marburg	Crimean-Congo	Hantavirus
Hepatitis A	California encephalitis	Rabies
Hepatitis B	Dengue	
Hepatitis C, D, E	Eastern equine	
Herpes simplex	Japanese B	
HIV	Powassan encephalitis	
Influenza	St. Louis encephalitis	
MMR	Western equine	
Poliomyelitis	Yellow fever	

In addition to nonspecific barriers like skin, respiratory epithelium, and gastric acidity, three main host-defense mechanisms combat most viral infections: (1) the production of specific antiviral antibody, (2) the development of specific cell-mediated immunity involving cytotoxic T cells and the nonspecific effector cells like natural killer (NK) cells, and (3) the proliferation of macrophages that restrict virus replication and dissemination and also destroy infected cells.

The typical viral infection is initiated when one or a very few number of virus particles are deposited in the respiratory, gastrointestinal, or genitourinary tract, or are injected percutaneously. Human viral infections may be classified according to mechanisms of pathogenesis. Many infections are limited to cells at the portal of entry, and thus dissemination does not occur. An example is adenovirus type 8 for conjunctivitis and several respiratory viruses. Other viruses, such as echoviruses and aseptic meningitis, spread hematogenously to distal sites. In other infections, viral replication in the secondary site produces a viremia that results in replication in still other sites. This happens with smallpox and measles. In these circumstances, rash may be a manifestation of primary or secondary viremia. Recent advances in antiviral chemotherapy have produced a number of specific antivirals that are effective for prophylaxis and treatment of certain viral diseases. Drugs such as trifluridine, amantadine, ribavirin, acyclovir, and interferon-alpha are available for use in the United States. The recent addition of a new class of protease inhibitors has shown significant results in treating and delaying the onset of symptomatic and asymptomatic HIV infection.

Explicit connections between climatic events and disease risk can be made in many instances, but in most areas, far more evaluation needs to be done. In the United States, for example, several scientists dispute whether climatic changes will result in the higher incidence of dengue fever in the Southwest. Independent of changing weather patterns, the Southwest has a solid health infrastructure that includes good sanitation with air-conditioned and screen-protected homes and workplaces. So factors that increase potential risk do not necessarily translate into increased cases.

OCCUPATIONAL RISK FACTORS

Travelers come in all sizes and itineraries, and travel activities usually fall into two main types: leisure or business. There is no typical traveler, but some general characteristics of the traveler, the route traveled, and the potential risks are fairly well understood. The archetypal traveler is male and in his early 40s. In business or occupational travel, the usual duration is one to three weeks. Frequently, overseas travel is for a more extended period. The business traveler usually has time to prepare for travel. The traveler generally chooses destination, mode of travel, and departure times, and typically stays in above-average accommodations. Often, travel is rapid, and travelers journey for long stretches with multiple stops. Frequently, leisure elements are combined with business, which may increase exposure to additional agent or environmental threats [8]. All these variables should be considered in determining the viral health risks. Travelers to developing countries should obtain advice on the ever-changing international health requirements and the epidemiology of diseases abroad. Detailed information on specific geographic areas can be obtained from the Centers for Disease Control and Prevention (CDC) through its publications or by calling the CDC International Travelers Hotline, 888-232-3299. The same information is also available via the Internet web site at *http://www.cdc.gov/travel/index.htm*. Different travel itineraries require varying kinds of travel advice.

Prevention and Control

Prevention is the key to effectively dealing with infectious disease. Infectious disease results from the interactions between factors associated with the host, agent, and environment. There are therefore several different components to an effective prevention program. Immunizations, personal protection, and engineering barriers to prevent exposure are just a few of the methods utilized to prevent viral exposure and infection. Methods of control attempt to modify these factors and ultimately depend on the epidemiology of each disease.

ADMINISTRATIVE CONTROLS

Controls on behavior in the workplace are primarily divided into two kinds: administrative and work practice. Administrative controls include rules and regulations, sometimes called *standard operating procedures (SOP)*, that prohibit smoking or eating in prohibited areas or the scheduling of high hazard activities when few workers are present. Almost all industry restricts those workers who do not have the proper training from working in areas where health and safety hazards exist. In a similar vein, SOPs that guide or control travelers' behavior during their journey are just as important in minimizing associated health risks. Unfortunately, individual travel histories and related health and medical histories are often neglected prior to travel. Depending on travel circumstances, administrative oversight can play a pivotal role in preventing or controlling viral diseases. A travel history that includes health status and immunization history should be reviewed and considered before travel commences. "Shot" records should be a mandatory item for all travelers. Ideally, this form of administrative SOP would be used to track who traveled when, where they went, and how well they medically tolerated the journey. Travelers with a history of irritable bowel symptoms, for instance, who had previously demonstrated poor tolerance when traveling to developing countries could selectively be restricted or at least advised and educated to use extreme caution when consuming the local cuisine.

SAFE WORK PRACTICES AND ENGINEERING CONTROLS

Engineering controls are the primary technique used to factor out the human element in most high-risk work practices in industry [7,8]. Worker awareness, education, and training are part of every basic in-house safety program required by OSHA. Yet despite intensive, reward-based safety programs, which may also use other incentives, accidents still happen. The safety industry has long recognized the importance of taking the man out of the loop in order to reduce accidents. While behavior research continues to find additional ways to motivate employees to remain safe in the workplace, it is frequently more cost effective to change the work practice rather than change the worker. Education, training, and supervision form the backbone of all workplace safety programs.

Education on the presence and avoidance of travel hazards, in conjunction with training on the desired practices, is necessary for workers to remain safe while traveling. Supervision is an important part of any industrial operation, but it is difficult to enforce compliance with company SOP when a business person is traveling. Whenever several travelers are together, one of the group should act as supervisor to enforce compliance with proper, safe work practices.

Historically, business travel involved face-to-face meetings to negotiate and close deals. Interestingly, the cyber age has provided an important alternative. The advent of the video teleconference (VTC) now allows business representatives to meet face to face in the comfort and safety of their own offices. Gone are the many inconveniences and health risks associated with international travel. From an epidemiologic perspective, the two largest risk factors associated with the leading causes of morbidity and mortality for travelers, cardiac events and motor vehicle accidents, can now be circumvented. The contribution that travel, beyond the daily commute, contributes to motor vehicle accidents and cardiac events can potentially now be eliminated. Even the mundane common-cold cycle can be short-circuited if business people no longer have to shake hands. The person-to-person spread of coronaviruses and echoviruses, primary harbingers of the common cold and the most common cause of worker absenteeism, can be completely avoided if there is no personal contact. Therefore, a company that historically has a high percentage of its lost work time related to travel injury or illness could consider utilizing VTCs as an administrative or engineering solution to their problem of lost workdays.

For those who do need to travel, the value of soap and water to combat the spread of infectious disease must not be underestimated. Especially viruses that are spread person to person can frequently be halted with good personal hygiene. Universal Precautions are a vital part of any successful hospital infection-control program. The proven effectiveness of hand washing in the clinical setting reinforces a significant work practice for the traveler as well. While it may be inappropriate to shake hands with latex gloves on, given the local customs of the country visited, attention to personal hygiene should never be compromised. Needless to say, the strongest warning and education to use full preventive measures should always be given to any traveler who decides to engage in any sexual activity abroad [13,14]. HIV and several hepatitis viruses are preventable if proper precautions are utilized. Abstinence is 100% effective in preventing the sexual transmission of infectious disease. While a "moral" approach may provide some additional educational benefit to enhance the traveler's knowledge of virally spread sexual disease, morality rarely works as well as a candid discussion and a condom.

PERSONAL PROTECTIVE EQUIPMENT

It is difficult to ensure that personal protective equipment (PPE) is both used and effective. In the industrial setting, the use of PPE is less desirable than engineering approaches in maintaining an effective illness and injury control program in the workplace. In the classic workplace, PPEs are used when the remaining hazardous worksites cannot be reengineered, because of high capital expenditure costs, for instance, or when further product substitution considerations are completely exhausted [8]. In the case of preventing and controlling travel-associated viral diseases, the use of PPE should be considered an essential first line of defense for all travelers, especially those who travel to developing countries. Secondary to immunizations, the use of PPE assumes a much greater importance for the business traveler than for the occupational worker in a factory. Although the company may exercise direct oversight of the assembly line worker for an eight- to 12-hour shift, the business traveler may be exposed for 24 hours a day to numerous health threats. Supervisory control over the host in a travel situation is very difficult. It is a daunting challenge to actively change the health risks posed by the agents or the environment in the 24-hour travel process. The critical importance of the proper use of PPE cannot be overstated when it comes to adding another potential barrier between the traveler and many infectious viral diseases.

Lessons learned about the effective use of PPE to prevent disease from infectious agents by the United States' and other nations' military forces during worldwide deployment are worth reviewing. Initially, geographic areas at risk of arbovirus or zoonotic diseases, such as Eastern Europe and Asia, are evaluated for endemnicity of disease. Once the local level of the threats is known, the proper countermeasures to protect the military traveler from the potential health threats are developed. While protective immunizations are used in several deployment scenarios, PPE always plays a leading role for isolating military personnel from many of the local health threats.

The principal approach to prevention of vector-borne diseases is avoidance. Wearing long-sleeve shirts, long pants, and hats minimizes exposed skin to arthropod attack. In addition, insect repellents can be applied to clothing, shoes, tents, mosquito nets, and other personal gear as needed. For years, the military has effectively utilized uniforms treated with insect repellents to ward off the bite of disease-carrying mosquitoes and ticks. Insect repellents should contain no more than a 30% concentration of DEET (diethyltoluamide). An accepted technique is to place travel clothing in a large plastic bag, add the insecticide to the bag, and then shake the contents for proper mixing. Permethrin-containing repellents (e.g., Permanone) may also be applied to clothing and bed nets. It is less toxic than DEET and usually lasts through several washings. Perhaps most importantly, all at-risk military personnel are given personal mosquito netting to isolate themselves from the vector before it can attack or bite its victim. As with all PPE, proper instruction and supervision in the use of the equipment is essential for its effective use.

EMPLOYEE EDUCATION AND TRAINING

Employee education, training, supervision, and now incentives compose the backbone of industrial prevention and control programs. The prudent employer should provide all employees with adequate training to warn them of hazards that are unique to their jobs. Various OSHA ACT standards require the employer to make sure that workers understand appropriate precautions. Specialized training is conducted for the proper use of the Material Safety Data Sheets (MSDS) and for those who operate special conveyances, such as forklifts, cranes, and power presses.

In the travel setting, a solid education program is even more critical. The majority of the more serious viral travel-related infectious diseases can be prevented by avoidance and good personal hygiene [15]. This is especially true for the prevention of sexually transmitted diseases (STDs) [14]. After an initial reluctance of employers to discuss STDs in the workplace, most companies now have an active education and nondiscrimination program. Despite these efforts, there is still widespread misunderstanding of the methods of HIV transmission. The transmission of HIV or hepatitis B in a travel environment is most directly related to inappropriate or unprotected sexual contact, exposure to blood products, or trauma [16]. For the unimmunized traveler, potential exposure to hepatitis should be treated with hepatitis B immune globulin and the appropriate hepatitis B vaccine. The schedule and dosage of administration vary, depending on the traveler's vaccination status and source of infectivity.

MEDICAL SURVEILLANCE

Effective control of infectious disease depends on the detailed knowledge of its epidemiology and an accurate assessment of its occurrence. These details are usually obtained through public health surveillance.

The term *surveillance* suggests merely the observation of occurrences, but feedback is just as important to a successful prevention program. Feedback encourages the cooperation of the reporting individuals and imparts important health information that may be helpful for the traveler. In the United States, the reporting of notifiable infectious disease to state health departments takes place on a weekly basis. These departments then consolidate the information and forward it to the CDC. The individual practitioner can read the consolidated report in the CDC publication *Morbidity and Mortality Weekly Report (MMWR)*. On the international level, WHO publishes the *Weekly Epidemiological Record* from all countries that have reporting mechanisms. The WHO strategy uses the existing international health infrastructure as a base to improve global surveillance, enhance the capacity of local and national health laboratories, foster applied research to address practical problems, and improve infectious disease prevention and control. WHO has a worldwide network of collaborating centers that assist in surveillance to recognize outbreaks and emerging infectious disease problems. Some of the specific targets that have been identified for early action are influenza and exotic viral diseases. The influenza network has more than 200 laboratories worldwide. These labs isolate and characterize influenza viruses in circulation and forward them to one of three WHO centers (located in Atlanta, Melbourne, and London), where the isolates are characterized genetically and antigenetically. Then, on a yearly schedule, a representative of the three centers meets in Geneva to decide on the composition of the influenza vaccine. This system has proved to be quite effective in matching the vaccine to the influenza strains in circulation that year. WHO has a network of 36 laboratories in 27 countries specializing in the surveillance of emerging viral infectious diseases from arboviruses and hemorrhagic fever viruses like *Hantavirus* and Ebola virus, respectively [6]. This system is still being developed and is not as sophisticated as the global influenza surveillance program.

BIOLOGIC TESTING

Classic biologic monitoring measures a chemical, its metabolite, a reaction product, or a biochemical effect in some suitable media (e.g., blood, urine, exhaled air). Although there are over 100 different chemicals that can be estimated in an individual by measuring the chemical in the blood, air, or urine, an infectious viral body burden is seldom measured by the same approach. Usually, baseline and postexposure biologic monitoring for possible exposure to infectious viruses compose an integral part of the specific (e.g., hepatitis, HIV, rubella) viral serologic testing program [17].

Before any biologic monitoring program is instituted, some scientific and practical issues should be considered. The program should be able to produce results that are meaningful and cost effective and are able to reduce the traveler's adverse health effects from the virus exposure. Ethical and social aspects should also be considered. Monitoring of test results should be kept confidential; workers should be encouraged to respect other's privacy; and participation in the monitoring program should be voluntary.

General biologic testing parameters for any monitoring program should include an analysis of the timing of the collection, the body site sampled, and the selection of a competent laboratory for testing. In performing biologic measuring for viruses, the timing of the collection is variable and should be based on the incubation periods of the suspected viral pathogen. The postexposure evaluation is also quite variable and should follow the same guidelines as outlined earlier in the epidemiologic consideration section.

Historically, more attention has been given to preparing travelers for their journey rather than to following up their exposure risks after the return home. The longer the stay away, especially overseas, the greater the need to establish a plan for the health evaluation and care for the returnee. Travelers who have resided for a month or more overseas should have a reentry heath evaluation [18,19]. A good history, with a concentration on any symptoms of fever or illness, should be elicited. The use of any over-the-counter medications, injections, or trauma requiring sutures is also an important consideration. Even possible exposure to endemic pathogens or vectors should be included in the standard post-travel health care evaluation.

Several simple laboratory tests should also be considered for medically screening the returning traveler. Once again, a threat-based approach should be utilized. Considerations should include location and length of travel as well as the presence and exposure to prevalent viral pathogens.

Interesting recent studies suggest that the efficacy of screening returning travelers for nonspecific viral infections, even those symptomatic for fever, to confirm a viral-specific diagnosis may be of little value. In a 1995 study of 195 international travelers returning to London with fever, Doherty and colleagues concluded that the routine serology is unhelpful in the investigation of patients with acute imported fever [20]. On the other hand, serologic testing for "specific viral" infections like hepatitis A, via IgM antibodies, and the dengue fever flaviviruses were indicated, based upon the travel factors reviewed in the history [21].

IMMUNIZATION AND PROPHYLACTIC MEASURES

Immunization provides classic primary prevention, and establishing immunity to infectious disease is one of the most important components of preparing the traveler for international travel [9,11,22,23]. A planned business trip provides an excellent opportunity to update adult immunizations. Selecting the right immunizations before travel can be challenging. Every business traveler should be current on their primary and booster vaccinations and also receive those immunizations that are unique to their travel requirements. Such routine immunizations include:

- Diphtheria.
- Measles.
- Mumps.
- Polio.
- Rubella.
- Tetanus.

It is important to minimize the risk of even mild illness in a travel environment. Not feeling well has a major impact on productivity and job efficiency in all workplaces, but the deleterious effect is often compounded in overseas travel because time zone changes may impart additional physiologic stress.

Immunization is not a replacement for other forms of primary prevention, including prudent behavior. A recent survey of more than 3,000 Swiss travelers who sought travel advice from the Swiss Tropical Institute Travel Clinic reported that 50% engaged in casual sex abroad with a partner from the host country. Even though the travelers shared a good knowledge base about the risks of HIV and other sexually transmitted diseases, 38% admitted to unprotected sex [16]. By contrast, in many situations, the traveler may not be able to avoid the risks associated with the activities of daily living in the temporary location. Travel to a developing country, for a long-term stay, especially in a rural location, with possible intimate human or wild animal contact is just one of the modifiers that place the traveler at an increased risk of infectious disease. Medical personnel, teachers, volunteers, and clergy are some of the high-risk occupations that should receive mandatory vaccinations before travel.

The kind and frequency of immunizations given are based on the risk of exposure during travel (Table 27-2). Risks vary from region to region of the world and with the presence or absence of epidemics or significant endemicity of disease. The decision to immunize depends on balancing the risk of acquiring the disease in question with the efficacy, cost, and complications of the vaccine.

Preparations are available for protection against measles, mumps, rubella, smallpox, yellow fever, rabies, hepatitis A, hepatitis B, and influenza [15,23]. Additionally, unlicensed and experimental vaccines are available from the CDC for some of the arthropod-borne viruses [24,25].

Passive immunization with immunoglobulin continues to play an important role in immunotherapy. The risk of reactions to human immune globulin (HIG) preparations is negligible, compared to the old pooled horse immunoglobulin. In many developing countries, however, the costs of HIG is prohibitive, and older animal immune globulin is sometimes used. The traveler is cautioned to check the source of any injectable vaccine while traveling in developing countries.

Preparations of gamma globulin specific for hepatitis B, rabies, and varicella-zoster viruses are used following potential exposure to the organism. Finding a supply of this immune globulin may be very difficult in the rural areas of developing countries [11]. Specific regimens for the administration of this immune globulin are covered in subsequent sections of this chapter.

Compliance with the use of the recommended routine, basic and geographically unique vaccines is critical to the success of an effective viral-disease prevention program. While protective netting, repellents, and hazard avoidance are mainstays of prevention, they are not totally effective [26,27]. Therefore, the proper tracking of each traveler's health and immunization record should remain current to ensure a comprehensive prevention program. Anyone who has ever planned or taken part in international travel can attest to the ongoing necessity of frequent monitoring for changing conditions. Unusual things may happen at any moment. Even the best-laid plans require some flexibility to meet the changing needs of the situation at hand. Proper planning for any travel scenario is an ongoing challenge.

Table 28-2
Geographically Important Immunizations for Unvaccinated Adults

Vaccine	Dose Schedule	Indications
Hepatitis A	1.0 mL at 0, 6–12 months	Travel to endemic areas
Hepatitis B	1.0 mL at 0, 1, and 12 months	Travel to endemic areas
Influenza	Annually	High-risk patients; travel to endemic areas
Japanese B encephalitis	3 doses, 1.0 mL subcutaneously, 1-week intervals	Residence or work in endemic areas
Rabies	0.1 mL intradermally days 0, 7, 28 or 1.0 mL tramuscularly days 0, 7, 28; booster every 2 years	Residence or work in areas endemic for animal rabies
Yellow fever	0.5 mL subcutaneously, booster every 10 years	Travel to endemic areas of Africa, South and Central America

METRICS TO ASSESS ADEQUACY OF PREVENTIVE MEASURES

The use of outcome data to measure the effectiveness of therapeutic variables has become more common in the practice of medicine. This focus on the *science* behind the treatment has become the engine of several clinical pathways and guidelines applied to mainstream clinical care delivery. Although the decision tree used to arrive at useful outcome data in complicated internal medicine cases can be very complex, its use to measure the positive benefit in primary prevention activity is more direct. In most travel scenarios, the viral-disease medical end game is simple—to record that no infectious morbidity or mortality resulted from the travel. The occurrence of any viral disease, posttravel, can ultimately be traced to a breakdown of prevention and control of the host-agent-environment interactive cycle [28].

Before any preventive program metric is developed, it should reflect the ultimate strategic vision or outcome desired by either the external customer employer or by the internal customer medical clinic. Few clinics or companies have the time or information system to collect data that does not provide a return on program effectiveness. The prudent metric program should track only those outcomes that have true clinical or administrative significance.

Metrics to assess the adequacy of prevention programs should be derived from looking at outcomes associated with the breakdown of any of the three elements of the epidemiologic triangle: agent, host, and environment. The actual metrics chosen should be able to measure the value of the prevention program for the individual, the company, or the travel clinic.

Any occupational or medical clinic that supports frequent international travel operations should develop metrics to ensure they have some outcome statistics to market the effectiveness of their preventive care [29]. The use of outcome data will command the respect and earn the loyalty of any company that benefits from a comprehensive prevention program.

Suggested metrics to measure the adequacy of host protection include items such as the following:

- Ensuring 100% currency on basic and geographically unique vaccines for all travelers.
- Documentation of 100% training on the local hazardous health risks before travel.
- Evidence of 100% education on the use of PPE.
- Documenting responsible behavior associated with the travel.

Suggested metrics for measuring the preventive adequacy of agent intervention include:

- Issuance of mosquito netting for all travelers (100%).
- Documentation of the use of insect repellents.

Environmental metrics to measure the adequacy of disease protection could include:

- Geographic review of 100% of pretravel viral health risks.
- Avoiding countries or locales with epidemic levels of disease transmission.

Whatever metrics are chosen, they should be germane to the focus of the prevention program and be measurable and remediable.

Symptoms and Signs

While it is beyond the scope of this chapter to review the over 400 hundred viruses that produce disease in humans, the majority of common and exotic viral travel-related diseases produce similar signs and symptoms on initial presentation. Fever, malaise, and myalgia are the frequent prodromal symptoms of any infectious disease process. These signs and symptoms may vary in intensity and duration, depending on the offending pathogen. Likewise, the development of sequelae, be they self-limiting or more fulminate, is directly dependent on the variability of the host and agent interaction.

The incubation period of significant travel-related viral diseases is quite diverse. Influenza can manifest symptoms in as little as 24 hours, while the classic symptoms of hepatitis B may take 45–180 days. Several other strains of viruses have variable incubation periods—from a few to several days for arboviruses to four to six weeks for the EBV in infectious mononucleosis.

A convenient way to review the significant viral infections that present important health risks to the traveler is to study the diseases by their primary mode of transmission, person to person, arboviral, or zoonotic. This approach allows for consideration of the efficient and efficacious use of resources to interrupt the agent-host-environment infection cycle.

PERSON-TO-PERSON ACUTE VIRAL RHINITIS

The common cold virus, also known as an upper respiratory infection (URI), is the most frequent cause of viral disease in humans and the single most common cause of absenteeism from work or school. Although typically self-limiting, the cold virus can significantly impact business travel with its bothersome symptoms. Rhinoviruses and coronaviruses cause 50% and 15%, respectively, of the colds in adults. With an incubation period of 12–48 hours, colds are readily passed from person to person, especially in a crowded setting. Susceptibility is universal. While the average number in adults is approximately 3.5 to 4.5 colds per year, the presence of children in the family plays a direct role in the number of infections in adult family members. In addition to the symptom of malaise, usually without fever, coryza, rhinitis, and lacrimation are prominent signs.

Prolonged travel, especially next to an ill passenger, presents a personal hygiene challenge for all travelers. Covering of the mouth for coughs and sneezes and the proper sanitary disposal of contaminated tissues and napkins are important steps to stop the spread of the virus. Diligent and frequent hand washing can also retard the transmission cycle. If space permits, the healthy traveler may want to relocate away from people with colds.

INFLUENZA

Protracted fever, cough, headache, and prostration, in addition to the common cold symptoms discussed above, often accompany an influenza infection. Cough is often severe and may be protracted. Other symptoms are typically self-limited and recovery can be expected in two to seven days. In terms of morbidity and mortality, influenza is clearly the most serious viral infection in adults. Serious complications include viral and bacterial pneumonia. The most common cause of bacterial superinfection is *Streptococcus pneumoniae* and to a lesser extent, *S aureus* [30]. Seasonal epidemics are frequently associated with an excess of over 10,000 deaths per year. Influenza warrants even tighter personal hygiene attention, since the virus has been shown to persist for hours in dried mucous. Crowded in-door spaces accentuate the transmission of the infectious airborne viral particles.

Three types of influenza virus (A, B, C) are recognized. Type A is associated with widespread epidemics and pandemics like the Spanish flu of 1918, the Asian influenza of 1957, and the Hong Kong strain of 1968. Type B is associated with regional or widespread epidemics, and type C is associated with sporadic cases and localized outbreaks. In temperate zones, epidemics usually occur in winter. In the tropics, they often occur in the rainy season. Outbreaks or sporadic cases may occur at any time. Virus type is determined by the antigenic properties of the two structural proteins. Vaccine components are based on the viral strains currently circulating as determined by international surveillance efforts.

During the early febrile period of the illness, laboratory confirmation can be made by isolation of influenza virus from upper respiratory secretions, washings in cell culture, or embryonated eggs. Direct identification of viral antigens in nasopharyngeal cells by FA test or ELISA or demonstration of a specific serologic response in acutely ill and convalescent patients also confirms the diagnosis.

Annual administration of the flu vaccine provides the most effective prophylaxis. Killed virus vaccines confer a protection efficacy of 70–80% in healthy young adults. A single dose suffices for those with prior exposure to influenza A or B viruses (all persons over 9 years old). Although routine immunizations are aimed at those with the greatest risk of serious complication or death and at health care workers generally, the vaccine should also be considered for those engaged in essential community services or travel-related business. The vaccine should be given yearly before influenza is expected in the community (November to March in the United States). For those traveling outside the United States, timing of immunization should be based on the different seasonal patterns of influenza in different parts of the world (April to September in the Southern Hemisphere and tropics).

Amantadine or rimantidine hydrochloride is effective in the chemoprophylaxis of influenza A, but not influenza B. The drug should be continued throughout the epidemic. It will not interfere with the response to the influenza vaccine.

Amantadine or rimantidine hydrochloride started within 48 hours of influenza illness and continued for three to five days has been shown to reduce the symptoms and viral titers in respiratory secretions. The usual adult dosage is 100 mg twice a day. During treatment, resistant isolates may develop, and close contacts may develop the illness despite prophylactic treatment. Overall, these antiviral medications are considered 70–90% effective.

VIRAL HEPATITIS A, B, C, D, AND E

Several distinct viral infections are grouped as viral hepatitides [31]. Typically, these viruses effect the liver and have similar clinical presentations. However, they do differ in etiology, epidemiology, immunology, and some clinical and pathologic characteristics. Their individual prevention and control vary greatly and thus are discussed separately. Personal hygiene remains the mainstay for primary prevention of hepatitis viral infections.

Hepatitis A

Hepatitis A (HBA) is prevalent worldwide and spread via contaminated food and water. To ward off infection, personal hygiene and proper sanitation is a must in endemic areas. The disease is more common in developing countries or areas where sanitation standards are low. Onset of symptoms is usually abrupt, with fever, malaise, anorexia, nausea, jaundice, and abdominal discomfort. The incubation period is 15–50 days, depending on the dose of pathogen. The average incubation is 28–30 days. Many infections are asymptomatic and mild, and often without jaundice, especially in the younger population. The average risk of contracting the disease in a developing country is 1% per month of time in the country. Although the case fatality rate is low (< 1/1,000), one study found that travelers who developed hepatitis A were off work a median of 33 days.

Nearly all international travelers should receive the hepatitis A vaccine. The inactivated-viral vaccine confers almost complete immunity 14–21 days after vaccination. A booster dose at six months provides 100% prolonged immunity for up to 10 years. A second option for protection from hepatitis is to use hepatitis A immune globulin (IG), which is about 85% effective in preventing clinical disease in persons exposed to hepatitis A. IG in a single dose of 2 mL should be given for exposures up to three months. For more prolonged exposures, 5 mL should be given and repeated every six months for prolonged stays in high-risk areas [32].

HEPATITIS B

Parenteral transmission—either apparent injury, like a needlestick or transfusion, or inapparent injury or sexual contact—is the usual mode of spread for hepatitis B virus (HBV) infection. Contaminated needles and blood products and unprotected sexual intercourse with an infected person are the most common causes of HBV in travelers. Onset of symptoms is typically insidious, with anorexia, vague abdominal complaints, nausea or vomiting, occasional arthralgias, and rash. Clinical jaundice is seen in only 30–50% of adults with acute hepatitis B, and fever may be absent or mild at most. The incubation period for HBV is 50–180 days (average 60–90 days).

HBV is worldwide in distribution, and the CDC recommends vaccination for all travelers who plan to spend more than six months in developing countries. This guideline should be expanded to include shorter stays in endemic areas, especially if activity is to result in intimate contact with local populations. Any traveler contemplating sexual intercourse while away should consider receiving the HBV vaccine and be counseled on the risk of other STDs as well. HBV vaccine is given as a three-dose series on months 0, 1, and 6. Effective antibody production is present in 90–95% of vaccine recipients. Because this dosing schedule is not very user-friendly for travel needs, an accelerated schedule can be used, with doses given at 0, 1, and 2 months and followed by a booster at 1 year. Specific guidance for postexposure treatment of potential HBV exposure appears in the treatment section of this chapter.

HEPATITIS C

Hepatitis C (HCV) often presents clinically with the same insidious onset as other hepatitis viruses. Approximately 75% of those infected have no symptoms and do not know they are ill. Anorexia, vague abdominal discomfort, nausea, and vomiting progress to jaundice in patients with HCV less frequently than in those with HBV. Ninety percent of cases of HCV in the United States occur posttransfusion from contaminated blood, and HCV accounts for 20% of all acute viral hepatitis. Parenteral transmission is also seen in intravenous drug users and hemodialysis patients.

HVC is worldwide in distribution, and transmission occurs by percutaneous exposure to blood and plasma derivatives. It is estimated, however, that percutaneous exposure only accounts for 50% of the cases of HCV in the United States. The incubation period for the disease is 14–180 days, most commonly 6–9 weeks. Approximately 85% of all persons with hepatitis C eventually develop chronic liver disease [33].

HEPATITIS D

Hepatitis D (HDV), or delta agent, is unique in that it appears only in concert with HBV infection. Onset of illness is abrupt, with signs and symptoms resembling those of hepatitis B. Occurrence is worldwide, but prevalence varies widely. HDV exists in epidemic or endemic proportion in populations where HBV is endemic (Russia, Romania, and southern Italy).

HDV has an incubation period of 14–56 days. HBV vaccination protects against infection with HDV, but HBIG, IG, and HB vaccine do not protect HBV carriers from infection by HDV.

HEPATITIS E

The clinical course of hepatitis E (HEV) is similar to HAV. Although, in general, it has a low case fatality rate like HAV, HEV infection in the third trimester of pregnancy has been linked to a 20% fatality rate from fulminating disease [34]. Therefore, pregnant travelers should receive special educational instruction on the risks of HEV infection.

HEV has been implicated in epidemics in India, Iran, Southeast Asia, Africa, China, and Mexico. The incubation period is 15–64 days, and more than 50% of HEV infections are anicteric. Preventive measures are the same as those for HAV, and personal hygiene and sanitation precautions are key to avoiding the risk of infection.

HERPES SIMPLEX

Herpes simplex virus (HSV) typically presents as a localized primary lesion with a tendency for latency and localized recurrence. HSV exists as two separate etiologic agents, HSV type 1 and 2, and usually produces two distinct clinical syndromes, depending on the portal of entry.

The primary infection with HSV 1 is mild, often inapparent, and occurs in early childhood. Reactivation of latent infection results in fever blisters and cold sores. HSV 2, genital herpes, occurs mainly in adults and is sexually transmitted via unprotected sexual activities with infected contacts. Because primary and recurrent infections can be asymptomatic, it is important to stress health education and personal hygiene measures for minimizing the transfer of the disease for the traveler. Both HSV types 1 and 2 may be transmitted to various sites by oral-genital, oral-anal, anal-genital contact. HSV 2 antibody is found in up to 60% of lower socioeconomic groups and persons with multiple sexual contacts. The use of oral, intravenous, or topical acyclovir or famciclovir has been shown to be effective in reducing the shedding of virus, decreasing pain, and accelerating the healing time in primary and secondary herpes infections.

ACQUIRED HUMAN IMMUNODEFICIENCY SYNDROME (HIV)

The clinical course and demographics of HIV disease are changing rapidly [35,36]. While it is beyond the scope of this book to summarize an international health concern that has volumes of literature dedicated to it, the worldwide occurrence of the retroviruses that cause HIV are an important health consideration for occupational travel. Suffice it to say that at-risk behaviors, including having multiple sexual partners and sharing drug paraphernalia, are the primary parenteral modes of contracting HIV infection. Therefore, personal protection and personal hygiene are paramount to stopping the transmission of the virus.

HIV is currently pandemic, with the largest proportion of infections reported in the Americas, Europe, Africa, and Southeast Asia. A global prevention and care program coordinated by WHO was initiated in 1987. Several countries have initiated a program for AIDS, HIV testing before entry by foreign travelers. The reader is referred to the CDC web site at *http://www.cdc.gov/travel* for current information of the geographic health risks and treatment modalities recommended for HIV exposure and infection [17]. The CDC also has an AIDS Hot Line at (toll free) 800-342-AIDS.

Even with the promise of multidrug therapies, which have turned the HIV infections from a perceived death sentence to a more manageable chronic illness, HIV infections and their manifestations as AIDS still remain a global threat. Worldwide, the AIDS epidemic grows unchecked in Third World countries that have little resources to combat the disease. Domestically, the face of HIV infection is also changing. HIV is now infecting populations that were untouched when the epidemic was just beginning.

POLIOMYELITIS

Flaccid paralysis occurs in less than 1% of patients with poliovirus infection. Greater than 90% of infections are inapparent or present with a nonspecific fever. Other accompanying symptoms include malaise, cephalgia, nausea, and vomiting. If the disease progresses to a major illness, severe muscle pain and stiffness of the neck or back typically occur. Major illness may or may not be accompanied by flaccid paralysis. In highly endemic areas, polio cases are routinely recognized by their clinical presentation. In countries with a low prevalence of infection, viral stool testing is frequently required for a definitive diagnosis. Polio remains primarily a disease of infants with an 80–90% attack rate in children less than 5 years old. Routes of transmission are person to person, and fecal-oral.

Aggressive vaccination practices have eliminated poliomyelitis in several parts of the world. The greatest risk for infection now exists in West and Central Africa and the subcontinent of India. Vaccination is recommended for all travelers who journey to developing countries or war-torn nations with major disruption of the sanitation infrastructure. Adults who have already received the primary vaccine series should receive a booster dose of the trivalent live, attenuated oral (OPV) or an injectable inactivated poliovirus (IPV) vaccine.

MUMPS, MEASLES, RUBELLA (MMR)

The primary concern for exposure to rubella is its attendant ability to produce fetal anomalies [34]. Congenital rubella syndrome (CSR) occurs in up to 90% of infants born to women who acquire rubella in the first trimester of pregnancy. The rubella virus is worldwide in distribution, and to prevent contracting this infection, pregnant travelers should adhere to proper immunization schedules before travel. Rubella has recently been reported among the crews and passengers of commercial cruise lines [37]. The more than 4 million seafarers who sail international waters are potentially at risk for rubella infection unless vaccine-preventable diseases are given to ship crews. Aside from CRS, rubella, measles, and mumps pose only a small, yet very preventable, infection threat for travelers.

EBOLA AND MARBURG VIRAL DISEASES

Ebola virus presents clinically with the sudden onset of fever, malaise, myalgia, and headache, followed by gastrointestinal disturbance and exanthem. Also known as *African hemorrhagic fever*, the hemorrhagic phase is often accompanied by hepatic insult, kidney failure, CNS involvement, and last, shock and multiorgan dysfunction. Lymphopenia, thrombocytopenia, and elevated liver function tests (LFT) are common laboratory findings. Marburg virus infections have a 25% case fatality rate, while the rate for the Ebola strain is often 50–90% [5,38].

For both Ebola and Marburg viruses, transmission is from person to person via parenteral contact with an infected individual. The Marburg causative viruses have been found in Germany and Yugoslavia after humans came in contact with African green monkeys from Uganda. Ebola strains have been discovered in Sudan, Zaire, and several other areas of sub-Saharan Africa. The incubation period is three to nine days for Marburg virus and two to 21 days for Ebola.

ARTHROPOD-BORNE VIRAL DISEASES

There are over 100 arboviruses that produce clinical and subclinical infections in humans. Most of these viruses are maintained in animal, zoonotic cycles, with humans as an incidental host. Infection in humans is usually secondary to an infected arthropod feeding on a blood meal and passing on the virus in the feeding process. However, in at least two instances, humans do serve as the principal source of viral growth and vector infection: dengue [39,40] and yellow fever [11]. Although the viral agents and their associated manifestations differ significantly, many of the agents share a common epidemiologic pattern in their transmission, the understanding of which plays a key role in the prevention of disease.

Arboviral disease typically produces four main clinical syndromes that vary by that part of the human host affected by the condition. Four different clinical syndromes have been described: (1) acute CNS illness with mild to severe meningitis, encephalitis, often progressing to coma and death; (2) hemorrhagic fevers, following acute febrile illness, associated with internal or external bleeding, shock, and a usually high case fatality rate; (3) polyarthritis and exanthem, variable fever with arthralgic sequelae lasting several weeks to months; and (4) acute benign fevers with variable rash that occasionally progress to CNS involvement or hemorrhage [40].

Arboviruses are typically unique to specific geographic sections of the globe. Their dependence on a specific vector limits the range and magnitude of the attack rates. Environmental conditions conducive to the propagation of the arthropod vector and the subsequent interaction of host and vector play a pivotal role in the prevalence of disease in certain areas [41,42]. Gaining a thorough understanding of this host, agent, and environment association, although challenging, affords the greatest opportunity to disrupt the infection sequence for travelers to high-risk areas. A few of the major, clinically important classes of arthropod-borne viral disease are described below.

Mosquito-Borne Encephalitides

Japanese (JE), St Louis (SLE), California (CE), Murray Valley (MVE), Jamestown Canyon

(JCE), Western equine (WEE), and Eastern equine (EEE) are just a few of the geographically determined mosquito-borne viral diseases of short duration that affect parts of the central nervous system (CNS), specifically the brain, spinal cord, and meninges [43]. Most infections are asymptomatic. Signs and symptoms include febrile headache or aseptic meningitis and are mild in the majority of cases. The acute onset of cephalgia, high fever, meningeal signs, disorientation, coma, or convulsions with spastic paralysis herald an infection of severe magnitude. Case-fatality rates vary from less than 1% to 60%, with JE and EEE among the highest. CNS complications, especially their sequelae, are age dependent and quite variable. EEE followed by SLE and Venezuelan equine encephalitis are the most significant contributors to CNS sequelae of retardation, spastic paralysis, and brain atrophy.

Transmission of these viral entities results from the bite of an infected mosquito. Several strains of mosquitoes are involved, and their geographic distribution determines the health risk to the traveler. Mosquitoes can be infected transovarially or can acquire the infection from wild birds, pigs, or small mammals. The usual incubation period is five to 15 days.

Tick-Borne Encephalitides

Far Eastern (FEE), Central European (CEE), and Powassan (PE) viral encephalitis clinically resemble the mosquito-borne infections, except that FEE often produces shoulder paralysis, focal epilepsy, and CNS sequelae. Case fatality rates vary, with PE having a 10% rate and a 50% likelihood of neurologic complications. Transmission of the disease to humans is by tick bite or the consumption of infected raw milk from goats and sheep. Areas of highest incidence are geographically related to the distribution and numbers of the infected tick vector. Typically, forests and rural areas present the largest risk for infection. The incubation period ranges from seven to 14 days.

Mosquito-Borne Viral Hemorrhagic Fevers

Yellow fever and dengue fever are two representative examples of mosquito-borne viral fever infections that are often clinically mild in their initial presentation, especially yellow fever, but may progress to life-threatening hemorrhage, especially dengue hemorrhagic fever (DHF) [44,45].

In yellow fever, within three to six days after being bitten by an infected mosquito, the human host acutely develops fever, chills, headache, backache, myalgia, nausea, vomiting, and sometimes prostration. Faget's sign, a slow, weak pulse in concert with high fever, and jaundice are early clinical findings. Renal changes of albuminuria and anuria may accompany leukopenia by the fifth day of infection. Most infections resolve at this time, and less than 5% are fatal. However, hemorrhagic symptoms often follow a short remission of the condition and there is onset of more serious sequelae such as mucous membrane bleeding, hematemesis, melena, and renal or liver failure. It is estimated that 20–50% of cases involving jaundice are fatal [38].

Yellow fever is spread by several different species of mosquito, depending on its native environment. *Aedes aegypti* is the common mosquito vector in the urban setting, while in the South American forests the genus *Haemagogus* provides the primary vector for the transmission of yellow fever. Humans play a key role in transmission of the disease in the urban setting by acting as an amplifying host for the mosquito vector. However, humans play no such role in the jungle environment.

Yellow fever is endemic to the tropical regions of Africa and South America. In Africa, the endemic zone extends through northern Angola, Zaire, and Tanzania. Once an area of high prevalence, the Central Americas have not reported a case of yellow fever for several years. Recent reinfestation of the *A aegypti* vector to the area has renewed the risk of urban yellow fever. To date, the disease has never been reported in Asia or the eastern coast of Africa.

Dengue fever is an acute viral febrile disease characterized by sudden onset of intense headache, myalgia, arthralgia, retro-orbital pain, anorexia, gastrointestinal upset, and rash [46]. The viral exanthem typically appears as a diffuse maculopapular eruption as the fever wanes. Leukopenia and lymphadenopathy are typical. The illness is self-limiting, and fatality is rare unless the disease progresses to DHF. Signs and symptoms of DHF include extreme lassitude, restlessness, diaphoresis, pallor, tachycardia, hypotension, and a narrow pulse pressure [47]. Hemorrhagic phenomena include scattered petechiae, easy bruisability, abdominal and thoracic effusions, and the ominous sign of GI hemorrhage. Case fatality rates can approach 50%, but with proper fluid replacement, rates should be less than 2%.

The four dengue fever viruses (dengue-1, -2, -3, -4 serotypes) are endemic to most of the tropics and all of Africa and have a much wider global distribution than yellow fever [48]. Dengue fever virus is highly endemic to Asia and has a presence in southwest Asia and the South Pacific. Transmission is primarily via the mosquito vector, *A aegypti*, which is typically a day-biting species. All four viral serotypes have been isolated in the Americas and found as far north as southern Texas [44].

Tick-Borne Viral Hemorrhagic Fevers

Crimean-Congo hemorrhagic fever (CCHF) presents suddenly with fever, malaise, headache, weakness, extremity and groin pain, and severe anorexia. Gastrointestinal symptoms of nausea, vomiting, and diarrhea may be present. Facial erythema is accompanied by hemorrhagic petechiae in the oropharynx. A fine petechial rash frequently appears on the trunk before extending peripherally. Hematuria and albuminuria are common, and bleeding from the gums, nose, lungs, uterus, or intestines appears in the more serious presentations of the illness. Once again, leukopenia and thrombocytopenia are common, especially with the hemorrhagic form of the disease. Case fatality rates may approach 50% but typically are much lower.

Transmission is primarily by infected ticks that acquire the virus from infected animals [41]. Nosocomial and tertiary person-to-person infections have been reported in medical family members. The disease is found in several areas of the former Soviet Union as well as in Albania, Bosnia, Bulgaria, Iraq, Pakistan, western China, and the tropical and southern regions of Africa.

ZOONOTIC VIRAL DISEASE

Hantavirus

Hantaviruses are found worldwide as infectious viral agents of rodents. Human disease results from secondary exposure to aerosolized rodent excreta. Two distinct human illnesses can result from viral exposure: hemorrhagic fever with renal syndrome (HFRS) and hantavirus pulmonary syndrome (HVPS) [49,50].

HFRS typically presents with fever, low back pain, headache, malaise, and anorexia with hemorrhage and variable renal signs. The clinical course of the disease includes five separate stages: fever, hypotension, oliguria, diuresis, and convalescence. Fatalities typically occur during the hypotensive and oliguric phases of the illness. In the severe form of the disease, the case fatality rate is close to 5%.

Several *Hantavirus* species exist, many associated with a specific rodent species. Distinct viruses are found in Asia, the Balkans, Russia, Brazil, Argentina, and the United States. The incubation period is estimated to be two to four weeks. Seasonal variation is linked to the increased number of infected rodents.

In the United States, HVPS was first recognized in 1993. Fever, myalgia, and gastrointestinal complaints are quickly followed by the abrupt onset of hypotension and respiratory distress. In 40–50% of the cases, the condition can rapidly progress to respiratory failure, cardiogenic shock, and death. Transmission is by aerosol exposure to rodent feces and urine, and although the disease has been found throughout North America, it occurs predominantly in the western states and Canada.

Rabies

Rabies is a disease primarily of animals: dogs, cats, wild carnivores, and bats. Human infection classically results from the bite or scratch of a rabid animal. The disease is almost always fatal; death results from respiratory failure after two to six days of the illness. Initial clinical findings include fever, headache, and malaise coupled with a profound sense of apprehension and excitability. The disease progresses to paresis and paralysis, spasm of the deglutatory apparatus, delirium, convulsions, respiratory paralysis, and death.

The rabies virus is found worldwide except in those countries that are free of rabies in their animal population [51]. Travelers at high risk include veterinarians, spelunkers, and those who handle wild animals. Long-term travel, in excess of two to four weeks, to highly endemic areas like Mexico, El Salvador, Guatemala, Peru, Columbia, Ecuador, India, Nepal, the Philippines, Thailand, and Vietnam significantly increases the risk of rabid animal contact. All travelers should refrain from petting or playing with wild and feral domestic animals. Those working in high-risk occupations in high-risk areas should receive rabies vaccine as pre-exposure prophylaxis. The immediate cleansing of bites with soap and water has been shown to reduce the risk of developing the disease substantially.

Differential Diagnosis

The clinical picture and routine studies associated with diagnosing viral infections are, for the most part, very similar. Often, the initial presentation of fever, malaise, and cephalgia mimic other infectious disease agents and some general health conditions. The clinician presented with preventing or treating a possible travel-related viral infection should always perform an in-depth review of the individual's health history and travel locations (see Table 27-1).

Many viral illnesses have clinical characteristics that aid in the diagnosis of conditions such as measles, mumps, chickenpox, and poliomyelitis. But even mumps can be a tricky physical diagnosis, since cases of lymphadenopathy are frequently mislabeled mumps. Additional considerations include other causes of parotitis-like influenza A, coxsackieviruses, lymphocytic choriomeningitis virus, and *Staphylococcus aureus.* Enlargement of the parotid gland may also be seen in patients with Sjögren's syndrome, sarcoidosis, thiazide ingestion, iodine sensitivity, tumor, and salivary duct obstruction.

Macupapular eruptions are central to several infectious disease processes. Enteroviral diseases are usually distinguished from measles and rubella by their summertime occurrence, absence of posterior auricular nodes, and their relatively short incubation period. The absence of significant coryza and conjunctivitis further distinguishes enteroviral exanthems from measles. Even the differential diagnosis of measles includes other possibilities like rubella, scarlet fever, infectious mononucleosis, secondary syphilis, drug eruptions, and toxic shock. Perhaps most important, a well-documented history of immunizations provides the greatest aid in making the correct diagnosis.

The mild form of yellow fever is not clinically distinguishable from other tropical fevers. Severe yellow fever simulates viral hepatitis, including HDV, other hemorrhagic fevers, leptospirosis, rickettsial fevers, malaria, and drug- and toxin-related hepatotoxins. The differential diagnosis for dengue fever includes all epidemiologically relevant diseases listed under arthropod-borne viral fevers and measles, rubella, and other systemic febrile illnesses that are accompanied by a rash.

When diagnosing arthropod-borne viral encephalitis, the most important consideration is differentiating it from other acute CNS infections caused by treatable nonviral organisms. In viral encephalitis, the early prodromata resemble influenza, dengue, or other influenza-like illnesses. Bacterial meningitis, especially partially treated or early-onset disease, can mimic viral encephalitis. Bacterial endocarditis, brain abscess, subdural empyema, and cerebral thrombophlebitis are often confused with viral encephalitis. Frequently, even some of the CSF findings of lumbar puncture are similar. Infections that cause meningoencephalitis—tuberculosis, cryptococcosis, histoplasmosis, coccidioidomycosis, rickettsial fevers, falciparum malaria, trichinosis, typhoid fever, and *Mycoplasma* pneumonia—must also be differentiated from viral encephalitis [12].

Acute meningoencephalitis may result from infections with other viruses, including herpes virus, HIV, mumps, rabies, influenza, and other exanthematous viral infections. Exposure history, presence of community or household illness, and seasonal occurrence are important clues to support a nonarboviral etiology. Although enterovirus encephalitis also occurs in summer, the presence of aseptic meningitis, rash, and pleurodynia help distinguish it. It is also important to diagnose herpes simplex encephalitis, since pharmaceutical treatment is available. Localized neurologic signs, positive CAT or MRI findings, and possibly a brain biopsy may be necessary to distinguish between herpes and arboviral disease.

Cerebrovascular accident is one of several noninfectious CNS conditions that may mimic viral encephalitis. St. Louis encephalitis, a classic disease of the elderly, has often been misdiagnosed as stroke. Subarachnoid hemorrhage and some metabolic conditions can produce the similar signs of meningismus, fever, headache, and other neurologic signs of viral hepatitis. Other differential diagnoses to consider are neoplastic and granulomatous diseases and a whole host of other unusual conditions such as Behçet disease, Reye syndrome, multiple sclerosis, and systemic lupus erythematosus.

Diagnostic Evaluation

Immunization history plays a key role in assisting the clinician when evaluating travel-related viral illness. Individuals who keep their travel vaccinations current should be immune from disease, since most vaccines provide more than a 90% protection factor by interrupting the agent-host-environment cycle. Other elements of the immunization history include a comprehensive review of the patient's travel history and possible exposures to animal or insect bites or environmental threats.

The physical examination and any further diagnostic tests should follow a risk-based model focused on the probability and need to diagnose a specific viral illness that is amenable to specific treatment protocols. Virus isolation is technically very difficult, and a thorough history and pertinent physical examination will significantly assist the clinician in quickly moving through the differential diagnosis. The proper use of antivirals requires that specific viral diagnoses be made. Viral diagnostic laboratories are expanding, and rapid reagent techniques are gaining acceptance. Readers are once again referred to their local state or CDC laboratory for current viral-testing specimen collection and testing capabilities.

The diagnostic evaluation of person-to-person, arthropod-borne, and zoonotic viral illnesses is as unique as the number of viruses that cause the conditions in question. Usually, routine blood, nasal secretions, urine, or spinal fluid testing—to obtain blood counts, protein levels, liver enzyme tests, or urinalyses—are helpful to initiate a general evaluation of the illness. Frequently, an enzyme-linked immunosorbent assay (ELISA), viral serology, or cell culture is needed to specifically identify the infectious agent. Specific diagnostic testing for the viral diseases covered in this chapter includes the following laboratory tests.

Positive results obtained by ELISA for specific IgG antibody suggests infection with Ebola-Marburg virus or one of several other viruses. The presence of positive IgM serology typically suggests more recent infection. ELISA antigen detection in blood, serum, or organ homogenates and the viral isolation in cell culture or suckling mice also are used to confirm the diagnosis. Ebola-Marburg virus testing represents an extreme biohazard, and any blood products should only be handled with the strictest precautions.

Several of the other viral diseases discussed in this section also require the use of ELISA, complement fixation (CF), hemagglutination inhibition (HAI/HI), fluorescent antibody (FA), or other serologic tests for precise pathologic agent identification. Cross-reactivity in testing is frequently seen in testing for arthropod-borne viral groups.

Although the specific diagnosis of rabies is usually post mortem, FA may make a presumptive diagnosis on frozen sections of skin from the posterior scalp. Another variation in testing is seen in the diagnosis of HIV, for which ELISA acts only as a screening test and the Western blot or indirect IFA is used as a confirmatory test.

Treatment and Rehabilitation

Recent advances in antiviral chemotherapy have produced a number of specific antiviral agents that are effective for prophylaxis and treatment. Both commercial and investigational vaccines and medications are available, and the reader is reminded to contact the CDC for the latest recommendations for therapies that are not listed below. Several travel-related viral diseases have specific treatment regimens, while there is no known effective therapy for others.

Primary prevention that includes avoidance of high-risk agents, environments, and behavior is the prudent approach to interrupting the infection cycle of travel-related viral disease. Primary immunization to induce passive immunity has previously been discussed.

Hepatitis B, HIV, and rabies present unique challenges for evaluation and treatment after incidental or purposeful exposure to suspected carriers of the disease. Products available for postexposure hepatitis prophylaxis include hepatitis B immunoglobulin (HBIG) and hepatitis B vaccine.

Hepatitis immune globulin (0.06 mg/kg or 5 mL for adults) in combination with hepatitis B vaccine should be started as postexposure prophylaxis for unimmunized individuals exposed to blood or other bodily fluid contact with hepatitis B infections or carriers. HBIG should be given within the first 24 hours after high-risk exposure. A complete decision tree on how to balance the risk of infection with the need to provide hepatitis B prophylaxis has been published by the CDC.

HIV, since its dramatic entry into the global village in 1981, has witnessed accelerated treatment modalities that are constantly being updated with new classes of antiviral medications [15]. Recent antiretroviral therapy has shown significant promise in slowing the progression of the infection in many cases. The goal of therapy is to improve survival and decrease morbidity by continuously maximizing suppression of HIV replication. Many clinical trials of anti-AIDS drugs are currently under way, and the reader is advised to contact the CDC for guidelines for current treatment options. The recent CDC guidelines for the prophylactic protection of those who may have been inadvertently parentally exposed to HIV-positive individuals, is recommended for a period of four weeks. Laboratory evaluation for antiretroviral adverse effects after two weeks of prophylaxis is also recommended. Current CDC-recommended HIV treatment regimens are available by contacting the CDC/AIDS Post Exposure Prophylaxis hot line at 888-448-4911 or by reviewing CDC guidelines [19].

The prevention and treatment of rabies after an animal bite or scratch consists of several steps, depending on the vaccination status of the animal and the human host. First, all bites and scratches should receive immediate and thorough cleansing with soap and water. This simple step is the most effective in reducing the risk of viral infection. Second, human rabies immune globulin (HRIG) should be infiltrated into the wound area, and third, a series of five 1.0 mL IM vaccine doses should be given on days 0, 3, 7, 14, and 28–35. The decision to start treatment typically depends upon the likelihood of the animal in question being positive for rabies. Tetanus prophylaxis and antibiotic treatment for bacterial wound infections are frequently required and should always be considered in any contact situation. Treatment for clinical rabies is supportive.

For the rest of the more serious viral-related diseases previously discussed, treatment is also mostly supportive. The clinical care for the more severe forms of yellow fever, Ebola-Marburg virus, and several other arthropod and zoonotic illnesses consists of intubation for respiratory support, coupled with close management of hemodynamic fluid shifts. The fatality rates remain high for these diseases, even when treated.

Occupational Considerations

For many careers, international travel has become a way of life. Any disease or illness that results from occupational travel should be considered for its work relatedness. Unless some unusually neglectful behavior is readily apparent, most conditions fall under workers' compensation. What were frequently called "shot clinics" in the past have now matured into specialty clinics for travel medicine that offer complete travel care for the occupational traveler [52]. Although the staffing and expertise of these clinics may vary, the emphasis on preventing illness by interrupting the agent-host-environment transmission cycle is critical to those who travel to high-risk areas of the globe [53,54].

Travel-related health risks vary significantly with the general health of the traveler and the location, duration, mode of travel, and local prevalence of pathogens. Descriptions of worldwide health risks for any country are now readily available on the Internet from several governmental and civilian sources. All occupational travelers should have the benefit of a current health and immunization review in addition to health-risk education pertinent to their routes and destinations. A second group of workers frequently overlooked but also requiring prevention are those who come in daily contact with international travelers [27,55]. Domestic staff may be the primary victims of imported influenza and other illnesses. Therefore, their health history and possible need for immunization or chemoprophylaxis should also be part of any comprehensive travel-related occupational medicine program.

References

1. LeDuc J. World Health Organization strategy for emerging infectious diseases. *JAMA* 1996;275:318–20.
2. Berkelman RL, Bryan RT, Osterholm MT, et al. Infectious disease surveillance: a crumbling foundation. *Science* 1994;264:368–70.
3. Beller M, Ellis A, Lee SH, et al. Outbreak of viral gastroenteritis due to a contaminated well: international consequences. *JAMA* 1997;278:563–8.
4. Lederberg J, Shoope RE, Oaks SC (eds). *Emerging Infections: Microbial Threats to the United States.* Washington, DC: Institute of Medicine, National Academy Press, 1992.
5. Schmaljohn C, Hjelle B. Hantavirus: a global disease problem. *Emerg Infect Dis* 1997;3:95–103.
6. World Health Organization. Emerging infectious diseases: memorandum from a WHO meeting. *Bull WHO* 1994;72:845–50.
7. Last JM (ed). *Maxcey-Rosenau Public Health and Preventive Medicine*, 13th Ed. Stamford, CT: Appleton & Lange, 1996.
8. LaDou J (ed). *Occupational and Environmental Medicine*, 2nd Ed. Stamford, CT: Appleton & Lange, 1997.
9. Nettlemann MD. Preparing the international traveler. *Gastroenterol Clin North Am* 1996;25:451–69.
10. Beeton S. Facts on travel health. *Community Nurse* 1996;2:49.
11. Benenson AS (ed). *Control of Communicable Diseases Manual,* 16th Ed. Washington, DC: American Public Health Association, 1995.
12. Bennett JC, Plum F (eds). *Cecil Textbook of Medicine*, 20th Ed. Philadelphia: Saunders, 1996. Pp 1739–42.
13. Mulhall BP. Sex and travel: studies of sexual behavior, disease, and health promotion in international travelers—a global review. *Int J STD AIDS* 1996;7:455–65.
14. Hawkes S, Hart G. The sexual health of travelers. *Infect Dis Clin North Am* 1998;12:413–30.
15. Mawhorter SD. Travel medicine for the primary care physician. *Cleveland Clin J Med* 1997;64:483–92.
16. Arvidson M, Kallings I, Nilsson S, et al. Risky behavior in women with history of casual travel sex. *Sex Transm Dis* 1997;24:418–21.
17. Centers for Disease Control and Prevention. Public Health Service guidelines for the management of healthcare worker exposure to HIV and recommendations for postexposure prophylaxis. *MMWR* 1998;47(RR-7):1–33.
18. MacLean JD, Libman M. Screening returning travelers. *Infect Dis Clin North Am* 1998;12:431–43.
19. Steffen R, Rickenbach M, Wilhelm U, et al. Health problems after travel to developing countries. *J Infect Dis* 1987;156:156–84.
20. Doherty JF, Grant AD, Bryceson ADM. Fever as the presenting complaint of travellers returning from the tropics. *Q J Med* 1995;88:277–81.
21. Strickland GT. Fever in the returned traveler. *Med Clin North Am* 1992;76:1375–92.
22. Thanassi WT. Immunizations for international travelers. *West J Med* 1998;168:197–202.
23. Innis BL, Snitbhan R, Kunasol P, et al. Protection against hepatitis A by an inactivated vaccine. *JAMA* 1994;271:1328–64.
24. Centers for Disease Control and Prevention. Yellow fever vaccine. *MMWR* 1990;39:RR-6.
25. Centers for Disease Control and Prevention. Inactivated Japanese encephalitis virus vaccine. *MMWR* 1993;42(RR-1):1–15.
26. Robertson SE, Hull BP, Tomori O, et al. Yellow fever: a decade of reemergence. *JAMA* 1996;276:1157–62.
27. Insect repellents. *Medical Lett* 1989;31:45–7.
28. Zenz C (ed). *Occupational Medicine*, 3rd Ed. St. Louis: Mosby, 1994. Pp 1088–113.
29. Travel medicine clinics growing. *Physicians Fin News* 1999;17:19–21.
30. Centers for Disease Control and Prevention. Update: influenza activity—United States, 1998–1999 season. *MMWR* 1999;48:25–7.
31. Judson P. Viral hepatitis: the alphabet soup of liver infection. *Indiana Epidem Newsletter* 1998;6:3–5.
32. Koff RS. Preventing hepatitis A infections in travelers to endemic areas. *Am J Trop Med Hyg* 1995;53:586–90.
33. Hepatitis C screening. *Indiana Epidemiol Newslett* 1998;6:8–10.
34. Samuel BU, Barry M. The pregnant traveler. *Infect Dis Clin North Am* 1998;12:325–54.
35. HIV/AIDS theme issue. *JAMA* 1998;280:3–95.
36. Centers for Disease Control and Prevention. HIV/AIDS surveillance report. *MMWR* 1996;8:3–33.
37. Centers for Disease Control and Prevention. Rubella among crew members of commercial cruise ships–Florida. *MMWR* 1998;46:1247–50.
38. Samaranayake LP, Peiris JS, Scully C. Ebola virus infection: an overview. *Br Dent J* 1996;7:264–6.

39. Schwart E, Mendelshon E, Sidi Y. Dengue fever among travelers. *Am J Med* 1996;101:516–20.

40. Shirtcliffe P, Cameron E, Nicholson KG, et al. Don't forget dengue: clinical features of dengue fever in returning travellers. *J R Coll Physicians Lond* 1998; 32:235–7.

41. Schwartz TF. Imported vector and rodent-borne virus infections—an introduction. *Arch Virol—Supplementum* 1996;11:3–11.

42. Gubler DJ. Arboviruses as imported disease agents: the need for increased awareness. *Arch Virol—Supplementum* 1996;11:21–32.

43. Dobler G. Arboviruses causing neurological disorders of the central nervous system. *Arch Virol—Supplementum* 1996;11:33–40.

44. Centers for Disease Control and Prevention. Imported dengue—United States 1996. *MMWR* 1998;47: 544–7.

45. Centers for Disease Control and Prevention. Dengue and dengue hemorrhagic fever in the Americas. *MMWR* 1988;37:7.

46. Gubler DJ. Dengue and dengue hemorrhagic fever. *Clin Microbiol Rev* 1998;11:480–96.

47. Karp BE. Dengue fever: a risk to travelers. *Maryland Med J* 1997;46:299–302.

48. Jelinek T, Dobler G, Holscher M, et al. Prevalence of infection with dengue virus among international travelers. *Arch Intern Med* 1997;157:2367–70.

49. Bartlett JG, Breiman RF, Mandell LA, et al. Community acquired pneumonia in adults: guidelines for management. *Clin Infect Dis* 1998;26:826.

50. Kahn AS, Khabbaz RF, Armstrong LR, et al. Hantavirus pulmonary syndrome; the first 100 U.S. cases. *J Infect Dis* 1996;173:1297–303.

51. Centers for Disease Control and Prevention. Rabies prevention—United States 1991. *MMWR* 1991;40(RR-3):1–19.

52. American medical news, *JAMA* 1998;42:23–4.

53. Blair DC. A week in the life of a travel clinic. *Clin Microbiol Rev* 1997;10:650–73.

54. Goldsmith MF. Health woes grow in shrinking world. *JAMA* 1998;279:569–71.

55. Shoemaker S. Overview: adult vaccine preventable diseases and recommended vaccination schedules. *Indiana Epidemiol Newslett* 1998;6:1–5.

Electronic Resources

1. Centers for Disease Control and Prevention. Travel information automated fax line 888-232-3299 (toll free). Available at *http://www.cdc.gov/travel.html.*

2. Centers for Disease Control and Prevention. Health information for International Travel 1996–97. Available at *http://ww.cdc.gov/travel/yellowbk/page180b.htm.*

3. Centers for Disease Control and Prevention. Health Information for International Travel 1996–97. Available at *http://ww.cdc.gov/travel/yellowbk/page 198.htm.*

4. World Health Organization. Available at *http://www.who.int.*

5. International Travel Healthline. Available at *http://www.travax.com.*

28 / Bacterial Travel-Related Infections

Alain J. Couturier and Karin E. Byers

As other countries have become increasingly accessible, Americans are traveling in greater numbers to remote areas of the world, where they may be exposed to infections that are endemic to those regions. It is estimated that more than 8 million North Americans travel to developing countries each year for vacations, study, business, or missionary activities. In order to prevent infections, travelers need to take specific precautions both before and during their travels. Clinicians must also be able to recognize illnesses that are associated with travel.

One third of persons who travel abroad develop travel-related illness. The most common illness is diarrhea, affecting up to half of the travelers from industrialized countries who visit the developing world. Health care workers, those working with animals, military personnel, and those working for prolonged periods of time in remote areas may be exposed to more unusual pathogens. This chapter provides an overview of the more common bacterial illnesses affecting travelers. Many of the diseases discussed are reviewed in greater detail in other chapters.

A number of things can be done to prevent illness when traveling. The most important considerations are immunizations, food and water precautions, and avoiding mosquitoes and ticks.

Immunizations

Travelers should be up to date on all of their routine immunizations, but they may require additional vaccinations. Some countries require yellow fever and cholera immunizations prior to entry. A list of the requirements for each country is available in *Health Information for International Travel*, published by the Centers for Disease Control and Prevention. An up-to-date version is also available on their web site at *www.cdc.gov/travel/index.com*. These vaccinations must be documented in the International Certificate of Vaccination and validated by a stamp issued by state health departments.

In general, inactivated vaccines can be given simultaneously at separate sites, but yellow fever and cholera vaccines may be less effective if administered within three weeks of each other. Vaccines commonly associated with local or systemic side effects, such as cholera or parenteral typhoid, may be more severe when administered at the same time. Theoretically, live virus vaccines may be less effective if administered within one month of each other. However, the oral polio vaccine (OPV) and measles, mumps, rubella vaccine (MMR) can be given simultaneously.

Live, attenuated vaccines should be avoided in persons who are immunocompromised or if a household member is significantly immunocompromised, including having an illness such as HIV, leukemia, lymphoma, generalized malignancy, or prolonged therapy with corticosteroids [1].

Yellow fever is endemic in areas of Africa and South America. The vaccine is required for protection against infection in these areas and may also be required to enter some of these countries or when leaving these areas to enter other countries. The vaccine is administered only at designated centers, and it must be documented in the International Certificate of Vaccination. It is a live, attenuated virus vaccine. It is contraindicated in persons with known allergy to eggs or egg products, infants less than 6 months of age, pregnant and lactating women, and persons who are immunocompromised. It is administered as one dose (0.5 mL subcutaneous injection), with a booster given every 10 years. This is discussed in greater detail in Chapter 27 [2].

Typhoid fever is endemic in much of the developing world. It can be prevented with food and water precautions in fastidious travelers, but the vaccine is suggested for most travelers. There are three typhoid vaccines available. The parenteral inactivated vaccine requires two doses given four weeks apart and a booster dose at three-year intervals. This vaccine is about 70% effective and is often associated with fevers, headaches, or significant local pain. The oral live, attenuated Ty21a vaccine is administered as one capsule every other day for a total of four doses. Because it is a live vaccine, the patient must not be taking antibiotics at the time of the vaccine. Like the inactivated vaccine, it is also about 70% effective and does not appear to have significant side effects. Boosters are required every five years. A parenteral polysaccharide Vi-antigen vaccine (Typhium Vi, Connaught Laboratories, Swiftwater, PA) is also available. A single doese provides protection for two years, and it is better tolerated than the two-dose parenteral vaccine [3,4].

The cholera vaccine is administered parenterally with a two-dose primary series. It is generally not recommended, even for persons travelling to cholera-epidemic areas such as South America, because the currently available vaccine is only 50–70% effective and lasts only a few months. Patients should be advised to follow food and water precautions to reduce their risk of contracting cholera or another infectious disease. New oral cholera vaccines, which appear to be more effective, are currently in development [2,3].

Hepatitis A is the most common dangerous infection for travelers, affecting up to 1 in every 50 susceptible travelers. The hepatitis A vaccination should be given two to four weeks before departure. There are now two vaccines available in the United States. Four weeks after the initial dose, the traveler should have protective immunity. Because of the long incubation period of hepatitis A, the vaccine may actually be effective if given later. However, it is recommended that if persons are traveling to high-risk areas before four weeks after the initial dose, they should also receive an injection of immune globulin (0.02 mL/kg) [3]. This subject is covered in greater detail in the Chapter 27.

Hepatitis B is appropriate for high-risk travelers, such as health care workers. It is usually given as three doses over six months. This is covered in Chapter 27.

Neisseria meningitidis epidemics frequently occur in sub-Saharan Africa during the dry season, between December and June. Outbreaks are also common among pilgrims going to Mecca, Saudi Arabia, during the annual Hajj. Many outbreaks are due to serotypes A and C, which are included in the quadrivalent polysaccharide vaccine. The vaccine is recommended for travelers going to sub-Saharan Africa, Nepal, parts of India, Mongolia, Saudi Arabia, and East and Central Africa. Saudi Arabia requires proof of immunization from all visa applicants. This vaccine is effective against serotypes A, C, Y, and W-135. Serotype B causes some outbreaks and is prevalent in the United States, but there is no effective vaccine [2,3].

Streptococcal pneumonia is not a disease that is limited to travelers, but it is still the most common cause of pneumonia, and resistant *Streptococcus pneumoniae* is more common in European countries than in the United States. Vaccination with the pneumococcal vaccine should be considered for those at increased risk for infection or for serious complications of infection. This includes those with chronic pulmonary disease, advanced cardiovascular disease, diabetes mellitus, alcoholism, cirrhosis, chronic renal insufficiency, CSF leak, and all of those older than 65 years of age. Persons in an immunocompromised state, such as those with splenic dysfunction or asplenia, multiple myeloma, lymphoma, Hodgkin's disease or HIV and those who have had organ transplantation should also be considered.

The influenza vaccine should also be considered for patients in the previously mentioned groups. While influenza occurs almost exclusively in the winter months (December to April) in the Northern Hemisphere, it occurs most often between May and September in the Southern Hemisphere. Influenza may not only cause morbidity and mortality due to the viral illness, but it may also predispose to secondary bacterial infections.

The tetanus and diphtheria vaccine should be given to all Americans, with a booster at 10-year intervals. If vaccinations are not up to date, travelers should be revaccinated prior to travel rather than risk needing the vaccine in areas where it may not be available or the safety of needles is in question. In recent years, there has been an outbreak of diphtheria in Russia and the new independent states of the former U.S.S.R., and travelers to these regions must be protected [3].

Food and Water Precautions

There are several commonsense rules for avoiding food-borne illness. Although many travelers are cautious about the source of their drinking water, it is easy to forget that ice, salad bars, and brushing teeth may be other sources of contaminated water. Boiling water is the most reliable method of purifying it for drinking. Water should be brought to a vigorous boil for 1 minute. When the altitude is above 2 km (6,526 feet), water should be boiled for 3 minutes, or a chemical disinfectant should be used [5].

Chemical disinfection can be performed with iodine or chlorine. Iodine is preferred, because the efficacy of chlorine depends on the temperature, pH, and organic content of the water. However, iodine cannot kill *Cryptosporidium* unless the water is allowed to sit for 15 hours before drinking it. Five drops (0.25 mL) of 2% tincture of iodine should be added to each quart or liter of water. If the water is cold or cloudy, the amount should be doubled. Alternatively, iodine can be added in the form of hydroperiodide tablets (e.g., Globaline, Porta-Aqua, Coghlan's). These should be added according to the manufacturer's instructions [5].

Filters provide protection against many organisms, but their efficacy is variable. Reverse-osmosis filters provide the best protection against bacteria, viruses, and protozoa, but they are expensive and cumbersome. The small pores in these filters may also become clogged quickly with cloudy water. Microstrainer filters with pores in the 0.1- to 0.3-μm range may effectively filter bacteria and protozoa, but they are not effective against viruses. If these are used, viruses may be killed with the addition of iodine or chlorine [5]. In general, drinks should be limited to carbonated and bottled soft drinks, beer, and wine. Bottled water *may* be safe, but it is sometimes bottled from a local source and thus may not be pure.

Travelers should be advised to avoid any food that may have been contaminated by water or food that is uncooked. Unpasteurized milk and milk products, such as cheese, should also be avoided. Food should be well cooked and eaten right after preparation. Even cooked food that has been allowed to sit at room temperature for several hours may not be safe, and it should be reheated. Only fruits and vegetables that the traveler can peel should be eaten. Homemade sauces and mayonnaise should be avoided. The general rule is "boil it, peel it, cook it, or forget it."

Prophylaxis can fall into the category of prevention, that is, food and water precautions or vaccines, or the use of specific agents. Drugs for prophylaxis are generally not necessary because diarrhea is generally self-limited. For those who do take prophylaxis, agents such as bismuth subsalicylate (Pepto Bismol) are preferred over antibiotics. Bismuth subsalicylate has been shown to decrease the incidence of traveler's diarrhea by 60% but must be used with caution in patients with aspirin allergy, renal insufficiency, or gout and in those who are taking anticoagulants, probenicid, or methotrexate. Because of the risk of salicylate toxicity, bismuth salicylate is also contraindicated in persons who are already taking aspirin. It should *not* be given to anyone with a viral syndrome because of the risk of Reye's syndrome. Travelers should be advised that it may turn their tongue or their stools black, and it may occasionally cause nausea or constipation. The usual dose is 2 ounces or two tablets four times per day. Because consuming this volume of the liquid can become cumbersome, it is easier for most people to take the tablets [5].

Prophylactic antibiotics are generally not recommended because of the risk of side effects, including drug allergies, photosensitivity, yeast vaginitis, or *Clostridium difficile* infection. If diarrhea occurs, it can be ameliorated quickly by a short course of antibiotics.

Diarrhea

Diarrhea is the most common travel-related illness, affecting 30–50% of travelers to developing countries [6]. High-risk areas include Latin America, Africa, the Middle East, and Asia. Intermediate-risk areas include most of the southern European countries and a few of the Caribbean Islands. Low-risk areas include Canada, northern Europe, Australia, New Zealand, the United States, and a number of the Caribbean Islands [5]. Greater than 80% of cases are due to bacteria, predominantly *Escherichia coli* [7]. However, because most traveler's diarrhea is a self-limited illness, it is usually not necessary to make a specific diagnosis. The duration of traveler's diarrhea, without treatment, is usually three to four days. Sixty percent of patients recover within 48 hours [8]. Ten percent of cases persist for longer than one week, and 2% for longer than one month. Approximately 2–10% have diarrhea accompanied by fevers, bloody stools, or both [5]. Table 28-1 lists the common causes of diarrhea.

When mild diarrhea occurs, it can be treated symptomatically with diphenoxylate (Lomotil) or loperamide (Imodium) and with an empiric three- to five-day course of antibiotics (Table 28-2). Travelers with fever or bloody diarrhea should seek medical care. Bloody diarrhea and abdominal pain suggest amebic dysentery (*Entamoeba histolytica*) or bacterial dysentery (*Shigella dysenteriae*, *Campylobacter jejuni*, or *Plesiomonas shigelloides*). If the medical history reveals recent antibiotic use, *Clostridium difficile* should be considered. Ingestion of raw or undercooked meat followed by bloody diarrhea suggests *E coli* 0157:H7, which may cause hemolytic-uremia syndrome.

If diarrhea is severe, patients may require oral rehydration. One of the best oral rehydration solutions is the WHO formula. This comes in packets that can be easily ordered. A homemade version would include 1 L of clean water, ½ tsp salt, ¼ tsp salt substitute (for potassium), ½ tsp baking soda (for bicarbonate), and 2–3 tbsp of sugar. Ingestion of glucose is important to promote water and sodium absorption from the gut. Too much glucose, however, can inhibit water absorption by its osmotic pull of water into the intestinal lumen. The ideal glucose concentration is 20 g/L. Apple juice, Gatorade, or cola drinks should be avoided because of their high sugar content.

One cause of traveler's diarrhea that deserves special attention is cholera. Cholera is endemic in more than 60 countries, and there has been a recent epidemic in Latin America. Fortunately, the disease rarely poses any risk to short-term travelers, since outbreaks are usually well localized and are not usually in areas near tourist attractions. It is caused by *Vibrio cholerae.* While most *V cholera* infections are asymptomatic or result in mild diarrhea, the infected individual may have profuse, watery diarrhea. Patients with severe disease can die in several hours if they are not properly treated. Early symptoms cannot be distinguished from other causes of traveler's diarrhea, and self-therapy is identical [9]. In severe cases, intravenous hydration and antibiotics may be necessary. Resistance to antimicrobials has been developing rapidly, but in most regions, traveler's diarrhea can be treated with tetracycline or doxycycline. Antibiotics decrease the duration of symptoms, the excretion of live cholera bacteria, and the volume of fluid lost, but they are not necessary for successful treatment.

Table 28-1
Bacterial Causes of Diarrhea

Noninflammatory	Inflammatory
Bacillus cereus	*Aeromonas hydrophila*
Campylobacter species	*Campylobacter* species
Clostridium perfringens	Enteroaggregative *E coli* (EaggEC)
Enteropathogenic *E coli* (EPEC)	Enterohemorrhagic *E coli* (EHEC)
Enterotoxigenic *E coli* (ETEC)	Enteroinvasive *E coli* (EIEC)
Salmonella species	*Plesiomonas shigelloides*
Vibrio cholerae	*Salmonella* species
Vibrio parahemolyticus	*Shigella* species
	Yersinia enterocolitica

Table 28-2
Drug Regimens for the Treatment of Traveler's Diarrhea

Drug	Adult Dose	Comments
Bismuth subsalicylate (Pepto Bismol)	20 mL or 2 tablets every 30 minutes for 8 doses	Maximum 240 mL (16 tablets) per day
Loperamide (Imodium)	2 caplets; then 1 caplet after each loose stool	Maximum 8 caplets (16 mg) per day
Ciprofloxacin (Cipro)	500 mg twice daily or 750 mg as one dose	Contraindicated in pregnant women and those under age 18
Ofloxacin (Floxin)	200 mg or 300 mg twice daily	Contraindicated in pregnant women and those under age 18
Trimethoprim/sulfamethoxazole (Bactrim, Septra)	One 160 mg/800 mg tablet twice daily	Increasing resistance among many enteric pathogens
Doxycycline	100 mg twice daily	Contraindicated in pregnant women and those under age 18

Prolonged diarrhea suggests a nonbacterial infection, such as *giardiasis*. In patients who have taken antibiotics, *C difficile* should be considered. Finally, not all diarrhea in travelers represents travel-related illness. If the evaluation does not reveal any pathogens and there is no response to empiric treatment, noninfectious causes of diarrhea, such as lactose intolerance or inflammatory bowel disease, should also be considered.

Respiratory Infections

Prolonged air travel and crowded conditions predispose travelers to respiratory infections. The low humidity of airplane cabins dries out mucous membranes, impairing an important defense mechanism. Also cabin air is recirculated during flights, which may promote the spread of airborne diseases, including tuberculosis. Restriction in close quarters during flights or upon arrival increases the likelihood of spreading other airborne illnesses, such as influenza, *Neisseria meningitidis*, and diphtheria.

The evaluation of respiratory infections in recent travelers is similar to that of patients presenting from the general population. Underlying illnesses and vaccination status must be considered. However, tuberculosis should also be considered, especially in travelers returning from areas where tuberculosis is prevalent or among those who had prolonged exposure to residents. Teachers, health care workers, volunteer relief workers, and students are at particular risk. Transmission has also occurred during travel on commercial aircraft [10]. If tuberculosis is suspected, chest radiography, sputum culture for common respiratory pathogens and *Mycobacterium tuberculosis*, and a tuberculin skin test should be obtained. If hospitalization is required, the patient should be placed in respiratory isolation until TB can be excluded. Treatment depends on the likelihood of multidrug-resistant TB.

Exposure to influenza depends on the time of year and the destination. Influenza can occur year-round in the tropics. In temperate regions of the Southern Hemisphere, influenza activity is greatest between May and September. Travelers may also be exposed to influenza during the summer, when traveling with large groups, including persons from parts of the world where the influenza virus is circulating.

Meningitis

In certain parts of the world, *N meningitidis* is an important cause of meningitis. It is endemic in the "Meningitis Belt," which stretches across sub-Saharan Africa to Northern India and Nepal. When an individual who returns from travel to any of these areas exhibits symptoms and/or signs of meningitis, the possibility of *N meningitidis* infection is an important consideration. However, many of the systemic illnesses discussed below may also present with severe headaches and, rarely, meningitis. Table 28-3 lists other systemic illnesses that also may have cutaneous manifestations.

Systemic Illnesses

Malaria must be considered in any traveler who returns with a systemic febrile illness. Malaria due to *Plasmodium falciparum* is a medical emergency. All febrile patients who have traveled to endemic areas must be considered to have malaria until proved otherwise. This disease is caused by a parasite and is discussed in greater detail in Chapter 30.

ENTERIC FEVER

Enteric fever is most often caused by *Salmonella typhi*, although it may also be caused by *Salmonella paratyphi*. Although typhoid and paratyphoid fever are acquired through the enteral route, diarrhea is not a common presenting symptom. Patients usually present with high fever, prostration, and abdominal pain. Enteric fever is most commonly seen in those who are returning from developing countries. Although immunization decreases the likelihood of contracting this infectious disease, it does not exclude the diagnosis, since none of the available vaccines offers 100% protection. Enteric fever may have an insidious or abrupt onset. The incubation period ranges from five to 21 days, depending on the size of the inoculum and the underlying health of the traveler. Presenting symptoms are nonspecific and may include fevers, diarrhea, abdominal pain, constipation, headache, anorexia, cough, and muscle pains. Approximately 5–10% of patients develop neuropsychiatric manifestations, which may include psychosis and confusion. Thirty percent of patients develop "rose spots." This is classically a salmon-colored maculopapular rash on the trunk. The lesions contain organisms that can be cultured from punch biopsy specimens.

Table 28-3
Common Systemic Bacterial Infections Associated with Skin Lesions

Bartonellosis
Brucellosis
Gonococcemia
Leptospirosis
Lyme disease
Meningococcemia
Rat-bite fever
Rickettsial infections
Syphilis
Typhoid fever

The diagnosis of enteric fever depends on the isolation of *S typhi* or *S paratyphi* from the patient. Cultures of blood, stool, urine, rose spots, bone marrow, and gastric and intestinal secretions may be useful. In more than 90% of patients, bacteria are isolated from blood, bone marrow, or intestinal secretions. If only blood cultures are performed, the sensitivity is 50–70%. Bone marrow cultures are 90% sensitive in making the diagnosis. Stool cultures are often negative.

Resolution of fever and most symptoms occurs in 90% of patients by the fourth week of infection without antibiotic therapy. However, weakness, weight loss, and debilitation may persist for months. If the infection is treated with antibiotics, symptoms usually resolve in three to five days. Reasonable antibiotic choices include beta-lactam antibiotics, chloramphenicol, fluoroquinolones, or trimethoprim-sulfamethoxazole [11].

RICKETTSIAL INFECTIONS

Rickettsial infections include the spotted fevers, typhus fever, and Q fever. This group of infections is characterized by the abrupt onset of fevers and headaches. Except for Q fever, vectors (usually ticks) carry these illnesses.

The spotted fevers are often recognized by the tache noire, or eschar, at the site of the tick bite. The disease is transmitted by a tick bite and is caused by various *Rickettsia* species. The initial symptoms are fevers, myalgias, and headaches. A tache noire may be identified by careful examination. Severe cases may resemble Rocky Mountain spotted fever and result in disseminated vascular infection.

Murine typhus, which is caused by *Rickettsia typhi*, occurs after inoculation of infected flea feces into a fleabite wound. The presentation is nonspecific; patients usually have fevers, headaches, chills, myalgias, and nausea. Only 18% of patients have a rash at the onset of illness, but 50% develop a rash during the course of their illness. Most of the clinical findings are due to vasculitis, which may affect any organ [12].

Scrub typhus is caused by *Rickettsia tsutsugamushi* and is transmitted by the bite of larval-stage trombiculid mites (chiggers). It is found in eastern Asia and the western Pacific region. The vector predominantly lives in scrub, which is the vegetation in the transitional area between forest and clearings. Awareness of the vector's habitat is important for both military personnel and local residents. If an eschar and regional adenopathy are present, this strongly suggests the diagnosis. Symptoms begin six to 18 days after the bite. The most prominent findings are fever, severe headache, and myalgias. Lymphadenopathy is common [13].

Q fever is caused by *Coxiella burnetii.* The important reservoirs for this infection are cattle, sheep, and goats. The organism can be shed in urine, feces, milk, or birth products. The incubation period is approximately 20 days, and symptoms usually include severe headache, fever, chills, fatigue, and myalgias. Unlike the cutaneous involvement associated with other rickettsial infections, rash is rare in patients with Q fever. When it does occur, it is generally due to an immune complex vasculitis, which may result from chronic disease [14].

Rickettsial illnesses can be treated with tetracycline, doxycycline, or chloramphenicol. Fluoroquinolones may also be useful.

LEPTOSPIROSIS

Leptospirosis is found worldwide. It is transmitted from exposure to the urine of infected animals. Rats are the most important source of infection. Leptospirosis usually causes a mild, self-limited disease and is a biphasic illness. Fevers, headaches, and myalgias characterize the first phase, a "septicemic" phase beginning seven to 12 days after exposure. The initial phase is followed by an immune phase, which is characterized by headaches, myalgias, and mild delirium. Patients may have conjunctival suffusion, hepatosplenomegaly, adenopathy, and a rash. During the septicemic phase, bacteria can be isolated from blood, cerebrospinal fluid (CSF), and most tissues. During the immune phase, the organism can still be found in the kidney, urine, and aqueous humor. The diagnosis is often made retrospectively with serologic tests. Treatment with penicillin, tetracycline, or doxycycline during the first few days of the initial phase may shorten the duration of fever and reduce the incidence of renal, hepatic, meningeal, and hemorrhagic complications. Severe disease, or icteric leptospirosis, results in fulminant hepatic failure, or Weil's disease, characterized by jaundice and renal failure.

BRUCELLOSIS

Brucellosis, or undulant fever, is found worldwide, especially in the Mediterranean basin, the Arabian Peninsula, the Indian subcontinent, and in parts of Mexico and Central and South America. It is caused by *Brucella* species and occurs after direct or indirect contact with animals, in particular cattle, goats, sheep, swine, and dogs. The disease is most commonly seen in abattoir (slaughterhouse) workers, veterinarians, livestock industry workers, and laboratory workers. Most commonly, bacteria enter the body through abrasions in the skin or after accidental inoculation into the conjunctiva. *Brucella melitensis* is often ingested in unpasteurized milk. Symptoms begin two to eight weeks after inoculation. Patients present with nonspecific symptoms of fevers, sweats, malaise, anorexia, headaches, and back pains. If brucellosis is not treated, the patient may develop an undulant fever pattern. Because it is a systemic disease involving the reticuloendothelial system, patients often have lymphadenopathy, splenomegaly, and/or hepatomegaly. Isolating the bacteria from blood, bone marrow, or other tissues can make the diagnosis. Alternatively, serologic tests can be used to make a presumptive diagnosis. Because of the high rate of relapse associated with use of a single drug, combination treatment is generally recommended. Doxycycline is given in combination with rifampin or an aminoglycoside. With appropriate treatment, most patients recover within weeks to months.

ANTHRAX

Anthrax, a disease of herbivores that come into contact with spores in the soil, is caused by *Bacillus anthracis.* In its spore form, *B anthracis* can persist for years. Anthrax is found worldwide but is endemic in South America, Central America, Iran, and Russia. It is spread to humans by direct contact with skin, inhalation, or ingestion. Contaminated animal hides and wool can be a source of infection. Ninety-five percent of infections are cutaneous, and 5% involve the respiratory tract. Gastrointestinal anthrax has also been reported in Third World countries [15]. In humans, cutaneous illness presents as a painless papule, usually on exposed areas of the head, neck, and arms. The lesion becomes vesicular with an ulcerated center and then develops the characteristic black eschar.

Pulmonary anthrax occurs when spores are inhaled. Wool sorters are at highest risk. This is a biphasic illness. The initial symptoms of malaise, fatigue, myalgias, fevers, and a nonproductive cough often resemble a mild upper respiratory infection. After two to four days, the patient may show some improvement, but this initial phase is followed by the sudden onset of severe respiratory distress. Patients soon become hypotensive, and death usually occurs within 24 hours.

Intestinal anthrax occurs after ingestion of contaminated food and results in nausea, vomiting, anorexia, and fever. Abdominal pain, hematemesis, and bloody diarrhea may also develop. With further progression, shock, cyanosis, and death may occur two to five days after the initial ingestion. Oropharyngeal infection, resulting in edema and tissue necrosis in the area of the cervical spine, may also occur. The main clinical features are sore throat, dysphagia, fever, regional lymphadenopathy, and toxemia. Most patients with oropharyngeal infection die [15].

Infected patients almost always have an apparent source of exposure. Anthrax bacilli can often be isolated from vesicular fluid or blood, and the serologic findings of a four-fold rise in acute and convalescent titers or a single titer greater than 1:32 confirm the diagnosis. Because 20% of cutaneous disease results in death, antibiotic treatment is important. Penicillin G is the drug of choice; erythromycin, tetracyclines, and chloramphenicol are alternatives. Excision of the lesion is contraindicated. Dressings removed from the lesion should be treated as biohazardous waste [15].

BARTONELLOSIS

Bartonellosis is caused by *Bartonella bacilliformis,* which is found only in river valleys of the Andes Mountains (Columbia, Peru, and Ecuador) at altitudes between 2,000 and 8,000 feet. The only proven vector is the sandfly. *B bacilliformis* organisms invade red blood cells and cause intravascular hemolysis and fever. The organism can then invade the reticuloendothelial system [16].

The acute form of bartonellosis, Oroya fever, occurs after an incubation period of about three weeks. Patients may present with anorexia, headaches, malaise, and a slight fever. In more severe cases, the initial presentation includes high fevers, chills, headaches, and confusion. Patients may become jaundiced because of rapid hemolysis. Other possible findings are myalgias, arthralgias, dyspnea, insomnia, delirium, and in terminal cases, coma. Generalized lymphadenopathy and thrombocytopenic purpura may also occur. If patients survive this stage, the convalescent stage begins. The organisms disappear from the red cells, and there is a decrease in fever and an increase in the number of erythrocytes. Intercurrent infection is common at this stage and may be an important cause of mortality [16].

The diagnosis can often be made by eosin/thiazine stain of blood smears during the acute phase. IgM antibodies may be present but are nonspecific. Treatment is with chloramphenicol, penicillin, or fluoroquinolones. Fever often disappears within 24 hours. Patients with severe anemia may require blood transfusions [16].

An eruptive cutaneous form known as *verruga peruana* may occur after resolution of Oroya fever, or it may occur without prior symptoms in those with previous episodes of bartonellosis. Joint pains and low-grade fever often present in the pre-eruptive stage. Nodules (verrugas) develop over a period of one to two months and may persist for months to years. The verrugas appear most often on exposed parts of the body. Cutaneous lesions vary from red to purple and appear in crops. Individual lesions may reach 1–

2 cm in diameter, and the organism may be cultured from the lesions. There is a variable response to antibiotics. Secondary infections may require surgery or antimicrobial therapy [16].

Prevention requires control of the sandfly. Dwellings may be sprayed with DDT and insect repellents. Use of bed netting is important [16].

MELIOIDOSIS

Melioidosis is caused by *Burkholderia pseudomallei*. This disease is endemic in Southeast Asia, with the largest concentration of cases in Vietnam, Cambodia, Laos, Thailand, Malaysia, Myanmar, and northern Australia. It has been reported in latitudes between 20 degrees north and south of the equator and has rarely been reported in the Western Hemisphere. In endemic areas, the organism is found in surface water, mud, rice paddies, and market produce. Clinical disease is rare except in northeast Thailand, where it accounts for 40% of deaths from community-acquired septicemia [17]. The disease can recur months or years after apparent cure, or it may break out after many years of latency. The clinical manifestations are variable. The most common presentation is acute pulmonary infection, but melioidosis may cause transient bacteremia, asymptomatic pulmonary infiltration, acute localized suppurative infection, septicemia, or a chronic suppurative infection. The disease should be suspected in persons returning from an endemic area if symptoms of respiratory failure or multiple pustular or necrotic skin or subcutaneous lesions develop, or if there is a radiographic appearance consistent with tuberculosis but no mycobacteria can be isolated. The diagnosis can be made by culturing the organism or by serologic testing. When treatment is necessary, it should be based on the results of susceptibility testing. Combination therapy is recommended for severely ill patients.

PLAGUE

Plague is caused by the bacterium *Yersinia pestis* (see Chapter 15). It is found worldwide, with most of the human cases reported from developing countries in Asia and Africa. Plague is primarily a zoonotic infection. Humans become infected from contact with rodents and their fleas. The most common presentation is bubonic plague, which is characterized by the sudden onset of fevers, chills, weakness and headache, and painful regional lymphadenitis. The most common site of lymphadenitis is the groin, but axillary and cervical buboes also occur. Buboes are 1–10 cm in length and are extremely tender. They occur in 90% of cases of plague. *Septicemic plague* is defined as plague without a bubo, which often progresses rapidly to shock. Patients with septicemic plague have high-grade bacteremia; a blood smear may reveal the characteristic bacilli. The case-fatality rate is 33%. Pneumonic plague is most often a secondary pneumonia in a patient with bubonic plague. It can also occur in cases of human-to-human contact. The pneumonia is necrotizing and is invariably fatal if antibiotic therapy is delayed by more than one day. Plague meningitis is a rare complication of inadequately treated bubonic plague; it results from hematogenous spread and has a high mortality rate [18].

The diagnosis of plague should be suspected in febrile patients who have been exposed to rodents or other mammals in the known endemic areas of the world. A diagnosis can often be made quickly with a smear and culture of a bubo aspirate. In patients with negative cultures, a fourfold or greater increase in titer or a single titer of at least 1:16 provides a presumptive diagnosis. Streptomycin is the drug of choice; tetracycline and chloramphenicol are effective alternatives [18].

Prevention depends on controlling rodent and flea reservoirs. Proper disposal of food and refuse, removal of unused outbuildings and woodpiles, and periodic treatment with pesticides are important. Buildings should be ratproof. In high-risk areas, the formalin-killed vaccine should be considered. This is given as a primary series of two injections, with a one- to three-month interval between them, followed by boosters every six months [18].

TULAREMIA

Tularemia is caused by *Francisella tularensis*. Although widely distributed, it is primarily a disease of the Northern Hemisphere. Rodents and lagomorphs are important reservoirs. Transmission to humans occurs after an insect bite, direct contact with contaminated animal products, or inhalation. High-risk occupations include veterinarians, farmers, sheep workers, hunters and trappers, cooks or meat handlers, and laboratory workers [19].

The incubation period for *F tularensis* is generally three to five days but may be as short as one day or as long as three weeks. Clinical symptoms usually start abruptly with fever, chills, headache, malaise, anorexia, and fatigue. Without treatment, fever lasts an average of one month, and adenopathy may persist for several months. The presentation is often classified as ulceroglandular, glandular, oculoglandular, pharyngeal, typhoidal, or pneumonic. Ulceroglandular disease is most common and is characterized by tender localized lymphadenopathy. The inciting skin lesion may appear before, with, or after the lymphadenopathy. It generally starts as a painful red papule and then undergoes necrosis, leaving a tender ulcer. Glandular disease is similar but without an apparent skin lesion. Oculoglandular tularemia occurs when the organism gains entry through the conjunctiva. Patients may have photophobia, excessive lacrimation, and a painful conjunctivitis, with small yellow conjunctival ulcers or papules in some patients. Typhoidal tularemia is a febrile illness without prominent lymphadenopathy. This form is the most difficult to diagnosis. Pneumonic tularemia presents with predominantly pulmonary symptoms. It may occur after inhalation or from hematogenous spread to the lung. The most common complication is suppuration of involved lymph nodes. Patients with severe disease may have disseminated intravascular coagulation, renal failure, rhabdomyolysis, jaundice, and hepatitis [19].

The diagnosis depends on clinical suspicion. *F tularensis* may be recovered from various sites in the body, and it is a significant risk to laboratory workers. The diagnosis can be confirmed with serologic studies. The drug of choice for treatment is streptomycin; gentamicin is a reasonable alternative. Use of tetracycline or chloramphenicol, which are only bacteriostatic, results in a high relapse rate [19].

The best preventive measure is avoidance of exposure to the organism. Wild animals should not be skinned or dressed using bare hands or when the animal appears ill. Gloves, masks, and protective eyewear should be worn. Wild game should be cooked thoroughly. Water that is contaminated by dead animals should not be used. When working in high-risk areas with large numbers of ticks, clothing that covers most of the body should be worn. Tick repellents should also be considered [19].

Sexually Transmitted Diseases

Medical professionals who care for travelers often underestimate exposure to sexually transmitted diseases (STDs). There is evidence that travel increases the risk of acquiring STDs, although this may be due to overall high-risk behavior of individuals who have casual sex during travel [20]. The prevalence of STDs is much higher in developing countries than in the United States. Those most likely to engage in unprotected sexual intercourse with a new partner while abroad are business travelers and young men traveling for long periods of time alone. Chlamydia and gonorrhea are the most common causes of urethritis in men and cervicitis in women. However, the differential for genital ulcerative diseases is fairly large, including syphilis (*Treponema pallidum*), chancroid (*Haemophilus ducreyi*), lymphogranuloma venereum (*Chlamydia trachomatis*) granuloma inguinale, donovanosis (*Calymmatobacterium granu-lomatis*).

Syphilis is generally categorized by phase: (1) an incubation period lasting about three weeks; (2) primary syphilis with a painless ulcer (chancre), regional adenopathy, and early bacteremia; (3) secondary syphilis, which is characterized by generalized mucocutaneous lesions and adenopathy; (4) latent syphilis; (5) in a small proportion of patients, tertiary syphilis, which most often involves the ascending aorta and the central nervous system (CNS).

Primary syphilis begins as a single painless papule, which quickly erodes and becomes indurated to form a smooth, painless ulcer without any exudate (chancre). During this stage, darkfield microscopy can be used to make the diagnosis. The chancre usually resolves within three to six weeks. Secondary syphilis begins two to eight weeks after the appearance of the chancre. During this period, the spirochete is widely disseminated. Macular, maculopapular, papular, and/or pustular lesions may appear on the body, including the palms of the hands and soles of the feet. Mucous patches may be seen in the mouth. Plaques, known as condyloma lata, may also be seen; these are highly contagious. There are often constitutional symptoms, and the CNS is frequently involved. Syphilis may then enter a latent stage without any clinical evidence of disease, but it may recur later as late syphilis or neurosyphilis.

In primary and secondary syphilis, the diagnosis can be made with darkfield microscopy. However, the diagnosis is most often made with serologic tests. These tests are not reliable in primary syphilis but are usually positive by the time a patient develops secondary syphilis. Screening is usually performed with one of the nonspecific tests: a rapid plasma reagin test (RPR) or venereal disease research laboratory test (VDRL). These tests are inexpensive, rapid, and convenient, but there are many false-positive test results. When results are positive, the diagnosis can be confirmed with one of the specific treponemal tests. These include the fluorescent treponemal antibody absorption test (FTA-ABS) or the *T pallidum* hemagglutination assay (TPHA). Penicillin is the drug of choice.

Chancroid is found worldwide and is associated with low socioeconomic status and poor hygiene. Only 10% of reported cases are in women. The incubation period is generally five to seven days. Lesions begin as tender papules that become pustular and then erode to form an ulcer. The typical ulcer is painful, nonindu-rated, ragged, and undermined with an erythe-matous halo. The base bleeds easily and may be covered with a necrotic exudate, which can be up to 20 mm in size. Approximately half of patients have inguinal lymphadenopathy that is unilateral and tender and may require drainage.

The diagnosis of chancroid is difficult to make clinically. A culture specimen should be obtained with a swab from the purulent ulcer base or by aspiration of the bubo. Gram staining may show large numbers of gram-negative coccobacilli. Patients with suspected chancroid should also be evaluated for syphilis because the infections may be difficult to differentiate, and patients may be co-infected. Most patients respond to treatment with erythromycin, azithromycin, ceftriaxone (unless they are co-infected with HIV), or amoxicillin/clavulonic acid.

Lymphogranuloma venereum (LGV) is endemic in Africa, India, Southeastern Asia, South America, and the Caribbean. The primary lesion appears three to 30 days after infection. It is a small papule or ulcer that produces few, if any, symptoms. Days to weeks later, patients develop lymphadenopathy and systemic symptoms, including fevers, headaches, and myalgias. Initially, the lymph nodes are discrete and tender and have overlying erythema; then the inflammation spreads into the surrounding tissue, forming an inflammatory mass (bubo). Abscesses, fistulas, or sinus tracts may develop within this mass. Rupture of the bubo occurs in one third of patients and relieves pain and fever, although sinus tracts may continue to drain pus for several weeks or months. As the disease progresses, fibrosis of the lymph nodes develops.

The clinical diagnosis of LGV rests on the presence of painless ulcers and matted unilateral lymph nodes. Unlike herpes, in LGV there is usually just one lesion, which is painful. Indurated margins and bilateral adenopathy suggest syphilis. Large ulcers that are multiple and extremely tender suggest chancroid. *Chlamydia trachomatis* can be recovered from bubo aspirates, genital tissue, or rectal tissue in one third of cases. Histopathologic changes in LGV, combined with serologic tests in an appropriate setting, are sufficient to make the diagnosis. Doxycycline or erythromycin is used to treat this infection. A fluctuant bubo may also require aspiration to prevent rupture and formation of sinus tracts.

Granuloma inguinale is a chronic, progressive ulcerative disease. It is most commonly reported in southeast India, New Guinea, the Caribbean, and parts of South America. It has also been recorded in Zambia, Zimbabwe, the Natal region of South Africa, Southeast Asia, and among aborigines in Australia. After an incubation period of eight to 80 days, a small painless papule or indurated nodule appears. This soon ulcerates to form a beefy-red, granulomatous ulcer with rolled edges and a characteristic satin like surface that bleeds easily. Multiple lesions may coalesce to form large ulcers, and new lesions may form from autoinoculation. The ulcers are painless, unless there is severe secondary infection. The disease spreads subcutaneously and may become destructive. In severe cases, patients may develop lymphedema with elephantiasis of the external genitalia. The diagnosis is usually made clinically and can be confirmed histologically by punch biopsy of the edge of active lesions or a crush preparation of granulation tissue. The demonstration of typical intracellular Donovan's bodies is the gold standard for making the diagnosis. Tetracyclines are considered the drugs of choice, but there are still treatment failures. Other options include trimethoprim-sulfamethoxazole, fluoroquino-lones, chloramphenicol, and aminoglycosides.

References

1. Centers for Disease Control and Prevention. *Health Information for International Travel 1996–1997.* Atlanta: CDC, 1997.
2. Jong EC. Immunizations for international travel. *Infect Dis Clin North Am* 1998;12(2):249–66.
3. Wolfe MS. Protection of travelers. *Clin Infect Dis* 1997;25:177–86.
4. Miller SI, Hohmann EL, Pegues DA. Salmonella (including *Salmonella typhi*). In: Mandell GL, Bennett JE, Dolin R (eds), *Principles and Practices of Infectious Diseases*, 4th Ed. New York: Churchill Livingstone, 1995. Pp 2024–6.
5. Centers for Disease Control and Prevention. *Health Information for International Travel 1999–2000.* Atlanta: CDC, 1999.
6. National Institutes of Health Consensus Conference. Traveler's diarrhea. *JAMA* 1985;253:2700–4.
7. Kozarsky PE, Lobel HO, Steffen R. Travel medicine 1991: new frontiers. *Ann Intern Med* 1991;115 (7): 574–5.
8. Hill DR, Pearson RD. Health advice for international travel. *Ann Intern Med* 1988;108:839–52.
9. Haburchak DR, Felz MW. Diseases associated with foreign travel. *Comprehen Ther* 1997;23(1):19–24.
10. Centers for Disease Control and Prevention. Exposure of passengers and flight crew to *Mycobacterium* tuberculosis on commercial aircraft, 1992–1995. *MMWR* 1995;44:137–40.
11. Miller SI, Hohmann EL, Pegues DA. Salmonella (including *Salmonella typhi*). In: Mandell GL, Bennett JE, Dolin R (eds), *Principles and Practices of Infectious Diseases*, 4th Ed. New York: Churchill Livingstone, 1995. Pp 2020–1.
12. Dumler JS, Walker DH. Murine typhus. In: Mandell GL, Bennett JE, Dolin R (eds), *Principles and Practices of Infectious Diseases*, 4th Ed. New York: Churchill Livingstone, 1995. Pp 1737–9.
13. Saah AJ. *Rickettsia tsutsugamushi* (scrub typhus). In: Mandell GL, Bennett JE, Dolin R (eds), *Principles and Practices of Infectious Diseases*, 4th Ed. New York: Churchill Livingstone, 1995. Pp 17340–1.
14. Marrie TJ. *Coxiella burnetti* (Q fever). In: Mandell GL, Bennett JE, Dolin R (eds), *Principles and Practices of Infectious Diseases*, 4th Ed. New York: Churchill Livingstone, 1995. Pp 1727–35.
15. Lew D. *Bacillus anthracis* (anthrax). In: Mandell GL, Bennett JE, Dolin R (eds), *Principles and Practices of Infectious Diseases*, 4th Ed. New York: Churchill Livingstone, 1995. Pp 1885–9.
16. Roverts NJ. *Bartonella bacilliformis* (bartonellosis). In: Mandell GL, Bennett JE, Dolin R (eds), *Principles and Practices of Infectious Diseases*, 4th Ed. New York: Churchill Livingstone, 1995. Pp 2209–10.
17. Chaowagul W, White NJ, Dance DAB, et al. Melioidosis: a major cause of community-acquired septicemia in northeastern Thailand. *J Infect Dis* 1989;159:890–9.
18. Butler T. *Yersinia* species (including plague). In: Mandell GL, Bennett JE, Dolin R (eds), *Principles and Practices of Infectious Diseases*, 4th Ed. New York: Churchill Livingstone, 1995. Pp 2070–8.
19. Penn RL. *Francisella tularensis* (tularemia). In: Mandell GL, Bennett JE, Dolin R (eds), *Principles and Practices of Infectious Diseases*, 4th Ed. New York: Churchill Livingstone, 1995. Pp 2060–8.
20. Arvidson M, Hellberg D, Mardh PA. Sexual risk behavior and history of sexually transmitted diseases in relation to casual travel sex during different types of journeys. *Acta Obstet Gynecol Scand* 1996;75:490–4.

29 / Helminthic Travel-Related Infections

Jeffrey G. Jones

Although helminthic infections receive relatively little attention in the United States, they represent a significant burden of suffering throughout the world. In fact, some authors estimate that up to 25% of the world's populace is infected with helminths. As the world rapidly becomes more accessible to more people, helminthic infections are becoming more common in the United States. Groups at special risk for these infections include international workers, students and travelers, migrant laborers, refugees, children of foreign adoptions, and the homeless. Environmental factors include substandard housing, crowding, breakdown of hygienic standards, and inaccessible medical care, all of which are risks for contracting helminthic infections.

Parasites in general, but worm infections specifically, are looked upon in the United States with abhorrence. Thus, there is a strong social stigma associated with these infections, which may or may not be warranted by their detriment to health. The practitioner must keep this in mind when working with patients who have these infections. Unlike many other types of infections, helminthic infections are often diagnosed primarily through microscopic detection of helminth eggs or larval stages. For this reason, the practitioner is encouraged to have ready access to a high-quality atlas of parasites [1].

The helminths are composed of three groups. The first includes nematodes, or roundworms. These may be intestinal, in the blood or tissues, or zoonotic. The second includes the trematodes, or flukes, and the third, the cestodes, or tapeworms.

Adult Nematoda Residing in the Human Gut

These are the most prevalent of all nematodes. They are found primarily in tropical and subtropical climates. In general, their presence reflects the sanitary and socioeconomic conditions of the environment. To varying degrees, these are all found in the United States and worldwide.

ASCARIS LUMBRICOIDES

Ascaris lumbricoides is the largest intestinal nematode, measuring up to 30 cm in length. This nematode has the appearance of an earthworm but is white or light pink in color. It is the worm that frequently causes panic in the individual who passes one in the stool or coughs up or vomits a worm.

The prevalence of human *Ascaris* infection, which, as previously mentioned, may occur worldwide, is thought to be greater than 1.3 billion. This corresponds to approximately one fourth of the world's population. Point prevalence varies widely according to geographic variations, but up to 95% of populations may be infected in parts of Africa [2]. Approximately 10.5 million disability-adjusted life years (DALYs) are lost due to *Ascaris* infection and its complications [3]. *Ascaris* infections are responsible for more than 20,000 deaths per year. Transmission is by oral contact with fecally contaminated soil. Occupational and environmental risk factors include work in and around soil, especially clay soil, as it is especially well suited for survival of the organism's eggs [4]. Workers who are exposed to sewage also are at risk for this infection, especially since eggs may survive treatment of sewage [5].

The life cycle begins when an infected human passes eggs with the feces into the soil, where they embryonate and become infective over a two- to four- week period [6]. They contaminate the environment and reach another human through oral form. Under the proper circumstances, eggs can survive in the soil for up to a decade [6]. The embryonated egg must be swallowed for the life cycle to be completed, because the egg needs the bile salts and alkaline enteric juices in order to go through its next stage of development [2]. The adult worm can live 12–18 months. After ingestion, the eggs hatch in the intestine. There is a phase of transit through the lung. The larval forms are then coughed up and swallowed, and the mature worm ends up in the small intestine. The worms then lay eggs, which are passed with the feces, thus completing the cycle.

Techniques involved in effective prevention of infection include hand washing and proper hygienic precautions when working around fecally contaminated soil. Engineering controls include hygienic disposal of human feces. Respiratory protection when working in dusty, fecally contaminated soils is the primary personal protective measure. Surveillance includes screening families who are at risk for this infection and examining stool samples for ova and parasites. This should be done with adequate time for the eggs to be in the stool after exposure (two to three months). Stool assessment for ova and parasite is generally thought to be most useful in assessing the adequacy of a preventive program.

Clinical Features and Diagnostic Evaluation

Most people with *Ascaris* infection are asymptomatic; others may develop vague abdominal discomfort. *Ascaris* may cause malnutrition through unclear mechanisms [7]. Occasionally, some people develop signs of obstruction as a result of a bolus of worms, which can produce a mechanical small bowel obstruction, especially in children [8]. Biliary colic, hepatitis, and pancreatitis are other possible presentations. Löffler's pneumonia, the complex of substernal burning, cough, dyspnea, and wheezing and rales during the larval migration through the lungs, may cause the brief appearance of perihilar infiltrates on chest radiograph. During this time, Charcot-Leyden crystals and larvae may be present in the sputum, and eosinophilia in the blood. If the patient is re-infected, the pulmonary phase may take on the appearance of an allergic asthmatic reaction [9]. Obstruction of the liver or pancreatic ducts may be present [10]. If a barium study is performed, one may see a thin column of barium in the worm's body [4]. Several stimuli, including anesthesia, fever, illness or ingestion of spicy foods, may cause the worm to exit via the mouth, nose, or rectum [6].

The infection is usually diagnosed through the identification of characteristic eggs in the stools, but sometimes the infection can be diagnosed by viewing an adult worm that the patient has passed. An ELISA serologic test is available but usually is not necessary.

Treatment

One must remember that medications are not active against migrating larvae [4]. Treatment options for adults are mebendazole (Vermox), 100 mg orally twice daily for three days or 500 mg as a single dose; pyrantel pamoate at a dosage of 11 mg/kg up to a maximum of 1 g; and albendazole as a single dose of 400 mg [11]. Drugs and dosages are the same for children. In high-transmission areas, periodic, age-targeted chemotherapy is cost effective [12,13] and has the greatest effect in decreasing DALYs [14].

ENTEROBIUS VERMICULARIS

Enterobius vermicularis, also known as oxiuriasis, seatworms, pinworms, or threadworms, is the most common helminth seen by primary care practitioners in North America. It is estimated that more than 290 million people are infected [10]. The infection is most commonly seen in children; adults are apparently less susceptible to the infection [2]. Transmission is by the fecal-oral route, and humans are the only source of the infection [15]. The eggs can be ingested in food, dust, and fomites or from environmental contamination. Autoinfection (anus-to-mouth transfer of eggs by fingers) permits the infection to continue indefinitely and to be amplified [4]. People who work in childcare or institutional settings are at increased risk for this infection. Once the eggs are in the environment, they are quite hardy; they are not killed by chlorination of water in swimming pools [4]. The infection is cosmopolitan in distribution. It is more common in temperate than in tropical climates, a somewhat unusual feature of distribution. The life cycle is human to human.

Prevention and Control

Administrative controls such as personal hygiene standards are critical to controlling this infection. The cleaning and trimming of fingernails of children is very helpful. Washing clothing and bedding on a regular basis also helps to kill the eggs, which may remain viable for up to 13 days under optimal conditions [4]. Hand washing is the primary personal protective measure. The use of gloves when dealing with the hygienic needs of children in an institutional setting is also warranted. Families who have this infection need to be educated that it is not considered evidence of poor hygiene and that reinfections are quite common. Surveillance of institutionalized children, along with periodic mass retreatment if infection continues to be a problem, is a reasonable option. Retesting children represents the best method of assessing adequacy of control and prevention.

Clinical Features

Eggs laid on the perianal skin become infective in approximately six hours [10]. The prepatent period, or time from egg ingestion to egg production by the female worm, is one to two months [15]. Retroinfection, in which the eggs actually hatch on the perianal skin and return to the large intestine through the anus, is possible. Pruritus ani, perianal eczema, dermatitis, insomnia, enuresis, gastrointestinal (GI) disturbance, genitourinary infections (in girls), and vulvovaginitis are all potential symptoms. The infection often causes intense itching secondary to the development of hypersensitivity to the worm proteins. The infection may also be asymptomatic; it rarely causes serious lesions. Females can develop inflammation of the genital tract, and *Enterobius* infection has been associated with cervicitis, endometritis, salpingitis, and oophoritis [16].

Diagnostic Evaluation

The diagnosis is generally made most easily from visualization of characteristic eggs on the "Scotch tape" test. In this test, the sticky side of clear cellulose tape is pressed up against the perianal skin and then attached to a microscope slide, where it is scanned under low power. The eggs are not generally seen in stools collected for ova and parasite analysis. During the night, adult worms, which are approximately 1 cm in length, may be visualized in the perianal area. Laboratory findings are usually not helpful unless there is tissue invasion, which is unusual but is associated with eosinophilia [4].

Treatment

Simultaneous treatment—treating the whole family—with either pyrantel pamoate, 11 mg/kg as a single dose up to a maximum dose of 1 g, mebendazole, 100 mg as a single dose, or, albendazole, 400 mg as a single dose, is effective therapy [11]. Treatment must be repeated two weeks after initial therapy. The doses are the same for adults and pediatrics.

TRICHURIS TRICHIURA

Trichuris trichiura, also known as *whipworm*, is the most common helminth in the Caribbean. Nine hundred million cases are thought to occur worldwide and are responsible for 6.4 million lost DALYs [3]. Although other species of *Trichuris* are found in animals, host specificity is generally the rule, and these are not usually zoonotic infections. Transmission is by the fecal-oral route. Embryonated eggs are usually ingested with food, fluid, or from fingers contaminated with soil that contains the eggs. The primary occupational risk factor is contact with soil. The infection occurs worldwide but has the highest prevalence in tropical and subtropical areas. It may be aggregated in certain populations or geographic areas [17]. The life cycle is human to environment (soil) to human.

Prevention centers around hygienic treatment of sewage so as to avoid introduction of the eggs into the food chain. This is especially important in areas where sewage is used as fertilizer. The eggs are relatively resistant to chemical disinfectants, making hygienic practices of key importance. Hand washing is the primary personal protective measure. Surveillance can be done by obtaining stools for ova and parasite analysis. Chemoprophylaxis in the form of group treatment (e.g., treatment of all school-age children in a geographic area) may be warranted in situations in which there is a high prevalence of infection. This results in improved growth and physical fitness of school children [18].

Clinical Features

The incubation period is two to three months from the time of egg ingestion until eggs are present in the stool, but symptoms may start before this time. The infection is usually asymptomatic, although there may be vague abdominal symptoms. Tenesmus, due to mucosal swelling of the rectal tissue, may occur, and protracted tenesmus occasionally causes rectal prolapse in very heavy infections in infants [19]. Also seen with heavy infection are bloody diarrhea, hemorrhagic ulcerations of the colon, perforation, and peritonitis. Chronic infection may be responsible for growth stunting and malnutrition in children. Rarely, a worm bolus can cause obstruction. The mucosal damage caused by *Trichuris* may facilitate invasion by other pathogens.

Diagnostic Evaluation

Differential diagnosis includes other intestinal parasites, including amebic dysentery, and inflammatory bowel disease. Diagnosis is made by identification of the distinctive bipolar-plugged eggs in the stool. Charcot-Leyden crystals may also be seen. Low-grade eosinophilia and iron deficiency anemia may be seen, especially if infections are heavy [19]. The erythrocyte sedimentation rate (ESR) usually remains normal.

Treatment

Treatment options include mebendazole, 100 mg orally twice daily for three days, or 500 mg orally in a single dose; or albendazole, 400 mg as a single dose [11]. Regimens are the same for adults and children.

HOOKWORM

Hookworm infections are caused by *Ancylostoma duodenale* or *Necator americanis* and are also called *tropical anemia* and *uncinariasis.* There is a geographic distribution of hookworm, with *N americanis* predominating in the Americas and sub-Saharan Africa and *A duodenale* usually occurring in Southeast Asia and the Mediterranean area [20]. There are exceptions to this generalization, however. The species can be microscopically differentiated by characteristic morphology of the head capsule, but they are clinically indistinguishable. Approximately 900 million people are infected worldwide. Because these worms feed on intestinal mucosa and blood, they are a common cause of tropical anemia and have a disproportionately high effect on lost DALYs (22.1 million DALYs lost) [3]. Although infectious larvae can penetrate intact skin, they usually enter through hair follicles. The larvae can survive in soil for several months under optimal conditions. Risk factors include walking barefoot or having other skin-to-soil contact. This sort of infection is common in people who work in crawl spaces or other shady, moist areas. The life cycle is from humans to humans via soil.

Prevention

Administrative requirements to wear shoes and avoid skin-to-soil contact are the best methods for preventing the infection in employees who work in contaminated areas. Sanitary disposal of human feces as an engineering control is warranted. Education regarding the risk factors for hookworm infection is helpful to reinforce the need to wear shoes.

Clinical Features

Symptoms may be seen one to two days after contact with the eggs. The time from skin penetration until eggs are passed in the feces is between four to six weeks. *Ancylostoma* organisms can also infect if ingested or through transmammary or transplacental passage [9]. The classic acute signs of infection are ground itch, in which a pruritic maculopapular rash appears at the site of skin penetration. The second type of presentation is pulmonary and is due to the migratory phase of the worms as they pass through the lungs. This presentation is similar to that seen in patients with *Ascaris* infection. Shortness of breath, mucus production, and occult blood in the sputum are common during this phase. The GI phase is usually associated with vague complaints, although a more severe GI phase, known as *Wakana disease,* may occur if large numbers of larvae are ingested. This causes nausea, vomiting, dyspnea, and eosinophilia [21]. A major clinical feature of hookworm is iron deficiency anemia, resulting directly from chronic blood loss. Since the adult worms may live up to 15 years, the blood loss is significant; often up to 0.26 mL of blood per day per worm may be lost. In people with low iron intake, even small numbers of worms may result in iron deficiency and anemia [22].

Diagnostic Evaluation

Diagnosis is made by visualization of eggs in the feces. Species cannot be determined by egg appearance, however. There is often a high level of eosinophilia that begins two to three weeks after skin penetration. Stools are often heme positive. Hypoalbuminemia is not uncommon.

Treatment

Treatment consists of medications to kill the worms and, afterward, iron replacement therapy. Effective regimens are mebendazole, 100 mg orally twice daily for three days or 500 mg as a single dose; pyrantel pamoate, 11 mg/kg up to a maximum dose of 1 g/kg for three days; or albendazole, 400 mg as a single dose [11]. The drugs and dosages are the same for children.

STRONGYLOIDES

Strongyloides infections may be caused by *Strongyloides stercoralis* or, rarely, *Strongyloides fulleborni.* Approximately 200 million infections occur worldwide. *Strongyloides* is one of three helminthic genera that can reproduce within humans. Transmission can occur either through the transdermal route after contact with fecally contaminated soil or sexually. Occupational groups at risk include those who have contact with soil, especially miners in temperate climates. The geographic distribution is worldwide [20], but the infection is especially prevalent in Southeast Asia and Brazil. There is an endemic focus in Appalachia, with approximately 3% of Kentucky schoolchildren [23] and 6% of Tennessee Veterans Administration inpatients [24] testing positive for this infection. *Strongyloides fulleborni* is seen only in Africa and Papua New Guinea.

Prevention

Systems to hygienically dispose of human feces are key to avoiding this infection. Also, it is necessary to avoid direct skin contact with contaminated soil and infected animals. Wearing gloves when handling patients with hyperinfection or autoinfectious cycles is preventive for health care workers. Surveillance of patients, especially before instituting corticosteroid or other immunosuppressive treatments, is critical, as it helps prevent hyperinfection and dissemination of the infection.

Clinical Features

The time from skin penetration until rhabditiform larvae appear in the feces is two to four weeks. As with hookworm, there may be an initial cutaneous phase, which is characterized by an itchy eruption at the site of larval penetration. Although uncommon, there may also be a pulmonary phase as larvae pass through the lungs. The gastrointestinal phase may be asymptomatic or cause mild-to-severe abdominal symptoms, including acute steatorrhea or weight loss. Autoinfective *Strongyloides* occurs when rhabditiform larvae transform into the infective filariform stages within the host and then reinfect the same host, either by penetration of the perianal skin or the bowel wall. These larvae then migrate through the tissues and the lung, after which they re-establish themselves in the intestine as new adult worms. This allows the infection to persist for years after the original exposure. If autoinfective cycles are present, migrating larvae may cause larva currens, serpiginous wheals surrounded by a flare. These wheals come and go in the course of a few hours and are usually seen on the trunk. Hyperinfection occurs when the body loses its defenses against the autoinfectious cycle and enormous numbers of filariform larvae reinvade the host. This is common if the host is taking corticosteroids, is malnourished, or is immunosuppressed. Curiously, HIV infection does not appear to predispose to strongyloides hyperinfection [25], in which diarrhea, paralytic ileus, gram-negative septicemia, peritonitis, pulmonary symptoms, and even brain involvement occur. Eosinophilia is not associated with hyperinfection. In compromised hosts, hemorrhage, inflammation, and necrosis of any organ may result.

Diagnostic Evaluation

The differential diagnosis includes other intestinal parasites, especially hookworm. Other causes of eosinophilic pneumonia and cutaneous larva migrans must also be ruled out. The diagnosis of *Strongyloides* infection is often difficult. Demonstration of larvae in the stool or duodenal fluid often requires concentration techniques for examining stool samples [26]. Fecal culture, in which stool is mixed with water and charcoal and left to incubate at room temperature, is often helpful [27]. Serologic diagnosis does have a high sensitivity [26].

Treatment

For adults and children, the treatment regimen is ivermectin, 200 mg/kg/day for one to two days [11,28]. An alternative is thiabendazole, 50 mg/kg/day in two doses up to a maximum of 3 g per day. This is given for two days and is likely to produce toxicity.

Adult Nematoda Residing in the Blood, Lymphatics, or Subcutaneous Tissue

This section discusses filarial infections, including guinea worm infection. The human filarial parasites infect up to 140 million people worldwide. There are great similarities in the life cycles, in that the infective larval stage is carried by an insect and the adult worm is found either in the lymph nodes, adjacent lymphatic vessels, or subcutaneous tissue. The microfilariae (MF) either circulate in the blood or migrate through the skin and can then be ingested by the appropriate arthropod, where they develop into the infective larvae, thus completing the cycle. The adults are long-lived, some living up to 20 years. The MF tend to live three months to three years. They differ in nucleoli patterns and presence of a sheath [1]. Filarial worms exhibit a trait known as periodicity. This implies that the MF are only present and active during certain times. These *periodicity* traits are shown in Table 29-1. The clinical manifestations of filarial worm infection develop slowly, and the clinical picture varies according to whether the individual has had previous exposure. Unexposed individuals tend to have more acute onset of symptoms.

Although there are eight types of filarial worms, it is useful to consider them according to their clinical presentation. Thus, they are discussed in this chapter as lymphatic filariasis, onchocerciasis, loa loa, *Mansonella*, and guinea worm infections.

LYMPHATIC FILARIASIS

Three filarial worms are associated with lymphatic filariasis: *Wuchereria bancrofti*, *Brugia malayi*, and *Brugia timori*. These three thread-like worms all live in the lymphatic channels or lymph nodes of the host and may remain alive for more than 20 years.

W bancrofti is the most widely distributed of the filarial worms. It is present in Africa, in portions of South and Central America, in the Caribbean basin, in Southeast Asia, and in the Pacific islands [20]. *W bancrofti* is estimated to have a prevalence of greater than 100 million people [29]. *B malayi* is present in China, India, Indonesia, Japan, Korea, Malaysia, and the Philippines. *B timori* has been described as present only in specific islands in Indonesia. Although the lymphatic filarial worms usually exhibit nocturnal periodicity, there are also subperiodic forms of both major types. This implies that the MF are present in blood at all times but are maximal in number in the afternoon. Humans are the natural reservoir for infection, although *B malayi* can be a natural infection in cats and monkeys. Risk factors for infection include geographic factors and mosquito exposure.

Prevention and Control

Any engineering or administrative interventions that lessen the risk for the presence of mosquitoes are likely to lessen the risk for lymphatic fi-

Table 29-1
Selected Traits of Filarial Worms

Species	Periodicity	Vector	Adult Location	Microfilaria Location	Sheath on MF
Wuchereria bancrofti	Nocturnal	Mosquito	Lymphatics	Blood	Present
Brugia malayi	Nocturnal	Mosquito	Lymphatics	Blood	Present
Brugia timori	Nocturnal	Mosquito	Lymphatics	Blood	Present
Onchocerca volvulus	None	Black fly	Subcutaneous	Skin, eye	Absent
Loa loa	Diurnal	Deer fly	Subcutaneous	Blood	Present
Mansonella streptocerca	None	Biting midge	Subcutaneous	Skin	Absent
Mansonella ozzardi	None	Biting midge, black fly	Subcutaneous	Blood	Absent
Mansonella perstans	None	Biting midge	Body cavities, mesentery, perirenal	Blood	Absent

larial infections. Personal protective measures, including the use of insect repellents and netting, are likely to be helpful in lessening the problem. Education about the relationship between mosquito bites and the disease is also likely to be helpful. Surveillance is generally helpful only for populations who are not routinely exposed. In the routinely exposed, the use of diethylcarbamazine (DEC), either alone [30] or with either ivermectin or albendazole [29], may be helpful in interrupting the transmission of the filarial worms in a community. For the person who is not routinely exposed, insect precautions, along with DEC chemoprophylaxis, may be a consideration [31]. DEC is usually considered only for those who will be in endemic regions for longer than one month.

Clinical Features

The usual incubation period for lymphatic filariasis is five to 18 months. Symptoms may occur prior to the appearance of microfilariae in peripheral blood. The range of time from infection to the appearance of symptoms is a minimum of one to three months to a maximum of years. Early symptoms tend to be related to dilatation of the lymphatics and thickening of the vessel walls, along with damage to valves within the lymphatic vasculature, and often consist of scrotal symptoms in men, lymphatic inflammation, and obstruction. Even asymptomatic patients may have lymphatic abnormalities, which show up only on lymphoscin-tigraphy [32]. Lymphangitis, lymphadenitis, orchitis, urticaria, and epididymitis all may occur. Filarial fever, which typically recurs six to 10 times per year and lasts for three to seven days at a time, is more common in native populations.

Tropical pulmonary eosinophilia is an uncommon form of acute filariasis that is associated with the rapid clearance of microfilariae as they pass through the lungs. Patients who have this syndrome are usually males (4:1 predominance) in their third decade of life. Clinical features of tropical pulmonary eosinophilia are paroxysmal cough, nocturnal wheezing, weight loss, fever, adenopathy, and extremes of peripheral blood eosinophilia. Chest radiography usually reveals increased bronchovascular markings. Pulmonary function studies show restrictive abnormalities, which may be accompanied by obstructive defects. If the disease is not treated, pulmonary damage may result in chronic fibrosis.

Chronic findings include lymphedema of the legs, arms, and scrotum. There may be associated hyperplastic changes of the skin or elephantiasis, which may predispose the patient to secondary bacterial infection. If the lymphatic vessels rupture into the renal pelvis, chyluria may occur.

Diagnostic Evaluation

Differential diagnosis of the lymphatic filarial infections includes deep venous thrombosis, infection, and trauma. Definitive diagnosis of the disease requires the demonstration of MF. This can be demonstrated in on blood and is usually done after some sort of concentration process such as filtration through a Nuclepore filter or in a 2% formalin solution (Knott's concentration technique) [33]. Most serologic tests are useful only for individuals who are not native to the endemic area, since native populations may have positive serology due to the exposure to infected mosquitoes but not actually have infection. Polymerase-chain-reaction-based assays for the lymphatic filarial infections are also available. Evaluation of the lymphatic function with lymphoscintig-raphy can provide information about lymphatic function. In males, evaluation of the scrotum by ultrasonographic techniques may reveal nodules, evidence of lymphatic dilatation, or even active worm motion. Since some individuals with filariasis are not microfilaremic, the diagnosis may sometimes need to be made on clinical grounds alone.

Treatment

Diethylcarbamazine is the treatment of choice for the lymphatic filarial infections. Pretreatment with antihistamines or corticosteroids may be required to decrease the possibility of allergic reactions due to disintegration of the microfilaria in these infections. If microfilaria are present in the blood, a slow increase in dosing is warranted. On day one, 50 mg is given orally, followed by 50 mg orally three times daily on day two. On day three, 100 mg orally three times daily is given. On days four through 14, 6 mg/kg/day is given in three divided doses [11]. These doses are identical for pediatric dosing. If no microfilaria are present, full doses can be given from the first day [11]. Ivermectin is useful for killing the microfilaria but does not kill the adult worms. Care should be taken to rule out *Onchocerca* infection prior to DEC treatment, as a potentially serious Mazzotti reaction could result. Treatment of the chronic lymphatic obstruction should be directed at management of the lymphedema, including measures such as limb elevation, support stockings, and local skin care. Surgical decompression may be necessary in severe cases of elephantiasis. Hydroceles may be drained or managed surgically.

ONCHOCERCA VOLVULUS

Onchocerca is a tissue-dwelling nematode, the microfilaria of which are found primarily in the skin and eye. Its prevalence has slowly decreased as a result of mass campaigns to destroy the larvae with insecticides as well as the use of chemotherapy to decrease the pool of filariae in human hosts. Transmission occurs as a result of the black fly (*Simulium* species).

The primary environmental risk factor is living or working in an endemic area. Geographic distribution of onchocerciasis tends to be in western Africa and some areas of eastern Africa. There is a small endemic area in Yemen and southwest Saudi Arabia. In the Western Hemisphere, onchocerciasis is present in Central and South America in selected foci [31].

The uses of vector control via insecticide spraying has been beneficial in some sites but is not suitable for broad control. The community-wide use of ivermectin has become the primary strategy used for control of onchocerciasis. This technique is thought to be most effective in breaking the transmission cycle worldwide.

Clinical Features

The incubation period of onchocerciasis is usually one to two years. Microfilariae usually first appear between three to 15 months after exposure. Adult worms can survive for up to 15 years. The microfilariae may persist for two to three years. Usual signs and symptoms include dermatitis, subcutaneous nodules, eye findings, and lymphadenopathy. The most common manifestation of the dermatitis is pruritus, which may be incapacitating and is usually generalized. With long-term infections, this dermatitis results in exaggerated and premature wrinkling of the skin, with loss of elastic fibers and epidermal atrophy. It may also result in hypo- or hyperpigmentation of the skin. This condition is sometimes called *leopard skin* [20]. Subcutaneous nodules are usually palpable and are commonly found over the lower back, the hips, and the iliac crests. The most serious clinical finding associated with onchocerciasis is the resulting visual impairment. This is usually seen in persons with moderate to heavy infections. Lesions can occur in all parts of the eye. The most common early finding is photophobia and conjunctivitis. In the cornea, so-called snowflake opacities are common [20]; these are caused by a tissue reaction to dead microfilariae in the cornea. Sclerosing keratitis is the most common cause of blindness in patients with onchocerciasis. Anterior uveitis and iridocyclitis are not uncommon and may result in secondary glaucoma. Following damage to the anterior segments of the eye, choroidoretinal lesions frequently occur, with resulting optic atrophy. Lymphadenopathy, particularly in the inguinal and femoral areas, is common. The enlarged nodes may become dependent, causing what is commonly called *hanging groin*. In persons with heavy infections, generalized weakness and loss of adipose tissue and muscle mass is common. This is partly responsible for the increased mortality in people who are blind as a result of onchocerciasis.

Diagnostic Evaluation and Treatment

Diagnosis involves identification of microfilariae in skin snips or of an adult worm from an excised nodule. In up to one third of cases, microfilariae are found in the blood or other body fluids. Slit-lamp examination frequently reveals microfilariae in the anterior eye chamber. Highly specific and sensitive serodiagnosis of the infection will soon be possible with the advent of recombinant onchocercal-specific antigens [34].

Treatment of onchoceriasis is aimed at avoiding permanent damage due to the infection and alleviating nuisance symptoms. Nodules, especially if present over the head, should be excised in order to lessen the chances of eye problems secondary to proximity of the adult worm. However, chemotherapy with ivermectin, remains the treatment of choice for onchocerciasis. For both adults and children, ivermectin as a single dose of 150 μg/kg is given initially and repeated in six to 12 months [11]. If one elects to kill the adult worms, suramin, a potent but potentially toxic macrofilaricidal agent, is an option [31]. Prior to the use of this medicine, ivermectin should be given (at the dose mentioned above) to reduce the microfilarial load.

LOA LOA

Loaiasis, also called *African eye worm* and *Calibar swelling*, is common in the rain forests of west and central Africa [31]. Transmission is through the bite of a deer fly, also called the *Tabanid fly*. The adult worms can live for longer than 10 years in their human hosts. People who work in the African rain forest are at risk for this infection. The life cycle is from human to human via the Tabanid fly (*Chrysops dimidiata* or *Chrysops silacea*).

Prevention

Because of the ample number of breeding places for this fly, control of the vector is difficult. Engineering controls, such as placing screens over windows, may be helpful. Personal protective measures, such as the use of insect repellents and wearing of long sleeves and pants, may also be helpful. In workers who are at high risk, weekly dosing with DEC at 300 mg per week has been shown to act as chemoprophylaxis for this agent [35].

Clinical Features

The incubation period for loa loa is one year or more. The infection and production of microfilariae (MF) are fairly well tolerated. The appearance of the adult worm in the subconjunctival eye space is a frequently disturbing aspect of this infection. Allergic complications tend to cause most symptoms. Localized pruritus and swelling are common. The swelling, also called *Calibar's swelling*, results from hypersensitivity and is migratory. Nephropathy is thought to be caused by immune complex mechanisms [36]. The brisk humeral and cell-mediated immune response, sometimes referred to as the *hyperresponsive syndrome*, may also cause episodes of inflammation or allergic symptoms, especially in expatriates [37].

Diagnostic Evaluation

Other filarial infections and gnathostomiasis are in the differential diagnosis. The diagnosis depends on the identification of the adult worm in the eye or identification of microfilariae in the blood. The infection is generally accompanied by high-grade eosinophilic and increased antibody levels, although the serologic tests are not reliable.

Treatment

Treatment includes surgical removal of the worm as it crosses the eye, if possible. The primary therapy is a DEC regimen, however. In patients with MF, pretreatment with antihistamines or corticosteroids may help to prevent allergic reactions related to disintegration of the MF, along with a slow increase in the DEC dose. The usual protocol for DEC is 50 mg on the first day, 50 mg three times daily on the second day, 100 mg three times daily on the third day, and 9 mg/kg per day in three divided doses on days four through 21 [11]. The schedule is similar in pediatrics, although it is 1 mg/kg the first day, 1 mg/kg three times daily the second day, and 1–2 mg/kg three times daily on day three. On days four through 21, 9 mg/kg/day in three divided doses are also used [11]. If no MF are present, full doses of DEC may be used from the onset. In cases of heavy MF (more than 2,000 MF per milliliter of blood), there is a risk of meningoencephalitis with treatment. This risk must be carefully weighed. Albendazole and ivermectin, although neither is FDA-approved, are shown to reduce MF loads, and albendazole may actually kill the adult worm [38].

MANSONELLIASIS

Mansonella species include *Mansonella streptocerca*, *Mansonella perstans*, and *Mansonella ozzardi*. These filarial worms are all transmitted by the biting midge (culicoides species), although *M ozzardi* can also be transmitted by black fly (*Simulium* species). The primary occupational or environmental risk factor is living or working in a geographic area where these midges or filarial worms are found. For *M streptocerca*, this area is the tropical forest belt of Africa. For *M perstans*, it is the center of Africa and northeastern part of South America. *M ozzardi* is restricted to Central and South America as well as selected Caribbean islands [31]. Humans act as the reservoir for these infections, and the life cycles are all similar, in that the human-to-human transmission is either the biting midge and, in the case of *M ozzardi*, the black fly. Humans are the hosts, but *M streptocerca* can also be found in nonhuman primates. Avoiding bites from the arthropod vectors is the principal method of prevention.

Clinical Features

Data on the incubation period for *Mansonella* infections are lacking. The usual signs and symptoms of *M streptocerca* are skin pruritus, papular rashes, and changes in pigmentation. Most individuals with this infection also have inguinal adenopathy. The parasites and resulting cutaneous symptoms tend to be present across the shoulders and upper torso [39]. Most patients with *M perstans* are asymptomatic, although a transient angioedema and pruritus, with swellings that are like the Calibar swellings of loaiasis, may occur. Fever, headache, arthritis, right upper-quadrant pain, and occasional pericarditis or hepatitis may occur. With *M ozzardi* infection, it is not clear whether the organism is truly pathogenic. Symptoms may be similar to those attributed to other *Mansonella* infections.

Diagnostic Evaluation

The differential diagnoses include other filarial infections, especially onchocerciasis. In cases of *M streptocerca*, because of the hypopigmented macules, one must also rule out leprosy. The diagnostic test of choice for *M streptocerca* is the skin snip, wherein the characteristic unsheathed microfilaria may be seen. In *M ozzardi* and *M perstans* infections, identification of the microfilariae in blood or other body fluids is usually sufficient for diagnosis.

Treatment

Treatment for *M streptocerca* infection is generally with diethylcarbamazine, which is usually effective. This is usually given as a dose of 6 mg/kg/day in divided doses for 14 to 21 days. As with other filarial infections, urticaria, arthralgia, myalgia, abdominal discomfort, and headache may occur in response to treatment. Ivermectin, 150 μg/kg as a single dose, may also be used [11]. For *M perstans*, mebendazole, 100 mg orally twice daily for 30 days, is the drug of choice [11]. For *M ozzardi*, DEC is thought to be ineffective. Ivermectin, 6 mg twice daily, has been reported to be effective in a single case report [40].

DRACUNCULUS MEDINENSIS

Dracunculus medinensis, or guinea worm, has rapidly declined in prevalence, secondary to global eradication strategies [41]. This worm, which normally resides in the subcutaneous tissues, is acquired through ingestion of contaminated water. The geographic distribution for this infection is the Sudan and western Africa. There are progressively fewer cases in the Middle East and Indian subcontinent. After a human (terminal host) ingests water containing *Cyclops* (intermediate host) infected with guinea worm larvae, the larvae migrate from the *Cyclops* and penetrate the human host's GI tract. Here, the larvae develop into adults and mate. The female worm then migrates to the subcutaneous tissues of the human host, usually toward the lower extremities, where a blister forms. The migration may take up to one year. When the human host enters a body of water, the blister breaks, releasing a large number of rhabditiform larvae, which may then infect more *Cyclops*, thereby perpetuating the worm's life cycle. Later, at the site of the blister on the human host, an ulcer forms, and it is from this ulcer that the worm emerges.

Prevention

Engineering provisions for safe water through water treatment, filtering, or drilled wells all serve to lessen the risk for this infection. Filtering individual drinking water with a 100-μm-pore-size filter is also an effective method of preventing the infection.

Clinical Features

The incubation period is usually about one year, or until the worm emerges. During this time, vague symptoms associated with the migration may occur. The infection is usually asymptomatic until just before the blister forms. Then, fever and generalized allergic symptoms such as wheezing, urticaria, and periorbital swelling have their onset. The emergence of the worm is associated with pain and swelling. Multiple worms may emerge. Aberrant locations of the worms are not unusual. Arthritis may result if a joint is infected. The ulcer that results from the emergence of the worm can easily become secondarily infected and can act as a portal for tetanus [42]. There is no protective immunity after being infected with the worm, and reinfection is common.

Diagnostic Evaluation

Diagnosis is usually clinical, based on the presentation of the adult worm as it emerges. One can identify the discharged motile larvae microscopically. Treatment is usually the gradual extraction of the worm by winding a few centimeters of it on a stick each day.

Treatment

Treatment with metronidazole, 250 mg orally three times daily for 10 days in adults, or 25 mg/kg/day (maximum dose, 750 mg) in three doses per day for 10 days in children, is thought to decrease the inflammatory response and facilitate worm removal [11]. Mebendazole, 400 to 800 mg/day for six days, is reported to kill the worm directly [11].

Zoonotic Nematodes

Zoonoses are infections in humans by parasites that usually live in animals. In the nematodes that follow, humans are dead-end hosts. It is for this reason that these nematodes do not mature into adults, but rather, cause problems because of their larval stages. A vast array of zoonotic nematodal infections occur, but only the most important ones are discussed in detail.

ADULT ZOONOTIC NEMATODES RESIDING IN THE GI TRACT

Capillaria philippinensis

Capillaria philippinensis, a parasite of aquatic birds that feed on fish, produces a clinical condition called *intestinal capillariasis*. This organism is unique in that it can reproduce within the host and, in this capacity, resembles the autoinfectious cycle of *Strongyloides*. The adult worms resemble those of *Trichonella*. Transmission is from eating raw or undercooked fresh water fish. The geographic distribution is primarily the Philippines and parts of Thailand. A few cases have been reported from other parts of Southeast Asia and the Middle East. The reservoir is thought to be aquatic birds, while fish act as intermediate hosts [43].

Prevention. The most important prevention technique is the avoidance of eating raw or undercooked fish. Hygienic methods for disposal of feces can help disrupt the cycle of reinfection of fish.

Clinical Features. The incubation period for intestinal capillariasis is thought to be approximately one month. The primary symptom is rampant diarrhea, which is associated with malaise, anorexia, and vomiting. With time, the severe diarrhea causes electrolyte disturbances, malabsorption, and protein-wasting enteropathy [44]. The chronic aspects of this disease—cachexia, congestive heart failure, and secondary bacterial infections—are thought to be responsible for its 10% mortality rate [45].

Diagnostic Evaluation. Characteristic laboratory findings include persistent eosinophilia and low albumin levels. Differential diagnosis includes *Strongyloides*, giardiasis, cryptosporidiosis, isosporidiosis, and the malabsorption seen in patients with tropical sprue. The diagnosis depends on finding eggs or living larvae in species. The eggs resemble those of *Trichuris.*

Treatment. Treatment includes replacement of fluid and electrolytes along with nutritional support. The treatment of choice is mebendazole, 200 mg orally twice daily for 20 days [11], although albendazole, 400 mg daily for 10 days, is also effective. The same regimens are used for pediatric patients. All infected patients should be treated because of the high risk of autoinfection.

Trichinella spiralis

Trichinella spiralis, the etiologic agent of trichinosis, is capable of infecting all mammals. Its prevalence in the United Sates is thought to be about 4% on the basis of autopsy studies [9]. This infection is unusual in that the L1 larva causes the pathology and is also the infectious form. Transmission occurs through ingestion of raw or undercooked infected meat. Risks for infection are dietary. If undercooked or uncooked pork, bear or horse are eaten, the risk increases. Geographic distribution is worldwide among meat-eating populations. It is less common in the tropics. The life cycle is animal to animal; humans are an incidental host.

Prevention. Administrative controls generally consist of cooking refuse that is fed to pigs, thus stopping the cycle of propagation caused by feeding meat scraps to pigs. Personal protective measures include adequate cooking of meat [46]. It may be prudent to avoid homemade sausage.

Clinical Features. The incubation period of trichinosis is 10–20 days. Early symptoms include diarrhea, vomiting, abdominal pain, headache, and fever. Later, during the migration phase, fever, blurred vision, facial edema, cough, and eosinophilic develop. This phase may last up to one month. The muscular phase, characterized by muscle pain, follows. If the myocardium is involved, myocarditis may occur and abnormal ECGs may be seen. CNS involvement may occur with petechial hemorrhages of the brain. One may also see petechial hemorrhages in the conjunctivae and under the nails.

Diagnostic Evaluation. Differential diagnosis includes allergic reaction, Katayama fever, visceral larva migrans, and eosinophilia-myalgia syndrome. The diagnosis is characterized by laboratory studies through massive eosinophilia (more than 5,000 cells/cubic mm), but a low ESR. The ELISA test is positive two to four weeks after infection. Muscle biopsy may show encysted larvae. Other laboratory findings include an elevated CK and LDH.

Treatment. Treatment consists of mebendazole, 200–400 orally three times daily for three days, then 400–500 mg orally three times daily for 10 days [11]; or albendazole. Early treatment kills the adults that reside in the gut. These are normally excreted over two to three months, so early treatment may help to avoid excessive production of larvae. Corticosteroids are often helpful for severe symptoms. The larval stages, which encyst in muscles as “nurse cells,” are difficult or impossible to eradicate but tend not to cause symptoms and eventually calcify and die.

Trichostrongylus Species

Trichostrongylosis, also called *pseudo-hookworm infection* [47], behaves much like the common hookworm. *Trichostrongylus* worms are found in a variety of herbivorous animals. Living or working around infected animals is a risk factor for this infection. Geographic distribution of the disease in humans is primarily in Asia, although it is also seen in Europe, Africa, and especially in rural Iran and Iraq. Animal infection is seen throughout the world. The life cycle is one of animal to animal via the environment. Humans act as incidental hosts, but the life cycle can be completed within humans.

Prevention. Ingestion of food or water contaminated with animal feces is the most common form of acquisition [4]; thus, hygienic food practices are preventive. As with hookworm, *Trichostrongylus* worms can penetrate skin, so wearing of shoes is also a wise preventive measure.

Clinical Features. The incubation period of trichostrongyloides is thought to be about three weeks. The disease is usually asymptomatic, although mild gastrointestinal symptoms may occur. In patients with severe infection, anemia or occult blood in the stool may also occur.

Diagnostic Evaluation and Treatment. Differential diagnosis includes infections with other intestinal parasites, especially hookworm. Diagnosis is based on the identification of eggs in the stool or duodenal aspirates. Stool culture to recover larvae is also a useful technique. For both adult and pediatric patients, treatment is with pyrantel pamoate, 11 mg/kg as a single dose (maximum of 1 g); mebendazole, 100 mg orally twice daily for three days; or albendazole, 400 mg as a single dose [11].

Oesophagostomum Species

The *Oesophagostomum* species are nematodes related to and resembling hookworms. Infection with these worms has a variety of synonyms, including *helminthoma*, *pimplygut*, and *nodular worm* [10]. Unlike hookworm, transmission is by the fecal-oral route and percutaneous infection does not occur. Close proximity with the zoonotic reservoirs of this infection is the risk factor. The geographic distribution is primarily Africa. The life cycle is generally animal to animal, although humans may also permit completion of the transmission cycle and transmit the infection to other humans [48]. The normal animal hosts are sheep, goats, pigs, and some primates. Although these infections occur worldwide, the primary area of human infection has been Africa.

Prevention. Prevention of this infection is primarily through personal protective measures such as hand washing prior to eating and hygienic food practices. Hygienic disposal of human feces is especially important in areas where human-to-human transmission occurs.

Clinical Features. Symptoms commonly occur two to three weeks after ingestion of eggs. Thirty to 40 days after ingestion, eggs may appear in the stool. The infection may be asymptomatic, although right lower quadrant abdominal pain and fever may occur. Complications of the infection include abscess formation, fistula formation, hemorrhage, and perforation.

Diagnostic Evaluation and Treatment. Characteristic laboratory findings include low-grade eosinophilia. Differential diagnosis includes tumors of the GI tract, ameboma, schistosomal granuloma, appendicitis, and ileocecal tuberculosis. The diagnosis is made by the identification of eggs in the feces, which strongly resemble hookworm eggs. Treatment includes surgical resection of the nodule or pharmacologic treatment with albendazole, 400–800 mg as a single dose, or pyrantel pamoate, 10 mg/kg given once or twice [49]. Uncommon zoonotic nematode infections in the GI tract are listed in Table 29-2 [1].

MARINE NEMATODES

Anisakiasis is the term given to infection with marine nematodes of the *Anosacchus* or *Pseudoterranova* genera. Common names include *herring worm*, *whale worm*, *cod worm*, and *seal worm*. Prevalence is tied to the frequency of eating sushi or sashimi and appears to be increasing with the growing popularity of these foods. Transmission is oral, through the ingestion of the larval form of the nematode in infected fish. Although most reported cases are from Japan, there has been an increasing number worldwide. The life cycle involves marine vertebrates and invertebrates. Hosts of the worm are marine mammals, including whales, seals, and dolphins. They pass eggs into the sea water, which are taken up by small crustaceans and progress through the food chain.

Table 29-2
Uncommon Zoonotic Nematode Infections of the Human GI Tract

Name	Geographic Location	Animal Host	Disease Diagnosis	Symptoms	Transmission
Genus *Physaloptera*	Africa	Primates	Eggs in feces	Similar to ascaris	Accidental ingestion of insects (intermediate host)
Gongylonema species	Worldwide	Ruminants, monkeys	Eggs in feces	Local irritation in GI tract	Accidental ingestion of beetle or cockroach
Ternidens diminutus	South Africa	Simian primates	Fecal culture; eggs	Similar to hookworm	Fecal oral
Macracanhirudinaceus thorhynchus	China	Wide range of vertebrates, especially pigs	Eggs in feces	GI symptoms, gut perforation, ulceration	Accidental ingestion of beetle
Moniliformis moniliformis	Worldwide	Wide range of vertebrates, especially rats	Eggs in feces	GI symptoms, ulceration, perforation	Accidental ingestion of beetle

Many kinds of fish have been implicated in carrying the larval stages.

Prevention. The primary preventive measure is avoidance of eating lightly cooked or raw fishes. The larval form can be killed by thorough cooking or freezing of fish. There are some species that have been relatively resistant to freezing, however. Professional sushi chefs can often identify the parasites and avoid them if they are pigmented [50].

Clinical Features. Although anisakiasis may be asymptomatic, the most common presentation is related to the attachment of the larval worm to the gastric mucosa. This results in severe abdominal pain, nausea, vomiting, and diarrhea one to 12 hours after eating the larva-infected fish. Since the larvae can attach anywhere in the GI tract, tingling sensations in the throat may be experienced secondary to attachment there. Intestinal infection usually produces symptoms (abdominal pain, nausea, and vomiting) one to two weeks after ingestion. The worm may become invasive and penetrate the gastric or intestinal mucosa, then migrate to the omentum, pancreas, liver, or lung. Characteristic laboratory findings includes eosinophilia and leukocytosis. Differential diagnosis includes noninfectious causes. The gastric form of anisakiasis resembles peptic ulcer disease, gastritis, or pancreatitis. The intestinal form resembles appendicitis, diverticulitis, or inflammatory bowel disease [51]. Diagnosis is usually based on clinical grounds, although upper GI or barium enema may reveal thread-like filling defects at areas of thickened or obstructed bowel wall [10]. Eggs and larval forms are not found in the feces. Treatment is through removal of the worm, usually by means of an endoscopic procedure. Occasionally, during surgery for presumed acute abdomen, a worm is discovered and removed.

CUTANEOUS LARVA MIGRANS

Also called *creeping eruption*, cutaneous larva migrans (CLM) is actually a distinctive type of dermatitis that results from infection with larval stages of various animal nematodes. The larvae are generally confined to the epidermal layers of the skin but may go deeper. This condition is most commonly caused by *Ancylostoma braziliense*, although a number of other nematodes may cause this syndrome (Table 29-3). Transmission occurs through contact with contaminated soil, and any occupation that requires frequent exposure to soil may be in danger of this condition. The condition is especially common on hands, feet, knees, and buttocks. There is no predilection for age, race, or gender. The organisms causing CLM are ubiquitous and endemic to geographic areas most hospitable to the larval forms, namely, those with warm, humid climates. The life cycle involves the passing of rhabditiform

Table 29-3
Causes of Cutaneous Larva Migrans

Organism	Animal Host	Location	Incidence
Ancylostoma braziliense	Cats, dogs	Skin	Most common
A caninum	Dogs	Skin	Common
A tubaeformis	Cats	Skin	Rare
Uncinaria stenocephala	European dogs	Skin	Rare
Bunostomum phlebotum	Cattle	Skin	Rare
Pleodora strongyloides	Free living	Skin	Rare
Anatrichosoma species	Monkeys, opossum	Skin, nasal and oral mucosa	Rare
Thelazia species	Dogs, rabbits	Conjunctival sac, cornea	Rare

larvae with the feces of infected animals. These develop in the soil through a series of molts into filariform larvae, which then enter a host through hair follicles or intact skin via digestive enzymes. Humans are dead-end hosts.

Prevention

Since it is quite difficult to dispose of animal feces, protection of skin from fecally contaminated soil is the most practical way of avoiding CLM. Wearing shoes is especially important.

Clinical Features

The usual incubation period for CLM is two to seven days. The syndrome usually includes a pruritic serpiginous papulovesicular lesion, which becomes linear, the tract lengthening daily. There may be associated wheezing and urticaria, especially if there has been previous sensitization. In these cases, vesicles and marked edema may be present. Some nematodes may invade deeper tissues. *Ancylostoma caninum* can cause an eosinophilic enteritis [52]. Eosinophilia is a characteristic laboratory findings.

Diagnostic Evaluation and Treatment

Although a biopsy is not usually necessary, it reveals a mild perivascular dermal infiltrate composed primarily of polymorphonuclear cells and eosinophils. On chest radiograph, one may see migratory pulmonary infiltrates in up to 50% of cases. The differential diagnosis includes cercarial dermatitis, scabies, cutaneous filariasis, human hookworm, and *Strongyloides*. Human hookworm tends to have a more transient ground itch. *Strongyloides*, which causes larva curens, is more routinely associated with urticaria, and its symptoms are more intermittent. The diagnosis of CLM is made on clinical grounds. For both adult and pediatric patients, treatment options are topical thiabendazole; ivermectin, 150–200 μg/kg orally as a single dose; or albendazole, 400 mg orally every day for three days [11].

VISCERAL LARVA MIGRANS

Visceral larva migrans (VLM) is a clinical syndrome caused by the prolonged wanderings of the larvae of various zoonotic nematodes as they migrate throughout the human body. Since the human is a dead-end host, the larvae never mature into adults. During their movements, the larvae produce inflammatory reactions, which can cause diverse clinical syndromes, depending on their location. This can be the viscera or the eye—ocular larva migrans (OLM)—the central nervous system (CNS)—neural larva migrans (NLM). The majority of cases of VLM are due to *Toxocara canus* and *Toxocara cati*, which are the common large round worms of dogs and cats, respectively. Other causative organisms are addressed separately. VLM is a common infection: Serosurveys suggest that 2–3% of the world's population is infected, primarily children and people with pica [4]. Transmission is through ingestion of embryonated eggs, either from contaminated soil or from foods contaminated with the eggs. This could be an occupational risk factor for people working in contaminated soils, but practically speaking, VLM is a disease of young children. The geographic distribution is worldwide, but larvae tend to survive best in warm, moist clay soils. Although the larvae cannot mature into adults in the human host, they may remain viable for up to 10 years.

Prevention

Preventive techniques include control of dog and cat feces. For parents, such techniques are keeping covers over sand piles, a favored place of defecation for cats, careful attention to worming of domestic pets, and avoidance of pet feces in play areas. Personal protective measures include hand washing and other means of avoiding transmitting contaminated fomites to the mouth. Education should include the danger of pica.

Clinical Features

The incubation period of visceral larva migrans is approximately one month. The signs and symptoms are quite variable, and the patient may be asymptomatic. The most common symptoms are fever, cough, wheezing, abdominal pain, myalgia, and a large and tender liver and/or spleen [53]. Other symptoms reflect the location of the larvae. If they are in the CNS, seizures and encephalopathy are possible complications. In the heart, myocarditis may occur. In the eye, OLM may cause leukochoria, strabismus, decreased visual acuity, and fundal mass.

Diagnostic Evaluation

Characteristic laboratory findings include a high-grade, persistent eosinophilia unless there is an isolated OLM, in which case there is no eosinophilia. Liver function tests tend to be elevated, and a liver biopsy usually reveals eosinophils and granulomas. IgG levels are elevated and there is leukocytosis. On chest radiographs, about one third of cases have an infiltrate. Differential diagnosis includes invasive helminth infections of any type. For OLM, it includes retinoblastoma; cases of OLM have resulted in enucleation because of an assumed diagnosis of retinoblastoma. Diagnosis is best made with the ELISA test, which is relatively sensitive and specific. Identification of larvae in the tissue may provide a diagnosis, but this is not routine. Note should be made that eggs and parasites are not found in the feces.

Treatment

Treatment often involves the use of corticosteroids to suppress the intense manifestations of the inflammatory reaction. The use of antihelminthic medications is somewhat controversial. Diethylcarbamazine (DEC), 6 mg/kg/day in three doses for seven to 10 days, is considered to be the drug of choice [11]. Albendazole, 400 mg orally twice daily for three to five days, and mebendazole, 100–200 mg orally twice daily for five days, are alternatives. Regimens are the same for pediatric patients.

BAYLISASCARIS PROCYONIS

Baylisascaris procyonis, the common raccoon roundworm, is an increasingly recognized cause of VLM, found primarily in North America [54]. The Baylisascaral syndrome differs from toxicara in that it is caused by more aggressive larvae and has a much greater likelihood of causing neurologic disease, especially in patients with heavy infections [55]. Clinical findings range from mild to devastating CNS involvement. This often develops quickly, over two to four weeks, and progresses rapidly. *Baylisascaris* can also cause subacute neuroretinitis. Unfortunately, the prognosis for patients with this disease is grave, with or without treatment, because of the extensive neurologic damage done by the time the diagnosis is made.

GNATHOSTOMA SPINIGERUM

Gnathostomiasis is most commonly caused by *Gnathostoma spinigerum*, although several other species may infect humans [56]. *G spinigerum* is a parasite that affects a variety of mammals, including cats, dogs and mongeese, and has intermediate hosts including cyclops, birds, freshwater fish, snakes, and frogs. This nematode is present throughout Southeast Asia (especially Thailand) and parts of South America. Humans become infected by ingesting the intermediate host and may develop subcutaneous swellings, ocular larva migrans, and eosinophilic meningitis. The acute phase generally begins one to two days after ingestion of the larvae. Systemic symptoms include nausea, vomiting, pruritus, urticaria, and abdominal pain. After three to four weeks, the chronic stage begins. It is characterized by symptoms caused by movement of the parasite through various tissues, including the skin, or more rarely, the central nervous system or eye. A migrating red rash, a sign of subcutaneous involvement, is the most common manifestation of this disease. Rarely, the worm migrates to the central nervous system, where it may cause a variety of CNS syndromes. Surgical removal may be used for cutaneous gnathostomes, but albendazole, 400 mg orally twice daily for 21 days [11], may be necessary to kill larvae not accessible to excision [57].

ANGIOSTRONGYLUS SPECIES

Angiostrongylus cantonensis results from the ingestion of the third-stage larvae of the rat lungworm. After ingestion, the larvae migrate to the brain, spinal cord, and eye, where they cause a variety of symptoms, depending on their specific location. They are generally acquired through the ingestion of uncooked or under-cooked slugs or snails or vegetables contaminated by the slime of these mollusks. The incubation period is usually two weeks. Patients often have a severe headache, stiff neck, and low-grade to moderate fever. A variety of paresthesias, paralyses, or cranial nerve palsies may occur [58]. With eye involvement, decreased vision, extraocular muscle paralysis, and exophthalmus may occur. Laboratory findings include eosinophilia of the cerebrospinal fluid and peripheral blood. Treatment is usually supportive. Surgery may be used to remove larvae that enter the anterior chamber of the eye. Corticosteroids are useful for severe meningitis. The drug regimen for adults and children is meben dazole, 100 mg orally twice daily for five days [11].

Angiostrongylus costaricensis is in many ways similar to *A cantonensis*. Its geographic distribution is Central and South America. The primary difference is that, after being ingested, the larvae tend to develop in the lymphatics of the abdominal cavity and then migrate to the mesenteric arteries, where they deposit eggs in the intestinal wall. This causes granulomatous and eosinophilic inflammatory reactions that manifest as a variety of gastrointestinal symptoms [59]. Infected individuals frequently present with acute abdomen. If the spermatic artery is involved, testicular necrosis may be a complication. Larvae and eggs are not found in the stool examination. Treatment is generally supportive, and surgery may be necessary if perforation or obstruction occurs. Mebendazole, 200–400 mg orally three times daily for 10 days, or thiabendazole, 75 mg/kg/day in three doses for three days (maximum of 3 g per day) are the pharmacologic treatments of choice [11].

ZOONOTIC FILARIAL INFECTIONS

Dirofilarial infections are common in animals. *Dirofilaria immitis* causes the dog heartworm, while other species of *Dirofilaria*, including *Dirofilaria tenuis* (in raccoons), *Dirofilaria repens* (dogs), and *Dirofilaria ursi* (bears) cause subcutaneous infections both in the host and in humans, who are incidental hosts. *D immitis* can cause a pulmonary dirofilariasis in humans, while the other species cause a subcutaneous dirofilariasis. *D immitis* is acquired in humans from the bite of a mosquito that has bitten an animal host. It is most common in the Americas, Australia, Europe, China, India, and Japan. The other *Dirofilaria* species have been reported on all continents. *D immitis* is apparently not rare in humans. Serosurveys suggest that up to 5% of people in the United States may be infected. The incubation period is two to three months. *D immitis* larvae occlude a small pulmonary artery, causing a sharply defined infarct. This tissue contains the worm, necrotic material, granulomas, and eosinophils. The tissue may calcify, allowing it to be seen on routine chest radiograph [60]. The clinical presentation is usually cough, chest pain, low-grade fever, and, rarely, hemoptysis. If eosinophilia is present, it is usually low grade. The differential diagnosis for *D immitis* primarily involves ruling out a tumor or a granuloma-producing infection. The diagnosis is usually made from surgical biopsy of the necrotic material, although fine-needle biopsy has been used in some cases. Treatment generally consists of surgical removal.

For the other species of *Dirofilaria*, the mosquito is also the vector, with the exception of *D ursi*, for which it is the black fly. Clinically, these other species tend to cause subcutaneous nodules, which are usually single [61]. Rarely, these parasites may be found in the eye. The diagnosis of the other *Dirofilaria* species is usually through biopsy. In all *Dirofilaria* infections, microfilaremia is absent in humans. Treatment is surgical removal.

NEMATODES OF OTHER ORGAN SYSTEMS

Dioctophyma renale is the organism responsible for giant kidney worm disease. This is a rare infection resulting from ingestion of the larval form in raw or undercooked fish or frogs. The ingested larvae penetrate the intestinal wall, enter the peritoneal cavity, and migrate to the kidney, where they destroy the kidney, leaving only the capsule. Cases have been reported in Asia, the Americas, and Europe. The usual animal hosts are minks and dogs, which shed eggs when they urinate. If urination is near bodies of water, the eggs are then ingested by an aquatic worm, which is in turn ingested by fish or frogs [10]. Proper cooking of seafood and frogs prevents the infection.

Clinical Features

The usual incubation time between ingestion of larvae and appearance of eggs in the urine is three to six months. Symptoms include flank pain, renal colic, and hematuria. Rarely, there may be a subcutaneous mass [62]. Urinalysis, which usually shows hematuria, is helpful in making the diagnosis. If the worm is a female, eggs can be identified in the urine. In the case of male worms, only surgical removal of the nematode makes the diagnosis. Treatment is surgical removal of the parasite.

Risk factors for infection with *Eustrongylus* species are similar to those for dioctophymiasis. In nearly all cases, patients have reported the curious habit of swallowing live bait minnows [63]. Clinical symptoms tend to start within 24 hours and consist of intense abdominal pain, which is often localized in the right lower quadrant. Appendicitis is generally suspected in these patients. During surgery, large blood-red worms are found in the peritoneal cavity. Anisakiasis is one of the differential diagnoses for both of these infections.

Capillaria hepatica, a rat-liver parasite, which is also found in a number of mammals, causes the disease hepatic capillariasis [2]. Humans may develop the infection after ingestion of embryonated eggs, which may be present in contaminated soil. The eggs hatch and the worms migrate to the portal circulation of the liver, where they are nourished by the liver tissue. If enough worms are present, the host may suffer liver failure and die. The parasite is common in rats, but reports of human infection are rare. They have been seen in Africa, the Americas, Asia, and Europe. Eggs are hardy, remaining viable in the soil for some months. Prevention requires food and drink hygiene.

Diagnostic Assessment

Incubation is usually three to four weeks, and symptoms include fever, a tender, enlarged liver, splenomegaly, and often a transient pneumonitis. Laboratory studies include eosinophilia and abnormal liver function tests. The diagnosis is made by biopsy of the liver for identification of the parasite or eggs [64]. The eggs are not found in the intestine. Unfortunately, no treatment has been developed. Prevention is a matter of food and drink hygiene.

Trematodes

All of the medically important trematodes, including blood flukes, intestinal flukes and tissue flukes, are in the order Digenea.

SCHISTOSOMA

Schistosoma, which are blood flukes, exist as separate sexes but live *in copula*. Schistosomiasis, also called *bilharziasis* or *swamp fever*, affects more than 200 million people worldwide. Globally, this corresponds to 4.5 million DALYs lost [3]. Transmission of *Schistosoma* can be either by drinking infested water or by invasion of intact skin by a motile aquatic form called a *cercaria*. A cercaria can penetrate intact skin and is transformed into a Schistosomum, which migrates through the lungs and systemic circulation, slowly finding its way to the portal venous system, where it matures into an adult and resides for years. Eggs excreted by these adults find their way back to the environment via feces or urine and hatch in the water, releasing miracidia, which penetrate the snail, which then develops over four to six weeks into a cercaria, thus completing the cycle. Each species of schistosoma has an associated species of snail. The main occupational and environmental risk factor is working in areas where freshwater ingestion or exposure is commonplace. Even brief exposures to infested waters, such as fording a stream or rafting [65], may result in schistosomiasis. Schistosomiasis occurs in more than 70 countries, but a distinctive geographic distribution of the major species is present. *Schistosoma mansoni* is the only species of schistosome that occurs in the Western Hemisphere, where it appears in parts of Brazil and Puerto Rico. It is widely prevalent in Africa. *Schistosoma japonicum* is common throughout Asia, including the Philippines, China, and Japan. *Schistosoma haematobium* is also widely distributed throughout most of Africa and extends into southern Europe and western Asia [66]. Humans are the definitive hosts for all of the major *Schistosoma* species, although monkeys and baboons may act as hosts for *S mansoni* and *S haematobium*. In the case of *S japonicum*, water buffalo and cattle also may serve as hosts.

PREVENTION

Hygienic handling of urine and feces and assurance of a safe water supply are most important methods of preventing schistosomiasis. The use of molluscocidal agents to eliminate snails may also be an important administrative practice. Personal protective measures include wearing rubber boots to prevent skin contact with fresh water. Niclosamide lotion applied to the skin is said to prevent cercarial penetration [9].

Clinical Features

The incubation period of schistosomiasis varies with the clinical presentation. Cercarial dermatitis may develop within hours of exposure. For the acute form of schistosomiasis, Katayama fever, incubation is generally between two to 10 weeks. For the chronic syndromes, it may take weeks to years for the disease to present. Clinical presentations are highly variable. Cercarial dermatitis is more common with zoonotic schistosomal infections, those that attack birds and small mammals, and does not produce other pathology. This dermatitis, which occurs in areas of skin not covered by bathing suits, results in a hypersensitivity reaction that causes a maculopapular pruritic rash. This condition is self-limited but can be treated with antihistamines and topical corticosteroids.

Acute schistosomiasis, or Katayama fever, occurs in a minority of patients. It resembles serum sickness and is probably mediated by immune complexes [67]. It usually occurs four to five weeks after skin penetration. The symptoms are quite variable but may include fever, sweats, cough with wheezing, abdominal pain, urticaria, headaches, and diarrhea. There may be hepatosplenomegaly and lymphadenopathy. Laboratory tests are positive for marked peripheral eosinophilia. This, along with the travel history, usually makes the diagnosis. At this phase, eggs are not present. Treatment is with praziquantel, as in the chronic disease (see page 518). The addition of corticosteroids is often warranted.

The chronic aspects of schistosomiasis are mediated by the granulomatous response to the eggs. Many eggs are trapped in the host and never reach the external environment. There are several types of reactions, including intestinal, hepatic, urinary tract, and ectopic egg syndromes.

Intestinal schistosomiasis is commonly seen in all types of chronic schistosomal infections. The primary symptoms relate to the associated enteropathy and accompanying protein and blood loss. Signs include the presence of pseudopolyps with focal areas of hemorrhage. Schistosomal appendicitis may also occur.

Hepatic lesions result from the body's response to the eggs in the liver, which is initially due to a granulomatous process but followed by a fibrotic response. The most severe of these conditions results in the clay pipestem fibrosis of Symmers [2], which causes portal hypertension and its associated complications. Liver function studies are usually normal until very late in the disease process. Liver changes can be detected by ultrasonography, which has been used successfully for field diagnosis [68]. With the advent of mass chemotherapy and public educational intervention, the most severe forms of the hepatic fibrosis are becoming more rare [69].

Urinary tract schistosomiasis is most common with *Schistosoma haematobium*. More than half of the *S haematobium* eggs are present in the urinary tract, and, as with other organ systems, the pathology results from the body's reaction to the eggs. This leads to hematuria, dysuria, secondary urinary tract infections, and obstructive uropathy. Because of this, simple urine dipstick tests have been valuable for field identification of patients at high risk for the infection [70]. Chronic urinary schistosomiasis correlates with bladder cancer [71].

Ectopic egg syndromes result from the embolization of eggs to other organ systems. Most serious of these is brain and spinal cord involvement. The brain is more commonly involved with *Schistosoma japonicum*, while spinal cord involvement (especially transverse myelitis) is most commonly due to *Schistosoma haematobium* and *Schistosoma mansoni* [10].

There is an association between schistosomiasis and salmonella infections that causes prolonged typhoid fever with accompanying chronic anemia and splenomegaly. This probably results from salmonella's presence in the schistosoma themselves and usually requires simultaneous antibiotic and antihelminthic treatment [72].

Clinical Features and Diagnosis

Characteristic laboratory findings include a marked eosinophilia early in the course of schistosomiasis, which may decrease with time. In the case of *S haematobium*, radiographs of the genitourinary tract show linear calcifications in the submucosa of the bladder and ureters. Differential diagnosis includes visceral larva migrans, liver flukes, the migratory phase of strongyloides, and other helminth infections in the acute stage. Diagnosis usually depends on identification of viable eggs in the stool, urine, rectal biopsy specimen, or other tissues. Serologic tests have traditionally been useful to detect a response to the schistosoma but not to distinguish active from inactive infections; however, newer technqiues may not have this problem [73]. Serologic tests are available through the CDC. The diagnosis can be especially difficult to make early, before eggs are produced.

Treatment

Treatment is with praziquantel. The dosage is a function of the type of schistosomiasis. *For S japonicum* and *S mekongi*, a dose of 60 mg/kg/day in three divided doses for one day is therapeutic in both adults and children [11]. For *S haematobium* and *S mansoni*, the dose is 40 mg/kg/day in two doses for one day for both adults and children [11]. Oxamniquine is an alternative treatment for *S mansoni* and may be preferable for treatment of patients in some areas of Africa, where praziquantel may be less effective [74]. In this case, the regimen for oxamniquine in adults is 15–60 mg/kg in a single dose. For pediatric patients, it is 20 mg/kg/day in two divided doses for one day. The dosage varies with the specific country of acquisition.

INTESTINAL TREMATODES

The intestinal trematodes, or intestinal flukes, are not highly prevalent throughout the world, although there are pockets where they are quite common [20]. The transmission of all of these flukes is similar in that the metacercarial stages are typically encysted in freshwater fish, mollusks, or aquatic vegetation. After ingestion, they take up residence in the intestine of the human host. The eggs generally pass with the feces where freshwater snails act as an intermediate host. Risk factors for infection are primarily dietary. Details about geographic distribution and other details of infections are presented in Table 29-4. There are a variety of other flukes of animals in Southeast Asia that have been reported to cause zoonotic infections in humans. When present, they tend to be asymptomatic or cause mild inflammatory changes with associated diarrhea and colicky pain. These intestinal flukes tend to have a short lifespan, and symptoms are limited. They include the following: *Pygidiopsis summa*, *Haplorchis species*, *Gymnophylloides seoi*, *Gentrocestus formosanus*, *Prosthodendrium molenkampi*, *Stellantchasmus falcatus*, *Phaneropsolus bonnei*, and *Neodiplostomum seoulense* [1].

Treatment for all these intestinal flukes is with praziquantel. For all but *Nanophyetus salmincola*,

Table 29-4
Intestinal Trematodes

Scientific/ Common Name	Geographic Location	Acquisition	Reservoir	Incubation	Major Disease Manifestations	Diagnosis
Fasciolopsis buski (giant intestinal fluke)	Southeast Asia, Indian subcontinent	Ingestion of water plants: water caltrop, water chestnut, watercress, water bamboo	Humans, pigs, dogs, rabbits	2–3 months until eggs in feces; symptoms may start earlier	Most asymptomatic; occasional appearance of worms in feces; in heavy infection, diarrhea and edema, even obstruction; impaired vitamin B_{12} absorption; may migrate to other organs	Detection of large operculate eggs in feces; eosinophilic leukocytosis
Echinostoma species	China, Southeast Asia, other scattered areas; high prevalence in Thailand	Ingestion of raw or undercooked fishes or mollusks; drinking water; water plants	Humans, mammals, birds	1 month	Abdominal cramps and pain, bloating, diarrhea, edema if heavy infection	Eggs in stool
Heterophyes heterophyes (dwarf fluke)	East and Southeast Asia, India, southern Europe (Spain), North Africa (Nile River delta), Turkey	Ingestion of raw or undercooked fish; salted or pickled fish also a risk	Birds, mammals	1–2 weeks	Most asymptomatic or mild diarrhea, cramps, nausea; rarely may migrate to heart or brain	Eggs in feces
Metagonimus yokogawai (Yokogawa's fluke infection)	East and Southeast Asia, former Soviet states, southern Europe, Balkan states	Ingestion of raw or undercooked freshwater fish	Birds, mammals	2 weeks	Most asymptomatic	Eggs in feces
Nanophyetus salmincola (salmon poisoning in dogs)	North America, eastern Siberia	Ingestion of raw or undercooked fish or roe; common in salmon; can survive in salted or smoked fish	Raccoons, skunks, dogs, foxes, coyotes, birds	1 week	Usually asymptomatic or mild episodic diarrhea, abdominal pain, bloating; may co-transmit *Neorickettsia helmintheca*, a rickettsia	Identification of eggs (number is small)
Gastrodiscoides hominis (Gastrodisciasis)	India, Southeast Asia, former Soviet states	Ingestion of aquatic vegetation	Humans, pigs	Unknown	Diarrhea in heavy infection	Characteristic eggs

the dosage is 75 mg/kg/day in three divided doses for one day for both adult and pediatric patients. For *N salmincola*, it is 60 mg/kg/day in three doses for one day [11].

LIVER FLUKES

Liver flukes have a life cycle similar to that of the other trematodes. It involves an appropriate freshwater snail as the first intermediate host, and either fish or contaminated water plants as the source of acquisition for humans. An exception to this generalization is *Dicrocoelium dendriticum*, for which a terrestrial snail is the intermediate host, and ants who eat the slime from this snail are the vector to humans [1]. Specific information about the liver flukes is provided in Table 29-5.

Treatment

Treatment for *Fasciola hepatica* in both adult and pediatric patients is bithionol, 30–50 mg/kg on alternate days for 10–15 doses [11]. An alternative is triclabendazole, 10 mg/kg, which is a veterinarian fasciolide but has been shown to be effective [75]. For the other liver flukes, the treatment is praziquantel, 75 mg/kg/day in three doses for one day, for both adult and pediatric patients [11]. For *Clonorchis sinensis*, an alternative treatment for adult patients is albendazole, 10 mg/kg/day for seven days.

LUNG FLUKES

Paragonimus westermani and other *Paragonimus* species are responsible for human lung fluke infections. Their life cycle is similar to other trematodes in that there is an obligatory snail intermediate host. The species are found in Southeast Asia and the Indian subcontinent. The other fluke species cause infections in the Americas, Asia, and Africa. The infection is acquired through ingestion of raw or undercooked freshwater crayfish, crabs, and shrimp. It may also be caused, although rarely, by the ingestion of undercooked wild boar meat. A variety of mammals serve as reservoirs, including foxes, tigers, pigs, cats, and dogs. Incubation for the pulmonary symptoms is generally six months, while for CNS symptoms, it can be 12 to 16 months. The lung findings usually start insidiously with cough, hemoptysis, and rusty sputum. Later, wheezing, fever, and pleuritic pain may appear [76]. Lung flukes have the radiographic appearance of tuberculosis and can present an especially confusing picture if they coexist with tuberculosis. The flukes may migrate to other areas, where they can cause a variety of symptoms. In less than 1% of patients, they migrate to the central nervous system. When this happens, eosinophilic meningitis, along with a variety of other neurologic symptoms, may occur. Migrating larvae can reach any part of the body, and subcutaneous masses are not uncommon. Peripheral eosinophilia is a common laboratory finding. Sputum may contain Charcot-Leyden crystals. Chest radiographs commonly show effusions, diffuse infiltrates, nodules, cavities, and calcifications [77], frequently resembling tuberculosis, except that the apices are usually spared. Diagnosis is made by identification of eggs in sputum, feces, pleural fluid, or cerebrospinal fluid; the eggs may also be present in the feces because of swallowed sputum. Serologic studies may also be useful. The treatment is praziquantel, 75 mg/kg/day in three divided doses for two days [11], or bithionol, 30–50 mg/kg/day on alternate days for 10–15 doses [11]. The regimen is the same for adults and children.

Cestodes

Cestodes are parasitic tapeworms that can be quite large and are composed of a head, or scolex, and a long segmented portion, the strobilia. The scolex, which is the only point of attachment to the host, uses suckers, hooks, or grooves for this purpose. The rest of the body, or strobilia, is composed of the segmented sections, the proglottids, which are anatomically independent and contain both male and female sex organs. These proglottids may also be independently motile. Cestodes tend to have a complex life cycle, consisting of adult and larval stages. The pathology of cestode infections depends on whether humans act as hosts for the adult or larval stage of the tapeworm. The larval stages tend to be associated with much more invasive and serious disease. In general, adult tapeworms do not cause many symptoms. The adult tapeworms discussed

Table 29-5
Liver Flukes

Scientific/ Common Name	Geographic Location	Acquisition	Reservoir	Incubation	Major Disease Manifestations	Diagnosis
Fasciola hepatica (sheep liver fluke disease)	Worldwide in sheep and cattle-raising areas	Contaminated water, watercress, dandelion greens, lettuce	Sheep, cattle	3–4 months	Live in bile duct; asymptomatic or mild fever, liver pain, diarrhea, jaundice, cholangitis, cholecystitis; may migrate to other sites such as brain, orbits, subcutaneous; rare pharyngeal fasciolitis if raw liver	Abnormal liver function tests; anemia if heavy; filling defect in biliary tree; eosinophilia; eggs in stool or duodenal aspirate; serologic tests
Fasciola gigantic	Southeast Asia and Africa	Contaminated water, aquatic vegetation	Herbivorous mammals, especially cattle	3–4 months	Human infection rare; similar to *F hepatica*	Serodiagnosis, large eggs in feces
Clonorchis sinensis (Oriental liver fluke)	China, Japan, Korea, Taiwan, Vietnam; not uncommon in shipped fish	Raw or pickled freshwater fish or crayfish	Many, especially dogs and cats	3–4 weeks	Early—fever, epigastric and RUQ pain, diarrhea, malaise Chronic—may be asymptomatic, cholecystitis, pancreatitis, cholangiocarcinoma	High-grade eosinophilia; increased alkaline phosphatase; identification of eggs in feces or duodenal aspirate
Opisthorchis felineus	Eastern Europe, especially Poland, western Russia; Philippines, India, Japan, Vietnam	Raw or pickled freshwater fish or crayfish	Many wild and domestic animals	3–4 weeks	Same as *C sinensis*	Same as *C sinensis*
Opisthorchis viverrini	Thailand, Laos	Raw or pickled freshwater fish or crayfish	Cats, dogs	3–4 weeks	Same as *C sinensis*	Same as *C sinensis*
Opisthorchis guayaquilensis	Ecuador	Raw or pickled freshwater fish or crayfish	Cats, dogs	3–4 weeks	Same as *C sinensis*	Same as *C sinensis*
Metorchis conjunctus (North American liver fluke)	Canada	Raw fish, especially white sucker			Abdominal pain, anorexia, liver function abnormalities	Eggs in feces
Dicrocoelium dendriticum	Europe, former Soviet states, North Africa, northern Asia, Far East, Western Hemisphere	Ingestion of ants harboring metacercariae; terrestrial snails are intermediate hosts	Sheep, deer, cattle, other herbivores		Usually mild GI symptoms; if heavy, biliary symptoms	Eggs in feces; ingestion of infected liver may result in spurious passage of eggs

in this chapter include *Taenia saginata*, *Taenia solium*, *Diphyllobothrium* species, *Hymenolepis nana*, *Hymenolepis diminuta*, and *Diplylidium caninum*.

TAENIA SAGINATA

The human is the definitive host for *T saginata*, the beef tapeworm. Cattle act as intermediate hosts and become infected by grazing in pastures contaminated with eggs from human feces. The disease occurs worldwide in beef-eating countries. Acquisition is through ingestion of cysticerci in raw or undercooked beef. This infection can also occur in reindeer and camels.

The incubation period after consumption of the cysticerci is usually 10–14 weeks, after which proglottids can be found in the stool. Symptoms may occur earlier than this and may include epigastric discomfort, weight loss, nausea, vomiting, and diarrhea. The most common complaint is the passage of motile proglottids through the anus [4]. The proglottids may be found in the perianal area, in underclothing, or in bedding. Usually, only one worm is present. It may live for 25 to 30 years in the human intestine. Eosinophilia is not usually prominent, although IgE may be elevated. If a gastrointestinal barium study is performed, one may see a ribbon-like defect. The diagnosis is made by identification of either proglottids or eggs in the stool. The Scotch tape test may be useful in detecting these forms. The eggs of *T saginata* are not morphologically distinct from those of *T solium*. For both adult and pediatric patients, the treatment of choice is praziquantel, 5–10 mg/kg as a one-time dose to kill the adult worm [11].

TAENIA SOLIUM

The life cycle of *T solium* is the same as that of *T saginata* [6]. The major distinction is that humans may also serve as the intermediate host, causing cysticercosis (see below). As with *T saginata* infection, usually only a single worm is present and causes little tissue reaction. The disease is widely distributed, but in the United States, it is primarily seen in immigrants from endemic areas [78]. Humans acquire the infection through ingestion of raw or undercooked pork that is infected with the cysticerci.

It usually takes eight to 12 weeks from ingestion of cysticerci to the presence of proglottids or eggs in the stool of the human. The worm usually does not cause symptoms, although vague gastrointestinal symptoms, including epigastric discomfort, nausea and diarrhea may occur [79]. Finding that proglottids or eggs in fecal specimens is diagnostic for *Taenia* infection. Laboratory technicians or anyone handling fecal specimens must exercise caution because eggs are infective and could cause cysticercosis if accidentally ingested. Treatment is the same as for that beef tapeworm.

DIPHYLLOBOTHRIUM LATUM

Diphyllobothritis, or fish tapeworm infection, may result from ingestion of a large variety of fresh or seawater fishes [10]. The human is the definitive host, although other fish-eating mammals can be infected. The distribution of the disease is determined by the temperature requirements of the water, which are some 15°C to 25°C. Specific copepods are necessary to act as intermediate hosts. Acquisition is through ingestion of raw or undercooked fish or fish products. Pickling, kippering, cold smoking, and air drying do not reliably kill the parasites.

It takes four to six weeks from ingestion of infected fish until eggs appear in the feces. The adult worm may live some 30 to 40 years. The infection is usually mild or asymptomatic, although if symptoms are present, they may be nonspecific, including abdominal pain, distention, flatulence, and diarrhea [80]. Rarely, megaloblastic anemia may result from vitamin B_{12} deficiency produced by the tapeworm's competition within the host for absorption of essential nutrients [81]. Also rare are complications resulting from mechanical obstruction. Diagnosis is made by identification of characteristic eggs or proglottids in the feces. Treatment for both adults and children is praziquantel, 5–10 mg/kg as a single dose [11].

HYMENOLEPIS NANA

Humans act as the definitive and intermediate hosts for the dwarf tapeworm, *H nana*. Acquisition of the infection is through the fecal-oral route due to food, water, or fomites or by accidental ingestion of infected arthropods. *H nana* is unique among cestodes in that it is able to autoinfect its host. Geographic distribution is worldwide, although infections are most common in conditions of crowding and poor hygiene. *H nana* is the most common tapeworm in the United States, at least in children [6]. The incidence of infection is quite high in institutions such as day care centers, orphanages, and institutions for the mentally impaired.

It generally takes two to four weeks after ingestion for eggs to appear in the stool. Because of the capacity for autoinfection, the infection may be sustained indefinitely. Symptoms are usually mild, if present at all. Severe infections may be noted in immunocompromised patients. Signs and symptoms of heavy infection include diarrhea, epigastric pain, nausea, vomiting, irritability, anorexia, weight loss, headache, and weakness. Eosinophilia may occur in up to 30% of cases. Diagnosis is based on identification of the characteristic eggs in the stool. The treatment is praziquantel, 25 mg/kg as a single dose [11].

HYMENOLEPIS DIMINUTA

Infection with *Hymenolepis diminuta*, the rat tapeworm, is rare [10]. Infection with *H diminuta* usually occurs in children and is acquired through ingestion of arthropods containing the infective cysticercoid stage—usually mealworms or grain beetles that infest food. Although the rat tapeworm is present worldwide, human cases are reported primarily in areas with poor rodent control.

It usually takes two to four weeks from ingestion of the larva until eggs appear in the stool. The disease is usually mild. If symptoms are present, they tend to be nonspecific, but eosinophilia does accompany infection. Diagnosis requires identification of the eggs in feces [82]. Treatment is the same as that for *H nana*.

DIPLYLIDIUM CANINUM

Didlylidium caninum is the organism that causes dipylidiasis, dog tapeworm infection, which occurs worldwide. It is a common tapeworm of cats as well as dogs. Humans act as an incidental host, after ingestion of flea- or lice-contaminated food or water containing the larvae. Most infections occur in infants or young children [83]. The infection is relatively rare.

It takes three to four weeks after ingestion until proglottids appear in the stool. The infection is usually asymptomatic or mild. The proglottids, which resemble cucumber seeds, may migrate from the anus to the perianal area. Diagnosis is made from identification of the proglottids or from eggs. Eggs may be seen in packets, which contain eight to 15 eggs [1]. Hooks may often be seen within each egg. Treatment is with praziquantel at the same dosage as that for *T saginata* (see p. 522).

UNCOMMON CESTODE PARASITES

A number of cestodal zoonotic infections may occur in humans. *Bertiella* species occur in monkeys and may be transmitted by mites, which serve as intermediate hosts. *Bertiella* infection usually occurs in humans who work closely with or live with monkeys [84]. *Mesocestoides* commonly cause infections in monkeys, foxes, raccoons, and rodents. Cases of this infection are occasionally reported throughout the United States as well as Europe and Asia [85]. *Inermicapsifer* species are primarily parasites of rodents but may be transmitted to humans through accidental ingestion of arthropod intermediate hosts [1]. The proglottids are passed in the feces and resemble grains of rice when dried. *Diplogonoporus grandis* is a whale tapeworm, but human cases have been reported in Japan. Marine fishes are thought to serve as intermediate hosts [86].

Larval Cestode Infections

CYSTICERCOSIS

Cysticercosis is the human infection with the larval stage of *T solium*, the pork tapeworm. In this infection, humans act as an intermediate host. Cysticercosis is a common cause of neurologic diseases, especially seizures, in many parts of the world. Areas with the most cases with cysticercosis include Central and South America, parts of Asia, and Africa. Southern and eastern Europe also have had some cases of this infection. The acquisition is through ingestion of eggs contaminating food or water or eggs on fomites [87]. Reverse peristalsis associated with vomiting could potentially allow eggs from intestinal parasites to reach the upper GI tract, where they could hatch and start the cysticercosis cycle. More commonly, humans acquire cysticercosis by ingesting eggs from their own feces as a result of lapses in personal hygiene.

The time from egg ingestion to the occurrence of symptoms is usually at least two years. During this time, embryos hatch from ingested eggs, penetrate the gut wall, and disseminate via the circulation. They may lodge in a variety of tissues but are most commonly found in subcutaneous tissue, brain, eye, and skeletal muscle. These cysticerci cause little host reaction while alive, but when they start to degenerate, they may provoke granulomatous changes and other pathologic reaction. Cysts in the muscles tend to calcify with time. Signs and symptoms of cysticercosis of the CNS, or neurocystercosis, are varied and include seizures, intracranial hypertension, alteration of mental status, neurologic deficit, meningitis, and encephalitis. Neurocysticercosis involving the spinal cord is not uncommon, nor is ocular involvement. Nodules may appear in the skin and soft tissues and are usually about 2 cm in diameter.

Radiographic evaluation may reveal calcified cysticerci in muscle. CT or MR scanning of the head will reveal the cysts, often appearing as ring-enhanced cystic lesions [88]. Blood studies with the enzyme-linked immunotransfer blot are highly specific [89], and peripheral eosinophilia is usually absent. Diagnosis is usually made by a combination of serologic tests or the biopsy of tissue.

Treatment of cysticercosis is generally with albendazole or praziquantel. In adults, the dosage for albendazole is 400 mg twice daily for eight to 30 days; in children, it is 15 mg/kg/day to a maximum of 800 mg, given in two daily doses for eight to 30 days [11]. The dosage for praziquantel is 50 mg/kg/day in three doses for 15 days in both adult and pediatric patients [11]. Concurrent corticosteroid administration is often used to blunt the inflammatory response to dying parasites, which might exacerbate neurologic findings. The treatment of patients with cysticercosis must be individualized, since the antiparasitic drug treatment of ocular or spinal cysts may cause irreversible sequelae. Surgical treatment may also be warranted, and management of symptoms with anticonvulsants or ventricular shunting may be necessary.

ECHINOCOCCOSIS

Echinococcosis, or hydatid disease, is caused by the larval stage of *Echinococcus granulosus.* In this infection, dogs are the definitive hosts; sheep, other animals, and humans may serve as intermediate hosts. Environmental and occupational risk factors for the disease are living and working closely with dogs. Acquisition of infection is through ingestion of infective eggs via food and water contamination or fomites. The infection is present on all continents but is concentrated in sheep-raising areas [90].

It usually takes several years from ingestion of eggs to manifestation of the disease state. Signs and symptoms vary with the number and size of cystic lesions, but they are usually related to mechanical pressure of the mass or to allergic reactions to the foreign proteins. Cysts commonly involve the liver and lung. Other sites, including the kidney, spleen, heart, bones, muscle and CNS, may be involved. Anaphylactic reaction may accompany leakage of cyst fluids. Laboratory studies show peripheral eosinophilia in approximately one third of patients. This is associated with leakage of fluid. Single or multiple lesions can be visualized by ultrasonography, CT, or other imaging techniques. Definitive diagnosis is usually made by microscopic identification of the parasite in surgically removed specimens. Serology is also useful.

Treatment of adults is usually albendazole, 400 mg twice daily for 28 days; the pediatric dose is 15 mg/kg/day for 28 days [11]. Surgical resection and other procedures may be necessary [91].

ECHINOCOCCUS MULTILOCULARIS

This infection, also called *alveolar hydatid disease*, is similar to *E granulosis*, but the resulting mass tends to grow more rapidly. The rapidly enlarging mass is invasive, and hematologic dissemination may lead to metastatic infection [90]. Often, the disease is inoperable by the time the diagnosis is made. Laboratory tests are usually unremarkable, and imaging studies usually show a solid mass with central cavitation. Surgical resection may be curative if diagnosis is made early. Albendazole may slow the progress of the infection [91].

ECHINOCOCCUS VOGELI

Echinococcus vogeli infection causes polycystic hydatid disease and is also similar to *E granulosis* infection. Human cases have been reported only in Central and South America. Clinical symptoms usually are related to a liver mass. Treatment is usually a combination of surgical resection and albendazole [92]. The severity of this infection is usually intermediate—between that of *E granulosis* and *E multilocularis* [90].

COENUROSIS

Coenuriasis is a larval tapeworm infection caused by one of several species of *Taenia*, including *Taenia multiceps*, *Taenia serialis*, and *Taenia brauni*. (Some authors believe that these parasites belong to the genus *Multiceps*.) In this infection, dogs are the definitive hosts, and sheep are usually the intermediate hosts, although humans may act as incidental intermediate hosts. The infection results from ingestion of the eggs from contaminated food, water, or fomites. Human infection is rare, although the tapeworm is common in areas where sheep are present. In sheep, the infection is called *gid* or *staggers* [10].

After ingestion, onchospheres escape from the eggs, hatch, and penetrate the intestinal wall. Then, they are hematogenously spread to various tissues, where they form cysts. Common sites of larval encystment include the CNS, eye, subcutaneous tissue, and muscle. The clinical features depend on the location of these cysts. When the CNS is involved, common symptoms include drowsiness, headache, vomiting, papilledema, seizures, and hemiparesis [93]. A variety of ocular findings are seen in response to encystment of the eye [94]. Subcutaneous coenuri may or may not be painful and are commonly confused with lipomas, ganglions, and neurofibromas. The diagnosis is usually made on the basis of microscopic identification of coenuri. If the eye is involved, slit-lamp examination may be used to make direct diagnosis. Eosinophilia is not usually a feature. Treatment generally involves surgical excision of the cerebral, ophthalmic, or subcutaneous coenuri. Medications do not appear to be useful [10].

SPARGANOSIS

Sparganosis is caused by larval infection with a *Spirometra* species, usually *Spirometra mansoni*. The definitive hosts for this infection are dogs and cats. There are two intermediate hosts, including a cyclops and a vertebrate. Humans may be incidental intermediate hosts; they usually acquire this infection through ingestion of cyclops-contaminated water; ingestion of larvae in undercooked frog, snake, poultry, or pork; or application of raw frog flesh as a poultice. Although the infection is common in animals, it is rare in humans [10].

The incubation period varies greatly, depending on the route of acquisition. The clinical features, although usually mild, relate to the number of parasites and the areas the larvae reach during migration. Migrations may be subcutaneous, ocular, or neural. One may see either nonprolifer-ative or proliferative sparganosis. Nonproliferative sparganosis is more common and is characterized by the presence of one solitary discrete lesion that contains the tapeworm [95]. Proliferative sparganosis tends to occur with *Spirometra proliferum* and is highly invasive. It tends to proliferate and metastasize throughout the body by a process of branching and budding. Dissemination can occur anywhere but is most common in the CNS, skeletal muscle, subcutaneous tissue, and internal organs [96]. The diagnosis is usually made by serologic tests and pathologic specimens. Treatment of nonproliferative cases is surgical excision of the entire sparganum. Drug therapy does not appear to be helpful. There is no effective treatment for proliferative sparganosis.

References

1. Ash LR, Orihel TC. *Atlas of Human Parasitology*, 4th Ed. Chicago: American Society of Clinical Pathologists, 1997.

2. Despommier DD, Gwadz RW, Hotez PJ. *Parasitic Diseases*, 3rd Ed. New York: Springer-Verlag, 1995.
3. Chan MS. The global burden of intestinal nematode infections—fifty years on. *Parasitol Today* 1997;13:438–43.
4. Wilson ME. *A World Guide to Infections: Diseases, Distribution, Diagnosis.* New York: Oxford University Press, 1991.
5. Bryan FD. Diseases transmitted by foods contaminated by waste water. *J Food Protein* 1977;40:45–56.
6. Juckett G. Common intestinal helminths. *Am Family Physician* 1995;52:2039–48.
7. Crompton DWT. Chronic ascariasis and malnutrition. *Parasitol Today* 1985;1:47–52.
8. Lowe JH. Abdominal complications of *Acscaris lumbricoides* infection in children. *Br J Surg* 1966;53: 510–21.
9. Leventhal R, Cheadle R. *Medical Parasitology: A Self-Instructional Text*, 4th Ed. Philadelphia: F.A. Davis Company, 1996.
10. Part VI, helminthic infections. In: Connor DH, Chandler FW, Schwartz DA, et al. (eds), *Pathology of Infectious Diseases.* Stamford, CT: Appleton & Lange, 1997. Pp 1305–1588.
11. Drugs for parasitic infections. *Med Lett* 1998;40:1–12.
12. Arfaa F. *Ascaris* and trichuriasis. In: Walsh JA, Warren JA (eds), *Strategies for Primary Health Care.* London: University of Chicago Press, 1986. Pp 178–88.
13. Thein-Hlaing, Than-Sar, Myat-Lay-Kyin. Control of ascariasis through age-targeted chemotherapy: impact of six monthly chemotherapeutic regimens. *Bull WHO* 1990;68:747–53.
14. Warren KS, Bundy DA, Anderson RM, et al. Helminth infections. In: Jamison DJ (ed), *Disease Control Prevention in Developing Countries.* Oxford University Press, 1993. Pp 131–60.
15. American Academy of Pediatrics. Pinworm infestation. In: Peter G (ed), *Red Book: Report of the Committee on Infectious Diseases*, 24th Ed. Elk Grove Village, IL: American Academy of Pediatrics, 1997. Pp 407–8.
16. Beckman EN, Holland JB. Ovarian enterobiasis—a proposed pathogenesis. *Am J Trop Med Hyg* 1981;30: 74–6.
17. Croll NA, Ghadiran E. Wormy persons: contributions to the nature and patterns of over-dispersions with *Ascaris lumbricoides, Ancylostoma duodenale, Necator americanus* and *Trichuris trichiura. Trop Geogr Med* 1991;33:241–8.
18. Stephenson LSM, Latham NC. Treatment with a single dose of albendazole improves growth of Kenyan school children with hookworm, trichuris and ascaris infections. *Am J Trop Med Hyg* 1989;41:78–87.
19. Gilman RH, Chang YH, David C, et al. The adverse consequence of having trichuris infection. *Trans R Soc Trop Med Hyg* 1983;7:432–8.
20. Peters W, Gilles HM. *Tropical Medicine and Parasitology*, 4th Ed. London: Mosby-Wolfe, 1995.
21. Yoshida Y, Nakanishi Y, Mitani W. Experimental studies on the infection mode of *Ancylostoma duodenale* and *Necator americanus* to the definitive host. *Jpn J Parasitol* 1958;7:102–12.
22. Stolzfus RJ, Albonico M, Chwaya HM, et al. Hemoquant determination of hookworm-related blood loss and its role in iron deficiency in African children. *Am J Trop Med Hyg* 1996;55:399–404.
23. Walzer PD, Milder JE, Banwell JG, et al. Epidemiologic features of *Strongyloides stercoralis* infections in an endemic area of the United States. *Am J Trop Med Hyg* 1982;31:313–9.
24. Berk SL, Verghese A, Alvarez J, et al. Clinical and epidemiologic features of strongyloidiasis: a prospective study in rural Tennessee. *Arch Intern Med* 1987;147: 1257–60.
25. Petithory JC, Derouin F. AIDs and strongyloides in Africa. *Lancet* 1987;1:921.
26. Conway DJ, Lindo JF, Robinson RD, et al. Towards effective control of *Strongyloides. Parasitol Today* 1995;11:420–4.
27. Koga K, Kasuya S, Khamboonruang C, et al. A modified agar plate method for detection of *Strongyloides stercoralis. Am J Trop Med Hyg* 1991;45:518–21.
28. Datrya A. Treatment of strongyloides with ivermectin compared with albendazole: results of an open study of 60 cases. *Trans R Soc Trop Med Hyg* 1994;88:344–5.
29. Ottesen EA, Duke BOL, Karam M, et al. Strategies and tools for the control/elimination of lymphatic filariasis. *Bull WHO* 1997;75:491–503.
30. Ottesen EA. Efficacy of diethylcarbamazine in eradicating infection with lymphatic-dwelling filariae in humans. *Rev Infect Dis* 1985;7:341–56.
31. Ottesen EA. Filarial infections. *Infect Dis Clin North Am* 1993;7:619–33.
32. Freedman DO, Almeida Filho PJ, Besh S, et al. Lymphoscintigraphic analysis of lymphatic abnormalities in symptomatic and asymptomatic human filariasis. *J Infect Dis* 1994;170:927–33.
33. McCarthy JS, Ottesen EA, Nutman TB. Onchocerciasis in endemic and nonendemic populations: differences in clinical presentation and immunologic findings. *J Infect Dis* 1994;170:736–41.
34. Zimmerman PA, Guderian RH, Aruajo E, et al. Polymerase chain reaction based diagnosis of Onchocercal volvulus infection: improved detection of patients with onchocerciasis. *J Infect Dis* 1994;169:686–9.
35. Nutman TB, Miller KD, Mulligan M, et al. Diethylcarbamazine prophylaxis for human loiasis, results of a double-blind study. *N Engl J Med* 1988;319:752–6.
36. Klion AD, Massougbodji A, Sadeler B-C, et al. Loiasis in endemic and nonendemic populations: immunologically mediated differences in clinical presentation. *J Infect Dis* 1991;163:1318–25.
37. Nutman TB, Miller KD, Mulligan M, et al. Loa loa infection in temporary residents of endemic regions: recognition of hyperresponsive syndrome with characteris-

tic clinical manifestations. *J Infect Dis* 1986;154: 10–4.

38. Klion AD, Massouboudji A, Horton JH, et al. Albendazole in human loiasis: results of a double blind, placebo-controlled trial. *J Infect Dis* 1993;168:202–6.
39. Meyers WM, Connor DH, Harman LE, et al. Human streptocerciasis: a clinicopathologic study of 40 African (Zairians) including identification of the adult filaria. *Am J Trop Med Hyg* 1972;21:528–45.
40. Chadee DD, Tilluckdarry CG, Doo R, et al. Ivermectin treatment of mansonellosis blanchisseuse, Trinidad, West Indies. *Ann Trop Parasitol* 1996;90:645–9.
41. Hopkins DR, Ruiz-Tiben E, Ruebush T, et al. Dracunculiasis eradication: March, 1994 update. *Am J Trop Med Hyg* 1995;52:14–20.
42. Centers for Disease Control and Prevention. Imported dracunculiasis—United States, 1995 and 1997. *MMWR* 1998;47:209–11.
43. Benenson AS (ed). *Control of Communicable Diseases Manual*, 16th Ed. Baltimore: United Book Press, 1995.
44. Watten RH, Beckner WM, Cross JH, et al. Clinical studies of *Capillaria philippinensis. Trans R Soc Trop Med Hyg* 1970;66:828–32.
45. Cross JH. Intestinal capillariasis. *Clin Microbiol Rev* 1992;5:120–9.
46. Most H. Trichinosis—preventable yet still with us. *N Engl J Med* 1978;298:1178–80.
47. Markell EK. Pseudohookworm infection—trichostrongyliasis. Treatment with thiabendazole. *N Engl J Med* 1968;278:831–2.
48. Krepel HP, Baeta S, Polderman AM. Human *Oesophagostomum* infection in northern Togo and Ghana: epidemiological aspects. *Ann Trop Med Parasitol* 1992;86: 289–300.
49. Krepel HP, Haring T, Baeta S, et al. Treatment of mixed *Oesophagostomum* and hookworm infection: effect of albendazole, pyrantel pamoate, levamisole, and thiabendazole. *Trans R Soc Trop Med Hyg* 1993;87:87–9.
50. Zvejnicks PA, Lichtenstein KA, Koneman EW. Luminal anisakidosis due *to Pseudoterranova decipiens. Clin Infect Dis* 1998;26:1222–3.
51. Bouree P, Paugam A, Petithory JC. Anisokidosis: report of 25 cases and review of the literature. *Comp Immunol Microbiol Infect Dis* 1995;18:75–84.
52. Prociv P, Croese J. Human eosinophilic enteritis caused by dog hookworm *Ancylostoma caninum. Lancet* 1990;335:1299–1302.
53. Schentz PM, Glickman LT. Current concepts in parasitology. Toxocaral visceral larva migrans. *N Engl J Med* 1978;298:436–9.
54. Glickman LT, Magnaval JF. Zoonotic roundworm infections. *Infect Dis Clin North Am* 1993;7:717–32.
55. Kazacos RR, Boyce WM. Baylisascaris larva migrans. *J Am Vet Med Assoc* 1989;195:894–903.
56. Rusnak JM, Lucey DR. Clinical Gnathostomiasis: case report and review of the English language literature. *Clin Infect Dis* 1993;16:33–50.
57. Anantaphruti MT, Nuamtanong S, Waikagal J. Effect of ivermectin on experimental gnathostomiasis in rabbits. *Trop Med Parasitol* 1992;43:65–7.
58. Koo J, Pien F, Kliks MM. Angiostrongylus (Parastrongylus) eosinophilic meningitis. *Rev Infect Dis* 1988;10:1155–62.
59. Loría-Cortés R, Lobo-Sanahuja JF. Clinical abdominal angiostrongylosis. A study of 116 children with intestinal eosinophilic granuloma caused by *Angiostrongylus costaricensis. Am J Trop Med Hyg* 1980;29:538–44.
60. Risher WH, Crocker EF Jr., Beckman EN, et al. Pulmonary dirofilariasis. *J Thorac Cardiovasc Surg* 1989; 97:303–8.
61. Weissman BW. Raccoon heartworms causing a facial mass. *South Med J* 1992;85:845–6.
62. Gutierrez Y, Cohen M, Machicao CN. Dioctophyine larva in the subcutaneous tissues of a woman in Ohio. *Am J Surg Pathol* 1989;13:800–2.
63. Wittner M, Turner JW, Jacquette G, et al. Eustrongylidiasis—a parasitic infection acquired by eating sushi. *N Engl J Med* 1989;320:1124–6.
64. Attah EB, Nagarajan S, Obineche EN, et al. Hepatic capillariasis *Am J Clin Pathol* 1983;79:127–30.
65. Stuiver PC. Acute schistosomiasis among Americans rafting the Omo River, Ethiopia. *JAMA* 1984;251:508–10.
66. King CH. Acute and chronic schistosomiasis. *Hosp Pract* 1991;26:95–106.
67. Bell DR. *Lecture Notes on Tropical Medicine*, 4th Ed. Oxford: Blackwell Science, 1995. P 224.
68. Friis H, Ndhlovu P, Kaondera K, et al. Ultrasonographic assessment of *Schistosoma mansoni* and *S haematobium* morbidity in Zimbabwean schoolchildren. *Am J Trop Med Hyg* 1996;55:290–4.
69. World Health Organization. Report of the WHO expert committee on the control of schistosomiasis, Geneva, November 8–15, 1991; WHO Technical Report Series; 1991.
70. Hammad TA, Gabr NS, Talaat MM, et al. Hematuria and proteinuria as predictors of *Schistosoma haematobium* infection. *Am J Trop Med Hyg* 1997;57:363–7.
71. Schwartz DA. Helminths in the induction of cancer. *Schistosoma haematobium* and bladder cancer. *Trop Geogr Med* 1981;33:1–7.
72. Rocha H, Kirk JW, Hearey CD. Prolonged salmonella bacteremia in patients with *Schistosoma mansoni* infections. *Arch Intern Med* 1971;128:254–7.
73. Valli LCP, Kanamura HY, DaSilva RM, et al. Efficacy of an enzyme-linked immunosorbent assay in the diagnosis of and serologic distinction between acute and chronic *Schistosoma mansoni* infections. *Am J Trop Med Hyg* 1997;57:356–62.
74. Stelma FF, Sall S, Daff B, et al. Oxamniquine cures *Schistosoma mansoni* infection in a focus in which cure rates are unusually low. *J Infect Dis* 1997;26:95–106.
75. Apt W, Aguilera X, Vega F, et al. Treatment of human chronic fascioloiasis with trictabendazole: drug efficiency

and serologic response. *Am J Trop Med Hyg* 1995;52: 532–35.

76. Singh TS, Mutum SS, Razaque MA. Pulmonary paragonimiasis: clinical features, diagnosis and treatment of 39 cases in Manipur. *Trans R Soc Trop Med Hyg* 1986;80:967–71.
77. Johnson RJ, Johnson JR. Paragonimiasis in Indochinese refugees. Roentgenographic findings with clinical correlations. *Am Rev Respir Dis* 1983;128:535–8.
78. Despommier DD. Tapeworm infection—the long and short of it. *N Engl J Med* 1992;327:727–8.
79. Richards R Jr, Schantz PM. Cysticercosis and tzeniasis. *N Engl J Med* 1985;312:787–8.
80. Turner JA, Sorvillo FJ, Chin J, et al. Diphyllobothriasis associated with salmon—United States. *MMWR* 1981;30:31–2, 37.
81. Nyberg W, Gräsbeck R, Saarni M, et al. Serum vitamin B12 levels and incidence of tapeworm anemia in a population heavily infected with *Diphyllobothrium latum*. *Am J Clin Nutr* 1961;9:606–12.
82. Hamrick HJ, Bowdre JH, Church SM. Rat tapeworm (*Hymenolepis diminuta*) infection in a child. *Pediatr Infect Dis J* 1990;9:216–9.
83. Ratiere CR. Dog tapeworm (*Dipylidium caninum*) infestation in a 6-month-old infant. *J Fam Pract* 1992;34:101–2.
84. Panda DN, Panda MR. Record of *Bertiella studeri* (Blanchard, 1891), an anaplocephalid tapeworm, from a child. *Ann Trop Med Parasitol* 1994;88:451–2.
85. Schiltz LF, Roberto RR, Rutheford GW, et al. *Mesocestoides* (cestoda) infection in a California child. *Pediatr Infect Dis J* 1992;11:332–4.
86. Nakamura N, Nakayama J, Shimazu T, et al. First two cases of diplogonoporiasis grandis from Nagano prefecture, Japan. *Jpn J Parasitol* 1993; 42:434–7.
87. Botero DB, Tanowitz HB, Weiss LM, et al. Taeniasis and cysticercosis. *Infect Dis Clin North Am* 1993;7: 683–97.
88. Del Brutto OH, Sotelo J. Neurocysticercosis: an update. *Rev Infect Dis* 1988;10:1075–87.
89. White AL Jr. State-of-the-art: neurocysticercosis: a major cause of neurologic disease worldwide. *Clin Infect Dis* 1997;24:101–13.
90. Kammerer WS, Schantz PM. Echinococcal disease. *Infect Dis Clin North Am* 1993;7:605–18.
91. WHO Informal Working Group on Echinococcosis. Guidelines for treatment of cystic and alveolar echinococcosis in humans. *Bull WHO* 1996;74:231–42.
92. Meneghelli UG, Martinelli ALC, Llorach Velludo MAS, et al. Polycystic hydatid disease *(Echinococcus vogeli)*: clinical, laboratory, and morphologic findings in nine Brazilian patients. *J Hepatol* 1991;14:203–10.
93. Pau A, Perria C, Turtas S, et al. Long-term follow-up on the surgical treatment of intracranial coenurosis. *Br J Neurosurg* 1990;4:39–43.
94. Ibechukwu BF, Onwukeme KE. Intraocular coenurosis: a case report. *Br J Ophthalmol* 1991;75:430–1.
95. Norma SH, Kreutnew A Jr. Sparganosis: clinical and pathologic observations in ten cases. *South Med J* 1980;73:297–300.
96. Nakamura T, Hara M, Matsuoka M, et al. Human proliferative sparganosis: a new Japanese case. *Am J Clin Pathol* 1990;94:224–8.

30 / Protozoan Travel-Related Infections

Cynthia R. Lewis-Younger

Protozoan parasitic diseases have assumed greater importance over recent decades, in part due to technologic advancements. The development of medical technologies that use immunosuppression or enhance the longevity of immunosuppressed persons, along with spread of the human immunodeficiency virus (HIV), has created a population of highly susceptible human hosts. The development of transportation technology has created a truly global economy, fostering the spread of HIV and increasing travel into areas where various protozoal diseases are endemic. With global distribution systems for food, technology has also changed the nature of food-borne illnesses. Large water-distribution systems have proved vulnerable to contamination. Several protozoans are newly recognized as important causes of outbreaks of food- and waterborne illnesses.

As a consequence of their occupation, workers may be exposed to protozoan diseases, especially workers such as laboratory personnel or animal handlers who come into close contact with the organisms or their infectious hosts. Business travelers may come in contact with contaminated food, soil, water, or vectors during travel to areas where protozoan diseases are endemic.

Protozoa are one-celled eukaryotes that live singly or in colonies [1]. About one fifth of the human parasite burden consists of protozoan species [2]. They are widespread throughout the environment and have been found in almost every environmental situation on earth [3]. Protozoa are extremely diverse. Protozoan species were among the first microscopic organisms identified. The "animalcule" described by Van Leewenhook is thought to have been a member of the genus *Giardia* [4].

The majority of identified pathogenic protozoans live in warm, humid environments. Thus, the majority of pathogenic protozoan diseases have been considered primarily tropical diseases. However, several of the protozoans identified as pathogens in the last 30 years are found in temperate regions of the world [3].

Among the protozoan species that are pathogenic, many have natural hosts other than humans. These species are primarily zoonoses and infect humans only sporadically, often when they enter the habitat of the natural host or vector. Other species are primarily opportunistic: They do not cause disease in most healthy humans. Recently, the number of immunosuppressed individuals has increased significantly. These individuals are at greater risk of acquiring and suffering severe effects of protozoan disease. They include patients infected with HIV, those with debilitating diseases such as malignancies, and those who are iatrogenically immunosuppressed.

Humans are a natural host for several pathogenic protozoa. Among this group of protozoans, humans may either be the primary host or one of several possible hosts. Pathogenic protozoans can be classified as either intestinal parasites, which are spread primarily through the fecal-oral route, or as tissue and blood pathogens. Tissue and blood pathogens may be spread by vectors, such as mosquitoes or flies. Protozoans have complicated life cycles that include both sexual and asexual reproductive forms [1]. Life cycles are not discussed in this chapter, but many references describe these in detail [3–5]. Different forms of protozoa may exist in hosts compared with those in vectors or even in different host species. Some form cysts that are environmentally stable.

Although previously considered as one phylum, protozoans probably represent several phyla [1]. Many of these organisms have been classified with various other phyla or classes, such as fungi. Recent advancements in molecular and cell biology, including genetics, have allowed further delineation of relationships between the species, but it is still unclear how many species exist and how these species are related [1,6]. For this reason, multiple names may be used and identification can be confusing. This chapter uses the classification scheme published by Garcia in 1997 [7].

Some of these parasites cause severe, perhaps fatal, diseases among otherwise healthy individuals. Even organisms that normally do not pose a threat can result in overwhelming infection in an immunocompromised person. In one Spanish study, 80% of cases of leishmaniasis occurred in immunosuppressed patients; 60% of these patients were HIV positive. These diseases have profound impacts worldwide. Malaria, caused by members of the *Plasmodium* genus, is found in 90 countries, and approximately 2.4 billion people are at risk. Between 300 and 500 million cases occur annually, resulting in 1.5 to 2.7 million deaths [1]. This chapter primarily focuses on protozoan diseases other than malaria. While less common in the United States, these diseases are important in many areas of the world.

Protozoan organisms have evolved sophisticated means for evading the host immune system. One is their complex life cycles, which include intracellular forms, antigenic variation and mimicry, and plasticity of the genetic material [1,8]. Treatment is available for some protozoan diseases, but not all, but it is often unsatisfactory or may have severe side effects. Protozoans' successful evasion of immune system defenses suggests that successful treatment may be long in coming [1]. Employing preventive measures may be the only way to prevent serious illness or death, both in workers and in the general public. Business travelers may be at a very high risk in some areas. Occupational and environmental health practitioners must be cognizant of these diseases and of effective preventive measures to protect worker populations.

Epidemiology

In spite of progress in controlling infectious diseases in developed countries, persons traveling to, or living in, tropical climates are still vulnerable to infectious diseases. Even those living in developed countries are not immune from the effects of infectious diseases. These diseases (e.g., HIV) have profound effects, cause great human suffering, and deplete scarce resources [9]. Protozoan diseases are among the diseases that significantly impact the world's population.

INCIDENCE AND PREVALENCE

The incidences and prevalences of many of these diseases are poorly known and probably underestimated. Many have poorly recognized or unrecognized mild forms as well as asymptomatic forms. Voluntary reporting and passive surveillance are likely to catch only a few of the outbreaks that actually occur [10]. Many of those who are most at risk have no access to medical treatment or reside in countries where public health resources are limited [9].

Intestinal Amebae

The intestinal amebae include several *Entamoeba* species, *Endolimax nana*, *Iodamoeba bütschlii*, and *Blastocystis hominis* [7]. Amebas are primitive animals that appear not to have significantly evolved beyond their early forms. The pathogenic forms need to be distinguished from the commensal forms, which may infect but do not cause disease in humans. Amebas that may cause infections in humans include *Entamoeba histolytica*, *Entamoeba coli*, *Entamoeba gingivalis*, *Endolimax nana*, and *Iodamoeba bütschlii*. Pathogenic forms are primarily intestinal parasites, although serious extraluminal and systemic diseases have been associated with some of them. *Dientamoeba fragilis* is included with the amebas in some classifications [3].

E histolytica is found throughout the world and has been implicated in infectious outbreaks in the United States [11]. Its worldwide incidence is unknown. Studies have suggested percentages ranging from 0.2% to 50%. Although its prevalence tends to be higher in tropical and subtropical regions, the pathogen can be found even in cold areas of the world. In the general population, its prevalence depends on sanitary conditions, population density, and socioeconomic status. This is especially true in the tropical and subtropical regions. Prevalence is higher in male homosexuals, apparently because of oral-anal sexual practices [3].

E nana, *I bütschlii*, and *E coli* are commensal organisms that inhabit the gut. They must be differentiated from the pathogenic organisms, *E histolytica* and *D fragilis*. The prevalence of *E nana* is estimated to be 10–20% worldwide. *I bütschlii* has an estimated prevalence of 8%, while that of *E coli* ranges from 10% to 30%. *E gingivalis* is also nonpathogenic but is chiefly present in tartar of teeth and in gums. Its prevalence is dependent on the condition of the teeth and gums. It is found in about 10% of healthy mouths, while it can be isolated from about 95% of people with gum disease and tooth decay [3].

Blastocystis is a common intestinal organism. There has been much debate about its classification, but it has recently been recognized as a protozoan. It is found in 10–20% of stool specimens. There is disagreement as to the ability of this organism to cause disease [12]; however, the organism has been isolated from individuals with prolonged diarrhea in whom no other cause has been found [13].

Intestinal Flagellates

The intestinal flagellates include *Giardia lamblia*, *Chilomastix mesnili*, *Dientamoeba fragilis*, *Trichomonas hominis*, *Enteromonas hominis*, and *Retortomonas intestinalis* [7]. Humans serve as hosts to both pathogenic and nonpathogenic flagellates. *D fragilis* is considered pathogenic and is estimated to have an incidence of about 4% [3]. Nonpathogenic species include *C mesnili*, *E hominis*, *T hominis*, and *R intestinalis*. The major pathogenic flagellate of the intestinal canal is *Giardia*. The flagellated intestinal protozoans have evolved several mechanisms that allow them to resist peristaltic movements in the intestinal canal. Within each species, there is marked morphologic variation. A single protozoan species may be parasitic in multiple vertebrate species. Most, if not all, vertebrates can serve as hosts to some form of flagellate [3].

Giardia inhabits the upper small intestine, where its trophozoites have a rich supply of cholesterol, which it is unable to synthesize [14]. In the United States, giardiasis is most prevalent in children under 5 years of age and women of child-bearing age [15].

Intestinal Ciliates

Balantidium coli is the only identified pathologic species included as an intestinal ciliate [5,7]. It is widely distributed in hogs and is found in other mammals [4,5]. Although it appears worldwide, its prevalence in humans is unknown [4].

Intestinal Coccidia and Microsporidia

This group includes *Cryptosporidium parvum*, *Cyclospora cayentanensis*, *Isospora belli*, *Sarcocystis* species, and Microsporidia (Enterocytozoon) [7]. Coccidians are small, round protozoa that are primarily intestinal parasites. Several of this group of protozoan species have been identified as human pathogens in the last 20 years. Among species found to cause disease are members of the microsporidian groups and of the following genera: *Toxoplasma*, *Cryptosporidium*, *Cyclospora*, *Isospora*, *Sarcocystis*, and *Eimeria* [3].

Pathogenic *Cryptosporidium* may include a number of species; however, *C parvum* is the species thought to be most often pathogenic in humans [3]. *Cryptosporidium* is highly infectious [16]. A study published by DuPont in the *New England Journal of Medicine* showed that one of five healthy volunteers who ingested a solution containing approximately 30 *C parvum* cysts became infected. Using logistic regression, Dupont estimated that the median infective dose was 132 oocysts [17].

Cryptosporidium has been found to be the cause of a number of outbreaks in the recent past. It is a common cause of diarrhea in travelers, day care centers, and in outbreaks of waterborne disease [3]. Surveys of seroprevalence in North America and Europe have indicated a lifetime prevalence of 25–35%, while in developing countries, the prevalence appears to be closer to 66–67% of the population [18]. Between 3% and 13% of persons with diarrhea who have recently arrived from developing countries are found to have *Cryptosporidium* [11]. About 2% of AIDS patients have cryptosporidiosis as their disease-defining illness. That percentage rises to 3.5% of children with AIDS [19]. *Cryptosporidium* causes severe enteritis in approximately 5% of AIDS patients [20].

Isospora belli is the only parasite in this group for which humans are the main host. It is rare but has been found throughout the world. *Isospora* has been associated with outbreaks of diarrhea in nursing homes in developed countries [11]. *Sarcocystis* has been found in striated muscle of infected humans, although these parasites are primarily found in other mammals and birds [3].

Cyclospora is also an identified cause of diarrheal disease [3]. The first known case was reported in 1977. Reports of outbreaks associated with food began in 1996 [21]. A total of 50 *Cyclospora*-related outbreaks were investigated, all of which were due to contamination of food imported from Guatemala [22]. *Cyclospora* is unlikely to be transmitted from person to person, because the excreted oocysts require days to weeks under favorable environmental conditions to become infectious [21]. The infective dose is not known, nor is the percentage of subclinical infection [22].

Microsporidia are considered by some to represent a unique phyllum of primitive eukaryotic obligate intracellular organisms. They are widely distributed in nature [23]. Microsporidia have long been implicated in diseases of small animals, insects, and invertebrates [3]. They have been recovered from rabbits, mice, hamsters, rats, dogs, and foxes [23]. In humans, infections appear primarily opportunistic. Surveys of serologic markers indicate that up to 43% of individuals have antibodies to the organisms. The rates were highest among patients with malaria and male homosexuals. In a Ghanian study, the rate of positive sera markers was 43% in malaria patients, compared with about 5% of patients with a variety of other illnesses, including typhoid fever, leprosy, toxoplasmosis, and toxocariasis, as well as some normals. Healthy Swedes with a history of travel to a tropical region had a prevalence rate of 12% [24]. Impaired cell-mediated immunity renders animals susceptible to microsporidiosis. Infections in AIDS patients or other immunosuppressed individuals may represent reactivation of a latent infection [23].

Blood or Tissue Sporozoa (Flagellates)

Plasmodium species (malaria) and *Babesia* species are blood sporozoa [7]. Malaria is a major disease in the tropical and subtropical areas of the world. The *Plasmodium* species that cause malaria are responsible for many cases of hemolytic anemia. For example, half a million cases of malaria occur annually in Brazil alone. Although the disease has been controlled in most of the country, it is still prevalent in the Amazon region. As in other countries, more drug-resistant parasites have been noted in the recent past [25]. Throughout the world, hundreds of millions of cases occur annually, with over a million deaths per year. The incidence is increasing, and the risk for travelers to malaria-prone areas is probably higher than 40 years ago, due to the emergence of drug-resistant *Plasmodia* [15].

Like the trypanosomes and malaria, *Babesia microti* affects the red blood cells [3]. Because humans are not the primary hosts, outbreaks occur primarily in localized regions. An endemic focus exists in the region of Long Island and Shelter Island, New York, and Nantucket, Massachusetts. A few infections with related organisms have been reported in the western United States, but these appear to be a different species not yet named [26].

Various species of *Babesia* have been identified, but humans with intact spleens cannot be infected by most of them. *Babesia divergens* and *Babesia bovis* are found in Europe and can infect humans [18]. *B microti*, found in North America, has been shown to cause hemolytic anemia even in people with intact spleens [3]. Of six patients with clinical babesiosis, all six patients had participated in outdoor activities. None were known to be immunocompromised, although two had taken corticosteroids [27]. A study of the prevalence of pathogenic organisms transmitted by the *Ixodes dammini* tick in a county where the disease is endemic revealed that *B microti* was found in five of 100 ticks as the sole identified pathogen. In four additional ticks, *B microti* was found along with *Borrelia burgdorferi* and the human granulocytic ehrlichiosis agent (HGE) [28]. Approximately 3–7% of the population living in the endemic area have serologic evidence of prior infection [18].

Blood or Tissue Flagellates

Trypanosoma and *Leishmania* are flagellates that infect blood and tissues [7]. Trypanosomes are pathogenic in mammals, including humans. They are transmitted by arthropod vectors. Like malaria, diseases caused by these protozoans are limited to the geographic distribution of their vectors [3]. *Trypanosoma brucei* causes sleeping sickness and affects about 55 million people in 36 countries [1]. *T brucei rhodesiense* is found in East Africa, from Ethiopia to Botswana. *Trypanosoma brucei gambiense* is found in Central and West Africa, spanning Central Africa from Senegal to Sudan and from Angola to Zaire. New methods of characterization have shown that the current nomenclature is not adequate and these organisms are sometimes grouped by isoenzyme (zymodemes) or antigen profiles (serodemes) [29].

T brucei gambiense causes Gambian, or mid-African, sleeping sickness. Gambian trypanosomiasis occurs in less than 1% of the population per year in endemic regions. Periodic outbreaks related to the populations and distributions of the vector species may occur [3]. The vectors are various species of the genus *Glossina*, or tsetse flies [29]. In endemic regions, the prevalence of infection in flies is between 2% to 4% [3].

Trypanosoma brucei rhodesiense causes East African sleeping sickness, or Rhodesian trypanosomiasis. In addition to humans, other mammals are also hosts for these organisms. Rhodesian trypanosomiasis occurs less frequently than Gambian trypanosomiasis [3]. In a population of 50 million, 1,000–2,000 new cases are diagnosed each year. The prevalence is less than 0.01% in endemic regions [29].

Trypanosoma cruzi causes Chagas' disease, or American trypanosomiasis. It has been reported in 21 countries. A population of 90 million people are at risk [1]. The prevalence is estimated at 16 million [30]. It has a number of vertebrate hosts, including domesticated and wild animals. Prevalence of this disease varies by region, but up to 50% of populations has been reported to be infected [3]. American trypanosomiasis causes more than 5,000 deaths per year in Brazil [25]. *Triatomine* bugs and 14 species of mammals have been found to host these protozoa in the United States, in locations as far north as Maryland. However, human infection in the United States is rare [3]. Only three cases of U.S.-acquired Chagas' disease (excluding iatrogenic exposure) have been reported, although the parasite is found in animals in the United States [30]. *Trypanosoma rangeli* is an organism that can be mistaken for *T cruzi*. It is not known to be pathogenic in humans or other animals. Several species, including dogs, monkeys, opossums have and anteaters, are known to be hosts [3].

Leishmania are also trypanosomes. *Leishmania* species been reported in 88 countries; the total estimated at-risk population is 367 million [1]. *Leishmania* are intracellular flagellates that have complex life cycles, with stages in both vertebrate and nonvertebrate hosts [3]; they cause both cutaneous and visceral disease patterns. There are a number of disease-causing species, which are grouped into complexes. The various disease complexes have a variety of transmission patterns. Two complexes are found in the Americas: the *Leishmania braziliensis* complex, which causes cutaneous and mucocutaneous disease, and the *Leishmania mexicana* complex, which mainly causes cutaneous disease [4].

Members of the *Leishmania donovani* complex are found in both the New and the Old World. This complex includes *Leishmania infantum* and *Leishmania chagasi*. Dogs and humans are the major hosts for *L donovani* and related causes of kala-azar. Those organisms cause visceral leishmaniasis, or kala-azar. The disease is also known as *black disease* and *dumdum fever*. As many as 10 subclinical cases occur in adults for every case diagnosed in children. The infection may be latent and become activated when an individual is immunosuppressed [3].

Canine leishmaniasis is caused by *L infantum*. The dog is the source. It was common in Israel before 1948, but no cases in dogs have been reported since 1955. Despite the lack of cases in the source animals, cases have been reported in humans. Four human cases were reported in 1980 and 1982. Between January 1996 and November 1996, 30 human cases were reported [31]. In the Americas, this disease is common among poor, malnourished children who live in semiarid regions [32].

Leishmania tropica, *Leishmania major*, and *Leishmania aethiopica* cause Old World cutaneous leishmaniasis. Other names include *Oriental sore*, *Aleppo*, *Bhagdad boil*, and *chronic relapsing cutaneous leishmaniasis.* These protozoa have various distributions in the Middle East, Africa, and the Mediterranean region. The disease is limited to the skin, and the primary hosts are rodents. Sandflies, which are vectors, transmit the disease to humans accidentally. Occasionally, however, person-to-person transmission can occur. In the past, these infections were transmitted on purpose by scarification for cosmetic reasons among certain Middle Eastern cultures [3].

A form of leishmaniasis, referred to as *viscerotropic leishmaniasis*, was reported in troops returning from the Persian Gulf. It was caused by *L tropica*, which more commonly causes cutaneous manifestations. Travelers to the Middle East who have unexplained illnesses of several weeks' duration should be screened, especially if the illness is associated with fever, lymphadenophathy, or other signs of reticuloendothelial involvement [33].

American leishmaniasis is also known as *mucocutaneous leishmaniasis*, *espundia*, *uta*, and *chiclero ulcer*. It is caused by *Leishmania mexicana* and *Leishmania braziliensis* complexes. Both cause ulcers either on the skin or mucous membranes. *Lutzomyia* sandflies are the vectors. Rodents and marsupials are the primary hosts. These diseases are found throughout the Americas, from southern Texas to northern Argentina. The Caribbean is free of the disease, except for the Dominican Republic [3]. All cases acquired in the United States have been reported from Texas [34]. Brazil has noted an increase in the incidence of leishmaniasis (cutaneous and visceral) over the last few years. The disease is increasing, not only among populations in recently cleared forest areas but also in populations of urban poor [25].

Other Body-Site Amebas and Flagellates

Amebas include *Naegleria fowleri*, *Acanthamoeba* species, *Hartmanella* species, *Balamuthia mandrillaris*, and *Entamoeba* species. Flagellates include *Trichomonas vaginalis* and *Trichomonas tenax* [7]. *B mandrillaris* has been isolated in AIDs patients [35]. *Naegleria* and *Acanthamoeba* are free-living amebas, which may rarely accidentally infect humans. They are often called *amphizoic amebas* [36].

Naegleria has primarily been associated with primary amebic meningoencephalitis (PAM) [35,36]. Most reported cases of PAM have occurred in previously healthy children or young adults who swam in freshwater lakes during the hot summer months [35,37]. Some had inhaled dust or soil that contained amebic cysts [35]. *Naegleria* is ubiquitous worldwide. It multiplies well at temperatures of 40 to 45°C and probably encysts below that temperature [36].

Acanthamoeba has been reported to cause meningitis rarely but in association with outbreaks of keratitis among contact-lens wearers who prepared their own lens solutions [3,38]. *Acanthamoeba* and *Balamuthia* are more commonly associated with granulomatous amebic encephalopathy. *Acanthamoeba* is also widespread in nature. The ameba is ubiquitous: It has been found in cooling towers, air conditioner filters, oceans, ponds, sewage, lagoons, rivers, dust, eyewash stations, and pipelines. It may be part of normal nasal and oral flora. The distribution of *Balamuthia mandrillaris* is not known [36].

T tenax is not pathogenic. *T vaginalis* is a pathogen of the reproductive system. Although primarily spread by sexual contact, transmission through contamination of toilet facilities and other items is believed to occur [3]. There are approximately 128 million cases reported per year. The disease is worldwide and essentially the entire human population is at risk [1].

Other Body-Site Coccidia, Sporozoa, and Microsporidia

Toxoplasma gondii is a coccidian species that causes 1.4 million cases of toxoplasmosis occur each year, with 310 deaths [39]. It is worldwide in distribution, and the entire human population is considered to be at risk [1]. Antibodies to the organism have been found in up to 75% in some populations, indicating chronic but asymptomatic infections. Although *Toxoplasma* rarely produces significant pathology in adults, it poses a significant hazard to the fetuses of women first exposed during pregnancy [3]. Up to 9,500 cases of congenital toxoplasmosis may occur each year [8].

The definitive host for *T gondii* is the cat. Human infections have been traced to ingestion of raw meat, contact with feline feces, and drinking water contaminated with oocysts. *T gondii* is now the most common cause of space-occupying intracranial lesions in AIDS patients [40].

Microsporidia genuses include *Nosema*, *Pleistophora*, *Encephalitozoon*, and *Microsporidium* [7]. Microsporidia found outside the GI tract include *Encephalitozoon cuniculi*, *Nosema bombycis*, *Amblyospora*, and *Thelohania* [3]. A member of the genus *Nosema*, of uncertain species, has been isolated from the eye of a previously healthy man who developed keratitis and iritis following a trip to the Caribbean and Central America [23]. Cases of AIDS patients with ocular microsporidia infection have been reported [41]. A new species, *Trachipleistophora hominis*, has been identified in the muscle tissue, nasal sinus cavities, and conjunctiva of a patient with AIDS [42].

Pneumocystis carinii (which may be reclassified as a fungus) is considered by many to be a sporozoan. Its exact classification is not determined. It is widespread in humans, rodents, and dogs as well as in other domestic animals. It is primarily an opportunistic infection and is known primarily for the infections it causes in AIDS patients, although previous reports of cases in institutionalized children, patients taking immunosuppressive medications, and those with debilitating disease, such as malignancy, have been reported [3].

TRANSMISSION FACTORS

Transmission by the Fecal-Oral Route

Pathogenic protozoans can be grouped as intestinal or blood/tissue pathogens. Among the protozoa transmitted via the fecal-oral route, the most common in the United States is *Giardia lamblia*. Since the 1960s, several species have been identified as causing disease through this pathway. *Giardia* can be established either by the fecal-oral route or waterborne route with as few as one trophozoite or 10 cysts. In addition to *Giardia*, protozoa transmitted through the fecal-oral route include *Cryptosporidium*, *Microsporidia*, *Isospora*, and *Cyclospora* [15].

Hand-to-mouth contact can spread infection. Because hygienic practices are generally worse in children, they are more prone to infection [3]. Inadequate hygienic practices in day care centers have led to several outbreaks in those institutions [15]. Contact with the fecal matter of cats transmits *Toxoplasma gondii* [39]. Food can be contaminated by food handlers with poor hygiene practices [10].

Transmission by Contaminated Food and Water

The fecal-oral pathway can be indirect. *Cryptosporidium* and *Giardia* cysts and oocysts are widely distributed in the environment [43]. They are responsible for most of the parasitic infections in the United States. Recent studies indicate that cryptosporidian oocysts are present in 65–97% of all surface waters that have been tested [19]. Sixty-two percent of water treatment plants following current United States guidelines had finished water that was positive for *Cryptosporidium* or *Giardia* at various points in time. *Giardia* was more effectively removed than *Cryptosporidium* [43]. All of the waterborne outbreaks in the United States have occurred in communities where the water systems were in compliance with state and federal regulations. Small numbers of oocysts can be detected in the tap water of 27–54% of communities [19].

Untreated surface water is more likely to be contaminated than groundwater because the soil essentially serves as a filter. When wells have been found to be contaminated, their construction or location was poor or they had been damaged [22]. In the United States, *C parvum* and *G lamblia* are the parasites that most commonly cause infections [10,16].

Cryptosporidium was associated with the largest waterborne outbreak in United States history, which occurred in Milwaukee [44]. Over 400,000 people became ill [45]. The attack rate was estimated at 52% [16]. For the period between January 1993 through 1994, one third of all reported waterborne outbreaks were found to be caused by *Giardia* [45]. The standard methods of chlorination used by the water treatment industry do not kill Cryptosporidia [22]. Levels of cysts found during outbreaks ranged from 0.6/100 L to 21/100 L. During non-outbreak times, levels averaged at 0.19/100L and rarely were above 1/100 L [46].

The major source of contamination of food and water is contact with human and animal feces [10]. Cross-contamination between water and sewer lines has resulted in outbreaks [3]. The actual pathogen is not always identified [47]. Improper sewage pipe installation or maintenance can lead to outbreaks of enteric pathogens [48,49]. Wastewater is commonly used for irrigation and aquaculture in many countries. Raw waste water increases the risk of diarrheal disease in children younger than 15 years, and in individuals with *Entamoeba histolytica* infection, compared to partially treated water [12].

Both *Cryptosporidium* and *Giardia* have been associated with outbreaks related to recreational water [49], causing about 70% of such outbreaks. Current methods for disinfection of water in swimming pools appear to be inadequate to kill these pathogens. *Giardia* is more easily destroyed than *Cryptosporidium*, which may take up to several days to be inactivated by current methods [45].

Most recreational water systems use sand-filter media, which cannot remove very small *Cryptosporidium* oocysts. One diarrheal bowel movement can contain enough oocysts to contaminate 100 million gallons of water. A single mouthful can contain enough oocysts to cause illness [22]. *Naegleria* is found in swimming pools and artificial lakes. Warm water in the summer and at power plant outfalls, as well as poor chlorination of swimming pools, facilitates growth of this organism [35].

There are many opportunities for contamination of food. All the food-borne illnesses have an animal reservoir and are therefore food-borne zoonoses. Changes in the way food is produced and distributed have contributed to changing epidemic patterns. Instead of isolated, localized outbreaks, widespread distribution of foods contaminated with low levels of infectious organisms has led to diffuse and widespread outbreaks [50].

Protozoa pathogens are environmentally stable and resistant to methods that are effective for bacterial control in foods. Almost any food source can serve as a vehicle for transmission. The organisms are able to withstand a wide variety of food-storage and processing methods [10]. *Giardia*, *Entamoeba*, and *Cryptosporidium* have all been associated with contaminated food as well as water [11,51]. Food and water can be contaminated either by sewage or by food handlers with poor hygiene practices. *Cryptosporidia* oocysts do not survive cooking, but beverages, green salads, and other foods that are not cooked or heated after handling may be contaminated by an infected food handler [19]. *Cryptosporidium* has been reported in unpasteurized apple cider [39,52]. *Isospora* is also believed to be transmitted by food [3]. Ingestion of raw or poorly cooked meat can transmit toxoplasma [3,39]. *T gondii* has been found in almost all food animals and occasionally on unwashed fruits and vegetables [39]. Approximately 50% of toxoplasmosis is due to transmission of the organism by contaminated foods [40]. In 1996, several outbreaks of cyclosporiasis were traced to Guatemalan raspberries. Outbreaks occurred where raspberries or mixtures of raspberries and other fruit were served [10,21,50]. It is believed that the berries were sprayed with a fungicide mixed with contaminated surface water. The outbreaks were related, resulting from the wide distribution of the contaminated food. As the world develops a global food economy, more of these outbreaks are anticipated [22].

Transmission by Vectors

Flies can serve as vectors for blood or tissue infections. Sandflies of the *Phlebotomus* (Old World) or *Lutzomyia* (New World) genuses are the important vectors of visceral leishmaniasis. *Phlebotomus* flies transmit Old World cutaneous leishmaniasis. American leishmaniasis is transmitted by *Lutzomyia* sandflies [3].

Members of the genus *Trypanosoma* in Africa are transmitted by the tsetse flies of various species. This includes *T brucei gambiense* and *T brucei rhodesiense*, the most common causes of sleeping sickness. Riverine tsetse flies transmit Gambian trypanosomiasis. *G palpalis* and *G tachinoides* are concentrated in areas of high humidity [29]. Woodland tsetse flies transmit *T brucei rhodesiense* [3]. *Glossina morsitans*, a woodland species, carries *T brucei rhodesiense*. Under normal circumstances, males are more prone to infection as a result of occupational exposure. Under epidemic circumstances, the *G morsitans* has been found to invade homes, and *Euphorbia* and *Lantana* thickets near homes. In these outbreaks, women and children have been infected more often than adult males [29]. Trypanosomes that infect other African mammals are transmitted by horseflies. It is not clear whether some of these other protozoa may also cause human disease [3].

In the Americas, the primary vector for *L chagasi* (*Lutzomyia longipalpis*) lives in and around homes and bites humans at night, especially around twilight [32]. Bugs of the Reduviidae family (*Triatoma magista*), also known as *reduviid* or *triatomine* bugs, transmit Chagas' disease to humans. They inhabit roofs of mud houses and carry *T cruzi* in their feces, passing fecal material when they bite. Parasites enter through the skin wound [53].

Insects other than flies may act as vectors. The deer tick, *Ixodes dammini*, is the vector that transmits *Babesia* in New England. In South America, *T cruzi* is transmitted by several species of reduviid bugs that have become adapted to living and breeding in homes, particularly thatch huts in less affluent and rural areas [3,30,53].

Host Factors Relating to Transmissibility

Many factors influence susceptibility. These include diseases that cause immunosuppression, aging of the population, and malnutrition. The elderly, children, childbearing women, and patients with HIV or AIDS are at increased risk for zoonotic infection [54]. Immunosuppression is an important host factor. People who are immunosuppressed or have a serious underlying disease are much more likely to be infected with a pathogenic organism [40]. Genetic factors have also been implicated in some diseases. Rates of genetic immunodeficiencies are relatively stable, but worldwide acquired immunodeficiency is rising. Use of immunosuppressive drugs in organ transplantation and cancer chemotherapy is also increasing. Residence in a long-term care facility is a major independent risk factor for death due to diarrheal disease. Fecal incontinence is a risk factor for infections spread by the fecal-oral route. Malnutrition is common among the general population in much of the world and among certain groups in the United States [40]. In South America, malnutrition is a major risk factor for *Leishmania chagasi* infection [32].

Protozoa may infect multiple species. Where humans share or invade the habitats of the primary species, they are at risk. Nonhuman primates are infected with close relatives of human pathogens. As human beings interact more closely with other host species, the opportunity for pathogen exchange increases. For example, malaria is transmitted to humans from nonhuman primates and vice versa [55].

Mammals less closely related also share protozoan infections. *Glossina morsitans*, a woodland species that carries *T brucei rhodesiense*, also feeds on game animals [29]. Trypanosomes have been found in bushbuck, hartebeest, other antelope, cattle, lions, and hyena [53]. *T cruzi* affects domesticated animals such as dogs and cats. It does not require human hosts [30]. *Giardia* may also infect mammals such as dogs, cats, and beaver [15]. The dog is the source for leishmaniasis caused by *Leishmania infantum* and *L chagasi* [3,31,32]. *Cryptosporidium parvum* is found in numerous mammals [16,19]. In one study, 10% of puppies in an animal shelter were shedding *C parvum* oocysts. Approximately 50% of dairy calves shed the oocysts, and the organism can be found on 90% of dairy farms [19]. Recent genetic studies have identified two strains, one of which is spread from calves to humans and back to calves [56].

Transmission from Person to Person

C parvum is believed to be commonly spread person to person, especially among day care attendees and workers. Intimate play and diaper-changing habits are believed to contribute [19]. A recent study using polymerase-chain-reaction technology identified a strain of *C parvum* that appears to be exclusively transmitted human to human [56]. Transmission of *Trypanosoma cruzi* can occur through breast feeding and across the placenta [23]. *Trichomonas vaginalis* is sexually transmitted [3].

Transmission Facilitated by Travel and Population Movements

Travel has been recognized as an important force in disease transmission. More people travel than ever before, the speed of travel is greater, and more people are able to reach remote, previously isolated areas. As a result, many pathogenic protozoans have been introduced into new areas. Fortunately, most introductions do not lead to disease. Organisms that have animal hosts, environmental limitations, arthopod vectors, or complicated life cycles are generally not as successful in becoming established as those organisms without such limitations. Social, political, climatic, environmental, and technologic factors have combined to make the current era a time of great risk for spread of infectious diseases [57].

Humans may transport pathogens, including microbiologic flora or vectors, in or on the body. The migration or dislocation of individuals and populations can lead to dissemination of protozoal diseases into regions where they have not previously been found [57,58]. Population movements may be migrations for social or economic reasons or due to the upheavals of war [58]. Human migrations have been a major source of epidemics throughout history [57]. For example, the first case of kala-azar in Malaysia due to *Leishmania donovani* was reported in 1993. The affected individual was a migrant worker from Bangladesh [55].

Often, people migrate into crowded, substandard living conditions that favor the spread of disease [58]. These may be permanent slum areas surrounding urban centers or temporary dwellings, such as refugee camps. Conversely, humans may migrate into the habitats of vectors or hosts. An epidemic of visceral leishmaniasis occurred among people migrating to a food distribution center, because of contact with the sandfly vector [57]. In the United States, movement of people into reforested areas has led to greater contact with deer and deer ticks [58].

Shipping and transportation of goods have resulted in the inadvertent transport of vectors or organisms. Airplanes have carried infective mosquitoes outside malaria-endemic regions, and human disease has broken out [41,57]. Food production and industries that use or process products of biologic origin can spread infectious parasites [58].

Recreational and business travel can lead to infections, although this is not a major portion of human movement [57]. Cutaneous leishmaniasis lesions have been reported in visitors to endemic areas [59].

Some migrations stem from stresses associated with pathogenic protozoa. Outbreaks of African trypanosomiasis have led to large-scale migrations of humans out of areas that are otherwise highly suitable. As a result, large parts of the endemic area have been depopulated [29].

Nosocomial and Iatrogenic Transmission

Medical interventions can transmit or cause reactivation of latent disease. Microorganisms may also emerge as pathogenic as a result of changes in the susceptibility of the hosts to infection. Among the possible causes of susceptibility is increased use of immunosuppressive drugs [40]. Transplant of human organs is associated with a large number of deaths due to spread of infectious organisms, including parasitic disease [54]. Chagas' disease has been transmitted through allotransplantation. Renal transplantation has been associated with reactivation of latent, including microbiologic, flora or vectors [53]. If xenotransplantation (animal to human) becomes a useful technology, the potential for new zoonoses exists [54].

Transmission of American trypanosomiasis by infected blood can occur [53,60]. Hemophiliacs have been infected [53]. A recent study estimated that the risk of acquiring American trypanosomiasis through blood transfusion ranges from 2 per 10,000 in Ecuador to 219 per 10,000 for Bolivia. About 20–30% of those who receive a transfusion with *Trypanosoma*-infected blood will develop Chagas' disease [61]. Migration of infected persons into nonendemic areas can threaten the safety of the blood supply. Cases of transfusion-associated Chagas' disease have been reported from both the United States and Canada [30]. Babesiosis also can be transmitted by transfusion [18,27].

OCCUPATIONAL RISK FACTORS

Working with Infected Populations

Working with infected populations or individuals or in a population with a high endemic rate of infection, increases the risk to the worker. Health care workers are at risk for a variety of infectious diseases, including protozoan diseases. The risk for particular diseases is determined by the local prevalence of the disease as well as by the precautions taken by health care workers. Day care workers are at higher risk for certain protozoan diseases [61]. Several outbreaks of *Cryptosporidium* in day care centers have been reported [62], and the presence of this pathogen appears to be increasing in these settings [16]. Pneumocystis may be spread by droplets from infected hosts during coughing [3]. *C parvum* infections have been reported in day care centers, with outbreaks including the staff caring for children in diapers. Health care workers have been affected in bone marrow transplant units, pediatric hospitals, and patient wards where HIV-infected patients are cared for [16].

Working with Animals or Animal Products

At a veterinary school, a total of 12 cases of human cryptosporidiosis in animal handlers was identified. All were previously healthy and had no known deficiencies in their immune responses. Of the 12 individuals, 10 had symptoms and two had none. All cases had demonstrated cryptosporidial cysts in fecal material [63]. Facilities that process animal products may also pose a risk to workers [61]. Hunting, which may include tracking, capturing, handling, transporting, preparing or consuming meat, offers a number of opportunities for transmission of infectious parasites. Necropsy also poses high risk. Bites and scratches have transmitted pathogens to animal handlers. Urine may serve as a source of both antigen and antibody for infections such as malaria [64].

Working in Research

Research involving protozoa or their hosts poses risks of infection for research workers. In the United States, laboratory personnel working with *T cruzi* are more likely to acquire the infection than is the general population [3].

Working Outdoors

Working in an occupation or participating in an avocation that is primarily conducted out of doors permits the entry of humans into habitats of vectors. Agricultural, forestry, and related industries pose risks to workers. Agricultural occupations and hunting are risk factors for babesiosis [65]. Occupational zoonoses may present significant hazards for agricultural workers in developing countries, even when those diseases are controlled [61]. Hunting, gathering honey or fuel, fishing, and farming adjacent to *Glossinia morsitans* habitats are risks for infection with *T brucei rhodesiense*. Washing, water gathering, and water transportation are activities conducted in the habitats of the riverine tsetse fly, increasing the risk of acquiring *T brucei gambiense* [29].

Working in Occupations that Require Travel

Working in an occupation that requires travel to areas where these diseases are endemic and/or where sanitation is poor increases the risk of infection. As indicated above, travel is a major risk factor for coming in contact with new pathogens. Unsanitary conditions, poor food sanitation and food handler hygiene, encountering new vectors, and unreliably disinfected water systems put travelers at risk [57].

Working with Biologic Wastes

Working with human or animal wastes or in waters that are contaminated by such wastes has been reported in some studies [61]. Other studies, however, have not substantiated a higher rate of protozoal infection in sewage workers. A study of sewage treatment workers and PCB exposure identified a higher prevalence of diarrhea and nausea among employees who worked in the dewatering process than among other workers, but none of these workers were tested for parasites. The study was limited by using self-reported data. It was not clear whether this was a point or period prevalence and what the comparable prevalence of those symptoms would be in the general population [66]. Professional divers who dived in sewage-contaminated water developed diarrheal illness. In 12 patients, five had *Entamoeba histolytica*, and seven had *Giardia lamblia* [67]. A study conducted in 1984 among sewer workers did not identify an increase in parasitic diseases in sewer maintenance workers but did indicate higher rates of stools positive for enteric parasites among street cleaners. Organisms tested for included *Entamoeba coli*, *Endolimax nana*,

Isospora, and *Giardia*. The authors of this article considered *Entamoeba coli* as nonpathogenic. There was no mention of testing for *Cryptospo-ridium*, *Toxoplasma*, or other species that might reasonably be expected to be found in waste water effluence or dusts from streets [68]. In 1988, an outbreak of cryptosporidiosis was reported in Los Angeles County among swimmers who swam in a pool. An individual was known to have defecated into the pool. Because of their frequent contact with contaminated water, lifeguards and swimming teachers had a high rate of disease [69].

Prevention and Control

No protozoan diseases are targeted for worldwide elimination over the next several years [70]. For the foreseeable future, they will continue to present challenges to occupational and environmental health professionals as well as public health officials. Because of the different routes of exposure, different methods for control and prevention are needed. Many of these necessitate public health interventions.

ADMINISTRATIVE CONTROLS

Maintenance of an adequate public health system is the most important administrative control for the prevention of protozoan diseases. These diseases must be controlled at the population level and they require active surveillance [58]. For example, trypanosomiasis rapidly reemerged in a country where surveillance was discontinued [29]. Effective control may require surveillance and characterization of the pathogen in wild-animal populations, which act as hosts [64].

Workers at higher risk can be reassigned to areas of lower risk. If acceptable or desired by the worker, pregnant women who work with cats can be reassigned during their pregnancies. Immunosuppressed individuals can avoid working with children in diapers. Recreational water facilities can require showering before entry into pools, exclude persons with diarrhea or incontinence, and restrict children that wear diapers or in the toilet training stage to certain pools [22].

Until their recovery, employees with diarrheal illness should not be allowed to work with nursing home residents or day care attendees or in dental offices, hospitals, clinics, or renal dialysis units. Children with diarrhea should be excluded from day care [22].

If travelers must enter endemic areas, they should avoid streams and waterholes during the warm season [22]. Travel during nighttime hours to areas of endemic sleeping sickness can prevent exposure to the tsetse fly vector that transmits Gambian trypanosomiasis [3].

SAFE WORK PRACTICES AND ENGINEERING CONTROLS

Appropriate work practices depend on the activities undertaken. Generally, these practices involve hygiene, to decrease contact with infectious organisms, and methods to decrease vector populations or the potential for contact with them.

General Hygienic Measures

Frequent hand washing is helpful in preventing a number of potential infectious diseases. Hands should always be washed thoroughly after any contact with animals or soil, after changing diapers, and before preparing or eating food.

Keeping pets or working with animals increases the risk of acquiring parasitic diseases. Immunosuppressed persons should avoid contact with fecal material of animals to prevent cryptosporidiosis. The risk is greatest for animals less than 6 months of age [19,22]. Pregnant women should not have cats. If cats are kept, they should be kept in homes where there are no rodents. Cats should be fed dry or canned cat food that is cooked. Litter boxes should be emptied daily by persons who are not pregnant. Children's sandboxes should be covered [3].

Day care facilities should require frequent hand washing by staff and clear separation of diapering and food handling areas and responsibilities. Overclothes and diapers should be of high enough quality to contain liquid fecal material. Diaper areas should be disinfected frequently and covered with disposable paper, and disposable gloves should be used when changing diapers. The diaper-changing area should be separated from the play and eating areas. During an outbreak, toys should be disinfected frequently, at least twice daily. Disinfection for *Cryptosporidium* can be accomplished with 3% hydrogen peroxide [22].

Measures to Prevent Food-Borne Parasitic Illness

In developing countries, food is often unsafe and travelers should take a few simple precautions. Raw fruits and vegetables, unpasterized milk or dairy products, and foods purchased from street vendors are often contaminated. Steaming hot foods and fruits that the traveler peels are usually safe [22]. In any country, travelers should avoid the ingestion of raw meat; meat should be cooked thoroughly. Hands should be washed with soap and water after handling meats, and fresh fruit should be washed before eating [71]. Commercial dishwashers should have a dry cycle that exceeds 113°F for 20 minutes, 122° F for five minutes, or 162°F or one minute [22].

Animal manure should not be used to fertilize orchards. Apples that have fallen to the ground should not be used for making unpasteurized products, such as cider. Fruits should be washed and brushed before they are pressed. Cider should be preserved with sodium benzoate and should be routinely pasteurized [52].

Measures to Prevent Waterborne Parasitic Infections

Effective environmental sanitation is the key to preventing infections with amebas and intestinal flagellates. Sanitary methods of sewage disposal are necessary. Cattle should not be permitted to enter watershed areas of major cities [54]. Water supplies must be safeguarded, because chlorination does not kill all amebas. Boiling water is effective, or water can be treated with iodine tablets to obtain an iodine level of 6 to 7 ppm at a pH below 7.5. Microfiltration can also be used to remove amebic cysts from the water [3,25].

Water that has been purified by boiling for one minute, has been distilled, or has been treated with special filters is safe from *Cryptosporidium*. Water filters labeled "reverse osmosis" will remove the oocysts. Filters that are labeled "absolute 1 micron" or "Standard 53" and "cyst reduction" or "cyst removal" have met the NSF criteria for removal of *Cryptosporidium* oocysts. Some, but not all, bottled waters are safe: Careful inquiries into the sources and processes of purification is required. Labels do not usually provide that information [19,22]. Ozonation is currently not effective, nor is charcoal filtration or ultraviolet light exposure. Filters that are advertised to remove *Giardia* will not necessarily remove cryptosporidia oocysts [19].

Chlorination does not kill *Giardia* cysts. Filtration or use of deep sources is necessary [15]. Potable-water systems should use different piping from sewage or sewage-effluent systems. Plumbing diagrams should be maintained, and experienced maintenance personnel should repair systems [48]. Outdoor water sources need to be protected from fecal material. People should not drink from hoses, because they are prone to back siphoning [72].

Water sources in other countries may be less reliable than those in the United States. Drinks, tap water, and ice may be contaminated, as may raw fruits and vegetables. Bottled and canned processed drinks, hot coffee, and hot tea are generally safe [22].

Water should not be consumed directly from lakes, rivers, ponds, or streams [22]. Contact lenses should not be used during swimming or engaging in water sports [47]. Immunosuppressed persons should not swim in natural bodies of water, public swimming pools, or recreational water parks [22]. Swimming pools, whirlpools, and hot tubs should be properly chlorinated to eliminate *Naegleria*. Levels of 1 mg/L of chlorine below 26°C, and 2 mg/L for temperatures between 26° and 28°C, and 3 mg/L for temperatures over 28°C are recommended for contamination control [36].

Vector Control

Vector control has proved effective in reducing vector-borne illnesses. Clearing of habitats and judicious use of pesticides can control the riverine and woodland species of tsetse flies. Avoiding unsanitary homes and control of triatomid bugs in the home can control American trypanosomiasis [3]. Tsetse flies have been controlled using glue-covered backpacks on plantation workers, and selective clearing of their habitats has reduced their population. *Glossina* have not shown any insecticide resistance. The residual organochlorine insecticides (DDT, dieldrin) have been used to reduce the fly population. Aerial or ground applications may be used but are not very effective in humid habits or where thickets are dense. Long-acting insecticides are used because the pupa can live longer than short-acting insecticides during colder parts of the year. Multiple applications of insecticides may be used in certain circumstances. Traps impregnated with pesticides have also been used and proved effective in reducing vector populations [29]. Fine mesh screens, treatment of screens with pesticides, and repellents can reduce exposures. Destruction of breeding grounds for sandflies can help reduce sources of infection for visceral leishmaniasis [3].

Immunosuppressed persons may need to conduct periodic inspections of hot-water tanks, air filters, plumbing systems, and in-line filters. Eyewash stations may also help avoid transmission [36].

Prevention of Iatrogenic and Nosocomial Transmission

Screening of blood for transmissible protozoa can reduce transmission of these parasites [3]. Screening of transplant donors and recipients may be necessary to prevent transmission or reactivation of latent infections [30].

Personal Protective Equipment. Workers' use of personal protective equipment (PPE) may help prevent protozoan infections. Disposable gloves should be used to change diapers or handle animal wastes [19]. Netting, head nets, leggings or long pants, and gloves can help prevent the bites of day-biting flies, although care must be taken not to increase the risk of dehydration and heat-related illnesses. Insect repellent is also useful to prevent fly bites [3,5,12].

Employee Education and Training. GENERAL MEASURES. Workers who may come in contact with protozoan diseases should be instructed about them and taught specific methods to reduce the risk of acquiring them. Because some diseases are fatal if not treated early, workers who may be required to enter areas of risk should be informed about signs and symptoms and about how to access medical treatment. Education is especially important for business travelers who must enter areas where public health and medical services are insufficient.

MEASURES TO PREVENT FOOD-BORNE AND WATERBORNE PROTOZOAN DISEASES. Food service workers need education and instruction about food safety techniques. Travelers to areas where food is not safe should be instructed to choose foods that reduce the risk of acquiring a food-borne parasite. Instruction should also be given for use of potable water and selection of safe beverages. In some instances, instruction in water decontamination procedures may be appropriate.

MEASURES TO PREVENT VECTOR-BORNE PROTOZOAN DISEASE. Employees need instruction on how to avoid insects when working in areas where vector-borne diseases are endemic, including not only the use of PPE such as netting and appropriate clothing, but also insect behavior and habitats.

Medical Surveillance. For most of these diseases, medical surveillance of individual workers is not indicated. Surveillance by public health agencies is useful, however, for following trends and identifying and responding to outbreaks. For example, serologic screening is useful in surveillance for mid-African sleeping sickness, but infected individuals are not helped by early identification of their disease. Routine testing of stool specimens is unlikely to identify asymptomatic carriers of *E histolytica* [3].

Immunization and Prophylaxis. PREEXPOSURE AND POSTEXPOSURE MEASURES. Currently, there are no vaccines available for preventing infection with protozoan diseases [3,73]. Attempts to develop a vaccine against cutaneous leishmaniasis have been attempted but, to date, have been ineffective [3].

Chemoprophylaxis for mid-African sleeping sickness has been attempted: Pentamidine injections were given at four- to six-month intervals. However, the practice appears to result in the development of drug-resistant strains of parasites and may mask early CNS symptoms. Prophylaxis should not be used for control of this disease under most circumstances but may be considered in certain individual cases of high exposure [3,29]. Currently, prophylaxis is recommended only for those who must work in the habitats of the vectors. Among these high-risk groups are tin miners and construction (road and rail) workers [29].

Prophylaxis is most useful for immunosuppressed individuals. Prophylaxis for pneumocystis pneumonia has been successful with trimethoprim and sulfamethozarzole 5 and 25 mg/kg/day, respectively, in two equal doses every 12 hours. This regimen has been continued up to two years. In addition, aerosolized pentamidine has been found effective in AIDS patients [3]. Enteric cyclosporidiosis in AIDS patients is treated with trimoxazole to prevent relapse [8].

COMPLIANCE. Consistent compliance with most of the preventive measures is difficult to obtain. Sanitation techniques can be a problem, particularly if cultural practices do not reinforce the need for cleanliness. Use of personal protective equipment may be bothersome and may exacerbate other risks, such as heat.

Metrics To Assess Adequacy of Preventive Measures. Standard methods for evaluating water quality include techniques that detect the presence of *E coli* and those that measure turbidity. Turbidity is water's cloudiness due to suspended particles in it is measured in nephelometric turbidity units (NTUs) [22]. Currently, purified material is examined by antibody-based immunofluorescence assay. After staining, the sample is examined by microscope with an ultraviolet light source. Fluorescence indicates a tentative identification. Positive identification is made by light microscope identification of sporozoites [22]. Monitoring is necessary to ensure that levels of environmental parasites are sufficiently low in public water sources. Large volumes of food and water samples are needed because of problems with identification [10].

The CDC recommends that all communities whose water utilities serve more than 100,000 should consider performing surveillance for oocysts. Smaller communities should also consider surveillance if they use unfiltered surface water or if water quality indices suggest filters are not adequately removing the oocysts. Recent evidence indicates that *Cryptosporidium* is removed best when the turbidity of water is consistently at 0.1 NTU or lower [22].

A new method is the polymerase chair reaction (PCR), which may help detect *Cryptosporidium* in water supplies and asymptomatic carriers [16]. Currently available methods for identifying oocysts from environmental media are not very sensitive [16,74]. Recovery efficiency is 5–20%, and the method is time and labor intensive. At least 1,000 liters of water must be filtered and concentrated. PCR technology, however, does appear promising as a measurement technology [74].

If outbreaks of diarrheal disease are suspected, a small case-control investigation, using between 10 and 20 cases and a similar number of controls, can determine if there is a predominate species [22]. It has been suggested that changes in the rates of over-the-counter diarrheal medications could be used to identify outbreaks of diarrheal disease [22].

Monitoring for food- and vector-borne diseases may be somewhat more difficult [75]. Rates of seropositivity can be used for a number of organisms, such as *T brucei gambiense.*

Symptoms and Signs

Parasitic diseases have a number of presentations. Many of them are self-limited; others may have severe acute and chronic effects. Chronic sequelae can occur in up to 2–3% of food-borne cases. About 80% of immunosuppressed patients with diarrheal disease die of the disease or its complications [8].

INTESTINAL AMEBAS

The clinical symptoms of amebic infections depend on the location and severity of the infection. The picture can be altered further by superimposed bacterial infections. Acute intestinal disease is a severe diarrhea characterized by numerous stools that contain blood, mucous, and intestinal lining. Abdominal pain, tenderness, and fever as high as 39°C may also occur. Patients may be dehydrated and toxic, with leukocytosis as high as 20,000/mm^3 and eosinophilia. Subclinical chronic lesions have persisted for years or have been associated with irritable bowel or colitis. Symptoms may be mild; vague abdominal pain, malaise, constipation, and mild diarrhea have been reported. Asymptomatic infections may also occur [3].

Most infections with *E histolytica* are intestinal. The infected individual may present either with acute or chronic dysentery. Appendicitis, intestinal perforation, hemorrhage, stricture, granulomas, and pseudopolyposis may occur. *E histolytica* may become systemic, most often causing multiple liver abscesses. Amebic abscesses have been found in the lung, pericardium, brain, spleen, genitalia, and skin [3].

Blastocystis is commonly found in stools of healthy people. It is not clearly a pathogen [3,12].

INTESTINAL FLAGELLATES

Giardiasis may be asymptomatic or may cause either acute or chronic intestinal symptoms. Acute symptoms are the most easily recognized and include diarrhea, abdominal pain, nausea, and weight loss. Some or all of these symptoms occur in 50–70% of individuals who are infected. Chronic infection can cause chronic diarrhea and steatorrhea, with malabsorption and weight loss [15]. Severe hypothyroidism can result from chronic infection. Elimination of the parasite results in return to normal thyroid function [8]. Diarrhea caused by *Giardia* does not contain blood or cause an increase in polymorphonuclear leukocytes, as would be expected in patients with other dysenteries [3]. The incubation period is between three to 25 days, with a median of seven days [76].

Intestinal Ciliates

Balantidium coli may be asymptomatic or may present as severe dysentery. Nausea, vomiting, and headache may occur and there may also be muscle weakness, insomnia, and weight loss. The symptoms may persist for weeks or months [5].

Intestinal Coccidia and Microsporidia

Isospora may be asymptomatic or may be associated with diarrhea. *Sarcocystis* might present with muscle pain, although this has not yet been described. Enteritis is the most common presenting picture for microsporidia, although both myositis and hepatitis have been reported [3].

Most patients with cryptosporidia present with diarrhea, with or without crampy abdominal pain. Low-grade fever, weakness, malaise and anorexia, moderate to severe nausea, and vomiting can occur in some individuals. About 10% of AIDS patients have infections of the hepatobiliary system. A small proportion of severely immunosuppressed individuals have respiratory symptoms [18]. *Cryptosporidium* has an incubation period of two to 28 days, with a median of seven days, while *Cyclospora cayetanensis* has an incubation period of one to 11 days, with a median of seven days [75]. Symptoms may remit and relapse [76], and may persist for up to two months [22]. In the immunosuppressed, the disease is chronic [8].

Blood or Tissue Sporozoa (Flagellates)

Like malaria, babesiosis is a hemolytic anemia. It presents with fever, weakness, jaundice, and hepatosplenomegaly. Up to 25% of red blood cells can be infected in patients with intact spleens, and even more in those without spleens [3]. Most infections are probably subclinical. Most infections have occurred in older individuals, asplenic persons, and those with underlying diseases. Cough and pulmonary edema can occur but are rare. Fulminant disease can lead to shock, multi-organ system failure- and adult respiratory distress syndrome [18].

Blood or Tissue Flagellates

Both forms of African trypanosomiasis cause a meningoencephalitis [54]. Gambian trypanosomiasis, also known as *mid-African sleeping sickness*, may be mild or may progress to chronic central nervous system disease [3,53]. A nodule or chancre may appear at the site of the bite five to 15 days after infection [54]. The acute phase presents as an irregular fever, headache, joint and muscle pains, and a rash. The patient may be hyperactive [3]. Insomnia, amenorrhea, infertility, impotence, pruritus, and edema may also occur [29]. The chronic symptoms include pronounced fever and headache, lethargy and disinclination to work, avoidance of others, melancholia alternating with mania, mental slowing, tremors or choreiform movements, gait abnormalities, and altered reflexes. These symptoms occur over a period of approximately one year and are followed by a terminal sleeping phase, in which the individual becomes more and more difficult to awaken [3]. Lung edema predisposes patients to secondary infections, which are often the proximal cause of death [29].

Rhodesian trypanosomiasis is more rapid and fatal, often causing death within a year of infection [3]. In individuals of European descent, this form may progress to death within two weeks of infection, instead of several months for the more typical form [29,53]. Personality and behavior changes may be the initial signs, followed by indifference, lassitude, and daytime somnolence. Extrapyramidal signs, particularly a slow gait and masked expression, may mimic Parkinson's disease [53].

Acute Chagas' disease may be subclinical, especially in children. It is undiagnosed in about 66–99% of infected persons. When it is symptomatic, fever and generalized adenopathy occur. If the upper face or eye is the portal of entry, a unilateral orbital edema and conjunctivitis known as *Romaña's sign* may occur. Some persons develop severe, acute encephalitis and myocarditis. A mild meningoencephalitis occurs, as does a severe meningoencephalitis that is accompanied by convulsions, contractures, and paralysis. The acute myocarditis or meningoencephalitis may be fatal. Immunocompromised persons may have severe acute neurologic syndromes that include both memingoencephalitis and mass lesions. This may represent reactivation of a latent infection and has been noted in persons with leukemia, lymphomas, Hodgkin's disease, renal transplants, and AIDS [3,53].

During the intermediate phase, hosts remain infected. Neurologic signs are absent. In 20–40% of these individuals, this phase progresses to chronic or late progressive disease. Cardiac and gastrointestinal complications may be delayed, leading to conduction disturbances, arrhythmia, sudden death, cardiac enlargement, heart failure, and thrombus formation causing embolization. Megaesophagus or megacolon can occur, due to infection of the autonomic nervous system. The age of onset is variable [3,53].

Maternal Chagas' disease may lead to miscarriage, prematurity, or babies who are small for their gestational age. The risk of maternal-fetal transmission is 2–10%. Congenital Chagas' disease presents with pancarditis, encephalitis, and gastrointestinal inflammation [53].

In visceral leishmaniasis, primary lesions are uncommon. Minute papules have been seen in infants, and dermal lesions of legs have been reported in Africa. The onset of the disease is insidious; fever is accompanied by sweating, weakness, and slow weight loss. A nonproductive cough and abdominal discomfort may be present and may continue for months. The disease may progress more rapidly in patients with high fever and chills. Fever, splenomegaly, and cachexia may be noted, most prominently in the thorax and shoulder area. Generalized adenopathy has been noted but is not usually prominent. Hyperpigmentation may occur, giving rise to the term *kala-azar* ("black disease" in Hindi). Leukopenia develops in patients with monocytosis and lymphocytosis, anemia, and thrombocytopenia. Red blood cells have a reduced life span, and erythropoiesis is affected. These effects, along with general debility, cause a susceptibility to secondary infection. Untreated, the disease is usually fatal within a year. Rapidly progressive infections have resulted in death within a few weeks. Chronic infections have been known to persist for years [3–5].

In rare cases, skin lesions containing large numbers of organisms develop months or years after recovery, causing post-kala-azar dermal leishmaniasis. This syndrome does not have systemic signs and responds well to treatment [3].

Viscerotropic leishmaniasis has been reported to include an acute syndrome with chills and malaise, mild hepatosplenomegaly, generalized lymphadenopathy, and gastrointestinal symptoms (nausea, watery diarrhea, and abdominal pain). No patients with viscerotropic leishmaniasis have had the marked hepatosplenomegaly, pancytopenia, hypergammaglobulinemia, and cachexia more typical of kala-azar [33].

Cutaneous leishmaniasis appears as a reddish and itchy papule that gradually enlarges and forms an ulcer. Wet types have a seropurulent exudate; dry types form a crusted scab. Systemic signs, which often include regional adenopathy, are absent. Lesions are not painful. Metastatic lesions may form [3].

American leishmaniasis is similar in appearance, except that the mucous membrane may be involved. Chiclero ulcer erodes the pinna of the ear in chicle workers. Lesions may metastasize. Mucous membrane involvement usually follows skin involvement, and may begin with nasal obstruction and bleeding. Pain and deformity can result, with erosion of the nasal septum, palate, or larynx. Leishmaniasis with mucosal features is called *espundia*. A diffuse type, characterized by multiple nodular lesions resembling lepromatous leprosy, may occur as a result of failure of the immune response [3].

Other Body-Site Amebas and Flagellates

After an incubation period of two to seven days, primary amebic meningoencephalitis (PAM) presents abruptly and is rapidly progressive. Headache, fever, pharyngitis, or nasal obstruction and discharge occur initially. Occasionally, the senses of smell and taste are distorted. Headache, vomiting, and fever may persist and be followed by drowsiness, confusion, and stiff neck. The patient may have convulsions. Deterioration to deep coma, without focal signs, occurs rapidly. Death usually occurs within one to two weeks after the onset of the first symptoms [53].

Acanthamoeba causes granulomatous amebic encephalitis (GAE) and develops mostly in chronically ill, debilitated, or immunosuppressed patients. Its onset is insidious. Mental abnormalities and meningeal signs are present. Localizing neurologic signs also occur. These are followed by coma and death. Some patients have ulcerative or nodular skin lesions [53].

Acanthamoeba keratitis causes severe ocular pain, photophobia, blurred vision, and conjunctivitis. The symptoms may wax and wane. If untreated, the keratitis progresses to corneal perforation, scarring and vascularization of the cornea, and sometimes even loss of the eye [36].

Other Body-Site Coccidia, Sporozoa, and Microsporidia

Toxoplasmosis is usually asymptomatic in adults but may have severe symptoms if the infection is acquired prenatally, when it can be fatal. Impairments are present in 80% of prenatally infected persons who reach 20 years of age [8]. Toxoplasmosis may also occur as an opportunistic infection in immunosuppressed adults, in whom it affects the central nervous system (CNS), apparently because of reactivation of latent infection. CNS symptoms may include headache, fever, lethargy, and altered mental status, with progression to focal neurologic deficits or convulsions [3,8]. Toxoplasmosis is the most commonly recognized cause of CNS infection in AIDS patients. Chronic toxoplasmosis has been associated with several personality disorders, which appear to result from the infection rather than being pre-existing. Cancer treatments can cause latent muscle infections to become reactivated, sometimes leading to death [8].

Microsporidial infections may be subclinical or latent. When lesions are found, they are granulomatous and may be widespread. Common sites are the intestine, brain, kidney, liver, muscle, ganglia, and small muscular arteries [24].

Pnemocystitis presents as pneumonitis. It occurs primarily in immunosuppressed individuals [3].

Differential Diagnosis

INTESTINAL AMEBAS

Amebic abscess causes clinical signs and symptoms consistent with its locations. If the abscess is in the liver, liver function tests may be normal or slightly elevated. Occasionally, the patient is mildly jaundiced. Other causes of liver abnormalities need to be excluded. These include viral hepatitis, bacterial abscesses, hydatid cyst, gallbladder infection, and cancers. If the lung is affected, the patient presents with chest pain and cough. Amebic abscess of the brain causes the clinical picture of a brain mass and thus must be differentiated from other space-occupying brain lesions, such as tumors [3].

INTESTINAL FLAGELLATES

Syndromes of acute onset of diarrhea must be differentiated from bacterial and viral causes that cause dysentery or diarrhea. Among possible nonprotozoan causes are *Salmonella*, *Shigella*, *Campylobacter*, *E coli*, and Norwalk virus [3].

INTESTINAL CILIATES

Syndromes of acute onset of diarrhea must be differentiated from bacterial and viral causes that cause dysentery or diarrhea. Among possible nonprotozoan causes are *Salmonella*, *Shigella*, *Campylobacter*, *E coli*, and Norwalk virus [3].

INTESTINAL COCCIDIA AND MICROSPORIDIA

Syndromes of acute onset of diarrhea must be differentiated from bacterial and viral causes that cause dysentery or diarrhea. Among possible nonprotozoan causes are *Salmonella*, *Shigella*, *Campylobacter*, *E coli*, and Norwalk virus [3].

BLOOD OR TISSUE SPOROZOA (FLAGELLATES)

Babesiosis should be considered in patients with hemolytic anemia who are from areas where *Babesia microti* is endemic [3].

BLOOD OR TISSUE FLAGELLATES

The differential diagnosis for trypanosomiasis includes syphilis, leishmaniasis, and malaria. Visceral leishmaniasis may have a clinical presentation much like that of malaria, typhoid fever, schistosomiasis, or lymphoproliferative disorders [4]. Clinical appearance of cutaneous leishmaniasis must be differentiated from nonspecific or bacterial tropic ulcers, sporotrichosis, atypical mycobacteriosis, yaws, South American blastomycosis, and syphilis [3].

OTHER BODY-SITE AMEBAS AND FLAGELLATES

The clinical picture of primary amebic meningoencephalitis (PAM) cannot be distinguished from acute bacterial meningitis. Granulomatous amebic encephalitis (GAE) must be differentiated from acute and chronic bacterial meningitis, TB, fungal or viral encephalitis, brain abscess, brain tumor, and other space-occupying lesions [36,54]. *Acanthamoeba* keratitis must be differentiated from herpesvirus, bacteria, and fungal eye infections [36].

OTHER BODY-SITE COCCIDIA, SPOROZOA, AND MICROSPORIDIA

Central nervous system toxoplasmosis must be differentiated from other causes of encephalopathy. Retinochoroiditis and uveitis can be caused by *Toxoplasma* but must be differentiated from other causes. *Pneumocystis* must be differentiated from other bacterial, viral, and toxic causes of pneumonitis [3].

Diagnostic Evaluation

HISTORY

Diagnostic evaluation should include a thorough occupational and environmental history. Depending on the circumstances, a history of travel, working with animals, working outdoors, known occupational exposures to infectious agents, or working with children in diapers might be important. Ingestion of raw or poorly cooked meats suggests exposure to *T gondii*. A history of close contact with cat or cat feces or having a sandbox in the yard can also indicate a likely exposure to *T gondii*. Living conditions such as residence in a thatched hut, residence in a house with an inadequate sewer system, and eating unusual foods may be pertinent. A history of travel to endemic areas of Africa can indicate risk for trypanosomiasis, especially if insect bites were noted. A history of visiting or residing in underdeveloped areas of South America can lead to a diagnosis of American trypanosomiasis [3]. In previously healthy children or young adults who have meningeal signs, it is important to obtain a history of water-related activities and exposures to dust, which might be associated with exposure to free-living amebas [53].

PHYSICAL EXAMINATION

The physical examination may yield several clues to the diagnosis of parasitic protozoan disease. However, most of these organisms cause enteritis and do not have specific findings. Hepatomegaly is seen in kala-azar [3–5].

IMAGING TECHNIQUES

Imaging techniques are useful in only a few cases of parasitic protozoan infections. CT and MRI scans may demonstrate single or multiple lesions in the basal ganglia or junctions of gray and white matter consistent with *Toxoplasma* infections [3]. During an outbreak, the possibility of *Pneumocystis* may be suggested by radiographic findings consistent with interstitial pneumonia. CT scans may show diffuse cerebral edema in cases of primary amebic meningoencephalitis. CT and magnetic resonance imaging (MRI) usually are not helpful in identifying granulomatous amebic encephalopathy, although focal lesions have occasionally been seen [36].

LABORATORY TESTS

Laboratory procedures are usually required to confirm the diagnosis of protozoan disease. Several procedures may need to be undertaken. Because these organisms frequently cannot be identified through routine laboratory testing, special care in collecting and processing samples is imperative.

Microscopic Stool Analysis

The laboratory examination for some protozoa is difficult. However, stool examination is crucial. In 1987, protozoan parasites were found in 20% of stools examined in state laboratories; *Giardia* comprised 7% [77]. Several outbreaks have been reported, which upon investigation were determined not to be true outbreaks. These pseudo-outbreaks have been due in part to increased surveillance for these diseases and in part to lack of experience in identifying these organisms. Samples in which emerging pathogens have been identified should be confirmed in a reference laboratory and with clinical confirmation before beginning treatment [78]. The organisms can be confused with commensal organisms, macrophages, or other cells and artifacts [3]. For example, *E histolytica* may be confused with other intestinal protozoa but is commonly confused with macrophages and leukocytes [79].

For enteritides, microscopic analysis of feces or tissues may be necessary to identify the causal organism. Microscopic techniques are the mainstay for identifying parasitic organisms. The development of new concentrating and staining techniques has aided the identification of many parasites [11]. Such techniques are necessary because the protozoa are usually present in low concentrations. Recovery is generally poor and is affected by water quality and the presence of particulate matter [10].

Fresh specimens are needed because trophozoites are fragile and do not survive environmental stresses. Often, repeated examinations are necessary, since the trophozoites and cysts may be difficult to find and identify [3]. Careful specimen collection, handling, and storage techniques are needed to maximize the likelihood of identifying the trophozoites or spores. Fresh bulk stools have to be mixed at a ratio of one part stool to three parts preservative. Two preservatives, 10% formalin and polyvinyl alcohol (PVA), must be used to preserve the morphology of the trophozoites and cysts. Stool specimens not yet preserved need to be refrigerated at 4°C. Freezing destroys the organisms and renders samples unusable [11]. Once stool has been preserved, its consistency cannot be determined; therefore, it is important to describe the original consistency of the stool, as this determines the success of identification in certain diseases [22]. Careful instructions from the laboratory about proper collection of samples is important.

E histolytica can be identified as trophozoites in liquid stools of patients with acute infection. It may also be identified from aspirated material and as cysts in formed stools of chronic patients and carriers. Trophozoites are active in warm, fresh stools and move by pseudopods. They have indistinct nuclei and often contain partially digested red blood cells. Cysts may contain between one and four nuclei, large chromatoidal bodies and diffuse glycogen mass. It is unusual to find cysts in persons passing fewer than 100,000 cysts per day [3].

Dientamoeba fragilis is a trophozoite with two nuclei. It resembles *Trichomonas* and can be found only in fresh stools that are either soft or liquid. While it appears circular at rest, in motion it is stellate, due to multiple, leaf-shaped pseudopods. *Endolimax nana* is also small but moves sluggishly, has a unique-looking nucleus microscopically, and forms cysts that contain four nuclei [3].

Giardiasis is diagnosed by identifying its cysts in formed stools or its trophozoites and cysts in diarrheal stools. In saline, *Giardia* has a distinct morphology, unlike other intestinal protozoa. It is a bilaterally symmetric, pear-shaped organism with a rounded anterior and a tapering posterior. A concave sucking disk covers about 75% of the ventral surface [3].

Cryptosporidium is identified by identification of its oocysts in stools, using a modified acid-fast stain. *Isospora* oocysts can be found in stools; most of the oocysts are not sporulated [3,18]. Specimens for identifying *Cryptosporidium* with acid-fast stains should not be preserved with polyvinyl alcohol [22]. *Cyclospora* oocysts can be identified in stool by examination of wet mounts and phase microscopy and modified acid-fast stains or by demonstrating autofluorescence with ultraviolet epifluorescense microscopy [21]. *Blastocystis* can be found in the stools. Autofluorescence of oocysts can be detected with a 330–380 nm UV filter. This mechanism enhances identification of the organism on wet mounts and stained slides [80].

Microscopic Tissue Examination

Some intestinal pathogenic protozoa are hard to recover from stool but may be found in tissues. Tissue examination is imperative for the identification of blood and tissue protozoan infections. Blood specimens need to be refrigerated at 4°C [11].

Cryptosporidium oocysts can be seen in small intestinal biopsies, respiratory tissue biopsies, or respiratory secretions by using the modified acid-fast stain [18]. Microsporidia are difficult to identify on hematoxylin and eosin (H&E) stained tissue sections. *Encephalitozoon* is gram positive, and some are acid-fast, but other microsporidia cannot be identified with these stains [24]. Although they can be identified with the H&E stain and paraffin section, the organisms are most easily identified by Giemsa stain of resin sections [81,82].

The trypanosomes that cause the African sleeping sicknesses can be identified in blood, lymph nodes, and bone marrow early in the disease course. In central nervous system disease, they can be identified in the cerebrospinal fluid. A drop of anticoagulated blood may reveal the organisms. They will be concentrated in the buffy coat of centrifuged blood. Rhodesian trypanosomiasis is easier to detect than Gambian [3].

Visceral *Leishmania* can be found in stained blood smears. Tissue scrapings or biopsies of cutaneous lesions may also reveal the *Leishmania* organism [3]. *Babesia* can readily be seen on Giemsa- or Wright-stained blood smears and appear similar to *Plasmodium falciparum* [18].

A fresh sample of anticoagulated blood, the buffy coat of centrifuged blood, or stained thick smears can reveal the presence of *T cruzi* within one or two months of the acute disease. In red blood cells, the appearance of *Babesia* is similar to that of malarial parasites, forming small rings with a darkly stained nucleus and little cytoplasm. However, little associated pigment in the red blood cells is noted [3].

Pathologic examination of tissue obtained by open lung biopsies can identify the *Pneumocystis* organism. In many cases, it may also be identified in fluid obtained by bronchoalveolar lavage. Therefore, bronchoscopy is indicated for evaluation. Brush biopsy and needle biopsy have been used with varying levels of success. Sections must be stained with toluidine blue or methenamine-silver to reveal the thick-walled cysts [3].

Cerebrospinal fluid should be examined in cases of suspected PAM or GAE. Amebas may be visualized as motile organisms in unstained wet preparations. Polymorphonuclear leukocytes will be seen, without bacteria. Glucose is normal or decreased. CSF smears can be stained with Wright or Giemsa stain. *Acanthamoeba* are larger than *Naegleria*, and their cysts have a wrinkled double wall in tissues. Brain biopsy may be needed for diagnosis, and tissues preserved in formalin and imbedded in formalin can be used [53]. H&E stains are usually sufficient. Fomori methenamine silver and PAS-H stains will detect the amebas [36].

Serologic Testing

A number of technologies exist to identify antibodies to pathogenic protozoa. Indirect fluorescent antibody (IFA) and enzyme-linked immunosorbent assay (ELISA) techniques are available commercially for some infections.

Immunofluorescent staining has traditionally been used to identify parasites in stool samples, which are then confirmed by light microscopy. The method is time-consuming and expensive, and laboratory personnel must be highly trained. Algae and debris may cross-react and interfere with the test reliability. Other methods are being developed [10].

Several commercial immunodiagnostic methods for cryptosporidiosis are available. Those methods vary in cost, sensitivity, and specificity [22]. One study determined that sensitivity for enzyme immunoassay (EIA) assays ranged from 98% to 99%, with 100% specificity. DFA results were 100% specific and sensitive [83]. Serologic tests are useful in diagnosing invasive amebiasis. IFA and ELISA methods are available for *E histolytica* and are positive in most cases of liver abscess and about 75% of several intestinal amebiasis. Most patients with subclinical disease or minimal tissue invasion do not have positive serologic test results [3]. The presence of *Toxoplasma* can be determined by the presence of IgG or IgM antibodies using ELISA, which is the most sensitive and specific test. Almost all AIDS patients with *Toxoplasma* have positive IgG, since the infection probably represents a reactivation of a latent infection. Responses are variable, and IgM cannot be found. Therefore, serial antibody determination is not useful [3]. Serologic tests can detect IgG and IgA antibodies to *Giardia* [84]. Commercially available EIA kits had 94–99% sensitivity and 100% specificity [83].

Cryptosporidium can be detected by fluorescent stain or ELISA testing [18]. Diagnosis is made by using acid-fast or immunofluorescence staining on fecal smears. The fecal sample may need to be concentrated. Immunosorbent assays have 83–95% sensitivity in diarrheal specimens but are less sensitive in testing formed stools [16]. Complement fixation, direct agglutination, and indirect hemagglutination or immunofluorescence can be used to diagnose *T cruzi*. ELISA tests are being introduced. Direct agglutinating IgM antibodies are present acutely [3].

Babesia can be confirmed by immunofluorescent antibody assays. Individuals with active infections generally have titers of 1:1,024 or greater [18]. IFA can identify recent *Babesia* infections, when parasites are no longer present. Serum IgG for *Leishmania* can be detected by ELISA, IFA, or direct agglutination [3].

Culture

Gambian trypanosomiasis cannot be grown in laboratory rats, although Rhodesian trypanosomiasis can be demonstrated that way. *T cruzi* can be cultured in appropriate media [3]. *Trypanosoma brucei* can be recovered through animal inoculation and culture techniques [53].

Leishmania can be recovered from bone marrow cultures in cases of kala-azar. Skin lesions can be cultured to identify *Leishmania*. One to two milliliters of blood inoculated into a hamster can produce babeosis [3].

Genetic Tests

Polymerase chain reaction (PCR) has been used to identify *Enterocytozoon bieneusi* in the stool of AIDS patients [85]. PCR also has promise as a technique to identify *Toxoplasma* DNA [3]. PCR methods have been developed to detect *Giardia* and *Cryptosporidium* [10].

OTHER PROCEDURES

Sigmoidoscopy may be helpful in establishing the diagnosis of intestinal amebiasis by identifying classic lesions, such as ulcers or petechial lesions. The diagnostic evaluation of protozoal diseases includes demonstration of and identification of the parasite in body tissue or fluids. On occasion, it is necessary to diagnose the presence of organisms by using response to a trial of therapy [3].

Intradermal skin tests for delayed hypersensitivity can identify infection with *Leishmania* species, although the test remains positive for a long time and cannot indicate when the individual was infected [3].

EEGs performed on persons with African trypanosomiasis are found to be abnormal. In the late stages of the disease, they show large slow-wave oscillations (delta waves) like those produced by normal sleep [53].

Low-level parasitemia has been demonstrated by using uninfected bugs to feed on patients suspected of having trypanosomiasis. This process is called *xenodiagnosis* [3].

Treatment and Rehabilitation

Treatment for many protozoal diseases is less than adequate. Adequate hydration and nutrition are important, particularly in the more chronic diseases. Treatment for severe dysenteries must include adequate hydration. Bland diets high in protein and vitamins are recommended, along with bed rest. Nutrition and prevention of secondary infection is also important in patients with infections of the blood and soft tissues [3–5].

INTESTINAL AMEBAS

For severe intestinal amebiasis, metronidazole (Flagyl) is used at a dosage of 750 mg three times daily for five to 50 days [3]. Paromomycin has been approved by the Food and Drug Administration for intestinal *Entamoeba histolytica* [29].

INTESTINAL FLAGELLATES

Quinacrine hydrochloride, 100 mg three times daily for five to seven days, is approved for the treatment of giardiasis. Metronidazole is also effective. Treatment for *Dientamoeba fragilis* consists of iodoquinol, 650 mg three times a day for 10 days, or tetracycline, 250 mg three times a day for seven days [3].

INTESTINAL CILIATES

Balantidium coli is treated with tetracyline, metronidazole, paromomycin, chloroquine, or iodoquine [4,5].

INTESTINAL COCCIDIA AND MICROSPORIDIA

Patients with *Isospora* infection may need only rest and a bland diet. Pyrimethamine and sulfadiazine (75 mg and 4 g, respectively) or trimethoprine and sulfamethoxazole (160 mg and 800 mg, respectively) may be used for 10 days in otherwise healthy patients. There is currently no therapy for crytosporidiosis. Apicidin is a fungal derivative that, in vitro, is antiprotozoal at very low levels against *C parum* and drug-resistant human malaria. Animal trials have demonstrated its efficacy against *P bergei*, and in the future, it may prove to be useful therapeutically [86]. *Cryptosporidium* in immunosuppressed patients can be treated with paromomycin [72]. Paromomycin is a nonabsorbable aminoglycoside. High concentrations of the drug can be achieved in target areas, and it has been shown to inhibit infection of human enterocytes in culture [29]. When *Cryptosporidium* cause pulmonary symptoms, there is no effective treatment [8]. *Cyclospora* is treated with a seven-day course of oral trimethoprim-sulfamethoxazole (TMP/SMX) at a dosage of 160 mg TMP and 800 mg SMX twice daily [21]. Treatment for individuals allergic to sulfa drugs has not been identified [77].

BLOOD OR TISSUE SPOROZOA (FLAGELLATES)

Chloroquine has been given to treat babesiosis but did not appear effective [3]. Quinine, 650 mg orally, and clindamycin, 300 mg intravenously every six hours, has been effective for severe cases of babesiosis [26]. Mild cases may require only supportive therapy. Exchange transfusion has been used in life-threatening cases, when more than 10% of RBCs are parasitized [3,18]. Combinations of pentamidine and trimethoprim-sulfamethoxazole or azithromycin and quinine have been used [18].

BLOOD OR TISSUE FLAGELLATES

Therapy for trypanosomiasis can result in a good prognosis if it is instituted early in the course of the disease. Once the disease has progressed to the central nervous system, however, there is less success. Pentamidine isethionate, 4 mg/kg intramuscularly for 10 days, suramin sodium, 100–200 mg intravenously as a test dose, and then 1 g suramin given intravenously on days 1, 3, 7, 14, and 21, is the regimen for early-stage trypanosomiasis. The test dose of 0.2 g of suramin is needed to prevent adverse effects in patients with onchocerciasis [29]. Suramin is the drug of choice for the treatment of East African sleeping sickness [3]. Both suramin and pentamidine are effective for blood and tissue infections but not for CNS infections. However, pentamidine should not be used for therapy if it has been used for prophylaxis [29].

Drugs to treat CNS trypanosomiasis are arsenical medications and thus are toxic. Late infections are treated with melarsoprol or tryparsamide [3]. Because of its toxicity, melarsoprol (Mel B) is indicated only for patients with CNS involvement [53]. *Trypanosoma* may be developing drug resistance which is suggested by the number of relapses that occur [3]. The dosage for melarsoprol is 2–3.6 mg/kg intravenously daily for three days, then 3.6 mg/kg intravenously daily for three days and repeated beginning days 10 and 21. Mel B is associated with a death rate of about 10% due to associated encephalopathy [29]. The dosage for tryparsamide is 30 mg/kg intravenously every five days up to a total of 12 injections. Both these drugs have serious side effects, but they are generally rare [3]. A new drug is available, which is useful only in the Gambian form of African trypanosomiasis [3]. Intensive supportive care is imperative and requires hospitalization, administration of iron and vitamins, a nutritious diet, and rest for five hours after injection of Mel B is recommended. Corticosteroids have been tried in patients with advanced sleeping sickness. Treated patients should have follow-up lumbar puncture every six months for several years to identify relapses [29].

T cruzi is intracellular, so treatment is not very effective. Nifurtimox is investigational but appears most effective. Benznidazole is available in South America. To be effective, these drugs must be used in the acute stages of disease, but they may cause serious side effects [3].

Treatment for kala-azar includes nutrition and treatment for secondary bacterial infections. Blood transfusions may be needed for severely anemic or bleeding patients. Pentavalent antimony (SB^{+5}) is the recommended treatment. The drug sodium stibogluconate (Pentostam) is used in the United States. The dose is 20 mg SB^{+5}/kg given intravenously or intramuscularly on a daily basis for 20 days. Relapse is common, especially in patients in Africa and India. Pentamidine, 4 mg/kg given intramuscularly three times a week to a total of 10–15 doses, or amphotericin B, 1 mg/kg intravenously every other day to a total dose of 1.5–2.0 kg may be given [3].

Healing of cutaneous leishmaniasis can occur slowly without treatment. Nonspecific measures may help prevent secondary infections [16]. Pentavalent antimony, if given in early stages of the infection, reduces the case-fatality rate [32]. Sodium stibogluconate, 15–20 mg/kg/day given intramuscularly or intravenously for 15–20 days, is the treatment of choice. Up to three courses can be given over six to eight weeks. Ketoconazole, 400–600 mg orally per day, is an alternative but is less consistently effective [3]. The same regimens are useful for American leishmaniasis. For this disease, amphotericin B is an alternative; the dosage is 0.25–1.0 mg/kg intravenously daily to a total dosage of 1.5–2.5 g for adults [3].

OTHER BODY-SITE AMEBAS AND FLAGELLATES

PAM caused by *Naegleria* has a very high case-fatality rate and usually does not respond to therapy unless started very early in the disease course. The drug of choice is amphotericin B [36,53]. In those who have survived, long-term sequelae have not been noted [36]. The drug of choice for *Acanthamoeba* neurologic infections is ketoconazole or sulfadiazine; however, most patients respond poorly because of their underlying conditions. Propamidine isethionate (Brolene) has been used for *Acanthamoeba* keratitis [36,53]. It has been combined with topical polymyxin B, miconazole nitrate, gramicidin, neomycin, or neosporin. Hypersensitivity to the mucin antibiotics is possible; thus poly-hexamethylene biguanide (PHMB), 0.02%, ophthalmic solution is the treatment of choice. PHMB has been proved effective in amebic keratitis that is not responsive to other drugs. In a clinical trial, five of six patients had resolution of their worsening keratitis. The PHMB solution was instilled in the eyes according to the severity of the infection. The frequency varied from every two hours to three times per day, and the duration of therapy ranged from one week to seven months. Early institution of therapy resulted in better response [87].

OTHER BODY-SITE COCCIDIA, SPOROZOA, AND MICROSPORIDIA

Symptomatic *Toxoplasma* infections are treated with pyrimethamine (Daraprim), 25–50 mg per day for three to four weeks, plus trisulfapyrimidine, 2–6 g daily [3]. *Microsporidium* infection has no known treatment, but albendazole has been tried [5].

One patient with *Trachipleistophora hominis* was treated with a combination of albendazole, sulfadiazine, and pyrimethamine and recovered [42]. Two patients with *Enterocytozoon bieneusi* were treated with octreotide, but only one responded [85].

The treatment of choice for pneumocystis is TMP/SMX, 120 mg/kg/day, every six hours for 14 days. Pentamidine isethionate, 4 mg/kg per day intravenously for 12–14 days, is an alternative. It can be given intramuscularly but often causes severe local reactions [88]. Supportive measures such as oxygen, antibiotics, and hydration therapy are important [3].

Occupational Considerations

Many occupations put workers at increased risk for contracting infectious diseases. Even some that would intuitively seem low risk, such as day care, have proved to be risk factors for parasitic disease. Individuals who are required to travel in the course of performing their job duties are at risk for acquiring protozoan diseases that are rare in the United States.

The majority of individuals who are symptomatic for protozoan diseases have self-limited enteritis. However, most of the pathogenic species of protozoa appear capable of causing severe health effects. These diseases represent costs not only of medical care, but also of lost productivity. Because treatment is not very effective in many cases, and because vaccines or other prophylactic medications are not available, the employer must rely to a great extent on employees' compliance in using personal protective equipment. Inevitably, some workers will contract these illnesses, however.

Occupational and environmental health practitioners should be familiar with the diseases that are likely to impact populations with which they work. As the world economy becomes more and more global, the number of cases and the importance of these diseases is likely to continue to increase.

References

1. Smith DF, Parsons M (eds). *Molecular Biology of Parasitic Protozoa.* New York: IRL Press, 1996.
2. Ashford RW. The human parasite fauna: towards an analysis and interpretation. *Ann Trop Med Parasitol* 1991;85(1):189–98.
3. Neva FA, Brown HW (eds). *Basic Clinical Parasitology.* Norwalk, CT: Appleton & Lange, 1994.
4. Despommier DD, Gwadz RW, Hotez PJ. *Parasitic Diseases.* 3rd Ed. New York: Springer-Verlag, 1995.
5. Garcia LS, Druckner DA. *Diagnostic Medical Parasitology.* 3rd Ed. Washington, DC: ASM Press, 1997.
6. Pieniazek NJ, Herwaldt BL. Reevaluating the molecular taxonomy: is human-associated *Cyclospora* a mammalian *Eimeria* species? *Emerg Infect Dis* 1997;3(3):381–3.
7. Garcia LS. Classification of human parasites. *Clin Infect Dis* 1997;25(1):21–3.
8. Lindsay JA. Chronic sequelae of foodborne disease. *Emerg Infect Dis* 1997;3(4):443–52.
9. Satcher D. Emerging infections: getting ahead of the curve. *Emerg Infect Dis* 1995;1(1):1–6.
10. Jaykus LA. Epidemiology and detection as options for control of viral and parasitic foodborne disease. *Emerg Infect Dis* 1997;3(4):529–39.
11. Lew JF, LeBaron CW, Gless RI, et al. Recommendations for collection of laboratory specimens associated with outbreaks of gastroenteritis. *MMWR* 1990;39 (RR-14):1–13.
12. Miller RA, Minshew BH. Blastocystis hominis: an organism in search of a disease. *Rev Infect Dis* 1988;10(5): 930–8.
13. Telalbasic S, Pikula ZP, Kapidzic M. Blastocystis hominis may be a potential cause of intestinal disease. *Scand J Infect Dis* 1991;23(3):389–90.
14. Lujan HD, Mowatt MR, Byrd LC, et al. Cholesterol starvation induces differentiation of the intestinal parasite *Giardia lamblia. Proc Natl Acad Sci—USA.* 1996;93(15):7628–33.
15. Mahmoud AA. "New" intestinal parasitic protozoa. In: Krausen RM (ed), *Emerging Infections.* San Diego: Academic Press, 1998.
16. Guerrant RL. Cryptosporidiosis: an emerging, highly infectious threat. *Emerg Infect Dis* 1997;3(1):51–7.
17. DuPont HL, Chappell CL. The infectivity of *Cryptosporidium parvum* in healthy volunteers. *N Engl J Med* 1995;332(13):855–9.
18. Kemper CA. Pulmonary disease in selected protozoal infections. *Sem Respir Infect* 1997;12(2):113–21.
19. Juranek DD. Cryptosporidiosis: sources of infection and guidelines for prevention. *Clin Infect Dis* 1995;21(suppl 1):S57–61.
20. Marshall RJ, Flanigan TP. Paromomycin inhibits *Cryptosporidium* infection of human enterocyte cell line. *J Infect Dis* 1992;165:772–4.

21. Outbreaks of Cyclospora cayetanensis infection—United States, 1996. *MMWR* 1996;45(25):549–51.
22. Centers for Disease Control and Prevention. *Cryptosporidium and Water: A Public Health Handbook.* Atlanta: CDC, 1997.
23. Shadduck JA, Meccoli RA, Davis R, et al. Isolation of a microsporidian from a human patient. *J Infect Dis* 1990;162:773–6.
24. Shadduck JA. Human microsporidiosis and AIDS. *Rev Infect Dis* 1989;11(2):203–7.
25. Momen H. Emerging infectious diseases—Brazil. *Emerg Infect Dis* 1988;4(1):1–3.
26. Epidemiologic notes and reports: clindamycin and quinine treatment for Babesia microti infections. *MMWR* 1983;32(5):65–6, 72.
27. Epidemiologic notes and reports: babesiosis—Connecticut. *MMWR* 1989;38(38):649–50.
28. Centers for Disease Control and Prevention. Prevalence of tick-borne pathogens in *Ixodes scapularis* in a rural New Jersey county. *Emerg Infect Dis* 1998;4(1):97–9.
29. Molyneux DH. Selective primary health care: strategies for control of disease in the developing world. VIII. African trypanosomiasis. *Rev Infect Dis* 1983;5(5):945–56.
30. Moncayo A. Chagas' disease: epidemiology and prospects for interruption of transmission in the Americas. *World Health Stat Q* 1992;45:276–9.
31. Shimshony A. Epidemiology of emerging zoonoses in Israel. *Emerg Infect Dis* 1997;3(2):229–38.
32. Arias JR, Monteiro PS, Zicker F. The reemergence of visceral leishmaniasis in Brazil. *Emerg Infect Dis* 1996;2(2):145–6.
33. Viscerotropic leishmaniasis in persons returning from Operation Desert Storm—1990–1991. *MMWR* 1992;41(08):131–4.
34. Gustafson TL, Reed CM, McGreevy PB, et al. Human cutaneous leishmaniasis acquired in Texas. *Am J Trop Med Hyg* 1985;34(1):58–63.
35. Martinez AJ. Free-living amebas: infection of the central nervous system. *Mt Sinai J Med* 1993;60(4): 271– 8.
36. Martinez AJ, Visvesvara GS. Free-living, amphizoic and opportunistic amebas. *Brain Pathol* 1997;7(1):583–98.
37. Primary amebic meningoencephalitis—North Carolina, 1991. *MMWR* 1992;41(25):437–40.
38. Acanthamoeba keratitis associated with contact lenses—United States. *MMWR* 1986;35(25):405–8.
39. U.S. Food and Drug Administration. *Food safety from farm to table: a national food safety initiative. Report to the President.* Washington, DC: USDA. May 1997.
40. Morris JG, Potter M. Emergence of new pathogens as a function of changes in host susceptibility. *Emerg Infect Dis* 1997;3(4):435–41.
41. Epidemiologic notes and reports: Microsporidian keratoconjunctivitis in patients with AIDS. *MMWR* 1990;39(11):188–9.
42. Field AS, Marriott DJ, Milliken ST, et al. Myositis associated with a newly described microsporidian, *Trachipleistophora hominis*, in a patient with AIDS. *J Clin Microbiol* 1996;34(11):2803–11.
43. LeChevallier MW, Norton WD. *Giardia* and *Cryptosporidium* in raw and finished drinking water. *J Am Water Works Assoc* 1995;87(9):54–68.
44. Mackenzie WR, Hoxie NJ, Proctor ME, et al. A massive outbreak in Milwaukee of *Cryptosporidium* infection transmitted through the public water supply. *N Engl J Med* 1994;331(3):161–7.
45. Surveillance for waterborne-disease outbreaks—United States, 1993–1994. *MMWR* 1996;45(SS-1):1–35.
46. Rose JB, Haas CN, Regli S. Risk assessment and control of waterborne Giardiasis. *Am J Public Health* 1991;81(6):709–13.
47. Fogarty J, Thornton L, Hayes C, et al. Illness in a community associated with an episode of water contamination with sewage. *Epidemiol Infect* 1995;114(2):289–95.
48. Starko KM, Lippy EC, Dominguez LB, et al. Campers' diarrhea outbreak traced to water-sewage link. *Public Health Rep* 1986;101(5):527–31.
49. Joce RE, Bruce J, Kiely D, et al. An outbreak of cryptosporidiosis associated with a swimming pool. *Epidemiol Infect* 1991;107(3):497–508.
50. Tauxe RV. Emerging foodborne diseases: an evolving public health challenge. *Emerg Infect Dis* 1997;3(4): 425–34.
51. Epidemiologic notes and reports: common-source outbreak of Giardiasis—New Mexico. *MMWR* 1989; 38(23):405–7.
52. Outbreaks of *Escherichia coli* O157:H7 infections and cryptosporidiosis associated with drinking unpasteurized apple cider—Connecticut and New York, October 1996. *MMWR* 1997;46(1):4–8.
53. Chimelli L, Scaravilli F. Trypanosomiasis. *Brain Pathol* 1997;7(1):599–611.
54. Meslin FX. Global aspects of emerging and potential zoonoses: a WHO perspective. *Emerg Infect Dis* 1997;3(2):223–8.
55. Lam SK. Emerging infectious diseases—Southeast Asia. *Emerg Infect Dis* 1998;4(2):145–7.
56. Peng MM, Xiao L, Freeman AR, et al. Genetic polymorphism among *Cryptosporidium parvum* isolates: evidence of two distinct human transmission cycles. *Emerg Infect Dis* 1997;3(4):567–73.
57. Wilson ME. Travel and the emergence of infectious diseases. *Emerg Infect Dis* 1995;1(2):39–45.
58. Morse SS. Factors in the emergence of infectious diseases. *Emerg Infect Dis* 1995;1(1):7–15.
59. Cutaneous leishmaniasis—Ohio. *MMWR* 1985;34(33): 515–6.
60. Schmunis GA, Zicker F, Pinheiro F, et al. Risk for transfusion-transmitted infectious diseases in Central and South America. *Emerg Infect Dis* 1988;4(1):5–11.

61. Dutkiewicz J, Jablonski L, Olenchock SA. Occupational biohazards: a review. *Am J Ind Med* 1988;14(5):605–23.

62. Epidemiologic notes and reports: Cryptosporidiosis among children attending day-care centers—Georgia, Pennsylvania, Michigan, California, New Mexico. *MMWR* 1984;33(42):599–601.

63. Human cryptosporidiosis—Alabama. *MMWR* 1982; 31(19):252–4.

64. Wolfe ND, Escalante AA, Karesh WB, et al. Wild primate populations in emerging infectious disease research: the missing link? *Emerg Infect Dis* 1998;4(2): 149–58.

65. Healy G. The impact of cultural and environmental changes on the epidemiology and control of human babesiosis. *Trans R Soc Trop Med Hyg* 1989;83(Suppl): 35–8.

66. Nethercott JR. Health status of a group of sewage treatment workers in Toronto, Canada. *Am Ind Hyg Assoc J* 1988;49(7):346–50.

67. Epidemiologic notes and reports: gastrointestinal illness among scuba divers—New York City. *MMWR* 1983; 32(44):576–7.

68. Clark CS, Linnemann CC, Clark JG, et al. Enteric parasites in workers occupationally exposed to sewage. *J Occup Med* 1984;26(4):273–5.

69. Epidemiologic notes and reports: Swimming-associated cryptosporidiosis. *MMWR* 1990;39(20):343–5.

70. Meeting summary: conference on global disease elimination and eradication as public health strategies, February 26, 1998. *Emerg Infect Dis* 1998;4(2):349–51.

71. Update: outbreaks of *Cyclospora cayetanensis* infection—United States and Canada, 1996. *MMWR* 1996;45(28): 611–2.

72. Outbreak of cryptosporidiosis at a day camp—Florida, Jul–Aug 1995. *MMWR* 1996;45(21):442–4.

73. Centers for Disease Control and Prevention. Update on adult immunization: recommendations of the Immunization Practices Advisory Committee (ACIP). *MMWR* 1991;40(RR-12):1–52.

74. Mayer CL, Palmer CJ. Evaluation of PCR, nested PCR, and flourescent antibodies for detection of *Giardia* and *Crytosporidium* species in wastewater. *Appl Environ Microbiol* 1996;62(6):2081–5.

75. Centers for Disease Control and Prevention. Surveillance for foodborne-disease outbreaks—United States, 1988–1992. *MMWR* 1996;45(SS-50):1–68.

76. Outbreaks of cyclosporiasis—United States, 1997. *MMWR* 1997;46(20):451–2.

77. Publication of CDC surveillance summaries. *MMWR* 1992;41(08):145–6.

78. Outbreaks of pseudo-infection with *Cyclospora* and *Cryptosporidium*—Florida and New York City, 1995. *MMWR* 1997;46(16):354–8.

79. Epidemiologic notes and reports: pseudo-outbreak of intestinal amebiasis—California. *MMWR* 1985;34(9): 125–6.

80. Berlin OG, Peter JB, Gagne C, et al. Autofluorescence and the detection of *Cyclospora* oocysts. *Emerg Infect Dis* 1998;4(1):127–8.

81. Peacock CS, Blanshard C, Tovey DG, et al. Histological diagnosis of intestinal microsporidiosis in patients with AIDS. *J Clin Pathol* 1991;44(7):558–63.

82. Simon D, Weiss LM, Tarowitz HB, et al. Light microscopic diagnosis of human microsporidiosis and variable response to octreotide. *Gastroenterology* 1991; 100(1):271–3.

83. Garcia LS, Shimizu RY. Evaluation of nine immunoassay kits (enzyme immunoassay and direct fluorescence) for detection of *Giardia lamblia* and *Cryptosporidium parvum* in human fecal specimens. *J Clin Microbiol* 1997;35(6):1526–9.

84. Ljungstrom I, Castor B. Immune response to *Giardia lamblia* in a water-borne outbreak of giardiasis in Sweden. *J Med Microbiol* 1992;36(5):347–52.

85. Velasquez JN, Carnevale S, Guarnera EA, et al. Detection of the Microsporidian parasite *Enterocytozoon bieneusi* in specimens from patients with AIDS by PCR. *J Clin Microbiol* 1996;34(12):3230–2.

86. Darkin-Rattray SJ, Gurnett AM, Myers RW, et al. Apicidin: a novel antiprotozoal agent that inhibits paracyte histone deacetylase. *Proc Natl Acad Sci—USA* 1996;93(23):13143–7.

87. Larkin DF, Kilvington S, Dart JK. Acanthamoeba keratitis with polyhexamethylene biguanide. *Ophthalmology* 1992;99(2):185–91.

88. Gorbach SL, Bartlett JG, Blacklow NR (eds). *Infectious Diseases.* 2nd Ed. Philadelphia: Saunders, 1997.

31 / Fungal Travel-Related Infections

Robert S. Rhodes

Fungal and other related diseases have not been considered important or significant health problems in the United States and other highly developed Western nations with advanced public health systems. Many studies reporting results of investigations of health problems in travelers do not include fungal diseases. In a study of 10,000 Swiss travelers, fungal diseases were not mentioned as a cause of significant health problems [1]. Travel publications, including those put out by the Centers for Disease Control and Prevention, private publishers, and the World Health Organization, make passing reference only to fungal skin infections of the feet [2–4].

The globalization of business and industry in recent years has brought with it significant concerns for business travelers and their families about a variety of health issues. Fungal infections and fungus-related diseases, as well as other health problems, must be included as concerns for the business traveler. The key to managing travel-related health problems is prevention, which requires a thorough understanding of the diseases that may cause these problems. Fungal and mold-related health problems, including those associated with both systemic and other mycoses, are addressed in this chapter [5].

Occupational medicine specialists and other occupational health professionals must become cognizant of implications for all traveling individuals for which they may be called upon to provide counsel and services in diverse parts of the world. They must utilize demonstrated successful methods to keep employees and their families healthy.

Concerns with skin and respiratory problems related to fungal agents or their spores vary significantly from the deserts of Mongolia to the villages and cities of China, the jungles of Central and West Africa; and the island nations of the Pacific. These concerns also vary significantly among the countries of South and Central America, Southeast Asia, and the various American states. The needs of specific individuals and their family members also vary, depending on many factors, including current health status, potential predisposition to certain types of health problems, immune status, environmental considerations, personal habits, and recreational factors.

This chapter provides a global focus that stresses recognition of the increased volume and mix of travelers at risk. It is not intended to provide in-depth, comprehensive coverage of all fungal diseases. Many excellent resources cover these areas. Work-related fungal disorders are covered in Chapter 13 of this textbook. This chapter discussion is divided into systemic mycotic infections and superficial mycoses.

Epidemiology

Fungal pathogens are outnumbered by their bacterial, viral, and parasitic counterparts as primary etiologic agents producing infections. In spite of this, they continue to be responsible for an increasing number of emerging infectious diseases. At present, individuals with suppressed immune function, such as acquired immunodeficiency syndrome (AIDS) and transplant recipients, represent increasingly large numbers of persons worldwide who are becoming infected with fungal agents [6–13]. A growing number of these are nosocomial (hospital-acquired) infections. Worldwide, significant isolated outbreaks of various fungal diseases continue to occur in persons with normal immune systems. Increasing numbers of travelers, including many in business along with family members, fall into some of these risk categories or behave, through their recreational and other activities, in ways that bring them in contact with agents that put them at risk [14].

During the 10-year period between 1985 and 1995, the U.S. National Institute of Allergy and Infectious Diseases more than quadrupled its funding of studies of mycoses. The actual funding increased from about $6.5 million in 1985 to almost $30 million in 1995 [15].

In a 1990 U.S. nationwide hospital survey, fungal-related disorders were found to be responsible for approximately 10.4% of nosocomial infections; 5.1% of surgical wound infections; 5.7% of lung infections; 18.7% of urinary tract infections; and 9.9% of all bloodstream infections [16]. A study of 814 heart transplant recipients revealed that 12% developed fungal or protozoal infections. Patients with invasive fungal infections had a 36% fatality rate, nearly three times higher than that for bacterial or viral infections (13%) [17].

Many fungi found on the skin or in the environment rarely cause infections except in individuals who are compromised immunologically, for example, *Aspergillus* among individuals receiving bone marrow transplants. One study reported that some 20% of 275 such individuals had developed nosocomial pneumonia secondary to *Aspergillus* and had a 95% fatality rate [18].

Pneumocystis carinii pneumonia, a protozoan infection, is the most frequently recognized opportunistic infection in patients with acquired immune deficiency syndrome (AIDS), presenting as the AIDS-defining illness in more than 50% of patients. However, fungal infections are increasingly being seen as the presenting infection in these patients [19].

Disease-causing fungi are characterized as either primary or opportunistic pathogens. Primary pathogens can, but do not always, cause disease in healthy people. Opportunistic pathogens, on the other hand, are generally harmless to healthy persons, causing serious disease only in people whose immune systems have been weakened or suppressed. The most common primary pathogens include *Coccidioides immitis*, *Histoplasma capsulatum*, *Sporothrix schenckii*, and *Blastomyces dermatitidis*. Opportunistic pathogens include *Candida* species, *Cryptococcus neoformans*, *Aspergillus* species, *Penicillium marneffei*, and *Trichosporon beigelii* [12,13].

Most systemic fungal diseases are not transmitted from person to person. These disorders are usually acquired by individuals coming in contact with the fungal spores through inhalation when they are aerosolized and scattered from their soil or other habitats (e.g., in dust). Some opportunistic fungi, however, are normally present on human skin and in the gastrointestinal tract and therefore present the potential for person-to-person transmission, particularly in hospital settings.

On a global basis, there are numerous reports, from medical centers worldwide, of increasing occurrence of fungal infections. These involve a variety of cases, mostly in individuals with suppressed immune systems. Increasingly, however, there are many instances in which a fungal infection of a serious nature—life-threatening or fatal—occurs when this is not the case. On the other hand, there are also frequent reports of fungal infections caused by organisms not usually associated with fungal infections [20,21].

Worldwide, the most common systemic fungal diseases are blastomycosis, coccidioidomycosis, and histoplasmosis; also common but to a lesser extent, primarily in the immunocompromised, are infections caused by *Candida albicans* or *Sporothrix schenckii*. These two have been more often associated with localized infections of the skin and mucous membranes [22–24].

The most common fungal diseases occurring among travelers are those associated with skin and nail disorders. Systemic infections occur much less often but are being reported more frequently as individuals at risk become better able to travel because of improved medical management of immunocompromised and related disorders.

Candida and *Aspergillus* species are significant, primarily causing skin problems and, in some instances, allergic phenomenon, but they rarely produce invasive disease in the absence of some type of pre-injury (as a secondary contaminant) or in individuals with a defect in their immune response.

SYSTEMIC MYCOTIC INFECTIONS

Coccidioidomycosis, blastomycosis, and histoplasmosis share a number of characteristics in their production of systemic mycotic infections. In countries where they are found, they all occur in relatively circumscribed geographic areas. Usually, their spores are present in soil, and aerosolization of this dry soil and their spores in moist areas makes the respiratory tract their usual route of entry. These organisms are dimorphic and exist in their natural state as mold/mycelium bearing infectious spores, which in the host evolve into yeast-like organisms that are pathogenic to tissue. The common route of entry is, as noted, the respiratory tract, although there have been reported cases with no obvious respiratory involvement, the initial lesion being present in deep soft tissue wounds or internal organs other than the lungs. These disorders all share manifestations and pathologic features that are similar to those of other granulomatous disorders such as tuberculosis and are frequently misdiagnosed initially as tuberculosis infection. Individuals with intact or normal cell-mediated immune response only rarely develop clinical findings or overt evidence of clinical infection. In most individuals who contract systemic blastomycosis, coccidioidomycosis, histoplasmosis, or involvement by *Aspergillus* or, rarely, *Candida albicans*, the most common route of entry is the respiratory tract [6,23,25–27].

The most common characteristic of these infections is production of a granulomatous inflammatory response. As systemic disorders, they closely resemble pulmonary tuberculosis and are often initially mistaken for it. These infections tend to be of greatest danger in individuals with poor immune response. In these persons, the disseminated disease occurs very readily. In other people, the disease is often contained and consists of focal or localized suppurative granulomatous lesions.

Coccidioidomycosis

Coccidioidomycosis, also known as *San Joaquin Valley fever*, *desert fever* and *desert bumps*, is caused by *Coccidioides immitis*. This dimorphic organism's natural habitat is desert soil and geologic and climatic areas with semi-arid conditions and moderate rainfall. It occurs in the San Joaquin Valley, southern Arizona, Utah, New Mexico, Nevada, southwestern Texas, areas of Mexico near the U.S. border, and Central and South America. The dust containing the spores can be airborne and thus transported many miles from areas in which it is usually endemic. Individuals handling such things as packages or other items containing the dust can be affected. Dust storms may carry the organism's spores many hundreds of miles from endemic areas. There is an increased incidence of this disorder associated with the rising incidence of AIDS and other immunocompromising disorders. Human-to-human transmission is not thought to occur. The disease's highest prevalence is in field and construction workers.

The health care systems in California and other southwestern states have begun to require reporting of coccidioidomycosis infections. During the 1980s, fewer than 500 cases of coccidioidomycosis were reported in the state of California each year. In 1991, that number jumped to 1,200. The following two years saw an even greater increase, with 4,516 and 4,137 cases reported in 1992 and 1993, respectively [27,28].

Blastomycosis

Blastomycosis is a systemic mycotic infection caused by the fungus *Blastomyces dermatitidis*. This disease is endemic in the southeastern and central portions of the United States and along some sections of the Mississippi and Ohio River Valleys as well as in central Canada, with the central United States being the most heavily endemic area in the world. It is also seen in Central America and many African nations. There has been no major effort at mapping this zone, using large skin testing groups, as was done with histoplasmosis. Distribution plotting has been based on individual case findings and case reports. In other parts of the world, scattered cases of infection in individuals who have never traveled to one of the endemic areas are reported. Blastomycosis occurs in persons of all ages but most often in young and middle-aged adults. Individuals who work outdoors or participate in extensive outdoor recreation are in the greatest danger of contracting this infection. Its natural habitat is moist soil, particularly near waterways where there are large amounts of organic matter, especially animal excreta. Infection generally occurs after inhalation of the organism's conidia have become airborne as a result of disturbance of soil or the materials containing the organism. The incubation period is approximately 45 days. There have been significant problems in developing a sensitive and specific skin-test antigen, thus making it difficult to do accurate mapping of subclinical disease occurrences. The absence of acceptable immunologic markers of remote subclinical disease means that the size of the subclinical case "iceberg" remains uncertain relative to clinically apparent and diagnosed pulmonary and extrapulmonary cases [6,23–31].

Histoplasmosis

Histoplasmosis, also called *Darling's disease* and *reticuloendotheliosis*, is caused by the dimorphic fungus *Histoplasma capsulatum*. This agent is found worldwide in soil, particularly soil that is contaminated by droppings from starlings, chickens, other birds, and bats. There are endemic areas in various parts of the world. The greatest endemicity in the United States occurs in the eastern parts of the country, the Ohio and Mississippi River Valleys, and Virginia and Maryland. Histoplasmosis is also endemic in other areas of North America and throughout Latin America. There are reported outbreaks of histoplasmosis, particularly in those areas contaminated with droppings from birds and bats. Several incidents have involved outbreaks among cave explorers in bat-infested caves; there has also been a widespread epidemic involving over 100,000 persons in Indianapolis, Indiana, that was associated with construction. In Japan, *H capsulatum* has rarely been isolated from the natural environment. Prior to 1993, only seven cases of histoplasmosis had been reported in Japan, and these included cases that were contracted in foreign countries. In 1994, histoplasmosis was diagnosed in a group of eight Japanese travelers who had been exposed to bat guano while exploring a cave in Manaus, Brazil, in March 1993. All eight had developed respiratory symptoms about 12 to 20 days after their exposure. The total length of time in the cave for the eight persons was approximately two hours, and seven of the eight developed abnormal symptoms, while five also developed nodular pulmonary infiltrates. All had serologic evidence of histoplasmosis. Travelers should therefore be aware of the significant threat of histoplasmosis infection when exploring bat-inhabited caves in any part of the world. Persons particularly at risk are those that vacation or work in areas such as caves, forests, or buildings heavily populated by birds and bats. This disease is frequently seen in farmers and construction workers. It is contacted by inhalation. Infection is usually of the lung and is preventable [14,22,30,32].

Sporotrichosis

Sporotrichosis is the fourth of the invasive endemic fungal infections and is caused by the agent *Sporothrix schenckii*. This dimorphic fungus is found worldwide in soil and decaying vegetation such as sphagnum moss, rose thorns, old rotted wood, and garden soils. It most often enters the body through direct contact with the skin, usually after having been inoculated into the lymphatic system following penetration by wood splinters or other similar woody substances, such as rose thorns containing the spores. This then produces the infection sporotrichosis. This systemic mycotic infection differs from coccidioidomycosis, blastomycosis, and histoplasmosis in that it is much wider in its international distribution. Although it may infect other organs of the body, it most commonly occurs as a granulomatous skin infection in non-immunocompromised individuals [33–35].

NONENDEMIC FUNGAL INFECTIONS

Almost all the nonendemic fungal infections are opportunistic infections that occur primarily in individuals with compromised immune systems. A variety of fungal infections are seen in susceptible individuals at risk, and travelers are no exception. In over two thirds of HIV-infected individuals with clinical disease, some type of pulmonary disorder is present. Fungal infections play a key role in producing infections in this group [36].

Opportunistic disorders include such conditions as aspergillosis, producing nonclostridial necrotizing soft-tissue infections with gangrenous necrosis of the skin and associated tissue.

Other opportunistic infections, caused by organisms such as the dimorphic fungus *Penicillium marneffei*, have also been reported. This organism is now an emerging agent, particularly among patients with immunodeficiencies in Southeast Asia, and is now being seen in individuals who have traveled to this region as well as those who reside there. *P marneffei* infection may clinically resemble tuberculosis, *Moluscum contageosum*, cryptococcosis, or histoplasmosis. This infection is also reported in increasing numbers of patients in southern China and the Middle East. *P marneffei* infection causes a disseminated progressive disease and is the third most common opportunistic infection in HIV-infected patients in the reported areas [37–39].

Scytalidium dimidiatum and *Lecythophora hoffmannii* are also rare agents reported in recent years as those involved in a number of infections in immunocompromised individuals in Australia and other countries. These pathogens have caused such disorders as chronic sinusitis, common skin lesions, lymphangitis, and lymphadenitis [21].

Scedosporium prolificans has been involved in cases of infection, trauma, or surgery in immunosuppressed individuals. Many of these cases have been reported from medical institutions in Spain; however, the infection has been noted in diverse areas of the world [40].

Travel-related fungal infections occur not only in adults but also in children. Travelers who have children must be aware of this. Children who are at risk, as well as normal, healthy children, may be susceptible not only to endemic fungal infections but also to opportunistic ones. Children may be infected at any age, from infancy to the teenage years. In some studies, many of these infections have been reported in patients in intensive care units, following surgery or chemotherapy, or in those with important underlying diseases including malignancies, prematurity, and congenital anomalies. Medical procedures that commonly put patients at risk include parenteral nutrition, endotracheal incubation, central venous cathetertization, and surgical procedures. In many of these cases, the individuals have received antibiotics. The infectious organism seen most often is *Candida albicans* [41].

SUPERFICIAL MYCOSES

Epidemiologically, fungal skin infections have the highest incidence of all fungal infections. Although the skin is generally resistant to infection and has many inherent protective mechanisms, including the tough barriers of protein and lipid in the stratum cornea and the underlying epidermis, some organisms have the ability to attach to skin cells and reproduce, resulting in infection under certain conditions. This is especially true when environmental conditions such as excessive moisture or skin inflammation cause, for unknown reasons, breakdown of the skin's protective mechanisms [42].

The most common skin infections worldwide are those caused by dermatophytes. These fungi can infect skin, nails, and hair. This group includes *Microsporum trichophyton* and *Epidermophyton* species. These fungi are classified as anthropophilic, zoophilic, or geophilic, depending on whether the source is human, animal, or soil. The most common cause of fungal skin infections in humans is contact with anthropophilic dermatophytes. The most common routes of transmission are direct contact with an infected person or exposure to infected skin cells disseminated in the environment. The fungal spores from these agents can survive for many months in the environment. When the spores are inoculated directly into breaks in the skin, they can germinate and subsequently invade the cutaneous layers. As for other fungal infections, the most easily infected individuals are those with impaired immune systems [42–44].

The infections caused by various species of anthropophilic dermatophytes are unique in their geographic distribution patterns. In Southeast Asia and the Middle East, *Trichophyton violaceum* is the most common cause of scalp infections, whereas in the United States, the agent most commonly associated is *Trichophyton tonsurans.*

Dermatophytosis is more commonly referred to as *ringworm* and is classified according to the site at which fungal involvement occurs. Areas include the scalp (tinea capitis), body (tinea corporis), bearded areas, (tinea barbae), face in general (tinea faciei), groin area (tinea cruris), feet (tinea pedis), nails (tinea unguium), and skin of the hands (tinea manuum). Dermatophytic skin lesions are characteristically circular scaly patches that are usually dry in appearance.

The zoophilic dermatophytes are those associated with exposure to, animals commonly infected with microsporum as well as *Trichophyton* species. They rarely affect humans, although human infection with zoophilic species have occurred after exposure to dogs, cats, horses, cattle, pigs, rodents, poultry, hedgehogs, and some other animals [42–45].

Dermatophytes cause fungal infections of keratinized tissues, such as skin, hair, and nails. This group of organisms is divided into three genera: *Trichophyton*, *Epidermophyton*, and *Microsporum*. It is important to confirm the clinical diagnosis of onychomycosis and other tinea infections prior to commencing therapy. The identity of the fungal organism may provide guidance in choosing an appropriate topical antifungal agent. Special techniques may be required to obtain the best yield of fungal organisms from a given site, especially the scalp and nails [45].

Prevention and Control

Prevention of the endemic mycoses continues to be a matter of great concern, particularly because of the increasing numbers of travelers that may be in an immunocompromised state. The same applies to opportunistic fungal infections. Needless to say, the most effective way to prevent infection with any of the described fungal agents is to avoid inhalation of conidia from the environmental source.

The traveler must be aware of the risk of visits to endemic areas. These include areas of Canada, the United States, Mexico, and Central and South America. Recreational or tourist areas, including caves and forests inhabited by large flocks of birds, must be treated with appropriate caution. Respiratory protection as well as other means of contact avoidance should be utilized, as indicated [14].

Prevention of infection by *Sporothrix schenckii* involves protecting the skin through the use of gloves and other mechanisms to prevent contact with potentially infected woody or fibrous material.

Health care institutions are potential sources of opportunistic fungal infections, particularly for immunocompromised individuals. High-risk travelers must be aware of environmental risks, take particular note of the status of care available at their destination(s), and understand risk-containment measures.

Prevention of dermatophytosis requires knowledge of the conditions predisposing to infection and the maintenance of strict personal hygiene, particularly in areas that have a hot, humid climate. If a person is known to be infected, coworkers and health care workers should avoid contact with potentially infected material and, again, exercise strict hygienic practices and isolation, if necessary. Hygiene involves both the skin in general and the feet and scalp in particular when outbreaks of tinea pedis or tinea capitis are likely. Topical foot powders assist in drying, and certain antifungal shampoos may be helpful in the prevention of these disorders. Education of at-risk individuals about avoidance of contact with sources of infectious organisms is crucial [42,44,45].

Medical surveillance for travel-related fungal diseases involves testing individuals who live in, or have traveled from, endemic areas. Medical surveillance for the dermatophytoses and other skin infections and superficial mycotic infections in travelers involves history taking, inspection of the involved skin, and diagnostic testing for the suspected pathogen when appropriate. In regard to travelers, biologic testing for fungal infections is often constrained by the lack of knowledge as to all places where the person has traveled and is somewhat limited to the clinical testing that is done as a part of the diagnostic process. The exception to this is evaluation of soil and environmental samples from suspected areas, soil, dust, and avian and bat droppings from suspected areas harboring the fungal spores [22,32,46–48].

The prevention of any of the fungal diseases requires education of the traveler about:

- The area to which the individual will be traveling.
- The potential for various exposures.

- The individual's susceptibility.
- Mechanisms for prevention and information about means of managing simple problems early if they cannot be completely avoided.

IMMUNIZATION AND PROPHYLACTIC MEASURES

At present there are no immunizations available to prevent any of the known fungal diseases, either systemic or cutaneous. Infection by some of the agents induces immune responses that provide some level of immunity. Immunization against dermatophytosis has been investigated, but to date, no wholly effective vaccine has been developed for general use.

The prevention of opportunistic mycoses is extremely difficult because these infections are facilitated by the compromised immunity of individuals usually infected. Attempts have been made to utilize oral or systemic antifungal agents to reduce the occurrence of some of the infections, particularly candidiasis. Success with this approach has been mixed, however. For example, one of the more common opportunistic infections in immunocompromised individuals (travelers included) is aspergillosis. There has been limited success in prophylaxis by utilizing controls in the environment of the individual exposed to aspergillosis in the hospital environment, in particular, laminar air flow. However, to date, there has been no significant success with the use of antifungal drugs. In the case of zygomycosis, similar problems and results as those associated with attempts to prevent aspergillosis have occurred [42,45].

In the case of the superficial mycoses tinea pedis and tinea capitis, the use of antifungal agents in creams and powders, along with maintaining good skin hygiene and other modalities, has been successful in helping to prevent occurrence in areas of high endemicity.

METRICS

Most mycotic infections are not reportable diseases in the public health sector, except for coccidioidomycosis in California. Therefore, widespread public health data do not exist to allow accurate assessment of the adequacy of preventive measures other than in specific clinical studies reported in the literature [12,16,27,44].

Symptoms and Signs

In the immunologically competent host, blastomycosis, cryptococcosis, and histoplasmosis (the three most common of the primary systemic mycoses), all exhibit a similar presentations namely one resembling acute respiratory infection with influenza-like symptoms. The affected individual, and frequently the physician, often mistake these fungal diseases for the flu or a respiratory illness. If a traveler who lives in an endemic area or has visited or vacationed in one of these areas presents with these types of symptoms, systemic mycosis should be included in the differential diagnosis [14]. Each of the endemic systemic mycoses may also present with other types of clinical findings.

BLASTOMYCOSIS

Blastomycosis, with low frequency, may present as:

- An illness resembling bacterial pneumonia, with acute onset, high fever, lobular infiltrates, and productive cough.
- Subacute or chronic respiratory illness resembling active pulmonary tuberculosis or lung cancer, with mass-like lesions or fibronodular granulomatous infiltrates.
- Rapidly progressive adult respiratory distress syndrome (ARDS), with high fever, diffuse infiltrates, and progressive respiratory failure [6,8,23].

In almost 60% of cases of acute pulmonary blastomycosis, lung consolidation is the most consistent finding on chest radiographs. Other findings on chest radiographs include presence of a mass lesion, intermediate-size nodules, a miliary pattern, solitary cavitation, fibrotic and cavitary changes, a pattern of interstitial fibrosis, diffuse alveoli involvement, and mixed alveoli and interstitial infiltration. Other radiographic findings include hilar adenopathy, postinfectious calcification, chest-wall invasion, and pleural effusion [49,50].

Cutaneous disease is the most common form of extrapulmonary involvement and may present as raised verrucous, encrusted lesions with serpiginous borders, most often located on the face or upper extremities. These lesions have small abscesses that are apparent when the superficial crusting is removed. Atrophic scarification is sometimes present. Bacterial superinfection may change the appearance of these lesions, but characteristically they are not painful, nor is pruritus significant. Chronic draining fistulas may also be associated with blastomycosis, but these are rare [25,51]. In most cases, cutaneous manifestations occur as a result of metastatic spread from the lungs. Primary cutaneous infection, when it occurs, is usually seen in laboratory workers or other individuals that come in contact with the fungus by direct skin contact, such as veterinary workers or autopsy staff.

Osseous, prostatic, and central nervous system complications are the next most frequent presentations, in descending order. Between 50% and 75% of patients with active, clinical blastomycosis have multiple organ-system involvement.

Central nervous system infection does not commonly occur in immunocompetent patients with blastomycosis. In immunocompromised hosts, however, it is a much more common presentation, and intracranial blastomycomas and other central nervous system manifestations are not uncommon in these individuals [7,10,25].

COCCIDIOIDOMYCOSIS

Coccidioidomycosis tends to develop into the previously described influenza-like illness approximately seven to 28 days after exposure to the arthrospores. This occurs in approximately 40% of immunologically intact individuals and in a much higher percentage of individuals with compromised immune systems. In most immunocompetent individuals, there are no symptoms; the only sign of infection is a positive skin test. Those who develop progressive disease often have a generalized macular erythematous rash that is particularly prominent on the inguinal folds and the palms and soles. This rash is especially common in young children. Clinical disease is alleged to be more common among individuals of African or Philippino descent, Native Americans, and white females. There are, however, no significant data to determine if this is related to some racial or gender differences or if there are socioeconomic, nutritional, or other factors that account for it. In most of the literature in which statistics are quoted, the information is not discussed in relationship to these factors [27,52–54].

Most individuals who develop clinical coccidioidomycosis present with erythema nodosum or erythema mutiforme, as well as flu-like illness. These skin signs appear to occur as a result of the development of cell-mediated immunity and are often considered to be positive prognostic indicators. Other findings include the presence of generalized joint pain, conjunctivitis, episcleritis, and pharyngitis. These findings in individuals who work, live in, or have recently visited areas where coccidioidomycosis is known to be endemic, dictate diagnostic testing for this disorder. Other common findings include severe pleuritis; about 5–10% of individuals with acute disease have pleural effusions. Early in the disease, the acute pneumonititis that appears is often associated with cavitary and cystic lesions in the lungs, usually followed in a short time by complete healing of all lesions. Serious long-term or permanent lung injury occurs in only about 5% of patients with symptomatic pulmonary disease. There have been some cases of coccidioidomycosis in which patients exhibit fulminate lung disease characteristic of adult respiratory distress syndrome (ARDS). Another concern is individuals with AIDS or other disorders in whom corticosteroid therapy has been started as adjuvant therapy for control of their disease. In these individuals, conversion of the coccidioidal infection into a rampant progressive disorder often occurs and is fatal. The same is true for patients who have coccidioidomycosis but are misdiagnosed as having some other disorder and placed on corticosteroids. The disease then becomes rapidly progressive, leading to severe complications or death. There is evidence to suggest that when coccidioidomycosis becomes a disseminated disease, the primary factor governing this occurrence is the individual host's ability to develop an adequate cell-mediated immune response. If this is absent, the disease frequently becomes progressive, resulting in a poor response to therapy and, ultimately, death of the individual [27,52,55,56].

The most serious extrapulmonary manifestation of coccidioidomycosis is the occurrence of meningitis. This occurs in approximately 30% of individuals who develop disseminated disease. The characteristic finding is a granulomatous meningitis completely encasing the brain with extensive involvement of the base of the brain, resulting in hydrocephalus and cranial nerve palsies. On occasion, aneurysms occur as a result of an associated vasculitits. These can rupture and result in subarachnoid hemorrhage. None of these central nervous system features are common in patients with coccidioidomycosis, however. As with other fungal disorders, skeletal problems can occur, although they are infrequent. They tend to be present in about 10–20% of individuals who develop disseminated disease [27,57].

HISTOPLASMOSIS

Histoplasmosis occurring as a primary disorder results from the inhalation of *Histoplasma capsulatum* spores, and 60–90% of such cases only either exhibit no symptoms or a complex of mild respiratory symptoms resembling those of the common cold. The next most serious group of symptoms are those that have been described for other primary fungal disorders. Usually, the presentation resembles an influenza-like syndrome. As with other fungal disorders, *erythema nodosum* and *erythema muti-forme* may also occasionally occur in the early stages. Individuals who develop significant symptoms resulting in laboratory work-up may have bilateral bronchial, pneumonia-like changes on chest radiographs, or there may simply be a single solitary pulmonary nodule or multiple pulmonary nodules. Regional lymphadenopathy is also a common finding, but pulmonary effusions are uncommon. Rarely, patients develop active cavitary lesions, with healing and scarring and other changes producing a process very much like tuberculosis. Some individuals have healed pulmonary lesions, which may be confused with lung carcinoma and result in unwarranted surgery.

Disseminated histoplasmosis develops in an extremely small number of individuals (estimated at less than 1 per 50,000 cases of primary histoplasmosis). Clinical disseminated histoplasmosis may have multiple organ-system involvement, including hepatosplenomagly, generalized lymphadenopathy, fever, night sweats, anorexia, weight loss, anemia, and leukopenia. These findings also may be confused with tuberculosis. In some individuals, adrenal insufficiency occurs as a result of adrenal gland involvement and subsequent development of full-blown Addison's disease. In most individuals with disseminated disease, there is also concomitant immunodeficiency of some type. This disorder can be extremely serious in individuals with AIDS, as often there is rapid development of rapidly progressive histoplasmosis and central nervous system involvement. Occasionally, histoplasmosis may be the prominent finding upon presentation in patients with AIDS. Other individuals with impaired immune systems, including those with childhood leukemia and those who have had organ transplantation or have a disorder for which they are receiving long-term immunosuppressive therapy, may be particularly predisposed to the development of disseminated histoplasmosis. Again, histoplasmosis should be suspected in individuals who have returned from travel into areas known to be endemic or who have been involved in activities such as recreation in areas suspected to be infested by bats or heavily populated by birds [14,17, 23,58–60].

SPOROTRICHOSIS

Sporotrichosis, a fungal infection caused by the organism *Sporothrix schenckii*, differs from other systemic mycosis in that it is most commonly acquired through spore implantation in the skin, resulting in a painless ulcer or a subcutaneous nodule that is raised and surrounded by pink-to-purplish discoloration. This lesion then often breaks down to become a necrotic chancre-like lesion. There is usually extensive involvement of the draining lesional lymph nodes. These become swollen, and some suppuration may occur. Most of these patients have localized pain or serious disability. A systemic response presenting as fever, night sweats, or weight loss may occur in some patients. In an extremely small number of patients, disseminated pulmonary infections have occurred. In this group, the infection commonly mimics tuberculosis and resembles the other systemic mycoses, with manifestations such as hilar adenopathy and cavitary disease. There is often an associated persistent pulmonary infiltrate. It is assumed that this occurs when the spores are inhaled via the respiratory route of entry. In individuals who develop disseminated sporotrichosis, the onset is usually insidious and is characterized by low-grade fever and other symptoms mimicking tuberculosis. The major targets of these infections seem to be bones and joints rather than other organs of the body. There is sometimes a multifocal form of arthritis, with knee, ankle, wrist, and elbow involvement being most common. It is extremely rare to see widespread dissemination, although involvement of skin, mouth, nasal mucosa, and the central nervous system may occur, especially in individuals with immune system deficiencies or advanced metastatic cancer, diabetes, alcoholism, or lymphoproliferative diseases (34–36).

Differential Diagnosis

SYSTEMIC MYCOSES

Infections caused by endemic fungi or other opportunistic organisms have been increasingly studied over the past 25 or more years. With increasing emphasis has come the recognition of significant differences between the various types of infections, the pathology associated with the specific causative organisms and, consequently, the ability to differentiate between them.

Just 25 years ago, some medical textbooks still referred to cryptococcosis and blastomycosis as the same disorder [61]. As pointed out above, there are in fact many similarities between the endemic mycotic infections in their clinical presentations, and in most instances they may all present with minimal clinical findings and transient respiratory symptoms, with the only evidence of infection in the form of serologic evidence or a positive skin test. When the diseases become manifest, there are clinical similarities among them, but there are also some distinctive differences. Diagnosis requires suspecting their presence and, most often, first differentiating between infection due to one of these agents and pulmonary tuberculosis, using a combination of radiography, skin testing, and culture of tissue samples. Often, these fungal infections must also be distinguished from cancer of the lung or other organs, as they are often misdiagnosed, sometimes resulting in unneeded surgery. It is also critical that a distinction be made, particularly in the presence of cryptococcosis and blastomycosis, so that treatment with corticosteroids does not ensue for a mistaken diagnosis of some other condition. Such improper treatment aids in the production of widespread dissemination and aggressive behavior of the infection.

It is important to be aware of a traveler's exposure, potential susceptibilities, and risks. Risk behavior among travelers is important, as this may sometimes determine the likelihood of their acquiring a fungal or mycotic disorder. In instances in which the agent is demonstrated, as for instance, in blastomycosis, the exact strain is of importance, and distinctions can be made, for example, between the African *Blastomyces dermatitidis* strain and those found in the United States and other parts of the world [51].

Definitive diagnosis of blastomycosis is made by the successful growth of the organism in culture. Sputum or pus from cutaneous lesions, biopsy material, or prostatic secretions are usually used in the culture process and inoculated into several Sabouraud's dextrose agar. The process usually requires approximately 30 days of growth at room temperature of 30°C. The growth samples are then treated, and diagnosis is made by examination, using the appropriate techniques and the light microscope. Exfoliative cytology using Papanicolaou's method is useful in the examination of pulmonary secretions from patients with respiratory involvement. Immunologic methods are also helpful in the diagnosis. These are addressed in more detail in the section following on biologic testing [6,23,62,63].

Coccidioides immitis may be diagnosed if the characteristic spherules can be demonstrated on direct wet mount preparation of pus or sputum. The endospores are classic and, if demonstrated, confirm the diagnosis. In addition, this agent is also easily cultured on Sabouraud's dextrose agar. Immunologic response to the organism is usually demonstrated within two to 21 days after symptoms appear, and skin testing with the antigen can confirm the presence of infection. Appropriate precautions should be taken with skin testing because of the potential for severe reaction, particularly if testing is done during a time when the lesions of *erythema nodosum* are present. Other laboratory tests, including testing for the presence of antibodies in the spinal fluid and cytology of the spinal fluid, are also helpful. In many patients with mild or asymptomatic disease, complement-fixation IGG antibodies may develop. If they do, they are also useful in confirming the diagnosis [26,55].

The diagnosis of histoplasmosis depends on the isolation of *Histoplasma capsulatum* in culture. The usual specimens to be cultured are sputum, blood, and urine. In disseminated disease, bone marrow and/or lymph-node biopsy culture and tissue sections are useful. Culture of blood from involved organs and particle sections from marrow aspirates may also be helpful. Serologic tests are probably more useful than *Histoplasma* skin tests. Additional discussion of serologic implications may be found in the following section on biologic testing [30,32,62,64].

The usual clinical presentation of sporotrichosis is an ulcerated nodule on the dorsal hand, followed by the appearance of similar cutaneous nodules that spread in a linear fashion along lines of lymphatic drainage. The definitive diagnosis of *Sporotrichosis* requires isolation of the organism on culture and subsequent microscopic examination for confirmation. Direct microscopic examination of pus and biopsy material is not usually helpful in making this diagnosis, and other demonstration of the characteristic cigar-shaped organisms in infected tissue is difficult. Biopsies of the lesions may hinder the healing process and spread the organism. Material should be aspirated from the suspected lesions and cultured on glucose neopeptome argar. This results in the growth of a brownish-black mycelium within a few days after inoculation if the patient has this infection. Antibody to *Sporothrix schencii* appears in the serum and cerebrospinal fluid and is useful for confirmation. *Sporotrichosis* must be distinguished from atypical microbacterial infections caused by *Microbacterium marinum*, which it may mimic [33].

SUPERFICIAL MYCOSES

Skin infections are prevalent worldwide but particularly in warm, tropical climates. Various bacteria cause the most common and potentially harmful skin infections; however, a significant number are caused by fungi and molds. Effective management requires differentiation between bacterial and fungal etiology and then identification of the specific type of fungus. The cutaneous lesions of secondary syphilis are quite varied and often affect the palms and soles. In the tropics, yaws, caused by *Treponema pertenue* or *Treponemici carateum*, must be considered in evaluating many skin infections. Fungal infections may be superficial or deep, and they are most common in hot, humid climates. The majority of superficial fungal skin infections are caused by dermatophytes and develop in a nonspecific fashion (particularly involving the groin and feet), since the presence of moisture, sweat, and heat promotes fungal growth. Dermatophytes may infect the fingernails and hands of those with frequent wet exposures. Superficial infections of the body or the groin are common; they appear as reddish, flat, ring-shaped lesions that are dry and scaly or moist and crusty. Deep fungal infections are more serious and promptly should be treated by a physician.

Tricophyton rubrum typically causes a dry, scaly, sometimes painful eruption of the palms, which for some unknown reason is characteristically present on only one hand of the affected individual, sparing the other. Evidence of *T rubrum* infection can usually be found elsewhere on the body, particularly the toenails and soles. Wet work dries the skin of the affected palm even further, exacerbating the symptoms, and the individual often notices improvement when the wet exposure is discontinued. A scaling eruption confined to the palm of one hand should immediately prompt examination of the feet and a search for fungus.

Zoophilic fungi (i.e., those with animal reservoirs) may specifically infect handlers of animals. Travelers should be cautious about adopting pets whose hygiene and general state of health are unknown. Zoophilic *Tricophyton mentagrophytes* may be carried by a wide range of animals and these frequently produce an intense inflammatory cutaneous reaction with pustule formation. Lesions caused by *Microsporum canis* (dogs and cats) more typically have a ringworm-like appearance. *T verrucosum* is acquired from infected cattle and may produce a deep inflammatory reaction on the neck, beard, or scalp. Diagnosis is established by demonstrating fungal hyphae on KOH examination of scales or hair from infected skin. Warm, moist environments may nonspecifically predispose travelers to several types of infections due to *Candida albicans.* As with dermatophyte infections, *Candida* infections may develop in intertriginous body surfaces (the groin, axilla, and inframammary skin). Infection of the fingernail folds (paronychia) can appear in virtually anyone whose hands are constantly exposed to moisture, and paronychia is often caused by *Candida*. The clinical appearance is a red, swollen, mildly to moderately painful nail fold, which does not suppurate with local destruction of cuticle. Erosive dermatitis from *Candida* infections occasionally occurs in the web spaces between the fingers. *Candida* in the form of groin infection and vaginitis may also occur as an infection in travelers who had sexual contact during their time away [45,47,65–67].

Specific points to keep in mind when evaluating suspected skin infections are:

- If the skin has tiny bumps or sores, with much itching between the fingers and the wrist, the individual may have scabies, not a fungus.
- If the skin has red scaly patches with itching between the toes or on the bottom of the feet, the individual may be suffering from a fungus infection, such as candidiasis.
- If the skin has pimples or sores, the individual may be suffering from a bacterial and not a fungal infection.
- If you cannot classify a skin infection into a specific category, then take biopsy samples of the skin and send them to a laboratory for examination and culture. Skin scrapings may also be used in some cases.

A diagnostic questionnaire may be useful in making differentiation between skin infections. When used, it should include these questions:

- Where are the lesions?
- How big are they and how many are there?
- Are the lesions symmetrical?
- What shape are the lesions, and what did the first one look like?
- What color are the lesions?
- Are the lesions flat or raised? Are they solid or fluid filled?
- Are the lesions wet or dry?
- What do the borders of the lesions look like?
- Do the lesions itch?
- How fast did the lesions develop?

Biologic Testing

Culture of body fluids and tissue for fungus continues to be the diagnostic mainstay for identifying specific systemic fungal diseases. It is important to note, however, that definitive identification by culture may require as long as four weeks. A presumptive diagnosis is frequently made on the basis of the characteristic histopathology and special tissue stains, including periodic acid-Schiff (PAS) and Gomori-methenamine silver (GMS). Skin tests with antigens such as *Histoplasma spherulin* generally have no role in the diagnosis of active disease. Serologic tests have limited value for most fungal diseases because of low specificity and sensitivity; however, there are exceptions, which include the latex agglutination test for cryptococcal antigens in patients with suspected cryptococcosis. The complement fixation and immunodiffusion tests for coccidioidomycosis and paracoccidioidomycosis are also useful. Serologic tests for the diagnosis of blastomycosis have had improved results with the use of immunoassay (EIA), utilizing A-antigen of *Blastomyces dermatitidis.* The standard serologic tests for diagnosis of histoplasmosis include the complement fixation test (CF), which is quite sensitive, and the immunodiffusion test (ID), which is fairly specific. Radioimmunoassay (RIA) is an experimental serologic test that is even more sensitive than CF but also less specific. Problems with the specificity of serodiagnosis continue to occur. At present, highly specific and sensitive serologic tests are not available for early and rapid diagnosis of candidiasis and aspergillosis, the two most common and clinically important opportunistic fungal diseases in immunocompromised hosts [24,44,68–71].

Investigational approaches that show promise in improving the diagnosis and monitoring of systemic mycoses include:

- Detection of unique fungal metabolites by gas liquid chromatography or antigen/antibody-based methods.
- Detection of immunodominant fungal antigens by radioimmunoassay, ELISA, latex agglutination, or immunoblot test.
- Use of molecular probes, e.g., polymerase chain reaction, to detect fungal DNA [68].

Drug Therapy

SYSTEMIC MYCOSES

At present, the five licensed antifungal drugs that are the most important and commonly used agents against the systemic fungal diseases are amphotericin B, flucytosine, and the three azole drugs (ketoconazole, itraconazole, and fluconazole). Ergosterol, the principal sterol in the fungal cytoplasmic membrane, is the target site of action of amphotericin B and the azoles. Amphotericin B, a polyene, binds irreversibly to ergosterol, resulting in disruption of membrane integrity and ultimately cell death. The azole drugs inhibit synthesis of ergosterol through an interaction with the cytochrome P–450 dependent enzyme, 14 alpha demethylase, necessary for the conversion of lanosterol to ergosterol. By contrast, flucytosine, an oral-fluorinated pyrimidine, inhibits both fungal DNA and RNA protein synthesis.

While these drugs are effective therapies for many of the systemic mycoses, including blastomycosis, candidiasis, cryptococcosis, histoplasmosis, and sporotrichosis, they are only minimally or moderately effective for aspergillosis, coccidioidomycosis, non-*albicans* candidiasis, and phaeohy-phomycosis caused by diatomaceous molds. Moreover, these drugs may involve other problems. Amphotericin B, considered by some authorities to be the "gold standard" because of its broad spectrum of activity and fungicidal action, is available only as an intravenous formulation in the United States, requiring continuous intravenous access, and is associated with significant dose-limiting toxicity, especially nephrotoxicity. Flucytosine also has the potential for considerable toxicity, especially affecting the bone marrow, liver, gastrointestinal tract, and skin. As a result, this drug has never been optimally utilized. Although development of the azole class of drugs is an important advance and offers effective and safe alternatives to amphotericin B and flucytosine for many of the systemic mycoses, the azoles are not ideal drugs. Only fluconazole is available as both an oral and intravenous formulation. Amphotericin B, flucytosine, and the azoles are potentially hepatotoxic. They may inhibit steroid hormone synthesis in humans and may also have the potential to interact with many classes of drugs (e.g., oral hypoglycemics, oral anticoagulants, phenytoin, cyclosporine, H_1 and H_2 receptor antagonists, rifampin), with serious sequelae. *Candida* species resistant to fluconazole are an increasing cause of concern in AIDS patients and other immunocompromised hosts exposed to fluconazole as a prophylacitc drug over extended periods.

The toxicity and other problems associated with the currently available antifungal drugs make development of new treatment approaches critical. Current efforts in antifungal drug development are focused on:

- Drugs with novel fungal cell targets.
- Investigational azole and allylamine drugs.
- Novel formulations of currently licensed drugs.

With regard to novel fungal cell targets, an important difference between fungi and mammalian cells is that the fungal cell envelope consists of a cell wall, composed primarily of three carbohydrates: glycan and chitin, mannoproteins, and the cytoplasmic membrane. By contrast, cell walls are not found in mammalian cells and other eukaryotic cells. Available evidence indicates that drugs which target fungal cell wall structures do not adversely affect mammalian cells; thus, the potential for toxicity of such drugs in humans is reduced.

Examples of investigational drugs that interrupt formation of the unique fungal cell walls include:

1. Nikkomycins, which inhibit chitin synthesis.
2. The echinocandin/pneumocandin/lipopeptide class, which inhibits glycan synthesis.
3. Pradimicins, which exhibit calcium-dependent binding to mannan (mannoprotein).
4. The investigational azole drugs, under development by several pharmaceutical companies, which have the potential to outperform the currently licensed azoles, ketoconazole, itraconazole, and fluconazole, in terms of broader spectrum of activity, increased efficacy, and less toxicity.
5. The allylamines, a new class of drugs, which inhibit squalene epoxidase, another enzyme in the biosynthetic pathway of ergosterol.

Novel formulations of currently licensed drugs are aimed at enhancing the efficacy and reducing the toxicity of the parent compound. There are two classes of drugs in this group. The first class is lipid formulations of amphotericin B, including liposomal amphotericin B (AmBisome), amphotericin B colloidal dispersion (Amphocil), and amphotericin B lipid complex (ABLC). Enveloping amphotericin B in liposomes or complexing the drug with lipids offers several advantages of the novel formulations over conventional amphotericin B, which is complexed in desoxycholate, a bile salt.

These potential advantages include:

- Up to a five- to 10-fold increase in daily dose of amphotericin B, thereby increasing the therapeutic index.
- Less nephrotoxicity, the major limiting toxic effect of conventional amphotericin B.
- Tropism for reticuloendothelial organs such as lymph nodes, liver, and spleen, where fungi typically are in contrast to the tropism of conventional amphotericin B for kidneys.
- Preferential binding of lipid-formulated drugs to fungal cell membranes, which may have efficacy in some patients who have failed or cannot tolerate conventional amphotericin B.

New oral and intravenous preparations of itraconazole represent a second class of novel formulations. Itraconazole, currently available only for oral administration, is a weak base that requires an acid environment for optimal solubilization and absorption. The bioavailability of itraconazole is increased when it is formulated in hydoxypropyl-beta-cyclodextrin, a cyclic oligosaccharide carrier molecule that increases the solubility of lipophilic compounds in aqueous solutions. Hydroxypropyl-beta-cyclodextrin itraconazole may be especially helpful in selected clinical situations, such as for AIDS patients with achlorhydria or receiving concurrent drugs that impair absorption, or critically ill hospitalized patients who cannot take oral medications [68,73–78].

Invasive fungal diseases are increasingly observed in immunocompromised patients, especially those with protracted granulocytopenia secondary to neoplastic disease or cytotoxic chemotherapy, transplant recipients receiving immunosuppressive drugs such as high-dose corticosteroids and cyclosporine, and AIDS patients with progressively declining CD4+ T cells and other perturbations in immune function. Current evidence indicates that adequate number and function of granulocytes, as well as intact cell-mediated immunity, are keys to successful outcome in patients with opportunistic yeast and mold diseases. Cellular immunity also plays an important role in the host's containment of the endemic mycoses. Far and away the most common fungal infection associated with HIV infection is *candidiasis.* This tends to produce mucosal topical infections, and local treatment may be enough to control them (generally a course of one to two weeks, rather than chronic suppression, for fear of eliciting resistance). Fluconazole-resistant *Candida* species may be an increasing problem. For cryptococcosis, the problem is complicated. Fluconazole is highly effective for chronic suppression but not effective for initial therapy. A short course of amphotericin B for two weeks should be followed by long-term azole suppression. Fluconazole appears excellent, but itraconazole may also be effective. For histoplasmosis, itraconazole appears to be the most advantageous drug, producing an excellent clinical response within two weeks [68,79].

Immunomodulators may become important adjuncts to therapy for systemic mycoses. Recent in vitro and animal in vivo data suggest a role in the management of fungal diseases for the expanding array of recombinant cytokines, especially interferon-gamma, the colony-stimulating factors, the various interleukins or interleukin antagonists, as well as for monoclonal antibodies passive immunotherapy. Trials of these agents performed in humans with fungal disease have been limited [68].

SUPERFICIAL MYCOSES (FUNGAL SKIN DISEASES)

Skin infections can often be treated by topical (surface) treatments alone. Sometimes, it is necessary to take systemic (internal) medications. The following major rules apply:

1. If the lesion is wet, treat it with a dry dressing; if the lesion is dry, treat it with a cream or ointment.
2. If the lesion oozes, itches, or stings, treat it with cold compresses; if the lesion is hot, treat it with elevation and warm compresses.
3. Begin with the least potent treatment; work up to the most potent treatment only if necessary.

Topical antifungal agents may be broadly divided into specific and nonspecific agents. The former include the polyenes, azoles, allylamines, amorolfine, ciclopirox, and butenafine. Generally, the topical agent is available as a cream, sometimes for use intravaginally. Less commonly, the formulation may be in the form of a powder, lacquer, spray, gel, or solution. Many of these agents have a broad spectrum of activity, including activity against dermatophytes, yeasts, and *Malassezia furfur*. Most superficial fungal infections can be treated only with topical agents. Ointments, lotions, and creams placed into the kit given to individuals should include tolnaftate, clotrimazole, miconazole, ketoconazole, Whitfield's (benzoic and salicylic acid) ointment, Castellani Paint, potassium permanganate (1:10,000 solution), and silver nitrate (1:400 solution). Any or all of these can be effectively utilized, as appropriate. Superficial dermatophyte infections (on the general body surface) may be treated with topical imidazole antifungal preparations. Infections of the palms, soles, and nails and deep inflammatory reactions on hair-bearing surfaces do not generally respond well to topical agents, and oral therapy (250–500 mg of microsize griseofulvin, or its equivalent, two times per day) is preferred. Oral ketoconazole also has been used for treatment of dermatophyte infections. Chronic paronychia may need to be treated for months. Sulconazole nitrate has been used effectively for the treatment of skin infections in tropical Africa [43,46,67,80,81].

References

1. Steffen R, Raeber PA. Risks for Travelers. *Med Trop* 1997;54(4Bis):423.
2. Centers for Disease Control and Prevention. *Health Information for International Travel 1997–98*. Atlanta: CDC, 1998.
3. Rose SSR. *International Travel Health Guide*. McNaughton and Gunn, 1993.
4. Wolf MS. Preparing employees for international travel. *J Occup Med* 1977;19(10):671.
5. Wilson ME, von Reyn CF, Fineberg HV. Infections in HIV-infected travelers: risks and prevention. *Ann Intern Med* 1991;114(7):582–92.
6. Bradshear RW. Blastomycosis. *Clin Infect Dis* 1992; 14(Suppl 1):SA2.
7. Wheat J. Endemic mycoses in AIDS: a clinical review. *Clin Microbiol Rev* 1995;8(1):146.
8. Myer KC, McManus DJ, Makai DG. Overwhelming pulmonary blastomycosis associated with the adult respiratory distress syndrome. *N Engl J Med* 1993;329: 1231.
9. Sarosi GA, Davies SF. Endemic mycosis complicating human immunodeficiency virus infection. *West J Med* 1996;164(4):335.
10. Pappas PG. Blastomycosis in the immunocompromised patient. *Semin Respir Infect* 1997;12(3):243.
11. Cooper CR Jr, McGinnis MR. Pathology of *Penicillium marneffei*: an emerging acquired immunodeficiency syndrome-related pathogen. *Arch Pathol Lab Med* 1997;121(8):798.
12. Duong TA. Infection due to *Penicillium marneffei*, an emerging pathogen: review of 155 reported cases. *Clin Infect Dis* 1996;23(1):125.
13. Nittayananta W, Chungpanich S. Oral lesions in a group of Thai people with AIDS. *Oral Dis* 1997;3(Suppl 1):S41–5.
14. Suzaki A, Kimura M, Kimura F, et al. An outbreak of acute pulmonary histoplasmosis among travelers to a bat-inhabited cave in Brazil. *Kansen Shogaku Zasshi* 1995;69(4):444.
15. National Institute for Allergy and Infectious Diseases. *Fungal Diseases—A Public Health Problem*. Fact sheet. Bethesda, MD: NIAID, 1996.

16. Beck-Sague CM, Jarvis WR, and the NNIS. Secular trends in the epidemiology of nosocomial fungal infections in the United States, 1980–1990. *J Infect Dis* 1993;167:1247–51.

17. Miller LW, et al. Infection after heart transplantation: a multi-institutional study. Cardiac Transplant Research Database Group. *J Heart Lung Transplant* 1994;13: 381–92.

18. Pannuti CS, et al. Nosocomial pneumonia in adult patients undergoing bone marrow transplantation. *J Clin Oncol* 1991;9(1):77–84.

19. *AIDS Surveillance Quarterly Update for Cases Reported through September 1994.* (NY State Department of Health).

20. Marriott DJ, Wong KH, Harkness JL, et al.: *Seytalidium dimidiatum* and *Lecthophora hoffmanni:* unusual causes of fungal infections in a patient with AIDS. *J Clin Microbiol* 35(11):2949–52

21. Marriott DJ, Huang KH, Aznar E, et al. *Scytalidium dimidiatum* and *Lecythophora hoffmanni*: unusual causes of fungal infections in a patient with AIDS. *J Clin Microbiol* 1997;35(11):2949.

22. Taylor ML, Perez-Mejia A, Yamamoto-Furusho JK, et al. Immunologic, genetic and social human risk factors associated to histoplasmosis: studies in the state of Guerrero, Mexico. *Mycopathologia* 1997;138(3):137.

23. Davies SF, Sarosi GA. Epidemiological and clinical features of pulmonary blastomycosis. *Semin Respir Infect* 1997;12(3):206.

24. Gueho E, Leclerc MC, deHoog GS, et al. Molecular taxonomy and epidemiology of *Blastomyces* and *Histoplasma* species. *Mycoses* 1997;40(3–4):69.

25. Bradsher RW. Clinical features of blastomycosis. *Semin Respir Infect* 1997;12(3):229.

26. Stevens DA. Coccidioidomycosis. *N Engl J Med* 1995;332(16):1077–82.

27. Centers for Disease Control and Prevention. Update: Coccidioidomycosis/California, 1991–1993. *MMWR*, 1994;43:421–3.

28. Baumgardner DJ, Burdick JS. An outbreak of human and canine blastomycosis. *Red Infect Dis* 1991;13:898.

29. Vaaler AK, Bradshear RW, Davies SF. Evidence of subclinical blastomycosis in forest workers in northern Minnesota and northern Wisconsin. *Am J Med* 1990;89: 470.

30. Bradsher RW. Histoplasmosis and blastomycosis. *Clin Infect Dis Suppl* 1996;2:8102.

31. Reder PA, Neil HB III. Blastomycosis in otolaryngology: review of a large series. *Laryngoscope* 1993; 103(1pt1):53.

32. Wheat J. Histoplasmosis. Experience during outbreaks in Indianapolis and review of the literature. *Medicine (Baltimore)* 1997;76(5):339.

33. Winn RE. Systemic fungal infections: diagnosis and treatment: I. sporotrichosis. *Infect Dis Clin North Am* 1988;2:899.

34. Heller HM, Fuhrer J. Disseminated sporotrichosis in patients with AIDS: case report and review of the literature. *AIDS* 1991;5:1243.

35. Vierira-Dias D, Sena CM, Orefice F, et al. Ocular and concomitant cutaneous sporotrichosis mycoses. 1997;40(5–6):197–201.

36. Crampuz A, Zimmerli W. HIV-associated lung diseases. *Schweiz MED, Wochenschr* 1997;127(42):1725–33.

37. Johnson MA, Lyle G, Hanley M, et al. Aspergillus: a rare primary organism in soft tissue. *Am Surg* 1998;64(2):122–6.

38. Cooper CR Jr, McGinnis MR. Pathology of *Penicillium marneffeii* an emerging acquired immunodeficiency syndrome-related pathogen. *Arch Pathol Lab Med* 1997;121(8):798–804.

39. Dong TA. Infection due to *Penicillium marneffei*, an emerging pathogen: Review of 155 reported cases. *Clin Infect Dis* 1996;23(1):125–30.

40. Baranguer J, Rodriguez-Tudela JL, Richard C, et al. Deep infections caused by *Scedosporium prolificans:* a report on 16 cases in Spain and a review of the literature. *Scedosporium prolificans* Spanish Study Group. *Medicine (Baltimore)* 1997;76:256.

41. Chiu NC, Chung YF, Huang FY. Pediatric nosocomial fungal infections. *Southeast A N J Prop Med Public Health* 1997;28(1):191.

42. Roth RR, James WD. Microbiology of the skin: resident flora, ecology, infection. *J Am Acad Dermatol* 1989;20:367.

43. Bottoni U, Dianzani C, Rossi ME, et al. Skin diseases in immigrants seen as outpatients in the Institute of Dermatology at the University of Rome La Spaienza from 1989 to 1994. *Aur J Epidemiol* 1998;12(2):201.

44. DeVroey C. Epidemiology of ringworm. *Semin Dermatol* 1985;4:185.

45. Macura AB. Dermatophyte infections. *Int J Dermatol* 1993;32:313.

46. Gupta AK, Einarson TR, Summerbell RC, et al. An overview of topical antifungal therapy in dermatomycoses: a North American perspective. *Drugs* 1998;55(5):645–74.

47. Abraham AG, Kulp-Shorten CL, Callen JP. Remember to consider dermatophyte infection when dealing with recalcitrant dermatoses. *South Med J* 1998;91(4):349.

48. Wolf R, Movshowitz M, Brenner S. Supplemental tests in the evaluation of occupational hand dermatitis in soldiers. *Int J Dermatol* 1996;35(3):173.

49. Brown LR, Swenson SJ, VanScoy RE, et al. Roentgenologic features of pulmonary blastomycosis. *Mayo Clin Proc* 1991;66(1):29–38.

50. Winer-Muram HT, Reuben SA. Pulmonary blastomycosis. *J Thorac Imaging* 1992;7(4):23.

51. Mercantini R, Marsella R, Moretto D, et al. Macroscopic and microscopic characteristics of an African *Blastomyces* dermatididis strain. *Macroscopic Mycoses* 1995;38(11–12):477.

52. Sondergaard J, Weismann K, Vithayasai P, et al. Ethnic and geographic differences and similarities of HIV/AIDS-related mucocutaneous diseases. Danida Study Groups. *Int J Dermatol* 1995;34(6):416.

53. Mahaffey KW, Hippenmeyer CL, Mandel R, et al. *Unrecognized coccidioidomycosis* complicating *Pneumocystis carinii* pneumonia in patients infected with the human immunodeficiency virus and treated with cortical steroids: a report of two cases. *Arch Intern Med* 1993;153:1496.

54. Masuda K, Kumamoto K, Machida T. A surgical case of right pulmonary coccidioidomycoses—with subcutaneous coccidioidomycosis in the left wrist. *Nippon Kyobu Geka Gakkai Zafshi* 1997;45(10):1770–3.

55. Standaert SM, Schaffener W, Galgiani JN, et al. Coccidioidomycosis among visitors to a *Coccidioides immitis* endemic area: an outbreak in a military reserve unit. *J Infect Dis* 1995;171(6):1672–5.

56. Oudiz R, Mahaisavariya P, Peng SK, et al. Disseminated coccidioidomycosis with rapid progression to effusive-constrictive pericarditis. *J Am Soc Echocardiogr* 1995;8(6):947–52.

57. Vincent T, Galgiani JN, Huppert M, et al. The natural history of coccidioidal meningitis: VA–Armed Forces Cooperative Studies, 1955–1958. *Clin Infect Dis* 1993;16:247.

58. Wheat J. Histoplasmosis in the acquired immunodeficiency syndrome. *Curr Top Med Mycol* 1996;7(1):7.

59. Wheat LJ, Batteiger BE, Sathapatayavongs B. *Histoplasma capsulatum* infections of the central nervous system: a clinical review. *Medicine (Baltimore)* 1990;69:244.

60. Wheat LJ, Connolly-Stringfield PA, Baker RL, et al. Disseminated histoplasmosis in the acquired immune deficiency syndrome: clinical findings, diagnosis and treatment, and review of the literature. *Medicine (Baltimore)* 1990;69:361.

61. Hart FD. *French's Index of Differential Diagnosis*, 10th Ed. Baltimore: Williams & Wilkins, 1973. P 327.

62. Davies SF, Sarosi GA. Serodiagnosis of histoplasmosis and blastomycosis (editorial). *Am Rev Respir Dis* 1987;136(2):254.

63. Davies SF, Sarosi GA. Role of serodiagnostic tests and skin tests in the diagnosis of fungal disease. *Clin Chest Med* 1987;8(1):135.

64. Davies SF. Serodiagnosis of histoplasmosis. *Semin Respir Infect* 1986;1(1):9–15.

65. Rosatelli JB, Machado AA, Roselino AM. Dermatoses among Brazilian HIV positive patients: correlation with the evolutionary phases of AIDS. *Int J Termalog* 1997;36(10):729.

66. Henseler T, Tausch I. Mycosis in patients with psoriasis or atopic dermatitis. *Mycoses* 1997;40(Suppl 1):22.

67. Schmeller W, Baumgartner F, Dzikus A. Dermatophytomycoses in children in rural Kenya: the impact of primary health care. *Mycoses* 1997;40(1–2):55.

68. The National Institute of Allergy and Infectious Diseases. *The Second NIAID Workshop in Medical Mycology: Molecular and Immunological Approaches to the Diagnosis and Treatment of Systemic Mycoses, Status and Limitations of Diagnosis and Therapy of Systemic Fungal Infections*, 1996.

69. Wheat J, Wheat H, Connolly P, et al. Cross-reactivity in *Histoplasma capsulatum* variety capsulatum antigen assays of urine samples from patients with endemic mycoses. *Clin Infect Dis* 1997;24(6):1169–71.

70. Bradshear W, Pappas PG. Detection of specific antibodies in human blastomycosis by enzyme immunoassay. *South Med J* 1995;88(12):1256–9.

71. Cunningham ET Jr, Seiff SR, Berger TG, et al. Intraocular coccidioidomycosis diagnosed by skin biopsy. *Arch Ophthalmol* 1998;116(5):674.

72. Mangiaterra M, Alonso J, Galvan M, et al. Histoplasmin and paracoccidioidin skin reactivity in infantile population of Northern Argentina (1). *Rev Insp Med Trop (Sao Paulo)* 1996;38(5):349.

73. Wheat J, Hafner R, Korzun AH, et al. Intraconazole treatment of disseminated histoplasmosis in patients with the acquired immunodeficiency syndrome. AIDS Clinical Trial Group. *Am J Med* 1995;98(4):336–42.

74. Wheat J, Merichal P, Vanden Bossche H, et al. Hypothesis on the mechanism of resistance to fluconazole in *Histoplasma capsulatum*. Antimicrobes agents. *Chemother* 1997;41(2):410–4.

75. Mirels LF, Stevens DA. Update on treatment of coccidioidomycosis. *West J Med* 1997;166(4):291.

76. Stevens DA. Adequacy of therapy for coccidioidomycosis (editorial): Comment. *Clin Infect Dis* 1997;25(5):1205–10.

77. Bradsher RW. Therapy of blastomycosis. *Semin Respir Infect* 1997;12(3):263.

78. Pappas PG, Bradsher RW, Kauffman CA, et al. Treatment of blastomycosis with higher doses of fluconazole. The National Institute of Allergy and Infectious Diseases Mycosis Study Group. *Clin Infect Dis* 1997;25(2):200.

79. Graybill JR. Treatment of systemic mycoses in patients with AIDS. *Arch Med Res* 1993;24(4):403.

80. Gugnani HC, Gugnani A, Malachy O. Sulconazole in the therapy of dermatomycosis in Nigeria. *Mycosis* 1997;40(3–4):139.

81. Brautigam M, Nolting S, Schopf RE, et al. Randomised double blind comparison of trebinafine and itraconazole for treatment of toenail tinea infection. *Br Med J* 1995;311:919.

III / Unique Problems and Settings

32 / Occupational Infections in Pregnant Employees

Lori Checkley

During the twentieth century, the number of women seeking employment outside the home has steadily increased. By the year 2000, women will constitute 45% of the Western world's work force [1]. As a result, the impact of occupationally acquired infections on pregnant women is a growing concern. About 3% of newborn infants have serious congenital malformations; fetal and neonatal infections contribute to only about 5% of these [1]. Infections during pregnancy can have devastating effects on the developing fetus and mother. While the majority of infectious exposures that pregnant women face are outside the workplace, certain occupations do increase the risk of acquired fetal infections. Obviously, some occupations, such as health care workers, day care workers, teachers and animal handlers, are at increased risk for exposure. However, any job that involves interaction between the employee and other people, animals, or biologic materials could potentially involve exposure to infections. For example, contact with crowds of people, either during work in a busy office or while traveling to work, increases exposure to common infections. Most people would not consider these exposures to be occupationally acquired.

Pregnant women, and those desiring to become pregnant, are generally protected from exposure to occupationally acquired infection by following the standard safety procedures used to protect all workers. Unfortunately, it must be kept in mind that workers often do not follow recommended workplace safety precautions [2]. Many times, a woman is unaware she is pregnant during a significant portion of the first trimester, which is the time of highest risk for development of congenital malformations due to exposure to teratogens of any type, including infectious diseases. Therefore, the strategy of removing pregnant employees from certain duties or increasing their protection at conception has a high failure rate in preventing fetal and neonatal infections [3]. The most effective strategy is to educate all workers to use standard safety procedures and to emphasize to reproductive-age women the fetal risks that can occur during the time period between conception and diagnosis of pregnancy.

Infection during the prenatal period can wreak havoc with the developing fetus in myriad ways. Possibilities include any of the well-known fetal syndromes, from congenital anomalies associated with rubella infection contracted during the first trimester to the more general disorders such as fetal malformation or miscarriage or preterm delivery, which may result from any significant maternal illness or fever [4]. Certain diseases have a higher virulence in the pregnant woman herself—for example, varicella, which has a higher morbidity and mortality in pregnant women [5]. In addition, even those diseases whose course is unaffected by pregnancy may have treatments that pose risks to the fetus, such as certain antimalarial medications. Some maternal illnesses, e.g., human immunodeficiency virus (HIV) and hepatitis B, have the potential to be passed directly to the baby either transplacentally or at the time of birth [6].

An exhaustive review of all possible occupational infectious exposures is beyond the scope of this chapter. The remainder of the chapter focuses on those specific occupations associated with increased risk to the pregnant woman, fetus, or neonate and the most common and significant infectious agents that may be involved.

Health Care Workers

Health care workers are obviously at high risk for occupational exposure to infectious diseases, since in the course of their work they are constantly exposed to infectious agents. Pregnant health care workers have special risks because of the potential transmission of infection to the developing fetus. Not only do health care workers routinely come into contact with people who are ill, but many of their job duties may expose them to highly concentrated infectious sources such as blood and body fluids. Included in this category are physicians, nurses, nurses' aides, respiratory therapists, phlebotomists, laboratory personnel, physical and occupational therapists, dentists and ancillary dental personnel, home health care aides, and others. Certainly, some of these occupations are at higher risk than others, but all entail caring for patients or some type of interaction with patients. Paramedics, emergency medical technicians, police, and firefighters also are at considerable risk for exposure to blood and body fluids when rendering aid to the ill or injured. Hospital maintenance workers and dieticians are at risk even though they do not perform direct patient care duties, as they are potentially exposed by their access to patient care areas, carelessly discarded needles, or contaminated waste.

There are three major modes of transmission of infectious microorganisms [7]. One mode is airborne, or respiratory, spread. The second is contact, either direct person-to-person contact with infectious materials, such as occurs in fecal-oral exposure, or indirect, for example, contact with contaminated equipment such as an endoscope contaminated with hepatitis B. Transmission via a common vehicle such as blood (as in HIV infection) or food (as in campylobacter or shigella infection) is the third category. The type of contact between the health care worker and the infected individual or contaminated object must be considered in order to determine if transmission of infection can occur [8]. Also, the susceptibility of the exposed individual is an important factor in determining the risk of infection to the pregnant health care worker and her fetus. Immunity can occur either by previous infection (e.g., varicella) or by vaccination (e.g., rubella). Therefore, for most infections, restrictions on the pregnant health care worker in caring for infectious patients is based on the worker's susceptibility to the particular infection, not pregnancy per se [8].

Some of the most common, and potentially serious infections that may be contracted in the health care setting are HIV, hepatitis B, hepatitis C, varicella, cytomegalovirus, enteroviruses, parvovirus, tuberculosis, measles, rubella, and influenza. Common strategies for prevention of most of these are use of Universal Precautions, vaccinations, and chemoprophylaxis, when available [9]. In the following paragraphs, concerns surrounding the pregnant health care worker and exposure to specific infections in the health care work environment are briefly discussed.

HUMAN IMMUNODEFICIENCY VIRUS

Pregnancy does not seem to increase susceptibility to HIV; therefore, risk of infection in the health care setting is not dependent on pregnancy status [8]. Risk of seroconversion to HIV-positive status is primarily determined by type of exposure. The exposure with the highest risk is deep puncture by a hollow needle contaminated with HIV-positive blood. Seroconversion following this type of exposure is estimated to be 0.3–0.5% [9,14]. Seroconversion after mucous membrane splash or cutaneous splash on nonintact skin is 0.1% and slightly less than 0.1%, respectively. The Centers for Disease Control and Prevention (CDC) had documented 51 confirmed cases of occupational transmission and 108 cases of possible transmission of HIV in health care workers by 1996 [15].

The Occupational Safety and Health Administration (OSHA) and CDC emphasize proper handling of blood and needles to prevent exposure [16,17]. These infection control practices should be universally followed by all employees, not just pregnant workers. In pregnant women, needlesticks and other types of HIV exposure should be handled in the same manner as exposures in any other employee [18]. In 1996, the

CDC issued recommendations for prophylaxis after occupational exposure to HIV, based on the type of exposure and source material [19]. For exposures with the highest risk, chemoprophylaxis with antiretroviral drugs is recommended.

The risk of vertical transmission of HIV to the fetus from an infected mother appears to be approximately 20–30%, depending on the study [8,10]. Transmission can occur in utero, intrapartum, or postpartum via breast milk [11–13]. Recent studies have clearly shown decreased vertical transmission of HIV to the fetuses of known HIV-positive women when azidothymidine (AZT) is administered during pregnancy [20,21]. Therefore, postexposure prophylaxis makes sense both from the perspective of preventing primary infection of the exposed worker and decreasing the rate of transmission to the fetus. In the case of lower risk exposures, such as contact of infected blood with intact skin, the decision regarding chemoprophylaxis should be made jointly by the worker and her health care providers after review of the potential for infection and the risk/benefit ration of antiretroviral therapy [3]. After a health care worker has an exposure to HIV, surveillance for seroconversion should be continued for a minimum of six months. Because of the rapid pace of research in HIV treatment and prevention, frequent changes in treatment protocols due to viral adaptations and the unfortunate lag-time inherent in the publishing of textbooks, physicians should periodically contact the CDC for the most up-to-date prophylactic regimen.

HEPATITIS B

Acute hepatitis B virus (HBV) is the causative agent in approximately 40–50% of viral hepatitis cases in the United States and occurs in about 1 in 1,000 pregnancies [22]. Pregnancy does not increase susceptibility to infection [3]. The incubation period for HBV averages four months; onset of clinical disease is manifested as nausea, vomiting, jaundice, right upper quadrant pain, and malaise. An estimated 5% of the U.S. population carries antibody evidence of past HBV infection and approximately 0.5% are chronic HBV carriers [23]. The long-term results of HBV infection are well documented: Five to 10% of adults infected with HBV develop chronic hepatitis with persistent infectivity, and 15–25% of those with chronic infection subsequently develop cirrhosis or hepatocellular carcinoma.

The overall rate of transmission of HBV from a mother with active infection to her fetus is unclear [23]. However, it is known that the rate if highest in the third trimester, occurring in approximately 75% of cases. How many of these are the result of infection at the time of birth rather than during gestation is unknown. Clearly, exposure to HBV is more likely to result in infection than exposure to HIV. For nonimmune health care workers, the risk of infection from needle puncture accidents involving HBV-contaminated blood is 20–40% [23]. Factors such as viral load, presence of HBV surface antigen, and E-antigen positivity influence the rate of transmission.

Any health care worker with exposure to blood, body fluids, contaminated needles, or equipment should be vaccinated with the HBV vaccine. Ideally, workers should be vaccinated as early as possible after deciding to embark on a career in health care. OSHA requires that the vaccine must be offered to all at-risk employees at the employer's expense [24]. Employees may refuse vaccination, but they must sign a waiver indicating their awareness of the risks of HBV infection. Pregnancy is not a contraindication for vaccination, as the vaccine contains no infectious material [25]. However, little data are available regarding its use in pregnancy and whether seroconversion rates may be lower for pregnant women [8]. Therefore, elective administration is usually delayed until after delivery. HBV exposure in pregnant workers is treated the same as that in nonpregnant workers: Protocols are based on the vaccination status of the worker and the HBV-surface antigen status of the exposure source.

HEPATITIS C

The prevalence of HBV in health care workers is declining as a result of widespread HBV vaccination; however, the prevalence of hepatitis C viral (HCV) infections is increasing [9]. Approximately 20–40% of acute viral hepatitis in the United States is caused by HCV. HCV is responsible for the majority of cases previously referred to as non-A, non-B hepatitis. HCV leads to chronic hepatitis in 50–60% of infections. The prevalence of HCV in the general population is less than 1% but may be as high as 18% in hospitalized patients [26]. Prior to 1990, the primary risk factors were intravenous drug use and blood transfusions, but currently 50% of those infected have no recognized risk factors. The estimated prevalence of HCV in health care workers is slightly higher than that in the general population [27]. The rate of HCV infection following needlestick has been estimated to be approximately 4%, using development of antibody to hepatitis C as a marker [9]. Pregnancy does not appear to increase susceptibility to infection, and the vertical transmission rate is highly variable in different studies [22] .

Aside from Universal Precautions for handling blood and body fluids, there is little to offer health workers, pregnant or not, to prevent hepatitis C infections. There is currently no HCV vaccine, and administration of globulin after HCV exposure has been ineffective [28]. Interferon is used as a treatment for chronic active hepatitis but is contraindicated in pregnancy. Surveillance for seroconversion following a blood or body fluid exposure should continue for six to nine months.

CYTOMEGALOVIRUS

Cytomegalovirus (CMV) is a member of the herpes family of viruses. Infection with CMV during pregnancy can either be primary or reactivation of a latent infection. Either form of infection can result in congenital infection in the fetus via transplacental passage of the virus [29]. Primary infection during pregnancy is riskier for the fetus than reactivation of latent disease. In women with a primary infection, congenital infection of the fetus occurs in approximately 40% of cases, while congenital infection of the fetus occurs in only 10% of the cases in which the mother has reactivation of latent infection [30]. Fetal sequelae as a result of congenital infection range from severe to clinically inapparent. Among infected infants whose mother had a primary infection in pregnancy, approximately 10–15% have clinically apparent disease at birth. Usually, infected infants of mothers with reactivation of latent infection have less obvious disease at birth [31].

Severe neonatal disorders are uncommon, but many organ systems may be involved. Defects include microcephaly, hydrocephaly, intracranial calcification, chorioretinitis, sensorineural hearing loss, thrombocytopenia with petechiae or purpura, fetal hydrops, hepatosplenomegaly, and intrauterine growth retardation [32]. Manifestations that may be initially overlooked include hearing impairment, developmental delay, and motor or dental defects. Vertical transmission to the fetus may occur at any time during pregnancy, but the worst fetal outcomes are usually associated with infection during the first trimester [32].

The exact mechanisms for transmission of CMV are not completely understood, but transmission is believed to require prolonged intimate contact with an infected individual or exposure to infected blood or body fluids [33]. Airborne transmission appears unlikely. The degree of risk that CMV poses in the health care workplace is unclear. The CMV seroconversion rate for nurses is not significantly different from that of other age-matched controls, and 30–85% of reproductive-age women are already seropositive due to previous infection [32].

The primary method of prevention of CMV transmission is scrupulous use of universal precautions. Currently, no vaccination is clinically available (although a live attenuated virus is under development) nor has postexposure prophylaxis proved effective [33]. Routine blood screening of pregnant health care personnel for the presence of CMV antibodies has not been generally recommended. If a pregnant caregiver is tending for a patient known to be shedding CMV, it is prudent to review the use of Universal Precautions. However, in the majority of cases, the exposure becomes apparent only after the worker has become infected and develops a mononucleosis-like syndrome.

Infection with CMV is suggested by any of the following blood test results: conversion from IgG-negative to IgG-positive status, a several-fold increase in antibody titers over 2–3 weeks, or the presence of CMV IgM. Unfortunately, it can be difficult to interpret these test results, as few people have documented previous IgG-negative status, IgM can persist for months after infection, and there may be cross-reactivity with other herpes viruses [3]. Blood culture will not differentiate between primary infection and reactivation of latent CMV infection. If infection is confirmed in the mother, fetal infection should be suspected if ultrasonography reveals fetal anomalies, as detailed above. Amniocentesis or fetal cord blood culture for CMV may be used to confirm infection; however, if the fetus appears normal, because of the low likelihood of significant anomalies and the lack of effective interventions available, these tests are unnecessary and most physicians would choose to observe without further testing. Treatment of pregnant women with symptomatic CMV is primarily supportive; the patient may require prolonged convalescence.

ENTEROVIRUSES

Echovirus and coxsackievirus are members of the nonpolio group of enteroviruses that can be vertically transmitted from mother to fetus if the mother is infected during pregnancy [34]. Infection tends to be seasonal, peaking in the third quarter of the year. Enteroviral infection in pregnancy is relatively common during periods of high prevalence in the community, but the majority of these infections are not associated with significant maternal or neonatal morbidity [35]. While it is postulated that mother-to-child transmission usually occurs during delivery or via the fecal-oral route after birth, transplacental infection may occur [36]. Intrauterine infection is associated with a slightly increased risk of fetal congenital heart and urological defects, and late-term stillbirths have been reported. Manifestations of neonatal infection may range from nonsymptomatic to overwhelming sepsis and death [35].

Hepatitis A is an RNA virus in the enterovirus family. It is responsible for about 35% of all cases of infectious hepatitis in the United States [22]. Among adults, the prevalence of anti–hepatitis A virus seropositivity is approximately 38%. Transmission is primarily via the fecal-oral route; it is unclear if transplacental infection can occur. Most maternal disease is self-limited and has no effect on the pregnancy.

There have been reports of transmission of enteroviral infections to health care workers, primarily to those in neonatal nurseries during times of community epidemics [36]. Probably the route of transmission is from infected mother to neonate to nurse via fecal-oral contamination. No treatment for enteroviral infections exists, but the observance of good hygiene and body fluid precautions should prevent infection from most occupational exposures. Hepatitis A IgG, administered during the virus's two-week incubation period, is effective prevention for 80–90% of exposures. Hepatitis A vaccine is available but is usually reserved for international travelers [37].

RUBELLA AND MEASLES

While vaccination in childhood has decreased the pool of susceptible adults, measles and rubella remain a concern because a significant number of women remain nonimmune [38,39]. Congenital measles and rubella result in well-described syndromes in affected fetuses, specifically disorders of the eyes, heart, and central nervous system.

The time at which the mother contracts infection is important: If maternal infection with rubella occurs during early pregnancy [38], up to 50% of neonates may be born with significant anomalies and miscarriages are more common. Defects occurring with infection after 20 weeks' gestation have not been described. Unfortunately, 20–50% of adult infections may be asymptomatic and thus fetal infection may not be suspected until the time of delivery [39]. Serologic testing is the preferred method of diagnosis: A several-fold rise in rubella IgG or the presence of IgM is considered a positive test result.

Health care workers should have rubella and measles immunity documented at the time of employment. Workers with inadequate antibody titers should be immunized, and postimmunization titers checked three months later [40]. Because of the theoretical risk of fetal infection from the attenuated live virus in the vaccine, pregnancy should be avoided for three months after vaccination [38]. Contact isolation is mandatory for all patients with rubella or measles.

Treatment for patients with rubella or measles is supportive. If infection is documented in the first trimester of pregnancy, the worker must be fully informed of the significant risks to the pregnancy and the fetus.

PARVOVIRUS

Human parvovirus B19 is the causative organism of erythema infectiosum (fifth disease) in children, aplastic crisis in patients with sickle cell anemia or hereditary spherocytosis, chronic anemia in the immunocompromised, and a transient, febrile, arthritis-like illness in otherwise healthy adults [8]. Parvovirus is spread via the respiratory route, and anyone working with young children (e.g., day care workers, teachers) and health care workers are at risk for occupational exposure. Approximately 50–81% of adult women show serologic evidence of prior infection and thus are not at risk for infection during pregnancy [41]. Community cases may be isolated or clustered (usually in the spring). A study of a 1988 school outbreak revealed approximately 20% of susceptible adults became infected [42]. Hospital studies have shown a transmission rate to susceptible caregivers of approximately 40% [43]. Humans are not susceptible to animal strains of parvovirus [3].

If a woman becomes infected with parvovirus during pregnancy, she develops viremia, which may transplacentally infect the fetus. Infection of fetal bone marrow may result in significant fetal anemia, possibly leading to hydrops, high output congestive heart failure, portal hypertension, and myocarditis. The result may be spontaneous abortion or stillbirth [3]. The first half of pregnancy appears to be the time of highest fetal risk. The rate of fetal infection when parvovirus is acquired during pregnancy is unclear. Several studies of the pregnancy outcomes of women with serologic evidence of infection during pregnancy generally showed a fetal death rate of less than 3% [3,44]. No congenital anomalies or long-term adverse effects are believed to be associated with maternal parvovirus infection when the fetus survives the initial infection; if the pregnancy proceeds to term, the neonatal outcome is usually unaffected [8,45].

Pregnant workers should not care for high-risk patients such as sickle cell patients in aplastic crisis, unless they are known to have immunity. Again, it is not uncommon for women to be pregnant quite some time before they are aware that conception has taken place, so strict infection control procedures should be followed by all employees in health care and child care. The contagious period predates the appearance of the hallmark rash; thus, the patient's appearance is not a "red flag" to apply special precautions. There is no vaccine available at this time, although one is in development [8].

In adults, diagnosis is made on the basis of acute and convalescent titers of antibodies to parvovirus B19. Clinically, many adults are asymptomatic; arthritis and malaise are most common in those who do show clinical symptoms [3]. Ultrasound diagnosis of fetal hydrops or unexplained elevation of maternal serum alpha-fetoprotein may suggest fetal infection [46]. Cord blood sampling can be obtained and tested for parvovirus by polymerase chain reaction or viral antigens tested by ELISA. Serologic testing for fetal parvovirus IgM is helpful if positive, but parvovirus IgM is usually not detectable in fetuses less than 20 weeks' gestation [46].

Ultrasound scans of the fetus six to 12 weeks after exposure and measurement of maternal serum alpha-fetoprotein levels may be useful. Treatment is mainly supportive for patients with parvovirus, as IgG has not shown to be helpful for postexposure prophylaxis or treatment of acute infection. If fetal hydrops is diagnosed, standard treatment for the condition can be considered. It should be borne in mind that the majority of fetuses suffer no adverse effects of maternal parvovirus infection.

VARICELLA

Varicella-zoster, a herpesvirus more commonly known as chickenpox, is spread by the airborne route. Less commonly, it can be contracted by contact with herpesvirus skin lesions. After infection, the virus replicates in the lymph nodes and then spreads hematogenously, appearing as the characteristic rash approximately 10–21 days after exposure [46]. Asymptomatic infection is unusual. The infected individual is most contagious the day prior to eruption of the rash and up to about five days after the rash appears, with the period of infectivity lasting until all lesions are crusted over [38]. Varicella-zoster is highly contagious, with attack rates for susceptible household contacts greater than 90%. After the initial infectious episode, the virus may lie dormant in the dorsal root ganglion and reactivate as shingles years later. In the United States, nearly all cases of varicella are seen in children; only 2% of cases occur after age 15 [47] and immunity after infection is lifelong. Therefore, relatively few women (approximately 5%) are susceptible to varicella-zoster infection during their reproductive years. The incidence of varicella in pregnant women is 1–5 in 10,000 [48].

Varicella infections in adults tend to be more virulent than in children, with varicella pneumonia, an uncommon complication in pediatric populations, occurring in 10–20% of adults [47]. Prior to the development of acyclovir, varicella pneumonia had mortality rates as high as 20%. Pregnant women, if they develop varicella pneumonia, seem to have a more severe course than the rest of the adult population [49].

The effects of maternal varicella on the fetus vary, depending on the time during pregnancy at which the infection is contracted. First-trimester infection is associated with a congenital varicella syndrome consisting of limb atrophy, ocular anomalies, and dermal scarring [47]. The incidence of this syndrome is variable but is usually less than 10%. Infection late in pregnancy but more than a week prior to delivery is probably the least worrisome, other than the potential impact of maternal complications, i.e., pneumonia, on the fetus. The worst outcomes are associated with infection of the mother five days prior to, and up to two days after, delivery [42]. The neonate may develop disseminated cutaneous or visceral disease and severe, life-threatening pulmonary involvement. This is probably a result of the infant's exposure to maximal viremic load and very little time for maternal antibody to be manufactured and cross the placenta.

Persons who do not have a certain history of childhood chickenpox should have varicella titers drawn, and if they are not immune, be vaccinated prior to beginning work in the health care field. Pregnant women should not be vaccinated, as the virus is a live attenuated strain and has the potential risk of infection [50]. If a nonimmune pregnant health care worker is exposed to varicella, she should receive varicella-zoster immune globulin (VZIG) as soon as possible, preferably within 96 hours of exposure [47]. Neonates born to mothers with active infection should also receive VZIG. Because of its longer history and better-known risk profile than the newer antiviral, acyclovir is the antiviral of choice. Acyclovir treatment during pregnancy is definitely indicated if the varicella-infected woman has pneumonia, and the majority of physicians would treat all pregnant women in the hope of preventing a more severe course [3]. It is not known if treatment in the first trimester reduces the incidence of congenital rubella syndrome [3]. The pregnant patient with varicella infection should be observed very closely for worsening of respiratory status and may require hospitalization in isolation.

TUBERCULOSIS

Tuberculosis (TB) infection results from inhalation of acid-fast bacilli that triggers a cell-mediated hypersensitivity reaction in two to eight weeks. This leads to a positive tuberculosis skin test and containment of the infection if the host is immunocompetent [51]. TB is re-emerging as a threat to health care workers: The number of reported cases has increased and multidrug-resistant strains of *Mycobacterium tuberculosis* have developed. Neonatal tuberculosis results from transplacental hematogenous spread, ingestion of infected amniotic fluid, or aspiration during delivery [52]. All of these scenarios are unlikely without extrapulmonary disease, generally found only in immunosuppressed individuals [3]. The lung and the liver of the fetus are the most likely to be affected, although widespread dissemination is possible. Obviously, an uninfected newborn would be at risk to contact TB from a contagious mother given the close contact between them.

No special restrictions are required for pregnant workers. Occupational safety guidelines for pregnant workers are the same as those for nonpregnant workers. All workers should follow OSHA guidelines for TB infection control. The CDC has outlined strategies for preventing work-related spread of TB [53,54]; these include worker education, medical surveillance of employees, special infection control measures, such as negative-pressure rooms, and standard infection control measures.

Pregnant workers with potential *M tuberculosis* exposure should undergo TB screening by Mantoux testing and clinical evaluation, just as any other exposed worker would. Pregnancy is not a contraindication to performing a skin test [3]. If a pregnant worker has converted to a positive status on skin testing, chest radiographic films should be obtained to evaluate the individual for active disease [55]. Radiography should be performed with the use of abdominal shielding. If the chest radiograph suggests active disease, confirmation should be obtained by sputum culture. If documented recent skin test conversion without active disease occurs during pregnancy, therapy should be considered on an individual basis [3].

Active tuberculosis during pregnancy should be treated. Instead of a four-drug regimen, usually only isoniazid, rifampin, and ethambutol are used, since streptomycin can cause ototoxicity in the fetus and the effects of pyrazinamide are unknown [3,51]. If the tuberculosis organism is multiple-drug resistant, then pyrazinamide might be considered. Therapy should last nine months, although all the drugs may not be used, depending on the resistance pattern of the organism. The pregnant woman should be placed on pyridoxine if she is taking isoniazid.

INFLUENZA

Influenza infection is common in the winter months, and most health care employers require or recommend vaccination of employees to prevent spread of the infection among ill or elderly patients. Vaccination is not contraindicated in pregnancy [56], although pregnancy does not seem to increase susceptibility to influenza or worsen the course and no adverse congenital effects, besides those associated with maternal fever, have been clearly described. It has been postulated that schizophrenia is more common in adults whose mothers were infected with influenza during their fetal life [3], but this remains controversial. Therefore, since influenza can largely be prevented or attenuated by vaccination and health care workers should be vaccinated to protect their patients, it seems prudent to advise that the practice of vaccination be extended to pregnant workers as well. Besides vaccination, prevention relies on good hygiene practices. Treatment for the pregnant woman with influenza is largely supportive, mainly acetaminophen for fever. The potential risks of amantadine to the fetus outweigh the benefits of its use by the pregnant woman for relief of flue symptoms.

ANIMAL CARE WORKERS

Veterinarians, veterinary assistants, farmers, zookeepers, slaughterhouse workers, laboratory animal attendants, and others who work around animals have exposure to the diseases animals carry, and women in these professions have the potential to acquire occupational infectious exposures during pregnancy. However, unlike health care and childcare, these fields are not generally dominated by women; many primarily employ men. Toxoplasmosis, brucellosis, Q fever, chlamydia, leptospirosis, and Lyme disease are among the most common zoonoses.

TOXOPLASMOSIS

Toxoplasma gondii is a common intracellular protozoan that causes disease in humans and animals. Cats act as the definitive host in human disease [57]. They ingest *Toxoplasma* cysts (usually by eating wild game), which then reproduce and shed noninfectious unsporulated oocysts in the cat's feces. Sporulation occurs in two or three days, depending to some degree on environmental conditions, and the infectious oocysts are viable for up to one year in the soil in which the cat defecates.

Occupational exposure to toxoplasmosis may occur in any job that involves contact with cats or their feces, including soil in which infected cats have defecated. Toxoplasmosis does not appear to be spread human to human in immunocompetent people; thus, health care workers caring for AIDS patients are not at increased risk [3]. Most toxoplasmosis infections are asymptomatic, but some individuals may develop a mononucleosis-like illness. Toxoplasmosis is difficult to confirm on clinical grounds. Definitive diagnosis requires the identification of *Toxoplasma* IgM antibodies or several-fold increases in *Toxoplasma* IgG antibodies on serologic testing.

Pregnancy does not increase susceptibility to toxoplasmosis or worsen the clinical syndrome [3]. Fifteen to 40% of adult women have antibodies to *Toxoplasma* [57]. The rate of infection in pregnancy is in the range of approximately 1 in 1,000 to 1 in 8,000 [58]. Of those women who do become infected during pregnancy, one third infect the fetus. Of fetuses infected transplacentally, only 10% develop congenital anomalies [59]. Common anomalies include microcephaly, impaired vision, deafness, and developmental delay. Rarely, congenital toxoplasmosis syndrome—rash, lymphadenopathy, jaundice, thrombocytopenia, hepatosplenomegaly, and intracranial calcifications—occurs. Transplacental infection is more common in the third trimester, but worse outcomes are associated with earlier infection [57]. Fetal infection can be suspected if ultrasonography demonstrates the previously mentioned anomalies. Definitive diagnosis of fetal toxoplasmosis requires demonstration of fetal IgM on serologic testing or culture of the organism from the amniotic fluid.

Wearing gloves when working with cats or cat feces can prevent occupational exposure. If litter boxes are routinely changed every 24 hours, the *Toxoplasma* organism cannot sporulate and become infectious. Pregnant workers with frequent exposure to cats should consider titers and if not immune should avoid working with cats, especially their waste, if possible [3]. It is worth noting that humans can be infected outside the workplace by eating undercooked meats or by contact with a pet cat.

Maternal treatment for toxoplasmosis is a two-month regimen of pyrimethamine and sulfadiazine with supplemental folic acid. Fetal outcomes have been shown to improve with maternal treatment [3].

Q FEVER

The causative agent of Q fever, a rickettsial infection, is *Coxiella burnetii.* Both wild and domestic animals are a part of the life cycle of the organism. Epidemiologic studies indicate infection is widespread in sheep, goats and cattle, although dogs, cats, and chickens are also infected [60]. The organism is shed in the urine, feces, and placental tissues of infected animals and may remain infectious for months in animal products, sand, or clay. Placental tissues seem to be particularly infectious [61]. Parturient ewes are the most likely source of infection for humans.

Usually, infection occurs by inhalation of infected aerosols. Incubation is two weeks to one month, followed by an acute febrile systemic illness, including fever, chills, myalgias, severe headache, pharyngitis, conjunctivitis, and nonproductive cough with chest pain [62]. Usually, no cutaneous eruptions are visible, unlike most rickettsial infections. Many patients with Q fever are asymptomatic. Cardiac involvement is rare but may be fatal. The illness usually resolves in two weeks but may have a relapsing course.

The pathologic role of *C burnetii* in human pregnancy is controversial. In sheep, cattle, and goats it is suspected of causing abortions, low birth weight, and prematurity [62]. Only a few cases of Q fever in pregnant women have been reported; reported complications have been transplacental infection of the fetus and fetal death [63,64]. Prudence dictates that pregnant women avoid contact with high-risk animals like pregnant ewes at work and away from the workplace and follow all recommended infection control procedures while at work.

Prevention of infection is difficult. In the research laboratory, male sheep or nonpregnant ewes should be used for experiments whenever possible. Q fever–tested stock is available and should be used, but it is more expensive and should not be relied upon as a guarantee of safety [62]. Appropriate air handling systems, protective clothing, including masks, gloves, and shoe covers, should be used. All facilities and equipment should be disinfected with bleach or hydrogen peroxide after use. All individuals working with sheep should observe standard microbiologic laboratory and animal management practices to limit exposure [61]. Treatment for pregnant women with Q fever is erythromycin for several weeks [62]. Vaccines are under development.

PSITTACOSIS

Chlamydia psittaci is an obligate intracellular organism that is the causative agent of psittacosis. Psittacosis is also known as parrot fever, ornithosis, or chlamydiosis. *C psittaci* has a broad range of hosts, including guinea pigs, rabbits, cats, lambs, calves, birds, and frogs [62]. In animals, there are many strains of the disease and diverse disease spectrums, including abortion. The organism is shed in the feces and, upon drying, produces a highly infectious aerosol. Humans with psittacosis may be asymptomatic or present one to two weeks postexposure with respiratory illness and systemic symptoms. Diagnosis is made on the basis of clinical features and serology.

In laboratories that work with birds, stock tested for *C psittaci* is available, but veterinarians, zookeepers, and animal breeders may potentially still have exposures. The data on psittacosis in human pregnancy is limited, although spontaneous abortion has been reported [3]. Treatment is erythromycin for at least three weeks. It is prudent for pregnant workers exposed to bird wastes to wear masks.

BRUCELLOSIS

Brucellosis is a systemic bacterial infection caused by infection with one of several *Brucella* species. Infection can occur through several different routes, including cuts in the skin, ingestion, or conjunctival contact with infected body fluids. Brucellosis is a disease of animals that is passed to humans by contact with their carcasses, blood, or body fluids [62]. At-risk occupations include ranchers, farmers, meat packers and laboratory workers. Diagnosis is based on laboratory culture or increasing antibody titers. Treatment for pregnant women with psittacosis is with trimethoprim/sulfamethoxazole for four to six weeks [3].

Brucella infection causes an increased risk of spontaneous abortion in animals, but because brucellosis in pregnant women is rare [3], the impact on human pregnancy is unclear. One small case series of six patients resulted in four normal deliveries, one spontaneous abortion, and one elective abortion [66].

Prevention of brucellosis is dependent on eradicating the disease in domestic animals through eliminating infected animals and vaccination of healthy animals. Pregnant women should avoid contact with animals suspected or known to be infected.

LEPTOSPIROSIS

Leptospirosis is a bacterial infection caused by *Leptospira interogans.* There are more than two hundred subdivisions of the species that infect dogs, cattle, swine, and rats, among others [62]. In animals, asymptomatic infection occurs in the renal tubules and the organism is excreted in the urine. In humans, *Leptospira* can penetrate mucous membranes or abraded skin and spread hemotogenously to all organ systems. Most patients have asymptomatic or mild infection. Incubation is one to two weeks and may have a biphasic course. Fever, headache, and myalgias occur first, followed by a brief respite and, subsequently, severe headache, nausea, vomiting, and abdominal pain. Weil's syndrome, a severe form of leptospirosis characterized by hepatic and renal dysfunction, while uncommon, may be fatal [62]. Diagnosis is made by culture or serology.

The disease course is unaffected by pregnancy, and there is no known teratogenic effect on the fetus [3]. For all workers, prevention of infection relies on vaccination of livestock and avoiding skin and mucous membrane contact with animal urine. Treatment for pregnant women with leptospirosis is penicillin [62].

LYME DISEASE AND EHRLICHIOSIS

Both Lyme disease and ehrlichiosis are caused by members of the bacterial family Rickettsiaceae. *Borrelia burgdorferi* (the causative agent of Lyme disease) and Ehrlichia are both tick-borne bacteria; specific regions of the country are noted to be endemic for Lyme disease and ehrlichiosis. Two types of Ehrilichiae cause illness in humans, one carried by the Lone Star tick and one by Ixodes [66]. Ixodes is also the vector for *Borrelia burgdorferi.* Because of their significant similarities to syphilis, these rickettsial diseases and their fetal effects are of concern.

Even in endemic regions of the country, antepartum ehrlichiosis and Lyme disease are rare [66,67]; pregnancy data is therefore rare, although there have been case reports of transplacental infections and congenital anomalies in fetuses and newborns of women with Lyme disease [67]. Larger epidemiologic studies are needed to resolve the question of fetal risks. There are no current recommendations for treatment of ehrlichiosis in pregnant women. The American Academy of Obstetricians/Gynecologists recommends 21 days of amoxicillin for pregnant women with Lyme disease [68].

Women at risk for either of these infections are those whose work requires them to be outdoors, especially in rural areas of the endemic regions for these ticks. Prevention of infection during pregnancy or otherwise relies on good tick control [69]—that is, avoidance of tall grass, bushes, and woods if possible. If avoidance of the tick's habitat is impossible, wearing light clothing, long pants with the cuffs tucked into socks, long-sleeved shirts, hats, and closed shoes help keep ticks off. Use of insect repellents may act as an adjunct to protective clothing. After returning from tick-infested areas, a careful inspection of the entire body should be performed and any ticks promptly removed. Ticks that have fed on a host for less than 24 hours are unlikely to transmit infection.

CHILDCARE WORKERS

Day care employees and preschool and elementary school teachers are exposed to young children and the diseases associated with children. Like nurses, the majority of these employees are women. Many of their exposures are relatively unremarkable, for example, upper respiratory infections, and viral gastroenteritis. However, rubella, varicella, and parvovirus B19 can have serious adverse effects. Recently, several hepatitis A outbreaks at schools have been widely reported in the media. Difficulties in controlling employee exposure must address the poor hygiene practices of young children and possible fomite transmission in these workplaces. Especially in day care settings, where diapers must be changed and food prepared, putting both the employees and children at risk of fecal-oral transmission of infections unless excellent hygiene is adhered to by everyone. Unlike a health care setting, a day care or school may not be aware of the risk of certain infections. Preventing exposure to rubella and varicella in the childcare setting is easy, as both have available vaccines. All women in the childbearing years should have their antibody titers checked and those without immunity should be vaccinated. These diseases are more common in health care workers and have been addressed in the previous section.

There are a wide variety of less common occupations that may put pregnant women at risk for occupationally acquired infection. For example, morticians are at risk for many of the same disease exposures as health care workers and should follow the same prevention and treatment strategies. Pregnant workers in a crowded office may be exposed to influenza or varicella and should take precautions like those for workers in the health care or childcare field.

In conclusion, reproductive-age women work in many types of jobs that involve potential exposure to infections. Most of these exposures can be prevented or minimized by the use of protective measures that are considered routine for all workers. Infection control for the pregnant worker should be an integral part of a comprehensive worker safety program; very few situations require special modification of the workplace or removal of the pregnant worker from her duties.

References

1. Kapadia LH. Women at work. *Br Med J* 1996;313: 1073–6.
2. Marquardt M, Lovelance K. Environmental and occupational health. In: *Essentials of Family Medicine*, 2nd Ed. Baltimore: Wilkins & Wilkins, 1993. Pp 39–50.
3. Chamberlain G. Work in pregnancy. *Br Med J* 1991;302:1070–3.
4. Riley LE. Varicella zoster virus. In: Gonik B (ed), *Viral Diseases in Pregnancy*. New York: Springer-Verlag, 1994. Pp 92–105.
5. Conningham FG, MacDonald PC, Gant NF, et al. Infections. In: *Williams Obstetric*, 19th Ed. East Norwalk, CT: Appleton & Lange, 1993. Pp 1281–98.

6. Brachman PS. Epidemiology of nosocomial infections. In: Bennett JV, Brachman PS (eds), *Hospital Infections*, 2nd Ed. Boston: Little, Brown, 1992. P 2.
7. Valenti WM. Infection control and the pregnant health care worker. *Nurs Clin North Am* 1993;28(3):673–86.
8. Swinker M. Occupational infections in health care workers: prevention and intervention. *Am Fam Physician* 1997;56(9):2291–300.
9. Stratton P. Human immunodeficiency virus. In: Gonik B (ed), *Viral Diseases in Pregnancy.* New York: Springer-Verlag 1994. Pp 128–55.
10. Maury W, Potts BJ, Rabson AB. HIV-1 infection of first-trimester and term human placental tissue: a possible mode of maternal-fetal transmission. *J Infect Dis* 1989;160:583–88.
11. Minckoff H, Mofenson LM. The role of obstetric interventions in the prevention of pediatric human immunodeficiency virus infection. *Am J Obstet Gynecol* 1994;171:1167–74.
12. Oxtoby MJ. Human immunodeficiency virus and other viruses in human milk: placing the issues in broader perspective. *Pediatr Infect Dis J* 1988;7:825–35.
13. Case-control study of HIV seroconversion in health-care workers after percutaneous exposure to HIV infected blood—France, United Kingdom, and United States January 1988—August 1994. *MMWR* 1995; 44:929–33.
14. Number of health care workers with AIDS rose in 1996. *Occup Safety Health Reporter* 1996;26:659.
15. Jackson GW. Virus. In: *Physical and Biological Hazards in the Workplace.* New York: Van Nostrand Reinhold, 1994. Pp 290–1.
16. U.S. Occupational Safety and Health Administration. Bloodborne Pathogens. OSHA Standard 29 CFR 1910, 1030.
17. Centers for Disease Control. Public health service statement on management of occupational exposure to human immunodeficiency virus, including considerations regarding postexposure zidovudine use. *MMWR* 1990;39(No RR-1).
18. Update: provisional Public Health Service recommendations for chemoprophylaxis after occupational exposure to HIV. *MMWR* 1996;45:468–80.
19. Connor EM, Sperling RS, Gelber R, et al. Reduction of maternal-infant transmission of human immunodeficiency virus type 1 with zidovudine treatment. Pediatric AIDS Clinical Trials Group Protocol 076 Study Group. *N Engl J Med* 1994;331:1173–80.
20. Centers for Disease Control and Prevention. U.S. Public Health Service Recommendations of the U.S. Public Health Task Force on the use of zidovudine to reduce perinatal transmission of human immunodeficiency virus. *MMWR* 1994;43:1–20.
21. Dinsmoor MJ. Hepatitis in the obstetric patient. *Infect Dis Clin North Am* 1997;11(1):77–91.
22. Benenson AS (ed). Control of communicable diseases manual: an official report of the American Public Health Association, 16th Ed. Washington DC: American Public Health Association, 1995.
23. Occupational Safety and Health Administration. Occupational exposure to bloodborne pathogens—final rule. *Federal Register* 1991;56(235):64004–182.
24. American College of Physicians Task Force on Adult Immunization, Infectious Diseases Society of America. *Guide for Adult Immunizations*, 3rd Ed. Philadelphia: ACP, 1994. Pp 25–32.
25. Davis GL. Hepatitis C virus infection among health care workers. *JAMA* 1996;275:1474.
26. Dawson GJ, Lesniewski RR, Stewart JL, et al. Detection of antibodies to hepatitis C virus in U.S. blood donors. *J Clin Microbiol* 1991;29:551.
27. Gerberding JL. Management of occupational exposures to bloodborne viruses. *N Engl J Med* 1995;332:441–51.
28. Nardiello S, Galanti B. Congenital cytomegalic disease: current possibilities and prospects of prevention. *Clin Ther* 1990;134:281–7.
29. Demmler G. Infectious Diseases Society of America and Centers for Disease Control: summary of a workshop on surveillance for congenital cytomegalovirus disease. *Rev Infect Dis* 1991;13:315.
30. Yow MD. Congenital cytomegalovirus disease; a new problem. *J Infect Dis* 1989;159:163.
31. Scott LL, Hollier LM, Dias K. Perinatal herpesvirus infections. *Infect Dis Clin of North Am* 1997;11(1):27–53.
32. Murph JR, Baron JC, Ebelhack CL, et al. The occupational risk of cytomegalovirus infection among day care providers. *JAMA* 1991;265:603–8.
33. Valenti WM. Selected viruses of nosocomial importance. In: Bennet JV, Brachman PS (eds), *Hospital Infections*, 2nd Ed. Boston: Little, Brown, 1992.
34. Modlin JF. Perinatal echovirus and group B coxsackievirus infection. *Clin Perinatol* 1988;15(2):233–46.
35. Garcia AG, Basso NG, Fonseca ME, et al. Congenital echovirus infection—morphological and virological study of fetal and placental tissue. *J Pathol* 1990;160(2):123–7.
36. Centers for Disease Control. Protection against viral hepatitis: recommendations of the Immunization Practices Advisory Committee (ACP). *MMWR* 1990;39:1.
37. American College of Obstetrics and Gynecology. *Rubella and Pregnancy.* ACOG Technical Bulletin No 171. Washington, DC: ACOG, 1992.
38. Peter G. *1994 Redbook: Report of the Committee on Infectious Diseases*, 23rd Ed. Elk Grove Village, IL: American Academy of Pediatrics, 1994. Pp 308–33.
39. Grossman JH. Rubella in Pregnancy. In: Mead PB, Hagen EW (eds), *Infectious Protocols in Obstetrics and Gynecology.* Montvale, NJ: Medical Economics, 1992. Pp 115–9.

40. Rodis JR, Vintaleos AM. Parvovirus. In: Gonik B (ed), *Viral Infections in Pregnancy.* New York: Springer-Verlag, 1994. Pp 196–214.
41. Gillespie SM, Carter ML, Asch S, et al. Occupational risk of human parvovirus B19 infection for school and daycare personnel during an outbreak of erythema infectiosum. *JAMA* 1990;263:2051–5.
42. Mead PB. Parvovirus B19 infection in pregnancy. In: Mead PB, Hager WD (eds), *Infectious Protocols for Obstetrics and Gynecology.* Montvale, NJ: Medical Economics, 1992. Pp 101–6.
43. Anderson LJ. Role of parvovirus B19 in human disease. *Pediatr Infect Dis J* 1987;6:711.
44. Gratacos E, Torres PJ, Vidal J, et al. The incidence of human parvovirus B19 infection during pregnancy and its impact on perinatal outcome. *J Infect Dis* 1995;171:1360.
45. Rodis JR, Vintaleos AM. Parvovirus. In: Gonik B (ed), *Viral Infections in Pregnancy.* New York: Springer-Verlag, 1994. Pp 196–214.
46. Riley LE. Varicella zoster virus. In: Gonik B (ed), *Viral Infections in Pregnancy.* New York: Springer-Verlag, 1994. Pp 92–105.
47. McGragor JA, Madinger NE. Varicella zoster infections in pregnancy. In: Mead PB, Hager WD (eds), *Infection Protocols for Obstetrics and Gynecology.* Montvale, NJ: Medical Economics, 1992. Pp 94–100.
48. Sever JA, White LR. Intrauterine viral infections. *Annu Rev Med* 1969;19:471.
49. Hams RE, Rhoades ER. Varicella pneumonia complicating pregnancy: report of a case and review of the literature. *Obstet Gynecol* 1965;281:139.
50. Centers for Disease Control and Prevention. Unintentional administration of varicella virus vaccine—United States 1996. *MMWR* 1996;45:1017–8.
51. Riley L. Pneumonia and tuberculosis in pregnancy. *Infect Dis Clin North Am* 1997;11(1):119–33.
52. Sanders CV, Hill MK. Tuberculosis in pregnancy. In: Mead PB, Hager WD (eds), *Infection Protocols for Obstetrics and Gynecology.* Montvale, NJ: Medical Economics, 1992. Pp 66–77.
53. Guidelines for the prevention of *Mycobacterium tuberculosis* in health care facilities. *MMWR* 1994;43(No RR-13).
54. Essential components of a tuberculosis prevention and control program. *MMWR* 1995;44(No RR-11).
55. Medchill MT, Gillum M. Diagnosis and management of tuberculosis during pregnancy. *Obstet Gynecol Surv* 1989;44:81–4.
56. Centers for Disease Control and Prevention. Prevention and control of influenzas, recommendations of the Advisory Committee on Immunization Practices (ACIP). *MMWR* 1994;44:1.
57. Algler LS. Toxoplasmosis and parvovirus B19. *Infect Dis Clin North Am* 1997;11(1):55–75.
58. Wong S-V, Remington JS. Toxoplasmosis in pregnancy. *Clin Infect Dis* 1994;18:853.
59. Sever JL. Toxoplasmosis in pregnancy. In: Mead PB, Hager WD (eds), *Infection Protocols for Obstetrics and Gynecology,* Montvale, NJ: Medical Economics, 1992. Pp 131–3.
60. Bernard KW, Parham GL, Winkler WG, et al. Q fever control measures: recommendations for research facilities using sheep. *Infect Control* 1982;3:461.
61. Ruppanner R, Brooks D, Morrish D, et al. Q fever hazards from sheep and goats used in research. *Arch Environ Health* 1982;37:103.
62. Fox JG, Lipman NS. Infections transmitted by large and small laboratory animals. *Infect Dis Clin* 1991;5(1):131–63.
63. Merrie TS. Q fever in pregnancy: report of two cases. *Infect Dis Clin Pract* 1993;2:207–9.
64. Raoult D, Stein A. Q fever during pregnancy—a risk for women, fetuses and obstetricians. *New Engl J Med* 1994;330(5):371.
65. Scoud M, Saade C, Awar G, et al. Brucellosis in pregnancy. *J Reprod Med* 1991;36:441–5.
66. Harkess JR. Ehrlichiosis. *Infect Dis Clin North Am* 1991;5(1):37–52.
67. Silver HM. Lyme disease during pregnancy. *Infect Dis Clin North Am* 1997;11(1):93–7.
68. American College of Obstetrics and Gynecology Committee Opinion. Lyme disease during pregnancy. *Int J Gynecol Obstet* 1992;39:59.
69. Buchstein SR, Gardner RP. Lyme disease. *Infect Dis Clin North Am* 1991;5(1):103–16.

33 / Occupational Infections in Laboratory Workers

Gregg M. Stave

Biologic laboratory research is conducted in academic, industrial, and governmental research settings. Scientists, technicians, and other personnel employed in these settings are potentially at risk for exposure to infectious agents and organisms. Exposures of concern include:

- The agent or organism being studied.
- Agents and organisms used in the course of the work.
- Recombinant viruses and organisms.
- Infectious hazards present in human- or primate-derived materials (including bloodborne pathogens).
- Zoonoses in research animals.
- Transmission of infection by use of shared equipment (e.g., conjunctivitis transferred by a microscope eyepiece).

This chapter addresses the epidemiology, prevention, and control of infections in research laboratories. Zoonotic infections are covered in Chapter 36. Occupational infections in research laboratories are addressed in Chapter 33.

Epidemiology

The diversity of settings and types of biologic research means that there is no broadly applicable epidemiology of risk. A substantial amount of laboratory research is conducted to study organisms such as *Escherichia coli* K-12 that have limited ability to cause illness or survive outside the laboratory; by contrast, other research is conducted specifically to study highly contagious and hazardous viruses and organisms.

There are no broadly based population studies of laboratory-acquired infections. Instead the literature contains reviews, case series, case reports, and findings from surveillance programs at specialized facilities [1–4]. Some published studies also fail to clearly differentiate between the research and clinical laboratory settings. Nonetheless, the literature contains sobering reports of thousands of cases of laboratory-acquired infections that have occurred during the twentieth century. An overwhelming percentage of the infections were reported prior to the past 20 years, although recent case reports clearly demonstrate that continuing vigilance is required. The most commonly reported laboratory-acquired infections are brucellosis, Q fever, typhoid, hepatitis, and tularemia. It is important to note that a documented laboratory accident had occurred in fewer than 20% of cases [4]. Determination of mechanisms of known or suspected exposure is instructive in developing prevention strategies and procedural guidelines for laboratories. Documented routes of exposure have included needlesticks, aerosol spray from syringes, lacerations from sharps and glassware, conjunctival exposure, mouth pipetting, and equipment failure. Recent case reports are illustrative.

SABIA VIRUS

While it is likely that many laboratory-acquired infections are not reported, there have been several notable recent publications. In 1994, a virologist working at the Yale Arbovirus Research Unit developed a serious illness following exposure to Sabia virus [5–9]. Sabia is an arenavirus that was discovered after an agricultural engineer in Brazil died from hemorrhagic fever. Subsequently, a laboratory technician in Brazil developed a severe nonfatal illness during efforts to isolate and characterize the agent. The physician scientist at Yale was most likely exposed following a centrifuge accident. After opening the centrifuge, the investigator noted liquid on the outside of one of the centrifuge bottles and also saw fluid at the bottom of the rotor. During decontamination and cleanup, he wore two pair of gloves but did not utilize respiratory protection, even though a powered air purifying respirator (PAPR) was available. During his hospital stay, substantial precautions were taken in an effort to prevent secondary spread. This incident received extensive coverage in the media and resulted in a threat to shut down the research facility. Improvements in laboratory procedures were implemented following the incident.

HANTAVIRUS

A less well-publicized laboratory exposure (to hantavirus) occurred in the United Kingdom [10]. The case presented as hemorrhagic fever, with associated renal syndrome. The hantavirus infection resulted from the handling of immunocytomas propagated in laboratory rats. In addition to the risk of infection presented by rats, rat immunocytomas and anti-immunocytoma serum should be recognized as potentially infectious.

BRUCELLA

A 1994 report from Spain provides another reminder of the importance of adhering to standard microbiologic practice [11]. Acute brucellosis occurred in four technicians handling strains of *Brucella* and the blood cultures from which they were isolated. No accidents had been reported; however, blood culture bottles were handled without use of a biologic safety cabinet.

SIMIAN IMMUNODEFICIENCY VIRUS

Another topic of current concern is simian immunodeficiency virus (SIV) [12–17]. SIV is a lentivirus that causes an AIDS-like illness in macaque monkeys and is used in the study of AIDS. SIV is genetically and antigenically related to HIV-2, and HIV-2 is now considered to comprise a strain or strains of SIV that have become endemic in some regions of Africa.

The first case of laboratory-acquired SIV infection most likely occurred through skin exposure [13,14]. A worker performed serology testing on clinical specimens from SIV-infected monkeys without wearing gloves, while suffering from a severe dermatitis of the forearms and hands. There was no history of percutaneous or mucous membrane exposure. Antibody testing demonstrated persistent seroreactivity to SIV and HIV-2, although no clinical illness was described.

Another reported case of possible SIV infection in a laboratory worker occurred in 1990 [12,14]. A technician in a research laboratory experienced a needlestick injury while drawing blood from an SIV-infected macaque. Antibodies to SIV were first detected three months following the exposure, and titers declined five months after exposure. No clinical illness developed. An effort to fulfill Koch's postulate by injecting blood from the exposed technician into a previously uninfected macaque failed to produce any evidence of SIV infection. It is possible that this worker experienced a transient infection with SIV. Alternatively, this incident may have occurred because of exposure to viral antigens, resulting in an increase in antibody titers but not an actual infection.

An anonymous survey conducted in 1992 by the National Institutes of Health (NIH) and Centers for Disease Control (CDC) to evaluate SIV seropositivity among SIV laboratory researchers determined that three out of 472 samples were positive [14]. Because of the anonymous approach and use of stored serum samples, it is not known whether either of the cases of SIV described above was represented in the study. More recently, Sotir and colleagues reported a similar study involving 550 workers who handled nonhuman primates and nonhuman primate materials at 13 North American research institutions [17]. Two participants were seropositive, one of whom had been previously reported in the literature. The other was known to have experienced a needlestick injury with an inoculum of SIV. Possibly of more concern than the reports of seroconversion was the description of their frequency of exposures. Of the 378 workers handling nonhuman primate-derived material in the laboratory, 66 (18%) reported an injury with needlesticks or sharps, and 64 (18%) reported a skin or mucous membrane exposure. Among the 257 who performed laboratory work with SIV, 15 (6%) reported a needlestick and 19 (7%) sustained a skin or mucous membrane exposure.

SYSTEMIC LUPUS ERYTHEMATOSUS

An intriguing paper provides a reminder that risk of infection may arise in the laboratory under unexpected circumstances [18]. A national study was conducted to evaluate the presence of antinuclear antibodies in female laboratory workers handling blood from patients with systemic lupus erythematosus (SLE). Antibodies to double-stranded DNA (anti-dsDNA) were higher in the high-exposure group than the low-exposure group. No differences were found in anti-ssDNA or anti-poly(dA-dC)poly(dG-dT). This finding led the study authors to postulate that a transmissible agent may exist in blood from patients with SLE.

Prevention and Control

Development of a program to address occupational infections in laboratory research necessitates a hazard assessment for the specific workplace. Prevention of laboratory-acquired infection should be considered to be a component of a comprehensive approach that addresses all workplace hazards, including chemical use and animal allergens. A prevention program should use a standard control strategy to prevent exposure through inhalation, ingestion, or skin penetration. Exposure can be eliminated through a combination of administrative, work practice and engineering controls, along with the use of personal protective equipment. Employee education and training is essential and medical surveillance may be advisable. Under some circumstances, immunization should be considered. Finally, a prevention program must incorporate postexposure evaluation and treatment.

ADMINISTRATIVE CONTROLS

Administrative systems need to be in place to ensure that hazard evaluations are performed and control strategies are in place. For all but the most innocuous settings, there should be a general inventory of potential biologic hazards, which is reviewed by occupational health and safety professionals.

Substitution is a sometimes neglected strategy for control of hazards. Whenever possible, a less hazardous substance or agent should be used in place of a more hazardous one.

Work involving recombinant DNA should be conducted according to the *Guidelines for Research Involving Recombinant DNA Molecules (NIH Guidelines)* [19]. While the guidelines must be followed by organizations receiving federal (NIH) funding to conduct recombinant DNA work, the guidelines represent "best practice," and should be considered in all settings. From the administrative oversight perspective, the guidelines make use of an Institutional Biosafety Committee (IBC) to review, approve, and oversee research.

SAFE WORK PRACTICES

Good microbiologic technique is the cornerstone of preventive work practices. The standard recommendations for work practices are described in the CDC/NIH publication *Biosafety in Microbiological and Biomedical Laboratories*, 4th Edition [1], generally referred to by its acronym, *BMBL.* Laboratory work is divided into four biosafety levels (BSLs). The higher the level, the greater the risk of exposure by the aerosol route. Each level has an associated set of recommendations for work practices, engineering controls (including facility design), and protective equipment, and each level builds on the requirements of the previous level. Basic work practices for all laboratory work includes (1) avoidance of mouth pipetting, (2) decontaminating work surfaces daily, (3) regular hand washing, (4) prohibition of eating, drinking, smoking, handling contact lenses, and applying cosmetics, and (5) restricting access to the laboratory. Anyone working in a microbiology laboratory should be familiar with all of the relevant recommendations in BMBL.

In some circumstances, particularly with recombinant DNA work, a higher level of work practices are used without using a higher level facility. So, for example, some work may be conducted using BSL3 practices in a BSL2 facility.

ENGINEERING CONTROLS

Engineering controls are the preferred method to prevent exposure to biologic hazards. The handling of potentially infectious agents should take place in a biologic safety cabinet (BSC). BSCs can be class I, class II (A or B) and class III. The correct cabinet must be chosen to prevent exposure depending on the type of work being done. Class I cabinets are needed for work with low to moderate risk agents. In a class I cabinet, room air flows into the cabinet and is ducted through a high-efficiency particulate air (HEPA) filter. Class II cabinets are the most commonly used in microbiologic and biomedical applications. The air circulating inside the cabinet has already passed through a HEPA filter, protecting the materials inside from contamination. With class IIA cabinets, the filtered air is recirculated in the work zone. Class IIB cabinets are connected directly to the exhaust system and can be used when the work requires use of volatile or toxic chemicals or radioisotopes. Class III cabinets provide total enclosure and are used for the most hazardous organisms.

Another form of engineering controls is designing room ventilation systems so that the laboratory is maintained at negative pressure relative to adjacent rooms. In the event of a spill, aerosols in a negative-pressure environment will not contaminate surrounding facilities.

PERSONAL PROTECTIVE EQUIPMENT

The use of personal protective equipment (PPE) is necessary when hazards cannot be eliminated through other control strategies. The most common forms of PPE include gloves and lab coats. Respirators are not used for most routine work, except with highly hazardous agents. However, respirators may be necessary for cleanup activities following a spill.

EMPLOYEE EDUCATION AND TRAINING

Laboratory employees must receive both general and specific training. General training should address principles of biosafety and waste handling. Specific education and training of employees should lead to a full understanding of the hazards of the materials with which they will be working and procedures for working safely with specific agents or organisms. Training should also incorporate the appropriate response to a spill, contamination, or exposure.

MEDICAL SURVEILLANCE

Medical surveillance begins with the preplacement evaluation. Specific areas of concern for biologic research include medical conditions that may make exposure more likely, such as dermatitis, or may result in heightened consequences from exposure, such as an immunocompromised state. While conditions identified at preplacement are not necessarily contraindications to work, they may require special precautions.

Periodic medical surveillance may be useful to detect the same types of conditions that are of interest at the preplacement evaluation. For some types of work, there may be value in performing testing for specific antibodies to agents being used in the laboratory. Testing can be done either at a periodic interval or at the completion of a specific work activity involving high titers of infectious material. While worth considering, periodic testing has limitations, including a lack of time specificity for the exposure. The value of periodic testing depends to some degree on the type of research being conducted. Antibody testing also raises sensitive issues, which may make some employees perceive the surveillance process as too invasive. For example, testing for herpes simplex virus or other viruses that may be considered to be sexually transmitted diseases, may be disquieting. Decisions about antibody testing should be made after considering the broad range of issues, and employees should be educated about the purpose of any testing program. Antibody testing may be more acceptable as a voluntary component of medical surveillance. However, once an exposure incident occurs, postexposure assessment is essential. Standing protocols should be developed so that immediate postexposure treatment can be initiated when appropriate.

A topic closely related to antibody testing is the use of serum banking. Serum banking is recommended for employees handling nonhuman primates and working with nonhuman primate-derived materials. In the event of an exposure incident or illness, frozen stored serum can be thawed and tested. In other settings, the value of serum banking is less clear. Efforts to maintain and track a serum bank should not be underestimated. Consent of the patient is necessary for tests conducted on stored samples, just as it is required for tests done on fresh samples, unless the tests are part of an anonymous survey.

IMMUNIZATIONS AND PROPHYLACTIC MEASURES

The most common vaccines administered to laboratory workers protect against tetanus and hepatitis B. Generally, when a vaccine is available to protect workers from a specific hazard, it is recommended as a component of the prevention program. However, the use of vaccinia vaccine for workers handling the vaccinia virus, has been the subject of some debate [20–23]. Advantages of vaccination include (1) protection from inadvertent inoculation, (2) protection against serious infection from exposure through the eye, and (3) protection against seroconversion to a foreign antigen expressed a gene inserted into a recombinant vaccinia virus. Disadvantages include (1) adverse effects of vaccination, including the risk of auto-inoculation in the eye, (2) the need to prevent secondary infection for a two-week period after inoculation, (3) false reassurance, causing workers to be less careful in their work, and (4) the possibility that immunized workers would not be able to take advantage of future vaccinia-based vaccines or gene therapy.

Another controversial issue is whether workers who decline recommended vaccinations or do not mount an adequate antibody response following immunization should be excluded from work with a specific agent. Some contend that exclusion is appropriate because of the increased risk to the individual from potential exposure. However, it should be recognized that immunization is only one component of a comprehensive prevention approach and that avoidance of exposure is the most critical issue. Additionally, the lack of availability of vaccines for most infectious agents that are used in laboratory research does not preclude working with these agents. Ultimately, in these circumstances, recommendations will depend on the specific facts and risks, and the employee should be a fully informed and active participant in discussions. Final recommendations must also be consistent with the requirements of the Americans with Disabilities Act (ADA).

References

1. Centers for Disease Control and Prevention, National Institutes of Health. *Biosafety in Microbiological and Biomedical Laboratories*, 4th Ed. (HHS pub. no. [CDC] 93-8395). Washington, DC: Department of Health and Human Services, 1999.
2. Pike RM. Past and present hazards of working with infectious agents. *Arch Pathol Lab Med* 1978;102:333–6.
3. Pike RM. Laboratory associated infections: incidence, fatalities, causes and prevention. *Annu Rev Microbiol* 1979;33:41–66.
4. Sullivan JF, Songer JR, Estrem IE. Laboratory-acquired infections at the National Animal Disease Center 1960–1976. *Health Lab Sci* 1978;15:58–64.
5. Barry M, Russi M, Armstrong L, et al. Treatment of a laboratory-acquired Sabia virus infection. *N Engl J Med* 1995;333:294–6.
6. Gandsman EJ, Aaslestad HG, Ouimet TC, et al. Sabia virus incident at Yale University. *Am Ind Hyg Assoc J* 1997;58:51–3.
7. Murphy FA, Johnson KM. An exotic viral disease acquired in a laboratory. *N Engl J Med* 1995;333:317–8.
8. Anonymous. Scientist tests the public trust. *Nature* 1994;371:1.
9. Ryder RW, Gandsman EJ. Laboratory-acquired Sabia virus infection (letter). *N Engl J Med* 1995;333:1716.
10. Lloyd G, Jones M. Infection of laboratory workers with hantavirus acquired from immunocytomas propagated in laboratory rats. *J Infect* 1986;12:117–25.
11. Martin-Mazuelos E, Nogales MC, Florez C, et al. Outbreak of *Brucella melitensis* among microbiology laboratory workers. *J Clin Microbiol* 1994;32:2035–6.
12. Khabbaz RF, Rowe T, Murphy-Corb M, et al. Simian immunodeficiency virus needlestick accident in a laboratory worker. *Lancet* 1992;340:271–3.

13. Khabbaz RF, Heneine W, George JR, et al. Infection of a laboratory worker with simian immunodeficiency virus. *N Engl J Med* 1994;330:172–7.
14. Anonymous survey for simian immunodeficiency virus (SIV) seropositivity in SIV-laboratory researchers—United States, 1992. *MMWR* 1992;41:814–5.
15. Essex M. Simian immunodeficiency virus in people. *N Engl J Med* 1994;330:209–10.
16. Langley RL. Simian immunodeficiency virus (SIV). In: Wald PH, Stave GM (eds), *Physical and Biological Hazards of the Workplace.* New York: Wiley and Sons, 1994. Pp 311, 312.
17. Sotir M, Swtzer W, Schable C, et al. Risk of occupational exposure to potentially infectious nonhuman primate materials and to simian immunodeficiency virus. *J Med Primatol* 1997;26:233–40.
18. Zarmbinski MA, Messner RP, Mandel JS. Anti-dsDNA antibodies in laboratory workers handling blood from patients with systemic lupus erythematosus. *J Rheumatol* 1992;19:1380–4.
19. National Institutes of Health. *Guidelines for Research Involving Recombinant DNA Molecules (NIH Guidelines).* Washington, DC: Department of Health and Human Services, 1998.
20. Centers for Disease Control. Vaccinia (smallpox) vaccine: recommendations of the Immunization Practices Advisory Committee. *MMWR* 1991;40:1–10.
21. Williams NR, Cooper BM. Counseling of workers handling vaccinia virus. *Occup Med* 1993;43:125–7.
22. Anonymous. Pros and cons of vaccinia immunization. *J Occup Med* 1992;34:757.
23. Ducatman AM. Vaccinia. In: Wald PH, Stave GM (eds), *Physical and Biological Hazards of the Workplace.* New York: Wiley and Sons, 1994:312–4.

34 / Occupational Infections in Health Care Workers

Marion Swinker

The health care industry is one of the largest in the United States, employing 7 million people in 1990 and projected to increase to 11 million workers by 2000. Hospitals employ about 50% of all health service personnel; 20% work in nursing homes and personal care settings and the remainder in outpatient settings [1]. The majority (75–80%) of health care workers are women. The overall rate of work-related injury and illness for these employees is 11.8 per 100 for hospital workers and 17.3 for nursing home and personal care facilities. This exceeds the average rate of 8.5 in private industry. The majority of injuries experienced by health care workers are due to musculoskeletal injuries, not infectious diseases. Existing databases may not adequately capture the incidence of infectious illness in health care workers [1]. The OSHA 200 log record-keeping system should capture seroconversion due to bloodborne pathogens exposure or workplace infection with tuberculosis, but many other infections are not unique to the health care setting or may not follow a recognized exposure event.

Individuals who work in health care are exposed to a variety of infections from patients (Table 34-1) and may spread their own infections to patients (Table 34-2). Routes of infection include direct contact with infected persons, respiratory or airborne spread, the fecal-oral route, transmission via fomites, and percutaneous sticks, cuts, or abrasions. The Occupational Safety and Health Administration's (OSHA) initiatives of the 1990s to protect health care workers from bloodborne pathogens and tuberculosis have received considerable attention because they carry the force of law: They mandate immunization, surveillance, and postexposure procedures. The routine infection control policies and procedures that health care workers follow are less well publicized but just as important in preventing infection. These include isolation precautions, appropriate handling of materials, disinfection and sterilization practices, waste disposal, immunization (Table 34-3) and, especially, proper hand washing, which contribute to the protection of workers and patients [2]. This chapter reviews some common infections of concern in the health care workplace. Recognition of the possibility of nosocomial spread of infection and prompt institution of control measures are critical to counteract spread.

In the hospital setting, prevention requires the cooperation of various departments such as infection control, employee health services, administration and human resources; all have an important role in the process. In smaller institutions or the outpatient setting, similar principles apply. With fewer resources, the employer is ultimately responsible for ensuring that personnel can be safe and productive and that regulatory requirements are met.

Tuberculosis

Tuberculosis is an infectious mycobacterial disease that may be characterized by pulmonary or disseminated caseous lesions. The disease course may be indolent or acute, depending on host characteristics. Infected sites may include the meninges, bones, genitourinary tract, larynx, skin, pleura, and peritoneum. Hospitals may be settings for nosocomial transmission of infection, especially when persons infected with human

Table 34-1
Occupationally Acquired Infections Encountered in Specific Groups of Health Care Workers

Groups Affected	Infections
Laboratory workers	*Neisseria meningitidis* infections, brucellosis, Q fever, hepatitis, typhoid fever, tularemia, tuberculosis, dermatomycosis, Venezuelan equine encephalitis, psittacosis, coccidioidomycosis, rickettsiosis, arenavirus infection
Animal workers[a]	Cryptosporidiosis, cutaneous larva migrans, toxocaral infection, lymphocytic choriomeningitis
Primate handlers	Simiam B virus infection, hepatitis A, yellow fever, Marburg virus infection, tuberculosis, simian immunodeficiency virus infection, shigellosis
Pregnant health care workers[b]	Rubella, parvovirus B19 infection, cytomegalovirus infection, varicella, echovirus infection, coxsackievirus infection
Pregnant veterinarians[b]	Brucellosis, tuberculosis, cryptococcosis, listeriosis, lymphocytic choriomeningitis, Q fever, toxoplasmosis, Venezuelan equine encephalitis
Pathology workers	Tuberculosis, human immunodeficiency virus (HIV) infection (?), hepatitis B, Creutzfeldt-Jakob disease, legionnaires' disease, Lassa fever, anthrax, group A streptococcal infection, tetanus, typhoid fever
Surgery workers	Hepatitis B, other infections caused by bloodborne pathogens (?)
Dentists	Hepatitis B, hepatitis C, herpetic whitlow, mumps, tuberculosis
Anesthesia workers	Hepatitis B, rhinovirus infection
Laundry workers	Smallpox, salmonellosis, hepatitis A, scabies, Q fever

[a] Includes veterinarians and animal laboratory workers.
[b] Incidence of infection is not increased, but infection poses a potential risk to fetal development.
Adapted with permission from Sepkowitz KA. Occupationally acquired infections in health care workers. Part II. *Ann Intern Med* 1996;125:917–28.

immunodeficiency virus (HIV) are treated in ward settings [3]. Data on TB transmission in health care overall are limited; most reports come from large, urban, acute care hospitals [3,4]. However, tuberculosis (TB) has historically been a risk for health care providers. The incidence of TB infection in health care workers varies widely, depending on factors such as the location of the facility, local prevalence of the infection, and patient population of the facility.

EPIDEMIOLOGY

The baseline prevalence of past TB infection in health care workers ranges from 1–28% [4]. After a known exposure, 4–70% of exposed workers may develop a positive skin test; higher risk is related to the performance of bronchoscopy [4,5]. Without a known exposure, the yearly conversion rate for health care workers averages 0.1–5.0% [4]. Nationally, from 1985 to 1993, the number of reported cases of tuberculosis increased by 14%, leading to increased concern and attention to control measures (Figure 34-1), which effected a subsequent decrease of 26% by 1997 [6]. The decrease in the number of cases occurred primarily in persons born in the United States; cases among foreign-born persons continue to increase. In 1997, six states (California, Florida, Illinois, New Jersey, New York, and Texas) reported 57% of all TB cases [6]. The Centers for Disease Control (CDC) guidelines for preventing the transmission of TB in health care facilities, published in October 1994, were adopted by OSHA to protect health care workers in lieu of development of a formal standard [7].

PREVENTION AND CONTROL

Using CDC guidelines, OSHA mandates that health care facilities conduct a risk assessment, perform skin testing for TB at least yearly [8], and develop isolation procedures for potentially infectious TB patients in hospitals and in some outpatient settings. The mandate includes screening patients for symptoms of active TB, removing them to isolation rooms as quickly as possible, and health care personnel's use of surgical masks to prevent their contracting infection through aerosolization of the patient's lung.

Table 34-2
Guidelines for Work Restrictions for Personnel with Infectious Diseases

Disease Problem	Relieve From Direct Patient Contact	Partial Work Restriction	Duration
Conjunctivitis, infections	Yes		Until discharge ceases
Cytomegalovirus infections	No		
Diarrhea[a]			
Acute stage (diarrhea with other symptoms)	Yes		Until symptoms resolve and infection with *Salmonella* is ruled out
Convalescent stage *Salmonella* (nontyphoidal)	No	Personnel should not take care of high-risk patients	Until stool is free of the infecting organism on two consecutive cultures not less than 24 hours apart
Other enteric pathogens[b]	No		
Enteroviral infections	No	Personnel should not take care of infants and newborns	Until symptoms resolve
Group A streptococcal disease	Yes		Until 24 hours after adequate treatment is started
Hepatitis, viral hepatitis A	Yes		Until 7 days after onset of jaundice
Hepatitis B, acute	No	Personnel should wear gloves for procedures that involve trauma to tissues or contact with mucous membranes or nonintact skin	Until antigenemia resolves
Chronic antigenemia	No	Same as acute illness	Until antigenemia resolves
Hepatitis C	No	Same as hepatitis B	
Hepatitis non-A, non-B	No	Same as acute hepatitis B	Periodic infectivity has not been determined
Herpes simplex			
Genital	No		
Hands (herpetic whitlow)	Yes	(**Note:** It is not know whether gloves prevent transmission)	Until lesions heal
Orofacial	No	Personnel should not take care of high-risk patients	Until lesions heal
HIV-Ab positive	Yes		Until their job activities have been reviewed to determine under what circumstances, if any, they may continue to perform exposure-prone procedures
Measles (active)	Yes		Until 7 days after the rash appears
Postexposure (susceptible personnel)	Yes		From the 5th through the 21st day after exposure and/or 7 days after the rash appears
Mumps			
Active	Yes		Until 9 days after onset of parotitis
Postexposure	Yes		From the 12th through the 26th day after exposure or until 9 days after onset of parotitis

(continued)

Table 34-2 (continued)

Disease Problem	Relieve From Direct Patient Contact	Partial Work Restriction	Duration
Pertussis (active)	Yes		From the beginning of the catarrhal stage through the 3rd week after onset of paroxysms or until 7 days after start of effective therapy
Postexposure (asymptomatic personnel)	No		
Postexposure (asymptomatic personnel)	Yes		Same as active pertussis
Rubella (active)	Yes		Until 5 days after the rash appears
Postexposure (asymptomatic personnel)	Yes		From the 7th day through the 21st day after exposure and/or 5 days after rash appears
Scabies	Yes		Until treated
Staphylococcus aureus (skin lesions)	Yes		Until lesions have resolved
Tuberculosis, pulmonary	Yes		Until receiving adequate therapy, proof of three consecutive daily negative acid-fast bacilli smears, cough is resolved
Upper respiratory tract infections[c] (high-risk patients)	Yes	Personnel with upper respiratory tract infections should not take care of high-risk patients	Until acute symptoms resolved
Zoster (shingles), active	No	Appropriate barrier desirable; personnel should not take care of high-risk patients	Until lesions dry and crust
Postexposure (asymptomatic personnel)	Yes		From the 10th through the 21st day after exposure or if varicella occurs, until all lesions dry and crust
Varicella (chickenpox)			
Active	Yes		Until all lesions dry and crust
Postexposure	Yes		From the 10th through the 21st day after exposure or if varicella occurs, until all lesions dry and crust

[a] Various agents may cause diarrhea.
[b] Generally, personal hygiene, particularly hand washing before and after all patient contact, will minimize risk of transmitting enteric pathogens to patients.
[c] High-risk patients with upper respiratory tract infections are neonates, young infants, patients with chronic obstructive pulmonary disease, and immunocompromised patients.
Adapted from CDC guidelines for infection control in health care personnel. *Infect Control Hosp Epidemiol* 1998;19:407–63.

Table 34-3
Immunizing Agents Strongly Recommended for Health Care Workers

Agent	Dosage Schedule	Indications
Hepatitis B (HB) recombinant vaccine	Two doses IM 4 weeks apart; third dose 5 months after second; booster doses not necessary.	**Pre-exposure:** HCWs at risk for exposure to blood or body fluids. **Postexposure:** See Table 35-5.
Influenza vaccine (inactivated whole-virus and split-virus vaccines)	Annual vaccination with current vaccine. Administered IM.	HCWs who have contact with patients at high risk for influenza or its complications.
Measles live-virus vaccine	One dose SC; second dose at least 1 month later.	HCWs born during or after 1957 who do not have documentation of having received 2 doses of live vaccine on or after the first birthday *or* a history of physician-diagnosed measles or serologic evidence of immunity. Vaccination should be considered for all HCWs who lack proof of immunity, including those born before 1957.
Mumps live-virus vaccine	One dose SC; no booster.	HCWs believed to be susceptible can be vaccinated. Adults born before 1957 can be considered immune.
Rubella live-virus vaccine	One dose SC; no booster.	HCWs who do not have documentation of having received live vaccine on or after their first birthday *or* laboratory evidence of immunity.
Varicella-zoster live-virus vaccine	Two 0.5-mL doses SC 4–8 weeks apart if ≥13 years of age.	For HCWs who do not have either a reliable history of varicella or serologic evidence of immunity.

From Immunization of health care workers. *MMWR* 1997;46(suppl):3–37, with permission.

Recognition of infectious tuberculosis may be difficult in HIV-infected patients. The use of respiratory protective devices, such as high-efficiency particulate (HEPA) filters or other approved masks or helmet-type powered air-purifying respirators (PAPR), is required to protect workers when they are caring for such patients. The masks, with the exception of PAPR, must be individually fitted to the worker. There are little or no data on the effectiveness of these devices overall or compared to surgical masks [8–10], and the cost-benefit estimates for their use may be high in low prevalence areas.

Multidrug resistant (MDR) strains of TB are an increasing concern: They are frequently seen in HIV-infected individuals and are associated with a high mortality rate. During 1997, among the 42 states reporting on drug sensitivities, 7.6% of isolates were resistant to isoniazid (INH), and 1.3% to both INH and rifampin [6]. Nearly half of all MDR cases are reported from New York and California. It is recommended that four drugs be used in the initial management of active TB if the frequency of isoniazid resistance exceeds 4% in the state; in 1998, the majority of states exceeded that threshold.

In hospitals where INH resistance occurs, there can be implications for employee's health practices. If a health care worker is exposed to drug-resistant TB and experiences a skin test conversion, the typical INH prophylactic regimen may need to be modified or supplemented, using a drug(s) to which the infecting organism will be susceptible.

HIV infection with low CD4 lymphocyte counts can lead to atypical presentations of TB, including extrapulmonary presentations, such as meningitis or abscesses. In addition, negative results of sputum testing may be found in the presence of pulmonary disease [12]. Thus, recognition of TB and institution of appropriate precautions may be delayed.

Bacille Calmette-Guérin (BCG) vaccine is not routinely recommended for preventive use in U.S. health care workers [11] but may be considered in unusual circumstances, e.g., for workers who

Figure 34-1 / Number of Persons with Reported Cases of Tuberculosis by Country of Birth—United States, 1986–1997. (From Tuberculosis morbidity—United States, 1997. *MMWR* 1994;43(suppl):1–132, with permission.)

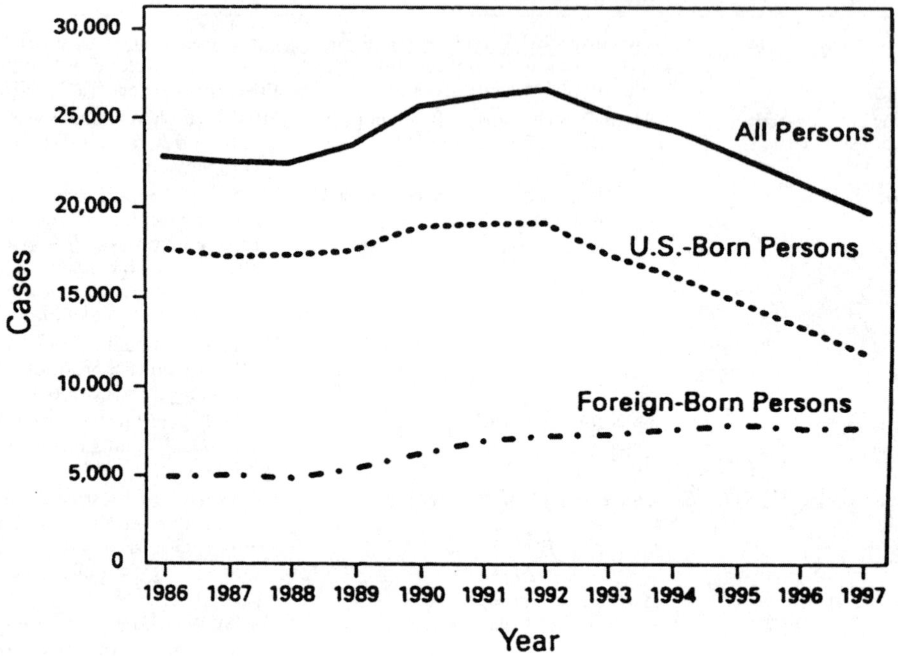

experience significant on-going exposure to multidrug-resistant TB (such as those who perform bronchoscopy), for whom INH prophylaxis could be ineffective.

MEDICAL SURVEILLANCE

Table 34-4 gives current interpretation guidelines for purified protein derivative (PPD) skin tests in health care personnel. All individuals with recent skin test conversions should be evaluated for INH prophylaxis after chest radiography is performed to rule out active disease. INH is typically given prophylactically for six months to adults, nine months to children, and 12 months to HIV-infected individuals. Preventive therapy should be considered for any health care worker who converts during yearly surveillance, regardless of age. HCW would typically meet the criteria for high risk: recent conversion and potential contact with active TB [7]. The risk of active infectious TB is about 3–5% within the first year or so after initial infection; another 3–5% may develop active infection at a time remote from acquisition. The ability of the host to contain the disease is diminished by conditions such as silicosis, HIV infection, diabetes, corticosteroid or immunosuppressive drug use, and gastrectomy [11].

Currently, CDC recommends that all health care workers (other than known reactors) be screened yearly with a skin test—more often for those at high risk of exposure. Individuals who have previously received BCG vaccine should be included in the screening. Testing is contraindicated only if the individual has experienced a large necrotic reaction to past skin testing. This is a change in practice, as many health care workers have previously been advised not to participate in skin testing because they have had prior BCG vaccination. Skin test reactions due to prior vaccination typically decline in severity with time, and the vaccine is not completely effective in preventing infection. During yearly surveillance, if a skin test response (induration) increases in size by 10 mm compared to the previous year's response, this suggests new infection rather than the effect of past BCG vaccinations. Essentially,

Table 34-4
Tuberculosis Skin Test Interpretation

1. An induration of ≥5 mm is classified as positive in:
   - Persons who have human immunodeficiency virus (HIV) infection or risk factors.
   - Persons who have had recent close contact[a] with persons who have active tuberculosis (TB).
   - Persons who have fibrotic chest radiographs (consistent with healed TB lesions).
2. An induration of ≥10 mm is classified as positive in all persons who do not meet any of the criteria above but who have other risk factors for TB, including high-risk groups[a] and high-prevalence populations.
3. An induration of ≥15 mm is classified as positive in persons who do not meet any of the above criteria.

[a] PPD skin-test results in health care workers (HCWs):
- The prevalence of TB in the facility should be considered when choosing the appropriate cutoff point for defining a positive PPD reaction. In facilities where there is essentially no risk for exposure to *Mycobacterium tuberculosis* (i.e., minimal- or very low-risk facilities, an induration ≥15 mm may be a suitable cutoff for HCWs who have no other risk factors. In facilities where TB patients receive care, the cutoff point for HCWs who have no other risk factors may be ≥10 mm.
- A recent conversion in a HCW should be defined generally as a ≥10-mm increase in size of induration within a 2-year period. For HCWs who work in facilities where exposure to TB is very unlikely (e.g., minimal-risk facilities), an increase of ≥15 mm within a 2-year period may be more appropriate for defining a recent conversion because of the lower positive-predictive value of the test in such groups.

Adapted from Guidelines for preventing TB transmission in health care facilities. *MMWR* 1994;43(suppl):1–132, with permission.

skin test results are interpreted no differently in BCG-vaccinated persons than in nonvaccinated individuals. In addition to skin testing, previous PPD reactors should be followed during yearly surveillance by interviewing them for reporting of symptoms. Repeat chest radiography should be reserved for those experiencing symptoms of chronic cough, fever, night sweats, and/or weight loss.

The 5-tuberculin-unit (TU) dose used in skin testing represents a compromise between sensitivity and specificity. The predictive value of a positive test is related to the prevalence of *Mycobacterium tuberculosis* in the population tested. In a population with a low prevalence of infection, i.e., 5–10%, the predictive value of a 10-mm skin test reaction (induration) is low, and the reaction is more likely due to nontuberculous mycobacteria than to TB. The area of cellular infiltration (induration) reflects the delayed, cell-mediated hypersensitivity response. Erythema, acute inflammation, vasodilatation or capillary congestion alone, without induration, does not constitute a positive skin reaction [13]. The skin hypersensitivity reaction begins to appear two to 10 weeks following infection with TB. A 1-TU test dose is sometimes used if there is the possibility of allergic reaction due to a humoral response or there is concern due to past BCG vaccination, but use of the 1-TU procedure is not standardized [10]. Ten percent to 25% of patients with active TB are nonresponders to PPD testing; other infections, malnutrition, drugs, and general debility (including HIV with CD4 lymphocyte counts less than 200) may contribute to false-negative results [13].

OSHA's current enforcement directives for inspectors mandate the use of two-stage testing for TB in all new employees who have not had a PPD skin test in the past year [14]. This procedure is used to detect a possible "boosting" effect, resulting when the first (negative) PPD leads to "recall" of the immune response. A larger reaction occurs if the test is repeated in one to three weeks, indicating past infection. This boosting effect can persist and lead to falsely considering the individual to be a recent seroconverter if enrolled in a yearly testing program. Boosting is most likely to occur in individuals over age 55 or in BCG-vaccinated individuals. In one study in Canada, the incidence of the boosting effect was noted to be 10% in BCG recipients and 2.5% in others [15]. In a group of U.S. medical students at the Uniformed Services University of Health Sciences, the incidence of the boosting effect was found to be 4.8%, but the BCG history was not obtained for the individuals in whom this occurred [16]. The boosting effect is also reported to be more common in areas with frequent cross-reactions due to nontuberculous mycobacteria [15].

The overall incidence of the boosting effect in health care workers is not known. In a high-prevalence area, a New York City hospital reports that 40% of new hires are PPD positive and an additional 10% are discovered by the two-step procedure [17]. Boosting was found to be most common in males, persons born outside the United States, and BCG recipients [18]. In other settings, the prevalence of the booster effect may be much lower—for example, in a tertiary care center in Eastern North Carolina, 0.6% of baseline preplacement skin tests were newly positive and an additional 0.4% were detected on two-step testing [19]. While rare, this boosting effect would falsely elevate the low yearly skin test conversion rate of 0.1% to 0.2% if not recognized [19]. CDC guidelines allow for decisions on the use of the two-stage test to be based upon institutional data on the incidence of boosting in the facility, but OSHA has chosen to enforce use of the two-step procedure for new employees, regardless of age, immune status, or facility experience.

In 1997, OSHA proposed its own TB standard [20], but it has not been adopted in final form. The final revised standard is expected to be promulgated in 2001.

Controversy surrounds the use of the TB skin test during pregnancy. There is no evidence that pregnancy affects the accuracy of the test, the test is safe and valid throughout pregnancy, and it has no known teratogenic effects [6], yet pregnant employees frequently refuse the PPD, based on the recommendations of their personal physicians. The basis of these recommendations is not clear.

DIAGNOSIS AND TREATMENT

A new PPD seroconverter should be questioned about symptoms and undergo chest radiography to rule out active disease. Prophylactic treatment should be considered, as previously discussed. Persons with active infection will need a 12-month course of therapy; for those without active disease, a six-month prophylactic course of INH, 300 mg per day, is 93–98% effective in preventing active TB. INH is frequently supplemented with pyridoxine, 25–50 mg, to prevent neurotoxicity. In states where MDR is seen, alternative prophylactic regimens, using a combination of drugs to which the organisms are likely to be sensitive, local health departments are a resource for the latest regimens. Individuals who are skin-test positive are usually considered to be at very low risk for subsequent reinfection with TB, but there are rare case reports of reinfection, presumably with a different strain of *M tuberculosis.* Reinfection is unlikely to result in active disease in the immunocompetent host [16,21].

The CDC guidelines recommend comparing the yearly skin-test conversion rates of clinical employees to those of non-patient-care employees (representing the community baseline) to assess the adequacy of preventive measures. Any skin-test conversions occurring in clusters or resulting from a known exposure should trigger a review of the adequacy of existing control measures.

Bloodborne Pathogens

HUMAN IMMUNODEFICIENCY VIRUS

HIV is a viral infection that progressively damages the immune system, eventually leading to acquired immunodeficiency syndrome (AIDS), first recognized in 1981. More than a dozen opportunistic infections and several cancers are considered relatively specific indicators of AIDS. The first report of HIV transmission via needlestick ushered in a new era of concern about occupational hazards in health care [1].

Epidemiology

By 1997, the CDC had documented 52 confirmed cases of occupational HIV transmission and 114 possible cases in health care workers [22]. Most of the cases were caused by percutaneous injuries with sharps. Nurses, physicians, and laboratory technicians are the workers who experience the majority of reported infections [12]. Overall, 18,000 health care workers have been diagnosed with HIV, but most infections resulted from non-work-related exposures.

Prevention and Control

Procedures that limit exposure to bloodborne pathogens, such as universal precautions and use of personal protective equipment, minimize exposure to HIV. When exposure does occur, postexposure prophylaxis should be considered. In 1996, the CDC issued guidelines for postexposure prophylaxis (PEP) of health care workers exposed to known HIV-infected blood or body fluids, using one to three antiretroviral agents, depending on the riskiness of the exposure [22]. These guidelines were updated in 1998 [23]. The risk of seroconversion following a needlestick with HIV-positive blood is generally estimated to be about 0.3%; it is 0.1% after a mucous membrane splash, and less than 0.1% for a cutaneous splash on nonintact skin. Among occupationally exposed health care workers, the risk of seroconversion increases in direct proportion to the quantity of blood with which the exposed individual comes into contact (e.g., a visibly bloody instrument or a hollow needle that had been removed from a vascular site), the depth of the wound (e.g., subcutaneous), especially if injection is involved, and the source patient's viral load (e.g., a patient with terminal AIDS) [22]. After exposure to HIV through blood or body fluids, surveillance for seroconversion should be continued for a minimum of six months, according to CDC guidelines. Rare instances of delayed seroconversion (within 12 months) have been reported and may be associated with simultaneous exposure to HCV and HIV [23].

The efficacy of zidovudine (AZT) in reducing the risk of HIV infection in health care workers is about 80% based on case-control studies [24]. The addition of two other drugs in high-risk exposures was based on clinical experience in treating HIV and is considered biologically plausible but is unsupported by data. Following the original guidelines, the cost of preventing a single case of HIV conversion was noted to be quite high in a setting of low HIV prevalence [25]. In addition to the direct costs of laboratory studies and antiretroviral drugs, there may be indirect costs. The majority of recipients of prophylactic treatment experience side effects (frequently nausea, diarrhea and myalgia; less commonly bone marrow suppression). Absences due to the side effects of prophylaxis or symptom-relieving drugs are not uncommon. In some centers, only a minority of workers are able to tolerate the full four-week course of PEP.

The new guidelines better define terms such as a *deep wound* or *large-bore needle* [23]. A recently published controlled study defines *large bore-needle* as larger than 18 gauge, and *high-risk patient* as one who, retrospectively, dies of terminal AIDS in the subsequent two months. *Deep wound* is defined as a "deep puncture or wound with or without bleeding," as opposed to a "surface scratch without bleeding" or "moderate skin penetration" [26]. This study reconfirmed zidovudine's efficacy in prophylaxis for exposed health care workers. When infection occurs, a deep wound was found to be associated with the greatest likelihood for infection (odds ratio = 15)—more than visible blood (OR = 10) on the object, vascular source (OR = 6), or terminal AIDS (OR = 4.8) [26].

The new CDC guidelines note that the majority of the documented HIV seroconversions in health care workers resulted from direct exposure to blood. Less often, cases were due to exposures to HIV concentrated in the laboratory or to potentially infectious body fluids other than blood. Eighty-seven percent of exposures were percutaneous and 10% mucocutaneous. While a low viral load in the source patient probably indicates a low viral titer exposure, the utility of the viral load measurement in defining risk of transmission is not known; HIV transmission from persons with a plasma viral load below the limits of detection has been reported [23].

The new guidelines provide an algorithm for treatment decisions using a matrix to characterize the riskiness of the exposure and the source patient (Figure 34-2). In low-risk situations, PEP may be unwarranted. If there is an increased risk of transmission, a three-drug regimen using zidovudine, lamivudine, and a protease inhibitor is recommended. In moderate-risk situations, in which HIV transmission is possible but has not been frequently observed, a two-drug regimen (zidovudine and lamivudine) is recommended. In low-risk circumstances, a two-drug regimen may or may not be offered at the clinician's discretion, but infectious risk is considered negligible. Exposure to tears, sweat, or nonbloody urine or feces is not considered HIV exposure and does not require evaluation for PEP.

Under the new guidelines, if the individual source patient cannot be identified or tested, decisions about PEP should be based on exposure risk and the prevalence of HIV in the local patient population. For the untested source patient, a history of intravenous drug use, sexual contact with a known HIV-positive partner, un-

Figure 34-2 / Determining the Need for HIV Postexposure Prophylaxis After an Occupational Exposure. (From Update: provisional Public Health Services recommendations for chemoprophylaxis after exposure to HIV. *MMWR* 1996;45:468–72, with permission.)

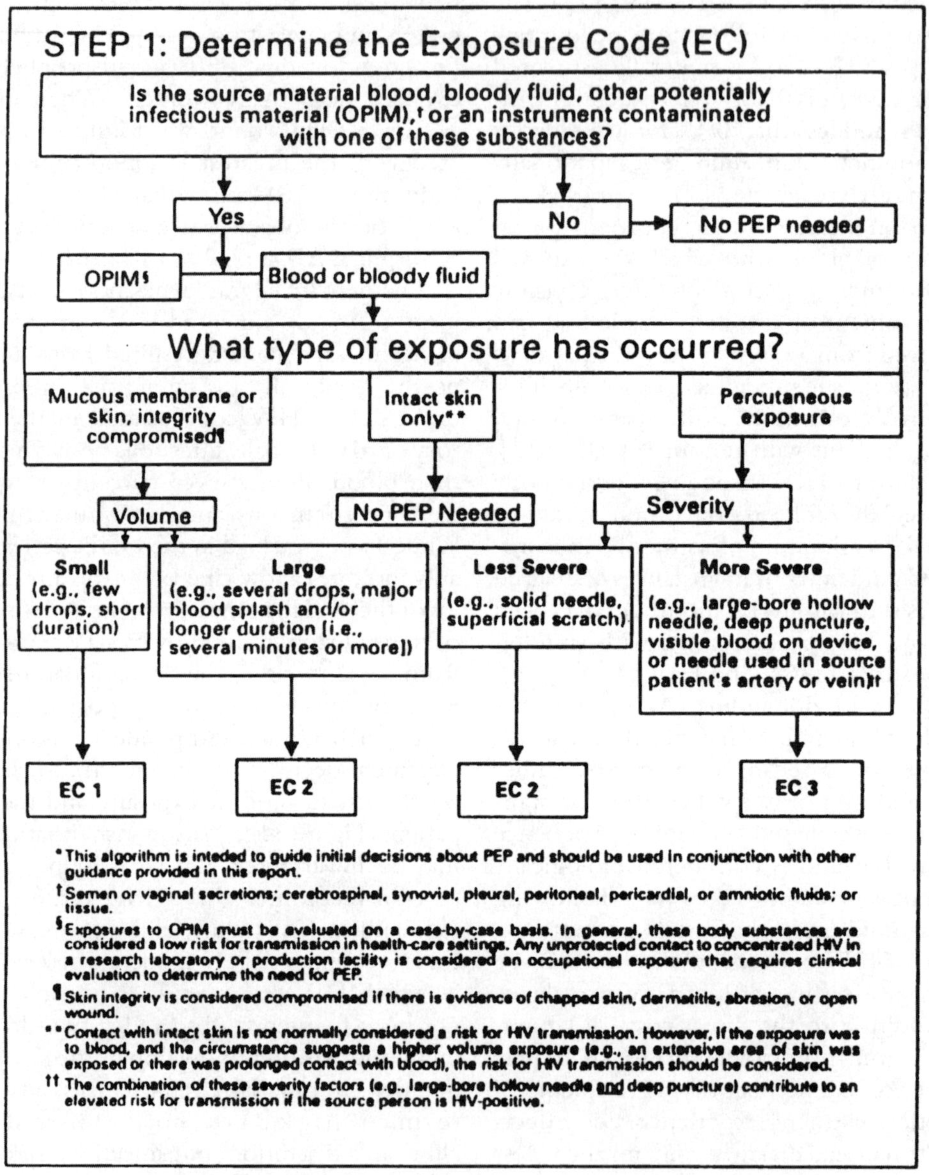

Figure 34-2 (continued)

STEP 2: Determine the HIV Status Code (HIV SC)

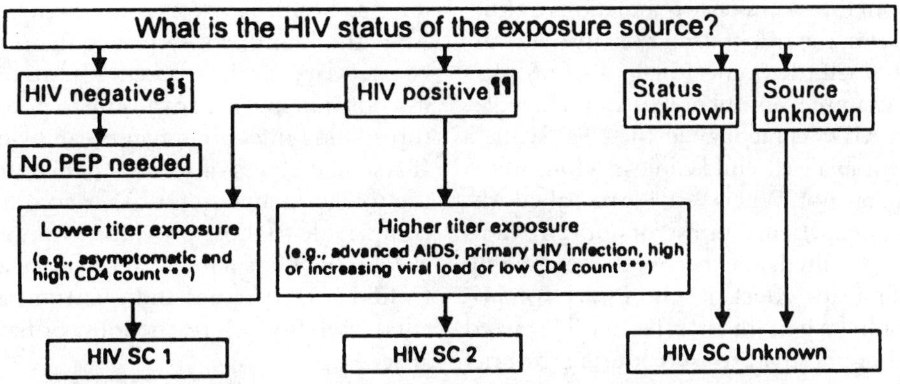

§§ A source is considered negative for HIV infection if there is laboratory documentation of a negative HIV antibody, HIV polymerase chain reaction (PCR), or HIV p24 antigen test result from a specimen collected at or near the time of exposure and there is no clinical evidence of recent retroviral-like illness.

¶¶ A source is considered infected with HIV (HIV positive) if there has been a positive laboratory result for HIV antibody, HIV PCR, or HIV p24 antigen or physician-diagnosed AIDS.

*** Examples are used as surrogates to estimate the HIV titer in an exposure source for purposes of considering PEP regimens and do not reflect all clinical situations that may be observed. Although a high HIV titer (HIV SC 2) in an exposure source has been associated with an increased risk for transmission, the possibility of transmission from a source with a low HIV titer also must be considered.

STEP 3: Determine the PEP Recommendation

EC	HIV SC	PEP recommendation
1	1	**PEP may not be warranted.** Exposure type does not pose a known risk for HIV transmission. Whether the risk for drug toxicity outweighs the benefit of PEP should be decided by the exposed HCW and treating clinician.
1	2	**Consider basic regimen.**††† Exposure type poses a negligible risk for HIV transmission. A high HIV titer in the source may justify consideration of PEP. Whether the risk for drug toxicity outweighs the benefit of PEP should be decided by the exposed HCW and treating clinician.
2	1	**Recommend basic regimen.** Most HIV exposures are in this category; no increased risk for HIV transmission has been observed but use of PEP is appropriate.
2	2	**Recommend expanded regimen.**§§§ Exposure type represents an increased HIV transmission risk.
3	1 or 2	**Recommend expanded regimen.** Exposure type represents an increased HIV transmission risk.
Unknown		If the source or, in the case of an unknown source, the setting where the exposure occurred suggests a possible risk for HIV exposure and the EC is 2 or 3, consider PEP basic regimen.

†††Basic regimen is four weeks of zidovudine, 600 mg per day in two or three divided doses, and lamivudine, 150 mg twice daily.

§§§Expanded regimen is the basic regimen plus either indinavir, 800 mg every 8 hours, or nelfinavir, 750 mg three times a day.

protected sex with multiple partners, or transfusion before 1985, might lead to a decision to implement interim PEP pending source testing, especially if the exposure is more than minimal in severity. In low-prevalence populations or low-risk exposures, the risk of drug toxicity may outweigh any small, theoretical benefit of prophylaxis. For example, an unknown-source needlestick in an AIDS clinic may justify PEP, while a similar event in a well-child clinic in a low prevalence area may not. When PEP is prescribed, clinicians with experience in use of antiretrovirals should be consulted, as expertise in recognizing and handling side effects is a necessary component. Prophylaxis is most effective if started within 1–2 hours after exposure, during the brief interval before systemic infection occurs. Animal studies suggest that treatment is most effective when started early and that prophylaxis may not be effective after 24–36 hours [27]. However, most authorities would not deny prophylaxis to persons with high-risk exposures, even after a 1- to 2-week delay, based on the assumption that it may represent early treatment rather than pure prophylaxis. In such situations, the baseline- and follow-up testing strategies may be adjusted to include HIV-RNA, DNA, or other antigen testing rather than antibody testing, since antibody formation lags behind infection by weeks to months. Expert consultation should be obtained for recommendations.

Treatment and Rehabilitation

In general, HIV-infected health care workers need not be restricted from routine patient care activities (see Nosocomial Bloodborne Pathogens Transmission, below). The Americans with Disabilities Act covers people who have AIDS or who are infected with HIV. The ADA prohibits any employer from discriminating against "physically handicapped" persons (or those perceived to be handicapped). The law took effect on July 26, 1992; employment provisions apply to businesses with 25 or more employees. Besides prohibiting discrimination, the ADA also requires employers to provide "reasonable accommodations" for workers with disabilities, defined as physical or mental impairment that substantially limits a major life activity. Such accommodations include flexible work schedules, restructuring the job, time off for medical appointments, more flexible sick leave, or job reassignment or transfer. Until immunosuppression occurs, as reflected by CD4 lymphocyte counts, the infected health care worker need not be restricted. After the immune system begins to fail, it may be necessary for the worker to be accommodated in a position in which exposure to potentially life-threatening infectious agents can be minimized. If systemic illness or general debilitation occurs, the worker may request other accommodations comparable to those provided to employees with chronic illness such as cancer or heart disease. Confidentiality issues and questions about benefits, disability, job restrictions, or flex time may arise.

Hepatitis B

Hepatitis B causes a spectrum of clinical illnesses ranging from anorexia, vague abdominal discomfort, nausea, and vomiting to jaundice or fulminating liver necrosis [28]. Only a minority of acute cases are recognized clinically.

EPIDEMIOLOGY

The risk factors for hepatitis B are well known, including intravenous drug use, sexual transmission, maternal-neonatal spread, exposure to blood or infectious body fluids via occupational blood exposure, or travel to endemic areas. In 30–40% of cases, the source of transmission is unknown [29]. One third of infections are asymptomatic; the majority experience flu-like symptoms, with or without jaundice, lasting weeks to months. A few may require hospitalization for acute symptoms

The sequelae of hepatitis B are well documented: Five percent of infected adults may develop chronic hepatitis with persistent infectivity, and the risk of eventual cirrhosis and hepatocellular cancer is 5–15% in those with chronic hepatitis [28,29].

It is estimated that 5% of the American population carries serologic evidence of past infection by hepatitis B virus (HBV) and that 0.1–0.5% of these are chronic carriers of the virus [28]. In the past, up to 30% of health care workers in high-risk areas such as dialysis units were infected by HBV. In 1990, the CDC reported 12,000 cases of hepatitis B in health care workers [30].

PREVENTION AND CONTROL

While there has been only a slight decline in the incidence of hepatitis B in the general population since 1985, there has been a 90% decrease in new cases in health care workers in the same time period [29]. This decrease is attributed to the widespread adoption of preventive immunization, universal precautions, and personal protective equipment like gloves, shields, and masks.

OSHA requires that hepatitis B vaccine be offered to all health care workers who are exposed to blood and body fluids in performing their job duties [31]. This protection should also be offered to persons who are not health care workers per se but are also at risk—for example, hospital housekeeping personnel who clean up blood spills or encounter needlesticks from improperly disposed syringes, or the plumbers and other maintenance personnel who dismantle drains where blood and body fluids are discarded. The risk of infection after percutaneous exposure ranges from 2%, if the source patient is hepatitis B E-antigen negative, to 30–40% if E antigen is positive [29]. Overall, the risk of infection is estimated to be 20–30% if percutaneous exposure occurs [32].

In theory, hepatitis B vaccination is highly effective: Ninety-five percent seroconversion rates were noted in initial studies [33]. In practice, however, it is less effective (73–88% seroconversion), especially in groups such as males, smokers, older individuals, and the very obese [34–36]. In health care workers, postvaccination testing is helpful if performed within one to six months of completing the vaccination series [37]. In occupationally exposed individuals, the results of postvaccine testing are useful in determining who needs additional doses as part of their initial series and who needs hepatitis B immune globulin (HBIG) after an exposure incident. An individual who initially seroconverted need not receive HBIG if exposed to a patient who is hepatitis B–antigen positive, even if the titer of antibody is undetectable at the time of the incident (Table 34-5). Antibody titers will decline with

Table 34-5
Recommended Postexposure Prophylaxis for Percutaneous or Permucosal Exposure to Hepatitis B Virus, United States

Vaccination and Antibody Response Status of Exposed Person	Treatment When Source Is		
	HbsAG[a] Positive	**HbsAg Negative**	**Source Not Tested or Status Unknown**
Unvaccinated	HBIG[b] × 1; initiate HB vaccine series[c]	Initiate HB vaccine series	Initiate HB vaccine series
Previously vaccinated:			
Known responder[d]	No treatment	No treatment	No treatment
Known nonresponder	HBIG[b] × 2 or HBIG[b] × 1 and initiate revaccination	No treatment	If known high-risk source, treat as if source were HbsAg positive
Antibody response unknown	Test exposed person for anti-HBs[e] 1. If adequate,[d] no treatment 2. If inadequate,[d] HBIG × 1 and vaccine booster	No treatment	Test exposed person for anti-HBs 1. If adequate,[d] no treatment 2. If inadequate,[d] initiate revaccination

[a] Hepatitis B surface antigen.
[b] Hepatitis B immune globulin; dose 0.06 mL/kg intramuscularly.
[c] Hepatitis B vaccine.
[d] Responder is defined as a person with adequate levels of serum antibody to hepatitis B surface antigen (i.e., anti-Hbs ≥10 mIU/mL); inadequate response to vaccination defined as serum anti-HBs < 10 mIU/mL.
[e] Antibody to hepatitis B surface antigen.
Adapted from Immunization of health care workers. *MMWR* 1997;46(suppl):23.

time; 60% of immunized individuals lose circulating antibody over 12 years [29]. An individual who has previously seroconverted should generate antibody if exposed [38]. While some authors question the cost effectiveness of postvaccine titers [39], their usefulness in health care workers seems clear in light of the frequency of exposures, the high rate of false-negative titers at the time of an exposure incident, the time pressure to obtain laboratory test results and administer HBIG within seven days, and the emotional factors associated with such an incident [36].

While some employees fail to seroconvert after a three-shot series, most subsequently convert after receipt of a second series of three doses. Up to 20% of individuals who do not respond to the original series will seroconvert when they receive a fourth dose, and 30–50% respond after a fifth or sixth [36]. If no antibody response occurs after six injections, no further vaccination is offered. Testing for the chronic carrier state (hepatitis B surface–antigen testing) (Table 34-6) or screening for alcoholism may be indicated in those who do not convert [40]. In one study, alcoholics as a group required larger vaccine doses to seroconvert [41]. Vaccine is injected into the deltoid muscle, as gluteal injection is associated with failure to develop antibody. The vaccine is very safe, although reports of anaphylactic reactions occurring once in 600,000 doses has been published [42]. At present, there is no recommendation for administration of routine booster doses of hepatitis B vaccine after the initial series.

The vaccine contains no infectious material, so its use in pregnant women is not contraindicated. Because there is not much data on its actual use during pregnancy, elective administration for general prevention is often delayed [42] but may be considered if an infectious exposure occurs during pregnancy.

Table 34-6
Interpretation of Hepatitis B Test Results

Test	Results	Interpretation	Recommendation
anti-HBsAg	Positive	Immunity to virus or vaccinated. Vaccine does not contain HBsAg or other parts of the virus.	
HBsAg anti-HBc	Negative Negative	Susceptible to infection/ never exposed to virus.	Consider vaccination.
HBsAg anti-HBc	Positive Positive or negative	Acute or chronic infection.	Conduct further evaluation.
HBsAg anti-HBc	Negative Positive	Multiple interpretations.[a]	Consider vaccination.
HBsAg anti-HBc anti-HBs HbeAg (Last 2 not part of screening)	Positive Positive Negative Positive	Carrier with chronic infection (if HBsAg positive 6 mos or more); highly infectious.	Refer for further evaluation. Consider interferon therapy.
HBsAg anti-HBc anti-HBs HBeAg (Last 2 not part of screening)	Positive Positive Negative Negative	Carrier with chronic infection (if HBsAg positive 6 mos or more); less infectious.	Refer for further evaluation. (Interferon therapy is contraindicated.)

[a] If an individual is positive for anti-HBc and negative for anti-HBs, there are four possible interpretations:
1. Recovering from acute HBV infection, with loss of HBsAg, but anti-HBs yet to appear (serologic window).
2. Immune to HBV, but anti-HBs never appeared or has fallen below the level of detection.
3. Chronic HBV infection, with low level of HBsAg that is undectable in serum.
4. False-positive anti-HBc, with susceptibility to HBV infection.

Interpretations 2 and 4 are the most common explanations for this serologic pattern.
Adapted from *Hepatitis C.* (Monograph.) Cedar Grove, NJ: American Liver Foundation, 1997, with permission.

Hepatitis C

As the prevalence of hepatitis B infection diminishes in health care workers, the relative proportion of cases of bloodborne hepatitis due to hepatitis C virus (HCV) is increasing. Hepatitis C constitutes the majority of what was previously termed *non-A, non-B hepatitis.* Since institution of screening of blood donors in 1990, the incidence of post-transfusion hepatitis C has fallen to less than 1%. Illegal drug use is the major risk factor today [43].

Hepatitis C leads to persistent infection, in 80–85% of cases, or to chronic hepatitis, in 50–60%. Progression of disease usually develops slowly over decades. Hepatocellular carcinoma is a late risk, developing after cirrhosis [44]. Clinically overt disease occurs in less than one third of acute infections [42]. Serum alanine aminotransferase (ALT) levels begin to rise several weeks after infection and usually remain elevated after acute symptoms, if any, have resolved [44]. One third of patients with chronic infection have normal ALT levels.

EPIDEMIOLOGY

Risk factors for infection include intravenous drug use (30–40% of cases) [45] or blood transfusion before 1990, but nearly half of infected persons have no recognized risk factors. Household contact or heterosexual activity may account for up to 10% of cases [42]. The estimated prevalence of hepatitis C virus (HCV) in health care workers is about 1–5% [45–47], with rates as high as 9% reported in oral surgeons [2]. Its prevalence is 0.1–2.0% in the general population but may be as high as 2–18% in hospitalized patients [47,48]. One third of patients with alcoholic liver disease are infected, as are 12–55% of patients with hepatitis B, 15–30% of renal dialysis patients, and 40% of transplant patients [43]. A New York City study found that among asymptomatic persons with mildly elevated transaminase levels, 58% were HCV positive, but the study cited references noting a 17% prevalence of HCV in similar circumstances in other locales [48]. The risk of HCV transmission from needlestick has been found to be roughly 4%, using the anti-HCV test for follow-up, or 10% using the more sensitive but less available RNA polymerase chain reaction (PCR) test [46].

PREVENTION AND CONTROL

If lapses in technique or disinfection procedures occur, nosocomial transmission of HCV is possible and has been reported [50]. Most cases of transmission to health care workers occur because of accidental needlesticks or sharps cuts. Conjunctival splashes have also been reported to result in seroconversion. Because no vaccine exists for HCV, universal precautions and use of personal protective equipment are the primary preventive measures.

TREATMENT

There is little to offer an HCV-exposed individual for prophylaxis, since gamma globulin is ineffective and interferon is used only for treatment. Due to the high risk of an HCV-infected individual's developing chronic hepatitis [43], some experts would initiate interferon when acute hepatitis develops, but this is not a universal practice. Surveillance for development of HCV after a verified blood or body fluid exposure incident should continue for six to nine months to detect anti-HCV. If available, the viral RNA test can detect viral antigen at two to four weeks, before anti HCV antibody develops at eight to 10 weeks, but in most situations, this does not affect the management of the employee. The CDC considers anti HCV the mainstay of hepatitis C diagnosis, but false-negative (5–10%) and false-positive test results may occur, especially the latter in populations with a low prevalence of HCV. The RNA PCR is recommended to confirm a positive anti-HCV test.

The conventional wisdom has been to counsel HCV-infected persons not to change sexual practices if they are in a monogamous relationship, due to the risk (5–10%) of sexual transmission [49]. However, because household spread of both HCV and HBV is fostered by sharing personal articles such as toothbrushes or razors, which may be contaminated with blood, infected persons should be advised against such practices.

Nosocomial Bloodborne Pathogens Transmission

EPIDEMIOLOGY

Occupational exposure to blood is a frequent event in health care. The rate of needlestick injuries among nurses is estimated to be 10–34%. Underreporting of such injuries is common: An estimated 30–60% of incidents are not reported [1].

Transmission of bloodborne pathogens from patient to health care workers is not uncommon, but there has been greater public concern about transmission from infected health care workers. There have been reports of transmission of HBV from surgeons [51], even those who were HbeAg negative [52]. Such reports support the use of postvaccination antibody titers to detect chronic carriers when they fail to seroconvert. In 1996, 34 verified cases of HBV transmission from provider to patient and one case of HIV transmission from a dentist were reported. Most of the cases of hepatitis transmission could have been prevented by vaccination. Among HIV- or HBV-infected patients, the risk of death due to an invasive procedure was estimated to be 2–24 per million procedures [53].

PREVENTION AND CONTROL

As universal precautions and needlestick prevention measures are increasingly implemented and effectively prevent percutaneous exposures [1], a relative increase in exposures due to skin and mucous membrane splashes may be observed. There is tremendous interest in devices to prevent needlesticks and other exposures to sharps, such as needleless infusion sets, retractable needle syringes, and puncture-resistant gloves.

In 1991, the CDC published recommendations related to HIV- or HBV-infected health care workers [32]. Subsequently, Congress mandated that each state implement CDC guidelines or their equivalent as a condition for continuing to receive federal public health funding. While all states have complied with this mandate, there is a fair degree of state-to-state variation regarding specific provisions. Some states mandate the reporting of HIV- and HBV-infected surgeons or others who perform infection-associated procedures, for review and possible limitation of their work practices. High-risk procedures are defined as digital palpation of a needletip in a body cavity and use of fingers, needles or sharps in a poorly visualized, highly confined area [32]. Local or state public health officials should be contacted to determine the applicable local regulations. The recommended work restrictions and reporting requirements have potential legal, ethical, risk management, and workers' compensation implications. There are many complex and unaddressed issues concerning their ramifications [54], leading surgeons and health care workers to be reluctant to report their exposure incidents.

At present there are no specific recommendations from the CDC or other authorities regarding restriction of health care workers with HCV, since the risk of its transmission appears to be very low and no current serologic test can reliably determine infectivity (Table 34-7) [46].

Bite Wounds

Human bites may occur in the health care setting and lead to skin infections or bloodborne pathogens transmission. Human bites can become infected with skin flora such as staphylococcus or streptococcus as well as anaerobes and other mouth flora such as *Eikenella corrodens* (associated with dental disease). Bite wounds of the hands are at increased risk for infection. A broad-spectrum antibiotic that will cover most potential pathogens (e.g., amoxicillin-clavulanate, ciprofloxacin, or cloxacillin) may be used for prophylaxis or treatment of infection [55]. If the worker's bite wound bleeds, the biter is clearly exposed to the employee's blood.

Questions also arise about the risk of transmission of bloodborne pathogens to the bitten health care worker. If the biter has bleeding gums or open mouth lesions, there is potential for transmission of bloodborne pathogens. Although saliva is not generally considered an infectious body fluid (unless visibly contaminated with blood), transmission of HBV via saliva alone has been reported [56]. Similarly, although HIV rarely exists in saliva, there have been isolated case reports of HIV transmission via bite wounds

Table 34-7
Interpretation of Hepatitis C Test Results

Test	Results	Interpretation	Recommendation
Anti-HCV (EIA-2)	Positive	Chronic hepatitis, chronic hepatitis C recovered, recent acute hepatitis C, or false-positive test	Further evaluation
Anti-HCV (EIA-2) ALT Supplemental test (RIBA-2)	Positive Normal Positive	Possible chronic HCV carrier; may have chronic hepatitis C infection	Further evaluation by HCV RNA PCR test
Anti-HCV (EIA-2) ALT	Positive Elevated	Presumed chronic hepatitis C infection	Further evaluation by HCV RNA PCR test; consider interferon therapy
Anti-HCV (EIA-2) ALT Supplemental test (RIBA-2)	Positive Normal Negative or indeterminate	Presumed false-positive anti-HCV test or recovered from hepatitis C infection	Further evaluation by HCV-RNA PCR test is RIBA-2 negative or indeterminate
Anti-HCV (EIA-2) ALT HCV RNA PCR	Positive Elevated Negative	Presumed false-positive anti-HCV test	Further evaluation for liver disease other than hepatitis C
ALT (no other symptoms)	Elevated	Possible fatty liver, chronic viral hepatitis, alcoholic liver disease, hemochromatosis, drug-induced liver injury, or other liver disease	Further evaluation

Definitions:
- *Anti-HCL:* antibody to hepatitis C virus.
- *ALT:* Liver enzyme released from liver cells that are injured (e.g., by virus, alcohol, fat, or drug).
- *RIBA-2:* Supplemental test to detect antibody to hepatitis C virus.
- *Indeterminate:* 1 of 4 antigens positive.
- *HCV RNA PCR:* HCV-RNA test by polymerase chain reaction (PCR) to determine whether the virus is multiplying.

Adapted from *Hepatitis C.* (Monograph.) Cedar Grove, NJ: American Liver Foundation, 1997, with permission.

[57,58]. While possible, the risk of transmission of HIV through saliva alone (or via biting) is considered so low as to be negligible. At present, CDC guidelines [23] do not recommend postexposure prophylaxis for HIV when a health care worker is bitten by an HIV-positive source if the source does not have bleeding gums, mucosal lesions, or other risk factors.

The risk for HCV infection via bite wound is presumed to be moderate—between the risk for HBV and that of HIV. Detection of the presence of HCV in saliva varies, depending on the study methods, timing, and population [59–61]. Currently, the decision regarding follow-up of a health care worker bitten by a HCV-infected patient is an institutional choice, pending better data.

Employee Skin Breaks and Lesions

Health care workers with rashes or nonintact skin, regardless of cause, may present a staffing dilemma. These workers can spread infections to patients if their condition results from a systemic or local infection. Broken skin may preclude the scrubbing necessary for participation in sterile procedures or work in special units in the hospital. If serous fluid is weeping from broken skin and cannot be covered, patients may be exposed to the employee's body fluid. Employee skin breaks present an entry route for a variety of infectious agents in addition to bloodborne pathogens. The algorithm in Figure 34-3 presents an approach to dealing with the complexities of employee skin breaks and lesions and is intended

Figure 34-3 / Restrictions for Health Care Workers with Skin Conditions (Rash or Nonintact Skin, i.e., Cuts, Sutures, Burns, Blisters, Deep Abrasions)

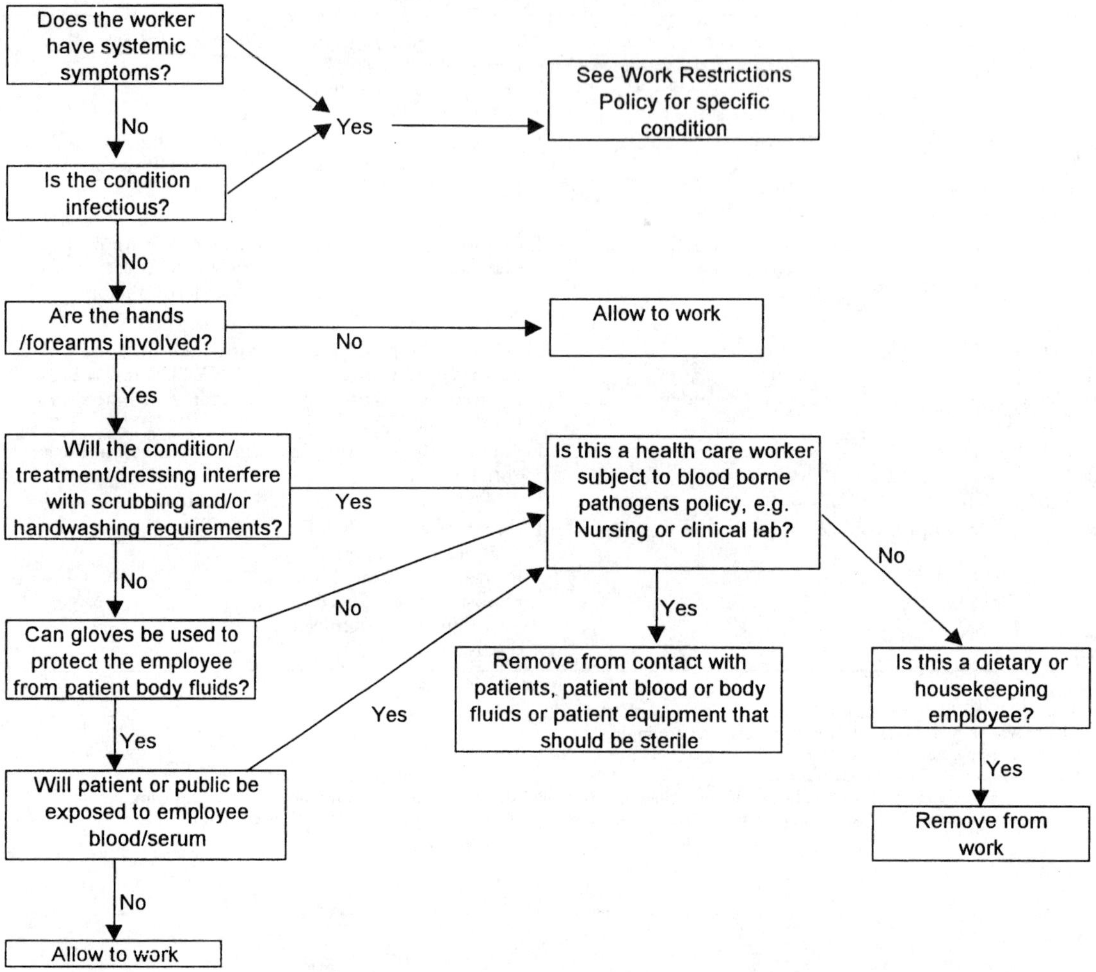

for use by unit managers in a tertiary care center. The specific approach used in any situation should, however, take into account actual work practices and estimation of employee and patient risk.

Patient Skin Infections and Infestations

Skin infections in patients put health care workers at risk. Tinea corporis may spread from patients to staff. Type I herpes simplex virus is a risk for nonimmune dentists, anesthetists, physical therapists, and nurses [2]. Patients can transmit ectoparasites like lice (*Pediculus humanis, P capitis, P pubis*, or *P corporis*), or scabies (*Sarcoptes scabei miti*) to health care workers.

The burrowing mites of scabies cause papular eruptions that itch, especially at night. In older children and adults, scabies lesions occur in interdigital folds, and centrally in skinfolds. In children under age 2, the eruption is more likely to occur as vesicles, on the head, neck, palms, and soles [62]. Scabies is readily spread by direct skin-to-skin contact, which may occur during bathing, lifting, or applying lotions. Even minimal contact with crusted scabies can result in mite transmission, even before the source is symptomatic. Incubation time can be four to six weeks, but a previously infected, sensitized individual may develop symptoms within one to four days of reinfection. A scabicide prescription is recommended for all health care workers after scabies exposure due to the high risk of infestation. Permethrin cream 5% is the current topical medication of choice [62]. Other options are crotamiton 10% and lindane 1% lotion. Contact precautions should be instituted when caring for infested patients prior to application of topical scabicide to their lesions. Routine cleaning of bed linens and upholstered furniture will help eliminate mites, but additional cleaning may be needed for crusted scabies [40].

Head lice are spread by hair-to-hair contact with infested persons; body lice can be spread by manual contact with the bed linen or clothing of infested persons, necessitating the use of gloves for such activities. Lice stay alive while on the host; when away from the host, their survival time ranges from one to two days for head lice to 10 days for body lice. Incubation time is six to 10 days, from laying of eggs until hatching [62]. Health care workers are treated only if infested and should be restricted from work for 24 hours after treatment [40]. Acquisition of pediculosis requires more intimate, direct, prolonged body contact than does scabies. Infestation may be treated with permethrin cream 1%, or malathion 0.5% or lindane 1% lotion.

Conjunctivitis

Infectious conjunctivitis in a health care worker can be an indication to restrict the worker from patient contact. There are many viral and bacterial causes of conjunctivitis (e.g., *Haemophilus influenzae*, *Streptococcus pneumoniae*, enterovirus, adenoviral pharyngeal conjunctival fever, chlamydial neonatal conjunctivitis), but nosocomial outbreaks due to such agents are rare [28]. In the health care setting, and in adults generally, adenovirus is of most concern because it can cause epidemic keratoconjunctivitis (EKC).

EPIDEMIOLOGY

EKC is spread by direct contact with infected eye secretions; outbreaks have been reported in eye clinics and medical offices [28]. The incubation time for adenoviral conjunctivitis averages five to 12 days. The virus is typically communicable from late in the incubation period to 14 days after onset of symptoms; viral shedding may be prolonged beyond 14 days [40].

PREVENTION AND CONTROL

To prevent the spread of EKC in clinics, thorough handwashing and high-level disinfection of instruments that come into contact with the conjunctiva or eyelids are recommended. Gloves should be worn to examine the eyes of patients with possible or confirmed EKC. Single-use strips, droppers, or applicators for should be used for application of ophthalmic medications. Health care workers with infectious conjunctivitis, whether AKC or purulent conjunctivitis, should be restricted from patient care while symptoms are present.

Varicella

Chickenpox (varicella) is an acute, viral disease characterized sudden onset of fever, mild constitutional symptoms, and skin eruption. The rash, which occurs in crops, is maculopapular for a few hours and then vesicular for three to four days, leaving scabs. Varicella-zoster virus is spread from person to person by the airborne route, direct contact with vesicular fluid or respiratory secretions, or by articles freshly soiled by these fluids.

EPIDEMIOLOGY

Varicella infection is most severe in adults, with a case fatality rate of 30 per 100,000 in the United States. Viral pneumonia is a frequent complication of varicella infection [28]. Children with acute leukemia, even those in remission, are at increased risk of disseminated infection, which is fatal in 5–10% of cases. Herpes zoster, or shingles, a localized outbreak of skin vesicles, results from reactivation of varicella virus, which lies dormant in the dorsal root ganglia years after the primary chickenpox infection [28]. Varicella virus is highly contagious, especially in the early stages of cutaneous eruption; herpes zoster has a lower rate of transmission. Both can cause chickenpox in seronegative contacts [28].

Exposure to varicella can be problematic for the nonimmune health care worker, as nosocomial spread is well recognized. If infected, the worker will be contagious for one to two days prior to the onset of the rash, at which time the virus can be spread to nonimmune or immunocompromised individuals [28]. Although rare, congenital varicella syndrome can cause low birth weight, cutaneous scarring, limb hypoplasia, chorioretinitis, cataracts, and other anomalies in newborns. Newborns of women in the first half of pregnancy are at greatest risk; if infected in utero, the risk for development of congenital varicella syndrome is 0.7–2.0% [63]. Nonimmune pregnant mothers who develop chickenpox near term can also transmit varicella to the newborn. This infection can be severe or fatal, as insufficient maternal antibody will have developed to protect the infant. Overall, premature or low-birth-weight infants and individuals with immune suppression or malignancy are at greatest risk for nosocomial infection. For these reasons, it is recommended that the nonimmune employee be removed from work days 10–21 following exposure, per CDC recommendations [40], or days 8–21, per recommendations of the American Academy of Pediatrics [64].

Most adults have developed immunity to varicella. A history of chickenpox is a very reliable indicator of immunity; 97–99% will be positive for antibody. Of adults with a negative or uncertain history, 71–93% are actually seropositive [63]. On the other hand, prior infection and antibody development is not 100% protective against reinfection with chickenpox or against recurrence as herpes zoster. When chickenpox occurs in immune persons, its morbidity may be mild and slightly atypical, with few lesions and minimal fever.

PREVENTION AND CONTROL

Varicella vaccine is recommended for use in health care workers who have no history of chickenpox and have tested negative for varicella antibodies [65]. Two injections are delivered four to eight weeks apart; 99% of recipients develop antibodies. While vaccine-induced immunity (like natural immunity) may still allow "breakthrough" infection to occur, disease will be mild and shorter in duration and will produce fewer lesions [66]. There is no indication for routinely removing healthy vaccinated workers from their patient care duties, as there is minimal risk of their transmitting the virus, unless a rash develops. From 1–5% of them may develop the varicella-like rash that sheds the virus at a low titer; the individual may then be removed from patient contact [29], especially if the skin lesions cannot be covered by clothing. The incidence of secondary transmission is less than 1%, with immunocompromised individuals at greater risk [63].

Routine postvaccination titers are not recommended but may be considered for health care workers following a varicella exposure. If no circulating antibody is detected, the titer may be repeated in five to six days, when an anamnestic humoral antibody response may boost the titer to detectable levels. Although the circulating antibody levels cannot reflect the activity of cellular immunity, employee furlough may be considered if circulating antibody does increase in response to the exposure. The effectiveness of postexposure immunization is not known [28], but may be of some value if administered within 96 hours [64].

Varicella vaccine contains live virus and is not recommended for pregnant women, HIV-positive individuals, or those with immunosuppression or malignancy. Vaccination should be delayed for five months following receipt of blood, plasma, immune globulin, or varicella-zoster immune globulin (VZIG) [63]. VZIG vaccination can prolong the incubation time for chickenpox to 28 days if the recipient has been recently infected with varicella. It is not recommended in the immunocompetent health care worker for whom the risk of infection is low, but if it is used, VZIG should be given within 96 hours of exposure [62]. For the immunocompromised, postexposure administration of acyclovir may be effective and is less costly than VZIG [63]. Moreover, VZIG is not recommended when immunocompromised patients are vaccinated [63].

Health care workers with localized herpes zoster should not care for immunocompromised patients until lesions are dry and crusted or unless the lesions are covered. Since the virus is transmitted by direct contact with lesions and by the airborne route, both contact and airborne precautions should be used by all health care workers caring for infected patients until all their skin lesions are crusted. Isolation of patients with varicella or disseminated zoster in a negative pressure room is recommended in addition to workers' use of masks and gowns to prevent spread of virus to other patients.

Pertussis

Over the past five years, the incidence of reported cases of pertussis (Figure 34-4) has increased beyond recent historic limits [67]. Pertussis, or whooping cough, can be a life-threatening infection in infants, but childhood immunization has eliminated much of the morbidity and mortality in young children. Immunity from vaccination wanes with time, and pertussis vaccine is not given to children older than 7 years of age; therefore, immunized adolescents and adults can be susceptible to infection and serve as a reservoir of infection to children. In adults, pertussis presents as a mild atypical respiratory illness, usually without the characteristic whooping cough. Of coughs lasting over one to two weeks, up to 25% have been attributed to pertussis [68]. It is estimated that 50 million adults are susceptible to pertussis and 20–60% of adults with pertussis infection are asymptomatic [69].

EPIDEMIOLOGY

Pertussis is frequently not diagnosed in adults due to the need for specific testing of nasopharyngeal secretions. While health care workers are not at substantially greater risk of infection than the general population [29], introduction of pertussis into the health care setting can be problematic. Mini-epidemics have occurred in hospitals where adults have transmitted the infection to pediatric patients. Infection is spread by direct contact with respiratory secretions; thus, hands-on caretakers can acquire the infection and

Figure 34-4 / Pertussis (Whooping Cough)—by Year, United States, 1966–1996. (From Selected notifiable disease reports. *MMWR* 1996;46:1021.

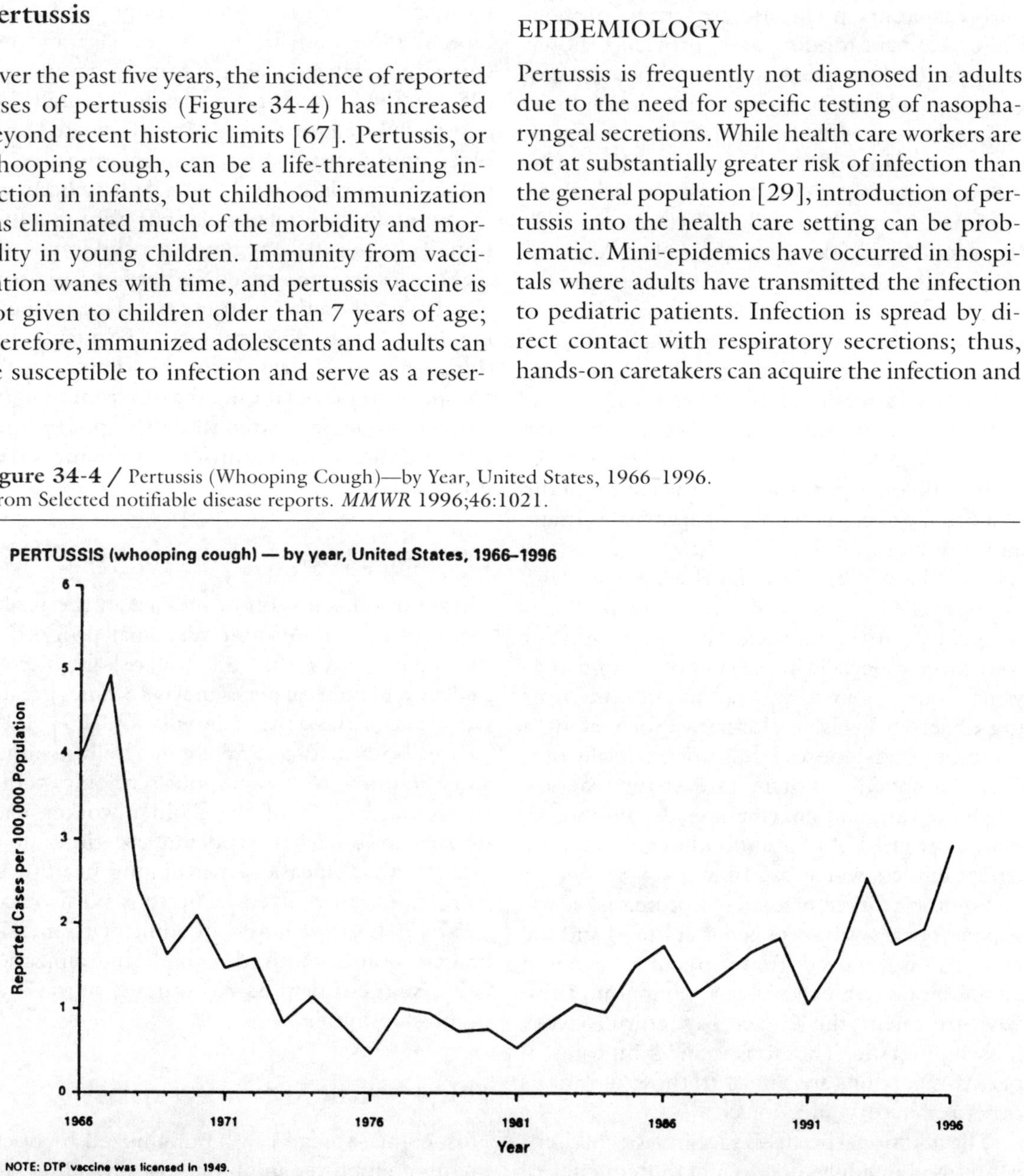

perpetuate the cycle. The incubation period for pertussis is six to 20 days and infection can last for four to eight weeks if untreated [28].

PREVENTION AND CONTROL

Isolation precautions to control droplet spread should be instituted for infected inpatients until five days of therapy have been completed. If an outbreak occurs in a health care setting, prophylactic treatment for direct care providers should be considered to break the cycle of spread, especially to children. For asymptomatic individuals, prophylaxis consists of a 14-day course of erythromycin, 500 qid, or trimethoprim-sulfamethoxazole, DS bid, started within three weeks of exposure [69]. The treatment dose and the prophylactic dose are the same. Azithromycin, 500 mg on day 1 and 250 mg daily for the next four days, is an alternative; the new macrolides may have fewer side effects, but there are fewer studies on their use. In one report, seven days of treatment for pertussis with erythromycin estolate was as effective as a 14-day course [70]. After paroxysmal cough develops, these antibiotics may not affect the course of the illness but will eradicate nasopharyngeal carriage and thus limit transmission.

Nasopharyngeal culture for *Bordetella pertussis* on Bordet-Gengou or Regan-Lowe media is helpful if positive, but organisms can be difficult to recover, especially in the later phase of paroxysmal cough. Direct-fluorescent antibody testing of secretions is an alternative for making a presumptive diagnoses but is not especially sensitive or specific. Polymerase chain reaction (PCR) testing and enzyme-linked immunosorbent assay (ELISA) for antibodies are more accurate but less widely available.

For the worker who is symptomatic, a nasopharyngeal swab specimen is cultured and the employee is removed from work and started on an antibiotic regimen. After a minimum of five days' treatment, the worker may return to work if asymptomatic. The nonspecific symptoms of pertussis in adults are similar to those of various other respiratory infections.

The traditional pertussis vaccine (for children) is not used in adults due to a high frequency of side effects. While not yet licensed for use in adults, the new acellular vaccine has been used effectively to terminate a persistent hospital outbreak when administered to employees [71], and an adult formulation of the vaccine is expected to be developed in the near future.

Measles

Measles is an acute viral disease characterized by fever, conjunctivitis, coryza, cough, and a red blotchy rash. Rash begins on the face and becomes generalized, lasting four to seven days [28]. In the United States, measles generally occurs in children too young to be vaccinated or in older individuals; pneumonia and encephalitis are potential complications. Outbreaks have occurred in immunized school populations prior to adoption of the two-dose regimen for children.

Measles is transmitted by large respiratory droplets via the airborne route and is highly transmissible during close contact. The incubation time is five to 21 days. Virus shedding from the nasopharynx occurs during the prodrome and for three to four days after the rash appears—for longer if the infected individual is immunocompromised.

EPIDEMIOLOGY

Although transmission of measles in the health care setting accounts for a very small proportion of total cases (less than 5%), the risk for measles infection in medical personnel is 13 times greater than that of the general population [29]. Individuals born before 1957 are generally assumed to be immune to measles, but serologic studies show that 5–10% of these older workers lack measles antibodies. In epidemic situations, up to one fourth of measles cases among health care workers have occurred in persons born before 1957 [29]. Overall, 40% of adults with measles had previously received a single immunization [72], suggesting possible waning of vaccine-induced immunity.

PREVENTION AND CONTROL

Nosocomial spread can be minimized by documenting employee immunity (or providing vaccine), identifying and isolating persons with fever and rash, and adopting precautions against airborne transmission when measles is suspected or proved. If exposed, a nonimmune health care worker should be furloughed from work from day 5 after first exposure until day 21 after the last exposure. If rash develops, the worker should be restricted from work for at least four days after eruption.

The CDC recommends a single dose of vaccine for workers born before 1957 if they lack evidence of immunity, e.g., are unvaccinated, have no history of disease, or lack serologic evidence of immunity. For those born in or after 1957, documentation of physician-diagnosed measles, two doses of vaccine after age 1, or serologic evidence of immunity is required [40]. Many adults immunized during childhood will need a second vaccine dose. Persons who received killed measles virus prior to 1968 should receive a second dose to protect against atypical measles [28]; it should be expected that they may have more reactions on repeat vaccination. Contraindications to the live attenuated measles virus vaccine include pregnancy (based on theoretical grounds), egg allergy marked by anaphylaxis, or immunosuppression, regardless of cause. Asymptomatic HIV infection is not a contraindication unless CD4-lymphocyte counts are suppressed [70]. During measles outbreaks, vaccination should be given within 72 hours after exposure, without prior serologic testing, to any adult who has not received two doses of vaccine, regardless of age or serologic status [29].

Anaphylaxis is a rare reaction to measles vaccine. There have been 30 reported cases of anaphylaxis per 70 million doses; urticaria and wheal and flare reactions are more common [42]. Egg allergy is a contraindication only when associated with anaphylactic reaction; unfortunately, skin testing for egg allergy has not been useful in predicting reactions [29]. Measles vaccine's efficacy is 95% with one dose and 99% with two. Measles vaccine prevents subacute sclerosing panencephalitis (SSPE) and does not increase its risk, even in those previously infected or vaccinated with live virus. Rarely, the measles mumps rubella (MMR) vaccine has been associated with thrombocytopenia within two months, at a rate of 1 in 30,000–40,000; a prior history of idiopathic thrombocytopenic purpura (ITP) is associated with increased risk [42]. To be fully efficacious, administration of this live virus vaccine should be delayed for at least five weeks after receipt of IgG.

Mumps

The age group at greatest risk for mumps infection is shifting from childhood to adolescence. This viral disease of the salivary and other glands can cause orchitis in 20–30% of postpubertal males and oophoritis in 5% of postpubertal females, but sterility is a rare complication [28]. Aseptic meningitis is a relatively common complication, but encephalitis is rare at 1–2 cases per 10,000. Pancreatitis occurs in 4% of cases [28].

EPIDEMIOLOGY

Outbreaks of mumps involving adolescents and young adults have occurred in hospitals and long-term care facilities [40]. Mumps virus is spread by contact with saliva or other respiratory secretions; the incubation period is 12–25 days, generally 16–18. Virus can be present in saliva for six to seven days prior to observable parotitis and for nine days after its onset. Infection is asymptomatic in about one third of cases.

PREVENTION AND CONTROL

Droplet precautions should be implemented and continued for nine days for inpatients when infection is recognized. Health care workers are considered immune if they have had physician-diagnosed mumps, received one dose of vaccine after age 1, or have serologic evidence of immunity. Most persons born before 1957 are considered immune. Nonimmune employees should be put on work restriction or furlough from days 12 through 26 postexposure or for nine days after onset of parotitis [29]. Although the failure of primary vaccine has been reported, it is about 95% effective.

Rubella

Rubella is a mild febrile illness; it is associated with a diffuse punctate, maculopapular rash in over half of cases. Encephalitis and arthralgia/arthritis are occasional complications in adults.

Rubella is most important because of its teratogenic effect on the developing fetus. Congenital rubella syndrome occurs in up to 90% of infants born to women infected during the first trimester. Fetal risk falls to 10–20% by the sixteenth week of gestation and is rare after week 20. Rubella during pregnancy is associated with intrauterine death, spontaneous abortion, or congenital malformations resulting in deafness, cataracts, congenital glaucoma, microphthalmia, mental retardation, cardiac defects or insulin dependent diabetes [28].

EPIDEMIOLOGY

Transmission of rubella from both male and female workers has occurred in the hospital setting. Rubella is less infectious than measles, but 10–15% of young adults may be susceptible, and about 6% of health care workers lack detectable antibody [29]. Transmission occurs through direct contact and nasopharyngeal droplets. The incubation period ranges from 12–23 days, with rash usually appearing at 14–16 days. Virus is shed from one week before to 5–7 days after appearance of the rash; individuals are most contagious while it is erupting.

PREVENTION AND CONTROL

Because of the frequency of subclinical, inapparent infections and the nonspecific nature of the illness, the clinical diagnosis of rubella is unreliable and a history of vaccination or serologic immunity must be obtained, even in health care workers born prior to 1957. Serologic screening prior to vaccination is not needed, as prior immunity does not increase the incidence of adverse reactions. Pregnancy is a contraindication to vaccination, and women are counseled to avoid pregnancy for three months following administration of vaccine, primarily on theoretical grounds. In cases in which pregnant women were inadvertently immunized, congenital defects have not been observed, so vaccination need not be considered an indication for abortion. The live, attenuated virus vaccine elicits an antibody response in 98–99% of recipients. Rubella vaccine is grown in human diploid cells, not in eggs; it may contain a trace of neomycin and thus so may be contraindicated in persons with anaphylactic allergy [73]. The CDC recommends that health care workers be immunized with MMR vaccine, if any single component is indicated, unless there is a specific contraindication to the combination.

Meningococcus

Meningococcal infection can lead to a wide spectrum of disease, including sepsis, meningitis, and pneumonia. Up to 5–10% of people in countries with endemic disease carry *Neisseria meningitidis* asymptomatically in the nasopharynx [28]. A small minority of individuals colonized with the bacteria progress to invasive disease.

EPIDEMIOLOGY

Group A organisms are found in subSaharan Africa and the Asian subcontinent. Group B has been the most common cause of disease in the Americas, and group C is equally common in the United States. Presently, serogroups B and C constitute 90% of endemic cases in this country [40]. Infection is ubiquitous, and disease occurs commonly in children and young adults, frequently among newly aggregated adults in crowded conditions such as barracks and institutions.

During sporadic endemic meningococcal episodes, the incidence of secondary community cases is low at 0.5 case per 100,000 per year. During outbreaks, this may rise to over 10 per 100,000 [74,75]. Persons at risk include household contacts, with a transmission rate of 7 per 1,000, or day care contacts, 4 per 1,000. Risk is fostered by close personal contact and direct exposure to oral secretions. The secondary transmission rate has been reported to be as high as 7% when individuals are exposed in a small closed space [76].

Nosocomial transmission from patients is uncommon. At-risk health care workers are those who have intimate, direct contact with oropharyngeal secretions of infected persons, e.g., during intubating, resuscitating, suctioning the airway, or examining the throat. After 24 hours of appropriate antibiotic therapy, patients may be considered noninfectious.

PREVENTION AND CONTROL

Droplet precautions should be implemented for patients with meningococcal meningitis or pneumonia, and masks and gloves used for the high-risk procedures involving oropharyngeal secretions. These precautions should also be considered during the evaluation of any child or young adult suspected of having meningitis, pending laboratory diagnosis. Patients with pneumonia and a productive cough have the greatest potential for spreading infection. Casual contact with infected persons, such as cleaning rooms or delivering trays, involves negligible risk of infection [40]. Pharyngeal colonization per se is not a risk factor for dissemination.

For health care workers who are intimately exposed to nasopharyngeal secretions without using appropriate precautions, postexposure prophylaxis should be administered, ideally within 24 hours, to eradicate possible pharyngeal colonization. *N meningitidis* has a short incubation time, typically three to five days; after 14 days following exposure, prophylaxis is of limited or no value [74]. Rifampin, 600 mg bid twice daily, is the traditional prophylaxis but cannot be used in pregnant women and may decrease the effectiveness of oral contraceptive medications. Ciprofloxacin, 500 mg PO once daily, can be used in adults but not pregnant women, and is reported to be 90% effective. Ceftriaxone, 250 mg IM, is 97–100% effective and may be used in pregnancy [75].

Laboratory personnel may also be at risk through handling respiratory secretions or blood specimens. Laboratory aerosolization of a respiratory specimen can transmit infection; thus, precautions should continue in the laboratory and with specimen handling. Prophylaxis for lab personnel should be considered after significant laboratory exposures.

Other types of bacterial meningitis do not have the same implications for health care workers. With *Haemophilus influenzae* meningitis, only children who are household or day care contacts require prophylaxis [75]; adult contacts are not at risk.

Influenza

Influenza may be transmitted by large airborne droplets or by aerosolization of small particles; the role of environmental or fomite transmission is unknown. The incubation time is one to five days. Individuals are most infectious during the first three days of illness; virus is shed prior to the onset of symptoms and for seven days thereafter.

EPIDEMIOLOGY

Individuals over age 65, those living in nursing homes or chronic care facilities, and those with chronic conditions, such as pulmonary or cardiovascular disease or diabetes, are at greatest risk [40]. In these groups, influenza can lead to secondary pneumonia and concomitant mortality. Nosocomial transmission can occur during community outbreaks, spreading among patients and staff and resulting in widespread absenteeism that may disrupt the effective operation of the health care facility [40].

PREVENTION AND CONTROL

Nosocomial infection can be prevented by instituting droplet precautions (requiring that health care workers use masks) when handling infected patients and by yearly administration of the influenza vaccine to health care workers. It is recommended that all health care workers be vaccinated, including pregnant women after the first trimester. Work-restriction policies should remove infected personnel from the delivery of patient care, especially in high-risk areas such as intensive care, neonatal, and transplant units. As it takes two weeks for immunity to develop, in anticipation of the peak flu season, the optimal time for vaccination is mid-October to mid-November [74]. Too-early vaccination may result in less-than-optimal protection by late spring.

During community epidemics, it may become necessary for health care facilities to isolate patients with influenza in negative-pressure rooms, restrict hospital visitors with febrile respiratory illness, and postpone elective surgery [77]. Obtaining culture specimens from employees via nasopharyngeal swabs or washings may be useful if there is not adequate community characterization of the influenza strains responsible for the epidemic. Culture and characterization of the virus may take five to seven days and will usually not change the management of the illness in the individual.

If nosocomial transmission of influenza A is documented, prophylaxis with the antiviral agents amantadine or rimantidine can be administered to unvaccinated staff, preferably in conjunction with vaccination. These drugs are 70–90% effective in preventing influenza [77], although less in individuals who are elderly or have chronic medical problems. These antiviral agents can also be used for treatment if instituted early in the course of the illness. Central nervous system side effects may occur in 5–10% of young healthy adults. Prophylaxis for the duration of the epidemic may be considered for workers for whom vaccination is contraindicated or who are immunosuppressed and expected to have poor antibody response.

During the 1997–98 flu season, the A/Sidney/OS/97(H3N2) strain was predominant [79]. The Sidney strain is notable in that the protection provided by the 1997–98 vaccine against this strain was low. Nonetheless, vaccination appeared to reduce death rates even when it failed to prevent influenza-like illness. The possibility of reduced effectiveness of vaccine against a particular strain emphasizes the need to use other adjunct control measures within institutions, including work restriction and isolation procedures, during epidemics.

Recent research suggests that flu vaccine may reduce overall rates of respiratory illness and absenteeism compared to placebo [80–82], justifying its use on a cost-effectiveness basis, even in healthy, low-risk workers. Side effects of the vaccine may include a mild local reaction in 25–50%, beginning the first day and lasting one to two days. Systemic reactions are less frequent (6% of adults), with fever, chills, malaise, and myalgia having their onset within six to 12 hours and lasting one to two days. Guillain-Barré syndrome has not been clearly associated with influenza vaccination since 1976. Anaphylactic hypersensitivity to eggs is a contraindication to flu vaccination [82].

Rabies

Rabies is an acute viral encephalomyelopathy, presenting with headache, fever, malaise, and other localized sensory changes and progressing to delirium, convulsions, and death. Routes of infections other than bites are frequently involved in the spread from zoonotic sources; 40% of cases have no identified source of exposure [83].

EPIDEMIOLOGY

In the United States, human rabies occurs infrequently but is almost always fatal. The incubation period is three to eight weeks but can be as short as nine days or as long as several years [28]. In 1996, three cases of rabies were reported in humans, and 6,982 cases in animals [84].

Rabies virus may be present in a variety of human fluids and tissues during the first five weeks of illness. In a majority of cases, virus is usually not found in urine, blood or serum, but rather in saliva or respiratory secretions [85]. Cerebrospinal fluid, brain tissue, skeletal muscle, skin, and peripheral nerve tissue also are frequent sites for virus isolation. Exposure of an open wound or mucus membrane to infected saliva is especially risky.

PREVENTION AND CONTROL

Although transmission of rabies from patients to health care personnel has not been documented, personal protective equipment (e.g., gloves, gowns, masks) should be used to avoid the potential hazard from saliva of patients who are coughing or unable to control secretions. A health care worker should be given prophylaxis if bitten, scratched, or stuck with a sharp or if mucous membranes or broken skin is splashed with infected fluid. Prophylaxis consists of immediate administration of human rabies immune globulin, 20 IU/kg, half infused into the wound and the other half given intramuscularly, and initiation of rabies vaccine series. Rabies vaccination consists of one dose injected into the deltoid muscle on days 1, 3, 7, 14, and followed by one dose anytime from day 28 to day 35. If the recipient has previously been immunized, only two booster doses of vaccine are needed after exposure.

Theoretically a bite or nonbite exposure to saliva could result in human-to-human infection, but there are no documented cases of such spread. The need for postexposure prophylaxis for health care workers caring for a patient with rabies should be assessed on a case-by-case basis to ascertain the level of actual risk. High-risk contact is percutaneous or mucus membrane contact with saliva, respiratory secretions, corneal tissue or tears, cerebrospinal fluid or urinary sediment, especially, with a bite, skin break, or percutaneous injury. Strategies to minimize exposure of health care workers and subsequent need for postexposure prophylaxis include early consideration of rabies in the differential diagnosis of progressive neurologic disease of unknown etiology or febrile encephalopathy, followed by prompt implementation of standard barrier precautions [84].

Pre-exposure prophylaxis is indicated for veterinarians and animal researchers using dogs, cats, or other carrier animals and for laboratory personnel involved in production of, or research using, rabies virus. Standard precautions and proper biosafety equipment should be used in the laboratory setting. Airborne spread does not occur unless there is centrifugation or other aerosolization of infected fluid or tissue. In these situations, respiratory and eye protection as well as gloves and gowns should be used, and a biosafety hood should be used if an aerosol is generated [29].

Gastrointestinal Infection

Nosocomial transmission of agents that cause gastrointestinal infection can occur through contact with infected individuals, consumption of contaminated food, water or beverages, or exposure to contaminated objects or environmental surfaces. Spread of infection to health care workers can occur via inadequate hand washing or inadequate disinfection or sterilization of patient care equipment and environmental surfaces.

EPIDEMIOLOGY

Airborne spread of Norwalk virus is postulated but not yet proved [29]. Laundry workers have been noted to be at increased risk for salmonella infection; *Helicobacter pylori* has a higher seroprevalence in endoscopists compared to general internists [2]. *Clostridium difficile* can cause hospital-acquired diarrhea and may be found on the hands of 14–50% of asymptomatic health care workers [2].

PREVENTION AND CONTROL

Personnel with acute gastrointestinal illness (i.e., vomiting, diarrhea, nausea, fever, and abdominal pain) should be excluded from work in patient care or food handling areas of a health care facility. Return to work is appropriate after symptoms resolve or, if a specific pathogen is involved, when cultures are negative [29]. Good personal hygiene is essential before and after contact with patients or food. Observance of standard contact precautions minimizes the risk of transmission.

Pregnant Health Care Workers

Occupational acquisition of infection is of special concern to female health care workers of childbearing age (Table 34-8). During pregnancy there are some cell-mediated immune system changes that permit fetal development, but these generally do not increase maternal susceptibility to infectious diseases [40]. Women health care workers should be encouraged to receive immunizations prior to becoming pregnant and to adhere to appropriate infection control practices (Table 34-8).

EPIDEMIOLOGY

Varicella infection may be more severe during pregnancy. Transplacental infection with parvovirus, varicella, or rubella may affect the fetus. Agents like cytomegalovirus, hepatitis B, influenza, and measles are transmissible to the fetus. Some drugs used to treat or prevent infections

Table 34-8
Pregnant Health Care Personnel and Risk Due to Occupational Exposures to Infectious Agents

Agent	Potential Effect on Fetus	Rate of Perinatal Transmission	Maternal Screening	Prevention
1. CMV	Hearing loss; congenital syndrome[a]	15% after primary material infection; symptomatic 5%	Antibody protects against clinical disease; routine screening not recommended	Standard Precautions
2. Hepatitis B	Hepatitis; hepatocellular cancer as adult	HBeAg pos. 90% HBeAg neg. 25%	Anti-HBsAg Anti-HBeAg	Vaccine (safe during pregnancy); Standard Precautions
3. Hepatitis C	Hepatitis	0%–15%	Anti-HCV; HCV RNA in reference labs	IgG no longer contains anti-HCV and is not recommended; Standard Precautions
4. Herpes simplex	Mucocutaneous lesions, sepsis, encephalitis; congenital malformations (rare)	Unlikely from nosocomial exposure; primary 33%–50%, recurrent 4%	Antibody testing not useful; inspection for lesions at delivery	Standard Precautions
5. HIV	AIDS by 2–3 years of age	8%–30%	Antibody by ELISA, Western blot; PCR	Avoid high-risk behaviors; consider postexposure prophylaxis following high-risk needlestick; zidovudine Intrapartum and postnatal for HIV-positive mothers and their babies; Standard Precautions
6. Influenza	Inconsistent	Rare	None	Vaccine (safe during pregnancy); Droplet Precautions
7. Measles	Prematurity; abortion	Rare	History, antibody	Vaccine;[b] Airborne Precautions
8. Parvovirus B19	Hydrops, stillbirth	Rare, 3%–9% maximum adverse outcome	IgM, IgG antibody prepregnancy; antibody protective	Droplet Precautions
9. Rubella	Congenital syndrome[a]	45%–50% overall; 90% in first 12 weeks	Antibody	Vaccine;[b] Droplet Precautions for acute infection; Contact Precautions for congenital rubella
10. Tuberculosis	Hepatomegaly, pulmonary, CNS	Rare	Skin test	INH ± ethambutol; Airborne Precautions
11. Varicella-zoster virus	Malformations (skin, limb, CNS, eye); chickenpox	Total 25%; congenital syndrome (0–4%)	Antibody	Vaccine;[b] VZIG within 96 hours of exposure if susceptible; Airborne and Contact Precautions

[a] Congenital syndrome: varying combinations of jaundice, hepatosplenomegaly, microcephaly, CNS abnormalities, thrombocytopenia, anemia, retinopathy, skin and bone lesions.
[b] Live-virus vaccines are given routinely prior to pregnancy.
From *Hospital Employee Health*, December 1997, with permission.

like TB may be contraindicated during pregnancy.

Cytomegalovirus (CMV) frequently causes a mononucleosis-like illness in students or young adults. CMV infection is most severe in infants infected perinatally and may result in central nervous system or liver impairment. The majority of fetal infections occur because of primary maternal infection but can be caused by reinfection or reactivation in the seropositive mother [40]. Women of childbearing age should be counseled regarding their occupational and nonoccupational risks. Infants, young children, and immunocompromised individuals may serve as reservoirs of infection. Virus is secreted primarily in urine, saliva, and respiratory secretions and may be found in blood. Personnel who provide care to high-risk patients have a rate of primary CMV infection similar to that in other health care workers (2–3%). Patient care personnel have no greater risk of acquisition of CMV than personnel who do not care for patients. The CDC concludes that the risk of occupational transmission of CMV to pregnant health care workers is no greater than the general public's risk [40]. Pregnant health care workers caring for infants and young children should follow standard precautions, including thorough hand washing. Work transfer is not indicated. If a health care worker is infected with CMV, work restriction is not required and standard precautions are indicated.

Human parvovirus B19 is also of concern to pregnant health care workers: In a nonimmune woman there is a possibility of fetal parvovirus infection and subsequent hydrops fetalis. An increase in the fetal death rate of up to 2–10% may be seen if parvovirus is acquired before the twentieth week of gestation; the highest risk of fetal infection occurs during the first 10 weeks of gestation. The virus infects erythroid precursors in the fetus, leading to severe anemia, hypoxia, and high-output cardiac failure. This can result in generalized edema and death. Parvovirus infection is common in adults; half have serologic evidence of past infection [86]. Exposure to human parvovirus B19 is common during community outbreaks, but 20% of adult and childhood infections are asymptomatic [87].

Parvovirus is associated with erythema infectiosum (EI), or Fifth's disease. The characteristic slapped-cheek rash is an immune manifestation that occurs after the constitutional symptoms; by the time the rash appears, the patient is no longer infectious. Immunosuppressed anemic patients can frequently be chronically infected with parvovirus. Most patients with hematologic disease (such as spherocytosis or sickle cell anemia) who present in transient aplastic crisis are infected with parvovirus [87]. These patients are potential sources of infection; the transmission rate ranges from 0% to 37% [88].

Current data on infection and fetal risk in health care workers suggest less cause for alarm than previously reported. In one hospital outbreak, rates of positive serologic tests (presence of IgM to B19) were similar in affected wards, control wards, and community controls, with a high rate of asymptomatic acquisition [88]. Nontransmission to susceptible health care workers from a chronically infected patient, even in the absence of isolation precautions, has been reported [89]. Overall, transmission in the hospital or laboratory is infrequently reported [90].

When viral infection is recognized, the risk of health care workers' acquiring human parvovirus B19 can be decreased by instituting droplet precautions (using masks) to avoid contact with respiratory secretions. Erythema infectiosum (EI) is noninfectious and there is no need for isolation. Patients with transient anemic crisis or chronic anemia and immunosuppression, such as in patients with AIDS or leukemia, should be considered infected and placed in isolation until serologic studies can be obtained [90]. Aplastic crisis is infectious for seven days after onset; chronic infection may persist for years. When acute infection occurs, IgM production begins within three days in 90% of those infected and declines after two to three months [87]. IgG appears in the blood of an infected person about 10 days after IgM.

The CDC recommends ensuring that pregnant personnel are aware of the risks associated with parvovirus infection and with the procedures to prevent transmission but states that pregnant personnel not be routinely excluded from caring for patients with B19. The 1997 *Pediatric Red*

Book states that "In view of the high prevalence of B19, low incidence of ill effects on the fetus and fact that avoidance of child care or teaching can only reduce and not eliminate the risk of exposure," exclusion of the pregnant woman from the workplace where EI occurs is not recommended [64]. The *Red Book* recommends that pregnant health care workers be informed of the potential risks and preventive measures to reduce infection, which include "nonparticipation" in the care of the high-risk patient [64].

Laboratory-Acquired Infections

The clinical pathology laboratory represents a unique health care environment, where potentially infectious specimens are manipulated in various ways. In the microbiology laboratory, pathogens are propagated and handled in concentrated form. Aerosol-generating procedures include pouring liquid cultures or supernatants, using automatic pipettes, mixing liquids with a pipette, spilling or breaking specimen containers, cutting or sawing through unfixed tissue, and homogenizing infected tissue. Aerosols may be inhaled directly or settle on environmental surfaces and be spread by direct contact.

EPIDEMIOLOGY

The laboratory work may be at elevated risk for hepatitis B, brucellosis, Q fever, typhoid fever, and chlamydia. Rare infections may be encountered, such as simian herpes B virus in primate research laboratories and the Creutzfeldt-Jakob disease in autopsies [91]. Potential exposure routes include percutaneous inoculation, skin breaks, inhalation, and mucous membrane or skin contact; however, only 18% of probable laboratory infections involve a known or identifiable incident [91].

There are data to suggest that clinical diagnostic laboratories have a lower incidence of laboratory-acquired infection than research laboratories, especially when the volume of specimens handled is considered. Laboratory workers do have a higher risk of infection than other hospital personnel. Not only are scientific and technical personnel at risk, but also the laboratory clerical staff, dishwashers, janitors, and maintenance personnel. Among public health and hospital clinical lab personnel, the annual incidence of laboratory-acquired infections has been calculated as 1.4 per 1,000 for public health, 3.5 per 1,000 in hospitals overall, and 2.7 per 1,000 and 4.0 per 1,000, respectively, for the persons who work directly with infectious agents in those laboratories [91].

In a review of laboratory-acquired infections from 1950–1974, over 4,000 laboratory-acquired infections were documented in the United States. The 10 most commonly reported infections were brucellosis, Q fever, hepatitis (especially hepatitis B), typhoid fever, tularemia, tuberculosis, dermatomycosis, Venezuelan equine encephalitis, psittacosis, and coccidioidomycosis [40].

PREVENTION AND CONTROL

As mentioned, standard laboratory procedures can generate respirable particles, and some agents such as *Francisella tularensis*, *Coxiella burnetii*, measles, and *Coxsackie virus* A21 have a very low infectious dose for humans. Inhalation of a small number of such organisms can lead to laboratory-acquired infection (Table 34-9). Generally, clinical laboratories operate at biosafety level 2, which is appropriate for handling most specimens and for inactivated specimens or fixed tissue. If aerosol-generating procedures are performed on potentially infectious agents, additional precautions should be used to protect against airborne diseases. These procedures would include using gowns, and respiratory protection (HEPA masks or PAPRA) and working under biological safety hoods [92] or adopting full biosafety level-3 procedures.

Because the infectious dose of 1–10 TB bacilli can be found in only 1- to 3-droplet nuclei, aerosol transmission of TB in the laboratory is possible. Specimens that can transmit the bacilli include sputum, gastric aspirate, bronchial lavage, cerebrospinal fluid, urine and caseous tissue lesions. Laboratory workers have 100 times the rate of TB infection as the general population, and workers in TB laboratories have an incidence 3–5 times that of laboratory workers generally [92].

Table 34-9
Infectious Dose for Humans

Disease or Agent	Dose[a]	Route of Inoculation
Scrub typhus	3	Intradermal
Q fever	10	Inhalation
Tularemia	10	Inhalation
Malaria	10	Intravenous
Syphilis	57	Intradermal
Typhoid fever	10	Ingestion
Cholera	10	Ingestion
Escherichia coli	10	Ingestion
Shigellosis	10	Ingestion
Measles	0.2[b]	Inhalation
Venezuelan equine encephalitis	1[c]	Subcutaneous
Poliovirus 1	2[d]	Ingestion
Coxsackie A21	18	Inhalation
Influenza A2	790	Inhalation

[a] Dose in number of organisms.
[b] Median infectious dose in children.
[c] Guinea pig infective dose.
[d] Median infectious dose.
From Fleming D, Richardson J, Tales J, et al. (eds). *Laboratory Safety*, 2nd Ed. Washington, DC: American Society for Microbiology, 1995, with permission.

There have been case reports of laboratory-acquired meningococcemia [93]. The CDC recommends that work involving high concentrations or aerosolization of *N meningitides* should be performed in a biosafety level-3 laboratory [93]. The tetravalent vaccine (covering types A, C, Y, and W135) can be used in laboratory workers who routinely deal with concentrated specimens or large quantities of meningococcal organisms, such as in research laboratories or vaccine production, but would not protect against type B organisms. Exposure in clinical laboratories is typically sporadic and involves small quantities of meningococcus. In 1991, the CDC recommended use of penicillin as prophylaxis for percutaneous exposure and rifampin for mucosal exposures in the laboratory [93].

Laboratory personnel are at greater risk of *Salmonella typhi* infection than are other health care workers. The incidence of infection has decreased in recent decades, but the occurrence of *S typhi* infection continues, especially in laboratories involved in proficiency testing or research. The typhoid vaccine is suggested for microbiology workers who regularly work with *S typhi*; either the oral or parenteral vaccine, with boosters given at appropriate intervals, can be used [40].

Malaria can be spread via needlestick or infected blood from open wounds. Leishmania is found in infected tissue and less commonly in blood. Trypanosoma can be acquired from handing cultures or blood specimens [94]. Toxoplasmosis can be acquired by a seronegative woman working with live organisms via percutaneous or mucus membrane exposure; it can also be acquired by handling infected human tissues. This is another agent with potential for causing congenital problems in the fetus.

Because some exposure risks are unique to laboratories, health care institutions need to ensure that lab personnel have adequate information regarding their risks and are supplied with appropriate personal protective equipment and biosafety cabinets. Separate laboratory safety policies and procedures detailing the safety equipment and precautions to be used should be developed.

Summary

The diseases previously discussed are just a few of the many infections that may cause problems in health care settings (Table 34-10). Health care

Table 34-10
Occupationally Acquired Infections Resulting from Airborne, Bloodborne, and Oral-Fecal Transmission

Infection	Attack Rate (%)[a]	Health Care Workers Most Affected
Airborne transmission		
Tuberculosis	20–50	Nurses, pathologists, laboratory workers, housekeepers
Varicella	4.4–14.5	All
Measles	NA	Physicians, nurses
Influenza	3.8–4.5	Nurses, physicians
Rubella	13	All
Mumps	NA	Pediatricians, dentists
Pertussis	43	All
Parvovirus	27–47	Nurses
Respiratory syncytial virus	42–56	All
Adenovirus	22–39	Workers in ophthalmology clinics, intensive care units, long-term care facilities
Bloodborne transmission		
Human immunodeficiency virus	0.1–0.4 (per needlestick)	Nurses, laboratory workers
Hepatitis B	2[b] to 20–40[c]	Nurses, laboratory workers, surgeons, dentists, dialysis unit workers
Hepatitis C	1.2–10.0 (per needlestick)	Oral surgeons
Cytomegalovirus	Very low	None
Ebola virus	High	Nurses
Simian B virus	High	Animal handlers
Creutzfeldt-Jakob disease	NA	None
Oral-fecal transmission		
Salmonella	5–20	Nurses, laundry workers
Hepatitis A	20	Neonatal nurses
Shigella	Low	Nursery nurses (?)
Cryptosporidium	31–67	Animal workers
Helicobacter pylori	Seroprevalence rate twice that of the general population	Endoscopy personnel
Clostridium difficile	Very low	None
Norwalk virus	30–50	Nurses, care attendants

[a] For airborne transmission, the attack rates are as reported for outbreaks; for bloodborne transmission, exposure-associated attack rates are given.
[b] In those who are negative for hepatitis B early antigen.
[c] In those who are positive for hepatitis B early antigen.
NA = Not available.
Adapted from Sepkowitz K. Occupationally acquired infections in health care workers. *Ann Intern Med* 1996;125:826–34, 917–28.

workers as a group are not at substantially increased risk for acquiring infections such as diphtheria, pneumococcal disease or tetanus, compared to the general adult population, and the Advisory Committee on Immunization Practices (ACIP) recommends that these immunizations be obtained from the individual's primary care provider rather than being included in employee health programs [29]. Laboratory personnel and animal researchers, however, may have a work-related indication for tetanus boosters.

Reducing the morbidity and mortality from some work-related infections became a federal issue with OSHA's initiatives regarding TB and bloodborne pathogens. Control measures can help to protect health care workers and their patients. These include immunization, work removal, work practices and use of personal protective equipment, and prophylactic antibiotics. Hand washing, vaccination, and prompt isolation of potentially infectious patients are cost-effective strategies to prevent occupationally acquired infection [2]. Effective infection control for the health care worker can be accomplished only when the employer and employee cooperate to use the full spectrum of administrative, educational, organizational, medical, physical, and behavioral measures to best advantage.

References

1. Rogers B. Health hazards in nursing and health care. *Am J Infect Control* 1997;25:248–61.
2. Sepkowitz K. Occupationally acquired infections in health care workers. *Ann Intern Med* 1996;125:826–34, 917–28.
3. Frieden T, Sherman L, Maw K, et al. A multi-institutional outbreak of highly drug-resistant tuberculosis. *JAMA* 1996;276:1229–35.
4. Bowden K, McDiarmid M. Occupationally acquired tuberculosis: what's known. *J Occup Med* 1994;36: 520–4.
5. Sbarbaro J. Tuberculosis: yesterday, today and tomorrow (editorial). *Ann Intern Med* 1995;122:955–6.
6. Tuberculosis morbidity—United States, 1997. *MMWR* 1998;47:253–7.
7. Guidelines for preventing TB transmission in health care facilities. *MMWR* 1994;43(suppl):1–132.
8. Weisman E. Engineering controls and tuberculosis. *Health Facilities Management* 1994;Feb:18–24.
9. Vesley D. Respiratory protection devices. *Am J Infect Control* 1995;23:165–8.
10. Adal K, Anglim A, Palumbo L, et al. The use of high-efficiency particulate air-filter respirators to protect hospital workers from tuberculosis. *N Engl J Med* 1994;331:169–73.
11. American Thoracic Society. Diagnostic standards and classification of tuberculosis. *Am Rev Respir Dis* 1990;142:725–35.
12. Sepkowitz K, Raffalli J, Riley L, et al. Tuberculosis in the AIDS era. *Clin Microbiol Rev* 1995;8:180–99.
13. Huebner R, Schein M, Bass J. The tuberculin skin test. *Clin Infect Dis* 1993;17:968–75.
14. Enforcement procedure and scheduling for occupational exposure to tuberculosis. *OSHA Instruction CPL 2.106*, February 9, 1996.
15. Menzies R, Belkes V, Rocher I, et al. The booster effect in two-step tuberculin testing among young adults in Montreal. *Ann Intern Med* 1994;120:190–8.
16. Manusov E, Bradshaw D, Fogarty J. Tuberculosis screening in medical students. *Fam Med* 1996;28:645–9.
17. Sepkowitz K, Feldman J, Louther J, et al. Benefit of two-step PPD testing of new employees at a New York City hospital. *Am J Infect Control* 1997;25:283–6.
18. Sepkowitz K, Fella P, Rivera P, et al. Prevalence of PPD positivity among new employees at a hospital in New York City. *Infect Control Hosp Epidemiol* 1995;16: 344–7.
19. Swinker M. Prevalence of positive PPD skin tests in two-step testing program at a teaching hospital in eastern North Carolina. *Infect Control Hosp Epidemiol* 2000;21:(1):39–40.
20. OSHA proposed rule for preventing occupational exposure to tuberculosis, Oct. 17, 1997. *Federal Register* Doc 97-27020.
21. Stead W. Management of health care workers after inadvertent exposure to tuberculosis. *Ann Intern Med* 1995;122:906–12.
22. Public Health Service guidelines for the management of health-care worker exposures to HIV and recommendations for postexposure prophylaxis. *MMWR* 1998;47 (suppl):1–39.
23. Update: provisional Public Health Services recommendations for chemoprophylaxis after occupational exposure to HIV. *MMWR* 1996;45:468–72.
24. Case control study of HIV seroconversion in health care workers after percutaneous exposure to HIV infected blood. *MMWR* 1995;44:929–35.
25. Forst L, Fletcher B. HIV prophylaxis for health care workers. *J Occup Environ Med* 1997;39:1212–8.
26. Cardo D, Culver D, Cielsielski C, et al. A case/control study of HIV seroconversion in health care workers after percutaneous exposure. *N Engl J Med* 1997;337: 1485–90.
27. National Center for Infectious Diseases. Management of Occupational Exposure to HIV, 1998. Available at *www.cdc.gov/ncidod.*
28. Benenson A (ed). *Control of Communicable Diseases Manual.* Washington, DC: American Public Health Association, 1995.
29. Immunization of health care workers. *MMWR* 1997;46 (suppl):3–37.
30. Protection against viral hepatitis; recommendations of the immunization practices advisory committee. *MMWR* 1990;30 (suppl):1–25.
31. OSHA Final Standard for Occupational Exposure to Bloodborne Pathogens, December 6, 1991. 29 *CFR* 1910.1030:64175-82.
32. Guidelines for prevention of transmission of human immunodeficiency virus and hepatitis B virus to health care and public-safety workers. *MMWR* 1989;38 (suppl):1–37.
33. Update on hepatitis B prevention. *MMWR* 1987;3 6:355.
34. Roome A, Walsh S, Cartter M, et al. Hepatitis B vaccine responsiveness in Connecticut public safety personnel. *JAMA* 1993;270:2931–34.
35. Wood R, MacDonald K, White K, et al. Risk factors for lack of detectable antibody following hepatitis B vaccination of Minnesota health care workers. *JAMA* 1993;270:2935–9.
36. Havlichek D, Rosenman K, Simms M, et al. Age-related hepatitis B seroconversion rates in health care workers. *Am J Infect Control* 1997;25:418–20.
37. Frymoyer C. Preventing the spread of viral hepatitis. *Am Fam Phys* 1993;48:1479–86.
38. Gerberding J. Management of occupational exposures to blood-borne viruses. *N Engl J Med* 1995;332:444–51.

38. Alimonas K. Prediction of response to hepatitis B vaccine in health care workers. *Clin Infect Dis* 1998; 26:566–71.
40. CDC guidelines for infection control in health care personnel. *Infect Control Hosp Epidemiol* 1998;19:407–63.
41. Rosman AS, Basu P, Galvin K, et al. Efficacy of a high and accelerated dose of hepatitis B vaccine in alcoholic patients: a randomized clinical trial. *Am J Med* 1997; 103:217–22.
42. Update: vaccine side effects, adverse reactions, contraindications and precautions. *MMWR* 1996; 45 (suppl):8.
43. Rosen H. Acquisition of hepatitis C by a conjunctival splash. *Am J Infect Control* 1997;25:242–7.
44. *Hepatitis C.* (Monograph.) Cedar Grove, NJ: American Liver Foundation. 1997.
45. Koff R, Wright T, Liang J. *Finding the Answers to Hepatitis B and C.* American Liver Foundation Progress, 1996. Available at *http://gi.ucsf.edu/ALF/pubs*
46. Centers for Disease Control. *Hepatitis Surveillance Issues and Answers.* (Report #14.) Atlanta: CDC. Apr 1996.
47. Davis G. Hepatitis C among health care workers. *JAMA* 1996;275:1474.
48. Salazar A, Hermogenes P, Yens D. Incidence of Hepatitis C in patients with chronic elevations of aminotransferases. *J Am Board Fam Practice* 1996;9:157–61.
49. Centers for Disease Control. *Hepatitis C Recommendations for Medical Evaluation and Counseling.* Atlanta: CDC, July 1994.
50. Esteban J, Gomez J, Marell M, et al. Repeated transmission of HCV from surgeon to patients during cardiac surgery. *N Engl J Med* 1996;334:555–60.
51. Transmission of hepatitis B to multiple patients from a surgeon without evidence of inadequate infection control. *N Engl J Med* 1996;334:549–54.
52. Heptonstall J. Transmission of hepaitis B to patients from four infected surgeons without hepatitis B antigen. *N Engl J Med* 1997;336:178–84.
53. Gerberding J. The infected health care provider. *N Engl J Med* 1996;334:594–5.
54. Lombardo L, Meyer J. Should hepatitis B-infected health care workers perform invasive procedures? *Occup Environ Med Report* 1997;11:41–3.
55. Carr MM. Human bites to the hand. *J Can Dent Assoc* 1995;61:782–4.
56. Richman K, Rickman L. The potential for transmission of human immunodeficiency virus through human bites. *J Acq Immun Defic Synd* 1993;6:402–6.
57. Khajatia R. Transmission of human immunodeficiency virus through saliva after a lip bite. (Letter). *Arch Intern Med* 1997;157:1901.
58. Anonymous. HIV transmission by a human bite. (news.) *Infect Control Hosp Epidemiol* 1996;117:707.
59. Numata N, Ohori H, Hayakawa Y, et al. Demonstration of hepatitis C virus genome in saliva and urine of patients with Type C hepatitis. *J Med Virol* 1993;41: 120–8.
60. Figueredo J, Borges A, Martinez R, et al. Hepatitis C virus but not HIV transmitted by a human bite. (Letter.) *Clin Infect Dis* 1994;19:547–8.
61. Detection of hepatitis C virus RNA in the cell fraction of saliva before and after oral surgery. *J Med Virol* 1995;43:223–6.
62. Herwaldt L, Pattinger J, Carter C, et al. Exposure work ups. *Infect Control Hosp Epidemiol* 1997;18:850–71.
63. Prevention of varicella. *MMWR* 1996;45(suppl):1–27.
64. Georges P (ed). *Red Book, 24th ed.* Elk Grove Village, IL: American Academy of Pediatrics, 1997.
65. Recommendations for the use of live attenuated varicella vaccine. *Pediatrics* 1995;95:791–6.
66. Varicella—related deaths among children—United States, 1997. *MMWR* 1998;47:365–7.
67. Selected notifiable disease reports. *MMWR* 1996;46: 1021.
68. Herwaldt L. Pertussis in adults. *Arch Intern Med* 1991;151:1510–2.
69. Weber D, Rutala W. Management of health care workers exposed to pertussis. *Infect Control Hosp Epidemiol* 1994;15:411–5.
70. Halperin S, Bortolussi R, Langley J, et al. Seven days of erythromycin estolate is as effective as fourteen days for the treatment of *Bordetella pertussis* infections. *Pediatrics* 1997;100:65–71.
71. Shefer A, Dales L, Nelson M, et al. Use and safety of acellular pertussis vaccine among adult hospital staff. *J Infect Dis* 1995;1171:1053–6.
72. Zimmerman R, Clover R. Adult immunizations. *Am Fam Phys* 1995;51:859–67.
73. Advisory Committee on Immunization Practices. Immunizations in medical education. *Am J Prevent Med* 1995;10(suppl):60–80.
74. Advisory Committee on Immunization Practices. Control and prevention of serogroup C meningococcal disease. *MMWR* 1997;46(suppl):1–8, 13–21.
75. Schwartz B. Chemoprophylaxis for bacterial infections. *Rev Infect Dis* 1991;13(suppl):S170–3.
76. Harrison L, Armstrong L, Jenkins S, et al. A cluster of meningococcal disease on a school bus following epidemic influenza. *Arch Intern Med* 1991;151:1005–9.
77. Centers for Disease Control. Guidelines for the prevention of nosocomial pneumonia. *MMWR* 1997;46 (suppl):1–79.
78. Centers for Disease Control and Prevention. Prevention and control of influenza. *MMWR* 1998;47(suppl): 1–79.
79. Influenza activity in the U.S., 1997–98. *MMWR* 1998;47:200.
80. Nichol K, Lind A, Margolis K, et al. The effectiveness of vaccination against influenza in healthy working adults. *N Engl J Med* 1995;333:884–93.

81. Campbell D, Rumley M. Cost-effectiveness of the influenza vaccine in a healthy working-age population. *J Occup Environ Med* 1997;39:408–14.

82. LaForce M, Nichol K, Cox N. Influenza: virology, epidemiology, disease and prevention. *Am J Prevent Med* 1994;10(suppl):31–41.

83. Human rabies—Michigan. *MMWR* 1983;32:159–60.

84. Human rabies and post exposure prophylaxis in health care workers. *MMWR* 1996;45:353–6.

85. Helmick C, Tauxe R, Vernon A. Is there a risk to contacts of patients with rabies? *Rev Infect Dis* 1987;9:511–8.

86. Dowell S. Turok T, Thorp J, et al. Parvovirus B19 infection in hospital workers. *J Infect Dis* 1995;172:1076–9.

87. Turok T. Parvovirus B19 and human disease. *Adv Intern Med* 1992;37:431–54.

88. Koziol D, Kurtzman G, Ayrib J, et al. Nosocomial human parvovirus B19 infection: lack of transmission from a chronically infected patient to hospital staff. *Infect Control Hosp Epidemiol* 1992;13:343–8.

89. Guerina N. Management strategies for infectious disease in pregnancy. *Semin Perinatol* 1994;18:305–20.

90. Summary of notifiable diseases, United States 1996. *MMWR* 1997;45(suppl):1–87.

91. Fleming D, Richardson J, Tules J, et al. (eds). *Laboratory Safety*, 2nd Ed. Washington, DC: Am Society for Microbiology, 1995.

92. Centers for Disease Control. Proposed Guidelines: Goals for Working Safely with *Mycobacterium tuberculosis* in Clinical, Public Health and Research Laboratories, 4/28/97. *www.cdc.gov/od/ohs.*

93. Laboratory-acquired meningococcemia—California and Massachusetts. *MMWR* 1991;40:46–55.

94. Herwaldt B, Juranek D. Laboratory-acquired malaria, leishmaniasis, trypanosomiasis and toxoplasmosis. *Am J Trop Med Hyg* 1993;48:313–23.

Additional Resources

- For information on the type and duration of isolation precautions needed for selected infections and conditions, please consult the CDC at *www.cdc.gov/ncidod/hip/isolat/isoapp_a.htm.*
- For recommendations on work restrictions for infected health care workers, refer to *Am J Infect Control* 1998;26:289–354.
- For more information on hepatitis, contact the American Liver Foundation at 1-800-GO- LIVER (465-4827), for the public; 1-888-4HEP-ABC (443-7222), for professionals.
- For more information on the Americans with Disabilities Act, contact the Office of the Americans with Disabilities Act, U.S. Department of Justice (202-514-0301).

35 / Occupational Infections in Sewage Workers

Robert P. Hurley

The sewage worker's occupational environment consists of large, open sewer drains, medium-size pipes, collection systems, various sewage treatment processes, all of which present various exposures. Sewage, compost, and waste water workers are exposed to a variety of biologic, chemical, metallic, and radioactive agents [1]. Concentrations of these agents vary widely, depending on the environment, season, country, and local public health standards [2]. In certain circumstances, almost any infectious disease can be acquired during the course of employment. Sewage work and infectious diseases have been shown to have a clear relationship [3]. The occupational physician may be asked to assess the causative nature of infection in a sewage worker, evaluate its relationship with work, and implement medical surveillance measures.

Sewage workers are exposed to infectious disease pathogens during various phases of waste treatment. Primary, secondary, and tertiary phases of treating the waste stream expose these workers to microorganisms that may be splashed on intact or abraded skin, mucous membranes, or clothing. Immersion of the body in waste water for short or prolonged periods of time increases the risk of disease from pathogenic and nonpathogenic organisms, and later stage treatment of sewage by aeration places sewage workers at risk of inhalation of bioaerosols. Handling of biosolids, which are spread on land for irrigation, fertilization or composting, increases the risk of ingestion, inhalation, or absorption of heavy metals or solvents.

In sewage, there are two classes of pathogens. The primary pathogens consist of bacteria, viruses, protozoa, and helminths. The other class comprises molds and fungi, particularly *Aspergillus* species. The presence, concentration, and ability of these pathogens to cause disease is determined by several factors:

- Prevalence of the pathogens in the population connected to the sewer system.
- Pathogen characteristics such as virulence, resistance to destruction during the sewage treatment process, and the ability of these organisms to survive and grow in sewage and sludge after treatment [4].
- Host factors such as immune competence and resistance.

Exposures to these pathogens have been associated with acute syndromes or chronic subtle illness. Inhalation of moist or dried bioaerosols may produce immune system dysfunction or allergic reactions. Zoonoses alone comprise over 160 diseases that are transmissible from vertebrate animals to man [5]. Because the availability of data is sparse and the prospects of well-controlled human studies pose unacceptable risks, quantification of risk for infectious diseases associated with sewage work has been elusive. This chapter focuses on the typical infections and exposures experienced by individuals employed as sewage workers.

Epidemiology

Sewage workers are exposed to a number of infectious agents. Bacteria, viruses, fungi, and substances derived from vertebrate animals are all found in the waste stream, and there is growing evidence to support that contention that infectious agents are important risk factors for health problems in sewage workers. Workers are exposed not only to known human pathogens but also to zoonotic infections associated with significant morbidity and allergic manifestations. Sewage compost workers are routinely exposed to several major pathogens such as gram-negative and endotoxin-producing bacteria. Although there is not a clear consensus among authors and studies, the pathogens that are likely to cause disease are *Leptospira interrogans*, *Legionella pneumophila*, hepatitis A and E, and the enteric viruses. *Aspergillus*, helminth, and protozoans also are significant pathogens to consider as possible causes of health problems in sewage workers.

The concentrations of pathogens vary by season, sophistication of public health measures, geography, and climate. In the United States, concentrations from facility to facility vary according to the process with which the waste is treated. Table 35-1 summarizes the relative concentrations of major pathogens in waste during the various stages of treatment.

BACTERIA

Leptospirosis

Leptospirosis, a zoonosis or anthrozoonosis, is a bacterial disease transmitted to humans that occurs throughout the world. Its severity ranges from an unnoticed subclinical condition to an acute septicemia that can be fatal. It is caused by the genus *Leptospira*, which has at least 12 genospecies. The bacterium can cause disease by any one of a large number of serologic types (serovars). The reservoirs of leptospirosis, the nonhuman carriers, excrete the bacterium in their urine.

Leptospirosis, or Weil's syndrome, was traditionally described as a disease caused by *Leptospira icterohaemorrhagiae*. However, leptospirosis is now recognized as a disease caused by various species of *Leptospira*, which comprises both pathogenic and saprophytic strains on the basis of DNA relatedness. Historically, the taxonomic classification of serovars and serogroups was based on serology using cross-agglutination with rabbit antisera and microscopic identification. This older taxonomic classification grouped pathologic species serologically as *L interrogans.* Nonpathogens were grouped as *L biflexa*. Significant reservoirs of leptospira infecting man have been the following serovars: *canicola*, found in dogs; *icterohaemorrhagiae*, associated with Norway rats; and *pomona*, found in cattle and swine.

The modern classification of *Leptospira* is based on genetic relationships of distinct species (genospecies). *Leptospiral serogroup* is the collective term for antigen-related serovars. Members

Table 35-1
The Relative Concentrations of Several Important Human Pathogens Found in Sewage. Density Levels of Organics in Raw Sludge and Septage[6]: × Average mean of organisms per gram of dry weight.)[7]

Organism	Primary	Secondary	Mixed	Septage
Total coliform count	1.2×10^8	7.1×10^8	1.1×10^8	1.4×10^8
Fecal coliform count	2.0×10^7	8.3×10^6	1.9×10^5	1.2×10^6
Fecal streptococci	8.9×10^5	1.7×10^6	3.7×10^{16}	6.6×10^5
Bacteriophage	1.3×10^5	NR	NR	NR
Salmonella sp.	4.1×10^2	8.8×10^2	2.9×10^2	5.1×10^{-1}
Shigella sp.	NR	NR	ND	NR
Pseudomonas aeruginosa	2.8×10^3	1.1×10^4	3.3×10^3	2.6×10^1
Parasites: ova/cysts × total	2.1×10^2	NR	$<5.0\ 10^1$	NR
Ascaris sp.	7.1×10^2	1.4×10^3	2.9×10^2	NR
Trichuris trichiura	1.0×10^2	$<1.0 \times 10^1$	0	NR
Trichuris vulpis	1.1×10^2	$<1.0 \times 10^1$	1.4×10^2	NR
Toxocara sp.	2.4×10^2	2.8×10^2	1.3×10^3	NR
Hymenolepis diminuta	6.0×10^0	2.0×10^1	0	NR
Enteric viruses	3.9×10^2	3.2×10^2	3.6×10^2	NR

NR = no data available; *ND* = none detected.

of any serogroup may belong to multiple species with DNA relatedness. At least 22 serogroups are based on, or share, major agglutinogens, and there are 250 different serotypes of *Leptospira* that have been identified. The species *borgpetersenii*, *inadai*, *interrogans*, *kirschneri*, *santarosai*, *weilii*, *faineii*, and *noguchii* include almost all of the pathogenic strains. The primary reservoir of leptospires is usually wild warm-blooded vertebrates, although some serovars appear to have adapted to domestic and potentially domesticated animals as hosts. There are significant occupational health concerns about leptospirosis, as the disease often causes acute and prolonged incapacity for work as well as loss of productivity. The costs of medical care, workers' compensation payments, and preventive measures to reduce these losses place financial strains on municipalities in which there are outbreaks of leptospirosis [8].

Legionella

There are more than 39 species in the Legionellaceae family and more than 61 serogroups [9,10]. *Legionella pneumophila* is responsible for about 90% of infections caused by members of this family. Other species of *Legionella* are *L micdadei*, *L longbeachae*, *L dumoffi*, and *L bozemanii*. *L pneumophilia* alone contains 14 serogroups, but the important pathogenic members are 1, 4, and 6, which account for most human infections. The natural habitats for *L pneumophila* appear to be rivers, streams, and polluted waters. The pathogen can survive wide ranges in temperature (0–63°C), a pH of 5.0–8.5, and reduced oxygen concentrations. The bacteria are chlorine resistant and therefore pass through the water treatment process and into the distribution system [11,12]. In natural aquatic environments, symbiotic relationships with amoebae and water bacteria are necessary for optimal growth of *Legionella* [13,14]. *Legionella* infect and then multiply within amoebae and ciliated protozoa. When the protozoan host ruptures, large numbers of *Legionella* are released [15,16].

The incidence of legionnaires' disease depends on the concentration of the organism, susceptibility of the individual, and intensity of exposure. Cigarette smoking, chronic lung disease, advanced age, and immunosuppression have been implicated as risk factors. Sewer systems, treatment plants, composting, and land dispersion provide *Legionella* species an excellent environment to breed and aerosolize. Currently, there is little documentation in the literature to support increased risk of infection from *Legionella* in the sewer worker population.

Transmission. Leptospirosis is transmitted by either direct or indirect contact with the urine of infected animals. The major routes of transmission to humans are exposure to urine-contaminated soil or water, namely by immersion in water or ingestion of contaminated food or water. Humans do not appear to be a reservoir, and person-to-person transmission is rare. Breaks in skin surfaces or abraded, macerated mucosal membranes are necessary for infection. Common source outbreaks have been associated with swimming in contaminated water.

The major form of *Legionella* transmission is inhalation of aerosols. The severe diarrhea associated with the disease and subsequent flushing of contaminated fecal matter into the sewage system places sewer workers at risk of exposure to high concentrations of the organism.

Occupational Risks. Infectious diseases that are capable of causing infection are present in sewage. Sewer workers are at particular risk, as they spend considerable time at work with parts of their bodies partially or totally immersed in water. This intimate, prolonged, chronic contact facilitates infection. The moisture, warmth, and alkaline to neutral pH favor the growth of *Leptospira*, *Legionella*, viruses, helminths, and protozoa. Risk correlations are not possible for most organisms because of the lack of control of the sewer environment and host factors. For example, leptospirosis host-serovar interactions are not possible because of the lack of available data. The infection, which was thought to be more common in tropical climates, is actually reported more often in temperate zones. Of the more than 2,000 cases that have been reported worldwide, 100 have occurred in the United States. Adding to the difficulty in characterizing leptospirosis is the fact that there has been a shift in the prevalence of the different infectious serotypes. In 1948, 90% of cases of leptospirosis were reported to be caused by *L icterohaemorrhagiae*, compared to

1978–1987, when only 32% were ascribed to that serotype. Presently, many serotypes may cause leptospirosis. In Table 35-2, we list many of the serovars associated with leptospirosis in the sewer workers' environment. It is important to keep in mind that any serovar may cause the myriad symptoms of this biphasic disease.

VIRUSES

Enteric Viruses

Hepatitis A. Hepatitis A (HAV), by the nature of its transmission, places sewage treatment workers at risk. As a small RNA virus of the Picornaviridae family, its genomic organization and replication is similar to that of polio. HAV is heat stable and can live for two weeks in feces [17]. It is viable at a pH of only 3 and can live for many years at –20°C. Formalin and heating to 100°C will deactivate HAV, but it is resistant to chlorine, hence its risk for sewage workers. Individuals who work in sewage treatment plants are at increased risk for HAV infection [18,19].

The most common mode of HAV transmission is person to person via the fecal-oral route. In sewers, its pathogenicity is significant. Sewers provide an ideal environment for growth of HAV because this environment enhances the virus' capacity to remain viable for long periods. HAV is endemic in the United States and there are periodic outbreaks. It has a higher incidence among Native Americans and Alaskan natives, and in Hispanic and Hasidic communities. Between 1990 and 1992, food- and waterborne outbreaks accounted for 4% of cases. The common-source food and waterborne epidemics have occurred with sewage-contaminated shellfish.

The prevalence of HAV antibodies in sewer workers has been shown to increase with age, yet this trend does not differ markedly from the general population [20]. Sewer workers greater than age 40 do have a statistically significant seropositivity rate compared to matched controls. The strongest correlation appears to be an association between seropositive status and the duration of sewage exposure. Among HAV-positive sewer workers, it has been shown that sewage exposure, increasing age, stay in an endemic area, or increased number of siblings were significant risk factors. Regression analysis of this data reveals an adjusted odds ratio of 2.15 for seropositivity to HAV among sewer workers compared to those not exposed to sewage [21].

Hepatitis E. In other parts of the world, hepatitis E (HEV) is a major cause of enteric non-A,

Table 39-2
Infectious Serotypes of *Leptospira*: Animal Hosts

Serovar	Human	Domestic	Wild
balcanica		C	
canicola	+	D[a], P, C	Skunk, raccoon
copenhageni	+	D	Raccoon, armadillo
fort-bragg	+	?	?
grippotyphosa		C, P	Mole, raccoon, fox, skunk, opossum, muskrat, leopard
georgia	+		Raccoon, opossum, skunk
hardjo	+	C[a]	
icterohaemorrhagiae	+	D, P, C	Rat,[a] mouse, fox, raccoon, muskrat, opossum, skunk, woodchuck, nutria, ape (zoo)
pomona	+	C,[a] P,[a] D, H, G	Skunk, raccoon, fox, oppossum, woodchuck, deer, mice, sea lion, armadillo
swajizak		C	

[a]Known major maintenance host.
M = man; *C* = cattle; *D* = dog; *P* = pig; *H* = horse; *G* = goat.

non-B hepatitis. In endemic areas, it may be the causal agent in as many as 60% of cases of sporadic viral hepatitis [22]. In 1980, Khuroo and Wong first described epidemics of non-A, non-B hepatitis contracted by exposure to contaminated water and thus likely to have been spread by the fecal-oral route [23,24]. In the 1980s, Balayan demonstrated that the entity now known as *hepatitis E* shared many of the viral characteristics of hepatitis A. Not only is it a nonenveloped, single-stranded RNA virus, but also shares other HAV characteristics such as having a fecal-oral route of transmission, point-source infectiousness, and the absence of persistent antibodies or a chronically active state. First identified in India, HEV now can be found in Mexico, the Middle and Far East, and northern and western Africa and Asia. The virus may cause a fatal fulminant hepatitis in the gravid female, especially in the third trimester.

Hantavirus. Hantavirus, first isolated in 1976, is known to infect rodents in many countries worldwide. Transmission to humans is from the saliva, urine, or feces of infected rodents. In humans, the virus is capable of causing severe illness characterized either by a hemorrhagic fever with renal failure or hemorrhagic pulmonary syndrome (HPS). The disease was initially known as *Korean hemorrhagic* fever. Recently, the World Health Organization has adopted the term *hemorrhagic fever with renal syndrome* to describe this disease. The hantaviruses are RNA viruses that belong to the family Bunyaviridae, of which there are four types associated with HPS: the Sin Nombre, Black Creek Canal, New York, and Boyou viruses. All are capable of causing HPS, yet nearly all reported cases have implicated the Sin Nombre virus. Newly characterized agents, such as Puumala virus, Seoul virus and Muerto Canyon virus, can all cause illness, but at this time the clinical syndromes caused by these agents appear to be less severe. The mortality rate of hantaviruses is about 5%. Muerto Canyon virus has been associated with a "hantavirus pulmonary syndrome," which clinically presents with fever and myalgia, followed by progressive pulmonary failure [25]. Clinically, the early presentation can be confused with leptospirosis (Weil's syndrome), although laboratory testing can differentiate between the two.

PARASITES

Parasitic diseases are a major health problem in the developing world. Many infections are acquired by eating feces-contaminated food or water. Others are acquired by arthropod vectors. The parasitic diseases can be divided into those caused by protozoa and those caused by helminths.

Protozoa

These single-cell organisms are divided into two classes: the systemic protozoa and the intestinal protozoa. The major agents that cause malaria, sleeping sickness leishmaniasis, and toxoplasmosis have not been described in the literature as risk factors for sewage workers. In countries where the parasites are endemic, sewer workers are assumed to be at risk for *Toxoplasma gondii* infection, as it is transmitted by the fecal-oral route. The protozoa that are known to cause intestinal diarrhea and are present in the sewage worker's environment in specific countries are giardiasis, cryptosporidiosis, cyclosporiasis, isosporiasis, and microsporidiosis.

In countries where solid waste and sewage are often the same, there are significant increases in parasitic infections in sewage workers. Stool samples taken from Indian sewage workers revealed 98% were positive for parasites. In comparison, the control group revealed a prevalence of 33%. Of those infected, the most frequent parasites were *Trichuris trichuria* (human whipworm) and *Ascaris lumbricoides* (human roundworm) [26].

BIOSOLIDS AND THE SEWAGE WORKER

The exposure to biosolids in sewer work depends on the treatment process at the particular sewage treatment facility. In order to reduce organisms and biologic oxygen demand, systems are designed utilizing criteria published in the *Federal Register.* Recommended treatment guidelines for biosolids can be found in Appendix B, 40 CFR, Part 503. There are five types of sewage treatment: aerobic digestion, biosolids air drying, anaerobic digestion, composting and lime stabilization.

In aerobic digestion, "biosolids are agitated with air or oxygen to maintain aerobic conditions . . . between 40-days at 20-degrees Celsius and 60-days at 15-degrees Celsius." The agitation of liquid, slurry, or desiccated material generates varying concentrations of bioaerosols.

Biosolids air drying entails the drying of biosolids on sandbags or in paved or unpaved basins for a minimum of three months. Storing of biosolids in an open basin results in little release if the material is liquid. When dry, considerable amounts of bacteria, viruses, and bacterial toxins can be dispersed by the wind for considerable distances. Sewage workers without masks may inhale high concentrations of dust and thus be exposed. In sludge treatment, high concentrations of toxins occur.

Anaerobic digestion is relatively safe, as the sewage is kept in containers under anaerobic conditions. However, when transporting this material, sewage workers are at risk for exposure.

Composting utilizes various techniques. Facilities are operated utilizing within-vessel, static-aerated pile or windrow composting methods. During this time, the temperatures of biosolids is raised to 40°C or higher and maintained for five days. Composting requires piles of biosolids to be turned repeatedly, often by machine in open air or occasionally in a closed environment. When moved, high airborne concentrations can occur within a closed facility. Outside, high concentrations may be moved by wind toward those working and living nearby the facility.

Lime stabilization is a crude method in which sufficient lime is added to biosolids to raise the pH to 12 after two hours of contact.

Sewage workers are at the highest risk of inhaling aerosolized pathogens when they are engaged in work near aerobic digestion, air-drying, and composting sewage-processing sites. To assess a worker's risk, data must be collected to support or refute allegations of high airborne levels of bioaerosols. The most useful representative sample of airborne organic content is volumetrically based data.

BIOAEROSOLS AND BIOSOLIDS IN THE WASTEWATER SETTING

Bioaerosols are airborne particulates that are comprised of living material, toxic products, or both. The major airborne pathogens are bacteria, viruses, fungi, and endotoxins. Waste water treatment workers who process biosolids such as sludge are primarily exposed to microbes, especially gram-negative rods. These exposures have been associated with symptoms such as fever and chest tightness [27]. Exposure to fungi such as *Aspergillus fumigatus (AF)*, which proliferates during waste water treatment, has been shown to be pathogenic to workers with impaired immune systems.

In waste water treatment plants, aerosols are created during phases in which materials are agitated. There are three forms of aerosols: liquid, moist, and dry. The concentrations of airborne biologic materials depend on facility design and prevailing environmental conditions. Sewage treatment workers may be exposed not only when participating in sewage treatment processes but also when working nearby, in unrelated job activities. In some communities, all three forms of biosolids are dumped on the land for fertilization and disposal purposes [28,29]. Irrigation or dumping of solid waste often occurs at night, ostensibly to maintain water content. Without the benefits of solar radiation, desiccation and decrease of the biologic load does not occur, and heavy concentrations of bioaerosols may be spread into respirable air. Homes and buildings can become contaminated if biosolids are dumped in or near a designated landfill or within close proximity of residential or business areas. The carpets, drapes, and "closed" ventilation systems of these contaminated structures offer excellent growing conditions for pathogens.

Dermal exposure to bioaerosols may cause irritant contact dermatitis, and respiratory tract infections may also occur [30]. The nasal passages and upper airways usually filter out large-size bioaerosol particles, ranging from 30 to 60 μm in diameter. These particles consist of organic and inorganic dirt, fibers, pollens, and mold spores. Smaller particles, in the 5-μm range, consist of hyphal fragments, pollen, and mold spores, which can land upon the mucosa or penetrate further into the lower airways. The smallest pathogens, such as bacteria, fungal spores and viruses, can be carried by inorganic matter as small as 1–5 μm and are considered truly respirable. In most persons employed in sewage work, the lungs are capable of inhaling very high numbers of spores or microorganisms without systemic effect or infection. Studies examining workers' exposure to sewage sludge and waste water in the United States and Sweden have revealed no increased risk of infection, except under extreme exposure conditions such as total body immersion in sewage water tanks and inhalation of water [31–33]. On the other hand, the EPA has stated that it is reasonable to assume that these bioaerosols have a systemic effect when inhaled [34].

Despite normal immunologic resistance to illness, *Aspergillus fumigatus* and other fungi have been shown to cause disease. These secondary or opportunist pathogens are especially prone to colonize individuals who are immunocompromised or otherwise debilitated by a pre-existing medical condition, such as severe viral infection or chemotherapy. Occasionally, *fumigatus* may cause widespread invasion of lung tissue, yet severe infections usually occur only in individuals who are immunologically incompetent.

BIOAEROSOLS AND BIOSOLIDS IN THE COMPOST SETTING

When processed properly, compost bioaerosols contain less than 20% moisture and are very friable. During normal handling, some of the biologic components may be released into the air [35]. Depending on the process or stage of waste treatment, workers may be exposed to a multitude of pathogenic organisms that are not destroyed in the sewage treatment process. Compost bioaerosols may contain actinomyces, other bacteria, fungi, arthropods, protozoa, and organic constituents of feedstock materials. Microbial products include endotoxins, microbial enzymes, B-1,3-glucans, and mycotoxins [35]. The compost contains not only biologically active organisms but also chemicals and heavy metals [36–42]. These primary and secondary pathogens are summarized in Tables 35-3, 35-4, 35-5, and 35-6.

Table 35-3
Bacterial Infectious Agents in Sewage

Bacteria	Reservoir	Disease/Comments
Aeromonas hydrophilia	M, F, SF, W	Gastoenteritis, gangrenous wound infections, pneumonia
Acinetobacter calcoaceticus	FL, W	Tracheobronchitis, pneumonia
Klebsiella pneumoniae	P, A, W	Endocarditis, LRT infections, ear infections
Enterobacter agglomerans cloacae	M	Opportunistic skin, respiratory, and urinary tract infections
Escherichia coli	M, DA, WA	Gastroenteritis
Staphylococcus	M	Skin and soft tissue infections: osteomyelitis: pneumonia; toxic shock syndrome; gastroenteritis; endocarditis
Streptococci	M, SW	Scarlet fever, pharyngitis, pneumonia; streptococcal toxic shock syndrome
Leptospira	R, DA, D, SW	Myocarditis, hepatitis, meningitis, conjunctivitis, lymphadenitis, pneumonia
Legionella pneumophila	S, W, PZ, AM	Pontiac fever, pneumonia
Salmonella sp.	M, DA, WA, B, RP	Enteric fever, enterocolitis (over 1,700 types)
S typhi	M, WA, SF	Typhoid fever
Shigella	M, I	Shigellosis, bacillary dysentery
Pseudomonas aeruginosa	S, W, P, A, PR	Endocarditis, respiratory infections

A = animals; *AM* = amoebae; *B* = bird; *D* = dog; *DA* = domestic animal; *F* = fish; *FL* = free living; *I* = insects; *M* = man; *P* = plants; *PZ* = protozoa; *R* = rat; *RP* = reptiles; *S* = soil; *SW* = swine; *SF* = shellfish; *W* = water; *WA* = wild animals.

Table 35-4
Viral Infectious Diseases Found in Sewage

Viruses	Disease	Reservoir	Comments
Adenovirus	Respiratory disease, conjunctivitis	M	31 types
Enteroviruses (nonpolio)	Gastroenteritis, heart anomalies, meningitis	M, WA	4 types (68–71)
	Entero 71 encephalitis		Polio-like paralysis
Coxsackie A, B	Myopericarditis B 1-5 HFM disease A16 + Entero 71[a] AHC disease A24 + Entero 70[b]	M	23 group A (A1–A24, except type A23) 6 group B (B1–B6)
Echovirus	Petechial exanthem, meningitis	M	31 types (1–34, except 10, 28, and 34)
Hepatitis A	Hepatitis	M, P	Myocarditis (rare)
Hepatitis E	Hepatitis	M	Not endemic in Europe or North America
Hantavirus	Sin Nombre virus	R	Pneumonitis with hemorrhage and shock
Parvovirus[c]	Gastroenteritis	M	
Poliovirus	Paralysis, meningitis	M	
Rotavirus	Gastroenteritis	M, DA	

[a]Hand foot and mouth disease.
[b]Acute hemorrhagic conjunctivitis.
[c]Parvovirus-like agents.
DA = domestic animal; *M* = man; *P* = primates; *R* = rat; *WA* = wild animals.

The most important biologically active material is *A fumigatus* (*AF*). AF is one of the most prevalent *Aspergillus* species on Earth. It is able to grow within a wide range of temperatures (12–50°C), relative humidity, and growth media [43]. Individual spores (conidia) are small (2 μm in diameter) and, if inhaled, can enter the lungs [35]. AF can cause dermal and mucosal irritation as well as inflammation and infection [44,45]. It is a common organism in the general environment, with levels up to several hundred spores per cubic meter having been reported [46]. In the aeration tank or compost row, the growth of *Aspergillus* can be impressive. Fortunately, studies have indicated that 250–500 feet from the compost site, the airborne concentrations of AF are at or below background concentration levels [47,48].

The organisms present in bioaerosols represent both true and opportunistic human patho-

Table 35-5
Fungal Infectious Diseases Found in Sewage

Organism	Disease	Comments
Aspergillus fumigatus	Bronchitis, endocarditis, aspergilloma, aspergillosis allergy	
Bronchopulmonary *Aspergillus candidus*, *A flavus*, *A niger*, *A terreus*	ABPA	Rare; usually occurs among immunosuppressed or immunocompromised
Cladosporium cladospoidies	Asthma, hyperactive airways	
Eurotimea amstelodam		
Histoplasma capsulatum	Histoplasmosis, pneumonia, disseminated disease, skin lesions	
Penicillium spinulosum		

Table 35-6
Protozoan and Helminths Found in Sewage

Organism	Disease	Reservoir	Comments
Protozoa			
Balanitidum coli	Balantidiasis	M, S	
Cryptosporidia spp.	Cryptosporidiosis	B, C, D, DA, F, RP, W, S, P	Gastroenteritis, may be chronic in immuno-compromised
Entaomoeba histolytica	Amebiasis	M	
Giardia lamblia	Giardiasis	B, F, RP, R, W, WA, M, DA	Diarrhea
Helminths			
Nematodes (roundworms)			
Ascaris lumbricoides	Ascariasis	M, SW	
Ancyclostoma duodenal	Ancyclostomiasis	M	Wakana disease Chronic anemia
Necator americanus	Necatoriasis	M	Mild CLM symptoms[a]
Ancylostoma braziliense	CLM[a]	C	Cat hookworm
Ancylostoma caninum	CLM[a]	D	Dog hookworm
Enterobius vermicularis	Enterobiasis	M	Pin worm
Strongyloides stercoralis	Strongloidiasis	M, D	Threadworm
Toxocara cati	VLM[b]	CA	Cat roundworm
Toxocara canis	VLM[b]	CA	Dog roundworm
Trichuris trichiura	Trichuriasis	M	Whip worm
Cestodes (tapeworms)			
Taenia saginata	Taeniasis	M	Beef tapeworm
Taenia solium	Taeniasis	M	Pork tapeworm
Hymenolepis nana	Taeniasis	M, R	Dwarf tapeworm
Echinococcus granulosis	HCD[c]	C, D, DA	Dog tapeworm (larval cysts)
Echinococcus multiocularis	ACD[d]	D, CA	Infected canines (larval cysts)

[a]Cutaneous larva migrans.
[b]Visceral larva migrans.
[c]Hydatid cyst disease.
[d]Alveolar cyst disease.
B = bird; *C* = cat; *CA* = carnivores; *D* = dog; *DA* = domestic animal; *F* = fish; *FA* = farm animals; *M* = man; *P* = plants; *R* = rat; *RP* = reptiles; *S* = soil; *SW* = swine; *W* = water; *WA* = wild animals.

gens. Although there is concern that airborne microbes may cause disease from inhaled mists or dried organic dusts, true infections are rare [35]. Despite a statistically significant exposure risk, the incidence of disease by inhalation is low [33, 47, 49]. Currently, the data do not support the contention of elevated risk in immuno competent individuals who handle or have ambient exposure to biosolid waste material.

Nonetheless, municipalities are increasingly looking to compost solid waste from their sewage treatment plants for use as fertilizer or for other uses. In 1994, there were over 200 sewage-sludge composting facilities, 17 solid-waste composting facilities, and over 3,000 yard-waste composting facilities in the United States [50]. With the increase in municipal composting, the exposure to bioaerosols of workers and residences nearby will increase as will health and safety concerns. Case studies from Silver Springs, Maryland; Westbrook, Maine; and Windsor, Ontario, support European data indicating that with current technology *Aspergillus* levels reach background levels at less than 500 feet. Furthermore, at the Silver Springs site, an employee surveillance program instituted in 1987 failed to reveal any adverse health effects related to AF during a five-year period [51]. Studies outside of the United States have documented small numbers of workers who experienced subjective symptoms such as nausea, headaches, and diarrhea. In these workers, endotoxins were thought to be the causative agent [47]. In 1983, Clark studied airborne gram-negative bacteria, endotoxins, and AF. Indoor as well as outdoor bioaerosol concentrations were assessed in mixing biosolid waste and sludge.

Airborne levels of gram-negative bacteria ranged from 0.0 to 3.7×10^5 CFU/m^3. Refuse hoppers, waste-processing areas, and screening areas had the highest mean airborne levels. Over one half of the bioaerosols was respirable, and endotoxin levels ranged from 0.001µg/m^3 to 0.042 µg/m^3. Rylander has studied exposure to aerosols of biologically active agents and endotoxins. In compost facilities, respirable dust levels ranged from 0.1 mg/m^3 to 12.0 mg/m^3. The compost screening areas generated the highest mean levels: 10.6 mg/m^3. The lowest levels were associated with the areas of storage for compost piles. Respirable levels of bacteria ranged between 50% and 60%, yet the data could not establish a dose-response relationship. Until safe standards are set, *it would be prudent to limit individuals working with aerosolized biosolid waste to concentrations no greater than 0.02–0.1 ug/m^3*, as this is the level sufficient to stimulate the mucociliary response of the upper and lower airways. For case definitions and evaluation protocols, please refer to Table 35-7.

BACTERIAL ENDOTOXIN, GLUCANS, AND MYCOTOXINS

Sewage processing and sewage composting are known to be occupations in which workers are exposed to endotoxins, glucans, and mycotoxins [44]. Gram-negative bacteria and their endotoxins are found in high concentrations in areas of biosolid processing. The literature supports the notion that dust in and of itself can cause changes in respiratory responsiveness and lung function [52]. Bacterial endotoxin is the outer layer of the cell walls of gram-negative bacteria. These walls form a heat-stable complex, which is released into the environment both during cell growth and after the cell dies [53]. In the airways, the bacterial cell walls are capable of stimulating macrophage activity, thus causing release of endotoxins. The endotoxins in turn increase the activity of the macrophages and escalate the inflammatory response [54,55].

Fungal cell walls contain the polymer B-1,3-glucan, a polysaccharide composed of glucose units. In the lung, these glucans depress macrophages, inhibiting their ability to function in response to endotoxins and other antigens [56,57]. Mycotoxins are the toxic metabolites of fungi excreted into the sewage by either the mycelium or spore. Generally speaking, the toxins are heat stable and of a low molecular weight and exhibit cytotoxic, mutagenic, teratogenic, carcinogenic, and/or immunologic properties [58].

INFLAMMATION AND INFECTION OF BIOAEROSOLS

Organic dusts affect the upper and lower respiratory tract as well as the dermal surfaces. Individual responses vary, and although symptoms are nonimmunologically mediated, often the presenting clinical picture suggests an immunologic or allergic response. Repeated exposures irritate the mucous membranes of the eyes, ears, nose, and throat [59]. Hyperreactivity of the airways and chronic bronchitis are the sequelae of heavy, repeated exposures. In the lung, increased activity of the macrophages and migration of neutrophils characterize the initial inflammatory response. Neutrophil activity and leakage from nearby capillaries, if severe, result in *organic dust toxic syndrome (ODTS)*. This nonallergic syndrome is characterized by fever, influenza-like symptoms, general malaise, and fatigue. Acute hemorrhagic pneumonitis has been associated with high levels of fungal spores (10^{9-10}/m^3) [60]. There is debate whether the mycotoxin or the glucan in the spores causes this. Asthma, although by definition an immunologic response, may well be mediated by antigenic properties associated with these agents. The most common fungal allergen spores are the saprophytic microfungi *Mucor*, *Rhizopus*, *Cladosporium*, and *Aspergillus.* Experimentally, it has been shown that 100 *Alternaria* and 3,000 *Cladosporium* per cubic meter of air can evoke allergic symptoms [61].

Infections caused by airborne microbial agents in, or on, organic dusts may occur. Pathogenic and opportunistic organisms may invade tissue disrupted by irritant mechanisms. Genetically sensitive individuals are at higher risk. Studies to date have not supported increased risk in individuals in the United States, and Sweden [62–64].

Secondary pathogens such as *Aspergillus fumigatus* may colonize and infect individuals who are immunocompromised or have underlying debilitating medical conditions. Diagnosis is not easily made. The organism is so common and readily inhalable, that isolation in the sputum is not considered diagnostic. Blood tests for circulating *Aspergillus* antibodies have detected elevated levels in healthy adults. Further allergy testing via skin prick, patch, or scratch testing is often unreliable, as commercially derived antigenic extracts are often contaminated with AF. Therefore, positive serologic testing is merely a marker of past exposure (Table 35-7).

There is little supportive evidence that *A fumigatus* and related species pose a risk to immunocompetent sewage workers or the general population. There is concern regarding immunocompromised individuals. The following strategy is important when evaluating the ill sewage worker. In the immunocompetent individual, the body's defense system is capable of clearing the exposure by a combination of cellular defense and the mucocilliary transport system. Unchecked, the pathways of infection are from (1) outer ear to inner, (2) nasal mucosa to meninges and brain, and (3) from lung to the bloodstream. Individuals with malignancies, those taking immunosuppressant medications, and those who have suffered trauma may be at increased risk for AF colonization. Individuals with abnormal lung function, such as those suffering from tuberculosis or sarcoidosis, may also be at risk for colonization. Saprophytic growth leads to the formation of "fungus balls," also known as *aspergillomas* or *mycetomas.* Despite mounting an antibody response, patients have mild symptoms early in the disease.

The immunodeficient individual is particularly at risk. Immune globulin disorders or immunodeficiency diseases occur in 1 in 500 individuals [65]. HIV increases the risk of contracting disease from both pathogenic and nonpathogenic organisms. Other at-risk individuals include those with genetically impaired immune system. Atopic individuals must be aware of the risks of sewage, both dry and moist. Airborne concentrations may be sufficiently high to increase symptoms in atopic individuals as well as sensitize nonatopic workers by constant exposure. The treatment and prognosis of these cases is on an individual basis.

The effects and reactions of sewer workers exposed to bioaerosols are often the same as those experienced by those in the "normal" environment. Under certain conditions, bioaerosol counts as high as 4.5×10^5 fungal spores/m^3 of air have been demonstrated in air samples from buildings [66]. Consequently, it is difficult to correlate measured levels of bioaerosols and ascribe a particular health effect based on data alone. Investigation of illnesses and alleged exposures must include site surveys and air sampling of exposure concentrations. The route of exposure as well as the immune condition, antigen sensitivity, and underlying diseases of individuals must be considered. Although a subjective matter, "annoyance" is often a large component of sewage workers' complaints and can be quantified by questionnaire. Rylander has set a threshold of 10%, "very annoyed," as an upper limit for emissions in densely populated areas. When the threshold has been exceeded, requests are made to reduce or eliminate airborne bioaerosols.

Prevention and Control

ADMINISTRATIVE CONTROLS

Management must keep the exposure to infectious agents at an acceptably low level. This can be accomplished only if there is a thorough understanding of the current sewage collection and processing systems in place. Administratively, one would attempt to control factors that expose sewer workers to a contaminated environment or animal hosts. Those charged with assuring health and safety need to provide support, leadership, and education in protecting the worker and his/her health. All outbreaks of waterborne disease should be investigated to characterize a potential common or point source. Individuals with a history of disorders of the liver or gallbladder or a past history of jaundice should be excluded from work with potentially hepatotoxic agents [67] including HAV, leptospirosis, protozoans, or organic chemicals.

For new sewage or sewage-composting facilities, preplanning and public involvement in the process is necessary for successful control. A large number of indoor air quality complaints, as well as illnesses, stem from external or outdoor sources. Preplanning of sewage facilities should

Table 35-7
Case Definitions for Diseases Caused by *Aspergillus Fumigatus*

I. Invasive aspergillosis
   A. *Aspergillus:* isolated by culture from a normally sterile site (blood or tissue); culture of sputum is not acceptable.
   B. Mycetoma (aspergilloma): diagnosed by sputum culture and chest or sinus radiography or CT scan.

II. Allergic bronchopulmonary aspergillosis
   A. Definitive diagnosis requires that *all* seven of the following criteria be met:
   B. Identification of possible cases requires that *five* of seven criteria be met:
      1. Asthma (evidence of reversible airflow obstruction defined by FEV 1/FVC < 0.70).
      2. Evidence of immediate skin reactivity, i.e., wheal and flare reaction, to *Aspergillus fumigatus* antigen using intradermal injection or "prick" test.
      3. The presence of aspergillus-specific IgE in serum.
      4. Quantitative serum IgE > 400 IU/mL or IgE > 250 IU/mL plus evidence of titer fluctuation with disease activity.
      5. IgG or precipitating antibody to *Aspergillus.*
      6. History of peripheral eosinophilia (absolute eosinophil count > 500 cells/mm^3).
      7. History of pulmonary infiltrates documented by chest radiography.

III. Acute allergic alveolitis (hypersensitivity pneumonitis)
   A. Fever and severe dyspnea four to six hours after exposure to a source of *Aspergillus* or episodic fever and dyspnea and high serum IgG precipitating antibodies to *Aspergillus.*
   B. At the time of symptoms, either diffuse micronodular infiltrates on chest radiograph or restrictive ventilatory defect documented by pulmonary function testing.
   C. A positive response to an inhalation-provocation test, using *Aspergillus* as the antigen.
   D. Lung histopathology with mononuclear inflammatory cell infiltrates in alveoli and interstitial spaces documented by lung biopsy.

IV. Asthma induced by *Aspergillus*: Criteria A, B, C, and D must be met for a definite case; criteria A, B, and E must be met for identification of a possible case.
   A. Recurrent or intermittent symptoms consistent with asthma, including wheezing, dyspnea, cough, or chest tightness.
   B. Documentation of reversible or variable airway obstruction (improvement of at least 10% in FEV 1 with use of a bronchodilator); at least 20% variability in serial peak expiratory flow rate (PEFR) measurements in a 24-hour period; positive inhalation challenge testing with methacholine or histamine (20% decrease in FEV 1 produced by five inhalations of 8 mg/mL or less).
   C. Temporal association between episode of asthma and known exposure to *Aspergillus.*
   D. Positive wheal/flare to *Aspergillus* or positive *Aspergillus*-specific IgE radioallergosorbent test (RAST) in absence of reaction to other allergens.
   E. Positive wheal/flare to *Aspergillus* or positive *Aspergillus*-specific IgE RAST.
   Note: Allergic asthma due to *Aspergillus* exposure usually occurs in atopic persons and is rarely due solely to such exposure. Allergic asthma occurs less often in individuals with *Aspergillus* exposure than those with hay fever.

V. *Aspergillus* sinusitis: Criteria A and B must be met.
   A. Isolation of *Aspergillus* species from sinus culture.
   B. Severe abnormalities on sinus CT scan.

VI. Allergies: While persons with sensitivity to aspergillus may have a skin test reaction or IgE levels to *Aspergillus* antigens, these tests alone are not definitive and the contribution to fungal exposure to allergy is difficult to evaluate. IgE skin testing correlates with biologic activity. RAST testing is an immunoassay and is less sensitive than skin testing. MAST testing evaluates antibody levels to a panel of antigens. Detection of antibodies in sera indicate exposure and are not diagnostic of an adverse health response.

consider their proximity to residencies and public facilities. Cities should regulate construction through the building inspection department to ensure that new buildings near sewage treatment areas are not constructed with "closed" ventilation systems. Those presently in operation should have periodic sampling to ensure that contamination has not occurred. Environmental studies of the meteorologic and topographic characteristics at the site and nearby the facility should be analyzed. New, upgraded or expanded sewage facilities require evaluation and installation of buffer zones or enclosures. Good management practices defined by state and federal legislation are primarily concerned with operational efficiency, pathogen reduction, and dust and odor control. In order to minimize bioaerosols and odors, current technology dictates the mechanization of sewage treatment and the method of handling materials.

As municipal solid-waste streams change, it is necessary to evaluate and eliminate volatile organic substances in sewage. Working with local industries and the board of health, periodic sampling of local biologic agents should be required. Dumping of illegal toxic wastes by industry, although banned by local, state, and federal statute, nevertheless occurs. Periodic unannounced sampling of all forms of sewage waste products is necessary to reduce risk to workers and ensure safe working conditions.

Depositing of treated or untreated sewage on land for agricultural or disposal purposes should undergo review. If this manner of dispersion is the only viable method of volume reduction, then it must be justified by agricultural studies supporting the benefits to soil and crops. Administrative issues that must be addressed if workers are exposed to land dispersion of sewage wastes are:

- What is the maximum rate of sludge application that will incur no harm to the soil?
- What crops can be most successfully cultivated on the treated areas on a rotational basis?
- Will the biologic agents, pesticides, nitrates, phosphates, organic solvents, and PCBs cause underground water pollution problems?
- What are the possible exposures to humans and animals to these wastes?

This "night soil," may contain multiple environmentally persistent agents; therefore periodic sampling of the sludge for pathogens and chemicals is necessary to protect the public health. The public health issue outweighs the purported benefit of this type of disposal [68].

SAFE WORK PRACTICES AND ENGINEERING CONTROLS

The occupational physician must understand the nuances of the job description of sewage workers in order to effect safe work practices. Those that work in *main drainage* are exposed to large intercepting sewers, pumping stations, and sewage disposal units. *Sewage systems* consist of pipes 20–60 cm in diameter. Brick and concrete sewers are 80–150 cm in height. *Compost systems*, open and closed, have special risks. The primary concern for composting is the inhalation of bioaerosols and derived products emitted by these facilities [35].

Evaluating engineering controls requires an understanding not only of the process but also of the environment. Physical and meteorologic characteristics impact workers and nearby public sectors, and topography and weather affect the operation of the compost facility. Some compost facilities are designed to distribute aerosols over large areas in order to decrease atmospheric concentrations. A wind map or information on daily prevailing winds should be used to schedule high release points to minimize concentrations of bioaerosols. If the plan is to keep the aerosols close to the facility, composting operations should be shielded from wind, and emission of aerosols kept below grade or at low release heights [69]. An undisturbed compost pile does not generate a significant amount of aerosolized microbes; therefore, those working in sewage composting or air drying of sludge should avoid churning it during windy conditions. Mechanical agitation as well as bulk movement has been shown to be a major source of airborne emissions. Reducing the size of the loads being moved or agitated as well as vigilance in dust control can minimize bioaerosol releases. Down-drafts onto dust-laden surfaces, as well as the mechanical agitation of wheels and tires of machines handling this material, increases bioaerosol releases. Attempts to reduce emissions may include changing the time of biosolid agitation and enclosing the facility to minimize site and off-site contamination. Monitoring of the temperature and moisture concentrations of bulking agents will help minimize formation of bioaerosols. Consideration of the amount of time that the compost "cures" may reduce the levels of bioaerosols, especially those of aspergillus. The use of filters has been suggested for odor control, but because of low emissions from static waste piles, there has not been adequate study of its effectiveness.

There has not been adequate dose-response modeling or quantitative risk assessment to assign safe levels of bioaerosol exposure. Differences in the response of the human immune system limit the ability to promulgate a minimum safe level. There is some dose-response literature regarding endotoxins, but the issue of testing humans for microbial agents may not be feasible. We rely on scarce studies and reports for guidance. As there are no widely recommended exposure levels for endotoxins, setting a time weighted average (TWA) or threshold limit should be considered [70]. There are recommendations that safe levels may be defined as those that do not adversely impact human health. The lowest concentration of endotoxin at which a pulmonary response has been detected is 10 ng/m^3 [71]. Palchack has recommended an eight-hour TWA exposure limit of 30 ng/m^3 for periodic industrial hygiene monitoring. This incorporates a 10-fold safety factor based on the median exposure associated with a 5% decrease in FEV 1 [72]. Rylander has set a threshold limit of 100–200 ng/m^3 for exposures to endotoxins, based on a documented decline in FEV 1, over one working shift [73].

Personal Protective Equipment and Practices

Although it is an admirable effort to institute environmental hygiene measures such as rodent control and work surface decontamination, the sewer environment is such that workers should assume that all waste and surfaces are contaminated. Since the environment is one in which exposure cannot be avoided, prevention centers around measures to physically protect the individual. Implementation of the use of personal protective equipment (PPE), waste management and treatment, and proper hygienic habits is essential.

First, all workers should be educated on a yearly basis to avoid prolonged or direct contact with sewage. Eliminating prolonged immersion by requiring workers to wear rubber boots and gloves, long pants, and protective eyewear will decrease exposure to skin, mucous membranes, and eyes. Personal protective equipment should include waterproof footwear, water-shedding aprons worn outside and over the boots or other clothing, and clear plastic face masks. In sewers, hot climates, and in areas requiring dexterity, impermeable protective equipment has been poorly accepted, but because pathogens often infect via wet, abraded or macerated skin, the use of water-proof boots by the sewer worker is an absolute minimum.

It is strongly recommended that sewage workers wash their hands prior to eating or smoking. After exposure, contaminated articles should be disposed of in an appropriate receptacle. Showering should also be required. Laundering of work garb using enzyme cleansing methods will eliminate pathogens and reduce complaints of dermatitis caused by traditional soaps and cleaners.

Respirators of an appropriate design should be utilized, especially when the worker is in confined spaces or when sampling has documented volatile chemicals in the waste stream. Regular worksite monitoring of benzene and other volatile organic solvents is recommended. For those working with compost sewage waste, protective face masks, which filter particle sizes of 1–5 μm, are recommended. Periodic examination of this equipment is necessary to ensure adequate protection. For those with special risks, such as those working in biofilter towers, the OSHA respirator medical evaluation questionnaire and physical examination are required upon assignment or transfer to a contaminated area. Fit testing and training in an ANSI/NIOSH-approved and appropriate-for-use respirator is also required for workers prior to their entry into contaminated areas. Individuals performing fit testing and training must be experienced and knowledgeable; the occupational physician should know the credentials of the person or company providing this service if it is not performed by the physician.

Proactive Preventive Measures in Developing a Prevention Program

Preventive measures for control of human infections vary, depending on sewage worker activity and local animal reservoirs. There are three important factors to consider when developing a prevention program.

- The exposed worker/individual: Minimize skin contact with sewage sludge, compost, and incinerator exhaust-fan residue and fly ash [74].
- The contaminated environment: (1) Ensure adequate ventilation for all sewage workers; (2) implement measures to minimize work-

ers' contact with bacterial aerosols, such as in aeration basins, especially if indoors; and (3) perform volumetric and biologic sampling around the sewage site at specified intervals to assess fluctuations and changes in pathogens.

- The animal shedder: The rodent is an important carrier of several diseases. In leptospirosis, it is the most common shedder. A rodent control and testing program should be investigated. The scope of eradication of this risk is more aptly addressed by sampling the population and assessing the shedder incidence. Antibiotics to eliminate the shedder state have not proved successful.

EMPLOYEE EDUCATION AND TRAINING

Individuals, whether working in a typical sewage treatment plant, state-of-the-art composting facility or near or at the point source of sewage, should be educated about the risks associated with exposures to sewage and biologically active agents. This education should take place upon hire, annually, or with job change or transfer. New employees should undergo training in the risks of exposure to *Leptospira*, *Legionella*, hepatitis A and E, and other common pathogens as part of job orientation. Education about signs and symptoms of organic solvent exposure and industrial and radioactive wastes should also be included.

Individuals working in processing of open compost, with or without agitation, aeration tanks, or downwind from other workers performing these activities should know the prevailing wind patterns. Records, for example, monthly wind arrows, should be kept to limit the concentration of exposure of bioaerosols and other pathogenic materials. Workers involved in operations that generate bioaerosols should be educated about personal risks as well as risks to their fellow workers and the population near the worksite.

RESCUE TRAINING

Training in rescue methods, practiced in coordination with the police and fire departments, is required on an annual basis to ensure worker safety.

PERSONAL-HEALTH EDUCATION

Cigarette smoking, chronic lung disease, advanced age, and immunosuppresssion put sewer workers at greater risk. Periodic health lectures and a viable wellness and employee assistance program may abate these risks.

PERIODIC MEDICAL SURVEILLANCE

An occupational and medical history as well as a completed OSHA Respirator Medical Evaluation Questionnaire should be obtained for all employees upon hire and annually. Special attention should be paid to the medical history; individuals with a past or present history of liver disease require special attention. Immunosuppressed individuals or those afflicted with HIV are at risk for progressive infections, extrapulmonary complications, bacteremia, and lung abscesses due to *Aspergillus* and *Legionella*. After initial assessment, a complete physical examination should be performed on an annual basis. Individuals who have, or are at risk for, pulmonary problems should be required by the employer or an occupational physician to undergo pulmonary function testing at the time of physical examination. Individuals in compost facilities are at increased risk for occupational asthma. Although data are sparse, it is recommended that one consider pulmonary function testing in settings of wet, slurry, or dry bioaerosol exposure [75]. It is prudent to document personal habits or other behaviors that may contribute to lung disease, such as smoking or use of marijuana. Passive exposure to cigarette smoke should not be overlooked. For workers exposed to high levels of dust, a baseline, periodic, symptomatic, and exit chest radiography should be performed. Often overlooked is the musculoskeletal system. Depending on the type of work, sewer workers are often in cramped, confined spaces that places stress on the joints and spine.

Routine or periodic blood and urine testing is not recommended for all individuals. Upon hire, only a baseline CBC, LFTs, and urinalysis are required in most situations. For individuals with the special risks mentioned above, testing should be on an individual basis. Although there is no clear consensus about risk, we recommend testing for hepatitis A antibodies upon hire or periodically, if hepatitis vaccination is refused by an individual.

Upon notification by the local board of health of a current infectious disease outbreak in the community or toxic spill into the sewage system, appropriate tests should be performed. Under these conditions, those with chronic liver disease, HCV or HBV and those who are not immunized against HAV or are immunocompromised should be excluded from work. At the time of periodic physical examination or upon notification of a toxic spill into the sewage system, special emphasis should be paid to the hematologic and nervous systems.

IMMUNIZATION AND PROPHYLACTIC MEASURES

Pre- and Postexposure Measures

Bacteria. Eradication of bacterial pathogens in the sewage workers' environment is not possible. Prophylaxis for leptospirosis can be provided by utilizing doxycycline, 200 mg, administered once weekly. This regimen has been shown to be effective and is indicated when the exposure is known to be of short duration and the attack rate is calculated to exceed 1%. Vaccinations for animals are available to protect them against illness but are not protective against leptospirosis and leptospiruria in humans. Transmission of infection to workers from immunized, asymptomatic animals shedding leptospires in their urine has occurred. Human leptospirosis vaccines have been utilized in Europe, Israel, Japan, and Italy; they are serotype-specific, require two or more doses 2–4 weeks apart, and must be repeated annually [76]. Acceptance of an early generation protein-free vaccine for humans, despite evidence of its effectiveness, has not been widespread.

Legionella is a known contaminate of the aquatic environment. The most cost-effective methods of primary and secondary prevention of legionellosis have not been identified. Development of preventive strategies is limited by the complex interaction of the environment, transmission, and animal hosts. The CDC has recommended culturing of environmental sources only in cases of documented legionnaires' disease. Biocides and hyperchlorination have been ineffective in eradicating the organism from cooling towers and have been marginally effective in reducing pathogen counts [77]. Hyperchlorination of influent or effluent sewage is not recommended. Chlorine breaks down at higher temperatures, the bacteria are resistant to chlorine, and corrosion of plumbing systems and the potential for chlorinated carcinogenic by-products are major disadvantages [78]. Methods for destruction of *Legionella* such as UV irradiation, copper-silver ionization, and superheat and flush are not plausible in the sewer environment. *Legionella* immunization that induces cell-mediated immunity is currently being tested in animal models [79–80]. It appears that vaccines for sewer workers would be cost efficient, depending on levels of exposure. For immunosuppressed individuals, erythromycin chemoprophylaxis has been protective against legionnaires' disease. However, colonization of the sewer environment, coupled with the low overall attack rate, renders this strategy seldom indicated.

Viruses. There are numerous reports from around the world that identify the incidence and prevalence of hepatitis A among sewage workers. In the United States, there are no protocols that advocate immunization for sewage workers against hepatitis A despite its intermittent presence in wastewater. In Singapore, a sharp decline in hepatitis A transmission was concomitant with improvements in environmental hygiene. In the United States, less than 1% of the population under 20 years of age possesses IG antibodies to HAV (anti-HAV). Forty percent (40%) of reported HAV cases are imported, most likely from Southeast Asia or the Indian subcontinent.

We recommend hepatitis A vaccination for all sewage workers documented to be HAV-antibody negative. After the risks and benefits of the vaccination are discussed with an employee and informed consent is obtained, vaccination should be performed utilizing standard guidelines. Individuals that accept the hepatitis A vaccination should receive a booster in six to 12 months, depending on the type of vaccine and the manufacturer. Vaccination should be performed prior to exposure to point-source sewage or during a known community outbreak of HAV. Currently, follow-up titers are not recommended nor required. In the future (10–15 years), titers may be necessary, however, to document individuals immune status. For individuals that refuse hepatitis A vaccination, there is no recommended biologic monitoring. Sewage workers have a higher conversion rate than controls and convert to a seropositive status based on several factors, as noted above.

Hepatitis E vaccination and treatment may be possible, as there are several recombinant vaccines currently under development and there is theoretical evidence of antiviral activity in available medications [81]. In areas where HEV is endemic, it may be possible to utilize pooled serum immune globulin to protect or modify the illness. In the United States, the processing of serum immune globulin does not contain these antibodies, so it is not reasonable to offer it to sewer workers or travelers to endemic areas. If vaccines become available, assessment of the relative risk of the sewer worker population and vaccination on a case-by-case basis will be necessary. Obviously, there is little need in the United States for this recommendation at present.

Current recommendations are that workers be current in their vaccinations for tetanus. These can be provided by the local occupational health clinic or the public health nurse if available. Individuals should have documented childhood polio vaccination. Currently, the CDC and ACIP have recommended splitting doses between injectable and oral dosing schedules. In the near future, an all-injectable schedule may exist. Individuals working in sewers may not be protected by their childhood oral polio immunization. It is recommended that all sewer workers receive a booster dose of injectable polio vaccine. Further boosters should be considered for workers in communities with known outbreaks or viral-culture-positive plates during periodic sampling. For determination of measles, mumps, and rubella (MMR) vaccination status, it is no longer considered adequate to rely on a personal or family recall of diseases. A single injection of the MMR vaccine is also considered inadequate. It is recommended that documentation of two MMR vaccinations are in the medical record prior to medical clearance. In countries with sporadic outbreaks of measles or rubella, documentation of titers are necessary prior to medical clearance to work with sewage.

Although few specific risks of sewer workers' exposure to hepatitis B virus (HBV) have been documented, it is now standard public health policy to vaccinate all health care workers and individuals under the age of 18. HBV vaccination is a prudent recommendation that can be accomplished either through the local board of health or private insurance. Sewer workers involved in point-source exposures should have HBV vaccination either offered to them upon hire or prior to exposure.

COMPLIANCE

Upon hire, review of immunizations by the physician should be performed. During the orientation period, the worker should be educated concerning the risks associated with sewage work, specifically the risks associated with the different processes in sewage treatment. In conjunction with the director of human resources and representatives of the workers' union, recommendations should be written into the employment contract to ensure worker safety. Occupational physicians in municipalities without public health officials or programs should work with state and local government to fund periodic antibody screening and vaccination programs. Many states have enacted centralized immunization databases. We recommend working with the local and state departments of health to document in a central location the vaccination status of municipal employees rather than keeping this information at a local level. In the future, individuals may access this information via the Internet utilizing personal identification number (PIN) technology. This will allow freedom of movement in the workplace without reliance on local practitioners or the board of health to document vaccination status. As always, medical confidentiality issues abound in regard to vaccination status and need to be clarified.

METRICS TO ASSESS ADEQUACY OF PREVENTIVE MEASURES

Working with the local health department or the department of waste water, a representative profile of pathogens should be developed. Utilizing this profile, the physician may monitor antibody responses to specific antigens from the known pool of pathogens.

Symptoms and Signs

Undiagnosed febrile illnesses in sewage workers should be reported to the local board of health or occupational physician for evaluation.

LEPTOSPIROSIS

Leptospirosis has an incubation time that may range from four to 19 days but is commonly seven to 10 days. The disease reveals biphasic tendencies, with the initial or febrile stage lasting around seven days, followed by the second (immune) stage lasting 0–30 days or more [82,83]. Many organ systems can be affected; therefore, the clinical presentation may vary. Mild flu-like symptoms or a fulminant course may ensue. In the initial stage, fever (39–41°C) of a week's duration or more is common. Individuals complain of anorexia, myalgia, headache, prostration, and retro-orbital pain. Often, there is profuse sweating. During the first 48 hours, bulbar conjunctival injection may be observed. Respiratory symptoms may be prominent. In the second stage, anorexia progresses to nausea and vomiting accompanied by either diarrhea or constipation. During this febrile period, ophthalmologic examination reveals papilledema, optic neuritis, and oculomotor paresis. Late manifestations include uveitis, which may occur from two weeks to one year after infection. Other neurologic symptoms, such as stiff neck and nuchal rigidity, are present. Lymphadenopathy that mimics mononucleosis is noted in roughly 50% of patients. For the remainder of afflicted individuals, glandular swelling is not prominent. Hemorrhagic manifestations may occur. The occurrence of liver and spleen enlargement, as well as jaundice and kidney involvement, depends on the severity of the infection and its stage.

LEGIONELLOSIS

Diseases attributed to *Legionella* species are legionnaires' disease, a potentially fatal form of pneumonia, and Pontiac fever, a self-limited, nonpneumonic illness. In patients with legionnaires' disease, pneumonia is the predominant clinical finding; symptoms may be mild (e.g., slight cough and fever) or severe (e.g., pulmonary infiltrates and multisystem failure). The incubation period is two to 10 days. Mild cough may progress to a productive one that is occasionally streaked with blood. Pleuritic or nonpleuritic chest pain accompanied by hemoptysis suggests pulmonary embolus. Diarrhea, which is watery rather than bloody, occurs in 20–50% of patients. Nausea, vomiting, and abdominal pain are experienced by 10–20%.

Pontiac fever has an incubation period of 24–48 hours; its attack rate is often more than 95%. Prominent symptoms are malaise, myalgias, fever, chills, and headache. In some cases, a nonproductive cough, dizziness, and nausea are present. Findings of chest radiography are normal, and with supportive care, complete recovery is the norm.

Hepatitis A and E are acute self-limiting illnesses. Patients often present with complaints of fever, malaise, jaundice, anorexia, and nausea. In children, hepatitis A is often mild. The illness is usually several weeks in duration, but cases of relapsing disease lasting as long as six months may occur. Fulminant hepatitis is rare and chronic infection is not known to occur. Hepatitis E is not distinguishable from other forms of hepatitis but may be fulminant in the third trimester of pregnancy.

Differential Diagnosis

The history of medical problems related to work with sewage does not make the job of diagnosing disease any easier. Sewer workers suffer less from nausea than referent groups and exhibit no significant difference in the prevalence of diarrhea, dyspepsia, or irritable bowel syndrome. There is some evidence to support increased risk for peptic ulcer disease, yet studies of associations with *Helicobacter pylori* and sewage work have not found this type of work to be a significant risk [35].

The clinical manifestations of leptospirosis are not pathognomonic and have been confused with many other diseases such as influenza, poliomyelitis, dengue, Q fever, and viral meningitis. Unless a physician has considerable clinical experience with leptospirosis, the diagnosis is usually made by laboratory analysis. Of the greater than 1,000 cases registered by the CDC since 1949, leptospirosis had been included in the differential diagnosis in only 25% [84]. The difficulty in making a timely diagnosis is often due to a locale's lack of laboratory procedures that would rapidly confirm the diagnosis in the important first stage. Therefore, a high degree of suspicion is warranted when sewage treatment workers present with fever.

Legionella infections, both Pontiac fever and legionnaires' disease, present nonspecifically. The following signs should raise the clinician's suspicions as to the diagnosis:

- Sputum gram stain, with increased neutrophils but few organisms seen on microscopic examination.
- Hyponatremia.
- Failure to respond to B-lactams (penicillin or cephalosporin) or aminoglycoside antibiotics.
- Exposure to potentially contaminated aquatic environments.

In the sewer worker, exposure to HAV, HEV, or leptospirosis may cause jaundice. When discharges of potent hepatotoxins from industry occur, HBV and HCV must be considered in the differential diagnosis of workers who become ill. Releases by industry of certain chemicals in sufficient quantities can cause toxic hepatitis. It is important not only to ask co-workers about unusual smells that have their onset within several days to two weeks of the onset of jaundice, but also to understand the types of industries and potential by-products of manufacturing that could be illegally dumped into the sewage system. Hospital emergency departments usually have the material safety data sheets (MSDSs) of local industry. When these are not available, the health and safety or industrial hygiene officer at the local plant can be a valuable resource in understanding the etiology of jaundice in sewage workers.

Hantavirus infection presents in several phases: the prodrome, followed by the cardiopulmonary and convalescent phases. The nonspecific prodromal symptoms include fever and myalgia lasting three to six days as well as headache, backache, and gastrointestinal symptoms. The disease becomes differentiated in the second stage, in which noncardiogenic pulmonary edema often accompanies shock. Those that have progressed to the second stage have a mortality rate that often reaches 50%.

Diagnostic Evaluation

Many diseases of sewer workers also afflict the general population. When confronted with an ill sewage worker, it is important to remember that sewage workers' illnesses often reflect the illnesses in the community at that specific period of time. A high degree of suspicion must be maintained if an early diagnosis is to be made for the typical pathogens that inhabit the sewage worker's environment. In addition, a thorough occupational history and an understanding of the sewage treatment process and conditions of exposure are paramount in making a timely diagnosis in the ill sewage worker.

LEPTOSPIROSIS

In patients with leptospirosis, routine laboratory testing reveals leukocytosis or leukopenia with a left shift. Urinalysis reveals proteinaceous casts with an increase in BUN and creatinine. Since leptospirosis can present with multiple symptoms, it is recommended that culture of the organism be obtained and grown. Culture media containing long-chain fatty acids, such as oleic acid or Tween with 1% bovine serum albumin as a detoxicant, are used. Optimum temperature for cultivation is 28–30°C. Most strains do not grow above 37°C. Small numbers of organisms are seen within two to three days, and cultures should routinely be examined weekly for up to three months. Blood cultures taken during the first acute phase of the infection (up to 10 days) usually are positive. Cultures may also be taken from CSF, urine and tissues, including autopsy specimens. To an experienced pathologist utilizing darkfield microscopy and thin specimen preparations, the organisms appear as motile, bright, beaded, rotating, thin rods, usually with one or both ends curved, against a black background. Phase-contrast microscopy is of limited value, as is staining of the organisms. Serologic typing requires reference antisera or serogroup/serovar-specific monoclonal antibodies. Gene probes utilizing polymerase chain reaction (PCR) are capable of detecting 10–10^3 leptospires in specimens. This method is particularly useful in the diagnosis of acute illness and identification of leptospires in cultured isolates [85–87]. Detection of antibodies in sera of infected individuals may be performed utilizing agglutination or enzyme-linked immunosorbent assay (ELISA) methodology. Of the two types of agglutination methods, most laboratories perform the microscopic (MAT) rather than the macroscopic agglutination test because it is sensitive and is read microscopically under darkfield. However, it is not without its disadvantages. The subjectiveness of the interpretation test results and the labor intensiveness of preparation may lead to errors owing to incorrect serovar choice and use of live cultures. Direct use of IgG or IgM testing is not available at present. ELISA technology has the advantages of precision, objectivity, ability to screen large numbers of sera specimens, reasonable cost, and ability to measure IgG and IgM antibodies. In terms of making the diagnosis, practically speaking, MAT and ELISA are preferable to culture.

LEGIONELLOSIS

Clinical studies have shown that it is not possible to differentiate legionnaires' disease from community-acquired pneumonia on the basis of signs, symptoms, routine laboratory tests, or radiographic findings. Since patients are otherwise unremarkable in the clinical presentation of this upper respiratory disease, specific laboratory tests are necessary to establish the diagnosis of legionellosis. Sewage treatment workers with potential exposures to *Legionella* who present with cough and fever should have a chest radiography. By the third day of the disease, the majority of patients with legionnaires' disease will have an abnormal radiograph. Classic findings are that of a predominantly unilateral lower-lobe infiltrate. The definitive method for diagnosis of *Legionella* infection is culture of respiratory secretions. Culture of secretions from both the infected individual and his/her environment is still considered the "gold standard" for diagnosis. *Legionella* organisms are best demonstrated by utilizing buffered charcoal-yeast extract medium enriched with alpha-ketoglutarate (BCYE-alpha). They cannot be isolated with routine clinical bacteriologic techniques. The limitations of culture include the lack of experience of many pathology laboratoriess in both the United States and other countries. A recent survey revealed that nearly two thirds of laboratories were unable to culture a heavy growth of *Legionella pneumophilia* from sputum. Often, sputum that may have culturable *Legionella* present is routinely discarded because it has too many squamous cells and too few polymorphonuclear cells [88,89].

Serologic tests have limitations in that a four-fold rise in antibody titers by IFA occurs in 70–80% of patients, yet seroconversion may take place two to three months after the onset of illness. A four-fold rise in titer does not confirm the diagnosis of legionellosis in patients with community-acquired pneumonia [90]. Acute- and convalescent-stage sera are required, as pneumonia due to other agents is nearly as likely to cause an acute rise in titer and delayed antibody response. Serology is therefore not helpful in making the immediate diagnosis. One would have to acquire a baseline titer and compare this with acute titers. However, this may be a reasonable approach in monitoring the sewage worker population, especially if the baseline antibody titers are low and episodic disease is prevalent.

Diagnosis of legionnaires' disease by direct fluorescent antibody (DFA) testing has the drawback of requiring large numbers of organisms to be present and very experienced laboratory technicians. The sensitivity of DFA testing is between 25–75% and its specificity is less than 95%. The specificity of polyvalent DFA reagents are probably lower than monoclonal reagents, leading some labs to advocate their exclusive use [91]. DFA is more likely to be useful when there are diffuse, multilobar infiltrates on chest radiograph. Commercially available urinary radioimmunoassay (RIA) testing is available for detection of *L pneumophila* serogroup 1. In infected individuals, its sensitivity is 60–80% and its specificity is nearly 100% [92]. Genus-specific DNA probe technology is available and is comparable in sensitivity and specificity to that of DFA testing. Utilizing this technique exclusively has resulted in the erroneous identification of outbreaks of legionnaires' disease based on false-positive test results. It is recommended that other confirmative methods be utilized in conjunction with this diagnostic method. PCR is a promising technology because it has the capability of identifying the organism in water [93].

VIRUSES

HAV and HEV quantifications can be obtained by monitoring IgM anti-HAV or IgM anti-HEV, respectively. Monitoring IgG antibody titers is also helpful. Hantavirus infection may be diagnosed by serology or PCR of tissue samples.

PARASITES

Routine stool samples for culture of ova and parasites should be required for all ill sewage workers with diarrhea.

Clinical Management and Rehabilitation

Recommendations for prevention and treatment are often predicated on the population and the type of sewer system in place. Occupational physicians may be asked to make recommendations regarding the health, safety, welfare, and treatment of these individuals. At present, a case-by-case approach is recommended, since there are few consensus guidelines to follow.

LEPTOSPIROSIS

The treatment of leptospirosis has traditionally utilized penicillin, streptomycin, tetracycline, cephalosporins, and macrolides with success. Tetracycline antibiotics, however, are leptospirostatic rather than leptospiricidal and are contraindicated in children, gravid women, and individuals with compromised renal function. Antibiotics must be administered within two to four days for optimal outcome. Since the presentation may include myriad symptoms, a high level of clinical suspicion should be maintained in this population of workers with febrile illnesses. For those who present with severe infection, admission to a hospital for supportive care, with particular attention to fluid and electrolyte status, is required. The patient should be monitored until afebrile for at least one week. Relapses are fairly common, especially in those that present late for treatment or diagnosis. Hemodialysis may be necessary for individuals with renal failure. For those traveling in areas where leptospirosis is endemic, doxycycline, 200 mg once weekly, appears to be protective.

LEGIONNAIRES' DISEASE

Legionella diseases have been traditionally treated with erythromycin, 2 g orally or 4 g intravenously daily. Early administration and appropriate dosage improves survival [94]. There is associated ototoxicity with the 4-g dose. Oral administration may be adequate for some patients, yet abrupt deterioration in "stable" patients with advanced disease may occur. The high percentage of patients with gastrointestinal symptoms makes oral administration and absorption of erythromycin difficult, however. The prudent practitioner initially treats patients with parenteral antibiotics. Since the macrolides and quinolones have shown superior in vitro activity to erythromycin, once the patient is stable (three to five days), oral therapy with this agent may replace parenteral, for a total treatment duration of 10–14 days in immunocompetent individuals. For patients with severe infections, rifampin is occasionally used concomitantly with erythromycin.

Convalescence from *Legionella* infection may take several months. Lingering problems such as shortness of breath and weakness are common. Pulmonary diffusing capacity defects, as well as reinfection in the immunocompromised, have been noted [95,96].

HEPATITIS A

Hepatitis A is best managed by vaccination and education of the worker about sanitation and hygiene. For infected adults, expedient diagnosis and supportive care are usually all that is needed. Hepatitis E is also best managed by education and prevention. Research has shown that ribavirin and alpha-interferon have activity against HEV, yet FDA protocols are not available at present.

HANTAVIRUS INFECTION

Hantavirus infection is also best managed by education and prevention of exposure to rodent excrement. When the diagnosis is made, admission of the infected individual to the hospital for monitoring and supportive care is required. Oxygen, as well as fluid and electrolyte management for shock, is critical for the survival of patients with this disease. The use of ribavirin has been suggested for treatment but has not received FDA approval.

References

1. Nethercott, JR, Holness DL. Health status of a group of sewage treatment workers in Toronto, Canada. *Am Ind Hyg Assoc J* 1988;49(7):346–50.
2. Elia VJ, Clark CS, Majeti VA, et al. Hazardous chemical exposure at a municipal wastewater treatment plant. *Environ Res* 1983;32:360–71.
3. Jonstone RT, Miller SE. Infectious occupational diseases. In: *Occupational Diseases and Industrial Medicine*. Philadelphia: Saunders, 1960. Chap 13, pp 252–61.
4. Langeland G. *Salmonella* species. In the working environment of sewage treatment plants in Oslo, Norway. *Appl Environ Microbiol* 1982;43(May):1111–5.
5. Cohen SH, Hoeprich PD. Environmental factors in infectious diseases. In: Hoeprich and Jordan (eds), *Infectious Diseases*. 4th Ed. Philadelphia: Lippincott, 1989. P 184.
6. Golueke CG. 1983 Epidemiology aspects of sludge handling and management. *Biocycle* 1983;24(3): 52–8.
7. Epstein E. Neighborhood and worker protection for composting facilities: issues and actions. In: Hoitink AJ, Keener HM (eds), *Science and Engineering of Composting Design: Environmental, Microbiological, and Utilization Aspects*. (Environmental Science and Engineering of Composting: International Symposium.) Worthington, OH: Renaissance Publications, 1993. Pp 319–38.
8. Faine S. Leptospirosis. In: Evans AS, Brachman PS (eds), *Bacterial Infections of Humans: Epidemiology and Control*. 3rd Ed. Chap 20, pp 395–420.
9. Brenner DJ. Classification of Legionellae. *Semin Respir Infect* 1987;2:90–205.
10. Dennis PJ, Brenner DJ, Thacker WL, et al. Five new *Legionella* species isolated from water. *Int J Sysat Bacteriol* 1993;43:329–37.
11. Kuchta JM, States SJ, McNamara AM, et al. Susceptibility of *Legionella pneumophila* to chlorine in tap water. *Appl Environ Microbiol* 1983;1134–9.
12. Muraca P, Stout JE, Yu VL. Comparative assessment of chlorine, heat ozone and UV light for killing *Legionella pneumophila* within a model plumbing system. *Appl Environ Microbiol* 1987;53:447–53.
13. Tison DL, Pope DH, Cherry WB, et al. Growth of *Legionella pneumophila* in association with blue-green algae (cyanobacteria). *Appl Environ Microbiol* 1980;39:346–59.
14. Stout JE, Yu VL, Best M. Ecology of *Legionella pneumophila* within water distribution systems. *Appl Environ Microbiol* 1985;49:221–8.
15. Rowbotham TL. Isolation of *L pneumophila* from clinical specimens via amoebae, and the interaction of those and other isolates with amoebae. *J Clin Pathol* 1983;36:978–86.
16. Feilds BS. Legionella and protozoa: interaction of a pathogen and its natural host. In: Barbaree JM, Breriman RF, Dufour AP (eds), *Legionella: Current Status and Emerging Perspectives*. Washington, DC: American Society for Microbiology, 1993. Pp 129–36.
17. Margolis HS. Diseases spread by close personal contact: In: Last JM, Wallace RB, et al. (eds), *Public Health and Preventive Medicine*. East Norwalk, CT: Appleton & Lange, 1992. Chap 7, pp 131–3.
18. Poole CJ, Shakespeare AT. Should sewage workers and careers for people with learning disabilities be vaccinated for hepatitis A? *Br Med J* 1993;306(6885):1102.
19. Jilg W. Adult use of hepatitis A vaccine in developed countries. *Vaccine* 1993;11(suppl 1):S6–S8.
20. De Serres G, Levesque B, Higgins R, et al. Need for vaccination of sewer workers against leptospirosis and hepatitis A. *Occup Environ Med* 1995;52(8):505–7.
21. Cadilhac P, Roudot-Thoraval F. Seroprevalence of hepatitis A virus among sewage workers in the Parisian area, France. *Eur J Epidemiol* 1996;12:237–40.
22. Nanda SK, Ansari IH, Acharya SK, et al. Protracted viremia during acute sporadic hepatitis E virus infection. *Gastroenterology* 1995;108:225.
23. Khuroo MS. Study of an epidemic of non-A, non-B hepatitis: possibility of another human hepatitis virus distinct from post-transfusional non-A, non-B type. *Am J Med* 1980;68:818–24.
24. Wong DC, Purcell RH, Sreenivasan MA, et al. Epidemic and endemic hepatitis A in India: evidence for a non-A, non-B hepatitis virus etiology. *Lancet* 1980;2:876–9.
25. Warner GS. Hanavirus illness in humans—review and update. *South Med J* 1996;89:264.
26. Bhide AD, Sundaresan BB. Street cleaning and waste storage and collection in India. In: Holmes JR (ed),

Managing solid wastes in developing countries. New York: John Wiley & Sons, 1984.

27. Rylander R, Andersson K, Belin L, et al. Studies on humans exposed to airborne sewage sludge. *Schweiz Med Wochenschr* 1977;107(6):182–4.
28. Linnemann CC Jr, Jaffa R, Gartside PS, et al. Risk of infection associated with a wastewater spray irrigation system used for farming. *J Occup Med* 1984;26(1): 41–4.
29. Mueller HE. [Hygienic aspects of agricultural land applications of wastewater and sewage sludge.] *Naturwissenschaften* 1985;72(5):238–48.
30. Nethercott JR. Airborne irritant contact dermatitis due to sewage sludge. *J Occup Med* 1981;23(11):771–4.
31. Clark CS, Rylander R, Larsson L. Levels of gram-negative bacteria, *Aspergillus fumigatus*, dust and endotoxin at compost plants. *Appl Environ Microbiol* 1983;5:1501–5.
32. Clark CS, Linnemann CC, Clark JG, et al. Enteric parasites in workers occupationally exposed to sewage. *J Occup Med* 1984;26(4):273–5.
33. Lundholm M, Rylander R. Work-related symptoms among sewage workers. *Br J Ind Med* 1983;40: 325–9.
34. Environmental Protection Agency. Non-cancer health and discomfort effects of poor indoor air quality. In: *Report to Congress on Indoor Air Quality*, Vol 2. (EPA publication 400/1-89/001C.) Washington, DC: EPA, Office of Air and Radiation, 1989.
35. Millner PD, Olenchock SA, Epstein E, et al. Bioaerosols associated with composting facilities. *Compost Sci Util* 1994;2(4):6–57.
36. Morse DL, Kominsky JR, Wisseman CL III, et al. Occupational exposure to hexachlorocyclopentadiene. How safe is sewage? *JAMA* 1979;241(2):2177–9.
37. Morgan RW, Kheifets L, Obrinsky DL, et al. Fetal loss and work in a waste water treatment plant. *Am J Public Health* 1984;74(5):499–501.
38. Martin JE, Fenner FD. Radioactivity in municipal sewage and sludge. *Public Health Rep* 1997;112(4):308–16.
39. Ikatsu H, Nakajima T, Okino T, et al. [Health care of workers engaged in waste water treatment. (1) The exposure conditions to organic solvents in workers engaged in waste water treatment.] *Sangyo Igaku* 1989;31(5):355–62.
40. Frost P, Camenzind R, Magert A, et al. Organic micropollutants in Swiss sewage sludge. *J Chromatogr* 1993;643(1–2):379–88.
41. Elia VJ, Clark CS, Majeti VA, et al. Hazardous chemical exposure at a municipal wastewater treatment plant. *Environ Res* 1983;32(2):360–71.
42. Baker EL Jr, Landrigan PJ, Glueck CJ, et al. Metabolic consequences of exposure to polychlorinated biphenyls (PCB) in sewage sludge. *Am J Epidemiol* 1980;112(4):553–63.
43. Millner PD. Effect of nutritional and non-nutritional factors on the growth of *Aspergillus fumigatus* (AF) and natural sources of airborne AF and thermophillic *Actinomycetes.* In: Sikora LS, Millner PD, Burge WD (eds), *Chemical and Microbial Aspects of Sludge Composting and Land Application.* (U.S. EPA Interagency Agreement Project AD-12-F-2-534.) Cincinnati, 1985.
44. Mattsby I, Rylander R. Clinical and immunological finding in workers exposed to sewage dust. *Occup Med* 1978;20(20):690–2.
45. Epstein E. Neighborhood and worker protection for composting facilities: issues and actions. In: Hoitink HAJ, Keener HM (eds), *Science and Engineering of Composting: Design, Environmental, Microbiological and Utilization Aspects.* (Environmental Science and Engineering of Composting: An International Symposium.) Worthington, OH: Renaissance Publications, 1993. Pp 319–38.
46. Aspergillosis and Composting Advisory Medical Panel, 4/4/94. Santa Clara County Public Health Department. Division of Disease Control and Prevention, 1994.
47. Lundholm M, Rylander R. Occupational symptoms among compost workers. *J Occup Med* 1980;22(4): 256–7.
48. Clark CS, Rylander R, Larsson L. Levels of gram-negative bacteria, *Aspergillus fumigatus*, dust and endotoxin at compost plants. *Appl Environ Microbiol* 1983;5:1501–5.
49. Clark CS, Linnemann CC, Clark JG, et al. Enteric parasites in workers occupationally exposed to sewage. *J Occup Med* 1984;26(4):273–5.
50. Goldstein N, Steuteville R. Biosolids composting strengthens its base. *Ciocycle* 1994;35(12):48–57.
51. Chesapeake Occupational Health Services. *Health Surveillance Program for Compost Workers: An Epidemiological Review. WSSC Site II.* Silver Spring, MD: COHS, 1991.
52. Carvalheiro MF, Peterson Y, Rubenowitz E, et al. Bronchial reactivity and work-related symptoms in farmers. *Am J Ind Med* 1995.
53. Windholz M, Budvari S, Stroumstos LY, et al. (eds). *The Merck Index*, 9th Ed. Rahway, NJ: Merck and Company, 1976. P 469.
54. Duncan RL Jr, Hoffman J, Tash BL, et al. Immunologic activity of lipopolysaccharides released from macrophage after the uptake of intact *E coli* in vitro. *J Immunol* 1986:136:2924–9.
55. Rylander R, Snells M-C. Endotoxins and the lung: cellular reactions and risk for disease. *Prog Allergy* 1983;33:332–44.
56. Rylander R. Experimental exposures to (103)-B-D-glucan. In: Sterling E, Bieva C, Collett (eds). American Society of Heating, Refrigeration, Air Conditioning, and Engineering. 1993. Pp 338–40.

57. Fogelmark B, Lacey J, Rylander R. Experimental allergic alveolitis after exposures to different microorganisms. *J Exper Pathol* 1991;72:387–95.

58. Ciegler A, Burnmeister HR, Vesonder RF, et al. Mycotoxins: occurrence in the environment. In: *Mycotoxins and N-nitroso Compounds: Environmental Risks.* Vol 1. Boca Raton, FL: CRC Press, 1981.

59. Richerson HB. Unifying concepts underlying the effects of organic dust exposure. *Am J Ind Med* 1990;17:139–42.

60. Creasia DA, Thurman JD, Wannemacher RW, et al. Acute inhalation toxicity of T-2 mycotoxin in the rat and guinea pig. *Fund Appl Toxicol* 1990;14:54–9.

61. Gravesen S. Fungi as a cause of allergic disease. *Allergy* 1979;34:135–54.

62. Clark CS, Bjoronson HS, Schwartz-Fulton J, et al. Biological health risks associated with the composting of wastewater treatment plant sludge. *J Water Poll Cont Fed* 1984;56:1269–76.

63. Clark CS, Rylander R, Larsson L. Levels of gram-negative bacteria, *Aspergillus fumigatus*, dust and endotoxin at compost plants. *Appl Environ Microbiol* 1983;5:1501–5.

64. Lundholm M, Rylander R. Occupational symptoms among compost workers. *J Occup Med* 1980;22(4):256–7.

65. National Institutes for Allergy and Infectious Disease. *Report of the NIAID Task Force on Immunology and Allergy.* Bethesda, MD: U.S. Department of Health and Human Services. National Institutes of Health, Sept 1991. Pp 84.

66. Hunter CA, Grant C, Flannigan B, et al. Mould in buildings: the air spora of domestic dwellings. *Int Biodeterioratino* 1988;24:81–101.

67. Stellman JM (ed). *Encyclopedia of Occupational Health and Safety*, 4th Ed. Geneva, Switzerland: International Labour Organization, 1998.

68. Bacon V, Dalton F. Professionalism and water pollution control in Greater Chicago. *J Water Poll Control Fed* 1968;40(9):1586–1601.

69. Millner PD, Marsh PB, Snowden RB, et al. Occurrence of *Aspergillus fumigatus* during composting of sewage sludge. *Appl Environ Microbiol* 1977;34:764–72.

70. Laitinen S, Kangas J, Kotimaa M, et al. Workers' exposure to airborne bacteria and endotoxins at industrial wastewater treatment plants. *Am Ind Hyg Assoc J* 1994;55(11):1055–60.

71. Castellan RM, Olenchock SA, Kinsley KB, et al. Inhaled endotoxin and decreased spirometric values. *N Engl J Med* 1987;317(10):605–10.

72. Palchack RB, Cohen R, Ainslie M, et al. Airborne endotoxin associated with industrial scale production of protein products in gram-negative bacteria. *Am Ind Hyg Assoc J* 1988;49:420–1.

73. Rylander R. The role of endotoxin for reactions after exposure to cotton dust. *Am J Ind Med* 1987;12:687–97.

74. Nethercott JR. Airborne irritant contact dermatitis due to sewage sludge. *J Occup Med* 1981;23(11):771–4.

75. Lees PSJ, Tockman MS. *Evaluation of Possible Public Health Impact of WSSC Site II Sewage Sludge Composting Operations.* (Report prepared for Maryland Department of Health and Mental Hygiene, Baltimore, Maryland.) Baltimore: John Hopkins University, School of Hygiene and Public Health, 1987.

76. Torten M, Marshall RB. Leptospirosis. In: Beran GW (ed), *Handbook of Zoonoses, Section A: Bacterial, Rickettsial, Chlamydial and Mycotic Diseases*, 2nd Ed., Vol 1. Boca Raton, FL: CRC Press, 1994. Pp 245–64.

77. Muraca PW, Stout JE, Yu VL. Environmental aspects of legionnaires' disease. *J Am Water Works Assoc* 1988;80:78–86.

78. Morris RD, Audet AM, Angelillo IF, et al. Chlorination, chlorination by-products, and cancer: a meta analysis. *Am J Public Health* 1992;82:955–63.

79. Blander SJ, Horwitz MA. Major cytoplasmic membrane protein of *L pneumophila*, a genus common antigen and member of hsp family of heat shock proteins induces protective immunity in guinea pig model of legionnaires' disease. *J Clin Invest* 1993;91:717–23.

80. Howitz MA, Marston BJ, Broome CV, et al. Prospects for vaccine development. In: Barbaree JM, Breiman RF, Du Four AP (eds), *Legionella: Current Status and Emerging Perspectives.* Washington, DC: American Society for Microbiology, 1993. Pp 296–7.

81. Twu J, Sherker AH, Fung K, et al. Inhibition of hepatitis E virus replication by ribaviron and human alpha-interferon in primary human hepatocyte explants. Presented at the 1993 International Symposium on Viral Hepatitis and Liver Disease, Tokyo, May 1993.

82. Turner LH. Leptospirosis I. *Trans R Soc Trop Med Hyg* 1967;61:842–55.

83. Dutkiewicz J, Jablonski L, Olenchock S. Occupational biohazards: a review. *Am J Ind Med* 1988;14:605–23.

84. Alexander A. Leptospirosis. In: Hoeprich PD, Jordan MC (eds), *Infectious Diseases*, 4th Ed. Philadelphia: Lippincott, 1989. Chap 84, p 816.

85. Letocart M, Baranton G, Perolat P. Rapid identification of pathogenic *Leptospira* species (*Leptospira interrogans*, *L borgpetersenii*, and *L kirschneri*) with species-specific DNA probes produced by arbitrarily primed PCR. *J Clin Microbiol* 1997;35:248–53.

86. Merien F, Perolat P, Mancel E, et al. Detection of *Leptospira* DNA by polymerase chain reaction in aqueous humor of a patient with unilateral uveitis. *J Infect Dis* 1993;168:1335–6.

87. Gravekamp C, van der Kemp H, Franzen M, et al. Detection off seven species of pathogenic leptospires by PCR using two sets of primers. *J Gen Microbiol* 1993;139:1691–1700.

88. Eldenstein PH. *Legionnaires' disease. Clin Infect Dis* 1993;16:741–9.

89. Ingram JG, Plouffe JF. Danger of sputum purulence screens in culture of *Legionella* species. *J Clin Microbiol* 1994;32:209–10.

90. Plouffe JF, File TM, Breiman RF, et al. Reevaluation of the definition of legionnaires' disease: use of the urinary antigen assay. *Clin Infect Dis* 1995;20:1286–91.

91. Eldenstein PH. Legionnaires' disease. *Clin Infect Dis* 1993;16:741–9.

92. Ingram JG, Plouffe JF. Danger of sputum purulence screens in culture of *Legionella* species. *J Clin Microbiol* 1994;32:209–10.

93. Matsiota-Bernard P, Pitsounni E, Legakis N, et al. Evaluation of commercial amplification kit for detection of *Legionella pneumophila* in clinical specimens. *J Clin Microbiol* 1994;32:1503–5.

94. Roig J, Carreres A, Domingo C. Treatment of legionnaires' disease: current recommendations. *Drugs* 1993;46:63–79.

95. Lattimer GL, Rhodes LV III, Salventi JS, et al. The Philadelphia epidemic of legionnaires' disease: clinical, pulmonary and serologic findings two years later. *Ann Intern Med* 1979;90:522–6.

96. Leverstein-van Hall MA, Verbon A, Huisman MV, et al. Reinfection with *Legionella pneumophila* documented by pulsed-field gel electrophoresis. *Clin Infect Dis* 1994;19:1147–9.

36 / Occupational Zoonoses

Roy L. DeHart

By tradition, zoonoses are diseases and infections that are naturally transmitted between vertebrate animals and humans. Afflictions caused by vertebrate-produced toxins or venoms, such as those of snakes and fish, are not within this definition [1].

For the purposes of this chapter, a broader definition of *zoonoses* has been developed that includes other pathogens and modes of transmission. For example, in order to be more inclusive, viral transmission from animals to humans by insect vectors (arbovirus) are included in this discussion. The four arbovirus families included are Bunyaviridae, Reoviridae, Togaviridae, and Flaviviridae.

A classification system, based on the life cycle of the infectious organism, has been devised.

- *Direct zoonoses*: Transmission between an infected vertebrate host and a susceptible host via direct or fomite contact or by mechanical factors. Examples are brucellosis, rabies, and tularemia.
- *Cyclozoonoses*: Requires more than one vertebrate host but no invertebrate hosts. Examples include echinococcosis, pentastomiasis, and taeniasis.
- *Metazoonoses*: An agent multiplies, develops, or both in an invertebrate host before transmission to a vertebrate host is possible. Examples include arbovirus, plague, and schistosomiasis.
- *Saprozoonoses*: For these infections to be transmitted, a nonanimal development site or reservoir, such as food, plants, soil or other organic material, is required. Examples include larva migrans and mycotic diseases.

Using the broader definition of *zoonoses*, there are nearly 200 organisms that produce a zoonotic disease [2]. These include prions, viruses, rickettsia, bacteria, fungi, protozoa, helminths, and arthropods. Tables 36-1 and 36-2 illustrate the variety of infections that are categorized as zoonoses [2–6]. Those that are more common and those with greater potential for adverse health outcome are described in more detail elsewhere in this volume. The majority of zoonotic diseases occur in the general population and are not limited to the work setting. For example, rabies, tularemia, plague, and hantavirus have a higher incidence due to activities of daily living than to exposures at work.

Epidemiology

Information on the actual incidence of these diseases in the general population is not available. Approximately 800 cases of psittacosis were reported to the Centers for Disease Control and Prevention (CDC) from 1987 through 1996 [7]. However, not all states require physicians to report cases of psittacosis. Most of these cases resulted from exposure to pet birds; 43% were among owners and bird fanciers, with only 10% reported to be among pet shop operators.

In the United States, 100–250 cases of brucellosis are reported annually. The majority of these cases involve workers who become infected as part of their job. Farmers and ranchers may be victims, but nearly 50% are abattoir workers [6]. A 25-year review of laboratory workers who acquired infections at the National Animal Disease Center illustrated the risk of zoonoses. During the review period, 128 cases caused by transmission from animals occurred. The investigations focused on 70 strains of bacteria, viruses, and mycotic agents. Infections are in descend-

Table 36-1
Bacterial and Viral Zoonotic Diseases Acquired from Animals

Disease	Mode of Transmission	Source
Anthrax	Contact Airborne	Cattle Sheep Goats Donkeys Wild herbivores Animal by-products Hides and furs Contaminated soil
Arbovirus encephalitis	Blood-sucking insects Mosquitoes Mites Lice Ticks	Birds Horses Mules
St. Louis encephalitis (SLE)		
Western equine encephalitis (WEE)		
Eastern equine encephalitis (EEE)		
Powassan encephalitis (POW)		
Bovine spongiform encephalopathy	Ingestion Contact (?)	Cattle
Brucellosis (bangs, undulant fever)	Contact Airborne Ingestion (milk, cheese)	Cattle Swine Goats Canines Buffalo Yaks
Cat-scratch disease	Contact	Felines Canines
Ebola hemorrhagic fever	Contact (?) Inhalation (?)	Unknown
Erysipeloid	Contact	Cattle Chickens Ducks Fish Pheasants Sheep Shellfish Swine Turkeys Crabs
Fish tank granuloma	Contact	Fish Fish tanks Crustacea
Hantavirus	Airborne	Deer mice Cotton rats
Infectious diarrhea	Fecal-oral	Cattle Felines Canines Chickens Rodents Sheep Swine
Influenza	Airborne	Swine Horses Birds
Leptospirosis	Contact Waterborne Inhalation Ingestion	Cattle Rats Foxes Raccoons Marsupials

(continued)

Table 36-1 (continued)

Disease	Mode of Transmission	Source
Lyme disease	Tick bite	Deer Dogs Mice Squirrels
Lymphocytic choreomeningitis	Airborne	Mice Hamsters
Marburg virus	Contact Inhalation (?)	Monkeys
Newcastle disease	Airborne	Poultry Other birds
Orf	Contact	Sheep Goats
Ornithosis (psittacosis)	Airborne Contact	Parrots Poultry Other birds Sheep Goats Cattle
Plague	Airborne Flea bite	Rats Prairie dogs Ground squirrels Chipmunks Mice Rabbits
Q (Query) fever	Airborne Contact Ingestion (milk)	Cattle Sheep Goats Rabbits Felines
Rabies	Contact (animal bite)	Canines Skunks Bats Raccoons Cattle Monkeys Felines Horses Most animals
Tularemia	Contact Bite Insect vector	Rabbits Hares Rodents Squirrels Birds

ing order of frequency: brucellosis, Q fever, typhoid, hepatitis, tularemia, tuberculosis, dermatomycoses, Venezuelan equine encephalitis, typhus, and psittacosis [8].

Leptospirosis was first described in 1983 among sewer workers. It continues to be work related, particularly among farmers and ranchers. Approximately 100 cases occur each year in the United States and between 1,500 and 2,000 worldwide [9].

The United States' reported incidence of selected zoonoses for 1997 is given in Table 36-3 [10]. However, not all states require reporting for each of these diseases, nor is there any data on the percent that may represent occupationally related disease.

Although some data are available on the epidemiology of zoonoses among workers, they are limited and may be misleading. The actual rates of these diseases among workers is unknown. Many of the infections are mild for most infected individuals or are mistaken for another illness (Q fever, Newcastle disease, leptospirosis, or histoplasmosis). Because the symptoms may mimic

Table 36-2
Fungal and Parasitic Zoonotic Diseases Acquired from Animals

Disease	Mode of Transmission	Source
Cryptosporidiosis	Water Fecal-oral	Cattle Sheep Rodents Fowl
Cutaneous larva migrans	Contact	Canines Fish Cattle Sheep
Echinococcosis	Ingestion Contact	Canines Sheep Goats Camels Horses
Histoplasmosis	Airborne	Poultry Birds Bats Soil
Ringworm	Contact	Canines Felines Poultry Swine Rodents Horses Cattle
Taeniasis	Ingestion	Beef Pork
Toxoplasmosis	Ingestion	Felines Birds Sheep Goats Some cattle
Trichinosis	Ingestion	Swine
Tuberculosis	Inhalation Ingestion	Cattle

other more common infections, such as the "flu," zoonotic diseases may be misdiagnosed. The reporting system, both in the United States and worldwide, is inconsistent, and rarely are the existing systems designed to identify occupational relevance. Without a comprehensive reporting system, the available incidence data are minimal at best. In order for a zoonotic disease to be reported, it must be entered in the surveillance system, but many of those infected, such as farmers and ranchers, are stoic and seek health care only when an illness becomes life threatening.

When considering the epidemiology of zoonotic diseases over time, the evidence supports the conclusion that the rate of human disease is decreasing. Improved sanitation in both the workplace and the community has reduced the opportunity for spread to humans. Vaccination programs for domestic animals (brucellosis and bovine tuberculosis) and the introduction of vaccine programs for wild animals (e.g., rabies) has increased herd immunity, lessening animal infection and thus reducing human exposure. Improved worker education and bloodborne pathogen training have reduced exposure for animal handlers, laboratory technicians, and veterinary personnel. In-house animal husbandry practices to reduce cross-infection has had a major role in the successful downward trend in the incidence of zoonotic diseases in agricultural workers.

Although the true overall incidence of zoonoses is unknown, a survey conducted in 1990 in Great Britain among farm workers re-

Table 36-3
Selected Zoonotic Diseases Reported in the United States in 1997

Disease	Number of Reported Cases
Anthrax	0
Cryptosporidiosis	1,963
Encephalitis	
California	120
Eastern equine	10
St. Louis equine	12
Western equine	0
Hantavirus	18
Plague	4
Psittacosis	37
Rabies	
Human	2
Animal	7,853
Rocky Mountain spotted fever	400
Trichinosis	9

From Provisional cases of selected notifiable diseases, U.S., cumulative, week ending Jan 3. MMWR 1998;46:1265–71.

ports that 15% indicated at least one infectious episode [5]. Worldwide, it is estimated that 500,000 cases of brucellosis occur in humans annually [11].

Occupations at Risk

Risk of zoonotic disease is highest among those occupations with direct and frequent contact with animals. Table 36-4 lists the most common occupations in which risk is increased [4,5]. Most episodes of zoonotic diseases are not unique to specific jobs but occur in situations of casual, infrequent, or unrecognized contact or exposure. Examples include rabies, arthropod-spread infections, hantavirus, and tapeworms. Workers in close contact with animals have the highest risk for exposure to zoonotic diseases; these are farmers, ranchers, veterinarians, animal research personnel, pet shop operators, and animal-product workers. Some workers, such as transport workers, out-of-door workers and sanitation employees, have only occasional but time-intensive exposure. A final group of individuals have only occasional or distant exposure: sports hunters, hikers, campers, tourists, and those who are simply in the wrong place at the wrong time.

Case Studies

BRUCELLOSIS

In six Middle East countries, there are nearly 100,000 human cases of brucellosis annually. The cost of current control activities for people and animals approaches $400 million yearly [12]. Ingestion of unpasteurized dairy products manufactured in developing countries continues to be a primary source of brucellosis. Cheese made from raw goat's milk is a particular problem.

LYME DISEASE

The 1975 epidemic of juvenile inflammatory arthropathy in Old Lyme, Connecticut, implicated the spirochete *Borrelia burgdorferi*. Since then, cases have been reported in 48 states, and the number reported annually has reached 16,000 [13].

HANTAVIRUS PULMONARY VIRUS SYNDROME

In May 1993, the New Mexico Department of Health was notified that two persons died within a week of each other from similar respiratory symptoms. In early June 1993, the CDC proved that a new hantavirus was the cause [14,15]. From May 1993 through July 1994, the CDC reported 83 confirmed cases, with 45 deaths. At least three viruses have been identified; Sin Nombre, Black Creek, and Bayou [16].

TOXOPLASMOSIS

Serologic testing established that one third of the U.S. population has evidence of toxoplasmosis postinfection. Serologic surveys of cats in the United States have demonstrated *Toxoplasma gondii* infections in 30–80% [17]. Human clinical disease has a low incidence and occurs only periodically.

CRYPTOSPORIDIOSIS

There have been more than a dozen reports of outbreaks of cryptosporidiosis in day care centers. Two recent waterborne outbreaks have been

Table 36-4
Selected Occupations with Exposure to Zoonotic Disease Classification

Agriculture	Health Services	Animal Products	Miscellaneous
Animal transporters	Animal control officers	Abattoir workers	Animal trainers
Breeders	Laboratory technicians	Butchers	Circus, carnival, and fair operators
Dairy workers	Refuge collectors	Furriers	Foresters
Farmers	Veterinarians	Hide processors	Game wardens
Animal groomers		Meat packers	Grass cutters
Poultry keepers		Rendering plant workers	Hunters
Ranchers		Stockyard workers	Line maintenance workers
Sheep shearers		Tanning workers	Military personnel
Shepherds		Wool workers	Pet shop workers
			Transport workers
			Trappers
			Wild life managers
			Wood cutters

documented. Fecal-oral transmission is from animals to humans; waterborne transmission has become a problem in Milwaukee, Wisconsin, where over 400,000 people became ill, and more recently in Sidney, Australia.

RABIES

Although only several cases of human rabies occur in the United States annually, the disease is of far greater concern worldwide. Each year, approximately 50,000 humans and millions of animals die from rabies worldwide. Respiratory transmission was implicated when two men who had been working in a bat cave died of rabies [18]. In the United States, the four wild animal groups responsible for dissemination are skunks, raccoons, foxes, and bats.

ANTHRAX

The work of Davaine, Koch, Pasteur and others identified anthrax as the first disease recognized to be caused by a microorganism. Anthrax was also the first bacterial disease to be prevented by a vaccine. Causes of human cases have been reported to be commercial products of animal origin, such as fur, shaving brushes, yarn, and lanolin oil [19]. Anthrax in humans is secondary to the disease in animals.

Q FEVER

In a European country, a shipment of cotton received from another nation was the source of the disease among those who handled the shipment. Evidence suggests that the cotton was contaminated by rodents during storage. In moving the shipment, the workers were exposed to cotton dust heavily contaminated with *Coxiella burnetii* [1].

TULAREMIA

A large outbreak of tularemia involving over 100 workers occurred in a sugar factory. This was related to mechanical washing of sugar beets that had been contaminated with field soil containing the causative organism, the bacillus *Francisella tularensis.* The beet-cleaning process suspended the infective organisms in an aerosol [1]. In most situations, transmission occurs by direct contact with an infected animal or by an insect bite from a tick, fly, or mosquito.

ARBOVIRUSES

This group of viruses causes a number of diseases, including encephalitis. The virus is transmitted primarily by mosquitoes; however, other biting insects, including ticks, have been implicated.

LEPTOSPIROSIS

As with many zoonotic diseases, there has been a reduction in cases of leptospirosis, due in large part to improved sanitation and better animal control. However, it remains a concern for sewage workers and others who work in water along rivers or estuaries. In Great Britain, employers usually provide workers with an information card to show to a physician if they develop symptoms [5]. Recreational water enthusiasts, such as water skiers and canoers, are considered at risk, although minor, due to their increased exposure.

Emerging Occupational Zoonoses

For most animal infections, transmission to humans does not occur or is rare. In some cases, although the human is infected, the result is a dead-end host and there is no further transmission. On rare occasions, although it has recently occurred more frequently due to greater human encroachment into the remaining jungles and rain forests of the world, the rate of species' jumping to humans has increased [20]. So has the severity of health effects on humans. The infections in humans caused by human immunodeficiency virus and Ebola hemorrhagic fever virus are examples.

VIRAL HEMORRHAGIC FEVER

A new family of viruses has been identified—the Filoviridae. This family includes Marburg virus, Reston virus, and two types of Ebola virus. Each produce a form of hemorrhagic fever. Marburg virus first appeared in 1967 among laboratory workers in Marburg, Germany, and nearly simultaneously in Bulgaria, Yugoslavia; these workers had been exposed to blood and tissue from African green monkeys. This outbreak produced 25 primary cases and six secondary cases of hemorrhagic fever. In subsequent years, further cases have occurred in African nations [21].

Ebola fever first appeared in two major outbreaks, which also occurred nearly simultaneously: one in Zaire and the other in Sudan in 1976. Over 500 cases, with exceptionally high mortality (88% in Zaire and 53% in Sudan) were identified. Although there have been extensive investigations, there is no convincing evidence of an association with monkeys. Marburg and Ebola viruses are identified with Africa, but the third, Reston virus, originated in the Philippines and was isolated from cynomolgus monkeys. The virus can infect humans, as was demonstrated when an animal caretaker working in a primate facility in Reston, Virginia, developed antibodies. This occurred during a devastating spread among the primates in the holding facility. Although a species jump occurred, the victim experienced few symptoms, and there were no secondary human cases identified. This outbreak became the centerpiece for Richard Preston's 1994 best seller, *The Hot Zone*. The CDC announced in April 1996 that two monkeys developed Reston fever at a primate quarantine facility in Texas. No human disease was reported, however.

Secondary transmission of Ebola virus infection to man appears to be caused only by direct contact with infected patients [22]. However, the primary route of transmission to humans remains speculative. The evidence suggests human contact with infected monkeys as a primary source of infection. Revised standards issued by the CDC recommend eye and oral nasal mask protection for health care workers treating viral hemorrhagic fever patients [23].

MONKEYPOX

Because of the similarities between smallpox and monkeypox, there is intense interest in the natural history of this disease. The first case of monkeypox was identified in 1970, and over the next decade only 55 cases were confirmed by the World Health Organization (WHO) in the forested areas of central and western Africa. It was initially believed that human-to-human transmission would die out by the tenth generation or so. However, new case reports from the Democratic Republic of the Congo have been increasingly reported by WHO [24]. Smallpox vaccination provides cross protection from monkeypox; however, with the increasing number of young people who have never been vaccinated, there is a growing population susceptible to monkeypox.

SPONGIFORM ENCEPHALOPATHIES

Since the identification of bovine spongiform encephalitis (BSE) in Great Britain in 1986, there has been renewed interest in spongiform encephalopathies' (SE) spread to humans. Several forms of SE have occurred in humans, including occupationally related infections. The two main forms are kuru and Creutzfeldt-Jakob disease (CJD). Occupational transmission of CJD from corneal grafting and neurosurgery has been related to cases of the disease in laboratory technicians, a neurosurgeon, an orthopedic surgeon, and a pathologist [5]. More recently, exotic ruminants in zoos in Great Britain were diagnosed with BSE around the time the disease was first identified, and later the disease has also appeared in domestic cats. The risk to human health from BSE has been carefully monitored. In 1995, a variant of CJD was first diagnosed in Great Britain. Studies of additional variant cases have subsequently established that these cases can be regarded as human BSE [25]. To date, the route of transmission appears to be limited to the food chain, that is, from ingestion of contaminated animal products. Other forms of contact with animals or animal products do not appear to represent an occupational hazard for contracting BSE, but the potential remains.

Prevention

In the industrial world, control of zoonoses is proving effective for most related diseases, but it continues to present major problems for developing countries. The expenses associated with vaccination and immunization programs, sacrifice of diseased animals, improved sanitation, and other control measures are not just barriers, but without international assistance, may be impossible for developing nations. Expenses related to animal reservoir controls can be expected to further increase.

The methodologies used in occupational medicine to control toxic or bloodborne exposures are applicable to protection from zoonotic diseases. Whenever possible, hazard should be reduced or eliminated. Whenever appropriate, vaccination should be provided for employees who are at risk. Personal protective equipment should be provided to those exposed to direct contact or aerosol spread of the zoonotic organism. Strict hygiene practices and work environments that are hygienically maintained, reduce the opportunity for exposure. As always, training and education is the foundation for effective preventive strategies. Finally, a continuous improvement program will help both the employer and employee to cross-check program implementation, be sensitive to a breakdown in procedures, and be vigilant for the introduction of a new "sentinel case."

Fortunately, most zoonotic transfers or species jumps do not result in sustainable infections, as the disease is usually species specific. However, there is no current method to predict the next new zoonotic pathogen or its virulence in humans.

For research and technical personnel who are working with zoonotic organisms, established work procedures, as prescribed by the degree of infectious hazard, need to be observed. These include the facility's isolation design, biohazard disposal methods, care of any cut or skin lesions, safe practices when working with sharps, scrupulous personal hygiene, and appropriate immunizations.

When zoonotic disease is suspected in humans, public health resources must be committed to investigate the source for the index case and to maintain surveillance for secondary cases. In the occupational setting, an index case should be considered a sentinel and require an investigation similar to the response of safety professionals following an accident or that of industrial hygienists after a toxic exposure.

The CDC is engaged in the development of a strategy for preventing emerging infectious diseases [26]. In part, this is driven by recent outbreaks of zoonotic diseases. For example, an avian strain of influenza that had not previously infected humans proved fatal to victims in Hong Kong in 1997 [27]. It was recognized that many emerging diseases are acquired from animals or are transported by arthropods. The prevention strategy includes (1) improved surveillance and response, (2) applied research, (3) enhanced training, and (4) prevention and control.

In the future, zoonotic diseases can be expected to continue to challenge mankind, both in the workplace and in the larger community. Occupational health professions, especially, must be well-versed in the prevention and the identification and management of zoonotic diseases.

References

1. Abdussalem M. Zoonoses. In: Parmeggian L (ed), *Encyclopedia of Occupational Health and Safety*, 3rd Ed. Geneva, Switzerland: International Labor Office, 1985. Pp 2344–6.
2. Gerberding JL, Holmes KK. Microbial agents and infectious diseases. In: Rosenstock L, Cullen MR (eds), *Textbook of Clinical and Environmental Medicine*, Philadelphia: Saunders, 1994. Pp 699–716.
3. Snashall D. Occupational infections. *Br Med J* 1996; 313:551–4.
4. Dieckhous KD, Garibaldi RA. Occupational infections. In: Rom WN (ed), *Environmental and Occupational Medicine*, 3rd Ed. Philadelphia: Lippincott-Raven, 1998. Pp 755–74.
5. Ellis CJ, Symington IS. Microbial disease. In: Raffle PAB, Adams PH, Baxter PJ, et al. (eds), *Hunter's Diseases of Occupations*, 8th Ed. London: Edward Arnold, 1994. Pp 545–76.
6. Franklin S, Pruitt R, Willoughby D, et al. Animal exposure risk: implications for occupational health nurses. *AAOHN* 1997;45:386–92.
7. Compendium of measures to control *Chlamydia psittaci* infection among humans (psittacosis) and pet birds (avian chlamydiosis), *MMWR* 1998;47:RR-10.
8. Miller CD, Songer JR, Sullivan JF. A twenty-five year review of laboratory-acquired human infections at the National Animal Disease Center. *Am Ind Hyg Assoc J* 1987;48:271–5.
9. Kaufmann AF, Perkins Bradley. Leptospirosis. In: Wallace RB (ed), *Public Health and Preventive Medicine*, 14th Ed. Stanford, CT: Appleton & Lange, 1998. Pp 360–2.
10. Provisional cases of selected notifiable diseases, U.S., cumulative, week ending Jan. 3. *MMWR* 1998;46: 1265–71.
11. Joint FAO/WHO Expert Committee on Brucellosis: Sixth Report. Tech Report Series No. 740. Geneva: World Health Organisation, 1986.
12. Corbel MJ. Brucellosis: an overview. *Emerg Infect Dis* 1997;3:213–21.
13. CDC. Lyme disease. *MMWR* 1994;44:459–62.
14. Marshall E. Hantavirus outbreak yields to PCR. *Science* 1993;262:832–6.
15. Duchin JS, Koster FT, Peters CJ, et al. Hantavirus pulmonary syndrome: a clinical description of 17 patients with a newly recognized disease. *N Engl J Med* 1994;330:949–55.
16. CDC. Hantavirus pulmonary syndrome. *MMWR* 1994;43:548–9.
17. Yaeger RG, Frenkel JK. Toxoplasmosis. In: Wallace RB (ed), *Public Health and Preventive Medicine*, 14th Ed. Stanford, CT: Appleton & Lange, 1998. Pp 364–7.
18. Constantine DG. Rabies. In: Wallace RB (ed), *Public Health and Preventive Medicine*, 14th Ed. Stanford, CT: Appleton & Lange, 1998. Pp 349–53.
19. Anthrax vaccine. *Med Newslett* 1998;40:52–3.
20. Murphy FA. Emerging zoonoses. *Emerg Infect Dis* 1998;4:429–35.
21. Childs J, Shope RE, Fish D, et al. Emerging zoonoses. *Emerg Infect Dis* 1998;4:453–4.
22. Johnson KM, Scribner CL, McCormick JB. Ecology of ebola virus: a first clue? *J Infect Dis* 1981;143:749–51.
23. Jaax N, Jahrling P, Geisbert T, et al. Transmission of Ebola virus (Zaire strain) to uninfected control monkeys in a biocontainment laboratory. *Lancet* 1995;346: 1669–71.
24. Breman JG, Henderson DA. Poxvirus dilemmas—monkeypox, smallpox, and biological terrorism. *N Engl J Med* 1998;339:556–9.
25. Pattison J. The emergence of bovine spongiform encephalopathy and related diseases. *Emerg Infec Dis* 1998; 4:390–4.
26. Centers for Disease Control and Prevention. Preventing emerging infectious disease: a strategy for the 21st century. *MMWR* 1998;47:RR-15.
27. Centers for Disease Control. Isolation of avian influenza viruses from humans—Hong Kong. *MMWR* 1997;46:1204–7.

37 / Globally Emerging Occupational Infections

Alain J. Couturier and Andrew Nickelson

The twentieth century revolutionized infectious disease health care through advanced research, vaccinations, antibiotics, improved sanitation, and preventive public health measures. Some people thought there would be an end to infectious disease because of these tremendous strides, but the euphoria was premature. New infectious diseases are emerging around the world, and old diseases, once considered to be controlled, are re-emerging (Table 37-1). *Emerging infectious diseases* are defined as "infections that have newly appeared in a population or have existed but are rapidly increasing in incidence or geographic range" [1].

Factors Causing Emergence

In 1992, the Institute of Medicine published a landmark report titled *Emerging Infections: Microbial Threats to Health in the United States* [2]. This report identified six factors that contribute to disease emergence. The factors identified were ecologic changes, changes in human demographics and behavior, increased international travel and commerce, advances in technology and industry, microbial adaptation and change, and breakdown in public health measures.

ECOLOGIC CHANGES

Ecologic changes are some of the most frequently cited reasons for disease emergence (Table 37-2). Specific factors include agriculture, dam building, deforestation/reforestation, and climate changes. Frequently, the underlying cause of the emerging disease is contact between humans and the natural reservoir of the disease. The impact of humans and the climate on the land causes changes in animal populations. Conversion of grasslands to maize cultivation favored a rodent that was the natural host of Junin virus, the cause of Argentine hemorrhagic fever [3]. Water can have a dramatic effect on disease emergence. Expansion of standing water by dams or flooding can increase the mosquito population in an area, leading to an increase in mosquito-borne diseases. In Mauritania in 1987, outbreaks of Rift Valley fever occurred in villages near dams on the Senegal River. Dam construction has also favored thriving of the snail host of schistosomiasis [4]. These events could have implications for the Three Gorges Super Dam on the Yangtze River in China [5].

DEMOGRAPHICS

Demographics have a role in emerging infections. Population movements because of war or urbanization have led to outbreaks. Isolated people might come into contact with a new, denser population and carry diseases that were once obscure and localized. The spread of HIV has probably been advanced by the movement of workers from rural areas to urban areas, with global pandemic results. Modern-day changes in human behavior such as intravenous drug abuse and sexual promiscuity have also contributed to HIV's increased incidence [1].

The movement of people across national borders has increased dramatically in the twentieth century. Mobile populations include leisure and business travelers, military personnel, long-term expatriates, and missionaries. It has been esti-

Table 37-1
Examples of Newly Recognized Infectious Diseases

Year	Microbe	Disease
1991	Guanerito virus	Venezuelan hemorrhagic fever
1992	*Vibrio cholerae* O139	New strain of epidemic cholera
1993	Sin Nombre virus	Adult respiratory distress syndrome
1994	Sabia virus	Brazilian hemorrhagic fever
1995	HHV-8	Associated with Kaposi's sarcoma
1996	Unknown (prion)	Variant of Creutzfeldt-Jakob disease
1997	Influenza A (H5N1)	Avian influenza

mated that in 1995 over 1.4 million tourists crossed international borders every day, an annual total of over 500 million people. Air traffic exceeded 2 billion passengers. Virtually any destination can be reached in 36 hours. This 36-hour window is well within the incubation period of many diseases [6,10]; new influenza strains can be spread throughout the world quickly. Malaria is among the more commonly diagnosed serious travel-related diseases in the United States [7].

Table 37-2
Factors Contributing to Emergence of Infectious Disease

Categories	Examples
Societal events	Economic impoverishment, war, population migration
Health care	Organ transplantation, widespread antibiotic use
Food production	Globalization of food supplies, changes in food preparation
Human behavior	Sexual behavior, drug use, travel, outdoor recreation
Environmental changes	Deforestation/reforestation, global warming, flood/drought
Public health infrastructure	Reduction of prevention programs, lack of trained personnel
Microbial change	Development of drug resistance, changes in virulence

From Centers for Disease Control. Addressing emerging infectious disease threats: a prevention strategy for the United States, executive summary. (Adapted.) *MMWR* 1994;43(RR-5):3.

INTERNATIONAL COMMERCE

International commerce has long been known to induce outbreaks of disease. Historically, trade along the silk route between Europe and Asia brought rats and, with them, the bubonic plague to Europe. Trade and movement of Chinese laborers to San Francisco probably brought the plague in 1900 to the United States, where it then spread to wild rodents [8]. Recently, cholera entered South America for the first time in this century; it was carried in the bilge water of an Asian freighter [9].

Technology has allowed food products from around the world to be delivered to U.S. supermarkets. Before 1996, Americans considered *Cyclospora* an exotic disease. It sometimes presented as diarrhea in returning overseas travelers. In 1996, a large outbreak of Cyclospora (1,465 cases) hit North America; raspberries from Guatemala were epidemiologically implicated as the vehicle of infection [11]. Medical technologic advances have given disease new entries into the human body. A 1997 Japanese investigation of patients with Creutzfeldt-Jakob disease, a form of transmissible spongiform encephalopathy, showed that a large number had received cadaveric dura mater grafts from a neurosurgical or orthopedic procedure. The overwhelming majority of these patients had a single brand of dura mater graft produced by batch processing. This meant the patients had received grafts created from a batch of multiple cadavers, increasing their risk of exposure [12].

NEW MICROBIAL VARIANTS

Microbes are constantly evolving. Viruses such as influenza constantly yield new variants. Regular epidemics are caused by antigenic drift: A change in the antigenic surface protein allows the virus to escape recognition by the immune system [13]. Evolution and adaptation is best demonstrated by the emergence of antibiotic-resistant microbes. The indiscriminate use of antibiotics has promoted the evolution of new strains of microbes that are not affected by traditional antibiotics. Examples include penicillin-resistant streptococcus and vancomycin-resistant enterococcus. Chloroquine is no longer adequate prophylaxis in most malarial regions of the world due to resistant strains of *Plasmodium falciparum*. People in areas of Southeast Asia are also resistant to sulfadoxine/pyrimethamine (Fansidar), a drug that is often used for temporary emergency treatment of malaria in the field [14].

Breakdown of public health measures is one reason for the re-emergence of many diseases. Diphtheria re-emerged in the New Independent States of the former Soviet Union. It began in the Russian Federation in 1990 and spread to all the New Independent States by 1994, resulting in 125,000 cases and over 4,000 deaths. The re-emergence of this disease is a direct result of the loss of diphtheria vaccine and antitoxin, which had previously been supplied by the Soviet Union. With the breakup of the Soviet Union, the New Independent States were left without resources to procure these medical supplies [15].

Hantavirus Around the World

Hantaviruses are carried by numerous species of rodents throughout the world. The genus *Hantavirus* of the family Bunyaviridae comprises at least 14 viruses, including those that cause hemorrhagic fever with renal syndrome (HFRS) and hantavirus pulmonary syndrome (HPS). During the Korean war, thousands of United Nations troops developed an acute, severe febrile illness that became known as *Korean hemorrhagic fever (KHF)*. The causative agent, Hantaan virus, was isolated in 1976 from the lungs of the rodent reservoir, the striped field mouse. KHF was noted to have characteristics of another illness well known in Scandinavia and European Russia called *nephropathia epidemica*. The Puumala virus was found to be the causative agent of nephropathia epidemica, and as suspected, it belonged to the same genus as Hantaan virus, *Hantavirus*. The host of the Puumala virus is the bank vole [19,20,31].

Although most cases of hantavirus may be linked to exposure to the bank vole or striped field mouse, several cases of HFRS were documented in urban settings. This led to the discovery of a third member of the *Hantavirus* genus, which was named *Seoul virus*. This virus causes a less severe form of HFRS. The hosts are commensal rats, in particular *Rattus rattus* and *Rattus norvegicus*, two species that have been carried worldwide by ships. Any port city that has an identified rat population is at risk for an outbreak of Seoul virus–induced HFRS. A study performed in Baltimore showed that 50% of adult *Rattus* are infected [30].

With several species of virus identified and each associated with a different species of host rodent, a search started for a New World *Hantavirus* disease. In the fall of 1992, the second of two successive El Nino events led to exceptionally heavy precipitation in the Four Corners region of the southwestern United States, and deer mice flourished. A cluster of unexplained deaths in humans in May 1993 led to the discovery of Sin Nombre virus and its characteristic disease, hantavirus pulmonary syndrome (HPS). Three other *Hantavirus* species indigenous to North America are known to cause HPS; they are listed in Table 37-3 [29].

In 1995, an outbreak of HPS caused by the Laguna Negra virus occurred in an agricultural community in Western Paraguay. At least 17 people were affected. The host was the vesper mouse. The original outbreak of HPS was followed by another outbreak in 1996 in southern Argentina; it affected at least 18 people in the Rio Negro province [24,28]. The causal agent was the Andes virus, and the rodent reservoir was the long-tailed pygmy rice rat. This outbreak also had possible human-to-human transmission: An adolescent patient in Buenos Aires apparently contracted the virus from her parents, who were infected in Patagonia [26]. Overall, five hantavirus species in South America are known to cause HPS.

Since the discovery of the disease-causing members of the *Hantavirus* genus, many new viruses have been discovered. Each new virus has a unique rodent host. The worldwide distribution of rodents known to harbor hantaviruses suggests great disease-causing potential. No arthropod vector such as the tick, flea, or louse has been discovered. Rodents appear to be lifelong hosts for hantaviruses and suffer no detectable

Table 37-3
Rodent-Associated Diseases

Species	Disease	Distribution	Reservoir
Arenavirus			
Junin	AHF	Argentine pampas	*Calomys musculinis*
Machupo	BHF	Bolivia	*Calomys callosus*
Guanarito	VHF	Venezuela, Portuguesa state	*Zygdontomys brevicauda*
Sabia	Unnamed	Brazil, Sao Paulo state	Unknown
Lassa	Lassa fever	Rural West Africa	*Mastamys natalensis*
Lymphocytic choriomeningitis	LCM	Worldwide	*Mus musculus*
Hantavirus			
Hantaan	HFRS	China, Russia, Korea	*Apodemus agrarius*
DOB	HFRS	Balkans	*Apodemus flavicollis*
SEO	HFRS	Worldwide	*Rattus norvegicus*
PUU	HFRS	Europe, Russia, Scandinavia	*Clethrionomys glareolus*
Sin Nombre	HPS	U.S., Canada	*Peromyscus maniculitis*
New York	HPS	U.S.	*Peromyscus leucopus*
Black Creek	HPS	U.S.	*Sigmodon hispidus*
Bayou	HPS	U.S.	*Orysomys palustris*
Andes	HPS	Argentina	*Oligoryzormys longicauditus*
HU39694	HPS	Argentina	Unknown
Lechiguanas	HPS	Argentina	*Oligoryzormys flavesens*
Juquitiba	HPS	Brazil	Unknown
Yersinia pestis	Plague	Asia, Africa, North America, South America, extreme southeastern Europe	Multiple species of rodents

Abbreviations: *AHF* = Argentine hemorrhagic fever; *BHF* = Bolivian hemorrhagic fever; *VHF* = Venezuelan hemorrhagic fever; *HFRS* = hemorrhagic fever with renal syndrome; *HPS* = Hantavirus pulmonary syndrome; *LCM* = lymphocytic choriomeningitis; *DOB* = Dobrava; *SEO* = Seoul; *PUU* = Puumala (17–20).

clinical effects. Humans acquire the virus by inhaling rodent excreta (e.g., feces, urine, saliva). It is also thought that transmission may occur from rodent bites, direct contamination of broken skin with rodent excreta, and possibly ingestion of contaminated food or water [25].

HANTAVIRUS WITH RENAL SYNDROME (HFRS) AND NEPHROPATHIA EPIDEMICA

Epidemiology

Each year, there are approximately 150,000–200,000 cases of HFRS; more than half occur in China. Russia and Korea are also major reporters of HFRS, with hundreds to thousands of cases. With the exception of the Seoul virus, the disease occurs predominantly in rural areas. The disease appears to be closely linked with the rodent host. The incidence of the disease varies with the size of the rodent population and frequency of human activities that bring people in contact with rodents. HFRS is a seasonal disease, although individual cases are seen year-round. In Asia, most cases occur in late fall and early winter and are often linked with agricultural activities associated with the fall harvest. In the Balkans, the peak incidence of HFRS is during the warmer months of late spring, summer, and early fall. The primary reservoir of the virus is the yellow-necked field mouse. The disease is more frequently reported in males and has a peak incidence among those ages 20–50 years. The occupations at greatest risk are farming, forestry, sheep herding, and military service involving field operations [19,20].

The milder form of the disease caused by the Seoul virus usually occurs year round. It is more common in men and in the age range of 20–50 years. The Seoul virus has been a problem in laboratory settings where otherwise normal lab rats have infected animal handlers and others in Japan, Korea, Belgium, France, and England.

Nephropathia epidemica, a variant of HFRS, was first described in northern Sweden in 1934. Major outbreaks were noted in Finland in World War II among Finnish and German troops. The distribution of the disease corresponds to the range of the rodent reservoir, the bank vole. The disease is also seasonal, peaking in late fall and early winter. There is a second peak that occurs in mid to late summer. The seasonality of nephropathia epidemica relates to the movement of bank voles into homes, barns, and outbuildings in the fall and winter and to the increase in outdoor human activity in the summer. The disease increases directly with the population of the bank vole, occurring mostly in rural areas. It primarily affects men between the ages of 20 and 40 [19,20,31].

Clinical Features

HFRS is a complex multiphasic disorder with a broad spectrum of clinical severity. Classic HFRS has five phases: febrile, hypotensive, oliguric, diuretic, and convalescent. The phases often overlap, blend, or do not appear at all. Prodromal symptoms are rare and the onset is typically abrupt. Presenting signs and symptoms include high temperature, chills, malaise, myalgias, headache, dizziness and anorexia, followed shortly thereafter by severe back and abdominal pain, often leading to the misdiagnosis of acute abdomen. Erythematous facial flushing is characteristic; it usually extends to the neck and upper torso and is accompanied by periorbital swelling and conjunctival, palatal, and pharyngeal injection. Petechiae are frequently present on the soft palate and axillae. As the disease progresses, the white cell count gradually rises and the platelet count begins to drop. Proteinuria becomes increasingly prominent.

Within a week, a period of hypotension ensues, beginning abruptly and coinciding with defervescence. The decrease in blood pressure may be accompanied by typical signs of shock. By this stage there is leukocytosis, thrombocytopenia, and massive proteinuria. This phase is usually brief but can be severe; one third of all deaths occur during this phase. The oliguric phase begins as the patient stabilizes hemodynamically. Pulmonary edema may occur. After three to seven days, the patient enters a period of diuresis. Urine output can be 5–6 liters per day, with corresponding electrolyte disturbances. Convalescence is usually prolonged; in some cases, it may take months. Severe HFRS occurs in the Balkan states and is similar to Hantaan virus disease. Patients with Seoul virus usually present with milder clinical disease, although in rare cases it can be fatal. The five phases are indistinct if apparent at all. The symptoms of nephropathia epidemica are even milder than those of Seoul virus, and asymptomatic cases are common.

HANTAVIRUS PULMONARY SYNDROME

Epidemiology

Hantavirus pulmonary syndrome (HPS) is the New World presentation of *Hantavirus* disease. HPS appears to occur more commonly in men than in women. Patients have ranged in age from 11 to 69 years. Lower socioeconomic status is a risk factor because of poorer housing conditions and increased agricultural activities. Outbreaks of HPS are related to the size of the rodent reservoir population. Activities such as cleaning around the home, hand plowing, and cleaning of feed storage areas or animal shelters increase the risk of acquiring the disease. Cleaning rarely used rodent-infested structures constitutes a special risk situation. In the United States, HPS is an occupational hazard to grain farmers, livestock specialists, field biologists, agricultural workers, mill workers, construction workers, utility workers, and feedlot workers [27]. These occupations may not prove to be at increased risk in South America, but theoretically they would involve increased exposure to rodents.

Clinical Features

HPS begins abruptly with fever and myalgia, headache, and backache. In some cases, abdominal pain, diarrhea, nausea, and vomiting are prominent symptoms in the first 24 to 48 hours. The febrile prodrome is followed by the cardiopulmonary stage. This manifests as increased shortness of breath, nonproductive cough, tachypnea, tachycardia, hypotension, and rales on auscultation. The patient can develop severe pulmonary edema, which almost always requires oxygen and frequently mechanical ventilation. Laboratory studies show a leukocytosis with a left shift, thrombocytopenia, hemoconcentration, elevated serum transaminase, markedly elevated serum lactate dehydrogenase levels, and moderately prolonged partial thromboplastin times. Resolution of the cardiopulmonary stage is heralded by diuresis.

DIAGNOSIS OF HANTAVIRUS

Diagnosis of hantavirus disease requires a high index of suspicion. Patients complaining of fever and myalgia along with abdominal pain should prompt the physician to inquire about rodent exposure in endemic areas. HPS is likely in patients with a compatible clinical history and an oxygen saturation level of less than 90%. Laboratory diagnosis is available by enzyme-linked immunosorbent assay (ELISA) studies for specific hantavirus IgG or IgM antibodies in the acute sera. Isolation and culture of the virus is difficult.

TREATMENT

Treatment of HFRS consists of close monitoring and attention to fluid status. Early hospitalization and bed rest are crucial. For patients with HPS, the goal of therapy is maintenance of oxygenation and tissue perfusion. Hantaviruses are susceptible in vivo to ribavirin. When given early in the disease, ribavirin has been shown to reduce mortality in HFRS. Ribavirin is also used in clinical trials to treat HPS, but confirmation of its effectiveness is still lacking [32].

PREVENTION OF HANTAVIRUS

The prevalence and ubiquity of rodent reservoirs make rodent control impractical. However, measures to minimize rodent exposure and infestation can be undertaken (Table 37-4). Isolation of patients with HFRS or HPS is unnecessary, but use of Universal Precautions is prudent. Physical barriers and respiratory protection should be used when clinical procedures or specimen processing is likely to produce an aerosol. There are no human vaccines against the New World virus strains; however, prototype vaccines are being tested for the Hantaan virus [21,22].

Table 37-4
Rodent Control Measures in the Workplace

Eliminate food sources:
- Store food and garbage in containers with tight lids.
- Clean floor and counters where food is used.

Prevent entrance of rodent into the workplace:
- Clear brush and grass from around foundations.
- Seal holes or use flashing around the base of buildings.

Use continuous trapping efforts.

Eliminate possible nesting sites:
- Elevate hay, woodpiles, lumber, and garbage cans.
- Locate them 100 feet away from the workplace.
- Eliminate junk or things that provide shelter for rodents.

Encourage rodents' natural predators: nonpoisonous snakes, owls, hawks.

When cleaning in an area infested with rodents:
- Wear rubber gloves.
- Do not stir up or breathe dust.
- Soak contaminated areas with disinfectant (e.g., bleach solution).
- Disinfect or dispose of gloves.

When working in the field:
- Avoid contact with rodents.
- Stay away from rodent burrows or nests.
- Avoid littering food.

South American Hemorrhagic Fever

EPIDEMIOLOGY

In 1958, Junin virus emerged as the causative agent of Argentine hemorrhagic fever (AHF). Three other members of the same family of viruses have subsequently been implicated in South American hemorrhagic fevers (SAHFs): Machupo virus, first isolated in 1963, which causes Bolivian hemorrhagic fever (BHF); Guanarito virus, first isolated in 1990, which causes Venezuelan hemorrhagic fever (VHF); and Sabia virus, first isolated in 1990, which is a causative agent of hemorrhagic fever in Brazil. All the viruses are members of the New World Tacaribe complex of the family Arenaviridae. Prominent Old World members are the prototype lymphocytic choriomeningitis virus and the Lassa virus. All the SAHF viruses are associated with a rodent reservoir and are transmitted to humans primarily by aerosolized virus found in rodent excreta [18,33].

AHF is the best characterized of the SAHFs and has an annual incidence of 100–4,000 cases. There is a seasonal pattern, with cases beginning in late summer and peaking in autumn. Male agricultural workers are at greatest risk for infection [34]. BHF began as an epidemic in 1963 and 1964 with the occurrence of more than 500 cases. A second outbreak occurred in 1971 in western Bolivia. In 1993–1994, several sporadic cases were confirmed in the Beni region [35]. There was one outbreak that showed intrafamilial transmission, that is, the potential of these viruses to be spread from person to person instead of from rodent to humans [37].

VHF was recognized in 1989 and found to be the causative agent in 104 cases of hemorrhagic fever between May 1990 and March 1991 in northwestern Venezuela [36]. Males were primarily affected, but cases included women and children. Sabia virus was recognized in an index case in 1990 in Sao Paulo State, Brazil. Two laboratory workers were subsequently infected while working with the virus. There are no other cases known [38,39].

CLINICAL FEATURE

The clinical features of SAHFs are similar. There is an incubation period of six to 16 days. The onset of symptoms is gradual; fever and malaise are the first symptoms noticed. Headache, myalgia, arthralgia, and dizziness appear next. Gastrointestinal symptoms are also frequently present. Neurologic abnormalities, including tremor of the tongue and extremities, disorientation, hyporeflexia or ataxia, may appear. Early signs are flushing of the face, conjunctival injection, and hypotension. These may give way to more severe signs such as petechiae, periorbital edema, pulmonary edema, and shock. Bleeding disorders, including bleeding of the gums, hematemesis and melena, occur in about half the patients. Severely ill patients may bleed from other mucosal surfaces. Leukopenia, thrombocytopenia, and proteinuria are always present within the first few days of illness [18].

DIAGNOSIS AND TREATMENT

The diagnosis of SAHF is strongly suspected on the basis of a history of rodent exposure, clinical signs and symptoms, laboratory abnormalities, and geographic location. SAHF can be confirmed by ELISA antigen or IgM detection. Arenaviruses are known to be susceptible to ribavirin, but no clinical trials have been done. Early clinical evidence shows it is useful in SAHF. Treatment is otherwise supportive.

PREVENTION

Agricultural workers are the occupation overwhelmingly at risk for SAHFs. Hospital workers caring for infected patients are also at risk. Other occupations in which contact with rodent excreta occurs should also be considered at risk. Therefore rodent control is the cornerstone of prevention (see Table 37-4). The potential for human-to-human transmission is evident, so strict isolation procedures should be used for all suspected hospitalized cases. The viruses are consistently aerosol infectious in the laboratory; thus, they are at biosafety level 4 precautions [40]. A live, attenuated vaccine has been developed for AHF and is being tested.

Plague

EPIDEMIOLOGY

Plague is an acute and often fatal disease caused by the bacteria *Yersinia pestis*. There have been two major outbreaks of plague in the past decade. The pathogen is present on every continent except Australia and Antarctica. Most cases are reported from developing countries. The principal reservoir for the pathogen is wild rodents, and it is transmitted to humans principally by fleas when an infected flea feeds on them. Rare cases are caused by direct contact with infected tissues or fluids or by inhalation of respiratory droplets from aerosolized infectious materials [42,43].

It is likely that plague is closely associated with natural cycles of rodent populations. In urban settings, epidemic disease usually erupts after the infestation of large numbers of peridomestic rats. An often observed "rat fall," in which rats inhabiting the roofs and walls of slum homes become sick and die, often precedes human outbreak. This was noted before the outbreak of plague in India during 1994 [44]. Plague occurs in settings of war and social upheaval and almost always occurs in settings of extreme poverty, poor sanitation, and/or the absence of rodent control. Cats have become increasingly important vectors because of their tendency to hunt rodents and bring them back to the home [45].

Workers at risk include hunters, trappers, field workers who routinely work with rodents in enzootic areas, and people who work in veterinary clinics [42,46–48].

CLINICAL FEATURES

Plague generally presents as a bubonic disease (75% of cases) after an incubation period of two to eight days. The symptoms are abrupt onset of fever, chills, weakness, and headache. Usually there is a history of animal exposure but not always a history of insect bites. Twelve to 24 hours after the fever, painful adenopathy (bubo) appears, usually in a single area. Most of the time the bubo is in the axilla, the groin, or the neck. Abdominal pain, nausea, vomiting, and diarrhea commonly occur. Pneumonic plague (20%) occurs after bacteremia spreads to the lungs. At this stage, the patient presents with a cough and thin, watery blood-tinged sputum and shortness of breath. Laboratory findings of plague are nonspecific, revealing only leukocytosis [8].

DIAGNOSIS

Diagnosis is made by exposure history, presenting complaints, and physical findings. If a bubo is present, it can be aspirated, stained, and cultured using Universal Precautions and being careful not to make an aerosol. Sputum can also be stained and cultured in pneumonic plague. Direct fluorescent antibody staining of isolated bacteria is confirmatory when available.

TREATMENT

Treatment of plague is with intramuscular streptomycin at 30 mg/kg per day in two divided doses. A full 10-day course is required. Tetracycline can be used as an alternative in doses of 2–4 g/day. Patients with pneumonic plague should be placed in respiratory isolation until 48 hours after antibacterial therapy has started. Primary contacts should be started on prophylactic trimethoprim-sulfamethoxazole or tetracycline. Bubonic plague patients are not infectious to health care workers [49].

PREVENTION

Prevention primarily is by rodent control measures (see Table 37-4). Hunters should always were gloves when handling animals. Veterinary clinic workers in enzootic areas should be educated about handling sick animals. Examination of cats with fever and lymphadenopathy or pneumonia should include gloves, mask, and protective eyewear [48]. People working with rodents should generally avoid handling sick or dead animals. Appropriate clothing should be worn and insect repellent containing DEET should be used on clothing and skin.

For laboratory personnel who routinely work with *Yersinia pestis*, a killed-bacteria vaccine is available. It is also appropriate for people who have regular contact with wild rodents, such as wildlife biologists, mammalogists, and ecologists. The vaccine is given intramuscularly in three divided doses: the initial dose followed by a dose at one month and six months. Booster doses must be given every six months to people who remain at high risk for exposure [42]. Travelers to plague-endemic areas are at low risk if they avoid rat-infested areas. Insect repellent on clothes, skin, and bedding should be used to reduce exposure to fleas. Short-term antibiotic prophylaxis for plague is rarely appropriate for travelers.

Dengue

EPIDEMIOLOGY

Dengue was first described in the late 1700s but gained importance as a disease during and after World War II. A global pandemic began in Southeast Asia and has increased in the past 17 years. Dengue, or "breakbone fever," is caused by four distinct serotypes of *Flavivirus.* This genus of viruses also claims yellow fever virus as a member. Two serotypes were recognized in World War II, and types 3 and 4 were recovered in the Philippines in 1956. Before 1956, dengue was associated with a favorable prognosis, but subsequently a new syndrome, dengue hemorrhagic fever–dengue shock syndrome (DHF-DSS), emerged in Manila. Since that time, more than 3 million children have been hospitalized and 57,000 have died from the disease. Each year there are between 25,000 and 500,000 cases of dengue worldwide; the case fatality rate is 1–5% [50–52,55].

The virus is transmitted to humans principally by the *Aedes aegypti* mosquito. The *Aedes albopictus*, or the tiger mosquito, is also a vector. *A albopictus* is primarily endemic to Asia but has recently been introduced in the Western Hemisphere [50,54]. Both mosquitoes feed by day. Currently, *A aegypti* is almost universally distributed between 30 degrees north and 20 degrees south latitude, and dengue has spread throughout this range. Most transmission occurs below 2,000 feet during the rainy season when mosquito populations are high. Factors in the emergence of dengue as a major world health problem are not well understood. Many countries with endemic dengue have no means to control mosquitoes, thus allowing dengue to spread. An increase in air travel, which rapidly moves serotypes and new strains of dengue around the world, might also be a factor. Furthermore, worldwide demographic changes, such as rapid urbanization and population growth, are contributing to substandard housing with inadequate water, sewage, and waste management. All of these factors are leading to increases in the *A aegypti* mosquito population [51].

At present, dengue is endemic to tropical and subtropical Asia, Africa, South America, and the Caribbean basin. Dengue has re-emerged in Texas, mainly along the Mexican border, where there have been more than 150 cases since 1986 [53]. Dengue is an important disease affecting military troops. It was first recognized in World War II but just recently proved to have been a major disease in American troops stationed in Somalia [56]. Travelers to endemic areas are at greatest risk, and more than 2,500 cases have been imported into the United States by travelers returning or visiting from endemic areas.

CLINICAL FEATURES AND DIAGNOSIS

The symptoms of dengue varies from patient to patient. After an incubation period of one to seven days, there is sudden onset of fever accompanied by frontal or retro-orbital headache. Some patients complain of backache. Myalgia and arthralgia appear soon after the fever, and a transient macular blanching rash may also appear. After the first day, nausea and vomiting may occur. Other symptoms include hypesthesia, anorexia, taste abnormalities, and lymphadenopathy. After the deferescence of the fever, second rash, spreading outward from the chest, may appear. This is a maculopapular rash lasting one to five days. A second temperature elevation may occur with the second rash. Diagnosis is made by clinical suspicion and/or by a rise in serum antibodies [50,52].

Dengue hemorrhagic fever more commonly affects children less than 15 years of age. There are four grades of DHF based on the severity; DSS is grade three. It probably has the same incubation period and starts with abrupt fever, malaise, vomiting, headache, and anorexia. This is followed by rapid clinical deterioration after two to five days. The patient has cold extremities, flushed face, diaphoreses, restlessness, irritability, and abdominal pain. There are often scattered petechiae, and spontaneous ecchymosis may appear. Bleeding at venipuncture sites is common. Respirations are often fast and labored, and the pulse is weak, rapid, and thready. The liver may enlarge. During the period of shock, about 10% of patients have gastrointestinal bleeding. A complete blood count shows a decreased platelet count and an increase in hematocrit value. After 24 to 36 hours, there is a convalescent phase; recovery may be rapid.

TREATMENT

Dengue fever is treated with bedrest, analgesics, and acetaminophen as an antipyretic. Salicylates should be avoided because of their adverse effect on blood clotting. DHF-DSS is a medical emergency requiring hospitalization. The patient's vital signs and hydration status should be evaluated and electrolytes must be monitored for imbalances. Close monitoring of the patient for at least 48 hours is essential to ensure that shock does not occur. Supplemental oxygen should be given to patients with labored breathing, and fluid replacement and electrolyte replacement is often necessary. If bleeding occurs, transfusion of blood or platelets may also be necessary.

PREVENTION

Dengue is mainly controlled by limiting the mosquito vectors and avoiding mosquito bites [58]. The *A aegypti* mosquito is well adapted to urban environments; it usually deposits its larvae in water containers such as flowerpots, tires, bird baths, and old cans. To limit larval environments in endemic areas, water containers should be cleared away, emptied, or covered. A thin layer of oil sprayed on the surface of water pools may prevent egg laying or hatching. Commercial larvicides can be added to water. Screens should be used on windows. In the field, personal methods of prevention, including protective clothing, mosquito repellent, and mosquito netting, should be used. DEET is the most effective mosquito repellent available for use on skin. Permethrin is another repellent that can be used to impregnate clothes, tents, and netting [57]. Vaccines are currently under development, but none has been approved for widespread use.

Venezuelan Equine Encephalitis

EPIDEMIOLOGY

Venezuelan equine encephalitis (VEE) virus was first discovered in 1936 in the brain of a horse that had died from a fatal encephalomyelitis. The first recognized human case occurred in Trinidad in 1944. A large epidemic occurred in the years 1962–1971, with outbreaks affecting Columbia, Ecuador, Venezuela, Peru, Central America, and Texas [59]. The most recent outbreak of VEE started in northwestern Venezuela in April 1995 and spread westward to Columbia [61]. This was the first outbreak in 22 years and it caused an estimated 75,000 cases in humans, 3,000 with neurologic complications and 300 fatalities. Approximately 8% of the area's equines may have died. Although horses had declined in population in Venezuela since the previous outbreak, donkeys had increased and many were unvaccinated, as were many other equines. Donkeys were probably the principal susceptible population of animals that amplified the disease.

VEE has primarily been a disease of equines, but it has been found in many enzootic wild mammals. Other domestic animal species that have been found to be infected are cattle, goats, pigs, and sheep. Humans might also play a role in amplifying the disease because there are high enough viral titers in an infected person to be retransmitted to a biting mosquito. The virus has also been isolated in the pharynx of humans, and direct human-to-human transmission is possible [60,62].

There are a variety of mosquito species that transmit the disease during an epidemic; *Aedes*, *Mansonia*, and *Psorophora* are the most important. Factors in the recent Venezuelan outbreak were heavy rains and flooding in a normally arid region, leading to a proliferation of *Aedes taeniorhynicus* and *Psorophora confinnis* mosquitoes. During an outbreak, all persons exposed to mosquitoes in the area are at risk. Farmers or ranchers with unvaccinated equines are probably at higher risk, although this has not been proved. Workers at risk for the enzootic infection are those that enter the rain forest or swamps. These include rubber tappers, forestry workers, and military personnel on jungle maneuvers [63].

CLINICAL FEATURES

VEE usually affects humans about two weeks after an outbreak in horses. Typically, the infection is a mild acute febrile illness without neurologic complications. It is manifested by abrupt onset of headache, fever, rigors, malaise, and myalgia. Other symptoms include nausea, vomiting, diarrhea, and sore throat. Uncommonly there is photophobia, seizures, mental confusion, tremors, and coma. Lymphadenopathy occurs in approximately one third of cases. The disease usually resolves after three to five days but may last eight days in severe cases. Like dengue, there may be a biphasic course and the patient may redevelop symptoms on days 6 through 9 [60,62,63].

DIAGNOSIS

Laboratory studies show a normal leukocyte count but elevated neutrophils. Leukopenia may occur by day 3 of the disease. Examination of a cerebrospinal fluid specimen may reveal pleocytosis with an increase in protein and normal glucose levels. Diagnosis is made by clinical presentation and suspicion of the disease during an outbreak. It can be confirmed by isolating the virus in a serum or spinal fluid specimen or by detecting IgM antibodies in a serum sample. These are likely not immediately available but can be used for surveillance.

TREATMENT AND PREVENTION

Because VEE is usually self-limited, treatment is primarily supportive. Presently there is no human vaccine to prevent the infection. For equines, there is a live, attenuated vaccine that rapidly conveys immunity. Horses and donkeys in particular should be targeted. Outbreaks can be controlled by quarantine, immunization of equines, and mosquito control [60,61]. For people in endemic areas, efforts should be made to limit exposure to mosquito bites: Windows should be screened; insecticides should be used as appropriate; and personal protection should be increased by using clothing that covers the skin, including a hat. Insect repellents can also be used.

Rift Valley Fever

EPIDEMIOLOGY

Rift valley fever (RVF) is an acute disease principally affecting livestock, buffalo, sheep, goats, cattle, and camels. RVF virus was first detected in Kenya in 1931. Since then, it has been the cause of several epizootics, including an outbreak in the period 1950–1951, when an estimated 100,000 sheep died. These epizootics usually coincided with heavy rains. Slaughterhouse workers and veterinarians exposed to the animals were noted to have a brief flu-like illness with occasional vision-impairing retinitis. The first fatal human cases of hemorrhagic fever with accompanying hepatitis were reported in South Africa during an epizootic of RVF [64,65,70]. In 1977, RVF spread to Egypt and caused a major epizootic and subsequent human epidemic. There were an estimated 18,000 human cases, with 598 deaths. The presumed spread of the disease from animal to man was by mosquito vectors. Major outbreaks of RVF then appeared in Mauritania in 1987, Egypt in 1993, Madagascar in 1990–1991, and northern Kenya and Somalia in 1997. The latest outbreak may have infected an estimated 89,000 people [66–68].

RVF virus is found in several species of mosquito, but the *Aedes* species may be the most important in human transmission. It may be also transmitted by other biting insects such as the sand fly [69]. The reservoir of the virus is unknown, but the virus does infect many species of vertebrates. Factors in the emergence of the disease are those that increase mosquito populations, including heavy rains, building of new dams, and increases in the density of an area's livestock [71].

Humans can also become infected with the virus if they are exposed to blood or other body fluids of infected animals. This can result from the slaughtering or handling of infected animals or through touching contaminated meat during food preparation. Sleeping outdoors at night in endemic areas is a risk factor for the disease, presumably because it exposes people to biting insects. Animal herdsmen, abattoir workers, and other animal handlers in endemic areas are thought to have an increased risk for infection. Veterinarians and slaughterhouse workers are probably at highest risk. Travelers to an area where an outbreak is occurring are also at risk [65,66].

CLINICAL FEATURES

The incubation period of RVF is three to six days. Most people with RVF have no symptoms or mild disease. The onset of disease is abrupt; patients complain of malaise, chills, weakness, headache, retroorbital pain, myalgias, and backache. High fever develops rapidly. Other complaints include anorexia, loss of taste, epigastric pain, weight loss, and photophobia. Findings on physical examination are nonspecific and include flushing and conjunctival injection. Often the temperature curve is biphasic: an initial elevation for two to three days, followed by remission and then a second febrile period. Convalescence is usually rapid; but approximately 1% of patients develop severe complications such as hemorrhagic fever, encephalitis, retinopathy, or hepatitis.

DIAGNOSIS

Diagnosis is made by clinical suspicion during an outbreak. Serologic studies confirm the diagnosis [64]. They show initially a normal leukocyte count, followed by leukopenia, a decrease in neutrophils, and an increase in band forms.

TREATMENT AND PREVENTION

There is presently no established treatment for RVF; only supportive measures are used. Ribavirin is being studied as a possible antiviral drug, and other studies are examining interferon, immune modulators, and convalescent-phase plasma. People can decrease the risk of contracting RVF by decreasing their exposure to mosquitoes. Vaccines are available for use in animals but can cause birth defects and abortions in sheep and provides only low-level protection in cattle. A live attenuated human vaccine is being developed [65].

Leishmaniasis

EPIDEMIOLOGY

Leishmaniasis, an endemic disease of the tropics and subtropics, is caused by a variety of protozoans of the *Leishmania* species. The infection is acquired through the bite of infected female sand flies, usually of the genera *Phlebotomus*, *Lutzomyia*, and *Psychodopygus*. Clinical manifestations of the disease vary from a benign self-healing sore to a fulminant visceral disease (kala-azar) that results in death [72].

An estimated 350 million people are at risk for the disease, and as many as 12 million are already infected [73]. The disease types were originally divided by geographic location, vector type and animal reservoir, leading to the terms *Old World leishmaniasis* and *New World leishmaniasis.* This original taxonomy has been replaced by DNA species typing, but this is rarely available at the time of diagnosis. Currently, leishmaniasis is categorized by the presentation of the disease as cutaneous, mucocutaneous, or visceral. The original rule of one species/one syndrome has recently been challenged by atypical presentations of leishmaniasis in a number of species (Table 37-5).

Outbreaks of leishmaniasis tend to occur when a group of susceptible hosts move into an endemic area, such as American soldiers who were sent to the Middle East in the Gulf War. They also occur when sand fly habitats are disturbed, which commonly occurs with the establishment of roads, farms, and villages in newly cleared forests. Animal reservoirs are often incriminated in infection, but full knowledge of transmission patterns is lacking. Peridomestic animals may be secondary hosts because they also provide blood meals for sand flies. Chickens, horses, and especially dogs have been implicated for increasing the chance of outbreaks. Dogs are particularly important in the Mediterranean, Brazil, and China, where they have been identified as the principal reservoir in some species of the disease [74]. Visceral leishmaniasis was previously known as a rural disease in Brazil, but migration of impoverished people to the suburbs who often bring along their animals has led to large urban outbreaks. In the early 1980s, there was a large outbreak of visceral leishmaniasis in Brazil that peaked in 1994 [75].

CLINICAL FEATURES

Presentation of the disease varies, depending on where it is contracted. Visceral leishmaniasis is predominantly a disease of adults in India, but in the Mediterranean and in Brazil, it is mainly a disease of children. The cutaneous form occurs primarily in Asia, the Mediterranean, South America, and Ethiopia. In Asia, the disease usually presents as the classic cutaneous sore, a closed, nodular, chronic skin granulosa that ulcerates with time. In Ethiopia, leishmaniasis presents as cutaneous lesions that remain closed but slowly increase in diameter. South America has a rapidly ulcerating form of the cutaneous disease. In Brazil, Venezuela, Ethiopia, and the Dominican Republic, there is a form that is disseminated over the skin and associated with anergy. This is called *diffuse cutaneous leishmaniasis.* Mucocutaneous leishmaniasis is predominantly limited to South America, although a form in the Sudan has been

Table 37-5
Leishmania Species and Their Usual Disease States

Species	Predominant Syndrome	Other Syndromes	Location
L donovani group	VL	PKDL	India, China, Africa
L donovani infantum		CL	Middle East, Mediterranean, North Africa
L donovani chagasi		ACL	Latin America
L donovani archibald		CL	Sudan, Kenya, Ethiopia
L major	CL		Middle East, Asia, Africa, India (subcontinent)
L tropica	CL	Viscerotropic VL	Mediterranean, Middle East, West Asia, India
L aethiopica	CL	DCL	Northeast Africa
L viannia group	ACL	MCL	South America, Central America
L mexicana group			
L mexicana mexicana	ACL		Texas, Mexico, Central America
L mexicana amazonensis	ACL	DCL, VL	Brazil, Amazon Basin, Trinidad, Venezuela, Panama
L mexicana pifonoi	ACL	DCL	Venezuela
L mexicana venezuelensis	ACL		Venezuela
L mexicana species	DCL	ACL	Dominican Republic

CL = cutaneous leishmaniasis; *ACL* = American cutaneous leishmaniasis; *MCL* = mucocutaneous leishmaniasis; *VL* = visceral leishmaniasis; *DCL* = diffuse cutaneous leishmaniasis; *PDKL* = post-kala-azar leishmaniasis.
Adapted from Evan TG. Leishmaniasis. *Infect Dis Clin North Am* 1993;1:529.

well documented. A chronic condition known as *post-kala-azar dermal leishmaniasis* occurs mainly in India but may be encountered in other areas such as Africa. In this presentation, papular or nodular lesions of the face and body follow the occurrence of clinical or subclinical visceral leishmaniasis [76].

Visceral leishmaniasis (also known as *kala-azari*) is characterized by fever, weight loss, weakness, and night sweats. Physical examination usually reveals a thin patient with hepatosplenomegaly. The name *kala-azar* means "black fever" because of the propensity for the skin to become dry and dark. Laboratory investigations show a normocytic, normochromic anemia. Pancytopenia is usual. Eight military personnel stationed in the Gulf region during the Gulf War developed atypical visceral disease called *viscerotropic leishmaniasis* [77]. The causative organism, *Leishmania tropica*, usually presents with a relatively benign cutaneous disease. None of the military patients had skin lesions, however. Four patients had acute fever, malaise and anemia, and two had predominantly gastrointestinal complaints. In addition, weight loss and splenomegaly were not as apparent as they are in classic cases of this visceral form of the disease [72].

DIAGNOSIS

The gold standard of diagnosis is identification of the *Leishmania* protozoa from a tissue sample. For cutaneous leishmaniasis, a punch biopsy is done at the leading edge of the lesion. Alternatively, a scalpel incision can be made along the leading edge and the exposed tissue and fluid scraped onto a slide or culture medium. Visceral leishmaniasis isolates are obtained from the spleen or the bone marrow. Splenic aspirates have a higher sensitivity, but bone marrow aspiration may be needed to rule out other diseases such as tuberculosis or lymphoma. Giemsa stain is used to detect the organism. Other methods of testing for leishmaniasis are not sensitive enough, although the future may see the development of some reliable new methods [76].

TREATMENT

Treatment for all forms of leishmaniasis is patient isolation and administration of pentavalent antimonials. The usual treatment for visceral leishmaniasis is 20 mg/kg/day in two divided doses for 28 days, given intravenously or intramuscularly. The antimonials are not marketed in the United States but can be obtained from the Centers for Disease Control and Prevention (CDC). Cutaneous lesions may alternatively be treated with seven doses of pentamidine, 2 mg/kg intravenously every other day, or with a topical mixture of paromomycin and methylbenzethonium. However, most cutaneous lesions resolve without specific therapy [78].

PREVENTION

Personal prevention of the disease is the cornerstone of control. People in endemic areas should avoid activities at dusk when sand flies are apt to bite: For example, military troops in the Amazon frequently shower in the afternoon. Insect repellents and suitable clothing are also helpful. Use of permethrin-impregnated mosquito netting to cover beds is also prudent. Brazil controlled its urban outbreaks of visceral leishmaniasis by rapid treatment of human hosts, spraying DDT in households where infection occurred, and by destruction of infected dogs. Rural endemic visceral leishmaniasis is much more difficult to control because of the sylvan reservoir [73,75]. Vaccines have been developed, but their effectiveness is uncertain. Any physician who suspects a Gulf War participant of cutaneous or visceral leishmaniasis should report the case to the Department of Defense to receive further information.

Filoviruses: Ebola, Marburg, and Reston

EPIDEMIOLOGY

Unknown until 1967, the filoviruses quickly captured the attention of the world because of the severe and often fatal results for people who contracted infection. Marburg virus, Ebola virus, and Reston virus are members of the RNA virus family Filoviridae. They can cause infection in humans and in nonhuman primates.

In 1967, a simultaneous outbreak of Marburg virus occurred in Germany and Yugoslavia among laboratory personnel working with green monkeys imported from Uganda. Of the workers who had contact with the monkeys, a total of 31 cases of viral infection occurred, 25 cases of primary infection and six cases of secondary; seven of the cases were fatal. Since 1967, only sporadic cases, mainly related to travel in sub-Saharan Africa, have occurred: two health care workers, one doctor and one nurse, all of whom cared for patients infected with Marburg virus. There was also one case of a laboratory scientist in Russia who contracted it while working with an isolate of Marburg virus [79].

A new member of this family of viruses, Ebola virus, emerged in Zaire in 1976. Named after the Ebola River, where it was first detected, the virus caused two large simultaneous outbreaks in Zaire and in western Sudan. There were more than 550 cases, with 340 deaths. The fatality rate was extremely high: about 90% in Zaire and 50% in Sudan. Many secondary cases occurred because of exposure to infected blood or other body fluids. The re-use of needles and syringes and the absence of barrier protection for health care workers amplified the disease. The disease was also noted to be transmitted through sexual contact. A second outbreak happened in Sudan in 1979; it involved 34 people, with 22 fatalities [80,81].

Ebola virus reappeared in Kikwit, Zaire, in April 1995 [82]. A male laboratory worker became ill and was hospitalized. Severe abdominal pain was a prominent symptom. Members of a medical and surgical team who were mobilized to care for him began developing symptoms about four days after they first had contact with the patient. Many of the health care workers had inadequate barrier protection while caring for the man. Overall, about 300 cases, with a case fatality of 79%, were identified. About one third of the cases occurred in health care workers. Because of the re-emergence of Ebola virus, an outbreak of hemorrhagic fever which started in 1994 in Gabon, Zaire, was recognized as Ebola. Gabon had three apparently individual outbreaks of the Ebola virus between 1994 and January 1997, accounting for 59 cases, with 44 deaths [83]. A nurse caring for one patient transferred from Gabon to South Africa in 1994 contracted the illness and died. An isolated case occurred in the Ivory Coast when a Swiss ethnologist did necropsies on chimpanzees that had died of unknown causes [84].

The filoviruses were considered to be a threat only in sub-Saharan Africa, but that belief was disproved in 1989 when an outbreak of hemorrhagic fever occurred among cynomolgus monkeys in Reston, Virginia [85–87]. The causative pathogen was recognized as a subtype of Ebola virus. The monkeys were traced to an export facility in the Philippines. Subsequently, other monkeys in Texas and Pennsylvania imported from this facility were identified as carrying Ebola virus. Later, in 1992, infected macaques were identified in Italy. The macaques had come from the same export facility in the Philippines. In Reston, Virginia, the virus seemed to be transmitted by aerosolization and not just by contact with body fluids. The Reston subtype of Ebola only caused disease in the monkeys but had a case fatality of 75%. No human illness occurred in the outbreak, but several workers showed serologic evidence of infection.

The history of Ebola virus in Africa suggests that the virus passes from nonhuman primates to man. Dead great apes were found in the forests during the time of several outbreaks. One outbreak was associated with butchering dead chimpanzees, and one index patient was a hunter who lived near the site where a dead Ebola virus infected chimpanzee was found [83]. Although nonhuman primates have been involved in almost all recognized outbreaks of filoviruses, it is unlikely that primates are the wild reservoir of the disease because their case fatality from the infection is too high. The true reservoir remains unknown.

CLINICAL FEATURES

The disease presents like many types of hemorrhagic fever. Following an incubation period of three to eight days, there is sudden onset of frontal headache, chills, fever, myalgia, malaise, and anorexia. Nausea, vomiting, and abdominal pain also are early symptoms, and pharyngitis, conjunctivitis, and oral ulcers are frequently present. Patients are often apathetic and may be disoriented. A maculopapular rash develops on the trunk around day 5. Bleeding from the mucous membranes, the skin, the gastrointestinal tract, and injection sites often is present, and bleeding from internal organs may occur. Patients frequently have thrombocytopenia and leukopenia, with a left shift early in the disease. Neutrophilia appears in later stages of the disease. Death occurs secondary to shock on days 6 to 16 of the illness. If the patient lives, which is rare, convalescence is prolonged, requiring many weeks [79,81].

DIAGNOSIS

The diagnosis of Ebola virus and Marburg virus is by serologic indirect immunofluorescence assay, which is rarely readily available. Although sensitive, this test is not specific, and other testing is frequently necessary to confirm the diagnosis. The unique structure of these viruses can be seen in properly prepared tissue samples under an electron microscope. Clinical diagnosis is very difficult, since many other diseases, such as malaria, yellow fever and other hemorrhagic fever viruses and rickettsial diseases, have similar signs and symptoms. Often, diagnosis is made by the failure of the patient to respond to treatment for the more common types of infections.

TREATMENT AND PREVENTION

No specific treatment exists. The patient must be supported for shock, multiple organ failure, and clotting disturbances. There is no vaccine available. When cases of filovirus disease are suspected or confirmed, person-to-person contacts should be limited and patients should be placed in isolation. All equipment needs to be sterilized after use [88]. Health care providers should use gowns, mask, gloves, and goggles when caring for patients, and all waste should be burned. The virus is easily destroyed by disinfectants; thus, all hard surfaces should be cleaned with a sanitizing solution. Early recognition and isolation of cases is the best means of prevention. The workers at greatest risk are health care workers in endemic areas, including nurses, laboratory workers, and physicians, but workers involved with the collection, transportation, or study of wild-caught primates are also at risk. Guidelines have been established by the CDC for handling primates during transit and quarantine (Table 37-6).

Influenza

EPIDEMIOLOGY

Symptoms of influenza—acute fever, cough, headache, myalgia, and malaise—have been documented for centuries, and the disease has been the chief suspect in as many as 31 recorded pandemics. Three have been recorded this century: in 1918, 1957, and 1958. The most devastating of the three pandemics was known as the Spanish flu: It killed more than 20 million people between 1918 and 1920. Between pandemic, there are yearly flu epidemics affecting millions of people. Influenza has three major types of virus: A, B, and C. Influenza A and influenza B are known to infect humans; generally, influenza B is less virulent. Both types constantly mutate and change their immunogenicity, and this is the reason new epidemics are constantly emerging and new vaccines are developed yearly [89–91].

The influenza virus has two features that allow it to constantly re-emerge: surface proteins and a constantly changing genetic mix in its swine reservoir. The surface proteins are recognized by the human immune response change over time as part of the naturally occurring evolution of the virus. This is relatively rapid and unpredictable and causes annual epidemics as new strains emerge. Sometimes a new species enters human. This occurs when influenza viruses that normally infect swine or water fowl are transmitted to humans. The new species is probably unlike any previous influenza and is immunologically distinct. Most of the time, transmission from animal to man is a dead end and the spread of the virus is halted. Sometimes, however, a novel virus can be spread from human to human leading to widespread transmission in an immunologically susceptible population. This is when the pandemics occur.

All species of influenza A virus are known to occur in wild water fowl. Molecular studies have linked the 1958 Asian flu and the 1969 Hong Kong flu with avian influenza viruses. Swine are susceptible to both human and avian influenza viruses and may serve as an intermediary host for the reassortment of influenza viruses. Swine influenza viruses are closely related to the influenza type that caused the Spanish flu of 1918. In 1977, the swine influenza viruses re-emerged in humans, spreading through Asia, Russia, and then on to Europe and North America. This was not considered a true pandemic, because it occurred almost exclusively in persons younger than age 20.

In May 1997, the index case of a new influenza virus in humans was reported [92]. A 3-year-old child, who had complications of Reye's syndrome, died from it in Hong Kong. Prior to this, the virus was known only to infect species of birds, including chickens and ducks. By the end of 1997, 15 additional cases were confirmed. There was no clear-cut evidence of human-to-human transmission; infection was believed to have come through contact with infected birds. The virus is deadly when it infects chickens, and thousands of chickens died in Hong Kong in the spring of 1997 after contracting it [94].

Epidemiologic serum testing of contacts with the child, health care workers, poultry workers, and pig farm workers have been completed. Very few contacts of the child showed detectable antibodies to the virus. Lab workers that handled the virus also had a very low prevalence of antibodies. Poultry workers showed the highest prevalence of antibodies: five of 27 workers tested. No pig farm workers had antibodies [93].

Influenza viruses are spread primarily by small-particle aerosols of virus-laden respiratory secretions that are expelled from an infected person when coughing, sneezing, and talking. Spread by direct contact may also occur. Historical records and epidemiologic records suggest the pandemics started in China. China also has a highly dense human population. Furthermore, swine and fowl are known to harbor species of influenza, and farming practices of China frequently put the animals in close proximity to one another. The exact mechanism of the pig-bird-human interaction is unknown.

Table 37-6
Summary of CDC Guidelines for Handling Nonhuman Primates

1. Personnel should be instructed of the hazards of handling primates.
2. Person working with the primates should not eat, drink, or smoke while handling the animals, crates, or items retrieved from the crates.
3. Access to the holding area should be restricted to essential personnel.
4. All staff in direct contact with animals should wear a gown, mask, and gloves when opening the crates, feeding the animals, or removing items from the crates.
5. Each animal should have a separate water bottle.
6. All waste from the animal including bedding and uneaten food should be treated with disinfectant before removal from the facility. All cages, feeding bottles, and items in contact with the animal should be disinfected between each use or before disposal. Glass items should not be used.
7. A separate needle should be used for each animal and autoclaved or incinerated after use.
8. Used needles should not be manipulated. A proper sharp instrument container should be located as close as possible to the worksite.
9. Nonquarantined animals should not be permitted in the quarantined area.
10. Management should keep records of any serious illnesses and notify the CDC if the worker had direct contact with the primates.
11. The physician caring for the worker should be informed that he/she has been exposed to primates.

Additional Guidelines During Transit

1. Workers transporting the crates should have elbow-length reinforced leather gloves, long-sleeve shirts, thick trousers, and sturdy footware.
2. The crates should have minimal sharp projections.
3. Crates should be separated from other animals and cargo by a physical or spatial barrier.
4. The animals should not be handled directly, if possible.
5. Management should have records documenting the removal of dead animals.The carcass must be placed in waterproof double bags and incinerated.
6. All injections administered to the primates should be documented.

Additional Guidelines for Nonhuman Primates During Quarantine

1. The facilities should be secure.
2. The facilities should be designed to be properly disinfected.
3. Staff should use protective clothing, gloves, and masks while in the holding area and should use fresh protective clothing when going from area to area.
4. Adequate equipment and space should be available for waste disposal and disinfecting equipment, clothing, and cages.
5. Animals should be handled while anesthetized or tranquilized.
6. Different lots of primates should not be mixed together.
7. Management should notify the Division of Quarantine, CPS, and CDC of any severe illnesses and deaths of recently imported primates.

Adapted from Centers for Disease Control. Update: Ebola-related filovirus infection in nonhuman primates and interim guidelines for handling nonhuman primates during transit and quarantine. *MMWR* 1990;39:22–4, 29.

CLINICAL FEATURES

The symptoms of influenza are well known: fever, chills, sore throat, headache, dry cough, myalgia, anorexia, and malaise [95]. The severity of symptoms is variable, ranging from mild rhinitis or pharyngitis to fatal viral pneumonia. Serious complications most often occur in the very old or the very young. People with chronic cardiac, pulmonary, or metabolic disease are also at higher risk for severe complications. Influenza is often separated from the common cold by the presence of fever higher than 38°C and the severity of the symptoms.

Usually, symptoms resolve within one week. Fever occurs early and peaks within 24 hours of onset, lasting one to five days. Viral pneumonia, which is one of the more serious complications, usually occurs within three to five days of the onset of symptoms and progresses rapidly. Patients may also have secondary bacterial infection, which typically occurs five to 10 days after the initial onset of symptoms and is the more common type of pneumonia during an influenza outbreak.

DIAGNOSIS

Since the symptoms are broad, clinical diagnosis is often impossible without knowledge of an influenza outbreak within the community. Secretions obtained from a swab or wash of the upper respiratory tract or from sputum can be collected in virus transport medium and sent to a laboratory for culturing. This usually takes three to five days and is considered the gold standard of diagnosis. Blood serum can also be tested for influenza antibodies.

TREATMENT

Treatment of influenza with antiviral medications can shorten the duration of the illness and decrease its severity if started within 48 hours of onset. Amantadine or rimantadine is prescribed at a dosage of 100 mg twice daily for adults. Usually antiviral therapy is reserved for patients with severe disease or at risk for developing complications. Treatment is stopped 24–48 hours after symptoms disappear, which is generally after three to five days of therapy. Secondary bacterial infections should be treated with appropriate antibiotics [95].

PREVENTION

When influenza strikes a community, it often begins abruptly, peaks in two to three weeks, and ends in five to eight weeks. School absenteeism is initially high; work absenteeism rises later. The most important method of prevention is yearly immunization with inactivated influenza virus [96]. Adult immunization is indicated for individuals over age 65, those suffering from chronic heart, lung, or metabolic disease, and those at risk for developing complications of the disease. Health care workers and household contacts of people are at high risk and should be immunized. Because the vaccines are derived from virus grown on hens' eggs, people with allergy to eggs should not be immunized. Most working adults would benefit from the vaccine because studies have shown it to be a cost-effective measure to decrease work absenteeism. Many companies pay or subsidize vaccines for their employees.

Frequent outbreaks of influenza in institutions that house people at high risk, such as nursing homes, indicate the need for prophylactic use of antivirals in health care facilities. All patients and staff should receive amantadine or rimantadine for the duration of influenza activity in the community, regardless of vaccination status. Other populations who should receive antiviral prophylaxis are individuals with immunodeficiency and those for whom the vaccine is contraindicated.

Certain farming practices may help prevent the entry of new subtypes of influenza into the community. Pigs, waterfowl, and humans are the principal variables in new influenza pandemics. Often, both pigs and poultry are raised on the same farm; they should be kept separated as much as possible. Feeding pigs the carcasses of dead birds should be avoided. Raising pigs under chicken houses has been observed in areas of influenza outbreaks, and this practice should be avoided. Influenza can be devastating to poultry. Since wild waterfowl carry influenza viruses, domestic poultry should be isolated from wild species. Keeping a few ducks near a chicken farm can have unfortunate consequences, since the domestic ducks can attract wild ducks. Live bird markets may be another place where waterfowl can infect domestic poultry, and these different types of birds should be kept isolated from each other [91].

Cholera

EPIDEMIOLOGY

Cholera is an acute disease characterized by watery diarrhea, vomiting, fever, and rapid dehydration. The world is currently in its seventh cholera pandemic since 1817. The burden of disease is enormous. Each year there are more than 6 million cases of cholera, causing approximately 600,000 hospitalizations and 120,000 deaths. The current causative organism is the bacterium *Vibrio cholera O1.* This biotype has also been labeled *El Tor.* The most recent pandemic emerged in 1961 and spread through Asia and Africa. In 1991 it reached Peru. Before 1991, South

America had been free of cholera for over a hundred years. After explosive epidemics in coastal Peru, cholera spread rapidly throughout South and Central America [97,100]. Several cases have appeared in the United States because of travelers returning with the disease, or in one case, from contaminated seafood served on a flight from Lima to Los Angeles [98]. In 1992, a new serotype of cholera, *Vibrio cholerae O139*, also called *Bengal variant*, emerged in Bangladesh and India along the Bay of Bengal. It is being monitored to see if it will become the eighth pandemic strain [99].

Cholera is spread by eating or drinking contaminated food or water. The organism exists naturally in coastal or brackish waters and can be found in water, plankton, and shellfish. This means raw seafood may be contaminated before it is harvested. Cholera may have been transported around the world by ocean currents and bilge water in transoceanic vessels [9]. In warmer summer months, the organism is more prolific, and the incidence of human infection increases. Infection occurs when a person ingests enough bacteria for some to survive the gastric acid of the stomach and colonize the small intestines. Since infected people shed the bacterium in their feces, cholera can infect other people that ingest contaminated food or water. Cholera spreads rapidly when there is poor sanitation, which exists in much of the developing world. In displaced populations, who have poor access to sanitation and clean water as well as poor nutrition, the risk of cholera increases dramatically. Refugees are constantly at risk.

In Asia, children are more at risk for developing cholera than adults, while in South America adult men are more at risk. It appears that cholera is endemic in Asia and prior infections convey some immunity toward subsequent infections. Although it is now endemic, it has just recently re-emerged in South America, where men appear to have more exposure. Known risk factors for the disease include drinking untreated water, eating uncooked foods such as raw fruits and raw vegetables, eating foods served by street vendors, drinks with ice, and eating seafood from endemic areas [100]. Close contact with an infected person is also a risk factor, but casual contact is not. Theoretically, fishermen harvesting shellfish should be at higher risk but this has not been statistically proved. Sanitation workers are at increased risk, as are refugees and relief workers caring for them. Health care workers that fail to maintain good hygiene have increased risk because of more exposure to contaminated stool. Travelers to areas of endemic cholera are also at risk.

CLINICAL FEATURES

The disease has varying degrees of severity. Patients may have no symptoms or mild diarrhea, or they may have severe, dehydrating diarrhea characterized by large volumes of nonbloody, rice-water stools. The latter is a life-threatening syndrome, and is often called *cholera gravis*. Other symptoms include fever, nausea, vomiting, muscle cramps, and signs of shock.

DIAGNOSIS

The diagnosis of cholera is made by a history of watery stools and exposure to contaminated water or food. The diagnosis can also be made presumptively during an outbreak. Culture of a stool specimen can confirm the diagnosis, but this is not necessary because there are available kits that detect the cholera antigen directly in the stool. However, cultures should be obtained and checked periodically during an outbreak to observe for shifting antibiotic sensitivity of the bacterium.

TREATMENT

The cornerstone of treating cholera is rehydration [101]. Patients are generally categorized into one of three groups: no dehydration or mild dehydration, moderate dehydration, or severe dehydration. Patients who are severely dehydrated have lost about 10% of their body weight in fluids and require intravenous rehydration. Lactated Ringer's solution or normal saline are the fluids of choice. Patients that are less severely dehydrated may be treated with oral rehydration solution (ORS). This is usually available in packets that are mixed with clean water. The solution may also be made from locally available ingredients and there are several different recipes. ORS should be given in amounts to cover continuing stool losses and replace about 5% of body weight. Antibiotics are also helpful in shortening the duration of the disease. A single dose of doxycycline, 300 mg, remains the treatment of choice in areas where cholera is sensitive to it. Ciprofloxacin is used for resistant strains in a single 1-g dose [102]. Children are treated with trimethoprim 5 mg/kg and sulfamethoxazole 25 mg/kg twice daily for three days.

PREVENTION

Cholera is prevented by improving the quality of water supplies and sanitation. In the developing world, the cost of building a proper infrastructure for good sanitation is prohibitive. Thus, prevention strategies shift to improving education about how the disease is spread, making water decontamination methods widely available, licensing and educating street vendors, and thoroughly cooking seafood (cholera may survive light cooking). Other high-risk foods such as raw vegetables and fruits should be avoided [100]. A killed cholera vaccine is available, but it is not used because of short duration of protection and a low level of protection. Other vaccines have been developed and are used in Europe for people traveling to endemic areas. One is a killed oral vaccine and another is a live, attenuated oral vaccine [97]. These are not available in the United States. Prophylactic antibiotics are used during tetracycline-sensitive cholera outbreaks. Members of the immediate household are treated with a single dose of doxycycline, 300 mg. Its use is strictly limited to household contacts because community-wide prophylaxis leads to rapid development of resistant bacterial strains.

Cryptosporidiosis

EPIDEMIOLOGY

Once considered to be only of veterinary importance, the parasite *Cryptosporidium parvum* has emerged as a worldwide cause of human disease. The first human case of *Cryptosporidium* occurred in 1976, and in the 1980s HIV epidemic, many immunocompromised patients developed enteritis caused by this organism [103]. The protozoan pathogen *C parvum* obtained wide media attention in 1993 when it caused a diarrheal outbreak of approximately 400,000 cases in Milwaukee, Wisconsin after contaminating the municipal water supply [106]. Most of the cases involved otherwise healthy, immunocompetent patients.

The protozoan can be transmitted through contaminated water or through food. One outbreak in Maine involved unpasteurized cider obtained from a contaminated cider press. The cider press had probably been contaminated by a calf that was found to be shedding oocysts on the same farm as the cider press [107]. Cows are known to be carriers of the disease and cattle handlers are at increased risk [105]. Several cases of animal-to-human transmission of *Cryptosporidiosis* have been documented. The disease is capable of infecting all mammals but occurs almost exclusively in mammalian newborns. Approximately 50% of dairy calves shed oocysts, and the parasite is present in 90% of dairy farms. Mammalian pets have been implicated, but there is a paucity of supporting data. However, one study showed that 10% of puppies in an Atlanta animal shelter were infected with the pathogen and were shedding oocysts [104].

Besides animal-to-human transmission, human-to-human transmission may occur and is one of the more common modes. Outbreaks have been seen in day care centers where some of the children are still in diapers; transmission can occur either from children to adults changing diapers or from children to other children through intimate play [109]. Nosocomial infections also may occur when medical care workers come in contact with an infected person. High-risk activities for these workers include bathing patients, changing soiled bedding, and emptying bedpans. Patients have also developed nosocomial infections in bone marrow transplant units, pediatric hospitals, and hospital wards with HIV-infected patients. Any sex practice that might involve fecal-oral contact also could cause transmission of the parasite [103].

The *C parvum* parasite is highly infectious. As few as 30 ingested oocysts may cause infection. It also has a high secondary attack rate: Household contacts of the patients in the Maine outbreak had a 15% secondary attack rate, and there was a 58% secondary attack rate in household contacts in an urban slum in Brazil [103]. Outbreaks have also involved swimming pools, wading pools, and water theme parks despite chlorinated water. *C parvum* is highly resistant to chlorination and standard chlorine levels are insufficient [108]. Pools must be disinfected with high concentrations of chlorine for long periods: Either 3 mg/L for 53 hours or 8 mg/L for 20 hours should be adequate [103,104].

CLINICAL FEATURES

Patients usually present with voluminous watery diarrhea, often accompanied by crampy abdominal pain (often after eating), weight loss, flatulence, and malaise. Nausea, vomiting, fever, and myalgias occur less commonly. The incubation period is two to 14 days. The severity of the illness usually correlates with the immune status of the patient. Clearance of the oocysts may lag behind clinical improvement by one to two weeks.

DIAGNOSIS

The diagnosis is made by detection of oocysts in fecal or intestinal biopsy specimens. There are several methods to detect the oocysts, including acid-fast staining, direct immunofluorescent antibody staining, and enzyme-linked immunosorbent assays (ELISA). The sensitivity and specificity of each method is under investigation. Both immunocompromised and immunocompetent patients generate IgG in response to *C parvum*, and serum immunofluorescent and enzyme-linked assays are available to detect these antibodies.

TREATMENT

There is no effective treatment for the disease. In immunocompetent individuals, it is a self-limited disease, although the associated enteritis can be severe. Treatment is supportive and consists of fluid and electrolyte management and antidiarrheal medications such as kaolin plus pectin (Kaopectate), loperamide, diphenoxylate, or bismuth subsalicylate (Pepto-Bismol). The infection is often chronic in immunocompromised patients and leads to wasting. No antibiotic regimen has shown proven benefit. Paromomycin can be tried at a dosage of 500–750 mg three to four times daily. Azithromycin, 1,200 mg twice a day for one day, then 1,200 mg daily for 27 days is an alternative to paromomycin [110].

PREVENTION

Many municipal water supplies are inadequate equipped to prevent contamination of *C parvum*. The exact risk of infection from municipal water is not known and probably varies from city to city. Boiling water for one minute before ingestion will kill the organism. Water that has been filtered through an "absolute" 1-µm or smaller filter will be free of oocysts. Certain activities and occupations put immunocompromised people at risk. They should avoid drinking from lakes or streams, swimming in fresh water, pools or water parks, and having unprotected contact with infected people or animals. Occupations at risk are dairy farmers, cattle farmers, veterinarians, sewer workers, swimming pool or water park personnel, day care workers, and health care workers [104]. Risk can be reduced by observing proper precautions for fecally transmitted disease. People with immunodeficiency might want to avoid some of these occupations because of the severe and chronic nature of *C parvum* infection if contracted in an immunocompromised state.

Cyclospora

EPIDEMIOLOGY

Cyclospora is a unicellular parasite previously classified as a cyanobacterium-like (blue-green algae) or a coccidian-like body. It was identified in 1870 but was not known to cause disease in humans. The first evidence that it might cause disease (cyclosporiasis) came in 1977 when it was isolated from the stool of three individuals in Papua, New Guinea. Two of the three were complaining of diarrhea. Throughout the 1980s, the organism was isolated in various stool samples, but its role in diarrheal disease went unrecognized.

This was partly because it had been classified by so many different identifiers. The first documented outbreak occurred in a hospital dormitory in Chicago [111]. For the next several years there were only isolated cases and small clusters. Then, from May to June 1996, there were over 1,400 cases reported in the United States and Canada. During the following year, there were over a thousand cases reported in the spring and summer [112,113].

Human infection occurs with ingestion of the oocysts. *Cyclospora* appears to have worldwide distribution [114,115]. The incidence of disease is seasonal, coinciding with the spring and summer months in North America and with the warm, rainy seasons in Nepal and Peru. *Cyclospora* infects all ages. Both immunocompetent and immunodeficient individuals can contract the disease. Travelers to the developing world have an increased risk of infection. People native to endemic areas appear to be less susceptible, suggesting that infection may induce some immunity. When excreted in feces, the oocysts take days to weeks to become infectious; thus, direct human-to-human transmission is unlikely. Several of the outbreaks were associated with a contaminated water source, although some of the water sources had adequate chlorination. An outbreak of food-borne *Cyclospora* occurred in 1996. Fresh raspberries imported from Guatemala were identified as the source of the outbreak [11]. Despite trying to limit importation of fresh raspberries to those grown at farms in Guatemala with acceptable water quality and sanitation, another outbreak associated with Guatemalan fresh raspberries occurred the following year. *Cyclospora* has also been transmitted in fresh basil and mesclun lettuce [111,112].

CLINICAL FEATURES

The symptoms of *Cyclospora* infection (cyclosporiasis) include diarrhea, fatigue, anorexia, nausea, weight loss, abdominal bloating and cramping, and gas. Also, fatigue is often a major complaint. The diarrhea is watery and there are frequent, often explosive stools. Myalgias and arthralgia may precede the diarrhea, and a low-grade fever may be present. Cyclosporiasis is usually a self-limited disease that lasts two to six weeks in untreated individuals. In immunocompromised patients, the disease is often prolonged and may be chronic or relapsing.

DIAGNOSIS

Diagnosis is made by isolating oocysts from a stool sample or an intestinal biopsy specimen; a simple acid-fast stain after centrifuge will detect them. When examined, the oocysts appear similar to *Cryptosporidia* in structure, but those of *Cyclospora* are larger. In addition, *Cyclospora* oocysts will autofluoresce under ultraviolet epifluorescence microscopy, and this is a useful technique to distinguish them from those of *Cryptosporidia*. Since the diagnosis of cyclosporiasis is often missed and the sensitivity of detecting *Cyclospora* from stool by the various methods is unknown, a solitary negative stool sample does not rule out this infection. Three or more stool samples should be collected and examined [115].

TREATMENT

Trimethoprim-sulfamethoxazole (TMP-SMX), 160 mg/800 mg twice daily for one week, is the treatment of choice for cyclosporiasis. HIV-infected patients receive the same dose four times a day for 10 days, followed by the same dose three times a week for secondary prophylaxis [116]. No other treatment has proved effective.

PREVENTION

To prevent infection, the usual food and water precautions should be observed in the developing world. In these areas, water should come from a protected, sanitary source or should be boiled before use; chlorination does not appear to prevent transmission. Food should be cooked before eating, and raw fruits and vegetables avoided.

People traveling to developing countries are at risk [114,115]. This includes business travelers, tourists, missionaries, relief workers, development workers, and military personnel. Health care workers are not at increased risk, since direct transmission from human to human is unlikely. Sanitation workers may be at increase risk: One case involved a man exposed to raw sewage, and *Cyclospora* oocysts were isolated from a sewage pipe in his home [117]. Since *Cyclospora* is a newly recognized pathogen, its increasing incidence in humans will likely increase physicians' awareness of the disease and prompt them to consider the diagnosis when a patient presents with gastrointestinal distress, especially when the history reveals recent travel in the developing world. Investigations are being conducted to develop a reliable diagnostic technique.

Transmissible Spongiform Encephalopathies

EPIDEMIOLOGY

There are a group of well-known but rare diseases caused by a protein particle called a *prion*. Before 1986, these diseases were known to occur in animals in the form of scrapies, chronic wasting disease, and transmissible mink encephalopathy and in humans in the form of Creutzfeldt-Jakob disease, Gerstmann-Straussler-Scheinker syndrome, and kuru. Another form, bovine spongiform encephalopathy (BSE), was identified in 1986 in the United Kingdom. Since it was first recognized, more than 170,000 cases in cows had been reported through the end of 1997. It came to be known as "mad cow" disease [118,119]. The source of the infection was determined to be the meat and bone meal used in cattle feed. The leading hypothesis is that cattle were fed a protein meal produced by scrapie-infected sheep carcasses. Alternatively, the disease may have spontaneously arisen in one or more cattle and the practice of feeding cattle parts to more cattle cause the spread of the disease. Kuru, another transmissible spongiform encephalopathy, is known to be transmitted by the cannibalization of infected human brains in the remote highlands of Papua, New Guinea [122].

The danger of BSE passing to humans was always known, and despite protective measures, a new variant form of Creutzfeldt-Jakob disease (CJD) emerged in Britain. An adolescent with CJD died in May 1995. No prior case involving so young a victim had ever been seen. Atypical pathology results confirmed that this was a novel form or new variant of CJD [120].

The question arose as to whether this was the human manifestation of BSE or classic CJD in a new presentation. Circumstantial testing strongly links BSE with new variant CJD (vCJD). A group of mice were inoculated with infectious particles of vCJD, and another group of mice with infectious material from BSE. The diseases that arose were quite similar in lesion profile and incubation period, suggesting that this is the same disease in cattle as it is in man. BSE is now the *probable* cause of vCJD, not just the *theoretical* cause [118]. Besides cattle, BSE has also been found in cats that received parts of cattle's central nervous system in their food and in several zoo animals that were fed parts of cattle, including the central nervous system [119]. The tissues likely to have the highest concentration are the brain, spinal cord, tonsil, spleen, thymus, and intestine (particularly Peyer's patches in the terminal ileum).

The etiology of classic CJD is unclear. Because the disease is worldwide, the incidence is constant at one case per million and no natural transmission pattern could be found, it is hypothesized that the disease arises from spontaneous generation of the prion protein particle by the host's DNA. Inoculation of monkeys with infected CJD tissue caused the disease, demonstrating that transmission of an infectious particle can play a role in the disease. Scrapies has been known to exist among sheep and goats in Great Britain and Europe for 200 years, but it has never before caused infection in humans. It was accidentally brought to the United States in 1947 and has gradually spread, especially among sheep of the Suffolk breed. The hypothetical fear is that scrapie has been transmitted from sheep to cattle, causing BSE, and that just recently it has made the leap to humans in the form of vCJD.

CLINICAL FEATURES

Patients presenting with vCJD are much younger than those with classic CJD. The duration of the illness is relatively long, lasting, on average, 14 months. The first manifestations are often psychiatric, and it can take six to seven months before neurologic signs appear. Frequently there are complaints of dysesthesias or pain in the extremities. Later signs resemble classic CJD, and patients demonstrate ataxia, dementia, and myoclonic, jerking movements.

DIAGNOSIS

The characteristic EEG changes in patients with CJD are not seen in those with vCJD. Magnetic resonance imaging (MRI) and tsting for 14-3-3 protein can be helpful in making the diagnosis. Early evidence suggests biopsy of the tonsil can make the diagnosis. Otherwise, diagnosis must be made by brain biopsy or postmortem examination.

TREATMENT

Currently, effective therapy is available, and treatment is limited to supportive measures [119]. Recommendations by the World Health Organization (WHO) concerning BSE and vCJD have centered on limiting the spread of the disease. No part of an animal that has prions should enter the food chain. Ruminant tissues should not be used in feed for ruminants. In addition, research and surveillance for TSE should be increased [121]. Presently, in the United States and Canada, there is no evidence of vCJD in humans and there are no cases of BSE in ruminants [123–125].

No cases of human-to-human transmission of vCJD have been seen. The likely source of vCJD is BSE-infected cattle parts, but the precise mode of entry into the human body is unknown. No increase in the incidence of the disease has been seen among farmers or slaughterhouse workers. Steps taken by Great Britain have made future food-borne infection extremely unlikely. Except for one case in France, no other country besides Great Britain has had a case of vCJD.

Classic CJD continues to occur rarely and sporadically. It has been known to spread iatrogenically through corneal transplants, contaminated electrode implants, dura mater grafts, and human growth hormone derived from pituitary glands. To limit this risk, the practice of pooling human growth and dura mater grafts has been discontinued [12]. Transmission by blood products is not known to have occurred but is another potential mode of transmission. Reports of 15 cases of CJD among histopathologic technicians, a surgeon, a pathologist, and an orthopedist that collected dura mata indicate that health care workers are at risk for nosocomial transmission [122].

The minimum requirements for decontamination are unknown, and the prion particle seems unusually resistant to conventional methods of sterilization. The CDC advises that percutaneous exposure to blood, cerebrospinal fluid, or tissue from an infected person should be immediately followed by irrigation of the wound with 0.5% sodium hypochlorite. Any skin contact with possibly infectious material should be followed by washing with 1 N sodium hydroxide, and mucous membrane contact should be followed by washing with soap and water. Medical instruments used on people infected with TSE should be incinerated when possible; otherwise they should be sterilized. Sterilization should be by steam autoclave for one hour at 132° C. The instruments should then be immersed in 1 N sodium hydroxide for one hour at room temperature. Finally, they should be immersed in 0.5% sodium hypochlorite for two hours at room temperature [126–128].

References

1. Morse SS. Factors in the emergence of infectious disease. *Emerging Infect Dis* 1995;1(1). Available at *http://www.cdc.gov/ncidod/EID/index.htm.*
2. Lederberg J, Shope RE, Oakes SC Jr. (eds). Institute of Medicine. *Emerging Infections: Microbial Threats to Health in the United States.* Washington, DC: National Academy Press, 1992.
3. Johnson KM. Emerging viruses in context: an overview of viral hemorrhagic fevers. In: Morse SS (ed), *Emerging Viruses.* New York: Oxford University Press, 1993. Pp 46–7.
4. UNDP/World Bank/WHO Special Programme for Research and Training in Tropical Diseases (TDR). *Tropical Diseases: Progress in Research, 1989–1990.* Geneva: World Health Organization, 1991. P 41.
5. Hotez PJ, Zheng F, Long-qi X, et al. Emerging and reemerging Helminthiases and the public health of China. *Emerging Infect Dis* 1997;1(1). Available at *http://www.cdc.gov/ncidod/EID/index.htm.*
6. Ostroff SM, Kozarsky P. Emerging infectious diseases and travel medicine. *Infect Dis Clin North Am* 1998;12(1):231.

7. Centers for Disease Control and Prevention. Malaria surveillance—United States, 1993. *MMWR* 1997; 46:27–47.
8. Palmer D. Plague. In: Gorbach S, et al. (eds), *Infectious Diseases*, 2nd Ed. Philadelphia: Saunders, 1998. P 1569.
9. Wachsmuth IK, Evins GM, Fields PI, et al. The molecular epidemiology of cholera in Latin America. *J Infect Dis* 1993;167:621–6.
10. Wilson M. Advice to travelers. In: Gorbach S, et al. (eds), *Infectious Diseases*, 2nd Ed. Philadelphia: Saunders, 1998. P 487.
11. Herwaldt BL, Ackers ML. (The Cyclospora Working Group.) An outbreak in 1996 of cyclosporiasis associated with imported raspberries. *N Engl J Med* 1997;336:1548–56.
12. Centers for Disease Control. Creutzfeldt-Jakob disease associated with cadeveric dura mater grafts—Japan, January 1979–May 1996. *MMWR* 1997; 46(45):1066–69.
13. Webster RG. Influenza. In: Morse SS (ed), *Emerging Viruses*. New York: Oxford University Press, 1993. Pp 37–45.
14. Wyler DJ. Plasmodium and babesia. In: Gorbach S, et al. (eds), *Infectious Diseases*, 2nd Ed. Philadelphia: Saunders, 1998. Pp 2413–6.
15. Centers for Disease Control. Update: diphtheria epidemic—New Independent States of the former Soviet Union, January 1995–March 1996. *MMWR* 1996; 45(32):693–7.
16. Centers for Disease Control. Addressing emerging infectious disease threats: a prevention strategy for the United States, Executive summary. (Adapted.) *MMWR* 1994;43(RR-5):3.
17. Vainrub B, Salas R. Latin American hemorrhagic fever. *Infect Dis Clin North Am* 1994;8(1):47–59.
18. Doyle TJ, Bryan RT, Peters CJ. Viral hemorrhagic fevers and hantavirus infections in the Americas. *Infect Dis Clin North Am* 1998;12(1):95–110.
19. Mertz GJ, Hjelle BL, Bryan RT. Hantavirus infection. *DM* 1998;44:3.
20. Schmaljohn C, Hjelle B. Hantaviruses: a global disease problem. *Emerging Infect Dis* 1997;3(2). Available at *http://www.cdc.gov/ncidod/EID/index.htm*.
21. Centers for Disease Control and Prevention. Prevent Hantavirus Pulmonary Syndrome. (Updated 6/24/98.) Available at *www.cdc.gov/ncidod/diseases/hanta/hanta.htm*.
22. Centers for Disease Control and Prevention. Hantavirus: Laboratory Information. (Updated 6/24/98.) Available at *www.cdc.gov/ncidod/diseases/hanta/labguide*.
23. Centers for Disease Control. Hantavirus pulmonary syndrome—southwestern United States: interim guidelines for risk reduction. *MMWR* 1993;42(No RR-11):1.
24. Levis L, et al. Genetic diversity and epidemiology of hantavirus in Argentina. *J Infect Dis* 1998;177:529–38.
25. Mills JN, Childs JE. Ecological studies of rodent reservoirs: their relevance for human health. *Emerging Infect Dis* 1998;4(3). Available at *http://www.cdc.gov/ncidod/EID/index.htm*.
26. Wells RM, et al. An unusual hantavirus outbreak in southern Argentina: person-to-person transmission? *Emerging Infect Dis* 1997;3(2). Available at *http://www.cdc.gov/ncidod/EID/index.htm*.
27. Zeitz PS, Graber JM, Voorhees RA, et al. Assessment of occupational risk for hantavirus infection in Arizona and New Mexico. In: *Abstracts of the 35th Interscience Conference on Antimicrobial Agents and Chemotherapy*. Washington, DC: American Society of Microbiology, 1995. P 190.
28. Centers for Disease Control and Prevention. Hantavirus pulmonary syndrome—Chile, 1997. *MMWR* 1997;46:949–51.
29. Khan AS, Khabbaz RF, Armstrong LR, et al. Hantavirus pulmonary syndrome: the first 100 U.S. cases. *J Infect Dis* 1996;173:1297–303.
30. Childs JE, Korch GW, Glass GE, et al. Epizootiology of hantavirus infections in Baltimore; isolation of a virus from Norway rats and characteristics of infected rat populations. *Am J Epidemiol* 1987;126:55–68.
31. Niklasson B, et al. Temporal dynamics of Puumala virus antibody prevalence in voles and of nephropathia epidemica incidence in humans. *Am J Trop Med Hyg* 1995;53:134–40.
32. Prochoda K, et al. Hantavirus-associated acute respiratory failure. (Letter.) *N Engl J Med* 1993;23:1744.
33. Vainrub B, Salas R. Latin America hemorrhagic fever. *Infect Dis Clin North Am* 1994;8(1):47–59.
34. Mills JN, Ellis BA, McKee KT Jr, et al. A longitudinal study of Junin virus activity in the rodent reservoir of Argentine hemorrhagic fever. *Am J Trop Med Hyg* 1992;47:749.
35. Centers for Disease Control. Bolivian hemorrhagic fever—El Beni Department, Bolivia, 1994. *MMWR* 1994;43:943.
36. Salas R, de Manzione N, Tesh RB, et al. Venezuelan haemorrhagic fever. *Lancet* 1991;338:1033
37. Kilgore PE, et al. Prospectives for the control of Bolivian hemorrhagic fever. *Emerging Infect Dis* 1995;1(3). Available at *http://www.cdc.gov/ncidod/EID/index.htm*.
38. Coimbra TLM, Nassar ES, Burattini MN, et al. New arenavirus isolated in Brazil. *Lancet* 1994;343:391–2.
39. Barry M, Russi M, Armstrong L, et al. Brief report: treatment of a laboratory-acquired Sabia virus infection. *N Engl J Med* 1995;333:294.
40. Centers for Disease Control. Update: management of patients with suspected viral hemorrhagic fever—United States. *MMWR* 1995;44:475–9.

41. Barrera Oro JG, McKee KT Jr. Toward a vaccine against Argentine hemorrhagic fever. *Bull Pan Am Health Organ* 1991;25:118.

42. Centers for Disease Control. Prevention of plague: recommendations of the ACIP. *MMWR* 1996;45(No. RR-14).

43. Chanteau S, Ratsifasoamanana L, Rasoamanana B, et al. Plague, a reeemerging disease in Madagascar. *Emerging Infect Dis* 1998;4(1). Available at *http://www.cdc.gov/ncidod/EID/index.htm.*

44. Centers for Disease Control. Human plague—India, 1994. *MMWR* 1994;43(38):689.

45. Edison M, Tierny LA, Rollag OJ, et al. Feline plague in New Mexico: risk factors and transmission to humans. *Am J Public Health* 1988;78:1333–5.

46. Centers for Disease Control. Human plague case—Bernadillo County, New Mexico. *MMWR* 1975; 24:90.

47. Centers for Disease Control. Human plague—Texas, New Mexico. *MMWR* 1981;30:137.

48. Kaufman AF, et al. Public health implications of plague in domestic cats. *J Am Vet Med Assoc* 1981;179:875.

49. Welty TK. Plague. *Am Fam Phys* 1986;33:159.

50. Ramirez-Ronda CH, Garcia CD. Dengue in the Western Hemisphere. *Infect Dis Clin North Am* 1994; 8:107–28.

51. Centers for Disease Control and Prevention. Information on dengue fever and dengue hemorrhagic fever. (Updated March 1998). Available at *www.cdc.gov/ncidod/disease/dengue.htm.*

52. Halstead SB. Dengue viruses. In: Gorbach S, et al. (eds), *Infectious Diseases*, 2nd Ed. Philadelphia: Saunders, 1998. Pp 2237–42.

53. Centers for Disease Control. Dengue fever at the U.S.–Mexico border, 1995; 1996. *MMWR* 1996;45:841.

54. Kouri G, Guzman MG, Valdes L, et al. Reemergence of dengue in Cuba: A 1997 epidemic in Santiago de Cuba. *Emerging Infect Dis* 1998;4(1). Available at *http://www.cdc.gov/ncidod/EID/index.htm.*

55. Gubler DJ, Clark GG. Dengue/dengue hemorrhagic fever: the emergence of a global health threat. *Emerging Infect Dis* 1995;1(55–7). Available at *http://www.cdc.gov/ncidod/EID/index.htm.*

56. Kanesa-thasan N, Gwong-Jen JC, Smoak BL, et al. Molecular and epidemiological analysis of degue virus isolates from Somalia. *Emerging Infect Dis* 1998;4(1). Available at *http://www.cdc.gov/ncidod/EID/index.htm.*

57. Schreck CE. Protection from blood-feeding arthropods. In: Auerbach PS (ed), *Wilderness Medicine*, 3rd Ed. St. Louis: Mosby, 1995. Pp 813–30.

58. Pan American Health Organization. *Dengue and Dengue Hemorrhagic Fever: Guidelines for Prevention and Control.* Washington, DC: PAHO, 1994. Vol. 12, No 3.

59. Pan American Health Organization. Venezuelan encephalitis. In: Proceedings of the Workshop Symposium on Venezuelan Encephalitis Virus. Washington, DC: PAHO, 1972.

60. Rivas F, Diaz LA, Cardenas VM, et al. Epidemic Venezuelan encephalitis in La Guajira, Columbia, 1995. *J Infect Dis* 1997;175:828–32.

61. Centers for Disease Control. Venezuelan equine encephalitis—Columbia, 1995. *MMWR* 1995;44: 721–4.

62. Weaver SC, Salas R, Rico-Hesse R, et al. Re-emergence of epidemic Venezuelan equine encephalomyelitis in South America. *Lancet* 1996;348:436–40.

63. Sanford JP. Arbovirus infections. In: Wilson JD, et al. (eds), *Harrison's Principles of Internal Medicine*, 12th Ed. New York: McGraw-Hill. Pp 727–8.

64. Peters CJ, Linthicum KJ. Rift Valley fever. In: Beran GW (ed), *Handbook Series of Zoonoses*, 2nd Ed. Baco Raton, FL: CRC Press, 1994. Pp 125–38.

65. Centers for Disease Control and Prevention. Rift Valley Fever Fact Sheet. (Updated 1998.) Available at *www.cdc.gov/ncidod/disease/rift valley fever factsheet.htm.*

66. World Health Organization. Emerging and other communicable diseases. Disease outbreaks reported, 28 January 1998: Rift Valley fever and hemorrhagic disease in Kenya and Somalia. Updated March 1998. Available at *www.who.ch/emc/oldnews.htm.*

67. Centers for Disease Control. Rift Valley fever—Egypt, 1993. *MMWR* 1994;43:693, 699–700.

68. Centers for Disease Control and Prevention. Rift Valley fever—East Africa, 1997–1998. *MMWR* 1998; 47:261–4.

69. Fontenille D, Traore-Lamizana M, Diallo M, et al. New vectors on Rift Valley fever in West Africa. *Emerg Infect Dis* 1998;4(1).

70. Johnson K. Viral hemorrhagic fevers. In: Morse SS (ed), *Emerging Viruses.* New York: Oxford University Press, 1993. P 54.

71. Monath TP. Arthropod-borne viruses. In: Morse SS (ed), *Emerging Viruses.* New York: Oxford University Press, 1993. Pp 143–4.

72. Evans TG. Leishmaniasis. *Infect Dis Clin North Am* 1993;7:527–46.

73. Report of the World Health Organization Expert Committee. Control of leishmaniasis. *WHO Tech Rep Ser* 1990;793:1.

74. Evans TG, McAuliffe IT, Vasconcelos IDAB, et al. Epidemiology of visceral leishmaniasis in Northeast Brazil. *J Infect Dis* 1992;166:1124.

75. Arias AR, Monteiro PS, Zicker F. The reemergence of visceral leishmaniasis in Brazil. *Emerging Infect Dis* 1996;2(2). Available at *http://www.cdc.gov/ncidod/EID/index.htm.*

76. Marsden PD, Warren JD. Leishmania. In: Gorbach S, et al. (eds), *Infectious Diseases*, 2nd Ed. Philadelphia: Saunders, 1998. Pp 2420–6.

77. Centers for Disease Control. Viscerotopic leishmaniasis. *MMWR* 1992; 41:131.

78. Gilbert DN, Moellering RC, Sande MA. *The Sanford Guide to Antimicrobial Therapy*, 28th Ed. Vienna, VA: Antimicrobial Therapy, 1998:87.

79. McKee KT. Marburg and Ebola viral diseases. In: Gorbach S, et al. (eds), *Infectious Diseases,* 2nd Ed. Philadelphia: Saunders, 1998. Pp 2258–60.

80. Breman JG, van der Groen G, Peters CJ, et al. International colloquium on Ebola virus research: summary report. *J Infect Dis* 1997;176:1058–63.

81. Centers for Disease Control and Prevention. Ebola virus hemorrhagic fever: general information. (Updated 5/28/98.) Available at *www.cdc.gov/ncidod/virfvr/ebolainf.htm.*

82. Sanchez A, Ksiazek TG, Rollins PE, et al. Reemergence of Ebola virus in Africa. *Emerging Infect Dis* 1(3). Available at *http://www.cdc.gov/ncidod/EID/index.htm.*

83. Georges-Courbet MC, Sanchez A, Chang-Yong L, et al. Isolation and phylogenetic characterization of Ebola virus causing different outbreaks in Gabon. *Emerging Infect Dis* 1(3). Available at *http://www.cdc.gov/ncidod/EID/index.htm.*

84. Le Guenno B, Formentry P, Wyers M, et al. Isolation and partial characterization of a new strain of Ebola virus. *Lancet* 1995;345:1241.

85. Centers for Disease Control. Update: Ebola-related filovirus infection in nonhuman primates and interim guidelines for handling nonhuman primates during transit and quarantine. *MMWR* 1990;39:22–4, 29.

86. Centers for Disease Control. Update: Filovirus infection in animal handlers. *MMWR* 1990;39:221.

87. Centers for Disease Control. Update: Filovirus infections among persons with occupational exposure to non-human primates. *MMWR* 1990;39:266–7, 273.

88. Centers for Disease Control. Update: management of patients with suspected viral hemorrhagic fever—United States. *MMWR* 1995;44:475–9.

89. Cox NJ, Fukuda K. Influenza. *Infect Dis Clin North Am* 1998;12(1):27–38.

90. Webster RG. Influenza. In: Morse SS (ed), Emerging viruses. New York: Oxford University Press, 1993. Pp 37–57.

91. Webster RG. Influenza: an emerging infectious disease. *Emerg Infect Dis* 1998;4(3). Available at *http://www.cdc.gov/ncidod/EID/index.htm.*

92. Centers for Disease Control. Isolation of avian influenza A(H5N1) viruses from humans—Hong Kong, May–December 1997. *MMWR* 1997;46:1204–7.

93. Centers for Disease Control. Update: isolation of avian influenza A(H5N1) viruses from humans—Hong Kong, 1997–1998. 1998;46:1245–7.

94. World Health Organization. Influenza A(H5N1). (WHO Fact Sheet 188, updated January 1998.) Available at *www.who.ch/emc/oldnews.htm.*

95. Smith CB. Influenza viruses. In: Gorbach S, et al. (eds), *Infectious Diseases*, 2nd Ed. Philadelphia: Saunders, 1998. Pp 2120–5.

96. Centers for Disease Control. Prevention and control of influenza: recommendations of the ACIP. *MMWR* 1997;46(no. RR-9).

97. Gotuzzo E, Cieza J, Estremadoyro L, et al. Cholera lessons from the epidemic in Peru. *Infect Dis Clin North Am* 1994;8:183–205.

98. Centers for Disease Control. Cholera associate with an international airline flight, 1992. *MMWR* 1992; 41:134–5.

99. Morris JG, Losonsky GE, Johnson JA, et al. Clinical and immunological characteristic of vibrio cholera O139 Bengal in North American volunteers. *J Infect Dis* 1995;171:903–8.

100. Tauxe RV, Mintz ED, Quick RE. Epidemic cholera in the New World: translating field epidemiology into new prevention strategies. *Emerging Infect Dis* 1995;1(4). Available at *http://www.cdc.gov/ncidod/EID/index.htm.*

101. Centers for Disease Control. Update: cholera—Western Hemisphere, and recommendations for the treatment of cholera. *MMWR* 1991;40:562–5.

102. Khan WA, Bennish ML, Seas C, et al. Randomised controlled comparison of single dose ciprofloxacin and doxycycline for cholera cause by vibrio cholera O1 or O139. *Lancet* 1996;348:296–300.

103. Guerrant RL. Cryptosporidiosis: an emerging, highly infectious threat. *Emerging Infect Dis* 1997;3(1). Available at *http://www.cdc.gov/ncidod/EID/index.htm.*

104. Juranek DD. Cryptosporidiosis: sources of infection and guidelines for prevention. CDC. Updated 5/28/98. Available at *www.cdc.gov/ncid/dpd/sources.htm.*

105. Peng MM, Xiao L, Freeman AR, et al. Genetic polymorphism among *Cryptosporidium parvum* isolates: evidence of two distinct human transmission cycles. *Emerg Infect Dis* 1997;3(4):567–73.

106. MacKenzie WR, Hoxie NJ, Proctor ME, et al. A massive outbreak in Milwaukee of *Cryptosporidium* infection transmitted through the public water supply. *N Engl J Med* 1994;331:161–7.

107. Millard PS, Gensheimer KF, Addiss DG, et al. An outbreak of cryptosporidiosis from fresh-pressed apple cider. *JAMA* 1994;272:1592–6.

108. Kramer MH, Herwaldt BL, Craun BF, et al. Surveillance for waterborne disease outbreaks—United States, 1993–1994. *MMWR* 1996;45:1–33.

109. Cordell RL, Addiss DG. Cryptosporidiosis in child care settings: a review of the literature and recommendations for prevention and control. *Pediatr Infect Dis J* 1994;13:310–7.

110. Gilbert DN, Moellering RC, Sande MA. *The Sanford Guide to Antimicrobial Therapy*, 28th Ed. Vienna, VA: Antimicrobial Therapy, 1998. P 86.

111. Huang P, Weber JT, Sosin DM, et al. The first reported outbreak of diarrheal illness associated with *Cyclospora* in the United States. *Ann Intern Med* 1995; 123(6):409–14.

112. Centers for Disease Control and Prevention. Update: outbreaks of cyclosporiasis—United States and Canada, 1997. *MMWR* 1997;46:521–3.

113. Centers for Disease Control. Update: outbreak of cyclosporiasis—northern Virginia–Washington, D.C.–Baltimore, Maryland, metropolitan area, 1997. *MMWR* 1997;46:689–91.

114. Soave R. Cyclospora: an overview. *Clin Infect Dis* 1996;23:429–37.

115. Soave R, Herwaldt BL, Relman DA. Cyclospora. *Infect Dis Clin North Am* 1998;12:1–12.

116. Pape JW, Verdier RI, Boncy M, et al. Cyclospora infection in adults infected with HIV: clinical manifestations, treatment, and prophylaxis. *Ann Intern Med* 1994;121:654–57.

117. Hale D, Aldeen W, Carroll K. Diarrhea associated with cyanobacterialike bodies in an immunocompetent host: an unusual epidemiological source. *JAMA* 1994;71:144.

118. Schonberger L. New variant Creutzfeldt-Jakob disease and bovine spongiform encephalopathy. *Infect Dis Clin North Am* 1998;12:111–21.

119. Pattison J. The emergence of bovine spongiform encephalopathy and related diseases. *Emerg Infect Dis* 1998;4(3). Available at *http://www.cdc.gov/ncidod/EID/index.htm.*

120. Will RG, Ironside JW, Zeidler M, et al. A new variant of Creutzfeldt-Jakob disease in the UK. *Lancet* 1996;347:921–5.

121. Centers for Disease Control. WHO consultation on public health issues related to bovine spongiform encephalopathy and the emergence of a new variant of Creutzfeldt-Jakob disease. *MMWR* 1996;295–6:303.

122. Asher DA. Transmissible spongiform encephalopathies. In: Gorbach S, et al. (eds), *Infectious Diseases*, 2nd Ed. Philadelphia: Saunders, 1998. Pp 2283–98.

123. Centers for Disease Control. Surveillance for Creutzfeldt-Jakob disease—United States. *MMWR* 1996;45:665–8.

124. Stratton E, Ricketts MN, Gully PR. The epidemiology of Creutzfeldt-Jakob disease in Canada: a review of mortality data. *Emerging Infect Dis* 1997;3(1). Available at *http://www.cdc.gov/ncidod/EID/index.htm.*

125. Holman RC, Khan AS, Belay ED, et al. Creutzfeldt-Jakob disease in the United States, 1979–1994: using national mortality data to assess the possible occurrence of variant cases. *Emerging Infct Dis* 1996;2(4). Available at *http://www.cdc.gov/ncidod/EID/index.htm.*

126. Jarvis WR. Precautions for Creutzfeldt-Jakob disease. *Infect Control* 1982;3:238–9.

127. Committee on Health Care Issues, American Neurological Association. Precautions in handling tissues, fluids, and other contaminated materials from patients with documented or suspected Creutzfeldt-Jakob disease. *Ann Neurol* 1986;19:75–7.

128. Brown P. Guidelines for high-risk autopsy cases: special precautions for Creutzfeldt-Jakob disease 1990. In: *Autopsy Performance and Reporting 1990.* Northfield, IL: College of American Pathologists, 1990. Pp 68–74.

38 / Emerging Microbial Diseases of the Indoor Environment

Elissa Ann Favata, Harry M. Neill, and Chin S. Yang

Exposure to microbiologic aerosols in the indoor environment has emerged as a significant health concern both in residential and occupational settings. Epidemiologic and case studies have revealed that 33% of indoor air quality problems are related to microbial contamination [1,2]. Because people in industrialized nations spend more than 90% of their time indoors, often with sole reliance on mechanical ventilation in airtight buildings, the potential for indoor air exposures has increased [3].

The principal indoor microbial contaminants of concern include fungi, bacteria, viruses and, less frequently, protozoa. Not only must intact microorganisms be considered as etiologic agents of disease, but so must their cell wall constituents (endotoxin and ß-[1→3]-*D*-glucan) and metabolites (mycotoxins and volatile organic compounds). These bioaerosols, which are airborne particles that are living or originate from living organisms, have an ubiquitous presence in life. However, health risks are posed by their presence when problematic environmental conditions (such as wetted porous building materials) provide an appropriate substrate for growth of mold and gram-negative bacteria, and building systems and occupant activities foster their amplification and dissemination. Microbiologic and epidemiologic studies have shown that sources of indoor moisture, elevated relative humidity, and mold growth on walls, in heating and ventilating systems and within wall cavities, are associated with bioaerosol contamination and adverse health effects in building occupants [4–12]. In the investigation of housing characteristics that led to microbiologic contamination in the Canadian community of Wallaceburg, Ontario, indoor moisture sources were found to be significant factors in mold levels and dust-mite antigen contamination [13]. Moreover, home or building dampness and flooding have been associated with respiratory, dermal, neurologic and constitutional symptoms, asthma, hypersensitivity pneumonitis, and other immunologic abnormalities [14–20].

The recognition of indoor sources of microbial growth and/or concerns regarding potential building-related health problems serve as sentinel events heralding the involvement of health professionals. When physicians are called upon to evaluate patients with health problems related to indoor microbial exposure, they are faced with multiple complex challenges. Clearly, the microbial source, transmission, and associated health outcome are shaped by the societal, technologic, and environmental conditions impacting human hosts, each of whom has individual susceptibilities. An appreciation of the dynamic interactions of these factors is essential to the understanding of indoor-air-quality problems.

Although the industrial hygiene paradigm of recognition, evaluation, and control/remediation can be simplistically applied in the assessment of indoor microbial contamination, a comprehensive systematic problem-oriented approach needs to be developed for each evaluation. This investigative strategy should follow the scientific method: data gathering and identification of the problems, both environmental and medical; hypothesis development; diagnostic testing; and remediation/control, followed by testing the effectiveness of intervention. However, despite an orderly approach, the investigation of indoor air microbiologic issues is fraught with many complexities, including:

- The knowledge base for understanding biologic aerosols and their pathophysiologic effect is still evolving. Moreover, the building occupant is most often simultaneously exposed to multiple environmental offending agents, microbial and nonmicrobial, and the effect of this mixture of exposures (i.e., synergistic, additive, or antagonist) is not yet known. Clinically, dose-response data is lacking.
- There are limitations of knowledge and technology regarding testing methods, microbiologically and clinically.
- Regarding interpretation of sampling data for bioaerosols, there are no quantitative guidelines that are analogous to chemical toxin threshold limit values or permissible exposure limits.
- Psychosocial issues associated with indoor air quality problems may not only affect the reliability of subjective information obtained during problem characterization, but also may interfere with problem resolution even after appropriate remediation/control measures have been carried out.

Along with the unique investigative strategies required for assessment of microbial contamination of the indoor environment, development of a similarly unique multidisciplinary collaboration of microbiologists, industrial hygienists, engineers, and health professionals is necessary. Members of this team utilize their individual expertise to cooperatively reach a full understanding of the indoor microbial exposure and its association with adverse health effects.

Clearly, while current knowledge regarding indoor microbial contamination and related diseases is evolving, health professionals and environmental consultants daily face complex "real world" problems. This chapter addresses indoor microorganisms, with specific focus on fungi and bacteria, namely their impact on health, both environmental and clinical evaluations, and finally, methods of remediation.

Microbial Sources, Agents, and Effects

Fungi and bacteria are ubiquitous in the natural environment. Some fungi and bacteria are soil-borne or associated with the root system or leaves. Many fungi and bacteria are inhabitants of fruits, produce, and foodstuffs. These fungi and bacteria, after becoming airborne, may be carried into building environments by air streams and become part of the indoor environment. In these indoor environments, the prevalent airborne fungi are similar to those detected outdoors, principally *Cladosporium*, *Penicillium*, *Aspergillus*, *Alternaria*, basidiomycetes and, less often, *Acremonium*, *Trichoderma*, *Drechslera*, and *Epicoccum* [2,21–23]. However, if conditions allow (for example, water damage of a building material substrate or excessive humidity), some fungal spores and bacteria, principally gram-negative organisms, may grow and develop into active colonies. These colonies may release more spores and bacteria and also microbial volatile organic compounds (MVOCs). Fungal spores are particularly problematic because they are known allergens [24,25] and may contain mycotoxins in both the viable and nonviable states [26]. Several fungi commonly found indoors have been reported to produce mycotoxins, including immunosuppressive chemicals, such as cyclosporin [27] and stachybotrylactones [28,29], and carcinogens, such as aflatoxins. In addition, gram-negative bacteria are known to release endotoxins, which are lipopolysaccharide components of their outer cell wall.

RESERVOIRS, AMPLIFIERS, AND DISSEMINATORS

Airborne microbial populations depend on the presence of a source or reservoir of the microorganism, a means for the microorganism to multiply (amplify), and a mechanism for dissemination [30]. Fungi and bacteria that grow indoors are saprophytes—that is, they may feed on organic nutrients in the environment or on building materials of an organic nature. Also, the available moisture content, expressed as water activity, is a critical factor affecting fungal growth indoors [31]. Paper and wood products are particularly susceptible to the cellulolytic fungi and bacteria. Species of Basidiomycetes, *Chaetomium*, *Chrysosporium*, *Stachybotrys*, and *Trichoderma*, all known producers of cellulases, are frequently detected and identified in water-damaged building materials. Fast-growing colonizers, such as species of *Acremonium*, *Aspergillus*, *Cladosporium*, *Penicillium*, and *Ulocladium*, are also commonly found on water-damaged materials. Further descriptions of other fungal growth factors can be found in several texts and reviews [25,32–34]. In addition, gram-negative bacteria, including species of *Acinetobacter*, *Methylobacterium*, *Pseudomonas*, and *Stenotrophomonas*, are common contaminants of water-damaged materials or stagnant water in building systems. Filamentous bacteria (Actinomycetes) occasionally grow indoors in wet and damp conditions.

Often, mechanical devices or structures in a problem building, such as contaminated humidifiers, water towers, or heating, ventilating and air conditioning (HVAC) ducts, may serve as both reservoirs and amplifiers, or amplifiers and disseminators, of indoor microorganisms [30]. There have been observations that mites and insects may be attracted to fungal growth and feed on fungal matter, potentially facilitating spore and bacterial dissemination. Also, dispersal of fungal spores and gram-negative bacteria may be increased by disturbances in a room caused by occupant activities or, to a greater degree, by building renovation. The risk for microbial-dissemination during the latter makes the decision regarding occupancy during building remedi-ation even more critical.

SPORE RELEASE, LONGEVITY, AND VIABILITY

Fungi reproduce by means of spores, which survive for a period until suitable ambient conditions provide an environment for germination, growth, and continued spore production and dissemination. Spore release may be active or passive, peaking during certain hours of the day or night [1,35]. Accordingly, results of air sampling (as well as the potential for occupant exposure) may vary, based on this periodicity of discharge. Exposure and sampling may also be complicated by (1) the extended viability of spores (conidia of *Penicillium* and *Aspergillus* have been reported to be viable for over 12 years [36]) and (2) the fact that some spores are viable but not culturable. Finally, although not all airborne fungal spores are viable, they are potentially allergenic and may contain mycotoxins [1]. It is generally recognized that this potential allergenicity depends on an individual's genetic composition and previous sensitization. In a moldy building, occupants are very likely to become sensitized due to repeated and possibly large-dose exposures. Therefore, it is important that both clinicians and environmental investigators recognize and identify the extent and types of mold growth in a contaminated building.

MYCOTOXINS

Many fungi are known to produce various secondary metabolites that are toxic to humans and animals. These principally nonvolatile, low-molecular-weight by-products of fungal metabolic processes are called *mycotoxins* [34,37–39]. A comprehensive review of mycotoxins is beyond the scope of this chapter, but the topic is fully addressed in many review articles [37,38,40–44]. The most frequently studied mycotoxins are produced by species of *Aspergillus*, *Fusarium*, *Penicillium*, *Stachybotrys*, and *Myrothecium* [45]. Historically, reports of mycotoxicosis in animals and humans have been principally associated with ingestion of moldy hay and grain and the recurrent health outcomes of immunosuppression and opportunistic infection. Other reported mycotoxin-related health effects have included interference with pulmonary macrophage function or macrophage death, release of mediators of inflammation, cardiovascular problems (e.g., tachycardia, hypotension), neurologic effects, and carcinogenicity [45]. (Aflatoxins, which are produced by *Aspergillus flavus* and *Aspergillus parasiticus*, are the most potent known natural carcinogens. Specifically, they cause liver cancer.)

Concern regarding indoor airborne mycotoxin exposure has stimulated interest in inhalation exposure. Although routes of exposure for mycotoxins include inhalation, dermal exposure, and ingestion, inhalation has been deemed the primary route of exposure for these and other bioaerosols. Moreover, evaluation of toxicity of doses delivered via varied exposure routes in animals has revealed that inhalation of a specific mycotoxin, T-2 toxin, has a toxic potency that is of an order of magnitude higher than that administered intravenously [46]. Because the majority of mycotoxins are nonvolatile, mycotoxin exposure via inhalation is most likely associated with spore inhalation. Many recent case studies of bioaerosol inhalation exposures have focused on one particular mycotoxin group, the trichothecenes, considered by many mycologists, biochemists, and toxicologists to be one of the most toxic chemicals produced by nature [47] and the most potent small-molecule inhibitor of protein synthesis. Several fungi, including *Memnoniella echninata*, *Stachybotrys chartarum*, *and* some species of *Trichoderma*, *Aspergillus*, and *Penicillium* are commonly found in water-damaged materials and have been documented to produce trichothecenes. However, it is important to note that most fungi have not been investigated for their toxigenic potential. Therefore, "non-toxigenic" fungi may be only temporarily classified as such.

Investigations of water-damaged residences and offices have revealed subjective health complaints, including headache; eye, nose, and throat irritation; cough; chest tightness; wheezing; diarrhea; dermatitis; focal alopecia; fatigue; malaise. Objective findings of pulmonary hemosiderosis/hemorrhage in infants and T-cell abnormalities have also been reported [6,20,48,49]. Although associations of these health outcomes with exposure to toxin-producing strains of *S chartarum* have been drawn, the actual role for exposures to this fungus and its mycotoxins, or to it in combination with other fungal and bacterial contaminants, requires further investigation [45].

MICROBIAL VOLATILE ORGANIC COMPOUNDS

Microbial metabolism produces not only mycotoxins, but also microbial volatile organic compounds (MVOCs). Actively growing fungi and bacteria (including actinomycetes) produce various MVOCs both by primary metabolism, which extracts energy from nutrient molecules for essential cell component use, and secondary metabolism, which is not essential to maintaining the life of an organism and requires extra energy. An extensive listing of MVOCs and their producers has been compiled from the literature [50]. Current interest in MVOCs is based on (1) use of their moldy odors and specific compounds as markers of microbial growth (even when not visible) and (2) their potential adverse health effects [50]. When attempting to evaluate microbial exposures, it must be understood that, like mycotoxins, MVOCs produced in a laboratory may differ from those produced in nature because of the lack of control of growth condition variables such as temperature, pH, oxygen content, age of culture, moisture, and nutrients.

The health effects associated with exposures to MVOCs have not yet been fully documented, investigated, or studied. However, there have been suggestions that MVOCs contribute to the symptoms and complaints of some building occupants, such as mucous membrane and respiratory tract irritation, exacerbation of asthma, cacosmia, and central nervous system symptoms of headache, inability to concentrate, and dizziness [50,51].

β-(1→3)-D-GLUCANS

Microbial cell wall constituents, such as β-(1→3)-*D*-glucan and endotoxin, have been associated with health problems of occupants of water-damaged indoor environments. β-(1→3)-*D*-glucan is a polyglucose polymer found in the cell wall of plants, fungi, and certain bacteria [52]; it is a potent immunomodulator [52–54]. Epidemiologic studies have linked glucan exposure with airway inflammation, headaches, and fatigue in occupants of damp buildings [52,55,56]. However, there is lack of clarity as to whether these building-related health effects were specifically due to glucan exposure, as opposed to exposure to a mixture of fungi and bacteria and their cell wall constituents and metabolites.

ENDOTOXIN

In the cell wall of gram-negative bacteria, endotoxin contains lipopolysaccharide as part of the complex (with protein and other lipids) and may be released from the bacterial cell wall in various complex forms during active cell growth, division, or death [57].

Similar to other bioaerosols, airborne endotoxin is ubiquitous outdoors, except perhaps during times of snow cover. Elevated levels of indoor endotoxin have been associated with contaminated humidifiers, water-damaged building materials, and industrial settings where organic dust or recirculated water-based or metalworking fluids have been aerosolized [58]. In the recreational setting, outbreaks of endemic granulomatous pneumonitis have been attributed to endotoxin exposure from an indoor swimming pool [59]. Although low-level endotoxin exposures have been associated with building-related symptoms and increased severity of asthma, the health outcome of inhalation fever, manifested as fever, malaise and respiratory inflammation (i.e., cough, chest discomfort), has been associated with exposure to higher levels of gram-negative bacteria and endotoxin in buildings [60].

In summary, regarding microbial sources and agents, in a water-damaged environment, various species of fungi and bacteria (particularly gram-negative bacteria) may proliferate. It is very likely that building occupants are exposed to mixtures of fungi (and their spores) and bacteria of various species, as well as to mycotoxins, MVOCs, endotoxin, and glucans. Health effects should therefore be assessed with the recognition of this complex exposure mixture.

Health Effects

BUILDING-RELATED SYMPTOMS AND ILLNESS

In considering the health effects associated with indoor air exposures, it is important to address some terms that are frequently encountered in the literature as well as in daily life. The term *sick building syndrome*, now referred to as *building-related symptoms (BRS)*, has been used to describe nonspecific symptoms that are not associated with a specific pollutant or source in the building but temporally occur when occupants are present in the "problem" building and diminish or cease when occupants leave. BRS do not conform to a specific objective diagnostic entity; the spectrum of symptoms may include headache; eye, nose and throat irritation; dry cough; nausea; skin dryness and irritation; dizziness; fatigue; difficulty concentrating; and sensitivity to odors. In contrast, *building-related illness (BRI)* is caused by a specific agent and conforms to a diagnosable disease. The current lack of objective environmental causal agents, physical findings, and diagnostic test results does not, however, diminish the importance of BRS. In fact, several studies have implicated airborne microbial cell wall constituents (endotoxin or ß-[1→3]-*D*-glucan) or microbial metabolites (mycotoxins or volatile organic compounds), along with inadequate ventilation and off-gassing from building materials, as potential causative factors in the development of BRS [61].

Another perspective on building-related health problems categorizes the health endpoints as (1) clinically evident diseases for which a causal link can be established to an indoor pollutant by specific diagnostic tests, (2) exacerbation of established disease, such as asthma, and (3) perceptions of indoor pollutant exposure and disease [62]. The first two are subsequently discussed. However, the last category is important to note, as the effect of these perceptions may often lead to significant stress in an individual occupant of a building or groups of occupants, which in turn, acutely or chronically may induce immune alterations and vulnerability to disease [63,64]. Also, stress can lead to psychological impairment, which may even become severe enough to disable the worker from employment and adversely affect his or her quality of life. Finally, such perceptions of exposure and disease may actually impede resolution of indoor-air-quality problems, despite the most well-intentioned and comprehensive evaluation and remediation. These significant consequences underscore the need for competence and professionalism on the part of the indoor-air-quality investigators and for full disclosure and continued communication by all involved in addressing indoor air problems.

EXPOSURE CHARACTERIZATION AND HOST FACTORS

Health risks that are potentially associated with indoor environmental contamination must be assessed by systematic review of (1) the contaminant source/agent, (2) the exposure of the building occupant, (3) the unique susceptibilities of the occupant (host), and (4) subjective and objective findings obtained during a comprehensive medical evaluation.

Bioaerosol exposures of the building occupant pose unique circumstances that are far different from exposures associated with chemicals, for which a more exact dose of exposure can be ascertained. Reliable and accurate bioaerosol sampling, analysis, and interpretation of data are essential to assessing environmental contaminants. However, the results obtained from bioaerosol sampling are subject to variability, depending on many ambient and temporal factors, including available nutrient sources, temperature, humidity, light sources, diurnal patterns of spore release, and activity in the sampling area (quiescent/active). Accordingly, the exact dose of a bioaerosol can rarely be measured, and bioaerosol sampling results are used as a surrogate for exposure dose [65].

The exposure of the building occupant to microbial contaminants can be further characterized by considering (1) the mode of bioaersol transmission and exposure routes (i.e., inhalation, mucosal, dermal, or ingestion), (2) variables affecting absorption (size of particles and chemical composition of offending agents, indoor activity of occupant and resultant respiratory rate, clothing worn, and use of respiratory and dermal protective equipment), and (3) the duration of exposure.

Host factors also influence an individual's response to a particular microbial exposure [66]. Pre-existing immune differences, such as allergic disorders or atopy, increase one's susceptibility to respond to environmental allergens. In a review of rhinitis and inhalant allergens, the predisposition to respond to environmental allergens was noted to occur in 13% of children when neither parent was atopic, in 30% if one parent or sibling was atopic, and in 50% if both parents were atopic [67]. Immunosuppression is also a well-known host factor that increases one's vulnerability to varied infections. Pre-existing nonspecific bronchial hyperresponsiveness is another host risk factor that may be exacerbated by exposure to particulates and irritants, such as fungal volatile organic compounds. Finally, investigation of exposure to *S chartarum* and the health outcome of pulmonary hemosiderosis or hemorrhage in infants less than 12 months of age, predominately males, revealed age and gender to be host risk factors [48,49].

SPECIFIC HEALTH ENDPOINTS

The adverse health effects associated with fungal and gram-negative bacterial cell wall constituents and metabolites have already been discussed, and general issues of building-related symptoms and health perceptions, as well as building-related illness, have been characterized. This section addresses specific health endpoints related to bioaerosol exposure in the indoor environment. These disorders, which have diverse pathophysiologic mechanisms and clinical manifestations, include hypersensitivity diseases, inhalation fever, infections, and toxic and irritant effects. (Toxic and irritant effects have been discussed in earlier sections that describe mycotoxins and MVOCs.) For all of these bioaerosol-exposure-related conditions, inhalation is the primary route of exposure and the lung is the target organ most frequently affected, although systemic adverse effects also may occur.

Hypersensitivity Diseases

Hypersensitivity disorders, including allergic rhinitis/sinusitis and asthma, and hypersensitivity pneumonitis, are among the most common bioaerosol-related diseases. Sensitization to an antigen is common to all and requires (1) genetic capability to respond to the antigen, (2) sufficient exposure to the antigen and immunostimulating substance, and (3) time for the specific immune reaction to occur [68].

Allergic rhinitis and asthma are type I (IgE-mediated) hypersensitivity diseases, which are associated with an inherited predisposition to react to antigen exposure with formation of IgE (atopy). Allergic rhinitis affects approximately 22% of the U.S. population [69,70] and accounts for 3.5 million lost workdays annually [71]. It clinically presents with nasal itching, irritation, and congestion; watery nasal discharge; sneezing; itching of the eyes, ears, and throat; and fatigue. Epidemiologic studies have noted comorbidity between allergic rhinitis and asthma, with allergic rhinitis having precedence. Asthma is diagnosed in up to 38% of patients with rhinitis [72]. Asthma is characterized by chronic airway inflammation and intermittent episodes of bronchospasm. A 60% increase in the incidence of asthma has been noted over the past two decades, with concomitant doubling of the mortality rate [73]. Both allergic rhinitis, which may be complicated by sinusitis, and asthma are triggered by exposure to allergens of microbial origin and multiple other allergens (e.g., dust mites, cockroach feces, and animal dander). Also, airways may respond with hyperreactivity to irritant chemical and particulate exposure.

Hypersensitivity pneumonitis, also known as *extrinsic allergic alveolitis*, is a spectrum of inflammatory, granulomatous, interstitial, bronchiolar, and alveolar pulmonary disease [74]. It is caused by continuous or repeated inhalation exposures, and sensitization to bioaerosols (i.e., bacteria, fungi, animal proteins [avian], and low molecular weight chemicals [isocyanates]). Onset usually occurs four to 12 hours after exposure.

In its acute form, hypersensitivity pneumonitis may present as recurrent bouts of fever, chills, malaise, shortness of breath, cough, chest tightness, and myalgias. Physical findings may be normal, nonspecific, or those of bibasilar crackles on lung auscultation, with chest radiographs revealing normal findings, diffuse patchy infiltrates, or a ground-glass appearance [74]. With continued chronic exposure, there is recurrent illness manifested as flu-like symptoms and insidious progression of cough, shortness of breath, and fatigue. Pulmonary function tests may reveal a restrictive pattern, with decreased diffusing capacity. Marked lymphocytosis, without eosinophilia or neutrophilia, is found on bronchoalveolar lavage, and the results of lung biopsy reveal inflammatory infiltrates at sites distant from granulomas [74]. Although the findings of specific precipitating antibodies may be positive and are evidence of an immunologic reaction, the presence of these markers does not imply their involvement in disease pathogenesis. In the chronic form of hypersensitivity pneumonitis, irreversible lung damage and associated gas exchange impairment may occur [62]. Several epidemiologic studies have linked hypersensitivity pneumonitis with exposure to microbial contamination of ventilation systems and, more recently, to endotoxin-containing respirable bioaerosol exposures at an indoor swimming pool [11,12, 16,59,75,76].

Inhalation Fever

Inhalation fever differs from hypersensitivity pneumonitis in that it is an acute, short-term, benign, self-limited reaction. It is produced by inhalational exposure to unrelated agents such as metal or polymer fumes or bioaerosols such as organic dusts or humidifier mists. The principal symptoms are fever, chills, myalgias, cough, headache, general malaise, and chest discomfort. Onset of symptoms usually occurs four to eight hours after exposure; symptoms subside within 12 to 48 hours if exposure does not continue. Also, there is a tolerance pattern—that is, symptoms diminish with repeated daily exposures. However, with prolonged absence and then return to exposure, the symptoms recur [77–79]. Physical findings, pulmonary function tests, and chest radiographs are usually normal, although an increased erythrocyte sedimentation rate and polymorphonuclear leukocytosis are common. In contrast to the bronchoalveolar lavage findings of lymphocytosis in patients with hypersensitivity pneumonitis, those of patients with inhalation fever reveal an increase in neutrophils. Treatment is symptomatic and there are no reported sequelae [62,77].

Infections

Infections due to indoor microbial contamination principally include legionellosis, tuberculosis, other airborne bacterial infections, airborne viral infections, and systemic fungal infections. Both legionellosis and tuberculosis are fully discussed in other chapters in this text and thus are not addressed here. Airborne viral infections, such as common colds, influenza, measles, varicella and rubella, and the airborne bacterial diseases of pneumococcal origin, are contagious diseases that are transmitted from person to person. The risk of their aerosol transmission is increased by recirculated air, low ventilation rates, and increased occupant density. Therefore, the prevention of viral and bacterial airborne infection can be enhanced by mechanical HVAC delivery of adequate ventilation that is appropriate to occupant density as well as by appropriate use of immunizations.

The health endpoint of systemic fungal infection is determined by the immune status of the host, coupled with predispositions for fungal exposure such as (1) location in endemic geographic areas, where moisture conditions foster specific fungal growth, (2) exposure to settings associated with fungal sources and dissemination, and (3) the size of the fungal inoculum. For example, the organisms *Histoplasma capsulatum* and *Coccidioides immitis* are both soil-borne fungi. However, the former organism flourishes in moist environments, such as the Mississippi River Valley, whereas *C immitis* is found associated with dry soil, mainly in the southwestern United States. Accordingly, there is an increased prevalence of infection of *H capsulatum* and *C immitis* in these respective geographic locations. Also, *Cryptococcus neoformans* and *H capsulatum* have been recovered from bird droppings and bat excrement. These organisms have been disseminated indoors through contaminated HVAC units and construction dusts as well as during maintenance activities, with resultant infections in building occupants [80–85]. Finally, an immunocompromised host is at increased risk for severe infection by *all* of the above fungi, as well as by the opportunistic, thermotolerant fungus *Aspergillus fumigatus* [86,87].

Evaluation

Microbial contamination of the indoor environment presents unique and complex issues that require a systematic problem-oriented approach for their complete assessment and resolution. A comprehensive investigative strategy is used to identify offending microbiologic agents and their sources, correlate medical findings with results and data of environmental investigation, and formulate medical treatment and environmental control in order to reduce or eradicate exposures. The fundamental components of this strategy are data gathering and identification of the problems, both environmental and medical; hypothesis development; diagnostic testing; and remediation/control, followed by testing for effectiveness of intervention. Further discussion of these steps can be found in the literature [88,89]. However, the essential details of this problem-oriented approach are as follows:

- Review of presenting problem and available records.
- Characterization of complaint (health and building conditions).
- Site investigation (evaluation of sources of biologic agents).
- Hypothesis formation.
- Evaluation of bioaerosol and environmental conditions.
- Medical evaluation.
- Interpretation of data.
- Recommendation of corrective measures.
- Remediation.
- Validation of effectiveness.

In order for the above approach to be effective in resolving the microbial indoor air problem, it is important that it be carried out by qualified professionals who are experienced in the investigation of microbial issues. A multidisciplinary collaboration of industrial hygienists, engineers, microbiologists, and environmental and occupational health professionals is essential for such evaluations. In addition, it is of significant value to include in the investigation of each specific indoor air problem, "building team members" who are affected by indoor air quality issues, such as occupants, facility managers and staff, administrators, owners, and designers. The multidisciplinary team of professionals needs to employ common sense and professional judgment in carrying out the problem-oriented approach and must also effectively communicate their findings, assessed risks, and remediation plans to those who are potentially impacted by the building problem.

In addition, formation of an indoor-air-quality task force composed of all "building team members," with involvement of the multidiscipinary professionals, for the purpose of defining the current problem and planning remediation collectively, with full disclosure of all information, improves the opportunity to resolve the indoor-air-quality problem. Not only can the indoor-air-quality task force address the psychosocial issues of trust and credibility, but also prospective primary and secondary preventive efforts can be designed, leading to improved future indoor air quality.

MEDICAL EVALUATION

The unique complexities related to indoor microbial contamination challenge environmental and occupational medicine physicians asked to evaluate potentially related health effects. Although the problem-oriented approach offers a framework for solution of bioaerosol problems, multiple difficulties arise when attempting to characterize exposure, document disease, identify causal linkages, and intervene and manage disease [90,91]. This applies to the evaluation of individuals as well as assessment of health risks of cohorts in a public health setting. Nevertheless, these limitations in knowledge and the technical difficulties related to exposure mixtures, dose-response data, characterization of health endpoints, and diagnostic testing must not impede physicians' assistance of patients. Clinical decisions must be made based on the current available evidence, professional judgment, common sense, and a true sense of caring for the patient's physical and mental well-being. Therefore, the medical evaluation should be approached as follows:

- The occupational and environmental medical history is the cornerstone of the evaluation. It characterizes the specific health complaints (nature, frequency, duration, their temporal onset and improvement, and relation to building location); building problems, particularly in areas that the patient occupies (e.g., evidence of leaks, stained ceiling tiles, moldy odors, mold growth, poor maintenance); occupational history, outlining work duties, exposures (e.g., microbials, chemicals, and particulates), personal protective equipment, and engineering controls employed; recreational and residential exposures; individual habits (smoking/tobacco/recreational drug use); past medical history, including pre-existing diseases (e.g., allergies, hyperreactive airways); medications; family history; and review of systems.
- A comprehensive, detailed physical examination is imperative.
- Diagnostic testing should individualized in accordance with the outcome of the history and physical examination and the suspect target organ possibly affected by the exposure. For example, if symptoms of building-related cough, chest tightness, and wheeze occur, peak flow measurements and, if possible, pre- and post-shift spirometry should be carried out.

  Regarding specialized laboratory tests, there are concerns regarding costs and the clinical use of tests with inadequately defined sensitivity, specificity, and predictive value. For example, in the case of suspected mycotoxin and chronic antigen exposure, immunologic (lymphocyte subset) abnormalities have been noted [20,92]. However, under normal physiologic conditions, taking into account the effects of smoking, stress, drugs, age, gender and diurnal variations, there is variability in the number and percentage distribution of immune system components in blood [63,64,93]. It is therefore the opinion of these authors that such immunologic tests should not be employed routinely in the clinical setting but rather should be included in investigational protocols addressing the health effects of bioaerosol exposure.
- Referral to subspecialists should be carried out as needed for further diagnostic testing and treatment, e.g., allergists for skin testing.
- Data obtained in the building investigation, e.g., bioaerosol sampling results, should be reviewed.
- After the above steps have been accomplished, the physician should define the diagnosis and establish whether a causal association between the disease and the building environment exists.

Pharmacologic treatment should begin as soon as a disease has been appropriately diagnosed. If a causal linkage between disease and exposure has been established, decisions about medical removal of the individual, and possibly other building occupants, need to be made on a case-by-case basis. In making these decisions, the following factors should be considered:

1. Character and severity of the health problem.

2. Extent and type of microbial contamination.
3. Specific risk factors of the individual, such as immunocompromised health status, age (infants less than 12 months old and the elderly), pregnancy, and past history of hypersensitivity disease or chronic inflammatory respiratory disease.
4. If remediation is planned, assessment regarding occupancy should depend on whether methods of containment would be adequate to prevent building occupant exposure.

- Finally, after both remediation and reoccupancy have occurred, surveillance of individuals with building-related illnesses should be conducted. Protocol components and surveillance duration should be uniquely determined to address the specific clinical issue.

ENVIRONMENTAL EVALUATION

Building Investigation

The first and most important step in approaching any potential microbiologic problem related to a building's structure is to have individuals experienced in the evaluation of microbiologic issues and building systems perform visual inspections of the structure and of the heating, ventilation, and air-conditioning (HVAC) system(s). This detailed visual inspection is the most important step of the environmental evaluation because all other decision making regarding sampling (type and number of samples to be collected), structural and HVAC evaluation methods, and assessment of potential health effects are primarily based on the investigator's initial visual findings. Interviews with building occupants may also impact sampling decisions.

Visual Inspection. The visual inspection should include, but not be limited to, the following:

- Interior and exterior of the structure to detect potential migration (pathways) of moisture.
- Identification of areas or sources, causes, and pathways of moisture migration (e.g., liquid flow, capillary action, condensation, HVAC system, structural).
- Identification of structure type. (Certain structural assemblies and materials are conducive to moisture migration and provide substrates for growth if wetted.)
- Location of crawl spaces, which contribute to moisture build-up and potential growth of microbes.
- Identification of areas of suspected growth of microbes for characterization sampling and delineation of potential remediation.
- Identification of areas of potential hidden microbial growth, e.g., wall, floor, and roof assemblies.
- Assessment of the mechanical hygiene (dirt, moisture carry-over from coils, condition of interior insulation and linings, and potential microbiologic amplification) of the HVAC system's air-handling units and portions of the air conveyance systems.

Interviews with Occupants. Interviews with the building occupants should be conducted concomitantly to gain a better understanding of the moisture history, the presence of characteristic odors in the structure ("musty," "earthy," "moldy"), and a general understanding of the potential health issues.

Structural and Mechanical Evaluation. Some components of the structural and mechanical evaluation may be conducted during the visual assessment. Measurement and evaluation should include the following:

- Review of structural and mechanical design drawings in relation to actual installation.
- Temperature and relative humidity measurements inside and outside the building and in the crawl spaces and structural assemblies, to check for potential condensation problems and moisture build-up.
- Moisture probe measurements for excess moisture in wall, floor and roof assemblies, as indicated by visual inspection and interviews.
- Use of smoke tubes or pressure measurement devices to identify potential pathways of air flow and moisture migration, e.g., from crawl spaces to occupied spaces.
- In addition to visual inspection, use of a fiberoptic boroscope to view the inside of the

ductwork and air-handling units for potential problems.

Finally, if indicated, professional mechanical and/or structural engineers should evaluate the structural assemblies and HVAC system design, operation, and maintenance for problems contributing to the moisture that could be causing microbiologic amplification.

Microbial Sampling, Analyses, and Interpretation

In addition to careful review of the building history and visual inspection by an experienced environmental professional, assessing indoor fungal and bacterial contamination requires bioaerosol evaluation by means of air sampling. Suspected contamination should be collected by source sampling and confirmed to be fungal or bacterial growth or both. This approach not only identifies the source(s) of contamination but also facilitates medical diagnosis and eventual remediation and control of fungal and bacterial growth.

Air Sampling. In a medically based investigation, both clinicians and environmental consultants should work together and decide what possible offending etiologic agents to sample. Air sampling for culturable fungi, fungal fragments, bacteria, endotoxin, or total spore counts is often used to determine microbiologic loading in a building and potential human exposure. However, it must be kept in mind that currently available air sampling technology is often carried out for a short period of time, and therefore the results usually do not reflect the temporal and spatial differences and fluctuations of airborne fungi and bacteria. Also, although sampling and testing for mycotoxins and fungal surrogates (e.g., ergosterol) are possible [94], these applications have not been widely used.

When planning for air sampling, the following issues must be considered: which sampler has better collection efficiency, what media to use, when and how long to sample, how many samples to take, what to compare a sample to, which microbiology laboratory to use, and what to do with the results.

A number of air samplers for culturable fungi and bacteria and for total spore counts are available. These samplers are widely used by allergists, industrial hygienists, and environmental professionals. Sampling for culturable fungi and bacteria includes passive techniques, such as the settling method, and volumetric samplers. The settling method favors larger spores and its usefulness is limited. There are many available volumetric samplers. Three commonly used samplers are discussed in the following paragraph. There are also air samplers for total spore counts. Sampling for culturable fungi yields results reflecting the identities and viability of spores. It may take one to two weeks for analysis. Results of total spore counts may be available in hours or in days. However, the viability of spores is not known and the identities of spores are presumptive at best.

The volumetric samplers for culturable fungi are the Andersen single stage N-6 impactor (Andersen N-6), the Reuter Centrifugal Sampler, and the Surface Air System sampler. (The Andersen N-6 is popular with industrial hygienists and environmental consultants.) Other models of these three samplers are also available. Several new samplers have been introduced over the last two to three years; however, these have not been scientifically evaluated and validated. All samplers of cultural fungi require a device containing nutrient media to receive fungal spores and bacteria and allow them to grow into colonies. Many different fungal and bacterial media are available. For the general fungal population, 2% malt extract agar (MEA) and rose bengal agar are often used. For specific fungi, such as *S chartarum* (*S atra*), cornmeal agar (CMA) or Czapek cellulose agar (CCA) is preferred. Other fungal media may be used if they are available. Bacterial media include tryptic soy agar (TSA), R2A agar, and nutrient agar.

One should keep in mind that the three commonly used samplers each collect "grab samples," usually for less than 15 minutes (most often for 1–8 minutes). Taking into consideration the spatial and temporal variability of airborne fungi and bacteria, it is necessary to obtain a sufficient number of samples in order to draw a more realistic picture of actual fungi and bacteria in the air.

Conclusions should not be based on only a few air samples.

For total spore counts, spores are collected either on a membrane filter or on grease-coated slides. Filter cassettes powered with industrial hygiene pumps can be used. The Burkard spore trap (available from the manufacturer in England or from distributors in the United States) and Allergenco samplers collect spores and particles on a grease-coated 1" × 3" glass slide. A disposable cassette has been recently introduced in the United States for the collection of airborne particles, including fungal spores. This new device is commercially called *Air-O-Cell* and has been widely used in conjunction with the Andersen sampler. Other sampling devices for total spore counts are also available. This sampling method is not suitable for collecting bacterial particles.

Airborne endotoxin is collected with an endotoxin-free polycarbonate, 0.4-μm pore-size filter cassette with a pump running at 2–4 L/min. An air volume of at least 240 L or higher is recommended.

Source Sampling. Neither fungi nor bacteria grow in the air; they originate on surfaces or in substrates. Many building materials, such as ceiling tiles, wallboard, wallpaper and soiled fiberglass insulation, are well-known substrates for fungal or bacterial growth, or both, when they become wet or retain moisture. Water stains, discoloration, mildew, or sooty growth are signs of fungal and/or bacterial growth. Wipe samples, taken with sterile swabs or bulk samples of the materials, should be collected for analysis. Reference samples from "clean" surfaces or from similar materials may be collected for comparison: Elevated fungal and/or bacterial levels dominated by one or two fungal types or by gram-negative bacteria are often indications of fungal or bacterial amplification.

To quickly confirm fungal growth on surfaces, a clear sticky tape can be used to remove "growth." The tape is then examined directly under a compound microscope. This procedure provides qualitative, descriptive results. Identification of fungi is possible if sufficient fungal characters are seen on the tape samples. This method is not suitable for bacterial sampling because bacterial cells are too small for detection by microscopic examination.

Environmental endotoxin is collected by vacuuming contaminated dust into an endotoxin-free polycarbonate filter cassette with a high volume pump. A measurable amount of dust (preferably 1 g or more) is required for proper endotoxin analysis. Water samples may be collected with an endotoxin-free 25-mL vial. When shipped to a laboratory for analysis, these samples should be packed in ice.

Sample Analyses. When selecting a microbiology laboratory, it is important that the laboratory professionals include a competent mycologist or a microbiologist with extensive mycology training. Not only can knowledgeable mycologists and microbiologists identify fungi and bacteria, but they also can identify the possible sources of various fungi and bacteria, their health implications, and effective control measures.

Air samples for environmental fungi and bacteria are generally incubated at room temperature (between 20–28° C). However, if detection of *A fumigatus* or other thermotolerant fungi and bacteria is the main reason for sampling, the incubation temperature should be 35–37° C. Enumeration and identification are usually completed in seven to 10 days.

After wipe or bulks samples are obtained, they are extracted, diluted serially, and inoculated onto fungal and bacterial media. No direct inoculation should be allowed, because environmental samples often include a mixture of fungi and bacteria. All samples should be incubated at the appropriate temperature range. For fungi in general, MEA and an additional medium should be used. MEA is the medium used by most mycologists to study and describe fungi in culture. For slow-growing fungi, such as *S chartarum*, use of a low nutrient medium, such as CMA or CCA, provides a better chance of recovery of this microorganism. For xerophilic fungi (fungi growing at low water activity), DG18 is the medium of choice. Many indoor fungal contaminants, including species of *Aspergillus*, *Eurotium* and *Wallemia*, are xerophilic. For culture of bacteria, TSA, R2A, or nutrient agar may be used. If sampling is performed for detection of thermophilic actinomycetes, incubation should be conducted at 45–55° C.

Samples taken for total spore counts using a membrane filter can be cleared, stained with biologic dyes, and examined and counted under a compound microscope at a magnification of 400× or higher. Samples applied to grease-coated slides can be stained and examined directly.

The current analytical method of choice for endotoxin is the *Limulus* amebocyte lysate (LAL) assay. Recent advances allow the LAL reagent to be specific to bacterial lipopolysaccharide (LPS) without the interference of glucan and other impurities. Several variations of the LAL method are commercially available, including the gel-clot, the turbidimetric assay, and the kinetic chromogenic method. The kinetic chromogenic method is much more accurate, sensitive, and reproducible than the gel-clot or turbidimetric method and has become the method of choice for endotoxin analysis [95].

Interpretation. Because there are no generally accepted numeric guidelines or standards for assessment of fungal and bacterial bioaerosol exposure in indoor environments, comparative sampling is necessary. For practical purposes, outdoor samples and samples taken from a nonproblematic location are collected as a reference for comparison. Although the American Conference of Governmental Industrial Hygienists (ACGIH) has provided numeric guidelines for interpretation of bioaerosol data in previous documents [96], the current 1999 publication does not support any existing numeric criteria for interpreting data on biologic agents from building material sources or air samples in nonmanufacturing environments [61]. In keeping with current recommendations put forth by ACGIH [61], interpretation of possible indoor fungal and bacterial exposures should focus on:

- Comparison of indoor versus outdoor concentrations.
- Comparison of species' composition indoors and outdoors (with accurate identification of fungal species, not just identification of genus).
- Detection of the presence of indicator species in the indoor environment (such as a toxigenic fungi, e.g., *Stachybotrys chartarum* or *Aspergillus versicolor*) that are uncommon outdoors.

In general, indoor fungal and bacterial concentrations should be similar to, or lower than, outdoor concentrations. Residential buildings are usually leaky and tend to have fungal and bacterial levels similar to outdoor levels. It must be kept in mind that comparison of indoor and outdoor fungal and bacterial sample results require both expert and commonsense consideration of factors, such as the seasonal outdoor conditions. For example, with snow cover, the indoor fungal concentrations in nonproblematic buildings may exceed the outdoor concentrations [61]. Indoor fungal and bacterial species composition should also be similar to outdoors. If significant levels of fungi and gram-negative bacteria are found only indoors, this often suggests indoor amplification of the fungi. Furthermore, the detection of some fungi in the air, even at low levels, may require further evaluation. The presence of slimy-spored toxigenic fungi, such as *S chartarum* or *Fusarium verticillioides* (also called *F moniliforme*), suggests an indoor contamination source. In addition, the consistent detection of some fungi, such as species of *Aspergillus*, *Paecilomyces*, *Penicillium* and *Wallemia*, may indicate water damage, excessive humidity, or fungal amplification. Finally, identification of a particular fungus in an indoor environment sample does not, in and of itself, allow the conclusion that the building occupants are being exposed to antigenic or toxic agents [61]. Such a conclusion requires careful consideration of the results of all components of environmental and medical evaluations and the use of professional judgment.

Additional concerns regarding bacterial bioaerosols are as follows:

- The presence of actinomycetes (especially thermophilic) indoors suggests an indoor source, as they are relatively rare outdoors.
- Indoor bacteria may contain large populations of human-shed bacteria such as *Micrococcus*, *Staphylococcus*, and *Streptococcus.* These bacteria have been identified on human skin and hair and in sinus and oral cavities. Elevated ambient levels of these gram-positive organisms may be reflective of high occupant density, poor building maintenance, or inadequacy of ventilation. They should be excluded when performing comparisons of indoor and outdoor bacterial populations.

- A predominance of gram-negative bacteria in air may suggest the presence and aerosolization of contaminated water [61].

Results of total spore counts often have limited use because they usually have low detection sensitivity and wide standard deviations, and the spores can only be presumptively identified. In practice, total spore counts are used to estimate the airborne spore load in a heavily contaminated environment. However, if spore counting and quantification procedures can be standardized and standard deviations can be greatly reduced, the total spore count method may be a better assessment tool for exposure to airborne fungal spores than culturable fungal sampling.

Results of wipe and bulk samples give strong indications as to whether a sample is contaminated or not. A contaminated sample often results in a pure culture or a mixture of no more than two to three fungi. A high fungal level dominated by one or two fungi is suggestive of fungal amplification in situ. Contaminated materials or surfaces can then be removed or disinfected. Samples with high bacterial levels suggest wet and damp conditions.

Although guidelines for a no-effect level for environmental endotoxin were proposed [97], the guidelines were based on data collected from agricultural and industrial settings. Whether the guidelines can be applied to the indoor environment remains to be decided. For practical purposes, comparative sampling and analysis of indoor and outdoor endotoxin levels, and of indoor complaint and noncomplaint areas, are recommended. In addition, ACGIH has recently proposed a comparison of endotoxin levels in the suspect contaminated environment with simultaneously determined background levels, using relative limit values (RLV). This comparison has been suggested because of the recognition that endotoxin levels that are 10- to 100-fold higher than background levels are frequently associated with adverse health effects. Therefore, remedial actions are recommended when endotoxin exposures exceed (1) the RLV action level (10 times background levels) in the presence of symptoms and (2) the maximum RLV (30 times background) in the absence of symptoms [61].

Remediation

It is of primary importance that conditions leading to indoor fungal and bacterial growth, particularly moisture infiltration or condensation, be corrected before the remediation of microbial contamination, or there is a risk of recurrence of such growth.

In general, removing microbial growth is accomplished by *source removal*, meaning that porous materials which are extensively contaminated are removed from the structure under controlled conditions. Nonporous materials with surface microbial growth should be cleaned and treated. During remediation, moisture should be kept at levels that do not support microbial growth. Documents such as books and contracts can be fumigated or freeze-dried in an isolated chamber, high-efficiency particulate air (HEPA) vacuumed (in some cases), or perhaps copied.

General containment procedures, based on the size of the area affected and the growth characteristics of certain fungi [98,99] have been proposed. Various types of controls are employed to prevent dust or spore transmission from the work areas and for protection of workers performing the remediation. Other factors, including but not limited to, the types and distributions of the organisms isolated, location of the proposed remediation in the building, and use/occupancy of the building with microbial contamination, need to be considered by the professional who is categorizing the extent of the contamination and identifying remediation work areas. These factors, along with professional judgment, may change the containment procedures and remedial techniques.

Basic remedial procedures or techniques are:

- Isolation (also called *source containment*).
- Removal of contaminated porous materials in a manner that creates as little dust as possible.
- HEPA vacuuming of surfaces, work areas, and containment areas.
- Washing of nonporous materials, work areas, and containment areas (with or without biocides).
- Quick and thorough dehumidification and drying of work areas and materials.

ISOLATION

Source containment can be as simple as the use of plastic bags for the removal of moldy ceiling tiles [61]. "Tent enclosures" (some of which are commercially available) can be constructed of polyvinyl chloride (PVC) pipes or wood frames, covered by two sheets of polyethylene sheeting, and transported for localized remedial efforts, i.e., for the removal of contaminated sections of dry wall or ceiling tiles. Large-scale containments must be employed for the remediation of extensively contaminated areas or materials; *critical barriers* (two layers of polyethylene sheeting), decontamination/air lock unit(s), and HEPA-filtered negative-air machines are used for these containments. The decontamination unit and an air lock are used for the transport of bagged debris from the work area and for worker decontamination. To prevent the dissemination of bioaerosols to adjoining areas, all containment should be kept under negative pressure by use of a HEPA-filtered negative-air machine.

HEPA VACUUMING

HEPA-filtered vacuums should be used to vacuum the work areas, nonporous materials, and areas immediately outside the containment of settled dusts. Contaminated materials should be double bagged, and the surfaces of the bags should be HEPA vacuumed and wiped clean prior to transport outside the containment. Before the containment is dismantled, each layer of the polyethylene sheeting and the remediation tools should also be HEPA vacuumed to rid them of settled dusts that may have been generated during the remediation process.

WASHING AND BIOCIDE USE

Washing, with or without biocides, should be conducted with the use of a minimal amount of water and a damp rag. The question that is often asked is whether biocides should be used in the remediation process or may ordinary detergent be employed. Some professionals discourage the use of biocides for remediation of fungal contamination because of the potential adverse health effects associated with exposure for cleanup personnel, the potential residual biocide exposure for eventual occupants of the building, and possible negative environmental effects. However, if biocides are used according to manufacturer's instructions and their purpose is well defined, they may prove a valuable adjunct to the other specified cleaning procedures [99]. Descriptions of classes of biocides and their properties are available in publications from the American Conference of Governmental Industrial Hygienists [61] and the American Industrial Hygiene Association [100].

Consideration of factors such as safety during biocide application, the potential presence of residual biocide, biocide's effectiveness against the microbial contaminant(s), and extent of use that is necessary helps determine if biocides should be used [61]. Certain states may have training and certification requirements for those who apply biocides. There are, however, some basic precautions to be taken when applying biocides [61]:

- Never apply biocides in occupied buildings.
- Never spray biocides in operating HVAC systems.
- Personnel who apply biocides must be trained and use appropriate personal protective equipment to protect against exposure via all potential exposure routes.
- The possibility of the presence of residual biocides must be minimized.
- Any remaining microbial growth or fragments of organisms should be removed, to the extent possible, by HEPA vacuuming.

DEHUMIDIFICATION AND DRYING

Because water may be used in the remediation process and the remediation may expose damp structural materials or crawl spaces, the moisture content of structural materials as well as the relative humidity should be controlled. Containment areas undergoing washing may require the use of dehumidification units and air circulation to dry the surfaces quickly and thoroughly. Moisture and humidity control is the best strategy for controlling microbial growth [101]. Therefore, the relative humidity at the surface needs to be controlled; an effective approach is to maintain relative humidity at surfaces below 60%. Locally wet surfaces resulting from leaks and condensation may support microbial growth and should be dried as quickly as possible, preferably before remediation begins.

HVAC SYSTEM REMEDIATION

The same basic procedures described above should be used for remediation of the HVAC system. Particular emphasis should be placed on the removal and disposal of contaminated porous materials, such as HVAC duct linings and sound dampening materials, as opposed to simply vacuuming or treating them with biocides and antimicrobial coatings. There are commercially available closed-cell duct linings that afford a strong, virtually nonporous surface and that may be used as replacement materials. Contaminated porous linings in HVAC systems should be cleaned to the bare metal under controlled conditions, using isolation, negative pressurization of the ducts, HEPA filtration of the discharge air from the ducts, and HEPA vacuuming of the air-handling unit and air conveyance system.

The same general precautions for the application of biocides (see page 711) apply to their use in air conveyance systems. Most important, biocides must not be applied to operating HVAC systems or systems to be operated soon after application. If so, the air conveyance system could act as a pathway and driving force to spread the biocide throughout the service area, potentially exposing occupants. Some professionals believe that additional research into the potential health impacts on occupants of a building after the application of biocides in ductwork is needed. The U.S. Environmental Protection Agency (EPA) publishes a document on residential duct cleaning [102] that underscores this need.

PERSONNEL: HEALTH CONCERNS

Personal Protective Equipment

Health and safety professionals and occupational health physicians should select the appropriate personal protective equipment (PPE) for personnel performing microbial remediation on a case-by-case basis [61]. Minimal protection may include the use of even an N-95 respirator approved by the National Institute for Occupational Safety and Health (NIOSH) and work gloves for the removal of even a small amount of contaminated materials such as a few ceiling tiles. Personnel working in containment areas, where extensive removal of materials is carried out, should use eye protection and complete dermal protection such as Tyvek, and an N-95 (half- or full-face) respirator or a type of respirator with even higher respiratory protection factors, for example, a powered air-purifying respirator (PAPR). If biocides are applied, the appropriate chemical cartridge should be used. A complete respiratory protection plan should be developed and implemented, including a medical monitoring component. Guidance for respirator selection and respirator program development is available from NIOSH, the Occupational Safety and Health Administration (OSHA), and the American National Standards Institute (ANSI).

Fitness-for-Duty Evaluations

A physician experienced in evaluating risks and clinical outcome of exposure to indoor microbial contamination should make the medical decision regarding an individual's fitness for remedial employment in such environments. Medical examinations should fully evaluate any pre-existing conditions that would render the employee more vulnerable to the adverse health effects of microbial exposures or that would be exacerbated by the use of protective equipment, such as allergy (rhinosinusitis and dermatitis), hypersensitivity pneumonitis, inhalation fever, asthma, hyperreactive airways, and immunosuppression. Individuals who are immunocompromised or have a history or hypersensitivity reactions to microbial contaminants should avoid working in such environments [98].

Summary

It is clear that excess moisture and elevated humidity in indoor environments have been associated with microbial contamination and adverse health effects, particularly respiratory problems. It is equally clear that this microbial contamination is composed of a mixture of fungi (their spores) and gram-negative bacteria, and their cell wall constituents and metabolites. In both the clinical and research settings, application of a systematic problem-oriented approach to complex indoor microbial contamination issues, utilizing the expertise of a multidisciplinary team of professionals, is the most effective strategy. As knowledge in this area of science evolves, it is essential for investigators to accurately and responsibly draw conclusions regarding associations between exposure to microbial mixtures and resultant disease. Moreover, causal linkages between *specific* microbial etiologic agents and health endpoints should be carefully established—that is, only when source and exposure evaluations have comprehensively addressed the multiple offending agents potentially present and when complete medical assessments have defined the health outcome to the extent possible.

Although the knowledge base concerning microbial contaminants in the indoor environment has advanced significantly within the past two decades, the quest for solutions to problems regarding characterization of exposure and associated disease needs to continue with vigor. Future large-scale epidemiologic investigations must therefore address this important subject both comprehensively and with attention to detail, yielding specific results that will aid in disease identification, treatment, and prevention.

References

1. Yang CS. Understanding the biology of fungi found indoors. In: Johanning E, Yang CS (eds), *Fungi and Bacteria in Indoor Air Environments: Health Effects, Detection, and Remediation.* Latham, NY: Eastern New York Occupational Health Program, 1995. Pp 131–7.
2. Lewis FA. Regulating indoor microbes. In: Johanning E, Yang CS (eds), *Fungi and Bacteria in Indoor Air Environments: Health Effects, Detection, and Remediation.* Latham, NY: Eastern New York Occupational Health Program, 1995. Pp 5–9.
3. *Report to Congress on Indoor Air Quality, Volume II: Assessment and Control of Indoor Air Pollution.* Pp 1, 4–14. EPA-400-89-001C. Washington, DC: U.S. Environmental Protection Agency, 1989.
4. Smoragiewicz W, Cossette B, Boutard A, et al. Trichothecene mycotoxins in the dust of ventilation systems in office buildings. *Int Arch Occup Environ Health* 1993;65:113–7.
5. Andersson MA, Nikulin M, Köljalg U, et al. Bacteria, molds, and toxins in water-damaged building materials. *Appl Environ Microbiol* 1997;63:387–93.
6. Croft WA, Jarvis BB, Yatawara CS. Airborne outbreak of trichothecene toxicosis. *Atmos Environ* 1986; 20:549–52.
7. Verhoeff AP, van Wijnen JH, Brunekreef B, et al. The presence of viable mould propagules in indoor air in relation to home dampness and outdoor air. *Allergy* 1992;47:83–91.
8. Hunter CA, Grant C, Flannigan B, et al. Mould in buildings: the air spora of domestic dwellings. *Internat Biodeterior* 1988;24:81–101.
9. Platt DP, Martin CJ, Hunt SM, et al. Damp housing, mould growth, and symptomatic health state. *Br Med J* 1989;298:1673–8.
10. Hodgson MJ, Morey P, Leung W-Y, et al. Building-associated pulmonary disease from exposure to *Stachybotrys chartarum* and *Aspergillus versicolor. J Environ Occup Med* 1998;40:241–9.
11. Bernstein RS, Sorenson WG, Garabrant D, et al. Exposures to respirable, airborne *Penicillium* from a contaminated ventilation system: clinical, environmental and epidemiological aspects. *Am Ind Hyg Assoc J* 1983;44:161–9.
12. Outbreaks of respiratory illness among employees in large office buildings—Tennessee, District of Columbia. *MMWR* 1984;33:506–13.
13. Lawton MD, Dales RE, White J. The influence of house characteristics in a Canadian community on microbiological contamination. *Ind Air* 1998;8:2–11.
14. Dales RE, Burnett R, Zwanenburg H. Adverse health effects among adults exposed to home dampness and molds. *Am Rev Respir Dis* 1991;143:505–9.
15. Strachen DP. Damp housing and childhood asthma: validation of reporting of symptoms. *Br Med J* 1988;297:1223–6.
16. Hodgson MJ, Morey PR, Attfield M, et al. Pulmonary disease associated with cafeteria flooding. *Arch Env Health* 1985;40:96–101.
17. Brunekreef B. Damp housing and adult respiratory symptoms. *Allergy* 1992;47:498–502.
18. Brunekreef B, Dockery DW, Speizer FE, et al. Home dampness and respiratory morbidity in children. *Am Rev Respir Dis* 1989;140:1363–7.
19. Waegemaekers M, Van Wageningen N, Brunekreef B, et al. Respiratory symptoms in damp homes. *Allergy* 1989;44:1–7.
20. Johanning E, Biagini R, Hull D, et al. Health and immunology study following exposure to toxigenic fungi (*Stachybotrys chartarum*) in a water-damaged office environment. *Int Arch Occup Environ Health* 1996;68:207–18.

21. Dungy CI, Kozak PP, Gallup J, et al. Aeroallergen exposure in the elementary school setting. *Ann Allergy* 1986;56:218–24.
22. Strachen DP, Flannigan B, McCabe EM, et al. Quantification of airborne moulds in the homes of children with and without wheeze. *Thorax* 1990;45:382–7.
23. VerHoeff AP, van Wijnen JH, Boleij B, et al. Enumeration and identification of airborne viable mould propagules in houses. *Allergy* 1990;45:275–84.
24. Pope AM, Patterson R, Burge H. *Indoor Allergens: Assessing and Controlling Adverse Health Effects.* Washington, DC: National Academy Press, 1993.
25. Gravesen S. Fungi as a cause of allergic disease. *Allergy* 1979;34:135–54.
26. Sorenson WG, Frazier DG, Jarvis BB, et al. Trichothecene mycotoxins in aerosolized conidia of *Stachybotrys atra. Appl Environ Microbiol* 1987; 53:1370–5.
27. Sakomoto K, Tsujii E, Miyauchi M, et al. FR901459, a novel immunosuppressant isolated from *Stachybotrys chartarum* no. 19392. *J Antibiot* 1993;46:1788–9.
28. Jarvis BB, Salemme J, Morais A. *Stachybotrys* toxins 1. *Natural Toxins* 1995;3:10–6.
29. Jarvis BB, Zhou Y, Jiang J, et al. Toxigenic molds in water-damaged buildings: dichlorogriseofulvins from *Memnoniella echinata. J Natural Prod* 1996;59:553–4.
30. Burge HA, Feeley JC. Indoor air pollution and infectious diseases. In: Samet JM, Spengler JD (eds), *Indoor Air Pollution: A Health Perspective.* Baltimore: The Johns Hopkins University Press, 1991. Pp 273–84.
31. Yang CS, Johanning E. Airborne fungi and mycotoxins. In: Hurst CJ, Knudsen GR, McInerney MJ, et al. (eds), *Manual of Environmental Microbiology.* Washington, DC: ASM Press, 1996. Pp 651–60.
32. Alexopoulos CJ, Mims CW, Blackwell M. *Introductory Mycology*, 4th Ed. New York: John Wiley & Sons, 1996.
33. Griffen DH. *Fungal Physiology*, 2nd Ed. New York: Wiley-Liss, 1994.
34. Kendrick B. *The Fifth Kingdom*, 2nd Ed. Newburyport, MA: Focus Information Group, 1992.
35. Lacey J. Aerobiology and health. In: Hawksworth DL (ed), *Frontiers in Mycology UK: CBI*, 1991. Pp 157–85.
36. Miller DJ. Fungi as contaminants in indoor air. In: *Proceedings of the 5th International Conference on Indoor Air Quality and Climate, Indoor Air '90.* Toronto, 1990. Vol 1, Pp 51–64.
37. Jarvis BB. Mycotoxins and indoor air quality. In: Morey PR, Feeley JC, Otten JA (eds), *Biological Contaminants in Indoor Environments.* Philadelphia: American Society for Testing and Materials, 1989. Pp 201–13.
38. Jarvis BB. Mycotoxins in the air: keep your buildings dry or the bogeyman will get you. In: Johanning E, Yang CS (eds), *Fungi and Bacteria in Indoor Air Environments: Health Effects, Detection, and Remediation.* Latham, NY: Eastern New York Occupational Health Program, 1995. Pp 35–44.
39. Miller JD. Mycotoxins. In: Rylander R, Jacobs RR (eds), *Organic Dusts: Exposure, Effects and Prevention.* Boca Raton, FLA: Lewis Publisher, 1994. Pp 87–92.
40. Ciegler A, Bennett JW. Mycotoxins and mycotoxicoses. *Bio Science* 1980;30:512–5.
41. Ciegler A, Burmeister HR, Vesonder RF, et al. Mycotoxins: occurrence in the environment. In: Shank RC (ed), *Mycotoxins and N-Nitroso Compounds: Environmental Risks.* Boca Raton, FLA: CRC Press, 1981. Pp 1–50.
42. Hendry KM, Cole EC. A review of mycotoxins in indoor air. *J Toxicol Environ Health* 1993;38:183–98.
43. Miller JD. Fungi as contaminants in indoor air. *Atmos Environ* 1992;26A:2163–72.
44. Sorenson WG. Aerosolized mycotoxins: implications for occupational settings. In: Johanning E, Yang CS (eds), *Fungi and Bacteria in Indoor Air Environments: Health Effects, Detection, and Remediation.* Latham, NY: Eastern New York Occupational Health Program, 1995. Pp 57–67.
45. Burge HA, Ammann HM. Fungal toxins and ß-(1→3)-*D*-glucans. In: Macher J (ed), *Bioaerosols: Assessment and Control.* Cincinnati: American Conference of Governmental Industrial Hygienists, 1999. Pp 24-1–24-13.
46. Creasia DA, Lambert RJ. Acute respiratory toxicity of the trichothecene mycotoxins, T-2 toxin. In: Beasley VR (ed), *Trichothecene Mycotoxicosis: Pathophysiologic Effects.* Boca Raton, FL: CRC Press, 1989. Pp 161–70.
47. Samuels GJ. Trichoderma: a review of biology and systematics of the genus. *Mycol Res* 1996;100:923–35.
48. Etzel RA, Montana E, Sorenson WG, et al. Acute pulmonary hemorrhage in infants associated with exposure to *Stachybotrys atra* and other fungi. *Arch Pediatr Adolesc Med* 1998;152:757–62.
49. Centers for Disease Control. Acute pulmonary hemorrhage/hemosiderosis among infants: Cleveland, January 1993–November 1994. *MMWR* 1994; 43:881–3.
50. Ammann HM. Microbial volatile organic compounds. In: Macher J (ed), *Bioaerosols: Assessment and Control.* Cincinnati: American Conference of Governmental Industrial Hygienists, 1999. Pp 26-1–26-17.
51. Flannigan B, McCabe EM, McGarry F. Allergenic and toxigenic micro-organisms in houses. *J Appl Bacteriol* 1991;79:61S–73S.
52. Rylander R. Microbial cell-wall constituents in indoor air and their relation to disease. In: Seppänen O (ed), *Indoor Air and Health: Causative Agents, Health Hazards and Risk Assessment.* Munksgaard/Copenhagen: 10th Medical Symposium of the Yrjö Jahnsson Foun-

dation Porvoo, Finland, August 1996, 1998 Suppl 4:59–65.

53. DiLuzio NR. Update on the immunomodulating activities of glucans. *Springer Semin Immunopath* 1985;8:387–400.
54. Fogelmark B, Sjöstrand M, Rylander R. Pulmonary inflammation induced by repeated inhalations of (1→3)-ß-*D*-glucan and endotoxin. *Int J Exp Path* 1994;75:85–90.
55. Rylander R. Investigations of the relationship between disease and airborne (1→3)-ß-*D*-glucan in buildings. *Mediators Inflam* 1997;6:275–7.
56. Rylander R, Norrhall M, Engdahl U, et al. Airways inflammation, atopy, and (1→3)-ß-*D*-glucan exposures in two schools. *Am J Respir Crit Care Med* 1998; 158:1685–7.
57. Rylander R, Snella M-C. Endotoxins and the lung: cellular reactions and risk for disease. *Prog Allergy* 1983;33:332–44.
58. Milton DK. Endotoxin and other bacterial cell-wall components. In: Macher J (ed), *Bioaerosols: Assessment and Control.* Cincinnati: American Conference of Governmental Industrial Hygienists, 1999. Pp 23-1–23-14.
59. Rose CS, Martyny JW, Newman LS, et al. "Lifeguard lung": endemic granulomatous pneumonitis in an indoor swimming pool. *Am J Public Health* 1998; 88:1795–800.
60. Teeuw KB, Vandenbroucke-Grauls CM, Verhoef J. Airborne gram-negative bacteria and endoxin in sick building syndrome: a study in Dutch governmental office buildings. *Arch Intern Med* 1994;154:233–5.
61. Macher J (ed). *Bioaerosols: Assessment and Control.* Cincinnati: American Conference of Governmental Hygienists, 1999.
62. Lambert WE, Samet JM. Indoor air pollution. In: Harber P, Schenker MB, Balmes JR (eds), *Occupational and Environmental Respiratory Disease.* St. Louis: Mosby, 1996. Pp 784–807.
63. Cohen S, Tyrrell DA, Smith AP. Psychological stress and susceptibility to the common cold. *N Engl J Med* 1991;325:606–12.
64. Herbert TB, Cohen S. Stress and immunity in humans: a meta-analytic review. *Psychosom Med* 1993;55:364–79.
65. Burge HA, Macher JM, Milton DK, et al. Data evaluation. In: Macher J (ed), *Bioaerosols: Assessment and Control.* Cincinnati: American Conference of Governmental Industrial Hygienists, 1999. Pp 14-1–14-11.
66. Brooks SM. Host susceptibility to indoor air pollution. *J Allergy Clin Immunol* 1994;94:344–51.
67. Naclerio R, Solomon W. Rhinitis and inhalant allergens. *JAMA* 1997;278:1842–8.
68. Rose CS, Kreiss K, Milton DK, et al. Medical roles and recommendations. In: Macher J (ed), *Bioaerosols: Assessment and Control.* Cincinnati: American Conference of Governmental Industrial Hygienists, 1999. Pp 8-1, 8-9.
69. Turkeltaub PC, Gergen PJ. Prevalence of upper and lower respiratory conditions in the U.S. population by social and environmental factors: data from the second National Health and Nutrition Examination Survey, 1976 to 1980: NHANES II. *Ann Allergy* 1991;67:147–54.
70. Nathan RA, Meltzer EO, Selner JC, et al. Prevalence of allergic rhinitis in the United States. *J Allergy Clin Immunol* 1997;99:S808–S814.
71. McMenamin P. The economic toll of allergic rhinitis and associated airway diseases. In: Spector SL (ed), *The Chronic Airways Disease Connection: Redefining Rhinitis.* Little Falls, NJ: Health Learning Systems, 1995. Pp 26–8.
72. Corren J. The impact of allergic rhinitis on bronchial asthma. *J Allergy Clin Immunol* 1998;101(suppl): S352–S356.
73. Kalimer M. Asthma deaths: a social or medical problem? *JAMA* 1993;269:1994–5.
74. Rose C. Hypersensitivity pneumonitis. In: Harber P, Schenker MB, Balmes JR (eds), *Occupational and Environmental Respiratory Disease.* St. Louis: Mosby, 1996. Pp 201–15.
75. Hodgson MJ, Morey PR, Simon JS, et al. An outbreak of recurrent acute and chronic hypersensitivity pneumonitis in office workers. *Am J Epidemiol* 1987;125:631–8.
76. Arnow PM, Fink JN, Schlueter DP, et al. Early detection of hypersensitivity pneumonitis in office workers. *Am J Med* 1978;64:236–42.
77. Rask-Anderson A. Inhalation fever. In: Harber P, Schenker MB, Balmes JR (eds), *Occupational and Environmental Respiratory Disease.* St. Louis: Mosby, 1996. Pp 243–58.
78. Merchant JA. Agricultural exposures to organic dusts. In: Rosenstock L (ed), *Occupational Pulmonary Disease: Occupational Medicine State of the Art Reviews.* Philadelphia: Hanley and Belfus, 1987. Pp 409–25.
79. Baur X, Behr J, DeWair M, et al. Humidifier lung and humidifier fever. *Lung* 1988;166:113–24.
80. Stobierski MG, Hospedales CJ, Hall WN, et al. Outbreak of histoplasmosis among employees in a paper factory—Michigan, 1993. *J Clin Microbiol* 1996;34: 1220–3.
81. Levitz SM. The ecology of *Cryptococcus neoformans* and the epidemiology of cryptococcosis. *Rev Infect Dis* 1991;13:1163–9.
82. Ajello L: Relationship of *Histoplasma capsulatum* to avian habitats. *Public Health Reports* 1964;79:266.
83. Emmons CW, Klite PD, Baer GM, et al. Isolation of *Histoplasma capsulatum* from bats in the United States. *Am J Epidemiol* 1996;84:103.
84. Centers for Disease Control. Histoplasmosis. *MMWR* 1995;44:701–3.

85. Rose CS. Fungi. In: Wald PH, Stave GM (eds), *Physical and Biological Hazards of the Workplace*. New York: Wiley, 1994. Pp 392–416.

86. Hajjeh RA. Disseminated histoplasmosis in persons infected with human immunodeficiency virus. *Clin Infect Dis* 1995; 21(suppl 1):S108–S110.

87. Ampel NM. Emerging disease issues and fungal pathogens associated with HIV infection. *Emerg Infec Dis* 1996;2:109–16.

88. Zampiello FA. Setting the stage for change. In: Johanning E, Yang CS (eds), *Fungi and Bacteria in Indoor Air Environments: Health Effects, Detection, and Remediation*. Latham, NY: Eastern New York Occupational Health Program, 1995. Pp 1–3.

89. Developing an investigation strategy. In: Macher J (ed), *Bioaerosols: Assessment and Control*. Cincinnati: American Conference of Governmental Industrial Hygienists, 1999. Pp 2-1–2-10.

90. Hodgson MJ. Clinical investigations of emerging diseases in patients and buildings: management of patients, exposure, and remediation. In: Johanning E, Yang CS (eds), *Fungi and Bacteria in Indoor Air Environments: Health Effects, Detection, and Remediation*. Latham, NY: Eastern New York Occupational Health Program, 1995. Pp 183–93.

91. Hodgson MJ. The medical evaluation. In: Seltzer JM (ed), *Effects of the Indoor Environment on Health, Occupational Medicine: State of the Art Reviews*. Philadelphia: Hanley and Belfus, 1995. Pp 177–94.

92. Canada Mortgage and Housing Corporation. *Moldy Houses: Why They Are and Why We Care*. Ottawa, Canada: CMHC, 1995.

93. Terr AL. Immunologic methods. In: Harber P, Schenker MB, Balmes JR (eds), *Occupational and Environmental Respiratory Disease*. St. Louis: Mosby, 1996. Pp 126–38.

94. Dillon HK, Heinsohn PA, Miller JD (eds). *Field Guide for the Determination of Biological Contaminants in Environmental Samples*. Fairfax, VA: American Industrial Hygiene Association, 1996.

95. Olenchock S. Airborne endotoxin. In: Hurst CJ, Knudsen GR, McInerney MJ (eds), *Manual of Environmental Microbiology*. Washington, DC: American Society for *Microbiology*, 1996. Pp 661–5.

96. American Conference on Governmental Industrial Hygienists. *Guidelines for the Assessment of Bioaerosols in the Indoor Environment*. Cincinnati: ACGIH, 1989.

97. Rylander R. Evaluation of the risks of endotoxin exposures: endotoxins in the environment. *Int J Occup Environ Health* 1997;3(Suppl):S32–S36.

98. New York City Department of Health, New York City Human Resources Administration, and Mount Sinai–Irving J. Selikoff Occupational Health Clinical Center. *Guidelines on Assessment and Remediation of* Stachybotrys atra *in Indoor Environments*, 1993.

99. Health Canada. *Fungal Contamination in Public Buildings: A Guide to Recognition and Management*. Ontario, Canada: Federal-Provincial Committee on Environmental and Occupational Health, Environmental Health Directorate, 1995.

100. American Industrial Hygiene Association Biosafety Committee. *Biosafety Reference Manual*, 2nd Ed. Fairfax, VA: AIHA, 1995.

101. Lstiburek J, Carmody J. *Moisture Control Handbook: Principles and Practices for Residential and Small Commercial Buildings*. New York: Van Nostrand Reinhold, 1994.

102. United States Environmental Protection Agency. *Should You Have the Air Ducts in Your Home Cleaned?* Document No. EPA-402-K97-002. Washington, DC: Government Printing Office, 1998.

39 / Biologic Warfare

Harold E. Hoffman and Tee L. Guidotti

Overview and History of Biologic Warfare

Biologic warfare is the use of biologic agents (1) to kill people for war or terrorism, (2) as a strategic weapon to threaten people, or (3) to deny the use of terrain to opposing forces. In the past, biologic agents were not considered practical for modern warfare because they were indiscriminate, difficult to control, and delayed in their effect. In recent years, however, small groups, whose apparent aim is to cause fear and confusion, have used them for apparently indiscriminate urban terrorism. There is some evidence that a few of these groups have attempted to engage in terrorist acts using biologic agents. Since these efforts are likely to continue, health professionals need to consider biologic warfare in disaster planning scenarios and in any unusual outbreak of disease. Many lives could be saved if health providers understand the biologic agents, prevention measures, modes of attack, early surveillance, and treatment. Considerable preparation is required for education, training, immunization, hazard identification, and treatment in the event of biologic warfare.

Biologic warfare is contrary to the basic principles of the medical profession, which are prevention and treatment of illness. Apparently, for this reason, physicians have been very reluctant to talk about it. The increasing risk of usage of these agents, especially by terrorists, has made it imperative to overcome this reluctance and to address the problem.

In ancient history, the Greeks and Romans condemned biologic warfare. Poisons were considered inhumane in warfare and were forbidden by the Manu Law of India around 500 BC [1]. A form of biologic warfare was used in the fourteenth century: Bodies of plague victims were catapulted into the city of Kaffa by the besieging Turks [2]. In 1763, blankets from a smallpox hospital were given to Native Americans in order to produce an epidemic of smallpox in a deliberate act of genocide [2]. The 1925 Geneva Protocol forbade the use of bacterial agents in war. Biologic warfare research has been conducted throughout the twentieth century, often for defensive purposes but sometimes covertly for offensive purposes. Research on biologic agents was conducted on human subjects in Japanese-occupied Manchuria before and during World War II, and there was release of infectious agents to the civilian population.

Development of biologic weapons is likely to continue into the future. These weapons pose a particular threat in the hands of small, unpredictable terrorist groups and countries with limited resources that feel under extreme military pressure.

Magnitude of the Threat of Biologic Warfare

Biologic weapons have low visibility, high potency, and high accessibility. Therefore, civilian and military populations have become concerned about this hazard. Although production requires some technologic expertise and is easy to conceal, the small quantities of material required and the difficulty of their detection facilitate transportation of biologic agents by security measures. Dispersion of biologic agents requires low levels of technology, modest financial resources, and minimal training. The most likely biologic warfare tactic is release of an agent into the air as a biologic aerosol, which would create a stable cloud of suspended microscopic particles of bacteria or viruses. For optimal attack advantage, aerosol particle size would be approximately 1–20 μm, generating particles that can remain suspended in the air for hours. When inhaled, these particles penetrate into distal bronchioles and terminal alveoli. Because the agents delivered in this form are undetectable by the human senses and cannot be monitored by available instrumentation, the target population would not identify an attack until health effects occurred. Agents might also be introduced into air conditioning systems or, conceivably, into the water supply, especially where infection controls are inadequate.

Tactically, a biologic warfare attack is not very efficient in the battlefield. The effects are delayed, whether mediated by infection or toxins, and this allows time for retaliation. The agents are dispersed in air and therefore may expose the attacker's own troops or population centers if there is a change in the direction of the wind. Highly communicable agents would interfere with the occupation of enemy positions and territory after the attack. However, these tactical limitations are less of a drawback for acts of terrorism, wherein randomness of position and the horrific effects on a population are used to foster confusion and distrust.

Compared to chemical warfare, very little is understood about biologic warfare. In 1990, just before the Gulf War, scientific knowledge was completely lacking regarding the possible effects of an attack using anthrax and botulism agents. The civilian population has few well-studied past experiences to guide efforts at prevention. One of the few of the actual deployments of biologic weapons occurred in Manchuria during its occupation by the Japanese Army in 1941. The activities of the infamous "718 battalion" are documented in a museum dedicated to the incident near Harbin, in Heilongjiang province. In addition to the rarity of actual deployments, the fact that delivery methods are constantly changing compounds the lack of understanding about biologic warfare and thus increases the magnitude of the problem.

Agents of Biologic Warfare

Biologic agents that could be used for warfare or terrorism include bacteria, viruses, rickettsia, and toxins of microbes, plants, or animals. Toxins are high molecular-weight compounds produced by organisms; they tend to act much faster than infectious agents. Diseases that may result from biologic warfare include anthrax, brucellosis, plague, Q fever, tularemia, smallpox, viral encephalitis, viral hemorrhagic fevers, botulism, and staphylococcal enterotoxin B (SEB) toxicity [1–7]. In the past three years, efforts have been made to disseminate information on biologic threats widely in the civilian community [4].

ANTHRAX

Anthrax is the biologic agent considered to be the greatest threat to civilian populations, due to its relative ease of manufacture and its lethality. It is caused by *Bacillus anthracis*, a gram-positive, spore-forming bacterium. Anthrax can be produced in large quantities and requires only such readily available resources as dairy farms and breweries. Anthrax spores can survive adverse environmental conditions and remain viable for decades. During a biologic attack, anthrax spores are dispersed through aerosolization and are inhaled by intended victims. In the lungs, the spores are phagocytized and transported to hilar and mediastinal lymph nodes. The spores germinate into vegetative (live bacteria) bacilli, producing a necrotizing hemorrhagic mediastinitis. Inhalational anthrax begins with fever, malaise, and fatigue. Usually within one to six days, inhaled anthrax spores cause fever, cough, and weakness [3]. Within two to three more days, respiratory failure and septicemia may develop. If untreated, inhalation anthrax has a mortality rate of about 95% [3]. Once symptoms occur, treatment is ineffective. Fortunately, a vaccine has been developed to ward off the effects of anthrax; it is given at 0, 2, and 4 weeks and at 6, 12, and 18 months [3]. A protective antibody response does not develop until seven days after the second dose [3]. If a course of vaccine was not given prior to the exposure, oral antibiotics, such as doxycycline or ciprofloxacin, are recommended for 30 days for prophylaxis after exposure [3].

BRUCELLOSIS

Brucellosis is caused by small slow-growing, gram-negative, non-spore-forming coccobacilli that are species of *Brucella*. These bacteria are highly infectious through aerosolization. Brucellae may survive for six weeks in dust and 10 weeks in soil or water. Organisms could be delivered in slurry by bombs or as a dry aerosol. No vaccine is available.

PLAGUE

Plague is caused by *Yersinia pestis*, which are gram-negative bacilli. After an airborne biologic warfare attack, widespread, rapidly progressive primary pneumonic plague would be the most likely presentation. The case in Manchuria during the Japanese occupation in 1941 involved plague and resulted in the death of many people. A vaccine has been developed, but it is not very protective.

Q FEVER

Q fever is caused by *Coxiella burnetii*, which is an intracellular rickettsia-like organism. The spore-like form can withstand heat and drying and can survive on inanimate surfaces for weeks or months. This organism can be disseminated by wind, inducing infection miles from the source. Chronic disease develops in less than 1% of acute infections, but fatigue may occur for months. The case-fatality rate of acute Q fever is low, even without treatment. A vaccine is available in some countries.

TULAREMIA

Tularemia is caused by *Francisella tularensis*, a small aerobic gram-negative coccobacillus. The organism can remain viable for weeks. A vaccine has been developed.

TOXINS

Botulinum toxins are proteins produced by the anaerobic bacteria *Clostridium botulinum*. The use of this agent is actually a form of chemical attack. Botulism toxin can be "weaponized" by aerosol generators, including simple spray cans. Botulinum toxin is the most toxic compound known. It acts by binding to the presynaptic nerve terminal at neuromuscular junctions and at cholinergic autonomic sites [4]. This interrupts neurotransmission to cause bulbar palsies and skeletal muscle weakness [4]. Bulbar palsies begin with dysarthria, dysphonia, dysphagia, and ocular symptoms such as blurred vision [4]. Skeletal muscle paralysis progresses from a symmetrical, descending weakness to respiratory failure [4]. Symptoms appear 12 to 72 hours after ingestion or inhalation of contaminated food [1]. Initial symptoms are nausea and diarrhea, followed by weakness, dizziness, and respiratory paralysis [1]. Antitoxin can sometimes arrest the process [1].

Staphylococcal enterotoxin B (SEB) is produced by *Staphylococcus* bacteria. Enterotoxins are excreted from the organism and have their major effects on the gastrointestinal tract. SEB is extremely toxic, rendering a high proportion of exposed people very ill within a few hours. In biologic warfare, dispersion would most likely be through aerosolization; SEB may incapacitate humans many miles downwind from release. SEB might also be used to sabotage food or water supplies. A vaccine cannot be developed for this toxin.

Viruses such as viral hemorrhagic fever could be more lethal than anthrax but are difficult to culture. Viruses disperse readily by aerosolization or water contamination. Viral hemorrhagic fevers are infections caused by a variety of RNA viruses. In infected individuals, vascular endothelium damage causes internal bleeding. These viruses are highly infectious by aerosolization and have a high morbidity and mortality. One example is the Ebola virus.

Variola virus causes smallpox. The smallpox vaccine is effective in preventing infection, but may no longer be readily available. Smallpox was eliminated in 1977, and all stores of the virus (except the military collections) have been destroyed.

Equine encephalitis viruses, which cause viral encephalitis, are highly infectious by aerosolization. These viruses can be produced in large amounts in inexpensive and unsophisticated systems, and they are relatively stable during storage. No vaccine is available.

Viruses and most vegetative bacteria (live, active bacteria, not inactive spores) cannot survive long in aerosol form due to ultraviolet light and other environmental challenges. This makes them poor biologic weapons for outdoor dissemination. In the dissemination process, vegetative organisms, in particular, are subject to damage and thus a subsequent reduction in their viability. Protective measures for these agents are being researched to maintain the efficacy of these agents. One possible type of protection is encapsulation of the agents.

Prevention

Prevention of biologic warfare is possible only by limiting the development and production of biologic weapons. A strong global moral consensus opposing biologic weapon development is required. The use of biologic agents needs to be considered a crime against humanity, and full deterrence must be sanctioned by the international community. Education is a vital factor because it increases awareness of the threat of biologic warfare and the necessity for prevention.

People and facilities capable of developing biologic weapons should be identified. Intelligence activities—namely close monitoring of groups and countries with biologic agent capability—is the key to prevention. Regulation of commercial orders for pathogens involves controls over shipments of pathogens. Institutions that reinforce positive behavior and values are essential. This means that institutions that are open and follow the international rules should be rewarded for their positive behavior.

Early detection and prompt management of biologic warfare attacks is important to mitigate damage. Suspicious outbreaks of disease and alleged biologic warfare attacks should be considered grave acts of aggression by the international community and investigated thoroughly. To improve surveillance, diagnostic methods, practical therapeutic agents, and response plans should be developed.

Countermeasures

Countermeasures for biologic warfare include intelligence and appropriate intervention, detection devices, epidemiologic identification of biologic attacks, and use of personal protective equipment, vaccines, diagnostic modalities, and treatments.

Defense against biologic warfare requires early and, preferably, advance knowledge of the organism used in an attack. For countermeasures to be effective, the organism needs to be vulnerable to medical intervention. The major risks to combatants in the 1996 Gulf War were thought to be anthrax spores and *C botulinum* toxin. Emerging diseases should be combated by (1) identifying baseline data on endemic diseases throughout the world, (2) rapid reporting of unusual outbreaks, (3) responses to contain disease, such as advice on trade and travel [1], and (4) global surveillance of disease outbreaks.

Active immunization may be useful for military forces, but civilian populations probably cannot be adequately protected in this manner. Immunization and treatment requirements need to be anticipated. (Anthrax vaccine was in limited supply during the Gulf War because the entire production was reserved for the military [5].)

Effective rapid diagnostic tests will not be available in the foreseeable future. Therefore, we need a "rough and ready" approach to be maximally effective in countering biologic warfare with available resources.

Although a large population cannot be fully protected from a biologic attack, the effects can be diminished with a preventive health program. In preparation for an attack, postexposure prophylaxis, disease treatment, and follow-up care must be in place.

Immunization can be performed against certain agents, with some agents requiring several inoculations over an extended period of three to twelve months. If vaccines are available, the causative agents must be determined quickly so relief workers can prepare and administer these agents. Unfortunately, vaccines are not available for many agents.

Prophylactic medications such as antibiotics are effective against some bacterial agents but are not effective against viruses. To prevent infectious disease, appropriate antibiotic therapy must begin within a few hours of exposure, before symptoms appear. Obviously, this is not possible in the event of a massive attack.

Personal protective equipment needs to be available to protect relief workers. Respirators or gas masks require filter canisters that have activated charcoal to remove simple organic molecules, such as nerve gas, by adsorption. The paper filter in the canister removes particulates larger than 0.3 μm in size. Large populations will not wear gas masks for long periods of time. Some people feel claustrophobic in them, and others with respiratory disorders cannot use them. In hot weather, people are not able to tolerate a mask for more than a few minutes at a time.

Clothing protects against contact with open wounds or broken skin. Protective shelter, in a closed room insulated with plastic and ventilated with filtered air, may be effective in airborne attacks but requires substantial preparation. Although sunlight and ambient temperatures destroy most agents, and surfaces can be decontaminated with disinfectants, anthrax spores survive for decades and are not easily killed.

Early detection systems are needed, but only rudimentary field units for a few specific agents are currently available. Electronic detection devices, when available, should be placed in high-risk locations, where an attack is likely. Medical detection involves the identification and reporting of suspicious diseases. Epidemiologic evaluation will determine a pattern of disease but is likely to come too late to affect the course of the biologic effects of attack.

Early identification of an organism used in a biologic warfare attack is vital. Through antibody-antigen reactions, *B anthracis* (anthrax bacterium), *Y pestis* (bubonic plague), botulinum toxin (the toxin of botulinum organisms), and staphylococcus enterotoxin B (released by certain staphylococcal bacteria) can be identified in the field [1]. A database of antibiotic resistance of the relevant biologic agent should be established.

Although clinical tests can reliably detect and identify a biologic agent, they are dependent on optimal procedures. During an attack, it is unlikely that there will be time for such tests or that the equipment will always be operational. In warfare or terrorist conditions, substances such as engine exhaust, dust, dirt, chemical fumes, and fuel residue may interfere with the tests.

In an acute situation, local resources can be overwhelmed, necessitating the establishment of resource networks. Available human and material resources should be identified in advance and processed or committed to provide help in a crisis. Diagnostic equipment usually requires electric power or temperature controls. Treatment personnel and medications will need to be brought into the situation from a distance.

In the event of a biologic warfare attack, the medical community needs time to determine resources, appropriate protocols and medications, and equipment requirements. Relief workers require preparation time for education and training, to assemble equipment and clothing, to become familiar with operational procedures, and to administer vaccines and prophylactic antibiotics. Typical crisis responses are characterized by incomplete documentation, poor compliance with protocols, and inadequate identification of equipment and specialized human resources. The civilian population cannot rely on the assistance of the military because it will be occupied with other matters. An example of good planning is the U.S. government's coordinated program of specialized teams to manage the consequences of an attack.

Most diseases resulting from biologic warfare present nonspecific signs and symptoms that could be misinterpreted as natural occurrences. Initially, a point-source outbreak of disease would likely occur. Individuals in the attacked population would come into contact with the agent at approximately the same time, with a peak incidence for the most likely agent occurring within hours or at most days. The health system should respond quickly with accurate diagnosis and speedy treatment. If an attack is suspected, military and civilian authorities should be notified immediately. The incubation period for a virus, bacterium, or toxin could be several days, but toxins require no incubation period.

In the event of an attack, a likely scenario would be the unnoticed release of a biologic agent. When widespread effects on the attacked population became apparent, the health system would need to quickly detect the disease outbreak and begin prompt treatment for large numbers of exposed people. The immediate task for health personnel would be to confirm the existence of an outbreak. Formulating a case definition in advance would help to determine the number of actual cases and the attack rate. Hysteria may be confused with actual disease; therefore, objective criteria should be used to document the number of people affected. One would need to determine if the disease rate was greater than the background rate of disease that normally occurs. This would include determination of unusual changes in disease occurrence or etiology. The next task is to determine the most likely causes.

In addition to the adverse health effects on the general population, biologic warfare agents would impact the health care system. A biologic terrorist attack could cause thousands of casualties requiring prompt medical attention. The biologic agent could also contaminate air, water, and food supplies, and the local health resources could be overwhelmed. An act of overt biologic warfare could result in hundreds of thousands or even millions of casualties. Patients would present in unprecedented numbers, overwhelming the medical resources.

Immediately after a suspected attack, investigators should evaluate if biologic weapons were used. Properly protected specialists would collect specimens from victims and the environment, with subsequent analysis of specimens done locally or sent to distant laboratories. After exposure but before symptoms arise, active or passive immunization and pretreatment with therapeutic antibiotics or antiviral drugs should be instituted.

The health risk to local military population and external relief personnel would need to be assessed. Preliminary advice would need to be provided to local administrative and health authorities, who would coordinate the emergency response but would be unlikely to have experience with the disease involved.

For relief organizations, rapid analysis of the situation and planning of the population treatment and relief is essential. Health care professionals and relief workers should be trained and immunized in advance to minimize their risk of acquiring disease from populations infected in an attack and of exposure to agents persisting in the environment from sources such as secondary aerosol inhalation and contaminated wounds.

After the onset of illness from biologic warfare, diagnosis of the disease, specific medical treatment, and general supportive care over the long term will be required. Health care workers need the protection of personal protective equipment and education about work practices, including the psychological reactions of survivors and health professionals as well as the medical management of victims.

Acknowledgment

H. M. Mottl of Dycor Industrial Research Limited provided insight and technical information on biological warfare.

References

1. Cole LA. *The Specter of Biological Weapons.* San Francisco: Scientific American, 1996. Pp 60–5.
2. Christopher GW, Cieslak TJ, Pavlin JA, et al. Biological warfare: a historical perspective. *JAMA* 1997;278(5):412–7.
3. Anthrax vaccine. *Med Lett Drugs Ther* 1998;40(1026):51–4.
4. Franz DR, Jahrling PB, Friedlander AM, et al. Clinical recognition and management of patients exposed to biological warfare agents. *JAMA* 1997;278(5):399–411.
5. Steffen R, Mellin J, Woodall JP, et al. Preparation for emergency relief after biological warfare. *J Infect* 1997;34:127–32.
6. Kadlec RP, Zelicoff AP, Vrtis AM, et al. Biological weapons control prospects and implications for the future. *JAMA* 1997;278(5):351–6.
7. Lundberg GD. Why should we be concerned about biological warfare? *JAMA* 1997;278(5):431–2.
8. Simon JD. Biological terrorism: preparing to meet the threat. *JAMA* 1997;278(5):428–30.
9. Sidell FR, Patrick WC III, Dashiell TR. *Jane's Chem-Bio Handbook.* Alexandria, VA: Jane's Information Group, 1999.
10. Tucker JB. National health and medical services response to incidents of chemical and biological terrorism. *JAMA* 1997;278(5):362–8.

Appendix: Internet Resources

Jay A. Brown

Centers for Disease Control (CDC)

http://www.cdc.gov/ncidod

The home page of the National Center for Infectious Diseases is the first place to go for current and authoritative information about occupational infections. The home page has links to subsites that index the following topics:

- Bacterial and Mycotic Diseases
- Viral and Rickettsial Diseases
- Parasitic Diseases
- Vector-Borne Infectious Diseases
- Hepatitis
- Emerging Infectious Diseases
- Travelers' Health
- Special Pathogens
- Hospital Infections
- Rabies

Other resources available through the CDC include:

- Biosafety Documents: *http://www.cdc.gov/od/ohs/biosfty/biosfty.htm*
- Morbidity and Mortality Weekly Reports (MMWR): *http://www2.cdc.gov.mmwr*

Occupational Safety and Health Administration (OSHA)

- Needlestick Injuries: *http://www.osha-slc.gov/SLTC/needlestick/index.html*
- Tuberculosis: *http://www.osha-slc.gov/SLTC/tuberculosis/index.html*
- Contracting Occupationally Related Psittacosis: *http://www.osha-slc.gov/dts/hib/hib_data/hib19940808.html*

Bug Bytes

http://www.ccm.lsumc.edu/bugbytes/

Bug Bytes is a production of the Infectious Diseases Section at the Louisiana State University (LSU) Medical Center in Shreveport. Each page succinctly describes a topic, including epidemiology, pathogenesis, clinical features, diagnosis and therapy, points to remember, and suggested reading. Occupational infections covered at this site include *Bacillus anthracis*; rabies; cat-scratch disease; hepatitis A, B, C, D, and E; tuberculosis; Rocky Mountain spotted fever; Lyme disease; and the ehrlichioses.

Medscape
http://id.medscape.com/Home/Topics/ID/directories/dir-ID.Library.html

Free registration is required to browse the Medscape site. Informative articles on brucellosis, tularemia, cat-scratch disease, Lyme disease, Colorado tick fever, ehrlichiosis, hepatitis C, coccioidomycosis, and many other occupational infections can be found on this index page. Use the search function or choose from one of the "hyperkeywords," including Fungal, Insect-borne Infection, Lyme Disease, Q Fever, Wound Infection, or Zoonosis. A review of animal bite wounds can be found at *http://www.medscape.com/SCP/IIM/1996/v13.n11/m1736.lutwick/m1736.lutwick.html*

Photos of Occupational Skin Infections

The following Internet addresses lead to the "best-on-the-web" images of occupational skin infections.

DERMATOLOGY, UNIVERSITY OF IOWA

- Herpetic Whitlow: *http://tray.dermatology.uiowa.edu/HerpWhit01.htm*
- Fish Tank Granuloma: *http://tray.dermatology.uiowa.edu/MMarin01.htm*
- Swimming Pool Granuloma: *http://tray.dermatology.uiowa.edu/MMarin03.htm*
- Cutaneous Leishmaniasis: *http://tray.dermatology.uiowa.edu/~Clara/Leish002.htm*
- Sporotrichosis: *http://tray.dermatology.uiowa.edu/Sporo001.htm* and *http://tray.dermatology.uiowa.edu/~Clara/Sporo004.htm*
- Cutaneous Larva Migrans: *http://tray.dermatology.uiowa.edu/LarvMi02.htm*
- Chromomycosis: *http://tray.dermatology.uiowa.edu/~Clara/Chromo004.htm*
- *Candida* Paronychia: *http://tray.dermatology.uiowa.edu/Onychomyco01.htm*

DERMATOLOGY ONLINE ATLAS

- Erysipeloid: *http://www.derma.med.uni-erlangen.de/bilddb/diagnose/deutsch/i027100.htm*
- Cutaneous Larva Migrans: *http://www.derma.med.uni-erlangen.de/acadermis/CASES/edn9607/v4/index.htm*

- Anthrax: *http://www.derma.med.uni-erlangen.de/bilddb/diagnose/englisch/i022000.htm*

NATIONAL INSTITUTE FOR OCCUPATIONAL SAFETY AND HEALTH (NIOSH)

- Anthrax, Sporotrichosis, Chromomycosis, and *Trichophyton verrucosum*: *http://www.cdc.gov/niosh/ocderm15.html*
- Herpetic Fingers, *Mycobacterium marinum*, Milker's Nodule, and Orf: *http://www.cdc.gov/niosh/ocderm16.html*

Other Useful Sites

MEDICAL MYCOLOGY RESEARCH CENTER
http://fungus.utmb.edu/f-atlas/medmyc.htm

From the index page, follow the links to information about chromoblastomycosis (chromomycosis), coccidioidomycosis, paracoccidioidomycosis (includes images of skin lesions and chest radiographs), and histoplasmosis.

AMERICAN LYME DISEASE FOUNDATION
http://www.aldf.com/

Information about Lyme disease (including the newly available Lyme vaccine), babesiosis, ehrlichiosis, Rocky Mountain spotted fever, and tick paralysis can be found here.

JEGHERS MEDICAL INDEX
http://www.neoucom.edu/DEPTS/JEGH/sumref1.html

Of historical interest, this article covers many of the pathogens that cause work-related infections.

TRAVEL HEALTH ONLINE
http://www.tripprep.com/

This is a helpful site for health professionals who counsel overseas travelers.

UNIVERSITY OF MARYLAND INFORM
http://www.inform.umd.edu/EdRes/Topic/AgrEnv/ndd/occsafe/INFECTIOUS_DISEASES.html

This document describes zoonotic infections of agricultural workers, including bovine tuberculosis, histoplasmosis, hydatidosis, Newcastle disease, Q fever, psittacosis, swine influenza, and tularemia.

PEPNET

http://epi-center.ucsf.edu/PEP/pepnet.html

Maintained by the Epidemiology and Prevention Interventions Center at the University of California, San Francisco (UCSF), and San Francisco General Hospital (SFGH), PEPNet provides current information about postexposure prophylaxis for preventing infection with HIV and other bloodborne viruses after exposure.

HAZ-MAP: A RELATIONAL DATABASE OF TOXIC CHEMICALS AND HAZARDOUS JOBS

http://www.haz-map.com/

Two pages on this site are devoted to occupational infections and occupational skin infections. Each page shows a comprehensive list of occupational infectious diseases and the associated high-risk jobs.

OCCUPATIONAL HEALTH BRANCH, DEPARTMENT OF HEALTH SERVICES, CALIFORNIA

http://www.ohb.org/rabies.htm

This site gives information on occupational exposure to rabies virus.

UNIVERSITY OF CALIFORNIA AT SAN DIEGO (USCD) BIOSAFETY HANDBOOK

http://www-ehs.ucsd.edu/bio4.htm

This site gives information on infectious agents and the laboratory worker.

SITES WITH LINKS TO OTHER INTERNET RESOURCES

- North Carolina Statewide Program for Infection Control and Epidemiology *http://www.unc.edu/depts/sicp/resource.html*
- Infectious Disease Association of California *http://home.idac.org/idac/idlinks.html*

KAROLINSKA INSTITUTET

- Bacterial Infections and Mycoses: *http://www.mic.ki.se/Diseases/c1.html*
- Viral Diseases: *http://www.mic.ki.se/Diseases/c2.html*
- Parasitic Diseases: *http://www.mic.ki.se/Diseases/c3.html*

Index